Current Issues in Nursing

Current Issues in Nursing

SIXTH EDITION

Joanne McCloskey Dochterman, PhD, RN, FAAN

Distinguished Professor
Chairperson, Organizations, Systems and Community Health Area of Study
Director, Center for Nursing Classification
College of Nursing
The University of Iowa
Adjunct Director of Nursing
The University of Iowa Hospitals and Clinics
Iowa City, Iowa

Helen Kennedy Grace, PhD, RN, FAAN

Formerly Special Assistant to the President
W.K. Kellogg Foundation
Battle Creek, Michigan

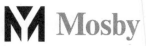

A Harcourt Health Sciences Company

St. Louis   London   Philadelphia   Sydney   Toronto

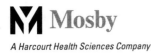

A Harcourt Health Sciences Company

Vice President, Nursing Editorial Director: Sally Schrefer
Acquisitions Editor: Michael S. Ledbetter
Associate Developmental Editor: Fran Murphy

Sixth Edition

Mosby, Inc.
A Harcourt Health Sciences Company
11830 Westline Industrial Drive
St. Louis, Missouri 63146

Printed in the United States of America

Library of Congress Cataloging in Publication Data

Current issues in nursing / [edited by] Joanne McCloskey Dochterman, Helen Kennedy Grace. — 6th ed.
　　　　p. cm.
　　　Includes bibliographical references and index.
　　　ISBN 0-323-01276-0
　　　1. Nursing. 2. Nursing—Social aspects—United States. 3. Nursing—Practice—United States. I. Dochterman, Joanne McCloskey. II. Grace, Helen K.
　　RT63.C87 2001
　　610.73—dc21

　　　　　　　　　　　　　　　　　　　　　　　　　00-048942

01　02　03　04　05　/　9　8　7　6　5　4　3　2　1

Contributors

Cynthia J. Abel, MSN, RN, CEN
Trauma Clinical Nurse Specialist, Rush-Copley Medical Center, Aurora, Illinois

Michelle Aebersold, MSA, RN
Clinical Nurse Manager, University of Michigan Hospitals and Health Center, Ann Arbor, Michigan

Tonia Dandry Aiken, JD, RN
Adjunct Instructor, Louisiana State University School of Nursing; A Founder and Officer, Health Care Mediators, Inc.; Attorney at Law, New Orleans, Louisiana

Carole A. Anderson, PhD, RN, FAAN
Professor and Dean, College of Nursing, and Assistant Vice President, Health Sciences, The Ohio State University, Columbus, Ohio

Ida M. Androwich, PhD, RNC, FAAN
Professor, Community and Administrative Nursing, Niehoff School of Nursing, Loyola University Chicago, Chicago, Illinois

Jo Ann Appleyard, PhD, RN
Medical Group Administrator, Kaiser Permanente, South San Francisco, California

Harriet Udin Aronow, PhD
Director of Research, Casa Colina Centers for Rehabilitation, Pomona, California; Assistant Researcher, School of Medicine, University of California Los Angeles, Los Angeles, California; Evaluator, Center for Healthy Aging, Santa Monica, California

Victoria Averhart, MS, RN, CS
Clinical Nurse Specialist, University of Michigan Health System, Ann Arbor, Michigan

Judith Gedney Baggs, PhD, RN
Interim Associate Dean for Academics and Associate Professor, School of Nursing, University of Rochester, Rochester, New York

Suzanne Bakken, DNSc, RN, FAAN
Professor of Nursing and of Medical Informatics, School of Nursing and Department of Medical Informatics, College of Physicians and Surgeons, Columbia University, New York, New York

Amy J. Barton, PhD, RN
Assistant Professor and Associate Dean for Practice, University of Colorado Health Sciences Center School of Nursing; Director of Advanced Practice, University Hospital, Denver, Colorado

Anne S. Belcher, DNS, RN, PNP
Assistant Professor, Environments for Health Department, School of Nursing, Indiana University, Indianapolis, Indiana

Suzanne Cushman Beyea, PhD, RN, CS
Director of Research, Association of periOperative Registered Nurses (AORN), Denver, Colorado

Marjorie Beyers, PhD, RN, FAAN
Patient Care Services Consultant, Barrington, Illinois; Formerly Executive Director, American Organization of Nurse Executives, Chicago, Illinois

Mary A. Blegen, PhD, RN
Professor, School of Nursing, University of Colorado Health Sciences Center, Denver, Colorado

Cheryl L. Brandi, DNSc, RN
Professor of Nursing, College of Nursing, Aichi Medical University, Aichi-ken, Japan

Vern L. Bullough, PhD, RN, FAAN
Distinguished Professor Emeritus, State University of New York, Buffalo; Professor Emeritus, California State University, Northridge; Adjunct Professor, Department of Nursing, University of Southern California, Los Angeles, California

Dorothy D. Camilleri, PhD, RN
Assistant Professor and Executive Associate Dean, Emerita, College of Nursing, University of Illinois at Chicago, Chicago, Illinois

Patricia T. Castiglia, PhD, RN, FAAN
Professor and Dean and Director, Kellogg Community Partnerships, and Co-Director, Kellogg Graduate Medical and Nursing Education Institute, College of Health Sciences, University of Texas at El Paso, El Paso, Texas

Helen M. Castillo, PhD, RN, CNA, FAAN
Professor and Dean, University of Texas Pan American;
Editorial Board Member, *Journal of Advanced Nursing*,
Edinburg, Texas

Linda K. Chase, MA, RN, CNAA
Administrative Associate, Children's and Women's Services,
Children's Hospital of Iowa, University of Iowa Hospitals and
Clinics, Iowa City, Iowa

Peggy L. Chinn, PhD, RN, FAAN
Professor, School of Nursing, University of Connecticut,
Storrs, Connecticut

June Clark, DBE, PhD, RN, RHV, FRCN
Professor of Community Nursing, School of Health Science,
University of Wales Swansea, Swansea, Wales, United Kingdom

Patricia Clinton, PhD, RN, ARNP
Clinical Assistant Professor, College of Nursing, University of
Iowa, Iowa City, Iowa

Mary C. Corley, PhD, RN
Associate Professor, School of Nursing, Virginia Commonwealth University, Richmond, Virginia

Mori Costantino, MS, RN
Doctoral Candidate, School of Nursing, University of
California, San Francisco, San Francisco, California

Perle Slavik Cowen, PhD, RN
Associate Professor, College of Nursing, University of Iowa,
Iowa City, Iowa

Susan L. Dean-Baar, PhD, RN, FAAN
Associate Dean for Academic Affairs, School of Nursing,
University of Wisconsin–Milwaukee, Milwaukee, Wisconsin

Betty Pierce Dennis, DrPH, RN
Chair, Department of Nursing, North Carolina Central
University, Durham, North Carolina

Donna Diers, MSN, RN, FAAN
Annie W. Goodrich Professor, School of Nursing; Lecturer,
Department of Epidemiology and Public Health, School of
Medicine, Yale University; Project Director, RIMS/Nursing
Office, Yale New Haven Hospital, New Haven, Connecticut

Joanne McCloskey Dochterman, PhD, RN, FAAN
Distinguished Professor of Nursing, Director, Center for
Nursing Classification, and Chair, Organizations, Systems, and
Community Health Area of Study, College of Nursing,
University of Iowa, Iowa City, Iowa

Katherine Dontje, MSN, RN, CS
Assistant Professor, College of Nursing, Michigan State
University, East Lansing, Michigan

Donna M. Dorsey, MS, RN
Executive Director, Maryland Board of Nursing, Baltimore,
Maryland

Joellen B. Edwards, PhD, RN
Professor and Dean, College of Nursing, East Tennessee State
University, Johnson City, Tennessee

Nancy Edwards, PhD, RNC
Assistant Professor, School of Nursing, Purdue University, West
Lafayette, Indiana

Joann M. Eland, PhD, RN, FNAP, FAAN
Associate Professor and Director of the Office of Information,
Communication and Technology, College of Nursing,
University of Iowa; Associate Director of Informatics,
University of Iowa Hospitals and Clinics, Iowa City, Iowa

Charlotte Eliopoulos, PhD, MPH, ND, RNC
Specialist in Holistic Chronic Care and President, Health
Education Network, Glen Arm, Maryland

Marilyn S. Fetter, PhD, RN, CS
Assistant Professor, College of Nursing, Villanova University,
Villanova, Pennsylvania; Editor, *MedSurg Nursing: The Journal
of Adult Health*, Pitman, New Jersey

Mohan Garg, ScD
Professor, Department of Medical Education, College of
Medicine, University of Illinois at Chicago, Chicago, Illinois

Barbara A. Given, PhD, RN, FAAN
Professor, College of Nursing, Michigan State University, East
Lansing, Michigan

Colleen J. Goode, PhD, RN, FAAN
Vice President Patient Services and Chief Nursing Officer,
University of Colorado Hospital, Denver, Colorado

Helen Kennedy Grace, PhD, RN, FAAN
Formerly Special Assistant to the President, W.K. Kellogg
Foundation, Battle Creek, Michigan

Victoria T. Grando, PhD, RN, CS, AP/MHCNS
Assistant Professor, Sinclair School of Nursing, University of
Missouri–Columbia, Columbia, Missouri

Cecelia Gatson Grindel, PhD, RN
Associate Professor, Georgia State University School of
Nursing, Atlanta, Georgia

Sheila A. Haas, PhD, RN
Professor and Dean, Niehoff School of Nursing, Loyola
University Chicago; President, National Federation of Specialty
Nursing Organizations, Chicago, Illinois

Ann Henrick, PhD, RN, FAAN
Lecturer, Centre for Nursing Studies, National University of
Ireland, Galway, Ireland; Formerly Clinical Associate Professor,
Niehoff School of Nursing, Loyola University Chicago, and
Clinical Nurse Specialist, Edward Hines Junior Veterans
Administration Hospital, Hines, Illinois

Jillian Inouye, PhD, APRN
Professor and Graduate Chair, School of Nursing and Dental
Hygiene, University of Hawaii, Honolulu, Hawaii

Lucille A. Joel, EdD, RN, FAAN
Professor, College of Nursing, Rutgers—The State University
of New Jersey, Newark, New Jersey

Gail M. Keenan, PhD, RN
Assistant Professor, School of Nursing, University of Michigan,
Ann Arbor, Michigan

Bette Keltner, PhD, RN
Dean, School of Nursing and Health Studies, Georgetown
University, Washington, D.C.

Karlene M. Kerfoot, PhD, RN, CNAA, FAAN
Senior Vice President for Nursing and Patient Care Services
and Chief Nurse Executive, Clarian Health Partners, Inc., and
Associate Dean for Clinical Practice, School of Nursing,
University of Indiana, Indianapolis, Indiana

Diane K. Kjervik, JD, RN, FAAN
Professor of Nursing and Director, Carolina Women's Center,
School of Nursing, University of North Carolina at Chapel
Hill; President-elect, American Association of Nurse Attorneys,
Chapel Hill, North Carolina

Jeanette C. Klemczak, MS, RN
Director, Faculty Clinical Practice, College of Nursing,
Michigan State University, East Lansing, Michigan

Mary Jo Kocan, MSN, RN
Clinical Nurse Specialist, University of Michigan Health
System, Ann Arbor, Michigan

Phyllis Beck Kritek, PhD, RN, FAAN
Florence Thelma Hall Distinguished Professor of Nursing and
Director, Doctoral Program in Nursing, School of Nursing,
The University of Texas Medical Branch at Galveston,
Galveston, Texas

Mary Krugman, PhD, RN
Director, Professional Resources, University of Colorado
Hospital, Denver, Colorado

Jody L. Kurtt, MA, RN, CNAA
Associate Director, Department of Nursing, Children's and
Women's Services, Children's Hospital of Iowa, University of
Iowa Hospitals and Clinics, Iowa City, Iowa

Susan Park Kyzer, MS, RN
Associate Consultant, The Center for Case Management, South
Natick, Massachusetts

Gerri S. Lamb, PhD, RN, FAAN
Associate Dean, College of Nursing, University of Arizona,
Tucson, Arizona

Judy Lee, CPM
Executive Director, The ARC of Las Cruces, Las Cruces, New
Mexico; President, MBA Management Consulting Group, San
Miguel, New Mexico

Judith M. Lewis, EdD, RN
Professor, College of Health Sciences, Touro University
International, Los Alamitos, California; Chief Executive
Officer, The Claremont Group, Claremont, California;
Professor Emeritus, Division of Nursing, California State
University, Dominguez Hills, California

Salima Manji Lin, MS
Manager, PricewaterhouseCoopers, Management Consulting,
Health Care, Chicago, Illinois

Sally Peck Lundeen, PhD, RN, FAAN
Professor and Interim Dean, School of Nursing, University of
Wisconsin–Milwaukee, Milwaukee, Wisconsin

Francene Lundy, MSA, RN
Director of Patient Care Services, University of Michigan
Health System; Adjunct Instructor, School of Nursing,
University of Michigan, Ann Arbor, Michigan

Meridean L. Maas, PhD, RN, FAAN
Professor; Chair, Adult and Gerontologic Nursing Area of
Study; Director, Doctoral Studies; and Senior Associate
Director, The Office of Research, College of Nursing, The
University of Iowa, Iowa City, Iowa

Peggy Jo Maddox, EdD, RN
Coordinator, Graduate Programs in Health Systems
Management, College of Nursing and Health Science, and
Director, Office of Research, Center for Health Policy, Research
and Ethics, George Mason University, Fairfax, Virginia

Beverly L. Malone, PhD, RN, FAAN
Deputy Assistant Secretary for Health, United States
Department of Health and Human Services, Washington, D.C.

Andrea Mengel, PhD, RN
Head, Department of Nursing, Community College of
Philadelphia, Philadelphia, Pennsylvania

Patricia Maguire Meservey, PhD, RN, FAAN
Professor, Bouvé College of Health Sciences, and Vice Provost
for Faculty and Budget, Northeastern University, Boston,
Massachusetts

Karen L. Miller, PhD, RN, FAAN
Professor and Dean, Schools of Nursing and Allied Health, University of Kansas, Kansas City, Kansas

V. Jane Muhl, PhD, RN
Associate Professor and Chairperson, Professional Program in Nursing, University of Wisconsin–Green Bay, Green Bay, Wisconsin

Fe Nieves-Khouw, MSN, RN
Faculty Associate, School of Nursing, University of Maryland; Coordinator, Clinical Practice Development, University of Maryland Medical Center, Baltimore, Maryland

Adele W. Pike, MSN, RN
Patient Services Manager, Visiting Nurse Association of Boston, Boston, Massachusetts

SueEllen Pinkerton, PhD, RN, FAAN
Associate Dean for Leadership in Practice, College of Nursing, University of Florida, Gainesville, Florida; Senior Vice President and Chief Nursing Officer, Shands Health Care/Shands Jacksonville, Jacksonville, Florida

Molly A. Poleto, BSN, RN, CHPN
Director of Community Education and Public Relations, The Community Hospice, Inc., Rensselaer, New York

Joan E. Predko, PhD, RN
Director of Outreach and Technology, College of Nursing, Michigan State University, East Lansing, Michigan

Marilyn J. Rantz, PhD, RN, FAAN
Professor, Sinclair School of Nursing, University of Missouri–Columbia, and University Hospitals Professor of Nursing, University of Missouri Hospitals and Clinics, Columbia, Missouri

Marilyn L. Rice, MPA, RN, CNAA
Health Care Consultant, Freeport, Illinois

Janet C. Ross-Kerr, PhD, RN
Professor, Faculty of Nursing, University of Alberta, Edmonton, Alberta

Marilyn L. Rothert, PhD, RN, FAAN
Professor and Dean, College of Nursing, Michigan State University, East Lansing, Michigan

M. Gaie Rubenfeld, MS, RN
Associate Professor, Department of Nursing, Eastern Michigan University, Ypsilanti, Michigan

Marla E. Salmon, ScD, RN, FAAN
Dean of Nursing and Professor of Nursing and Public Health, Nell Hodgson Woodruff School of Nursing, Emory University, Atlanta, Georgia

Barbara K. Scheffer, MS, RN
Associate Professor, Department of Nursing, Eastern Michigan University, Ypsilanti, Michigan

Donna Young Schmidt, MS, MBA, RN
Senior Clinical Consultant, Computer Sciences Corporation, New York, New York

Jill Scott, PhD, RN
Associate Director of Nursing, Area Health Education Center, and Assistant Professor, School of Nursing, University of Colorado Health Sciences Center, Denver, Colorado

F. Michael Seefeldt, PhD
Associate Professor, Department of Medical Education, College of Medicine, University of Illinois at Chicago, Chicago, Illinois

Kathleen Rice Simpson, PhD, RNC, FAAN
Perinatal Clinical Nurse Specialist, St. John's Mercy Medical Center, St. Louis, Missouri

Mechem Slim
Undergraduate Nursing Student, School of Nursing and Health Studies, Georgetown University, Washington, D.C.

Carolyn Smeltzer, EdD, RN, FACHE, FAAN
Partner, PricewaterhouseCoopers, Management Consulting, Health Care, Chicago, Illinois

Deborah Smith, MS, MBA, RN, CEN, CNAA
Assistant Administrator, Patient Services, OSF St. Joseph Medical Center, Bloomington, Illinois

Debra Smith, MSN, RN
Evaluation and Development Coordinator, Human Services Division, Indian Health Services, Cloquet, Minnesota

Linda S. Smith, DSN, RN
Founder of the United States–Russian Nurse Exchange Consortium, Racine, Wisconsin; Assistant Professor of Nursing, Oregon Health Sciences University, Klamath Falls, Oregon

Ann Solari-Twadell, MSN, MPA, RN
Director, International Parish Nurse Resource Center, Advocate Health Care, Gurnee, Illinois

Janet K. Pringle Specht, PhD, RN, FAAN
Assistant Professor, College of Nursing, The University of Iowa, Iowa City, Iowa

Dulcelina Albano Stahl, PhD, RN, CNAA, LNHA
President and Chief Executive Officer, D.A. Stahl & Associates, Northbrook, Illinois

Nancy A. Stotts, EdD, RN
Professor, School of Nursing, University of California, San Francisco, San Francisco, California

Gail W. Stuart, PhD, RN, CS, FAAN
Professor, Colleges of Nursing and Medicine, Director of
Doctoral Studies, and Coordinator of Psychiatric–Mental
Health Graduate Program, Medical University of South
Carolina, Charleston, South Carolina

M. Elaine Tagliareni, MS, RN
Professor and Independence Foundation Chair, Community
Health Nursing Education, Community College of
Philadelphia, Philadelphia, Pennsylvania

Teruko Takahashi, PhD, RN
Dean and Professor of Nursing, College of Nursing, Aichi
Medical University, Aichi-ken, Japan

Geraldine J. Talarczyk, EdD, RN
Associate Dean for Academic Affairs and Associate Professor,
College of Nursing, Michigan State University, East Lansing,
Michigan

Marita G. Titler, PhD, RN, FAAN
Director of Nursing Research, Quality and Outcomes
Management, Department of Nursing Services and Patient
Care, University of Iowa Hospitals and Clinics, Iowa City, Iowa

Linda M. Titus, MSN, RN, CNAA
Nursing Director, Acute and Extended Care, Veterans
Administration Connecticut Healthcare System, West Haven,
Connecticut

Sheila Dinotshe Tlou, PhD, RN
Professor of Nursing, Department of Nursing Education,
University of Botswana, Gaborone, Botswana

Sara Torres, PhD, RN, FAAN
Chair and Associate Professor, Behavioral and Community
Health Nursing, School of Nursing, University of Maryland,
Baltimore, Maryland

Toni Tripp-Reimer, PhD, RN, FAAN
Professor and Associate Dean for Research, College of Nursing,
University of Iowa, Iowa City, Iowa

Cayce P. Truong, MBA
Manager, PricewaterhouseCoopers, Management Consulting,
Health Care, Chicago, Illinois

María Mercedes D. de Villalobos, MSN, RN, PGAS
Titular and Emeritus Professor, Faculty of Nursing,
Universidad Nacional de Colombia Sede Bogotá, Coordinator
of Latin American Network for Nursing
Bogota D.C., Colombia

Patricia Hinton Walker, PhD, RN, FAAN
Dean and Professor, School of Nursing, University of
Colorado, Denver, Colorado

Maria R. Warda, PhD, RN
Assistant Dean, School of Nursing, University of California,
San Francisco, San Francisco, California

Kay Weiler, JD, MA, RN
Formerly Associate Professor, College of Nursing, University of
Iowa; Vice President, CompleWare Corporation, Iowa City,
Iowa

Robert H. Welton, MSN, RN
Faculty Associate, School of Nursing, University of Maryland;
Coordinator, Professional Development, University of
Maryland Medical Center, Baltimore, Maryland

Rita M. Williams, MSN, NP-C, PA-C
Curriculum Coordinator, Primary Care Associate Program,
Department of Family and Community Medicine, Stanford
University School of Medicine, Palo Alto, California; Nurse
Practitioner and Physician Assistant, Primary Care Associates,
Daly City, California

Ruth Williams-Brinkley, MSN, RN
Senior Vice President, Performance Management, Catholic
Health Initiatives, Louisville, Kentucky

Donna Zazworsky, MS, RN, CCM
Adjunct Faculty, College of Nursing, University of Arizona;
Program Director, Home Health and Outreach, St. Elizabeth of
Hungary Clinic, Tucson, Arizona

Polly Gerber Zimmermann, MS, MBA, RN, CEN
Instructor, Department of Nursing, Harry S Truman College;
Associate Editor, *Journal of Emergency Nursing*, Chicago,
Illinois

Margo R. Zink, EdD, RN, CNAA
Consultant, Johns Hopkins Home Care Group, and
Independent Home Healthcare Consultant, Baltimore,
Maryland

Laurie Zoloth, PhD
Professor of Social Ethics and Director of Jewish Studies
Program, California State University, San Francisco, San
Francisco, California

Mary Zwygart-Stauffacher, PhD, RN, CS, GNP/GCNS
Professor and Chair, Department of Nursing Systems,
University of Wisconsin–Eau Claire, Eau Claire, Wisconsin;
Geriatric Nurse Practitioner, Nursing Home Services, Red
Cedar Clinic/Mayo Health System, Menomonie, Wisconsin

Preface

Welcome to the sixth edition of *Current Issues in Nursing.* Previous editions of this book were published in 1981, 1985, 1990, 1994, and 1997. The purpose of this edition, as with past editions, is to provide a forum for knowledgeable debate on the important issues that concern all of today's nurses so that intelligent decision making can occur.

Given the rapidity of changes in the health care environment, we believe that a book like this that attempts to describe and discuss all the current issues in nursing is important. In periods of rapid change, decisions must often be made quickly. With many issues confronting such a large and diverse profession, there is danger that decisions will be made without full knowledge or without sufficient opportunity to discuss and debate. Or worse yet, issues may be ignored and decisions not made. The chapters in this book provide excellent information and thoughtful comment on the important issues currently facing the nursing profession.

As in the previous editions, the issues are identified and addressed in sections. In this edition we have 12 sections: Definitions of Nursing; Changing Information; Changing Education; Changing Practice; Quality Improvement; Governance; Health Care Systems; Health Care Costs; Role Transitions; Cultural Diversity; Ethics, Legal, and Social Issues; and International Nursing. As a new feature of this edition, we have grouped all the chapters about nursing in other countries in the last section on international nursing. In previous editions, beginning with the third, the international chapters were at the end of each section. Following the format of the fifth edition, the chapters in the section on changing practice focus on changes and issues in specific areas of specialty practice.

In the first edition, we had 75 chapters, in the second 84, in the third 89, in the fourth 103, in the fifth 92, and in this edition 85. We made a conscious attempt in the fifth edition and in this edition to reduce the number of chapters as the size of the book was beginning to be unmanageable. Of the 85 chapters in this edition, 4 are reprints from the fifth edition, 41 are updates from the fourth edition, and 40 are totally new. Most of the updated chapters are so much revised that they are not comparable to the previous version. All of the chapters are original pieces written for this book, and none, to our knowledge, have been published elsewhere.

Among the *new* content topics for this edition are evidence-based practice, international distance education, collaborative institutional approaches to education, outcomes management, patient satisfaction, contracting for services, reimbursement models for nurse managed centers, complementary therapies, reimbursement for alternative providers, finance skills for nurse managers, nursing of Native Americans, nursing of Asians and Pacific Islanders, caring for those with dementia, and health care in Africa, Japan, and Latin America. We have kept the fourth edition format of Section One, Definitions of Nursing, whereby the section overviews the facts and issues about specific groups of nurses and serves as an introduction to the rest of the book. Chapters in this section overview the roles of staff nurses, clinical nurse specialists and nurse practitioners, nurse executives, faculty members, and researchers. Section Four, Changing Practice, addresses issues in numerous specialties: ambulatory, community, and emergency nursing, gerontological nursing, hospice nursing, adult health/medical-surgical nursing, parish nursing, perinatal nursing, perioperative nursing, and psychiatric nursing. These chapters are among the most exciting in the book and demonstrate the impact of health care changes on nursing. Section Ten, Cultural Diversity, looks at changes and nursing issues in specific cultures: African Americans, Asians and Pacific Islanders, Hispanics/Latinos, and American Indians. The information in these chapters should help nurses provide culturally sensitive care for an increasingly diverse population. Section Twelve includes chapters about nursing in Africa, Canada, Great Britain, Japan, Latin America, and Russia. The comparison of nursing and related issues in selected countries around the globe is helpful to all of us.

Each section begins with an *overview* where we briefly introduce the section and "overview" each of the chapters in it. The sections' overviews, which highlight some of the important points in each chapter and raise some related issues, assist readers in selecting chapters for in-depth reading.

Following the overview is a *debate* chapter, in all but the international section, featuring the pros and cons of one of the problematic issues in nursing. A listing of the titles of debate chapters in the edition gives some idea of the scope of the issues:

- What Is Nursing?
- Nursing Theory, Nursing Research, and Nursing Practice: Connected or Separate?
- The Century Ahead: Old Traditions and New Challenges for Nursing Education
- Moving the Care: From Hospital to Home, from Nurses to Whom?
- Can Quality of Care Be Maintained in a Managed Care System?
- The Increasing Use of Unlicensed Assistive Personnel (UAP): The Erosion and Devotion of Nursing
- From a Medical Care System for a Few to a Comprehensive Health Care System for All
- Controlling Health Care Costs: Regulation vs. Competition
- Collaboration Between Nurses and Physicians in the 21st Century: What Is It? Does It Exist? Why Does It Matter?
- Why Isn't Nursing More Diversified?
- The Ethics of Health Care Reform: Should Rationing Strategies Target the Elderly?

In the first edition the debate chapters were a result of master's students' participation in an issues course at the University of Illinois College of Nursing. The chapters were based on actual oral debates that took place in class. For each debate a small group of students (anywhere from two to five) was asked to choose a topic, make up a reading list for advance distribution, and present all sides of the issue in a debate format to the rest of the class. Each group was instructed to stress the facts and research findings and to be as creative in presentation as they could. The approach was intellectual, but the mood was fun. Several groups conducted their own surveys of class knowledge and opinions prior to class. Others dressed for and acted out parts. For example, in one class there was a physician's assistant and a nurse practitioner who dressed exactly alike in their lab coats and stethoscopes, and in another the students played the

parts of nursing deans to argue out the merits of a PhD or a DNSc program.

Each group was required to state their debate topic in a debate form; the same topic could lead to several debates. For example, the topic expanded role resulted in one group in a debate entitled "Should Nurses Practice Dependently, Independently or Interdependently?" and another group's debate was entitled "Nurse Practitioners or Physician Assistants?" In a 2-hour course, 1 hour was allocated for the debate presentation and 1 hour for questions and debate with the rest of the class.

Some of the class debates were written up and were published in the first edition. In ensuing editions we have kept the same format, as we think debates are an excellent teaching mode for this content. Students who debate the material as well as their audience are involved in sorting out the complicated issues surrounding the debate. Many times just knowing all the facts leads to effective decision making; other times, it leads to the knowledge of what further research is needed before effective decision making can occur.

The bulk of the book is composed of *viewpoint* chapters. In these, authors give their own view and critical analysis of one particular aspect of the section's general topic. Viewpoints are those of the authors and may involve their taking a controversial stand, presenting a case study or results of some research, reviewing the past and current status of a topic, or outlining problems and future directions. The viewpoint chapters differ from the debate chapters, as the words viewpoint and debate differ: the viewpoint chapters, for the most part, offer only one side or segment of an issue. It is hoped that the viewpoint chapters provide material and ideas for other debates, that readers will agree or take issue, that after reading a viewpoint they will be stimulated to think and seek out more information. It is impossible to list all the many viewpoints here, but a sample list of titles will, we hope, make you eager to read these and more.

- Clinical Nurse Specialists and Nurse Practitioners: Who Are They, What Do They Do, and What Challenges Do They Face?
- Benchmarking: A Tool for Management Decision Making
- Critical Thinking: What Is It and How Do We Teach It?
- Alternative and Complementary Therapies: An Overview and Issues
- The Problems with Health Care Customer Satisfaction Surveys
- Shared Governance Models in Nursing: What Is Shared, Who Governs, and Who Benefits?

- Business Coalitions in an Electronic Age: Surviving in Local and Global Markets
- Cost of Home Care for Persons with Disability
- Conflict and Collaboration: Relationships and Challenges
- Finally We Have Arrived: Men in Nursing
- Just Managing: Ethical Obligations and the Managed Health Care Marketplace

This edition of *Current Issues in Nursing,* as did others in the past, offers a fairly complete analysis of all of today's important nursing issues. Careful reading, thought, and debate today can result in good decisions, actions, and achievements tomorrow. We hope you will enjoy the work of many talented contributors who collectively represent the diversity and wisdom of nursing.

Joanne McCloskey Dochterman
Helen Kennedy Grace

Who Is This Book For?

This book is appropriate for several audiences. First, it is an ideal book to use in a senior level undergraduate or graduate level issues course. Faculty who are teaching courses designed to help associate degree and diploma RNs make the transition to the university will also find this particularly useful. A teacher using this book could easily have her class orally present the debates written here or could structure a whole new set of debates using the readings as source material.

Second, it is a good book to use as a core book for a graduate curriculum. There is something here that will fit with most graduate nursing courses. For example, the section on changing information is useful in theory and informatics courses, the section on education for education courses, the sections on practice, quality improvement, and health care systems for advanced practice and nursing administration courses, the section on governance and role transition for leadership classes, and so on. By picking and choosing from the numerous viewpoints, every class in the graduate curriculum can benefit from the use of this book. By using one text throughout the curriculum, there is financial savings for the individual student and consistency in expectations from the faculty.

Third, the book is an excellent source of information about nursing and about the issues confronting the profession. The chapters are written by experts in the area and include many well-known nursing leaders. The book is stimulating and invigorating, and the challenges within will revitalize and energize the reader. It would make a good gift for a new RN or for a nurse going back to graduate school.

Acknowledgments

For help with the sixth edition, we wish to thank the following:

- Jennifer Clougherty, Program Associate at the University of Iowa, who completed with her usual competency and cheerfulness the administrative detail work related to the book. Thank you Jen.
- Michael Ledbetter and Thomas Eoyang, Editors at Mosby, who helped us plan this edition and work our way through the process. Thank you Michael and Thomas.
- Fran Murphy, Developmental Editor at Mosby, and Mary Espenschied, Copy Editing Supervisor, who did a great job preparing the book's manuscript for publication. Thank you Fran and Mary.
- Our authors for taking the time from busy schedules to think and write about their topics in an interesting and helpful manner. This book is only as good as their contributions.
- Our readers in the United States and other countries for their continued support and enthusiasm. We hope that this edition continues to meet your needs.
- Our immediate families who continue to be our main strength. Thank you Bruce, Dan, Michelle, and Meg and Elizabeth, David, and Peter.

Joanne McCloskey Dochterman
Helen Kennedy Grace

Contents

Section Four
Changing Practice

Section Five
Quality Improvement

Section Twelve

International Nursing

Section One

Definitions of Nursing

The Richness of Nursing

JOANNE McCLOSKEY DOCHTERMAN, HELEN KENNEDY GRACE

Nursing is a profession with rich career opportunities. In the past, nursing was viewed primarily in terms of direct patient care roles, mainly in hospitals. As the health field is changing, so are the roles of nurses and the places in which they work. Nearly 50% of nurses now work in settings outside of hospitals. As care is moving into community settings and patients return to their homes after very brief hospital stays, the context of care has changed. Hospice care, home care with intensive treatment protocols, and nursing home care for the elderly are examples of this changed context. In addition to nurses in direct practice roles, the opportunities for nurses as faculty members, researchers, and administrators in a variety of systems are expanding.

Not only is the organizational context of practice changing, but also the forms of practice are shifting. Increasingly nurses are developing their own group practices and working in new forms of collaboration with physicians. For example, many obstetricians/gynecologists now incorporate nurse midwives as practice partners. Whereas in the past, nurses' roles have been defined primarily in relationship to practice and practice settings, the "business" world of health care has opened up new opportunities for nursing in the management of health care. Nursing educational programs are beginning to forge partnerships with schools of business for nurses who want to build careers in the "business" side of nursing. The new world of information technology is opening up other vistas. Monitoring of patient care through use of computer technology is another example of a potential career track for nurses merging nursing knowledge with that of information-communication expertise.

Traditionally, nurses in the past tended to develop career paths opportunistically. Hopefully, in the future, persons entering the field will first be knowledgeable about the opportunities for career development in the field and have more clearly delineated career paths to a variety of opportunities within nursing that are matched by a com-mensurate reward system. This first section serves as an introduction to some of the potential career fields for nursing. Subsequent sections introduce other possibilities.

Perhaps no other profession has been so obsessive in defining its field as nursing. Diers differentiates dictionary definitions that record common usage from legal definitions that serve to regulate and establish the boundaries for the field. Because medicine was first to develop a regulatory framework that is so broad that "practically anyone's work including a mother's may be captured within it," all other professions have had to contend with this "first mover" effect and build their definitions in ways that are not duplicative. Thus defining the field of nursing is a political process rather than an intellectual and logical exercise. Instead of diagnosis and treatment of disease, which would be squarely in the medical domain, nursing has defined itself as diagnosing and treating human responses to actual or potential health problems. The evolvement of Social Policy Statements by the American Nursing Association is traced. Noting that Nightingale defined a nurse "as any person in charge of the personal health of another" and that Henderson wrote, "the unique function of the nurse is to assist the individual sick or well, in the performance of those activities contributing to health or its recovery (or to a peaceful death) that he would perform unaided if he had the necessary strength, will or knowledge," Diers commented that these are statements about what nurses *do,* not what nursing *is.* A further challenge is that of defining advanced practice nursing, which Diers describes as growing up outside of the professional organization. Whereas the nursing organizations and the nursing theorists continue the conceptual debate, the world of practice is pressing another set of questions. The challenge for the future will be "what patient outcomes can legitimately be claimed as effects of nursing"? The burden of proof will be squarely on nursing to validate its worth based on outcomes, including the cost-effectiveness of nursing interventions.

Turning specifically to hospital nursing, Grando traces the history of nursing in hospitals. The hospital of today presents formidable challenges to nursing related to the greater intensity of care required and the sophisticated technology in the care setting. The declining proportion of nurses practicing in hospital settings, the aging of the nursing population, and the lag in diversifying the nursing profession to match that of the general population are some of the challenges. Increased specialization and cross-training of nurses, delegation of tasks to assistive personnel, and the need to accelerate nursing work such as patient teaching create increased pressure on nursing in hospital settings. In addition to traditional roles, nurses are assuming greater responsibility for management of patient care as case managers and discharge planners. Within this context, nurses in hospital settings live with the constant fear of health risks in the workplace, such as the danger of being infected with HIV or hepatitis C by needle prick, and the relatively new phenomenon of violence in the workplace. Hospital nursing is responding favorably to these challenges.

Some form of nurse specialization has been in place over a long period of time. Henrick and Appleyard trace the origins of clinical nurse specialists and nurse practitioners. Clinical nurse specialists were developed primarily in hospital settings related to areas of specialty medical practice and acuity of care. Clinical nurse specialty areas developed around intensive care, for example, and in medical, surgical, and obstetrical specialty areas. As medical practice has become increasingly specialized, so has nursing in its clinical specialty areas. In contrast, nurse practitioners primarily practice in ambulatory settings and perform as generalists rather than as specialists. Current efforts are under way to merge the clinical nurse specialists with nurse practitioners under one council, The Council of Nurses in Advanced Practice. A major issue related to advanced practice nursing is the degree of independence of the nurse, and concerns for the degree of *supervision* of practice by medicine, in contrast to the preference of nurses for *collaboration*.

Just as care has changed, the roles of nurses in management are changing. Traditionally, nurse managers were limited to the management of nursing services. Responsibilities of nurse executives have broadened in scope. Pinkerton defines their role, "they are concerned with maximizing the quality of patient care, maximizing the professional satisfaction of the nursing staff, meeting the cost-effectiveness goals of the organization, and participating in long-range strategic planning, including nursing. They are clinical and business leaders in the or-

ganization. They know how to coordinate care and the cost of such care." At a time when the opportunities for nurse executives are increasing, programs to prepare nurses in the field of administration are declining. The current nursing shortage presents a formidable challenge for nurse executives, who are pushed by hospital executives who tend to see the solution to the problem as bringing additional assistive personnel into the care setting, the "slice and dice" approach. Pinkerton advocates that nurse executives have a clear set of standards and a "line they will not cross" in compromising patient care. Pinkerton ends with a case study in which the dilemmas facing nurse executives are clearly illustrated.

Anderson opens her discussion of faculty roles by raising the question, Who is the faculty? and then answering the question by noting that it depends on the three types of educational programs in nursing. Faculties at the associate degree level and in diploma schools of nursing are primarily teachers and clinicians, whereas those teaching in baccalaureate and higher degree programs are part of the university and its culture. Scholarly work in the form of research is an expectation. Yet only 50% of nursing faculty hold a doctorate, considered to be the basic preparation for research work. This lack of doctorally prepared faculty puts nursing in a marginal position vis-à-vis other faculty in the university. Anderson then goes on to describe the role of faculty in teaching, research, and service. The challenges facing nursing education relate to the danger of a culture of mediocrity because of weak doctoral programs, concerns for bridging the chasm between clinical practice and education, and the dominance of the profession by women, which puts it in a weak position within academia. The marginal status of all academic women is compounded in nursing. The general aging of the nursing population, particularly nursing faculty, and younger nurses' interests in pursuit of clinical work rather than in becoming faculty are noted as serious problems for the profession.

Ending this section, Stott addresses the role of nurse researchers. Nurse researchers "seek to understand the science of care through systematic investigation." Pathways to research careers are outlined. Successful researchers are adept at problem definition, and their expertise in research methods permits them to gather data to address the problem. Ability to attract funding for research, grant-writing skills, publishing research results, and participating in scientific discourse are talents integral to the role of a researcher. Particular challenges are the tendency for nurses to be overly critical of others whose substantive content or research methodologies differ from their own, the dependence on others for generating a caseload of research subjects, and the limited funding available to support nursing research.

In this changing kaleidoscope of nursing the challenge is that of keeping grounded in the positive traditions of the past—concern for the well-being of patients and participation in the here-and-now complex problems of providing cost-effective quality care—while shaping health policy for a future that will fully actualize the potential of nursing.

CHAPTER 1

What Is Nursing?

DONNA DIERS

Nursing does not suffer from lack of attempted definition.

In this chapter, the search for definition is examined. The intent is not to resolve the question by providing a new definition nor to debate old ones. Rather, the purposes, parameters, and consequences of this search are examined with a beady eye. Why define nursing? To what end?

If we do not know what nursing is, how can we justify teaching it or studying it or making decisions about it in a policy framework?

DICTIONARY DEFINITIONS

Dictionaries are published reports of common usage, and only that. In the first edition of the *Random House Dictionary* (1966) for example, the verb, "to nurse" means to foster or cherish ("to nurse one's meager talents"); to treat or handle with adroit care ("to nurse one's nest egg"); to bring up, train, or nurture; to clasp or handle carefully or fondly ("to nurse a memento"); to preserve ("to nurse a drink") (p. 990). "Nurse" suggests attendance and service; its antonym is neglect.

Note that these definitions are of the transitive verb form. Because the word *nursing* derives from it, there is no definition of "nursing." In the noun form in this dictionary, a nurse is "a person, especially a woman [sic] who takes care of the sick or infirm; a woman who has the general care of a child or children; a woman employed to suckle an infant; or any fostering agency or influence." A delightfully obscure meaning in billiards says a "nurse" is the act of maintaining the position of billiard balls in preparation for a carom.

Since dictionaries record common meaning, that meaning can and does change. It is encouraging to note

that in the 1995 *Random House Collegiate Dictionary,* the first meaning of "nurse" is now, "a person formally educated in the care of the sick or infirm, especially a registered nurse," surely progress even if they have not learned to capitalize the title.

The purpose of dictionary definitions is simply to record common usage, not to distinguish nursing from anything else or to isolate core concepts. There is no political agenda for dictionary definitions, except to the extent common meaning reflects the perspective of those who write the definitions and the common usage.

Encyclopedia definitions of nursing, which are really descriptions, are uneven in their grasp of the field. "Nursing: The Practice of Nursing" is in a section called "Medicine: Related Fields" in the 1999 CD-ROM version of *Encyclopedia Britannica.* Although the discussion of nurse practitioners acknowledges their global practice, the evolution of this advanced practice role is attributed to a World Health Organization policy paper in 1978. By that time the training and employment of nurse practitioners were 12 years old or so. That section also ends with the notion that "specially trained nurses can save the physicians' time" (www.eb.com).

DEFINITION IN THE LAW

Legal definitions in nurse practice acts exist to protect the public and to protect the *title*. These laws define (more or less vaguely) authorized practice and qualifications for using the legal title registered nurse (or licensed practical [vocational] nurse, advanced practice registered nurse, or nurse-midwife, depending upon state law). Licensing laws and their definitions are regulatory. They do not protect the nurse's practice from the challenge of practicing medicine without a license nor malpractice, although with clever legal assistance the language of practice acts may be used to *win* a court case.

Practice acts are interpreted by state agencies and

Suzanne Boyle, RN, MSN, and Joan Rimar, RN, MSN, doctoral students at the Yale University School of Nursing, made valuable comments toward this revision.

boards of nursing by interpretive statements, in regulations or declaratory rulings, and by ad hoc interpretations by the board or staff in court or less formally. For example, performing a genital examination in a case of suspected child abuse or first-assisting at surgery may be within the authorized advanced practice of nursing in one state but not in another, depending on how expert and liberal the interpreter and the law are. Further refinement of definitions of nursing come from attorneys general rulings when requested by the board of nursing or another state agency. The extent to which attorneys general understand modern nursing practice or consult with practicing nurses will determine how conservative or liberal an interpretation of the nurse practice act will emerge.

North Carolina was the first state to pass a licensing law (1903), and like many subsequent acts in other states, it was intended to protect the title, not to define the practice. The early statutes were certification laws, permissive rather than mandatory, and in general permitted anyone to perform legally the functions of a nurse, even for compensation, but only those who were licensed could use the RN title (Hadley, 1989).

New York was the first state to incorporate a definition of nursing, in 1938. The New York State Nurses Association (NYSNA) argued that "No practice can be controlled unless it is defined" (Driscoll, 1976, p. 46). The control that was sought was over unlicensed or otherwise unqualified individuals who were trading on the title "nurse" and, it could be assumed, taking work away from those who could demand higher wages because of the license.

In this regard, nursing is not different from other licensed professions including medicine. Licensure is usually sought by the profession to protect its own interests, as a study by Andrews (1983) of medical licensure laws often amusingly points out. By defining medicine very broadly, practically anyone's work including a mother's may be captured within it. See, for example, the Michigan definition of medical practice:

> "Practice of medicine" means the diagnosis, treatment, prevention, cure or relieving of a human disease, ailment, defect, complaint or other physical or mental condition, by attendance, advice, device, diagnostic test, or other means, or offering, undertaking, attempting to do, or holding oneself out as able to do, any of those acts. [Andrews, 1983, p. 21, citing Michigan Comp. Laws, 1980]

Medical licensing laws were written long before those of any other profession. The "first mover" advantage has meant that all other personal health care professions have had to contend with the fact that medicine defined the territory first (Safreit, 1993).

The act of defining the work of a profession within the law, then, is a political act and the resulting definitions must be read in that context. A compelling instance is the way in which the notion of diagnosis has been inserted into nursing practice acts. Idaho slipped the diagnosing function into its practice act first by legislating an exception to the part of the statute that prohibited unauthorized diagnosis and treatment (Bullough, 1980). It was New York, however, that redefined nursing:

> The practice of the profession of nursing . . . is defined as diagnosing and treating human responses to actual or potential health problems through such services as casefinding, health teaching, health counseling and provision of care supportive to and restorative of life and well-being. [Driscoll, 1976, p. 59]

The New York State Nurses Association was advised by its counsel that the diagnostic privilege was the sine qua non of independent practice (Driscoll, 1976, p. 59). The "human responses" phrase slips around "disease," which is central to medical practice acts. As a legislative memorandum (drafted by NYSNA) that accompanied the original bill notes,

> Inclusion . . . of the diagnostic function would authorize the nursing practitioner to make *nursing diagnoses, not* medical diagnoses. Whereas the diagnostic function as an intellectual process is central to the practice of any number of professions, including medicine and nursing, the *focus* of this function varies among these professions. For example, the focus in medicine is the nature and degree of pathology or deviation from normalcy; within nursing the focus is the *individual's response* to an actual or potential health problem and the nursing needs arising from such responses. [Driscoll, 1976, p. 61; italics in original]

Thus the attempt to broaden the definition of nursing to include diagnosis had, on the advice of one person, to consider the reality of physician opposition to *independent* practice, and what emerged was a semantic sleight of hand. The political reality was the need to build a fence between medicine and nursing; the problem is that this very real concern translates to defining the core of nursing in a way ("human responses") that limits expansion and economic progress. Once "diagnosis" was defined as a nursing function, then obviously there had to be a taxonomy of things nursing could name or diagnose that were not the same as "medical" diagnoses. Thus nursing diagnosis began as a political movement. The rich intellectual history of the work of classifying nursing is a topic for another book.

As advanced nursing practice roles evolved, a crazy quilt of state license laws followed. These are usefully summarized every year in the January issue of *Nurse Practitioner*. The newest wrinkle in this patchwork is the proposal for "multistate" licensure for advanced nursing practice, originally entered into debate by the National Council of State Boards of Nursing (NCSBN) in 1997 (Minarik & Price, 1999). The notion was that states, through their legislatures, would enter into mutual recognition contracts such that licensure in one state would be accepted as licensure in another, much as driver's licenses, banking regulations, and water usage are presently governed across state lines. A competing proposal by the American Nurses Association suggests a "uniform practice act" as a template for state law. Either proposal would require state legislatures, lobbied by their nursing constituencies, to act. Minarik and Price argue in favor of the template proposal, noting that whereas practice act language can be guided by templates, the regulatory processes to implement state practice acts vary wildly from state to state. They suggest that a less politically difficult step could be writing uniform education and certification requirements into acts for advanced practice registered nurses. Negotiating practice act language brings out the opposition forces, generally in medicine, whose lobbying power may outweigh nursing's bravest attempts. Nurses in many states have sat through public hearings in which naive legislators questioned whether it was "legal" for a nurse to use a stethoscope or whether a physician needed to see and confirm every time the red throat the advanced practice nurse called "pharyngitis."

These battles in advanced nursing practice are now so familiar that they can be called what they are: incursions into physician "autonomy," economic challenges, turned into language about patient safety. The examples are so numerous that the interested reader is referred to the American Medical Association's web site for continuous updates. The hits to that web site probably increased exponentially with the publication of the first randomized controlled clinical trial of nurse practitioner (NP) and physician primary care in the *Journal of the American Medical Association*'s first issue in 2000 (Mundinger et al., 2000). That high-profile study concluded that primary care delivered under similar circumstances of practice (private or not) and clientele by NPs and doctors of medicine (MDs) produced similar results.

The landmark case *Sermchief v. Gonzales* (1983) turned on the language of the nurse practice act in Mis-

souri, which was close to language suggested by the ANA's model practice act at the time. In *Sermchief* the Supreme Court of Missouri determined that the acts of two family planning nurse practitioners did indeed constitute the practice of nursing under Missouri law, including prescribing under standing orders and protocols, overturning a ruling by the circuit court. In arriving at this decision, the court did its own research and noted that many states had by then revised their nurse practice acts to broaden nursing's function. The court explicitly refused to "draw the elusive line between medicine and nursing," saying that the "hallmark of the professional" is knowing the limits of one's knowledge (Wolff, 1984, p. 26).

The legal challenges to the definition of nursing may also bring into question a particular act or task. One interesting case in Texas that went all the way to the U.S. Supreme Court cracked open a door that swings both ways for nursing. In *Irving Independent School District v. Tatro* (1984) the Supreme Court ruled that performing clean intermittent catheterization did not require a medical license and could be performed by a school nurse or "other qualified person." The background of this case illuminates why the context of definition is important. The Tatros are parents of a child with spina bifida. They wished their child, who is fine apart from this neurological problem, to go to public grade school, but the child required catheterization every 4 hours. Under federal law— the Education for all Handicapped Children Act of 1975 (PL 94-142)—with provisions that bind the states, public education systems must provide free, accessible education for handicapped children but are not obliged to provide health services (diagnosis, evaluation) by a licensed physician, which services were thought to be expensively beyond the intent of the law. The Court explicitly interpreted clean intermittent catheterization as "a simple procedure that can be performed in a few minutes by a layperson with less than an hour's training" (p. 883). Thus the Irving School District was obligated to arrange for the provision of this service so that Amelia Tatro could benefit from free public education. Advocates for disabled persons hailed the decision as broadening the provisions of the law and making education available even when a special service was required. Some in the nursing community cheered that catheterization was interpreted not to need physician supervision. Others were concerned that if this one task could be performed by a layperson, the school nurse's definition of practice was compromised (Vitello, 1987). This piecemeal task-oriented interpretation of what is or is not nursing has contemporary consequences, as we shall see later.

Courts will use professional association statements when confronted with cases alleging violations of practice acts. Thus it is well to consider how professional association "definitions" evolve.

DEFINITIONS BY PROFESSIONAL ASSOCIATIONS

The publication and wide distribution of the American Nurses Association monograph *Nursing—A Social Policy Statement* (1980) has had the effect of codifying a definition of nursing based on that of New York state: "Nursing is the diagnosis and treatment of human responses to actual or potential health problems" (ANA, 1980, p. 9), as if there were some national consensus. The slippage from one political agenda in one state to ANA's own agenda underscores the need to examine definitions according to their purpose. The purpose of the ANA document was to define the nature and scope of nursing practice to serve as a basis for ANA policy regarding credentialing and establishment of qualifications for entry into nursing practice (ANA, 1980, p. v). ANA has another agenda, however, which is to position the Association to speak to and for all kinds of registered nurses, resisting the notion of a second license for specialized practice. Having lost the second license battle, as suggested in the previous section, ANA's support of a uniform advanced practice act template can be seen as an organizational fallback.

In spite of the publication of the *Social Policy Statement* and its new language in 1980, in 1981 the ANA's suggested language for nurse practice acts did not mention "human responses" nor "actual or potential health problems." The purpose for these statements is different, however. The *Social Policy Statement* was exactly that, a statement of organizational policy cast as more general policy. The suggested language for state law is much more operational, because law always is. Thus in keeping with the agenda above, the suggested language read:

The practice of nursing means the performance for compensation of professional services requiring substantial specialized knowledge of the biological, physical, behavioral, psychological and sociological sciences and of nursing theory as the basis for assessment, diagnosis, planning, intervention and evaluation in the promotion and maintenance of health; the casefinding and management of illness, injury or infirmity; the restoration of optimum function; or the achievement of a dignified death. Nursing practice includes but is not limited to administration, teaching, counseling, supervision, delegation, and evaluation of practice and execution of the medical regimen including the administration of medications and treatments prescribed by any person authorized by state law to prescribe. Each registered nurse is directly accountable and responsible to the consumer for quality of nursing care rendered. [ANA, 1981, p. 6]

The "accountability to the consumer" language was a direct attempt to remove physician supervision or direction from suggested practice act language.

By 1990, ANA's suggested language had changed in an interestingly subtle way. Now, "the practice of nursing means the performance of services for compensation in the provision of diagnosis and treatment of human responses to health or illness" (ANA, 1990, p. 8). This change from "health problems" in the *Social Policy Statement* to "health and illness" broadens the target of nursing practice and still slithers away from boldly stating that nurses diagnose and treat disease (a "human response" to health could . . . er . . . be disease). The 1990 version also widens nursing's scope to include case management, establishing standards of practice, directing practice, and collaboration, again following from ANA's wish to be representative of all nurses.

By 1995, new forces within nursing advocating for redefining nursing without using medicine as the standard had produced revisions to the *Social Policy Statement* that included new language about healing and caring (ANA, 1995, p. 6):

[N]ursing philosophy and practice have been influenced by a greater elaboration of the science of caring and its integration with the traditional knowledge base for diagnosis and treatment of human responses to health and illness. As such, definitions of nursing more frequently acknowledge four essential features of contemporary nursing practice:

- Attention to the full range of human experiences and responses to health and illness without restriction to the problem-focused orientation
- Integration of objective data with knowledge gained to form an understanding of the patient's or group's subjective experience
- Application of scientific knowledge to the processes of diagnosis and treatment
- Provision of a caring relationship that facilitates health and healing

Jean Watson comments that the internal political work in nursing to tilt definitions away from diagnosis and treatment toward caring and healing led to nearly irreconcilable differences. She and other "postmodern" nursing theorists propose that there is damage done by the diagnosis and treatment process and that alternative approaches to healing and caring could bring about a revolution in the healing professions and their definitions. The interested reader is urged to mine this new wave of nursing thinking, best exemplified in Watson's book (Watson, 1999).

NIGHTINGALE AND HENDERSON

A careful examination of Florence Nightingale's and Virginia Henderson's "definitions" of nursing is in order because they are so often consulted when the nature of nursing is in question.

In *Notes on Nursing—What It Is and What It Is Not* (1859/1946), Florence Nightingale wrote, "I use the word nursing for want of a better" (p. 6) and "a nurse means any person in charge of the personal health of another" (p. 79).

Miss Nightingale wrote *Notes on Nursing* as a kind of Red Cross handbook for home nursing, to explain the laws of the human body as she understood them and thus how the nursing functions could affect health and comfort. She wrote to make conscious the implicit knowledge that women in particular had, especially of diet and cleanliness, so that all women who "nursed" could be better prepared. But she was also writing a political treatise to enlist others in her ideas.

The often-quoted "definition" of nursing comes late in the book in a discussion of what medicine or surgery can do and what nature can do (better) if just left alone:

> It is often thought that medicine is the curative process. It is no such thing; medicine is the surgery of functions, as surgery proper is that of limbs and organs. Neither can do anything but remove obstructions; neither can cure; nature alone cures. [p. 74]

And then, "what nursing has to do . . . is put the patient in the best condition for nature to act upon him" (p. 75). But this is not a definition of nursing. Read in context, it is a somewhat off-handed statement of nursing's function or goal in the context of Miss Nightingale's notions about the causes of illness and her reservations about medicine with its suspicious germ theory.

Virginia Henderson's definition is of the unique *function* of the nurse, which she deliberately calls not a definition but a "personal concept" (Henderson, 1991):

> The unique function of the nurse is to assist the individual sick or well, in the performance of those activities contributing to health or its recovery (or to peaceful death) that he would perform unaided if he had the necessary strength, will or knowledge. And to do this in such a way as to help

him gain independence as rapidly as possible. [Henderson, 1961, p. 2]

Miss Henderson is careful to say in the immediately following sentences that this is not all there is to nursing, and thus this definition was never intended to define either the entire discipline or the entire field of practice. The statement is about the *unique* function of the nurse, "this aspect of her work . . . she initiates and controls; of this she is master" (Henderson, 1991, p. 21). For Miss Henderson, this unique function is the core of nursing that must be protected. "No one . . . should make such heavy demands on another member [of the medical team] that any one of them is unable to perform his or her unique function" (p. 42).

In these activities, the nurse is, and, as Miss Henderson argues, should be, an independent practitioner, "able to make independent judgments as long as he, or she, is not diagnosing, prescribing treatment for disease, or making a prognosis, for these are the physician's functions" (p. 22). Reflecting on these statements 30 years later, Miss Henderson (1991) revised her emphasis:

> Today I see the role of nurses as givers of "primary health care," as those who diagnose and treat when a doctor is unavailable, even as the midwife functions in the absence of an obstetrician. Nurses may be the general (medical) practitioners of tomorrow. [p. 33]

> The modification in my concept of nursing since I wrote in 1966 suggests a different emphasis. . . . I recognize now, as I think the majority of health care providers recognize, that registered nurses . . . are the major providers of primary care. Obstetrical nurses, or midwives, have been universally recognized worldwide as the providers of primary care for mothers and newborns. They diagnose and treat as well as "care." [p. 98]

Both Nightingale's and Henderson's definitions go not to what nursing "is" but rather to what nurses *do*. That is a distinction to keep in mind as we dig deeper into the definitional trench.

THEORIES AND DEFINITIONS

This is neither the time nor the place to analyze fully the various theoretical perspectives on nursing that might constitute another source of definition. That work has been done (and done and done again) and is usefully summarized by Afaf Meleis (1991) and Leslie Nicoll (1992).

Most of the work on the nature of nursing in theory was done by the first wave of nurses either seeking or profiting from doctoral degrees in education or in other disciplines, since there were few doctoral programs in nursing. Most of the theorists came of nursing age before there was the degree of specialist immersion now common in practice. Further, the nursing theories emerged at a time when nursing was moving rapidly into the universities. It was important for nursing faculties to justify what was particularly and peculiarly nursing. Thus the search for ways of conceiving of nursing and its knowledge that would mark it as intellectual and as different from simply "applied" anything else (Wald & Leonard, 1964). What resulted was what Virginia Henderson actually advocated—personal conceptions—but those conceptions were not about the work or the practice of nursing, they were about the *discipline*.

These were the content theories: Martha Rogers' "science of unitary man"; Sr. Callista Roy's adaptation theory; Dorothea Orem's theory of self-care deficits, and so on. These theories were really conceptual models, as Fawcett (1980) points out, and they all had the same domains: person, environment, health, and nursing. "Nursing" was more or less the glue that held the whole thing together, often without much specificity as the theories dealt more with the nature of human beings in sickness and health than about what we are supposed to do about sickness and health. Thus, for Martha Rogers, the goal of nursing is to "strengthen the coherence and integrity of the human field and to direct and redirect patterning of the human and environmental fields" (Rogers, 1970, p. 122). And nursing is simply the "learned profession" that does that, whatever that is. For Imogene King, nursing is called for when individuals cannot function in their roles and is "a process of human interaction between nurse and client whereby each perceives the other in the situation and, through communication, they set goals, explore means and agree on means to achieve goals" (King, 1981, p. 144).

The purpose of these grand theories or conceptual models was to develop the discipline, particularly the academic part of the discipline, to provide some structure to the research, and perhaps to stake out turf that would be uniquely nursing, not in opposition to medicine, but as different from applied social science. There was, however, a less-than-explicit agenda that if we would all just do the research guided by whatever conceptual model under whatever theoretical emphasis, when it was all added up we would know what nursing *is*.

The grand theories can be contrasted to another set of "practice theories" that evolved about the same time. The ones most often cited are Ida Orlando's (1961, 1972), Ernestine Weidenbach's (1964), and Joyce Travelbee's (1966). There are two important differences between the grand theories and these: these are about *practice*, not about the nature of the discipline, and their authors were all nurses prepared in specialist or advanced practice (Orlando and Travelbee in psychiatric nursing, Weidenbach in nurse-midwifery).

With the possible exception of Travelbee, these latter theorists did not even attempt to define nursing. For them there is an assumption that we know what nursing is, we just need to understand what within it works, that is, produces desired changes in patient state. The purpose of the theories here was to guide practice and practice-based research, not to fight the definitional battles. For these theorists, nursing was already an independently practicing profession, as their experience in specialized practice roles had taught them. The present effort to create categories of nursing intervention (Iowa Intervention Project, 1995; McCloskey & Bulechek, 2000) follow from the ideas of practice theory, if not explicitly from the theorists. The developing taxonomy of nursing interventions is about practice and the relationship of nursing work to patient outcomes, not about definitions of nursing or nursing diagnoses.

ADVANCED PRACTICE AS A DEFINITIONAL PROBLEM

When nursing roles began to expand beginning in the 1960s with critical care, nursing's outer boundaries, which no one had worried much about before, both loosened and sharpened, again depending on the purpose of definition.

Expanding the nursing role was made legitimate by the *Report of the Secretary's Commission to Study the Extended Role of Nurses* (1971) chaired by Rozella Schlotfeldt. This report defined "primary care" as first contact, continuing, and coordinated care that nurses surely could provide. The expansion of nursing's boundaries was a twofold expansion: into independent functioning without physician direction, and into providing services, especially physical examination, diagnosis, and treatment that had been "formerly medicine" (Diers & Molde, 1983).

By this time, nurse-midwives and nurse anesthetists were already firmly established in primary practice roles (Diers, 1992), but with much the same internal and external controversy about whether what they did was "really" nursing. Martha Rogers was moved to write that nurse practitioners ought to just admit that they were filling in for doctors (Rogers, 1975); her argument was not that nurses should not do this work, but that it should be acknowledged as nursing. Loretta Ford (1982) has written poignantly of the discrimination both from nursing and medicine against her pediatric nurse practitioner program.

Ford was clear from the beginning that the nurse practitioner role grew from a base in community health nursing in which nurses had long functioned independently and managed illness alone. Very soon, research showed that nurses could do the work, and over time, enough evidence accumulated to conclude that the performance of nurse practitioners, in productivity and quality, was at least equal to if not better than that of physicians (Brown & Grimes, 1993; Office of Technology Assessment, 1986; Safreit, 1993).

Yet questions remain about whether the work of advanced practice, as it has come to be called (Cronenwett, 1995), is delegated medical functions or within nursing's boundaries. The definitional question, however, is a political and legal one, not a conceptual one, and it is increasingly becoming an economic question as well. The growing recognition that primary care is interdisciplinary or shared practice is raising subtle questions about nurses' "playing doctor" (Fairman, 1999).

Nurse practitioners grew up in an era of physician shortage, so it was all right for nurses to substitute. When there is a need, it is okay for nurses to do almost anything, as even Virginia Henderson wrote. Where there is competition, challenges to the definition of nursing surface and are difficult to defend against because the problem is not whether this is nursing but whether we ought to get paid for it.

Advanced practice nursing grew up outside of the professional organization (ANA) for the most part because ANA's priorities have been occupied by economic and general welfare and entry into practice. Without the strong leadership of a national organization representing the breadth of nurse practice roles, both the roles and their definitions have had to turn to the legal system or to specialized nursing associations. In the United States the regulation of practice is done state by state and there are now over 50 specialized nursing associations, many of them quite professional with journals, newsletters, annual conventions, lawyers, and lobbyists. There is such a patchwork of nursing specialties that it has become a political problem for nursing at the federal level. It is not the lack of definition that has led to this confusion, however, it is the absence of leadership from a professional association consumed with other issues.

OTHER DEFINITIONAL CHALLENGES

In the 1990s the challenge to the definition of nursing practice came from the managed care environment and the consulting firms, which advised hospitals that the fragmentation of patient care in more than 600 categories of hospital workers, as well as the downtime for professional nurses, could be fixed if only hospitals would realize that a good deal of what nurses do (and have to do) is not "really" nursing. Of course not. It does not require a license to call a physician to question a medication order (but it requires knowledge of clinical care) or to get the housekeeping department to mop a floor (but that requires knowledge of the system of care).

The argument goes that there are any number of tasks that nurses do (or did) that could be done by others because the tasks do not, of themselves, require a nursing license. Adding up tasks is not the way to define the work that registered nurses do or the way to define the discipline. By themselves, tasks are just that, but this is not about tasks or nursing work; it is about trying to decrease hospital expenses by substituting lesser prepared and lower paid personnel for professional nurses by breaking nursing tasks into pieces that can then be passed to others. By 2000, it was becoming fairly clear that this rabid reengineering had unfortunate consequences in nursing enrollments, morale, and perhaps hospital quality (Kovner & Gergen, 1998). The projected cost savings were generally not achieved. Nurses felt victimized and angry, and a level of suspicion of administrators often remained (Shindul-Rothschild, Berry, & Long-Middleton, 1996).

One potential benefit of the reengineering madness was to put the bright policy spotlight on the relative paucity of evidence about the effects of nursing skill mix (proportion of licensed to unlicensed personnel) on patient outcomes. The Institute of Medicine issued a crucial study calling for targeted research on the relationship between nursing "input" and patient outcome (Institute of Medicine, 1996). This topic will likely be the definitional challenge of the early years of the new century. This time, however, the question is different. It is no longer what nurses *do,* or what the discipline *is,* but what patient outcomes can legitimately be claimed as effects of nursing. Choosing such outcomes provokes fascinating debates in research teams. It is not hard to find agreement that decubitus ulcers and falls are an effect of nursing, or rather of lack of nursing. But is length of hospital stay an effect of nursing, as some would argue (Czaplinski & Diers, 1998)? To believe that, it is necessary to believe that the "definition" or conceptualization of nursing includes the possibility not only of caring for the sick, but of tending the entire environment within which care happens. Physicians may admit patients, but nurses get them out.

USES OF DEFINITION

It should be clear that there is no one agreed-upon definition of nursing with respect to the work, the discipline, the profession, or the public image. There is not one for any other discipline either if one probes deeply enough. Why then do we worry so much about definition in nursing?

It should also be clear that different purposes require different approaches to definition.

If the purpose is to define nursing in order to guide research, then an operational definition—and outline of the work—is in order.

If the purpose is to change the law, than a definition that will fit existing law and that is politically feasible is required.

If the purpose is to convince Congress or a state or federal agency of the value of nursing, definition is irrelevant; data on increasing access to care, decreasing cost, and improving outcomes will make the case, and those who do it—nurses—win.

If the purpose is to explain what nursing is to a lay audience, then no definition will work, because what the audience will relate to is a description of the work, not a definition.

[W]hen a person says, "I am going to *nurse* my cold," he hastens to arrange the environment so that he can be as free as possible from stress and takes all means at his disposal to increase his comfort. On the other hand, when he says, "I am *doctoring* my cold," we know that he is not only relying on his own inner natural resources, but also on the products of medical science—pills, inhalers and the like. [Orlando, 1961, p. 5]

That description works better than definition because everyone has had a cold. People who have never nursed have no way to understand what the work is like and what it takes to do it, it is so personal and intimate a service and so fiendishly difficult to describe.

Finally, if the purpose is to explain to one's extended family what one does for a living as a nurse, one might start with Virginia Henderson's translation of her own "personal concept":

[The nurse] is temporarily the consciousness of the unconscious, the love of life for the suicidal, the leg of the amputee, the eyes of the newly blind, a means of locomotion for the infant, knowledge and confidence for the young mother, the [voice] for those too weak or withdrawn to speak. [Henderson, 1964, pp. 63-64]

REFERENCES

American Nurses Association. (1980). *Nursing—A social policy statement.* Kansas City, MO: Author.

American Nurses Association. (1981). *Suggested state legislation.* Kansas City, MO: Author.

American Nurses Association. (1990). *Suggested state legislation.* Washington, DC: Author.

American Nurses Association. (1995). *Nursing's social policy statement.* Washington, DC: American Nurses Publishing.

Andrews, L.B. (1983). *Deregulating doctoring.* Emmaus, PA: People's Medical Society.

Brown, S.A., & Grimes, D.E. (1993). *Nurse practitioners and certified nurse-midwives: A meta-analysis of studies on nurses in primary care roles.* Washington, DC: American Nurses Publishing.

Bullough, B. (Ed.). (1980). *The law and the expanding nursing role* (1st ed.). Philadelphia: FA Davis.

Cronenwett, L.R. (1995). Molding the future of advanced practice nursing. *Nursing Outlook, 43,* 112-118.

Czaplinski, C., & Diers, D. (1998). Effect of staff nurse specialization on length of stay and mortality. *Medical Care, 36*(12), 1626-1638.

Diers, D., & Molde, S. (1983). Nurses in primary care: The new gatekeepers. *American Journal of Nursing, 83,* 742-745.

Diers, D. (1992). Nurse-midwives and nurse anesthetists: The cutting edge in specialist practice. In L.H. Aiken (Ed.), *Charting nursing's future: Nursing in the '90's* (pp. 159-180). Philadelphia: Lippincott.

Driscoll, V.M. (1976). *Legitimizing the profession of nursing: The distinct mission of the New York State Nurses Association.* Albany, NY: Foundation of NYSNA.

Fairman, J. (1999). Playing doctor? Nurse practitioners, physicians, and the dilemma of shared practice. *The Long Term View, 4*(4) (Massachusetts School of Law, Andover).

Fawcett, J. (1980). A framework for analysis and evaluation of conceptual models of nursing. *Nurse Educator, 5,* 10-14.

Ford, L.C. (1982). Nurse practitioners: History of a new idea and predictions for the future. In L.H. Aiken (Ed.), *Nursing in the 1980's: Crises, challenges, opportunities* (pp. 231-248). Philadelphia: Lippincott.

Hadley, E.H. (1989). Nurses and prescriptive authority: A legal and economic analysis. *American Journal of Law and Medicine, 15,* 245-300.

Henderson, V.A. (1964). The nature of nursing. *American Journal of Nursing, 64,* 62-68.

Henderson, V.A. (1961). *Basic principles of nursing care.* Geneva: International Council of Nurses.

Henderson, V.A. (1991). *The nature of nursing: Reflections after 25 years.* New York: National League for Nursing.

Institute of Medicine. (1996). *Nursing staff in hospitals and nursing homes: Is it adequate?* Washington, DC: National Academy Press.

Iowa Intervention Project. (1995). Validation and coding of the NIC taxonomy structure. *Image, 27,* 43-49.

Irving Independent School District v. Tatro, No. SC 3371. S. Ct. (1984).

King, I.M. (1981). *A theory for nursing: Systems, concepts, process.* New York: Wiley.

Kovner, C., & Gergen, P.J. (1998). Nurse staffing levels and adverse events following surgery in US hospitals. *Image, 30*(4), 315-321.

McCloskey, J.C., & Bulechek, G. (Eds.). (2000). *Nursing interventions classification* (3rd ed.). St Louis: Mosby.

Meleis, A.I. (1991). *Theoretical nursing: Development and progress* (2nd ed.). Philadelphia: Lippincott.

Minarik, P.A., & Price, L.C. (1999). Multistate licensure—for advanced practice nurses? *Nursing Outlook, 47*(2), 95-96.

Mundinger, M.O., Kan, R.L., Lenz, E.R., Totten, A.M., Tsai, W.Y., Cleary, P.D., Friedewald, W.T., Siu, A.L., & Shelanski, M.L. (2000). Primary care outcomes in patients treated by nurse practitioners or physicians: A randomized trial. *Journal of the American Medical Association, 283*(1), 59-68.

Nicoll, L.H. (1992). *Perspectives on nursing theory* (2nd ed.). Philadelphia: Lippincott.

Nightingale, F. (1859/1946). *Notes on nursing—What it is and what it is not.* Philadelphia: Lippincott.

Office of Technology Assessment, US Congress. (1986). *Nurse practitioners, physician assistants and certified nurse-midwives: A policy analysis.* Washington, DC: U.S. Government Printing Office.

Orlando, I.J. (1961). *The dynamic nurse-patient relationship.* New York: G.P. Putnam's Sons.

Orlando, I.J. (1972). *The discipline and teaching of nursing process.* New York: G.P. Putnam's Sons.

Random House dictionary. (1966). New York: Random House.

Random House collegiate dictionary. (1995). New York: Random House.

Rogers, M. (1970). *An introduction to the theoretical basis of nursing.* Philadelphia: Lippincott.

Rogers, M. (1975). Euphemisms in nursing's future. *Image, 7,* 3-9.

Safreit, B.J. (1993). Health care dollars and regulatory sense: The role of advanced practice nursing. *Yale Journal on Regulation, 9*(2), 417-488.

Secretary's Commission to Study the Extended Role of Nurses. (1971). *Extending the scope of nursing practice* (DHEW Publication No. HSM 73-2037). Washington, DC: U.S. Government Printing Office.

Sermchief v. Gonzales, 660 S.W.2d 683 (1983).

Shindul-Rothschild, J., Berry, D., & Long-Middleton, E. (1996). Where have all the nurses gone? Final results of our patient care survey. *American Journal of Nursing, 96*(11), 52-57.

Travelbee, J. (1966). *Interpersonal aspects of nursing.* Philadelphia: Lippincott.

Vitello, S.J. (1987). School health services after *Tatro. Journal of School Health, 57,* 77-80.

Wald, F.S., & Leonard, R.C. (1964). Towards development of nursing practice theory. *Nursing Research, 23,* 309-313.

Watson, J. (1999). *Postmodern nursing and beyond.* New York: Churchill Livingstone.

Weidenbach, E. (1964). *Clinical nursing: A helping art.* New York: Springer.

Wolff, M.A. (1984, February). Court upholds expanded practice roles for nurses. *Law, Medicine & Health Care,* 26-29.

Staff Nurses Working in Hospitals

Who Are They, What Do They Do, and What Challenges Do They Face?

VICTORIA T. GRANDO

Hospital nursing in the United States has a long and diverse history. It began in the late 1700s, when hospitals were mostly charitable institutions that served the sick-poor. By the 1800s, many hospitals were dirty, vermin-infested places that frequently spread disease. The nurses that worked in these marginal institutions had no formal training and were typically from the "dregs of female society." But this grim picture quickly changed with the establishment of hospital training schools of nursing in 1873 (Kalisch & Kalisch, 1995; Melosh, 1982; Reverby, 1987).

Upper-class women reformers, acting from both a sense of religious and class stewardship (the belief that the wealthy were entrusted to provide for the sick, poor, and the working class), sought to improve the care in hospitals in the late 1800s. To this end they established nurses' training schools for women of good moral character that incorporated bedside training and strict discipline. These reforms were very effective. Soon hospitals, staffed by student nurses, were clean environments in which patients received good care and became well. As a result of the improved care by student nurses and the increasing sophistication of medicine, the numbers of hospitals grew drastically, increasing from 200 in 1870 to over 4,000 in 1910 (Ashley, 1976; Flood, 1981; Melosh, 1982; Reverby, 1987).

Hospitals continued to be staffed largely by student nurses until the late 1920s.[1] In the 1930s, about 36% of graduate nurses worked for hospitals as directors, supervisors, head nurses, and instructors. Private duty nurses were also working more in hospitals. By 1928, some estimate that perhaps as much as 60% of private duty nursing was being done within hospitals. Private duty nurses working in hospitals held a variety of roles. Some worked for surgeons, some cared for the difficult patients, and others did general duty nursing for individual patients. But as the 1930s progressed, hospitals began to hire staff nurses. This shift resulted from numerous factors including nursing leaders' pressure to close inadequate schools of nursing, decreased enrollments in nursing schools, the continued increases in number of hospital beds, and the depression that rapidly brought about the collapse of home nursing. Moreover, graduate nurses unable to get private duty work were willing to work for low wages and sometimes for simple room and board. Thus hospitals increasingly began to hire graduate nurses to meet their increasing staff needs. In fact, paying staff nurses under these arrangements was often less expensive than educating students (Flood, 1981).

Hospital staff nursing as we know it today took shape by the early 1940s. Although many hospitals still relied heavily on student labor from their schools of nursing, the number of paid staff nurses was increasing.[2] By 1945, 49% of all registered nurses (RNs) were employed in hospitals as administrators, supervisors, head nurses, and staff nurses. Nurses worked in a variety of inpatient clinical areas including communicable diseases, tuberculosis, operating room, orthopedics, pediatrics, medicine, surgery, psychiatry, obstetrics, and gynecology, as well as in outpatient departments (American Nurses Association [ANA], 1946). After the mid 1940s, nurses' roles became

---

[1]During this period graduate nurses worked both as private duty nurses in patients' homes and as public health nurses. Some served as administrators in hospitals.

[2]In 1945 most schools of nursing were hospital-based diploma schools of nursing.

increasingly complex as new advances were made in surgery and medical technology and as physicians delegated various medical roles to nurses: Nurses became responsible for caring for critically ill patients in emergency rooms, recovery rooms, cardiac intensive care units, and premature infant centers. They provided complex care for patients recovering from open-heart surgery, receiving hemodialysis, and on respirators. Nurses took over intravenous care, participated in codes, supervised nurses aides, and conducted group therapy.

As these clinical advances were occurring, nurses faced numerous challenges. The end of World War II began a long period of nursing shortages. This added to the stress of nurses working 44- to 48-hour weeks, split shifts, and overtime without extra pay. Moreover, wages were low. Indeed, some questioned why nurses continued to work at all (Brown, 1948). Gradually through the efforts of the ANA and local nurses across the country, wages and working conditions improved (Grando, 1997, 1998, 2000).

HOSPITAL STAFF NURSES: TODAY'S PROFILE

Hospital staff nursing today in some ways mirrors hospital staff nursing of the past, but in other ways it is facing new horizons and challenges. Hospitals continue to employ most working RNs. The number of nurses working in hospitals had gradually increased to about 65% of all nurses by the 1960s and remained fairly constant until recently (Grando, 1994; ANA, 1985). At present, 59.6% of all employed nurses work in hospitals, and this number is projected to decrease to 52.8% by 2008 (Bureau of Labor Statistics, 2000). In 1992[3] most hospital nurses worked full time (70%) for an average of 41.6 hours a week, just slightly less than nurses did half a decade ago. Nurses working in hospitals are younger. In 1992, 84% of all registered nurses 30 years old or younger worked in hospitals, whereas only 50% of nurses over 50 worked in hospitals. Most hospital nurses work in general medical and surgical units (40%), but many work in acute care units such as critical care (18%), operating rooms (7%), and emergency rooms (8%). A little over 30% of hospital nurses work in specialty areas such as pediatrics, newborn nurseries, obstetrics and gynecology, and psychiatric units (ANA, 2000a).

To get a better understanding about who staff nurses are, we need to look at the current demographics of RNs

in the United States in 1996.[4] It was estimated that there were 2,558,874 people licensed as RNs. Of these, 82.7% were currently employed as RNs, and 60% were working in hospitals. Nursing continues to be a profession in which women predominate; however, the number of men in nursing is increasing steadily. It is estimated that the number of male RNs in 1996 was 5.4%, which is a substantial increase from the 3% in 1980. Moreover, in 1996 nearly 12% of newly licensed RNs were men (National Council of State Boards of Nursing [NCSBN], 2000). About 10% of RNs come from racial or ethnic minorities: 4.2% were African American; 3.4% were Asian or Pacific Islander; 1.6% were Hispanic; and 0.5% were Native American. Again, when one looks at the numbers of newly licensed RNs, one sees steady change: 5.5% were African American; 6% were Asian or Pacific Islander; 3% were Hispanic; and 0.8% were Native American (NCSBN, 2000). Most employed RNs (58.4%) had less than a baccalaureate degree: 31.8% had a baccalaureate as their highest degree; 9.1% had a masters as their highest degree; and 0.6% were doctorally prepared. The average salary of a full-time RN in 1996 was $42,000, which was an 11% increase over RN salaries in 1992 (Health Resources and Services Administration [HRSA], 2000a).

The aging American nursing work force is another important issue that is receiving increased attention. In 1992 only 11% of nurses were 30 years of age or younger, a 20% decrease since 1988. This trend for fewer young nurses, added to other recent statistics, gives cause for concern. The average age of RNs has steadily increased over the past 20 years. In 1996 it had risen to 44.3 years of age, and the mean age of newly registered nurses was 30.48 years (ANA, 2000a; HRSA, 2000a, 2000b; NCSBN, 2000). Moreover, some predict a high retirement rate for nurses in the next 10 to 15 years as those who came into nursing in the 1950s and 1960s leave the profession (American Association of Colleges of Nursing [AACN], 2000). These statistics clearly show an aging nurse work force. This trend stems from three related societal forces: increasing job opportunities for women, more individuals choosing nursing as a second career, and the declining attractiveness of nursing as a career.[5] These factors work together to keep young people from choosing nursing as

---

[3]The most current information we have on hospital nurses comes from the 1992 National Sample of Nurses (ANA, 2000a).

[4]The most current information we have on registered nurses is from the March 1996 National Survey of Registered Nurses (HRSA, 2000a).

[5]This is related to increased publicity of the many work-related problems such as forced overtime, understaffing, and increased workloads connected to hospital downsizing.

a career and bring older people into the profession. These nursing labor trends, added to the aging of the current nursing work force, are certain to influence hospital supply needs in the future.

HOSPITAL STAFF NURSES: TODAY'S ROLES

It is anticipated that in the near future the hospital will remain the primary employer of RNs. An important trend in hospital care that is shaping nurses' roles is the increased complexity of care rendered in hospitals. This is related to increased patient acuity, increased technological and medical advances, and shorter hospital stays. These changes have led to several shifts in nurses' roles within hospitals, including subspecialty roles within traditional nursing specialties, increased delegation of traditional nursing duties to unlicensed assistive personal, and increased cross-training of nurses. How these changes affect nurses depends largely on where they work. For nurses working in large hospital centers, increased specialization is common, but at the same time they are also expected to become cross-trained in related areas. In small rural hospitals, however, nurses are often called upon to be generalists, to be competent in caring for an older person with a cardiac condition as well as in emergency room treatment of an injured child.

Within hospitals, nurses are caring for sicker, often older patients for shorter periods of time with ever more sophisticated technology. To meet this challenge, hospital staff nurses require expert clinical and communication skills to:

1. Monitor and care for their patients
2. Counsel their patients' families
3. Interface and collaborate with other health care providers as part of a health care team
4. Keep up with rapid technological advances
5. Effectively use information systems to manage patient care
6. Participate in clinical research.

Nurses in this new era are assuming greater responsibility in the management of acutely ill patients in hospitals. Today hospital staff nurses run codes, monitor patients in induced comas and paralysis and on complex ventilation and intravenous systems, and provide crisis counseling to patients and their families. This has led to numerous acute care specialties with many subspecialties such as nurses working solely with diabetic patients or heading IV teams. To meet these new challenges, today's staff nurses have to anticipate events, make sound assess-

ments, evaluate unexpected findings, make decisions at the point of care, and set standards and quality measures (Benz, 1990; Porter-O'Grady, 1999). In response to these increased responsibilities, many nurses are becoming certified in their specialty area and taking the next educational step to becoming advanced practice nurses, including both clinical nurse specialists and acute care nurse practitioners.

Patient teaching is taking on new dimensions as hospitals shift to shorter patient stays. No longer do nurses have the luxury of longer stays in which to teach patients who will go home after long hospital stays. Nurses have to teach patients and their families how to manage at home even though the patient has had little time to recuperate and regain strength. For example, it is not uncommon for patients to be sent home from outpatient surgery only an hour or two after awakening from anesthesia. This makes it imperative that nurses be able to effectively and quickly instruct the patients and their families about how to cope with their complex health condition and their early discharge. Short stays make patient education a challenge for another reason. During short hospital stays families often do not have enough time to assimilate all they need to know because of their high anxiety level. Explaining to the family, who are often still in a state of crisis, about their loved one's state of health and the complex procedures they are receiving is a difficult challenge.

Today's hospital nurses increasingly have to supervise and delegate nursing duties to unlicensed assistive personnel (Fisher, 1999; King, 1999). Hospital nurses have been supervising assistive personnel since the 1930s. It was not uncommon during the severe nursing shortages of the late 1940s and early 1950s for nurses to delegate many nursing duties to nurses' aides, including giving medications (Grando, 1998, 2000). For today's staff nurses, this is a complex process. To delegate nursing duties,

1. Staff nurses need to know exactly what is allowed under their state practice acts; for example, they should not delegate nursing assessments and judgment.
2. Staff nurses need to be the ones who train the unlicensed assistive personnel to perform the tasks or to monitor the patients so that they know exactly what the assistant can do.
3. Staff nurses need to develop protocols for the unlicensed assistive personnel to work under.
4. Staff nurses need to supervise the care given (King, 1999).

Nursing case management is a new role for hospital nurses. It emerged in the late 1980s in response to unpredictable patient outcomes, poor quality care, high health care costs, and the advent of prospective payment system. Hospital-based nurse case management has proved to be an effective way to improve patient outcomes, reduce fragmented hospital services, and prevent unnecessary hospital days. Currently four models of nurse case management are being practiced. Utilization nurse case managers blend traditional utilization review with a focus on reimbursement and discharge planning. Insurance-based nurse case managers act as liaisons between the hospital administrators and the insurance providers. They deal with a wide range of health plan benefits to assure continuity of care and cost containment by focusing on utilization of resources, benefits management, and discharge planning. Another nurse case management model is a primary nurse case manager. They assume 24-hour accountability for their patients; they collaborate with their patients' health care team; and provide direct care. The newest nurse case management model is the advanced practice nurse case manager. In this role the nurse case manager identifies populations at risk and develops an interdisciplinary team to work at developing a coordinated service plan (Wayman, 1999).

Hospital nurses are assuming a greater responsibility for patient discharge planning also. In the era of hospital downsizing, fewer social workers are available to help with discharge planning. Thus nurses are taking a greater role. As a result, hospital nurses have to be knowledgeable about available community resources. This is especially important when patients are discharged early. The services these patients receive at home are increasingly complex, as more high technology is available for home use.

HOSPITAL STAFF NURSES: TODAY'S CHALLENGES

Staff nurses face many challenges, some of which are being revisited from nursing's past. Hospital nursing staff shortages that result in overwork, work-related stress, and mandatory overtime is one challenge that nurses have faced before. Nursing has had numerous periods of short staffing, and often the forces causing these shortfalls are similar. Today's hospital staff shortage has many underlying causes that have been seen before, such as drops in student enrollment, cost cutting by hospitals, and increased job opportunities for women. However, there are some aspects to the current nursing shortage that are different. The present aging of the nursing labor force is one. We not only are faced with fewer persons coming into nursing but also are losing more nurses to retirement. Another aspect of the current nursing shortage is the failure of nursing to

increase nursing's diversity; 90% of nurses are of Euro-American origin compared with roughly 72% of that heritage in the general population. It appears that the United States will not have enough nurses to meet government projections for needs in 2008 and that it is unlikely the percentage of nurses from the many minority groups in our nation will increase (Bureau of Labor Statistics, 2000; Trossman, 2000).

Health risks at the workplace have new aspects that create major challenges for today's hospital nurses. Nurses are being assaulted from many different fronts. The risks from needle sticks are especially troublesome. Although nurses have faced the threat of infections transmitted from patients before, the threats nurses face today are different. The danger of being infected with a deadly disease such as HIV or hepatitis C is shockingly real. It is estimated that health care workers receive from 600,000 to 1 million injuries from needles and sharps every year and that at least 1,000 of them contract a serious illness (ANA, 2000b). This is not the same as a time-limited situation such as the influenza outbreak in 1918-1919; this is the stress of working day in and day out with the knowledge that an accidental slip of a needle can be life changing and ultimately deadly. Another health-related threat increasing nurses' stress is the sensitivity many are developing to latex, which is found in many more areas of a hospital than just in latex gloves (Trossman, 1999).

The last major challenge facing hospital staff nurses is workplace violence. Workplace violence is increasing across the nation, and the health care industry is no exception. Hospitals and nursing homes account for 64% of workplace violence, and health care workers have a 16 times greater risk of sustaining a fatal injury on the job than the general population has (ANA, 2000c; Smith-Pittman & McKoy, 1999). The ANA reports they are receiving more reports from members who have been touched by workplace violence. Workplace violence is becoming a concern for all hospital nurses, not just those who work in emergency rooms or in psychiatric units (ANA, 2000c).

Hospital staff nurses are facing today's challenges with courage, professional competence, and commitment. They are striving in the face of numerous obstacles to improve the quality of patient care at the same time that they are responding to changes of new technology, increased responsibility, hospital downsizing, and managed care. Hospital staff nursing today, still one of nursing's major practice areas, continues to help move the profession forward as it did in nursing's past.

REFERENCES

American Association of Colleges of Nursing. (2000). *Nursing school enrollments decline as demand for RNs continues to decline* [On-line]. Available URL: *www.aacn.nche.edu/Media?NewsReleases/2000feb17.htm*.

American Nurses Association (Eds.). (1946). *Facts about nursing: A statistical, 1946.* New York: Author.

American Nurses Association (Eds.). (1985). *Facts about nursing: 84-85.* Kansas City, MO: Author.

American Nurses Association. (2000a). *Nursing facts: From the American Nurses Association* [On-line]. Available URL: *http://www.nursingworld.org/readroom/fsdemogr.htm*.

American Nurses Association. (2000b). *Nursing facts: From the American Nurses Association, needle injury* [On-line]. Available URL: *http://www.nursingworld.org/readroom/fsneedle.htm*.

American Nurses Association. (2000c). *Real news: Art imitates life: TV show, "ER," highlights threat of workplace violence* [On-line]. Available URL: *http://www.nursingworld.org/pressrel/2000/pr0209.htm*.

Ashley, J.A. (1976). *Hospitals, paternalism, and the role of the nurse.* New York: Teachers College, Columbia University.

Benz, H.G. (1990). *Critical care nursing: A holistic approach* (5th ed.). Philadelphia: Lippincott.

Brown, E.L. (1948). *Nursing for the future: A report prepared for the National Nursing Council.* New York: Russell Sage Foundation.

Bureau of Labor Statistics. (2000). In: *National industry-occupational employment matrix* [On-line]. Available URL: *http://stats.bls.gov/oep/nioem/empiohm.asp*.

Fisher, M. (1999). Do your nurses delegate effectively? *Nursing Management, 30*(5), 23-26.

Flood, M.E. (1981). *The troubling expedient: General staff nursing in United States hospitals in the 1930's, a means to institutional, educational, and personal ends.* Ann Arbor, MI: University Microfilms International, No. 8211927.

Grando, V.T. (1994). Nurses' struggle for economic equity: 1945 to 1965. *Dissertation Abstracts International, 55*(09B), 3815. (University Microfilms International No. 9504017).

Grando, V.T. (1997). ANA's Economic Security Program, the first 20 years. *Nursing Research, 46,* 111-115.

Grando, V.T. (1998). Making do with fewer nurses in the United States, 1945-1965. *Image, 30,* 147-149.

Grando, V.T. (2000). Hard day's work, institutional nursing between 1945-1950. *Nursing History Review, 8,* 169-184.

Health Resources and Services Administration. (2000a). *Notes from the National Survey of Registered Nurses, March 1996* [On-line]. Available URL: *http://158.72.83.3/bhpr/dn/survnote.htm*.

Health Resources and Services Administration. (2000b). *Basic workforce report executive summary* [On-line]. Available URL: *http://158.72.83.3/bhpr/dn/bwrepex.htm*.

Kalisch, P.A., & Kalisch, B.J. (1995). *The advancement of American nursing* (3rd ed.). Philadelphia: Lippincott.

King, B.A. (1999). Working with the new staff mix. *RN, 58*(6), 38-41.

Melosh, B. (1982). *The physician's hand: Work culture and conflict in American nursing.* Philadelphia: Temple University.

National Council of State Boards of Nursing. (2000). *Demographic data newly licensed RN and LPN/VNs* [On-line]. Available URL: *http://www.ncsbn.org/*.

Porter-O'Grady, T. (1999). Technology demands quick-change nursing roles (Guest editorial). *Nursing Management, 30*(5), 7.

Reverby, S.M. (1987). *Ordered to care: The dilemma of American nursing.* Cambridge: Cambridge University Press.

Smith-Pittman, M.H., & McKoy, Y.D. (1999). Workplace violence in healthcare environments. *Nursing Forum, 34*(3), 5-13.

Trossman, S. (1998, January/February). Diversity: A continuing challenge. *The American Nurse, 1,* 24-25.

Trossman, S. (1999, May/June). When workplace threats become reality. *The American Nurse, 1,* 12.

Trossman, S. (2000, January/February). Nurses fight short staff on several major fronts. *The American Nurse,* 1-2.

Wayman, C. (1999). Hospital-based case management: Role clarification. *Nursing Case Management, 4,* 236-241.

Clinical Nurse Specialists and Nurse Practitioners

Who Are They, What Do They Do, and What Challenges Do They Face?

ANN HENRICK, JO ANN APPLEYARD

Specialization has been articulated as "a mark of the advancement of the nursing profession" (American Nurses Association [ANA], 1992b, p. 21). The clinical nurse specialist (CNS) and nurse practitioner (NP) roles were developed in response to this advancement; the profession needed clinical practitioners who could focus on a specific segment of the whole of nursing, seeking in-depth knowledge and advanced skills in a defined area of practice (ANA, 1992b, p. 21).

Historically, there are two significant differences between the prototype CNS and NP: the primary reasons for their coming into existence and the educational requirements for their respective roles (Elder & Bullough, 1990; Hockenberry & Hodgson, 1991). On the other hand, they share a common element: a continuing commitment to clinical practices—a practice that demands expert knowledge and skill and includes the direct and continuous care of sick patients as well as health promotion for clients who are well.

Major related issues that currently affect the CNS and NP are being debated, such as (1) their merger (of sorts) into one entity, (2) the regulatory process that legitimizes their advanced practice, (3) prescriptive authority, and (4) compensation for their services. This chapter profiles the CNS and NP,[1] identifying their impact on the health care system and discussing related concepts and issues.

This chapter is an update of a chapter in the 4th edition of *Current Issues in Nursing* authored by Margaret Stafford and JoAnn Appleyard entitled "Clinical Nurse Specialists and Nurse Practitioners."

[1]The ANA lists 25,000 to 30,000 NPs and "about" 40,000 CNSs with advanced degrees.

HISTORICAL ORIGIN OF THE CLINICAL NURSE SPECIALIST

There have always been "specialists" in nursing who acquired specialized knowledge and skill through practice and on-the-job instruction. During the 1930s and 1940s, many nurses also attended short-term postgraduate educational programs sponsored by hospitals and became the specialists in their particular fields (Donahue, 1985; Hamrick, 1989). The modern CNS emerged, however, in response to the recognized need to improve the quality of patient care and the clinical *practice* of professional nursing, primarily in the acute care setting (Berlinger, 1973; Georgopulous & Christman, 1970; Koetters, 1989; Padilla, 1973; Reiter, 1961; Vaughan, 1968).

Nursing care had deteriorated seriously during and immediately after World War II, due in large part to the dramatic decrease in the number of registered nurses (RNs) practicing in hospitals (Sample, 1987). Many nurses returning from the war used the GI bill to go back to school and become teachers or administrators, and a number of nurses were no longer content to work in the paternalistic environment of the hospital, where low salaries and substandard working conditions were the norm (Donahue, 1985).

The "quick fix" (replacing RNs with less-qualified health care providers) to the acute nursing shortage and substandard patient care failed to address the nurses' concerns. Despite emerging technology and increased complexity of care, hospitals continued to use wartime measures to fill the gap: volunteers became paid nurses' aides and vocational (practical) nurses were introduced to provide the major portion of the direct care for patients (Berlinger, 1973; Donahue, 1985;

19

McClure, 1990; Reiter, 1966; Stafford, 1988). Team nursing was introduced, but it further fragmented patient care and frustrated the RNs, who continued to leave the hospital (Donahue, 1985). The RN felt devalued because others with less education and professionalism took over the nursing care of patients, while the professional nurse "nursed" the desk. In addition, the development of shortened programs in hospital diploma schools as well as associate degree programs in community colleges contributed little to the recognized need for increased knowledge and skill at the bedside.

In 1947, a National Nursing Council (representing the ANA and other health care organizations) obtained a grant from the Carnegie Foundation and commissioned Esther Lucille Brown to study and determine how professional nursing schools could meet the demand for nursing services. One result of the study was Brown's (1948) publication *Nursing for the Future,* in which she strongly proposed that basic schools of nursing be a part of universities and colleges but that

> provision for the development of some specialists within clinical nursing has been viewed in this report as necessary, if the base on which nursing service rests is to be strengthened, and if the profession is to look forward to a sound healthy development. [Brown, 1948]

The now famous Williamsburg Conference of nurse educators, which put into motion the first master's prepared psychiatric CNS (National League for Nursing, 1958), followed this report. In 1961, Frances Reiter presented a paper enunciating her concept of the nurse clinician, which is virtually synonymous with the CNS of today: "one . . . who consistently demonstrates a high degree of clinical judgement and an advanced level of competence in the performance of nursing care in a clinical area of specialization" (Reiter, 1961).

During the 1960s, publications expressing the need for clinical nursing to keep abreast of the knowledge explosion in both technological and behavioral sciences (Berlinger, 1973) flourished. Federal funding was obtained to support this "need," and by the early 1960s programs to prepare CNSs were in place in many areas of clinical practice (Hoeffer & Murphy, 1984). In 1966, a change in the structure of the ANA to include divisions of clinical practice gave further impetus to the development of master's-prepared clinicians (Donahue, 1985; Hoeffer & Murphy, 1984).

PROFILES OF THE CLINICAL NURSE

The criteria for specialists in nursing practice were identified in the ANA's *Social Policy Statement* as "a nurse

who, through study and supervised practice at the graduate level (master's or doctorate), has become expert in a defined area of knowledge and practice in a selected clinical area of nursing" (ANA, 1980). Hamrick and Taylor (1989) suggest that the development of this "expert" results from a "complex and emotional process." Their study describes seven identifiable phases of development but indicates that movement from phase to phase occurs in a highly fluid, individual fashion (Hamrick & Taylor, 1989). For purposes of this discussion, the focus is on the experienced CNS who has reached an advanced phase of practice and has successfully integrated the various components of the role.

Organizational Placement of the Clinical Nurse Specialist

Although CNSs work primarily in institutional settings, typically in staff positions, many and varied organizational arrangements have been described in the literature (Sample, 1987). The advantages and disadvantages of "line" versus staff accountability have been discussed elsewhere (Baird & Prouty, 1989; Hamrick, 1989), and are not dealt with here other than to present a bias predicated on years of successful experience as a CNS in a staff position and dialogue with CNSs in line positions. The success of this staff role, however, is contingent on reciprocal trust and respect and, as identified by Brown (1989), a sharing of responsibility and authority between the CNS and the person to whom he or she is accountable administratively.

Regardless of organizational placement and reporting mechanisms, the CNS usually works from a "home base" and is available for consultation from other units (Koetters, 1989). Many CNSs have clinical faculty appointments and some full-time faculty members carry part-time CNS appointments. The common element, however, is the direct and continuous involvement with patients and families with emphasis on a nursing versus a medical care model.

Functions of the Clinical Nurse Specialist

Expert clinical practice is the sine qua non of the CNS. Practice (i.e., actual ongoing experience with patients and families) provides the content and directs participation in various subroles such as clinical research, consultation, teaching, and leadership and administration (Hamrick, 1989). This concept is exemplified by the following CNS leaders with excerpts from their activities. These examples, gleaned for the most part from personal contact and interaction, are not intended to be all-inclusive but rather to provide the reader with some insight into what Fralic (1988) refers to as "nursing's precious resource."

• Nancy Burke is a CNS in psychiatric mental health nursing. She maintains a private practice, is a consultant to the department of psychiatry in a university hospital, has an adjunct appointment in the college of nursing, and maintains a collaborative practice with her psychiatrist husband. Her activities include liaison work with family members of hospitalized patients, seeing them in the hospital and office, and calling them at least weekly to keep them apprised of the patient's progress and involving them as indicated in the plans for therapy. As a certified psychodramatist, Nancy conducts four psychodrama groups per week. In her group at the university, she has medical residents, nursing students, and myriad others as participant observers, "who never fail to get involved."

• Kristin Kleinschmidt is an arrhythmia CNS in a large cardiology practice that encompasses three private hospitals. Her well-honed skills as teacher, provider of high-level comprehensive follow-up care for persons with complex arrhythmias, cardiac pacemakers, and automatic internal cardiac defibrillators, as well as consultant to nurses, physicians, and others who care for these patients, serve her well in her new role. Kris works in collaboration with two electrophysiology cardiologists to give complete care to these patients. In her practice, which is outpatient focused, Kris assesses patients independently and in collaboration with the physicians to provide patients with the best possible outcomes and an enhanced quality of life.

• Donna Murphy is a diabetes CNS whose practice has a dual focus in both the outpatient and inpatient arenas within the hospital. Donna acts as a mentor to staff nurses caring for persons with diabetes, helping these nurses to feel more confident in their roles as caregivers, teachers, and coaches of new as well as seasoned diabetics. Occasionally she will act as consultant in the care of a hospitalized diabetic patient with complex human responses to this illness. Donna works with nurses throughout the hospital to upgrade standards of care and gives regular group inservices to update nurses on the latest research in diabetic care. Donna has a diabetic self-management education clinic within the outpatient setting. She works outside the specialty endocrine clinic focusing on those patients cared for by the generalist physician. Her practice centers on coaching, teaching, and performing high-level assessments of these patients, helping them to monitor their own progress and effecting positive patient outcomes.

• Kathleen Perry functions in a hospital-based home care program, giving nursing care to four or five elderly patients and their families on an ongoing basis. She has explored and studied the diagnostic statement, Knowledge Deficit, a recurring problem for this patient population. She likewise has identified the potential for serious negative patient outcomes in the presence of caregiver stress, a phenomenon she currently is addressing as a PhD candidate in nursing. She believes her involvement as a clinical preceptor offers students a "knowledge embedded in practice" that enhances their ability to function in the CNS role. Kathy advises staff nurses in her agency on ethical and professional issues as they move forward in their state nurses' association's professional bargaining unit activities.

• Joyce Waterman Taylor is a CNS emerita in neuroscience. Joyce has not only implemented all of the subroles in a highly qualitative fashion, but she has also expanded and incorporated additional competencies. She believes strongly that primary nursing ("my patient, my nurse") is the way to improve care for all patients and to provide job satisfaction for nurses. In all of her work settings, she has introduced and taught the concepts of primary nursing within a holistic framework. For Joyce, collaborative practice also is an article of faith; she consistently develops and nurtures collaborative relationships with physicians and other disciplines. Her widely published work on the outcomes of care and outcome standards led to her appointment to several national and local committees and task forces. Joyce has been singled out by her peers and colleagues as the quintessential CNS.

ORIGINS OF THE NURSE PRACTITIONER ROLE

The 1960s were characterized by social change, including a political emphasis on health care as a right for all citizens. Access to all levels of health care services was seen as a particular problem, and the NP role was developed to help meet the demand for primary care services. The first formal education program for NPs was established in 1965 at the University of Colorado School of Nursing to prepare RNs to deliver primary care to children in underserved communities (Ford & Silver, 1967; "Interview with Co-founder of Nurse Practitioner Movement," 1995). By 1975, practitioner programs had proliferated, and NPs were being trained in a variety of medical fields, including obstetrics and gynecology, internal medicine, pediatrics, geriatrics, and family practice. During that first decade, educational programs tended to be nondegree certificate programs that were 1 year or less in length. Many of these programs were funded by the federal government in an effort to prepare more primary care providers for underserved populations. Since 1975, the number of nondegree programs has decreased substantially, and most NPs are now educated in graduate programs leading to a master's degree in nursing (Office of Technology Assessment [OTA], 1986).

National certification for NPs was first established in the mid-1970s by the National Certification Board of Pediatric Nurse Practitioners and Nurses. The ANA (American Nurses Credentialing Center) soon followed suit, establishing national certification for NPs in gerontology, pediatrics, adult health, family health, and school health. NPs in neonatology, obstetrics, and gynecology are certified by the National Certification Corporation for Obstetric, Gynecologic, and Neonatal Nursing Specialties. Most NPs today are certified by one of these national organizations. Increasingly, certification is a requirement for employment, and in some states, it is a requirement by the state licensing board.

Who Are Nurse Practitioners and What Do They Do?

Nurse practitioners are educated to perform a broad spectrum of primary care interventions, including health assessment, risk appraisal, health education and counseling, diagnosis and management of acute minor illnesses and injuries, and management of chronic conditions. Although most NPs work in primary care settings such as physicians' offices, health maintenance organizations, and community or public health clinics, increasing numbers are employed in hospitals, nursing homes, schools, colleges, industrial settings, and home health agencies (OTA, 1986). In all of these settings, NPs provide the essential health care services described above with emphasis on health promotion and disease prevention activities (Lewis & Resnik, 1985).

Taking into account the basic primary care practice divisions of internal medicine, pediatrics, family practice, obstetrics and gynecology, and geriatrics, NPs tend to perform as generalists rather than as specialists in terms of clinical practice. This means that they focus on broad health concerns within a given division of practice rather than concentrating on a particular body system or a set of related diseases. Exceptions to this are NPs who work as employees or as partners to physicians in specialty practice. In these specialty settings, the roles of NPs and CNSs are quite similar and may be considered interchangeable.

Specific Role Issues for Nurse Practitioners

The literature on NPs is voluminous, and a review by Koch, Pazaki, and Campbell (1992) categorizes five major topics: NP roles, educational issues, evaluation, legal issues, and the evolving health care crisis. One major concern that has been debated repeatedly over the past 20 years is whether NPs function as physician substitutes or as nurses in advanced practice roles (Bates, 1974a; Bates, 1974b; Edmunds, 1979; Edmunds & Ruth, 1991; "Interview with Co-founder of Nurse Practitioner Movement," 1995; Mauksch & Rogers, 1975; Weston, 1975). The differences between physician and nursing roles involve issues of nursing autonomy as well as paradigm disparities about the nature of health care (Allen, 1977; "Interview with Co-founder of Nurse Practitioner Movement," 1995).

Historically, nurses have tended to view their focus as "caring," while physicians have directed their efforts toward "curing" (Linn, 1974). Traditionally, nurses have assisted physicians in the cure of patients by following orders and using their nursing skills and knowledge to care for patients and their families. Caring involved activities such as bathing, feeding, and providing skin care and passive exercise for a bedridden patient. It also involved listening, counseling, teaching, and coordinating interventions from multiple health care providers. Curing involved specific activities directed toward the diagnosis and treatment of disease. When nurses followed physician orders in carrying out diagnostic tests or in administering treatments to patients, they were participating in the curative aspect of health care. When they assessed and provided for patient and family needs for emotional support and health teaching or guidance, they were participating in the caring component.

The historical view was that nursing practice was both dependent on medical practice and independent from it, and the independent functions tended to be those on the caring end of the continuum. Thus nursing autonomy was more related to caring interventions than to curative ones. The development of advanced nursing practice roles has changed this circumstance. NPs perform interventions aimed at curing acute minor illnesses and injuries daily. While carrying out these interventions, they assess their patients' responses to their health problems and initiate appropriate teaching and counseling to help them manage treatment plans and prevent recurrences or secondary problems.

As indicated earlier, caring and curing are not mutually exclusive concepts. Rather, they are part of a continuum, and both physicians and nurses carry out activities in these arenas. Both caring and curative interventions are necessary in primary care, and there is convincing evidence that NPs effectively combine these practice components in their roles (Leininger, Little, & Carnevali, 1972; Simborg, Starfield, & Horn, 1978; Yedida, 1981). Although NPs carry out health care activities that used to be primarily in the physician's domain, they are performing these activities as nurses with significant emphasis on the responses and needs of the whole patient and his or her family.

THE CLINICAL NURSE SPECIALIST AND NURSE PRACTITIONER IN TRANSITION
Merging the Two Councils

Several studies, papers, and intense dialogue with members of the ANA's CNS and NP councils have elucidated more similarities than differences between the CNS and NP (Forbes, 1990; Forbes, Rafson, Spross, & Kozlowski, 1990; Hockenberry & Hodgson, 1991; Kitzman, 1989; Sparacino & Denand, 1986). Thus, the two councils merged into a single Council of Nurses in Advanced Practice (Pokorny & Barnard, 1992). The educational requirements (master's or doctorate) and role development now are well established (ANA, 1980), and although the issue of a singular title at this time is still being debated (Kitzman, 1989), the concept of both groups being identified as advanced practitioners is widely accepted (Forbes et al., 1990).

Regulation and Reimbursement Issues

The inconsistencies of the regulation and professional certification of nurses in advanced practice prompted the National Council of State Boards of Nursing (NCSBN) in March 1992 to propose a second license for nurses seeking reimbursement and prescriptive authority (NCSBN, 1992). The profession's historical view (which is still valid) is that the responsibility and accountability for defining specialty nursing practice and its qualifications rest with the profession (ANA, 1980; "Interview with Cofounder of Nurse Practitioner Movement," 1995). Formal meetings between the NCSBN and the ANA continue to take place to examine alternative mechanisms (other than licensure) to regulate *advanced* practice.

In addition, the ANA is completing a deliberate process with organized nursing through the Nursing Organization Liaison Forum and other specialty organizations to revisit *Nursing: A Social Policy Statement* as it pertains specifically to specialization (ANA, 1992a; Cronenwett, 1992; Pokorny & Barnard, 1992). It is incumbent on all advanced practi-

tioners to be involved actively and cohesively in the ANA's and the state nurses' associations' collaborative efforts to:

- Protect the public's and nursing's autonomous control of advanced nursing practice
- Increase the adherence of nurses in advanced practice to national standards of certification and peer review
- Introduce requirements for uniform mandatory reimbursement to reflect adequately advanced practitioners' worth
- Eliminate barriers that restrict consumer access to services of qualified advanced practitioners
- Build a national and state database on advanced practitioners including their scope of practice, location, cost, and the outcome of this care (ANA, 1992a).

CURRENT MANDATES AND CHALLENGES

Barriers to NP and some CNS practice are substantial because of the overlap between traditional medical and nursing functions. This is especially true in settings in which nurses attempt to provide comprehensive primary care services. During the past 30 years, 49 of the 50 states have recognized the nurse practitioner title. Tennessee is the only state in which advanced practice nurses function under a broad nurse practice act (Pearson, 2000). By 2000, NPs in all 50 states had some legal authority to prescribe medications, but the language varies widely (Pearson, 2000). In many states NPs may prescribe independently all kinds of drugs, including controlled substances. Recently, many states have amended their nurse practice acts to permit NPs to receive and dispense drug samples as well (Pearson, 2000).

The issue of independence is a major problem for both NPs and physicians. From the inception of the NP role, it was intended that some of the interventions involving diagnosis and treatment of disease be carried out in collaboration with physicians or, as organized medicine asserts, *under physician supervision.*

The independent practice of nurses is a politically charged arena, with organized medicine firmly against all efforts of nurses to be recognized as independent health care providers who receive direct reimbursement for their services. When regulatory agencies and state and federal legislative bodies use the term *supervision* rather than *collaboration* to describe the interdependent relationship between physicians and nurses, organized medicine can claim that nursing practice is completely dependent on medical practice and that physicians should receive all direct reimbursement for health care services delivered by nurses outside of institutional settings. Nurses must continue to work diligently to educate legislators, regulators, and the public about the independent aspects of nursing practice that are defined broadly in all nursing practice acts. It is also necessary to remind these groups that nurses do practice under their own licenses and that nurses' licenses are not contingent on physicians' licenses.

An operational definition of the concept of collaboration was adopted in 1992 by the ANA Congress on Nursing Practice:

> Collaboration means a collegial working relationship with another health care provider in the provision of (to supply) patient care. Collaborative practice requires (may include) the discussion of patient diagnosis and cooperation in the management and delivery of care. Each collaborator is available to the other for consultation either in person or by communication device, but need not be physically present on the premises at the time the actions are performed. The patient-designated health care provider is responsible for the overall direction and management of patient care. [ANA, 1992b, p. 104]

This definition should be used as a basis in all discussions or negotiations in which the issue is "physician supervision" of nursing practice.

The individual accomplishments of CNSs and NPs are a prelude to their potential collective positive impact on the health care of individuals and families and on health care policy in general. To this end, they must sustain and enhance their significant roles in the following initiatives:

- State and local health care reform efforts
- Federal government's agenda to improve the effectiveness and appropriateness of health care services through their Agency for Health Care Policy and Research
- Nursing's taxonomy development and related scientific studies

It is likewise crucial that nurses in advanced practice (1) continue to demonstrate their cost-effectiveness in cost-driven hospital and clinic environments, (2) increase their presence in extended care or nursing home facilities, (3) advance theory- and research-based clinical practice models that demonstrate a high quality of patient care and reflect measurable, nurse-sensitive patient outcomes, and (4) help other health professionals, health care consumers, and public servants recognize the contribution being made by nurses in advanced practices (Donovan, 1985; Wright, 1990).

REFERENCES

Allen, M. (1977). Comparative theories of the expanded role in nursing and implications for nursing practice: A working paper. *Nursing Papers, 9*(2), 38-45.

American Nurses Association. (1980). *Nursing: A social policy statement.* Kansas City, MO: Author.

American Nurses Association. (1992a). *House of Delegates report: 1992 convention, Las Vegas, Nevada* (pp. 235-240). Kansas City, MO: Author.

American Nurses Association. (1992b). *House of Delegates report: 1992 convention, Las Vegas, Nevada* (pp. 104-120). Kansas City, MO: Author.

Baird, S.B., & Prouty, M.P. (1989). Administratively enhancing CNS contribution. In A.B. Hamrick & J.A. Spross (Eds.), *The clinical nurse specialist in theory and practice* (2nd ed., pp. 262-264). Philadelphia: Saunders.

Bates, B. (1974). Doctor and nurse: changing roles and relations. *New England Journal of Medicine, 283*(3), 129-134.

Bates, B. (1974). Twelve paradoxes: A message for nurse practitioners. *Nursing Outlook, 22*(11), 686-688.

Berlinger, M.R. (1973). The preparation and roles of the clinical nurse specialist. In J.P. Riehl & J.W. McVay (Eds.), *The clinical nurse specialist: Interpretations* (pp. 100-107). New York: Appleton-Century-Crofts.

Brown, E.L. (1948). *Nursing for the future.* New York: Russell Sage Foundation.

Brown, S.J. (1989). Supportive supervision of the CNS. In A.B. Hamrick & J.A. Spross (Eds.), *The clinical nurse specialist in theory and practice* (2nd ed., pp. 285-298). Philadelphia: Saunders.

Cronenwett, L.R. (1992, July 14). *A report to CNAP members from the chairperson, Congress of Nursing Practice.* Kansas City, MO: American Nurses Association.

Donahue, M.P. (1985). *Nursing: The finest art.* St. Louis: Mosby.

Donovan, C.T. (1985). Clinical nurse specialist practice in an acute care setting. In K.E. Barnard & G.R. Smith (Eds.), *Faculty practice in action.* Kansas City, MO: American Academy of Nursing.

Elder, R.G., & Bullough, B. (1990). Nurse practitioners and clinical nurse specialists: Are the roles merging? *Clinical Nurse Specialist, 4*(2), 78-84.

Edmunds, M. (1979, September/October). Junior doctoring. *Nurse Practitioner,* 8-46.

Edmunds, M.W., & Ruth, M.V. (1991). NPs who replace physicians: Role expansion or exploitation? *Nurse Practitioner, 16*(9), 46, 49.

Forbes, K.E. (1990). Merge!!! *Momentum, 8*(31).

Forbes, K.E., Rafson, J., Spross, J.A., & Kozlowski, I. (1990). The clinical nurse specialist and nurse practitioner: Core curriculum survey results. *Clinical Nurse Specialist 4*(2), 63-66.

Ford, L.C., & Silver, H.K. (1967). The expanded role of the nurse in child care. *Nursing Outlook, 15*(8), 43-45.

Fralic, M.E. (1988). Executive development, nursing's precious resource: The clinical nurse specialist. *Journal of Nursing Administration, 18*(2), 5-6.

Georgopulous, B., & Christman, L. (1970).The clinical nurse specialist: A role model. *American Journal of Nursing, 70*(5), 1030-1039.

Hamrick, A.B. (1989). History and overview of the CNS role. In A.M. Hamrick & J.A. Spross (Eds.), *The clinical nurse specialist in theory and practice* (2nd ed., pp. 3-18). Philadelphia: Saunders.

Hamrick, A.B., & Taylor, J.W. (1989). Role development of the CNS. In A.B. Hamrick & J.A. Spross (Eds.), *The clinical nurse specialist in theory and practice* (2nd ed., pp. 6-39). Philadelphia: Saunders.

Hockenberry, E.M., & Hodgson, W. (1991). Merging advanced practice roles: The NP and CNS. *Journal of Pediatric Health, 5*(3), 158-159.

Hoeffer, B., & Murphy, S. (1984). Specialization in nursing practice. In *Issues in professional nursing practice, part 2* (pp. 1-5). Kansas City MO: American Nurses Association.

Interview with Co-founder of Nurse Practitioner Movement. (1995). *Nurse Practitioner News, 3*(4), 8-12.

Kitzman, H.J. (1989). The CNS and NP. In A.B. Hamrick & J.A. Spross (Eds.), *The clinical nurse specialist in theory and practice* (2nd ed., pp. 379-394). Philadelphia: Saunders.

Koch, L.W., Pazaki, S.H., & Campbell, J.D. (1992). The first 20 years of nurse practitioner literature: An evolution of joint practice issues. *Nurse Practitioner, 17*(2), 62-71.

Koetters, L. (1989). Clinical practice and direct patient care. In A.B. Hamrick & J.A. Spross (Eds.), *The clinical nurse specialist in theory and practice* (2nd ed., pp. 107-123). Philadelphia: Saunders.

Leininger, M.M., Little, D.E., & Carnevali, D. (1972). Primex the professional nurse, responsible, accountable, reaching out and taking an active, frontline position in primary health care. *American Journal of Nursing, 72*(7), 1274-1277.

Lewis, C.E., & Resnik, B.A. (1985). Nurse clinics and progressive ambulatory patient care. *New England Journal of Medicine, 277*(23), 1236-1241.

Linn, L.S. (1974). Care vs cure: How the nurse practitioner views the patient. *Nursing Outlook, 22*(10), 641-644.

Mauksch, I.G., & Rogers, M.E. (1975). Nursing is coming of age . . . through the practitioner movement. *American Journal of Nursing, 75*(10), 1834-1943.

McClure, M.L. (1990, October 14-15). Introduction. In I.E. Goertzen (Ed.), *Differentiating nursing practice into the twenty-first century.* Selected papers from the 18th annual meeting and 1990 conference of the American Academy of Nursing, Charleston, SC. Kansas City, MO: American Academy of Nursing.

National Council of State Boards of Nursing, Inc. (1992). *Position paper on the licensure of advanced nursing practice, May 18, 1992.* Chicago: Author.

National League for Nursing. (1958). *The education of the clinical specialist in psychiatric nursing.* New York: Author.

Office of Technology Assessment. (1986). Nurse practitioners, physician assistants, and certified nurse-midwives: A policy analysis. *Health Technology Case Study 37,* Washington, DC: U.S. Congress.

Padilla, G. (1973). Clinical specialist research: Evaluation and recommendations, conclusions and implications. In J.P. Riehl & J.W. McVay (Eds.), *The clinical nurse specialist: Interpretations* (pp. 283-334). New York: Appleton-Century-Crofts.

Pearson, L.J. (2000). Annual update of how each state stands on legislative issues affecting advanced nursing practice. *Nurse Practitioner, 25*(1), 16-68.

Pokorny, B.E., & Barnard, K.E. (1992). AAA to revise nursing statement. *The American Nurse, 24*(5), 6.

Reiter, F. (1961). Improvement of nursing practice. In J.P. Riehl & J.W. McVay (Eds.), *The clinical nurse specialist: Interpretation.* New York: Appleton-Century-Crofts.

Reiter, F. (1966). The clinical nursing approach. *Nursing Forum, 5*(l), 39-44.

Sample, S.A. (1987). Justifying and structuring the CNS role within a nursing organization. In A.B. Hamrick & J.A. Spross (Eds.), *The clinical nurse specialist in theory and practice* (2nd ed., pp. 251-260). Philadelphia: Saunders.

Simborg, D.W., Starfield, B.H., & Horn, S.D. (1978). Physicians and non-physician health practitioners: The characteristics of their practices and their relationships. *American Journal of Public Health, 68*(l), 44-48.

Sparacino, P., & Denand, A. (1986). Specialization in advanced nursing practice [editorial]. *Council of Primary Health Care Nurse Practitioners–Council of Clinical Nurse Specialists Newsletter, 4*(2).

Stafford, M.J. (1988). Margaret Stafford. In T.M. Schorr & A. Zimmerman (Eds.), *Making choices, taking chances: Nurse leaders tell their stories* (p. 330). St. Louis: Mosby.

Vaughan, M. (1968). Difficult task: Defining role of the clinical specialist. *Hospital Topics, 5*(18), 93-94.

Weston, J. (1975). Whither the "nurse" in nurse practitioner? *Nursing Outlook, 23*(3), 148-152.

Wright, J.E. (1990). Joining forces for the good of our clients. *Clinical Nurse Specialist, 4*(2), 76-77.

Yedida, M.J. (1981). *Delivering primary health care nurse practitioners at work.* Boston: Auburn House.

Nurse Executives

Who Are They, What Do They Do, and What Challenges Do They Face?

SUE ELLEN PINKERTON

In this chapter, I intend to outline several problems facing nurse executives. The purpose is to provide a basis for continued discussion, to stimulate readers to think through the issues, and to motivate them to seek further information and dialogue.

NURSE EXECUTIVES: WHO ARE THEY?

The title "nurse executive" is fairly new in the language of the nursing profession. The title may be used for both deans of colleges of nursing and vice presidents for nursing, but in this chapter the focus will be on nurses who fill the role of vice president for nursing or chief nursing officer (CNO) in acute care facilities or hospitals.

Nurses in this role were known historically as superintendents and directors. Since the late 1970s and early 1980s as the impact of the nursing department or division on the business of the hospital became more apparent and valued, the title of vice president came into wider use, giving administrative parity (and higher salaries) to nurses. As vice presidents, nurses are also identified as chief nursing offices and nurses-in-chief to maintain parity with physicians.

NURSE EXECUTIVES: WHAT DO THEY DO?

Because the role of CNOs is broad, their preparation must be correspondingly broad. They are concerned with maximizing the quality of patient care, maximizing the professional satisfaction of the nursing staff, meeting the cost-effectiveness goals of the organization, maintaining relationships, and participating in long-range strategic planning, including nursing. They are clinical and business leaders in the organization. They know how to coor-

dinate care and the cost of such care. They can contribute to the growth of the organization and control patient outcomes. Smart chief executive officers (CEOs) know this and place nurses in a variety of positions. Are nurses promoting this talent? Is the nursing profession preparing leaders for nursing in the future?

As part of their business role, nurse executives expect to be included in planning, development, and decision making. It is still not unusual, however, for nurse executives to be excluded from such business activities as planning for new services, despite the fact that they will be expected to support the services by providing competent nursing staff. Nurse executives who are consistently excluded from such decision making but yet are held accountable for nursing and patient-related outcomes eventually must confront the CEO or president with a rationale for inclusion. If a satisfactory resolution is not reached, the CNO must decide whether to leave or remain in the position. To stay is to support a system that may not value nursing contributions or to support a system that uses these tactics as a subtle devaluation of nursing participation and contributions. A CNO who stays may also miss an opportunity to develop business skills, which may mean restricting job mobility.

In some cases the CEO or president in the acute care setting values only the clinical contribution of the CNO and prefers to have executives prepared with a business background make business decisions. During the 1980s it was not uncommon for CNOs to be asked by the CEO to return to school to get a master in business administration (MBA) degree. The thinking was that the nurse executive needed an MBA to contribute to the business growth of the acute care facility. Although some colleges of nursing offered joint nursing administration/business degrees, many nurses completed business degrees only. In fact, some hospital administrators told nurses a master's degree in nursing was a waste of time and only a business degree was of value. Nursing administration programs diminished in popularity in the late 1980s, mainly because of the emphasis on business degrees. They enjoyed a short span of growth in the mid 1990s but now are on the decline again, this time apparently because of the popularity of practitioner programs. Nurses have concluded that if they are going to study for an advanced degree in nursing, practitioner roles provide more job security than nursing administration roles.

Today, many nurses believe that opportunities for nurse managers, directors, and CNOs are diminishing as a result of the "right sizing" and the use of fewer nurses in management and administration positions. In fact, more nurses are now being appointed to such positions. The increase is due to the problems stemming from a lack of professional growth and development of the nursing staff, which has affected patient outcomes and patient satisfaction.

Many nursing directors and CNOs have moved into a variety of health care administration jobs including hospital director, chief operating officer, human resource officer, and CEO. Will this also have an impact on the professional growth of nursing? If there are no longer CNOs with advanced degrees in nursing administration, who will create care environments that promote the generation of nursing knowledge? Will there be a void in input from the practice arena, leading to knowledge built mainly on theory and research and excluding practice? Traditionally, new nursing knowledge was an amalgam of all three areas. What is the necessary commitment of colleges of nursing in assuring a balance in knowledge generation? What is the necessary commitment of colleges of nursing in succession planning for CNO leadership by providing academic programs in nursing administration/leadership? Are colleges of nursing faculty using ethically based principles when they require a practice focus in elective courses and research rather than encouraging nursing administration to include business courses and administrative research?

NURSE EXECUTIVES: WHAT CHALLENGES DO THEY FACE?

The biggest challenge facing nurse executives is the nursing shortage. The current shortage is predicted to be long lasting because there are so many forces at work increasing the demand for nurses as the supply diminishes.

Forces increasing demand include (1) population growth, especially of the over-100 age group who need more care as they age because of the increased onset of illnesses and diseases, (2) an increase in chronic illness that requires more caregivers, and (3) advances in technology that require more skilled caregivers (nurses) to operate the technology and provide the complex care required as a result of the implementation of such technology (transplants). The decreasing supply of nurses is due to (1) a preference by women, traditionally the majority of nurses, for careers such as law, pharmacy, and medicine, (2) a decrease of nursing faculty resulting in limitations put on nursing school enrollments, (3) a decline in growth of wages for nurses, and (4) the aging of the registered nurse (RN) workforce. The number of RNs younger than 30 years in 1980 was 25%; in 1996 it was 9% (Buerhaus, 1999).

How should CNOs address the nursing shortage? Should they look for more roles to carve out of nursing, joining the "slicing and dicing" club (Pinkerton, 1999)? Should they try to take the issue to the policy level and seek government investment in faculty positions, in financing undergraduate education, and in attracting more minorities and men to nursing (both currently underrepresented groups) (Buerhaus, 1999)? Should nurses contribute to the American Hospital Association's (AHA) political action committee (PAC) or to the American Nurses Association's (ANA) PAC, which often support opposing candidates?

Should CNOs rely on national media campaigns to eventually change the image of nursing, especially negative images related to working hours and shift work? Will younger generations be driven by altruism to enter nursing or will they remain true to their generation, seeking jobs that give them stock options in dot.com companies?

Can the American Organization of Nurse Executives (AONE) rally support for the nursing profession? The results of focus groups reported nurses as protectors of the patient and the main conduit for information and reassurance in a frightening situation. Nurses were also cited as having a special relationship with the public and remain a strong symbol of quality (AHA, 1998). This information, however, has not been a focus for recruitment or support of nursing, especially from the AHA or AONE. Where is nursing leadership making an impact on factors that can address the nursing shortage? How should such effort be organized? Which professional organization should nurse executives support?

Are the nursing profession and its leadership still functioning as an oppressed group? Susan Roberts (1983) in her classic article "Oppressed Group Behavior: Implications for Nursing" purports that dominate groups, which in hospitals are hospital administrators (CEOs) and physicians, control and influence outcomes for subordinate groups such as nursing. The way to move groups out of the oppressed status is through deliberate and active nursing leadership. Which brings us back to the question of current and future leadership of nurse executives. Are leaders supported? Is leadership united? Are we educating nurses as future leaders and future nurse executives?

Embedded within the challenge of the nursing shortage, besides the challenge of leadership, are the challenges of relationships with hospital CEOs and physicians. The relationship with hospital administrators has already been explored to a limited extent in this chapter. There are other issues, however, that can lead to hospital administrator support or lack of it for the nurse executive.

How much can a nurse executive learn during her or his interview for a position? Can the nurse executive get a sense of the support for nursing that the CEO demonstrates to the hospital board of directors? Does this really say anything about the CEO's support of nursing in daily operations? Is there a balance of discussions about financial and quality issues at the board of directors meetings? Does quality, when discussed, mean only medical care or does it include nursing care? Should the CNO be a voting member of the board of directors? Should this be negotiated before hire? What issues should a CNO consider in her or his decision to leave?

Each nurse executive needs to have a "line" that he or she will not cross as the nurse leader in the organization. When that line is crossed, the nurse executive must resign. But what if leaving creates a worse situation for nursing staff and patients than remaining does for the nurse executive? Is the line of no return related to variance in staffing? Will the nursing shortage create situations intolerable for CNOs? Is the line related to a continual devaluation of nursing? Is it related to sexual harassment by the CEO? Is it related to substance abuse by the CEO? Where does the nurse executive find colleagues with whom to discuss such situations?

The other embedded relationships in the nursing shortage are the relationships with physicians. What does it mean when a CNO addresses a group of physicians who won't give her or him eye contact? Do physicians really want collaborative relationships with nurses? What are the generational differences among physicians that impact relationships with nursing? How much support should the CNO expect from the CEO in creating productive nurse/physician relationships? How strong should the relationship be between the CNO and the medical chief of staff?

SUMMARY

In all of the issues put forward, nursing leadership by the CNO is key, especially when the outlined situations occur in hospitals. The structures of hospitals and the nursing profession, however, are complex. Where does the CNO begin? Does it matter if a CNO focuses only on her or his hospital organization to promote change? Will CNO leadership in her or his own hospital somehow impact another hospital? Should a CNO focus on creating excellence in her or his own hospital to attract and retain nurses and not worry about other hospitals? Should the CNO abandon worrying about the direction and future of the nursing profession, essentially becoming isolated in her or his own environment? If not, how will we connect as a profession to assure the continued development of nurse leaders and CNOs?

Will the spirit that nurses have always had be a central rallying point? Will the government through policy development help promote the continued growth of nursing? How should CNOs be involved?

There is plenty to do. How will we organize to do it? How will we get it all done?

CASE STUDY

Ann Mason has been a vice president for 14 years. This is her second position as CNO, having been very successful in her first position, which she left to take up the challenge of being a CNO in an academic health center with a college of nursing.

In her role as CNO, she is seen as a team player, and has had responsibility for departments other than nursing. The nursing staff is unionized, but the union has not been very active until just recently.

Ann is very loyal to nursing. Actually, she is passionate about nursing. She has a PhD in nursing and is anxious to work in partnership with the college of nursing on research and knowledge generation.

In her daily operations, Dr. Mason holds people accountable for their actions. She has been successful in putting a shared governance model in place, and recently extended the model from nursing to include all departments.

Dr. Mason has a productive relationship with the medical staff. She is respected for her knowledge and actions. The quality of care is seen by physicians to be excellent. Ann is responsible to physicians, including them in decision making and working with them in collaborative partnerships. As part of the shared governance model, she established physician-nurse committees.

One week ago, Dr. Mason was told to make some budget cuts that would affect nursing practice at the bedside. She feels the cuts into her budget are too deep. The vice presidents in operations take a slice-and-dice attitude about nursing, feeling Ann needs to divide the work among lesser-paid employees to achieve the cost savings.

Staff nurse reactions are starting to reach Dr. Mason. She thinks the staff feel she might be selling them out to a form of work redesign. Her communication through the nurse managers is strained at this point because of their fear and what seems to be immobility and paralysis on their part.

As Ann ponders the situation, she suddenly remembers the whimsical idea CNOs often entertain in tough situations: Is it time for me to leave and open my own boutique???

Should Ann leave or stay? Why? If she stays, what should her plan be for making her points to the administration? What elements can she use to make her points in a counter-proposal (Kritek, 1994)? If her request for reconsideration is denied, should she rally the staff nurses and the physicians?

How will she deal with the gap between staff nurses and the CNO? How can she convince the staff nurses *she* is not the enemy? What are the long-term implications of involving other persons in the response to the request for budget cuts? Will it be seen as the CNO and her allies against the CEO and administration?

If she gets a positive response to her request, how will Ann work with administration to keep them updated about the needs of nursing at the bedside? Does she risk stepping over the hospital "loyalty" line in favor of the nursing profession? How as a CNO does she keep a balance?

If Ann decides to leave, what are some likely scenarios for the future of the staff nurses and for patient care? Will it make any difference if she leaves? Is a decision to leave one of self-interest? How will she know if she is staying because she is afraid to leave? How can Dr. Mason get a good estimate of her own power in the organization?

REFERENCES

American Hospital Association. (1998, January). *Reality check II.* Chicago: Author.

Buerhaus, P.I. (1999, April 16). *Trouble in the nurse labor market? Recent trends, outlook for future employment and earnings, and prospects for a severe and sustained RN shortage.* Presented to the University Health System Consortium Chief Nursing Officer Council, Chicago, IL.

Kritek, P.B. (1994). *Negotiating at an uneven table: Developing moral courage in resolving our conflicts.* San Francisco: Jossey-Bass.

Pinkerton, S.E. (1999). The nurse executive: Slicing and dicing nursing. *Journal of Professional Nursing, 15,* 327.

Roberts, S.J. (1983). Oppressed group behavior: Implications for nursing. *Advances in Nursing Science, 5*(4), 21-32.

Nursing Faculty

Who Are They, What Do They Do, and What Challenges Do They Face?

CAROLE A. ANDERSON

WHO ARE THE FACULTY?

The correct answer to the question, Who are the faculty teaching in nursing programs? is, Well that depends. Because the profession has at least three types of basic nursing programs located in very different kinds of parent institutions with very different expectations of faculty, there isn't a single *typical* faculty member. Nursing education is located in hospital-based diploma programs, community junior colleges, senior colleges, and universities. But the differences don't stop there because within the colleges and universities are many types of parent institutions, ranging from small liberal arts colleges to the most research-intensive universities with large graduate programs. The profile of the faculty in each of these nursing programs and within baccalaureate and graduate programs is quite different. How different they are, however, is difficult to discern because current data are not readily available describing the faculty profiles in *other than* baccalaureate and graduate programs.

The most recent data for faculty teaching in diploma and associate degree programs are from 1992 (National League for Nursing [NLN], 1992, 1995), and these data are only quantitative. There are no data on other demographic characteristics, for example, age or academic preparation. Also, no professional associations of associate degree programs collect this kind of information on faculty. Only the American Association of Colleges of Nursing (AACN) publishes an annual survey of the type and characteristics of faculty teaching in baccalaureate and graduate programs (AACN, 1999). Some inferences, however, can be made from these data about the academic profile of faculty teaching in other programs.

The most significant characteristic that distinguishes

nursing faculty is the possession of a terminal doctoral degree, which is the entry-level credential for faculty teaching in colleges and universities and also increasingly in community and junior colleges. Yet in 1999 only half (50.1%) of these faculty possessed a doctorate (AACN, 1999). Although this is a 35% increase since 1978, when only 15% possessed a doctorate, it still falls far short of being comparable to the percentage of faculty with doctorates in other academic disciplines. Given this profile, it is safe to assume that few faculty teaching in associate degree and diploma programs are doctorally prepared.

Given the historical development of nursing education, with its origins in hospital-based programs followed by the slow movement into higher education, which was followed by an explosion of programs in community and junior colleges in the 1970s, it is not surprising that the faculty teaching in all of these programs look quite different from their academic colleagues.

Because the mission of diploma schools and community and junior colleges is teaching, it may be appropriate for these schools to be staffed by faculty who lack the doctorate. But this has many serious implications for faculty teaching in colleges and universities. In these institutions, nursing programs are seriously compromised because their faculties are so dissimilar from other faculty on campus. Furthermore, within the nursing unit itself the faculty are split into two factions—those with and those without the doctorate—a divisive and provocative arrangement.

Parent Institutions

As colleges and universities have increased their requirements for research and scholarship, non-doctorally prepared faculty find it increasingly difficult or impossible to gain tenure, a concept that is irrelevant to diploma and associate degree faculty. A unit's strength is in part measured by its tenure density. A unit with few tenured or tenure-eligible faculty is always vulnerable to changes within the institutions, the most dramatic being closure.

Colleges and universities have become increasingly competitive and rely more heavily than ever on reputational standings (although most deny their importance). Research and scholarly productivity are important variables in determining reputation. These contributions come primarily from doctoral faculty because doctoral education is the perquisite preparation for research and scholarship. Also, most nondoctoral faculty have heavy undergraduate teaching assignments, making scholarship difficult to accomplish.

Because nursing faculty on the whole are not as fully and comparably prepared as faculty in other academic disciplines, they *de facto* occupy a marginal social status in the university. Consequently they are not full participants in the life of academe and are denied membership in a group that represents the diversity of the institution. Many, knowing that they are less qualified than their colleagues, tend to isolate themselves in their own department or college and become further removed from valuable sources of information and opportunities to influence campus decisions.

Higher education is uniquely characterized by its system of faculty governance. Colleges and universities are, in their essence, a collection of people: the faculty and students. The lifeblood of the institution is the faculty because it is they who generate the reputation and attract the best students and whose opinions guide the course of action within the institution. Faculty who do not fully participate in this governance are, by definition, set apart from institutional life. To the extent that this is true for nursing faculty, the program is rendered vulnerable because it lacks a strong, fully empowered faculty.

Internal Conflicts

The fact that nursing faculty do or do not possess doctorates defacto creates a class system within the nursing program. Historically, those faculty with doctorates teach in the graduate program if there is one, and those without teach in the undergraduate program. Or, in those institutions with baccalaureate programs only, the distinction might be made between the amount of undergraduate *clinical* teaching each group does. Regardless of the type of program, distinctions are usually made, and these distinctions create what amounts to internal *social class* dif-

ferences. This makes for interesting and at times divisive interactions in which one group typically believes itself to be *second-class citizens*. Yet ironically this group teach the very students who are the potential leaders, the feeders into the master's and doctoral programs.

Nationwide, 88% of graduate programs in nursing offered nurse practitioner programs (AACN, 2000). The number of programs has been increasing every year, creating challenges for recruiting nurse practitioner faculty who are also doctorally prepared. Most nurse practitioners are prepared with a master's degree, and that degree is one that prepares the graduate for direct clinical practice, not teaching or research. Graduate education, both at the master's and doctorate levels, should have a strong basis in research, either utilization or training. Yet faculty without the doctorate lack the basic knowledge to be able to teach that content or to evaluate the extant research to guide clinical knowledge.

WHAT DO FACULTY DO?

In differing proportions faculty teach, conduct research, publish, and provide service to the institution and the profession. To accomplish these varied tasks, faculty need to acquire the very best graduate education. Ideally they should also possess the desire to develop and further strengthen a set of personal characteristics that Schoenfeld and Magnon (1994; in a delightful and enormously useful book called *Mentor in a Manual*) identify as being necessary to succeed in academe. These characteristics include knowledge (information, data, theories, concepts, facts); skills (technical, scientific, communication, information retrieval, analysis and synthesis); insight (wisdom, vision); and values (Schoenfeld & Magnon, 1994).

Teaching

A successful teacher possesses a thorough command of the subject matter being taught, which requires that faculty must strive continuously to expand their knowledge base in a world of rapidly changing information. This requires a commitment to continuous learning that goes beyond rhetoric to the investment of substantial time, energy and money in one's own development as a teacher. For nursing faculty, that includes staying abreast of contemporary clinical practice.

Successful teachers are those who convey a liking and deep respect for students that in turn creates an environment that is conducive to learning. Good teachers are able to present material in an objective and well-organized manner, convey a sense of excitement for the material, and stimulate students to want to learn more. Successful teachers vary their teaching methodologies according to the characteristics of the class (e.g., large lecture, seminar), understand and use state-of-the-art teaching methods, and evaluate student learning in an objective manner. The very best teachers truly enjoy teaching and their students and have learned to balance their teaching duties with their other responsibilities. Teachers also help students through the advising process to identify their interests and make decisions about their futures.

Research and Scholarship

Some institutions claim teaching to be their primary and almost exclusive mission, which means that very little, if any, research or scholarship is required of faculty. Certainly this is true for faculty who teach in diploma schools or associate degree programs. In liberal arts colleges, the focus historically has been on teaching. However, even these institutions are increasingly requiring at least a modest level of research and scholarship. Junior faculty are wise to devote considerable effort in determining the precise expectations for teaching, research, and scholarship to be used as a guide for setting priorities.

Research training is the primary objective of doctoral education. Although nursing typically has required knowledge of the research process as part of the required courses in the master's program, the depth of knowledge and skills necessary to actually conduct research are acquired in a doctoral program. Research in nursing is focused on the development of knowledge that provides the foundation for clinical practice. Consequently, nursing research should focus on clinical phenomena. In 1988, the National Center for Nursing Research (NCNR) was established within the National Institutes of Health (NIH) to provide nursing with increased access to federal support for research. In 1993, NCNR's status was upgraded to an institute (National Institute of Nursing Research [NINR]) within the NIH (NINR, 1994).

In 1991 the U.S. Surgeon General published *Healthy People 2000,* the objectives for the nation's health for the year 2000. The degree to which these objectives have been met and new health challenges constitute the newly published *Healthy People 2010.* Essentially, this document outlines the nation's most pressing health care problems and sets out objectives to improve the nation's health. These objectives serve as guiding principles for the delineation of research priorities within the NIH (including the NINR). Nursing research has the potential to make significant contributions to this agenda, and nursing faculty need to focus their research programs in these areas as a way of establishing nursing as a research discipline

capable of making a difference in the lives of those for whom we care: our patients.

Service

Faculty provide service to the nursing department or college, the parent institution, and the profession itself. This service takes many forms but a major mechanism for the provision of service is through a system of faculty governance that is typically operationalized through a committee structure.

In its simplest form, faculty governance is the authority and control possessed by the faculty to make decisions about curriculum, degree requirements, subject matter and methods of instruction, student policies as they relate to the educational process, and faculty status including appointments, promotion, and tenure. Faculty governance is a critical part of the faculty role and one that should not be taken lightly because it is, in its truest sense, the heart of the university.

Faculty contribute to the profession in a variety of ways. Faculty are members of professional organizations and provide service to them in the form of membership on committees and boards. Faculty also provide continuing education through different organizations that serve the profession.

Nursing faculty may also provide service to the institution through clinical practice. Such service may be part of the faculty role, but it may also be undertaken on a volunteer basis. The extent to which faculty do or do not practice affects their credibility as teachers. Unfortunately, many nursing faculty have become far removed from the realities of contemporary practice, which diminishes not only their teaching ability but also their research because they are not well positioned to identify relevant and significant clinical problems to investigate. This reality is one of the most important challenges facing nursing faculty today.

Although service is an expected part of the faculty role, faculty must guard against spending too much time doing it. Committee work can be very seductive and can also consume inordinate amounts of time. Faculty must remember that their *primary* mission is teaching and research and strive to limit their service activities not only to that which is expected but also to that which informs their teaching and scholarship.

CHALLENGES FACING NURSING FACULTY
The Landscape of Higher Education

The greatest challenge facing nursing faculty in colleges and universities is to become full participants in the academy by contributing fully to the goals of the institution through teaching, research, and service. Nursing faculty need to design and teach in excellent academic programs that are based on a knowledge of higher education and its standards, the discipline of nursing, and the needs of a health care system of both today *and* tomorrow.

Nursing, as a relative newcomer to higher education, can ill afford the risk of mediocre or poor-quality educational programs. The new millennium continues a time in which higher education faces particularly difficult fiscal challenges. In this type of environment only the very best will survive. Decisions will be made at the highest levels to preserve quality programs that will, in the long run, preserve and enhance the institution. Nursing programs in major research universities may be particularly vulnerable because their research profile usually does not parallel that of their colleagues. Furthermore it is apparent that the associate degree is *really* the entry level for nursing, since these associate degree programs constitute 60% of all nursing programs.

In the mid-1980s nursing programs were faced with dramatic declines in enrollment. In response to these declines many nursing programs very quickly designed a variety of program offerings as a means of attracting students, thereby preserving themselves. Many of these programs are quite innovative and long overdue, but many also challenge commonly accepted educational standards. As much as these can, in the short run, preserve nursing programs, they will contribute to their demise in the long run if they lack quality that is comparable to that of the parent institution. As an example, Leininger (1985) writes of her concern that doctoral programs in nursing may reflect a culture of mediocrity. Her concern derives from the fact that there has been a rapid proliferation in the number of doctoral programs but that many of them lack sufficient numbers of qualified faculty, are without a foundation of faculty research, and suffer from unstable leadership. Leininger's concerns, to the extent that they are true, should raise considerable alarm because the products of these programs are our future faculty. A culture of mediocrity will handicap them enormously in their ability to fulfill a faculty role.

In a paper discussing the strengths and limitations of doctoral education in nursing, Anderson (2000) presents data detailing the uneven quality of existing programs using commonly accepted quality benchmarks for students, faculty, and the curricula. In addition to the qualitative measures, there is concern about the increasing numbers of programs with steady enrollment and decreasing numbers of graduations (AACN, 2000). Without well-prepared faculty the quality of our educational programs will suffer.

Nursing faculty need to learn the norms that guide faculty work, particularly those related to self-governance. Faculty must become knowledgeable by reading widely and regularly about higher education (e.g., *Chronicle of Higher Education*), fully understanding the goals of their own institution, and knowing its system for advancement (knowing what is expected). Faculty especially must understand that colleges and universities are a meritocracy and that the *products* of their teaching, research, and scholarship are what are valued and rewarded.

Bridging the Clinical Practice–Education Schism

Because nursing is a clinical discipline, nursing faculty must make substantial efforts to bridge the historical schism between nursing service and nursing education. Collaborative efforts contribute to the enhancement of quality in both sectors. Nursing faculty must also increase and keep their knowledge of clinical practice current to design and implement high-quality programs, especially at the baccalaureate and master's levels.

Finding ways to stay abreast of current clinical practice, improving the practice environment, and keeping clinical skills current while also teaching, especially undergraduate clinical courses, is challenging for all faculty but particularly for those who teach in major research universities. Because these universities define themselves by their heavy involvement in research, their standards for promotion expect faculty to be active scholars and researchers. For many years, nursing faculty were treated as an exception to this requirement, but this is no longer true. Doctorally prepared faculty must develop and maintain programs of research and scholarship. However, this becomes very difficult to do if a faculty member is assigned to undergraduate clinical teaching on a regular basis. The time commitment is just too great. New models must be developed that utilize other types of instructional personnel. Such models include teaching assistants, clinical faculty, clinical specialists, and staff nurse preceptors. The challenge is to find a way to utilize doctoral faculty effectively in the teaching of undergraduates without burdening them with the direct clinical supervision aspect of that teaching. Nursing's success as a research discipline is unequivocally linked to meeting this challenge.

Female Dominance

Nursing has always been and continues to be a profession dominated by women. In a very real sense, nursing as a profession can be viewed as a microcosm of women's issues in this country. Women's history is nursing's history. Nursing's development both as a profession and as an academic discipline has been shaped by this powerful fact. Yet, ironically we in the profession do not often directly address this issue and how it influences our professional development and behaviors. Furthermore, nurses do not consistently identify with the goals, objectives, and strategies of the women's rights movement. Additionally, rarely do nurses use a feminist paradigm to analyze issues and circumstance. Rather, the tendency is to think more parochially, viewing situations in a particular or local context rather than to analyze events or situations in light of women's deemed social status.

The most recent data on women in higher education (Chronicle of Higher Education, 1999) indicate that although the number of women faculty is growing, women represent only about one third of the total college and university faculty, with 42% of them at the entry, assistant professor level. Compared with their male colleagues, women are clustered in the lower academic ranks, a smaller percentage achieve tenure, and they earn lower average salaries at every rank. The most disheartening fact is that precious little has changed in this profile over the last 20 years. The overall conclusion is that it is still difficult for women to succeed in the academe. Why?

On the basis of a review of relevant research, Tierney and Rhoads (1994) describe women faculty as being caught in a "revolving door" phenomenon as a result of such things as inadequate anticipatory socialization, weak mentoring, fewer networking opportunities, divergent priorities, and additional demands, especially families.

Aisenberg and Harrington (1988) studied two groups of academic women: those who were off the academic track and tenured women. They found similar themes in both groups, which depicted an experience of professional marginality and of exclusion from the centers of professional authority. Taken together, the stories reveal a continuum of outsideness—literal in the case of the deflected women but nonetheless real for the tenured women as well (Aisenberg & Harrington, 1988, p. xii).

Central to Aisenberg and Harrington's explanation of what happens to academic women is what they call the "marriage plot," which defines marriage as being the goal for all women and, in turn, the ways in which a woman should behave in order to meet her goal. Because this has been the paradigm for women for so long, it has been argued that women cannot ignore it or rid themselves of it as a guide for their behavior and as a measure of their success (Aisenberg & Harrington, 1988). As a result, women, like men, face the same overall task of becoming expert professionals, but women must also deal with a whole set of other demands and expectations that relegate the pursuit of a woman's career secondary to her other roles of wife and mother as well as to her male partner's career.

This conflict is carried into the daily lives of many female faculty, and they find themselves faced with a continuous struggle rooted in the desire to be "womanly" as society defines "woman" and "successful" as her profession defines "success." Couple this personal conflict with the reality that the typical academic institution's policies and practices, the very fabric of the culture of higher education, have been crafted by and for men. The result is a climate in which women find it difficult to thrive and achieve. Recent studies on various campuses across this country attest to a climate that makes it difficult for women to advance within professorial ranks and to high-level administrative posts that offer the opportunity to influence policy and improve the climate.

In a profound way then, this marginal status for academic women is compounded for nursing faculty who do not possess the same credentials as other women faculty. Quite realistically their disenfranchisement and marginality are made even greater.

Interesting behavior patterns emerge when individuals who are dominated by groups that deny them membership are placed in positions without power and influence. Anger, resentment, and distrust are common, as is a sense of futility and frustration and diminished pleasure derived from one's work. At times these sentiments generate negative behaviors, such as a sense of entitlement, the so-called "queen-bee syndrome," and generalized anger and hostility to compensate for the oppression. Men react to these discomforting behaviors in negative ways that cause them to isolate women further.

Because nursing faculty are predominately women, slightly different patterns of behavior emerge internal to the academic unit. In many ways these patterns parallel those described above: doctorally prepared faculty are the "privileged class," and nondoctorally prepared faculty are marginalized and made ineligible for membership in the elite group. To the extent that this situation exists then, negative behaviors are directed toward one's female colleagues and students. Master's-prepared faculty are often motivated to pursue doctoral education to gain membership in the more prestigious group. But they do so later in life, which seriously truncates their academic career.

The Aging Professoriate

Probably the most serious challenge facing nursing education today is the aging of the faculty. In 1999 the mean age for all full-time nurse faculty was 49.7 years and the median age was 51 years (AACN, 1999). Compounding this problem is the fact that the average age of the doctoral graduate is mid-40s. It is true that the number of doctoral programs has increased substantially, but enrollment and graduations have been static (AACN, 2000). The essence of the situation is that large numbers of current faculty will be retiring within the next 10 to 15 years and there are insufficient numbers in the pipeline to replace them.

Further compounding this problem is the increasing numbers of nurses preparing to be nurse practitioners and the attractive clinical positions that await them after graduation. It seems that fewer and fewer nurses are interested in doctoral education (which prepares them for academic roles) or teaching. It is not clear why this is, but it is a fact.

As the number of faculty decrease, nursing schools will be faced with decreasing enrollments and increasing workloads, which will further diminish the opportunity for scholarly work and create undesirable working conditions, which in turn will make an academic career an unattractive option for many. In fact, one author recently described the situation as one in which nursing faculty may be one generation away from extinction (Brendtro & Hegge, 2000).

Nursing's History

Nursing faculty are challenged to develop insight into their own history as nurses, faculty, and women and to confront the conflicts derived from each to be successful in their careers and personal lives. As identified by Schoenfeld and Magnon (1994), traits related to achievement in a faculty role include integrity, maturity, will, self-discipline, flexibility, confidence, endurance, decisiveness, coolness under stress, initiative, justice, compassion, sense of humor, creativity, humility, and tact. Developing these characteristics and traits may present substantial challenges for nursing faculty because some are counter to traits that are considered desirable for women and because models are lacking for others that have not been part of nursing's culture.

Finally, nursing faculty must actively pursue the elimination of those historic policies, practices, values, and norms that interfere with their personal goals as well as goals for excellence. Examples of practices that need elimination include large, cumbersome committee structures; commitment to the *process* of education at the expense of the *product;* teaching facts rather than principles and concepts; harsh and punitive treatment of students contributing to a reputation for "eating our young"; the absence of a norm for postdoctoral training; devaluing undergraduate instruction; and, finally, team teaching that makes it difficult for individuals to develop strong pedagogical skills and a sense of accountability and responsibility.

Being a faculty member is not an easy job. It requires the very best that one has to offer. It also affords a wealth of opportunity especially to shape the future of the profession and to contribute in meaningful ways to the solution of major health care problems. Becoming a faculty member is not for everyone. It should be reserved for the very best, brightest, and most promising. Nursing students, the future of the profession, deserve no less.

REFERENCES

Aisenberg, N., & Harrington, M. (1988). *Women of academe: Outsiders in the sacred grove.* Amherst, MA: University of Massachusetts Press.

American Association of Colleges of Nursing. (1999). *1998-1999 faculty salaries.* Washington, DC: Author.

American Association of Colleges of Nursing. (2000). *1999-2000 enrollment and graduations.* Washington, DC: Author.

Anderson, C.A. (2000, July/August). Current strengths and limitations of doctoral education in nursing: Are we prepared for the future? *Journal of Professional Nursing, 16*(4), 191-201.

Brendtro, M., & Hegge, M. (2000, March/April). Nursing faculty: One generation away from extinction? *Journal of Professional Nursing, 16*(2), 97-104.

Chronicle of Higher Education: Almanac issue. (1999, September). Washington, DC: The Chronicle of Higher Education.

Leininger, M. (1985). Current doctoral nursing education: A culture of mediocrity or excellence? In J.C. McCloskey & H.K. Grace (Eds.), *Current issues in nursing education* (2nd ed., pp. 219-235). St. Louis: Mosby.

National Institute of Nursing Research. (1994). *Nursing research at the National Institute of Health: Fiscal years 1989-1992.* Bethesda, MD: Author.

National League for Nursing. (1992). *Nursing data review: 1992.* New York: Author.

National League for Nursing. (1995). *Nursing data review.* New York: Author.

Schoenfeld, A.C., & Magnon, R. (1994). *Mentor in a manual* (2nd ed.). Madison, WI: Magna.

Tierney, W.G., & Rhoads, R.A. (1994). *Faculty socialization as cultural process: A mirror of institutional commitment.* (ASHE-ERIC Higher Education Rep. No. 93-6). Washington, DC: The George Washington University School of Education and Human Development.

CHAPTER 6

Nurse Researchers

Who Are They, What Do They Do, and What Challenges Do They Face?

NANCY A. STOTTS

Nurse researchers are scientists who seek to find answers to questions through methodical observation and experimentation. They design studies, participate in the conduct of research, and disseminate findings at professional meetings and in peer-reviewed journals.

Nurse researchers seek to understand the science of care through systematic investigation. The work they do is quite diverse. The design of the studies ranges from qualitative to quantitative research; it encompasses interviews, epidemiological surveys, controlled clinical trials, and laboratory experiments. The topics addressed by their research are broad and divergent, reflecting the vast scope of the practice of nursing as well as the rich heritage of nursing in both the biological and the social sciences. Nurse researchers study individuals, families, and communities as well as the health care delivery system. Nurse researchers also are basic scientists who work in the laboratory. There is a great deal of variety in the cluster of persons who call themselves nurse researchers and in the nature of their work.

This chapter is designed to introduce you to the world of nurse researchers. It will answer the following questions: Who are nurse researchers? What do they do? What challenges do they face?

WHO ARE NURSE RESEARCHERS?

In the most encompassing definition, *nurse researchers* are nurses who participate in the systematic study of topics related to nursing. They seek to develop the science behind evidence-based practice and understand the fundamental cellular and humanistic laws that have implications for health and illness.

Most nurse researchers begin their careers as staff nurses and progress up the clinical ladder. Several pathways lead to the role of the nurse researcher. Some have always dreamed of being a faculty member in a school of nursing and research is an integral part of that role in major institutions. Others realize they cannot progress in the clinical nursing arena because they do not want to take on administrative responsibilities and so turn to research as a way to progress in nursing. Another group is overcome with a desire to understand "why" and "what is the mechanism," and they use research to find the answers. A fourth group just happens into a job and falls in love with the work of research.

Doctoral preparation is required to be a scientist in nursing as well as most other disciplines. Usually the degree obtained is a doctor of philosophy (PhD) with a major in nursing or a doctor of nursing science (DNS or DNSc). Some nurses earn a PhD in another discipline (e.g., statistics) or in an allied field such as education. In the purest sense the PhD is designed to prepare a researcher, and the DNS is conceptualized as preparing an advanced clinician, parallel to the doctor of medicine (MD) but with the substantive focus being nursing; however, in practice there often is little difference between the curriculum in the PhD program and that in the DNS program. Doctorally prepared nurses are prepared to carry out all aspects of the research process. They have been taught and have actually carried out the process of conceptualizing a problem, formulating a question or hypothesis, designing the study, collecting the data, analyzing the data, and reporting the findings. This process is encompassed in their dissertation research.

Usually as nurses progress through the academic system, they begin to learn the research process by working initially as a research assistant. Classically the research assistant is an undergraduate or graduate student who is working for a faculty member, doing a library search as the basis for the literature review, collecting data, or entering data into the computer for later analysis. In the most ideal world, the research assistant is an integral member of the research team, learning both process and content through this paid position.

The next level of researcher is a research nurse. This nurse usually is master's-prepared and is hired to collect data, direct and coordinate data collection, or to carry out all aspects of the research that have been planned by the researcher who wrote the grant. The term *project director* is used for the research nurse who assumes responsibility for implementing the research study.

Coinvestigators are researchers who have expertise in a specific area and share in the responsibilities of conceptualizing and conducting the study. They are asked to participate because they have substantive expertise (e.g., social support) or exceptional knowledge in a particular research method (e.g., phenomenological research) or are recognized for understanding analysis technique (e.g., survival analysis). There may be one or more coinvestigators on a grant, depending on the nature of the project and the expertise of the various team members. Consultants also have expertise is a specific area, but their contribution is more circumscribed than that of a coinvestigator.

The leader of the research team is the principal investigator, the person who is responsible for seeing that the grant is written and ultimately for its scientific conduct. This means that this researcher needs to bring the team together, define their roles, see that the conceptual work is completed, and later see that the study is conducted and the data are analyzed. The tone for how the team works together is set by the principal investigator. The research team may be run with a democratic or autocratic style; one approach is not better than the other, they just produce different dynamics and each style has its own strengths and limitations. The principal investigator also initiates discussions about authorship of articles and plans with team members the nature of publications and order of authorship. This proactive negotiation sets a tone for fairness and parity in the team. When students are part of the research team, their contributions and roles needs to be addressed in the negotiations.

It is important to recognize that many research teams are interdisciplinary. The nurse may be the principal investigator, a coinvestigator, or have any of the other roles described. It is a rich experience to work on an interdisciplinary team, especially when all members of the team leave their titles behind and bring the full measure of their expertise to the research.

Thus, nurse researchers are nurses who do research. They usually are doctorally prepared. They may design and conduct the entire project or be responsible for only a portion of the research. They are found performing surveys, interviews, clinical trials, evaluation research, and laboratory research. They function with a variety of titles and roles and the work they accomplish is diverse and reflects the heterogeneity of nursing. The role a specific researcher occupies depends on the nature of the study, the various personalities of the team members, the expertise of the researcher, and timing or serendipity.

WHAT DO NURSE RESEARCHERS DO?

The research process outlines the type of thinking and activities in which nurse researchers engage. For a study to take place, a problem needs to be identified and the researcher must have sufficient interest and expertise in the problem to address it. Seasoned researchers have an identified area of research and know the literature in that substantive area. Often they have a long list of questions that they would like to answer. They need only time and funding to address them.

Knowledge of funding sources is an integral part of the role of the researcher because without funding, research productivity is limited. One important source is the National Institute of Nursing Research, which is part of the National Institutes of Health. There also are grants from foundations and professional organizations. Each has its own priorities, funding limits, and application process. In the library are books that specifically address funding sources, and increasingly those data are available by computer on the World Wide Web. The contracts and grants department in some universities also provides assistance in understanding the multiple sources for financial support for research. A specific funding source is usually targeted early in the proposal development process so that the specific criteria for a given funding source are incorporated into the proposal.

Writing the grant involves analyzing the literature to understand what has been done in the field. Normally, the researcher critically analyzes the literature and puts the proposed study in the context of work that has already been reported. Reviewing the literature also helps in the development of the study procedures because using established approaches and instruments increases the accuracy of the data obtained in the study. When a new area of study is embarked upon, often pilot work needs to be undertaken. The process for grant application for pilot work is the same as applying for a major grant; however, because pilot work usually can be done more inexpensively, the sources of funding may be different from those used for a larger grant.

A crucial aspect of grant writing is the development of a budget. This involves determining the costs for conducting the research. The researcher must "step through" the entire research process and estimate costs for personnel, equipment, data collection tools, data analysis, and reporting. While this sounds relatively easy to do, it is a sophisticated skill that requires knowledge of the population. For example, in calculating staff costs, one item to consider is recruitment of subjects. The researcher must know the number of subjects who meet the study criteria and have some estimate of how many will consent and in what time period. The researcher also must include in the calculation the number of subjects who will consent and later drop out or die. Part of the consideration is also how sick the potential subjects are, the amount of burden that the study imposes, and what the subject will gain by participating. All these factors need to be considered when calculating the amount of time it will take to recruit subjects and the level of personnel required to do the job.

Thus far the general activities of the nurse researcher have been discussed. It is important to recognize that what the nurse researcher does is determined in part by the researcher's employer. Researchers are employed by colleges and universities, by industry, or they may be self-employed and work by contract or do consultation.

In the college or university community, researchers serve in the academic series or the research series. The person in the academic series classically is in a tenure-track position where research or creative work is one criterion for progression in rank. Research needs to be completed, but time also needs to be devoted to teaching, professional competence, and university and public service. Thus most nurse researchers in the academic series do not do research solely. The nurse researcher who is in the academic series is usually on "hard money" (i.e., university or college funds), and grant funding is used to offset a part of his or her salary so release time is available to conduct the study. It also is important to realize that some colleges and universities allow their faculty little time to devote to research, and participation in research depends on the school's philosophy and how it is implemented.

In the research series the researcher is hired specifically to conduct her or his own studies or to be employed on someone else's research. Persons in the research series are

funded entirely on grant money or "soft money." Successful nurses in this series are flexible and creative because their position lasts as long as the research is funded.

Nurse researchers employed by industry often are hired because they bridge the gap between clinical practice and the basic sciences. They often are responsible for the clinical research testing of the company's products. These researchers often are responsible for locating places to conduct the studies, identifying a principal investigator, setting up multisite studies, insuring that the protocol is conducted consistently, and that findings are recorded in a manner that allows for analysis by site as well as for clustering of data across settings. Often the nurse researcher employed by industry must understand the requirements of the U.S. Food and Drug Administration for testing new products, so that the protocol developed and data gathered will meet the scrutiny required for ultimate approval of the product.

Nurse researchers who are self-employed contract with others who need their specific services. The type of services offered and the cost vary widely. Some do primarily data analysis, others assist with design of the study, and others combine their substantive nursing expertise (e.g., cardiovascular nursing of adults) with research skills. Their income depends on developing a set of clients with ongoing needs or being so well known that new clients are consistently referred to them.

Thus, in summary, nurse researchers are prepared to actualize all aspects of the research process. They may be responsible for the entire study or a portion of it. They may work in academia or industry or may be self-employed. There is much heterogeneity in what nurse researchers do.

WHAT CHALLENGES DO NURSE RESEARCHERS FACE?

Nurse researchers face a myriad of challenges. Among these are defining why nursing research is important to nursing practice; developing intradiscipline respect for nurse researchers whose substantive focus or research methods differs from their own; continuing to define the discipline of nursing through nursing research in a changing health care arena; gaining access to subjects because most nurse researchers do not have their own caseload; and obtaining funding in a world of shrinking fiscal resources.

Both within and outside of nursing there is limited appreciation of the need for nursing research. Research in nursing has been viewed as an activity of nursing students, one of the hoops to jump through to graduate rather than as being important to the development of the discipline and practice of nursing. This conclusion does not seem overwhelmingly surprising because in the past, few nurses have conducted research. Only recently have researchers in nursing been recognized for their program of research. Drew and colleagues' work in electrocardiography (Drew, Wung, Adams, & Pelter, 1998) is an example of important nursing research with significant clinical implications. Interdisciplinary work is illustrated in the work of Kathleen Puntillo and Martha Neighbor in pain assessment in ethnically diverse emergency room patients (Puntillo & Neighbor, 1997), Virginia Carrieri-Kohlman and associates' research is in the area of dyspnea in patients with chronic respiratory disease (Carrieri-Kohlman, Gormley, Douglas, Paul, & Stulbarg, 1996), and Nancy Stotts and colleagues' work in pressure ulcer risk assessment (Stotts, Deosaransingh, Roll, & Newman, 1998). One of the challenges nurse researchers face is to show their worth to clinical practice.

Within the nurse researcher community, there seems to be a lack of support for nurse researchers whose substantive content or research methods differs from one's own (Murdaugh, 1999). There are battles between quantitative and qualitative methods and between bench research and clinical studies. Although some of it is honest discussion in an effort to understand by comparing and contrasting, it often is divisive and detracts from nursing research. A kindlier and broader minded approach that encourages understanding of differences and appreciation of the types of knowledge that can be produced with different approaches would allow nurse researchers to focus their energies on generating research rather than defending their substantive content or research method.

Another challenge for nurse researchers is to continue to define the discipline of nursing through research in a changing health care arena. The nature of nursing is changing due to economic forces. Less expensive care may not be better care. Nursing has not done a good job of defining its unique contribution to health care, and the discipline is in jeopardy of being destroyed in this period when interventions are being tightly linked to outcomes. It would behoove nurse researchers to attend to this serious issue so nursing as a discipline and practice can continue to exist.

Nurse researchers seldom have their own caseload of patients, and when it is time to recruit subjects for studies, access to patients of other providers may be a challenge. In this instance, access to patients is dependent on the openness of the patient's primary physician to having the subject studied and the collaborative relationship that the nurse researcher has established. Other considerations that affect access to patients are the numbers of studies being conducted at a given site, the direct potential financial benefit of the study to the health care team, and whether the researcher is seen as someone who might "steal" patients from the primary care physician's practice.

Another challenge is limited funding. Money available from the National Institutes of Health for nursing studies is limited. When funds are limited, nurse researchers compete directly with each other and with scientists in other institutes. The benefit of research to the consumer needs more emphasis to help leverage funding from both the public and private sectors. One approach to this is to focus for a period on translational research, in which the emphasis is on research utilization and the effects research findings have on outcomes. There must be a fine balance between creating knowledge and findings ways to use it, however, and funding for the pipeline of knowledge must not be sacrificed for immediate utilization.

Thus nurse researchers face many challenges in their work. Knowing what the challenges are assists the researcher in consciously devising approaches to mitigate them in order to focus their energies on generation of knowledge.

SUMMARY

Nurse researchers are a hearty group of nurses who seek to develop an understanding of the basis for clinical care. For the most part they are doctorally prepared persons who initiate or participate in all phases of the research process. They are engaged in diverse research methods, and their substantive content addresses the full life span and the health and illness spectrum as well as the health care system. Nurse researchers face numerous challenges in their daily work. It is critical, however, to recognize that their work is pivotal to the profession and discipline because it lays the foundation of the future of nursing.

REFERENCES

Carrieri-Kohlman, V., Gormley, J.M., Douglas, M.K., Paul, S.M., & Stulbarg, M.S. (1996). Exercise training decreases dyspnea and the distress and anxiety associated with it. Monitoring alone may be as effective as coaching. *Chest, 110*(6), 1526-1535.

Drew, B.J., Wung, S.F., Adams, M.G., & Pelter, M.M. (1998). Bedside diagnosis of myocardial ischemia with ST-segment monitoring technology: measurement issues for real-time clinical decision making and trial designs. *Journal of Electrocardiology, 30*(Suppl), 157-165.

Murdaugh, C.L. (1999). Relationship of research perspectives to methodology. In A.S. Hinshaw, S.L. Feetham, & J.L. Shaver (Eds.), *Handbook of clinical nursing research* (pp. 61-70). Thousand Oaks, CA: Sage Publications.

Puntillo, K.A., & Neighbor, M.L. (1997). Two methods of assessing pain intensity in English-speaking and Spanish-speaking emergency department patients. *Journal of Emergency Nursing, 23*(6), 597-601.

Stotts, N.A., Deosaransingh, K., Roll, F.J., & Newman, J. (1998). Underutilization of pressure ulcer risk assessment in hip fracture patients. *Advances in Wound Care, 11*(1), 32-38.

Section Two

Changing Information

Data, Information, Knowledge

JOANNE McCLOSKEY DOCHTERMAN, HELEN KENNEDY GRACE

In order for us to move forward as a scientific discipline we must generate data about patient encounters and the different systems of health care delivery. These data can then be organized in ways that yield information, and the information in turn can be organized, explored, and tested to confirm what we know or to reveal new knowledge. The links between practice, research, and theory are data links, and our science is only as good as our data and what we do with it. This section deals with some of the new advances in this area of information management.

The first chapter in this section is a well-reasoned and thought-provoking debate about the relationships among nursing theory, nursing research, and nursing practice. After defining the terms, Blegen and Tripp-Reimer discuss the advantages and disadvantages of three positions. First, nursing theory, research, and practice should be kept as separate categories; second, the three categories should be closely connected; and third, the categories should be separate with bridges between them. They indicate their choice of the third position with middle range theory providing the connecting bridges. This position is now a real possibility because of the development of taxonomies of diagnoses, interventions, and outcomes that provide the "skeletal framework for nursing knowledge." This clear overview of the relationships among theory, research, and practice should provide good debate and discussion among all those interested in knowledge generation and use.

The link between knowledge development and the computer is explored in the next chapter. Bakken and Costantino provide a thorough overview of the challenges related to transforming nursing data into knowledge. The authors begin by addressing the question of why traditional automated nursing systems have not fostered the development of nursing knowledge. They review the development of standardized nursing terminologies and the evolution of standards for data exchange in information systems. The role of informatics in fostering knowledge development in nursing is reviewed through the system design framework of the National Commission on Nursing Implementation Project. The framework's four types of information system processes (data acquisition, storage, transformation, and presentation) are reviewed. Several examples are given that illustrate the interaction among information and information processes. These include data mining and knowledge discovery techniques for analysis of data repositories. The authors conclude that technological building blocks such as standardized terminologies and integrated systems are necessary but not sufficient for the development of nursing knowledge. Computer competencies related to the acquisition, organization, and analysis of large repositories of clinical data are required. The chapter ends with the formulation of three questions that demonstrate the evolution of nursing knowledge through the documentation of nursing care. Overall, the chapter illustrates the central role of the computer in building nursing science.

Using data, rather than tradition, to guide practice is referred to as evidence-based practice, the subject of the next chapter by Goode and Krugman. The authors begin their chapter by reviewing the history of the movement. In nursing this began as research utilization in the 1970s but the term was not understood by other disciplines and it did not address patient preferences. The evidence-based practice movement was begun in England in the early 1990s and has been dominated by medicine. Evidence-based practice in nursing is more recent. The authors present a multidisciplinary model they and their colleagues have developed. The main source of evidence constitutes a research core, but nine other sources of non-research evidence supplement the research core: patient record review, quality improvement and risk data, standards, infection control, patient preferences, clinical expertise, benchmarking data, cost-effective analysis, and patient's pathophysiology. Patient preferences can override all other sources. The authors review each type of evidence and include numerous web addresses to help locate evidence. They conclude that it is still unclear what best evidence is. This is a helpful chapter that will clarify a recent and growing movement in health care: using the best evidence to improve care practices.

One type of evidence is benchmarking, which is defined by Lin, Truong, Smeltzer, and Williams-Brinkley in the next chapter as the continuous process of comparing measures of services and practices against those of excellent competitors in order to improve practice in an organization. In this era of the Internet and rapid access to information, the consumer is empowered and desires comparison information on quality. According to the authors, successful health care organizations increasingly rely on benchmarking to improve quality and maintain a competitive advantage. The authors discuss three types of benchmarking: internal, competitive, and functional. They also overview the four phases of the benchmarking process: planning, analysis, integration, and action. It is most typical to benchmark performance measures (e.g., length of stay, total expense, number of patient days), but these measures do not indicate how one organization achieved better results. Thus benchmarking on, for example, treatments and medications administered, surgeries performed, and room maintenance services is also recommended. The authors say that benchmarking provides guidance and direction for change to improve practice, but users need to define measures carefully to be consistent with their objectives and needs. A list of reminders for the successful use of benchmarking is included. The chapter is a good overview of one popular data management tool that health care organizations are using to improve services.

The next chapter by Predko addresses the important topic of distance technology. Offering health care via distance technology (telehealth) can facilitate consumer access and convenience. Predko says that the challenge in telehealth is maintaining and improving quality while keeping costs reasonable and improving access. In her chapter she addresses the use of distance technology in education, practice, and research. Throughout the chapter she poses numerous challenging questions, for example: Should future growth at universities be in traditional classes or in telecommunication? How are the roles of teachers and students changed by distance education? What types of data are important to support clinical decision making and are worth monitoring? How can we assure equitable distribution of home care technology? Predko reviews the progress made by nursing as demonstrated in the various position statements on distance education issued by nursing's professional organizations. She

overviews the benefits, disadvantages, and barriers to the use of distance technology in education, practice, and research and makes recommendations for teaching distance education courses based on her personal experience. While the health care industry lags behind other industries in the use of information systems, nursing has emerged as a leader in the use of distance technology. Predko urges nurses everywhere to continue to increase their knowledge and skill in distance technologies. Her chapter is a great overview of the state of the art in this area.

The final chapter in the section, by Eland, presents a vision of information exchange in a future that is not so distant. This chapter is a good companion to the previous one. Eland logs us on to a computer using a retinal eye identification security system. Courses are available via the Internet, and most students are enrolled as distance learners. They can select courses from any university in the world. Libraries are electronic, and office hours are conducted via a Web camera. On-line texts are complete with moving video clips of actual clinical situations hyperlinked to related topics. The video clips are also used by family members who need to learn complicated procedures. Providers communicate with distant colleagues and provide consultation over the Internet. Research is conducted over the Internet, with immediate access to the data for analysis. As you read Eland's vision, ask yourself what has to happen to make the vision a reality. Do you like all of her vision? What part would you change? How does the vision change the nature of the university? How does it change the role of the nurse?

While nursing has made tremendous progress in the area of the use of distance technology and information management, we still have work to do to create a preferred future. Some of the challenges include better preparation of nurses with computer skills, the need to teach clinical decision-making skills in a more systematic way, continued integration of distance technology, the need for widespread use of standardized languages for documentation of care, and integration of nursing data in state and national databases. Although we will continue to conduct and value single research studies that collect small samples of data, we must also begin to collect data in standardized forms on the computer for each patient encounter. These data can be aggregated across units and facilities and connected with other data to build large sample sizes that can be used for sophisticated data analysis. Practitioners and researchers must work together to generate and analyze the data and then to improve practice based on what we learn. This is the computer age. We have made progress but still have much to do.

Nursing Theory, Nursing Research, and Nursing Practice

Connected or Separate?

MARY A. BLEGEN, TONI TRIPP-REIMER

In the last century, nursing progressed from a largely "on-the-job training," temporary occupation for unmarried women to one in which its members were fully educated and licensed, highly respected, and integral to the conduct of the health care professions. In the last half of the 1900s, nursing science developed rapidly and the knowledge that underpins the nursing profession grew at an amazing speed. In this new millennium, we must keep the momentum going and continue building this knowledge through all available avenues.

As nurse leaders examined the developing knowledge, they expressed concern about the divergent patterns that nursing knowledge development were forming. Knowledge was developing separately in three areas: practice knowledge, knowledge based in research or science, and theoretical knowledge. While most nurse scholars called for integrated knowledge, the development processes continued separately (Conant, 1967; Fawcett, 1978a; Fawcett & Downs, 1992; Jacobs & Huether, 1978). The concern about the lack of knowledge integration leads to the proposition addressed in this chapter: Should nursing knowledge be developed in three separate areas or as one seamless whole?

Nursing practice is the "performance of services for compensation in the provision of diagnosis and treatment of human responses to health or illness" (ANA, 1990). The knowledge that nurses use while engaging in practice comes from many sources and is learned initially in the courses taken during undergraduate education. These courses are carefully selected from all disciplines: biophysical sciences, social sciences, humanities, and finally nursing science. The courses in nursing science present knowledge based in other disciplines and knowledge generated by nurses. This nursing knowledge tends to be practical and is applied as soon as possible in a clinical setting. Nurse educators work diligently to present knowledge based in research and organized around a conceptual framework or nursing theory. Articles in nursing education encourage faculty to include nursing research and to use nursing theories. These exhortations emphasize the existing separateness of practice, research, and theory.

Nursing research is the conduct of systematic studies to generate new knowledge or confirm existing knowledge. The fact that nursing research is not often informed by theory and is seldom applied in nursing practice has been lamented for some time. While optimistic about the increase in application of research findings, most authors point to significant barriers to research utilization (Baessler et al., 1994; Carroll et al., 1997; Coyle & Sokop, 1990; Pettengill, Gillies, & Clark, 1994; Titler, 1997). The idea of applying knowledge from research in practice implies the crossing of a boundary. This boundary is composed in part of difficulties finding, reading, understanding, and preparing the research for application. Another part of the boundary between research and practice is the different orientations of nurses who conduct research and those who care for patients directly. The orientation of nurse researchers leads them to increase the validity of the general knowledge produced by their studies by removing or controlling the influence of unique individual characteristics of each patient or subject and the setting. Nurses oriented to practice must focus on those individual characteristics to provide care that truly meets each patient's needs. These different perspectives and tools continue to keep knowledge from research separate from knowledge used in practice until a nurse takes pieces of the knowledge from one arena and uses it in the other.

Nursing theory, on the other hand, is also portrayed as connected to neither practice nor research. Three reviews of research articles conducted to identify the nursing theory underpinning the research found that few of the studies were related to nursing theory. Silva (1986) found that 53 of the 62 research articles she reviewed were not tied to nursing theory. Moody et al. (1988) found that only 3% of clinical research articles actually tested nursing theory. More recently, Fawcett (1999) reviewed all articles published in 1998 in *Research in Nursing and Health* and *Nursing Research* and noted that only 3% were guided by recognized nursing theories. Some of the inattention to theory-testing research comes from the researchers themselves; however, it is increasingly recognized that the older "grand" theories of nursing's recent past are not testable (Acton, Irvin, & Hopkins, 1991).

Many conceptual models emerged in the late 1960s to early 1980s as efforts to define the discipline and foster curricular reform. Although these models were historically essential in nursing's articulation of its identity, they evolved parallel to, rather than interwoven with, research (Blegen & Tripp-Reimer, 1994). These models were statements of nursing philosophy and ideology but did not present knowledge that could be applied directly in practice. They were separate from the world of nursing practice and were neither developed from research nor tested through research. Nursing theory as a type of knowledge in that era was often considered by both practitioners and researchers to be too abstract to be useful. As others have noted, nurses seemed to believe that, in order to be theory, the knowledge needed to be obscure and lack immediate use and meaning (Levine, 1995). Therefore, theory was relegated to a place separate from other types of nursing knowledge. When the grand theories of this era were used, they were most often superimposed on educational, clinical and research environments with little regard to the fit. While the models are still selected by schools and hospitals as organizing frameworks, they do not drive practice, nor do they serve as frameworks for significant research programs.

In the 1980s, following Yura and Torres' (1975) National League for Nursing survey of curricular commonalities in baccalaureate schools of nursing, nursing scholars identified four common constructs (man-human, health, society-environment, and nursing) and declared that the metaparadigm of nursing had been established (Fawcett, 1978b; Flaskerud & Halloran, 1980; Newman, 1984). Scholars gratefully accepted this paradigm for nursing, in large part because perspectives in the philosophy of science had made achievement of disciplinary status contingent on having a paradigm. However, as Downs admonished, "To say that the metaparadigm of nursing is person, environment, health and nursing is to say virtually nothing at all" (Downs, 1988, p. 20). At its best, the metaparadigm of four central concepts provided a rationale and mechanism for the discipline to move beyond the conceptual models. Even after the identification of the nursing paradigm, nurse practitioners and researchers continued for the most part to ignore nursing theory in their work.

This chapter addresses several questions regarding the categories of nursing knowledge. Are the three categories still separate, and if so, is that situation inevitable? What are the advantages of keeping these categories separate? What are the advantages of connecting them? Can the three categories be separate and still useful? To stimulate debate, we present three positions: (1) keep the categories separate, (2) closely connect them, and (3) keep them separate but structure the knowledge with built-in bridges.

KEEP THE THREE CATEGORIES SEPARATE

Each category of nursing knowledge will develop most fruitfully when tended carefully with full focus on one primary category. Nurses with interest and skills in each of the three areas have different perspectives. Nursing practice focuses on specific unique patients with immediate needs in concrete situations. Researchers, however, must carefully control the unique features to produce findings that can be applied across settings to many patients. Theorists focus on general abstract knowledge that may or may not be directly applicable in practice or tested in research at any given time. Their job is to develop the metanarrative of nursing; to articulate the patterns of knowledge, naming, defining, and relating concepts and patterns; to sketch boldly the phenomena of nursing and nursing care; and to clarify how nursing is a unique discipline (Reed, 1995).

Most nurse theorists, researchers, and practitioners currently have highly developed skills in only one of these areas, and knowledge in each category is developing well. Continuing in this manner will produce the knowledge needed and will use the currently developed skills and abilities efficiently. Therefore, the first position is to continue doing what has been successful for the past 30 years.

If the categories of knowledge are kept separate, we must continue to develop the mechanisms to carry nursing theory both to practitioners to inform their practice and to researchers to guide their work. That is, a boundary-spanning role must be developed for persons who move and translate knowledge from each category to nurses working in the other categories. Initially, nurse educators would fill this boundary-spanning role by organizing the knowledge learned by beginning students around nursing theories and capturing the knowledge available from existing research and using it to support nursing practice knowledge. New curricular developments attempt to do just that (Walker & Redman, 1999).

After nurses complete their basic education, they must then rely on boundary-spanning activities in the form of continuing education, workplace facilitators, and publications for practicing nurses. Doctorally prepared clinical nurse researchers often facilitate the application process in practice arenas (Titler, 1997). Publications providing practitioners with nursing theory and current research findings would also assist in these efforts. Several publications have recently made valuable contributions in this area, e.g., *Applied Nursing Research, Clinical Nursing Research, Nursing Scan in Administration, American Journal of Nursing, MedSurg Nursing, Dimensions of Critical Care Nursing,* and the *Online Journal of Knowledge Synthesis for Nursing.*

Research utilization methods have been developed by nurses over the last two decades to provide this boundary-spanning role (Burns & Grove, 1997). While this type of activity is greatly needed by many applied professions, nurses are unique in constructing these methods in great detail. The profession has responded eagerly to this approach. Research utilization projects, often conducted by groups of staff nurses with advice and consultation from nurse research experts, have developed intervention protocols successfully for use in practice (Titler et al., 1994). The research utilization process is an example of successful boundary spanning across the knowledge categories of research and practice. More recently, evidence-based practice efforts have drawn knowledge from theory and practice traditions as well as empirical research to build guidelines and protocols for practice (Goode & Piedalue, 1999).

To reach across the categories of theory and research, boundary-spanning persons will need to identify theoretical developments that need testing and form research questions that need study. Research findings that inform theory development must be communicated back to the theoreticians. Practice problems without current solutions, or with questionable current solutions, must be identified and delivered to researchers for study. Researchers generally take on the role of boundary spanners themselves. That is, they have attempted to frame their research with theory and to derive research questions from practice. As previously noted, however, this has not been totally successful.

Keeping the categories of knowledge separate would allow the continuation of the present pattern of development, with which nursing has made great strides. Practitioners use practice knowledge as they provide care. Theoreticians focus on development of broad abstract statements of what nursing is and does, while researchers discover and develop knowledge from nursing's specific perspective. To facilitate fruition of each category separately and to use this knowledge in practice, boundary-spanning persons are needed to package and deliver knowledge from nurse theorists to researchers and practitioners and back. Basic and continuing nursing education, research utilization, evidence-based practice, and specialized publications have all functioned to span the boundary between research and practice. To facilitate continued progress in this mode, we must find efficient ways to span the boundaries between theory and practice and between theory and research.

CATEGORIES MUST BE CLOSELY CONNECTED

The professional discipline of nursing must have a body of knowledge that is unique, coherent, and as seamless as possible. There must be one unified body of knowledge that belongs to nursing. This knowledge must be organized by theoretically identified concepts, patterns, and relationships; the statements of this knowledge must be generated from and tested by systematic research; and knowledge needs must be identified in practice and generated knowledge applied immediately to practice. Anything less than full connectedness will continue the current pattern of separateness and the ongoing necessity for the special roles of boundary spanners.

Models for accomplishing this connectedness have been described. The ideal model brings together academic researchers, nurse theorists, and practicing nurses to identify knowledge needs, to carry out research projects, to create and refine theory, and to bring research findings systematically into nursing practice. Three subtypes can be identified. The first is the researcher-practitioner collaboration. Two examples of this model come from northern California and involve collaboration among several health care agencies and nurse research experts (Chenitz, Sater, Davies, & Friesen, 1990; Rizzuto & Mitchell, 1988). Another example comes from the Midwest and describes a collaborative research project that began as a utilization project, became a research conduction project due to the lack of adequate base for interventions, and concluded as the results of the research were used and evaluated in practice (Blegen & Goode, 1994).

The second type of collaboration is the theorist-practitioner model. Examples of this kind of collaboration are found in discussions of implementation of the conceptual models. The language and focus of a conceptual model are implemented through the nursing documentation and organization of a hospital or other patient care facility. Unfortunately, it is difficult to analyze the success of these efforts. How can we determine whether implementing model A or model B in a hospital leads to better outcomes? Real world problems are too complex to conclude unequivocally that the model implemented resulted in the changes specified and that the changes enhanced patient outcomes. Fawcett (1999) suggested that nursing needs two dominant provider types, which she labels nurse scholars. The first type, prepared in nursing doctoral (ND) programs, would integrate research and practice in caring for individual clients. The second type, prepared in doctorate of philosophy programs (PhD), would integrate nursing theory and practice with groups of patients.

The third type of collaboration is the researcher-theorist group, which most often evolves from an exploratory qualitative approach to research: the grounded theory approach. Yet another suggestion for increasing the connectedness of the production and use of knowledge is offered by Boyd (1993). The nursing practice research method features the relationship between the nurse researcher-as-clinician and the patient. The research process is collaboration between nurse and patient; it is therapeutic to the patient and leads to development of the nurse. It can be questioned whether the knowledge produced by these efforts is generalizable beyond the setting and patients involved in the project. Even researchers from the "perceived" view call for the creation of knowledge that can be used by all nurses, i.e., knowledge that is generalizable (Schumacher & Gortner, 1992). The greater the need for knowledge that is generally useful by all nurses, the less this approach will be satisfactory.

There are no examples of models combining all three knowledge areas. While needed—and this need is often discussed in published literature—no working models have been described. One recently suggested approach may be able to facilitate this. Theories can be "tested" using means other than traditional empirical research methods. Silva and Sorrell (1992) suggested that there are four approaches to testing theory: verification through correspondence with empirical research, testing to verify through critical reasoning, testing through verification of personal experiences, and verification through assessment of problem-solving effectiveness. If a theory were tested with all these approaches, it would clearly increase the connectedness between practice, theory, and research. However, theory testing using any one of these four methods also involves advanced skills that many practicing nurses either do not have or have little time to use. If the theories being tested with personal experience or problem-solving effectiveness were closer to practice and more narrow in scope than the grand theories, the possibility of practicing nurses carrying out these tests is more likely than if the theories were conceptual models or grand theories.

While collaboration is generally to be recommended and is essential if we set out to develop one coherent, seamless body of knowledge, there are limitations to the extent of collaboration that can actually take place. It is difficult to cross the differing perspectives of the persons involved. Practitioners focus on individual and unique patients; researchers focus on systematically collecting knowledge that transcends the individual subjects from whom they collect data; and theorists focus on general and abstract concepts and relationships among them. A great deal of time and effort must be expended to enhance communication among collaborators.

This highly connected approach to nursing knowledge would put to rest the problem of separated areas of knowledge; however, working in teams that draw persons from multiple settings consumes a great deal of time and other resources. With a highly connected approach to nursing knowledge creation and use, the boundary-spanning activities encompassed by research utilization would no longer be needed. This would release some resources for use in the collaboration needed for the success of the connected approach. At this point in time, the actual success of this model is questionable.

ESTABLISH STRONG CONNECTIONS BETWEEN SEPARATE CATEGORIES

Nursing knowledge must be separated by type of knowledge (action-oriented specific practice applications, controlled systematic and narrow research findings, and abstract and general theory) and by the perspectives of the nurses associated with each category. The development and the use of nursing knowledge are facilitated by keeping these separate and allowing clear and concentrated application of the different approaches used for each type. However, we need stronger connections than are presently provided by the boundary-spanning activities discussed in position one. These connections should be structural and intrinsic to the knowledge itself rather than dependent on boundary spanners. If the knowledge developed was closer to practice, amenable to research testing, and built around structures intrinsic to the discipline of nursing, we would then have the best of all worlds: separateness for development and connectedness for application.

The best solution for keeping the three separate categories more closely connected is to use middle-range theory as the connecting point. Middle-range theory, when developed from research and thoughtful consideration of practice and tested by other research projects, does represent the most valid and useful type of knowledge available in nursing and other disciplines (Lenz, Suppe, Gift, Pugh, & Milligan, 1995).

Middle-range theory provides the means of articulating general knowledge, confirmed by the specific results of research projects, to nurses in clinical practice. When middle-range theory is used to guide research and knowledge development, the theorist and researcher are either the same person or two persons focusing on the same carefully delineated topic. The scope of knowledge within the topic area is narrower than the grand theories and the metaparadigm concepts. The restriction of scope allows for far more precision and depth than the grand theories and conceptual models have allowed. This precise, in-depth and focused knowledge can then be used to inform and guide practice in specific and useful ways. Each middle range theory is more narrow and precise, and yet, as midrange theories develop, they will eventually produce a body of knowledge that covers a broad range of nursing activities.

Theories of the middle range were first suggested by the sociologist Robert K. Merton. The discipline of sociology also initially developed large theories attempting to differentiate sociology from other disciplines and to explain all of social phenomena with one effort. Merton (1967) responded by suggesting middle-range theories and differentiating them from the grand theories. Middle-range theory can be used to guide empirical inquiry because it lies between the minor working hypotheses that evolve in abundance during day-to-day practice and the all-inclusive systematic efforts to develop one unified theory that would explain all behavior. It is intermediate to the general theories, which are too remote from specific classes of behavior to account for what is observed, and to those detailed orderly descriptions of particulars

that are not generalized at all. Middle-range theory, according to Merton, involves abstractions, but they are close enough to observed data to be expressed in propositions that permit testing with systematic research.

Merton suggested that the search for the perfect grand theory led to a multiplicity of philosophical systems in sociology and, further, to the formation of schools, each with its own cluster of masters and disciples. Nursing perhaps has fallen to a similar fate. That is, we became differentiated from other disciplines but also became internally differentiated not in terms of specialization, as in other sciences, but in terms of schools of philosophy, held to be mutually exclusive and largely at odds. It is time to refocus from discussing these larger philosophical systems to producing knowledge that explains patient-related phenomena and helps in the choice and evaluation of interventions.

Merton further described the middle-range orientation as one that involves the specification of ignorance. Rather than pretend to have knowledge when it is, in fact, absent, the work on middle-range theories expressly recognizes what must yet be learned in order to lay the foundation for more knowledge. It does not begin with the task of providing theoretical solutions to all the urgent practical problems of the day, but addresses itself to those problems that might now be clarified in the light of available knowledge and to the identification of problems about which we know very little.

Our major task is to develop middle-range theory for the general advancement of nursing knowledge and to provide closer connections among theory, research, and practice. A large part of what is now described as theory consists of general orientations toward the discipline, suggesting types of variables that theories must take into account, rather then clearly formulated, verifiable statements of relationships between specified variables. We have many concepts but few supported propositions relating them, many points of view but few confirmed theories. It is time to move on.

To make use of the knowledge provided by middle-range theories, practicing nurses would need some grasp of research methods but they would not have to read and critique directly the often complex reports of research methods and findings. In addition, practicing nurses would not have to attempt to apply the global, highly abstract grand theories to everyday practice. Middle-range theories, developed and tested by research, would contain much more specific descriptions of human responses to health and illness and the nursing interventions applicable to these responses. Although understanding the theory and deriving specific nursing actions would be necessary, these activities would not be as daunting with theory developed in the middle range as they are with the grand theories.

Some boundary-spanning activities would still be needed. While the knowledge articulated with middle-range theories is much closer to practice, it still must be located and critiqued. Nurse educators and group leaders for evidence-based practice projects could provide this necessary assistance. Their job would be much easier with theory in the middle range that had been tested systematically by researchers. Knowledge built in this way is more easily synthesized: the cumulation of knowledge across individual studies occurs as part of the process of conducting research and testing a theory. Persons actively engaged in evidence-based practice could provide an additional service by formally feeding back to the researchers the evaluation of practice guidelines and protocols. This would provide a test of pragmatic usefulness for the knowledge.

Recent developments in nursing knowledge could provide other strong bridges connecting the three categories of nursing knowledge. In the last decade of the 20th century, more of the theoretical work has been in the middle range. Some of these middle-range theories, however, were drawn from other disciplines and did not cohere naturally within the practice discipline of nursing. While these theories were used to support nursing research, they did not fit as well within the practice arena. Liehr and Smith (1999) list five approaches to developing middle-range theory. We suggest that recent developments in nursing knowledge structures provide another way to ground these theories within the discipline.

Developments in the structure of nursing knowledge (the taxonomies for nursing diagnoses, interventions, and outcomes) hold great promise for capturing the middle-range theories within a thorough and extensive framework of nursing knowledge. The Iowa Intervention Project has advanced even beyond the taxonomy of interventions and has identified a three-dimensional structure underlying these interventions (Tripp-Reimer, Woodworth, McCloskey, & Bulechek, 1996). Classes of interventions were characterized along four factors that were then related to the dimensions. The dimensions indicated principal elements describing patient needs and setting characteristics that nurses use in selecting the interventions, and four factors characterized the interventions available. Combined, these produce three descriptive categories. The first dimension nurses might use in selecting interventions is the *intensity of care* dimension;

and the groups of interventions range along two bipolar factors: healthy self-care to provider illness care and continuous routine care to sporadic emergency care. The second dimension describing intervention selection is *focus of care* and the interventions range from individual independent to system collaborative. The third dimension is *complexity of care* and includes two groups of interventions: continuous routine to sporadic emergency and high-priority difficult to low-priority easy. These three dimensions and the factors within them could serve as the framework for guiding development of middle-range theories describing nurses' decision making in the selection of interventions.

The taxonomies of nursing diagnoses, interventions, and outcomes provide a full skeletal framework for nursing knowledge. This skeleton can be filled in with middle-range theories, the impetus and context for which would be clear. Theories would suggest explanations and predictions of relationships between diagnoses of actual or potential health problems, nursing interventions chosen to deal with these problems, and the patients' eventual outcomes (Blegen & Tripp-Reimer, 1997). Each theoretical linkage would need to be tested in systematic research studies. The theories and the framework itself would be modified as this research progressed.

To bring about the close connections among theory, research, and practice using middle-range theories, nurses from each perspective must understand and appreciate the uniqueness of each perspective and the need to communicate across all perspectives. Researchers must accept the responsibility of truly testing the middle-range theories. That is, not only must their research be guided by the theory, but their results must be used explicitly to develop and modify the theory. In addition, the researchers must ensure that the theory is described comprehensively and is useful to practitioners. Nurse theorists must work to develop theories that are testable by researchers and that can be applied by practitioners. This knowledge, confirmed by research, could be incorporated into educational programs. Nurse educators would need to continually update their grasp of current research and the state of the knowledge pertaining to these middle-range theories.

Even with well-grounded theories in the middle range, nurses may still need assistance in applying the knowledge in practice. As other disciplines have found, the time lapse from discovery of knowledge to full application is often quite long. This assistance could be less extensive and formal than the current research utilization process is. If research specifically tests middle-range theories and if the process of replication and extension is followed systematically, the knowledge would accumulate naturally and be directly applicable in practice. Furthermore, if these middle-range theories are organized around knowledge structures as closely tied to practice as the taxonomies currently under construction, and if they are indexed using the standardized languages, they will be readily found and immediately pertinent.

Nurse educators and nurses formulating evidence-based practice guidelines are important to the goal of incorporating nursing knowledge produced by theory building and testing in practice. However, nurses in practice must accept the primary ongoing responsibility of seeking out the most current developments in a theory and either applying it in practice or communicating to the researchers and theorists the reasons why it cannot be applied. Nurses in clinical practice provide the final test of the theories and the frameworks that organize these theories.

SUMMARY

We presented three positions in answering the opening questions. First, the three categories of nursing knowledge should be kept separate to facilitate full development of each unique type, and boundary-spanning activities must be enhanced to ensure that the knowledge developed in each area is communicated to nurses working in the other areas, particularly in nursing practice. In the second position, we argued that the three categories must be closely connected in order to have a body of knowledge that is coherent and seamless. To achieve this goal, new methods of conceptualizing, testing, and applying knowledge must be developed. Third, while nursing knowledge must be separated for the full focused development of each category, the connections between the categories must be strengthened by building bridges within the structure of the knowledge itself. These bridging structures are middle-range theory and the taxonomies of nursing knowledge currently under construction.

This third position was built on the recognition that the perspectives of theoreticians, researchers, and practitioners are different, and these differences are strengths that should be used well. This position also recognizes that the three categories must be closely connected and suggests both structural connections and continued use of boundary-spanning activities. Nursing theory, nursing research, and nursing practice would then be both separate and connected.

REFERENCES

Acton, G.J., Irvin, B.L., & Hopkins, B.A. (1991). Theory-testing research: Building the science. *Advances in Nursing Science, 14*(1), 52-61.

American Nurses Association. (1990). *Suggested state legislation.* Washington, DC: Author.

Baessler, C.A., Blumberg, M., Cunningham, J.S., Curran, J.A., Fennessey, A.G., Jacobs, J.M., McGrath, P., Perrong, M.T., & Wolf, Z.R. (1994). Medical surgical nurses' utilization of research methods and products. *Medical Surgical Nursing, 3*(2), 113-121.

Blegen, M.A., & Goode, C. (1994). Interactive process of conducting and utilizing research in nursing service administration. *Journal of Nursing Administration, 24*(9), 24-28.

Blegen, M.A., & Tripp-Reimer, T. (1994). The nursing theory–nursing research connection. In J. McCloskey & H.K. Grace (Eds.), *Current issues in nursing* (4th ed., pp. 87-91). St. Louis: Mosby.

Blegen, M.A., & Tripp-Reimer, T. (1997). Implications of nursing taxonomies for middle-range theory development. *Advances in Nursing Science, 19*(3), 37-49.

Boyd, C.O. (1993). Toward a nursing practice research method. *Advances in Nursing Science, 16*(2), 9-25.

Burns, N., & Grove, S.K. (1997). *The practice of nursing research: Conduct, critique, and utilization* (3rd ed.). Philadelphia: Saunders.

Carroll, D.L., Greenwood, R., Lynch, K.E., Sullivan, J.K., Ready, C.H., & Fitzmaurice, J.B. (1997). Barriers and facilitators to the utilization of nursing research. *Clinical Nurse Specialist, 11*(5), 207-212.

Chenitz, W.C., Sater, B., Davies, H., & Friesen, L. (1990). Developing collaborative research between clinical agencies: A consortium approach. *Applied Nursing Research, 3*(3), 90-97.

Conant, L.H. (1967). Closing the practice-theory gap. *Nursing Outlook, 15*(11), 37-39.

Coyle, L.A., & Sokop, A.G. (1990). Innovation adoption behavior among nurses. *Nursing Research, 39,* 176-180.

Downs, F. (1988). Doctoral education: Our claims to the future. *Nursing Outlook, 36*(1), 18-20.

Fawcett, J. (1978a). The relationship between theory and research: A double helix. *Advances in Nursing Science, 1*(1), 49-62.

Fawcett, J. (1978b). The "what" of theory development. In *Theory development: The what, why, how* (pp. 17-33). New York: National League for Nursing.

Fawcett, J. (1999). The state of nursing science: Hallmarks of the 20th and 21st centuries. *Nursing Science Quarterly, 12*(4), 311-318.

Fawcett, J., & Downs, F. (1992). *The relationship of theory and research* (2nd ed.). Philadelphia: F.A. Davis.

Flaskerud, J.H., & Halloran, E.J. (1980). Areas of agreement in nursing theory development. *Advances in Nursing Science, 31*(1), 1-7.

Goode, C.J., & Piedalue, F. (1999). Evidence-based clinical practice. *Journal of Nursing Administration, 29*(6), 15-21.

Jacobs, M.K., & Huether, S.E. (1978). Nursing science: The theory practice linkage. *Advances in Nursing Science, 1*(1), 63-73.

Lenz, E.R., Suppe, F., Gift, A.G., Pugh, L.C., & Milligan, R.A. (1995). Collaborative development of middle-range nursing theories: Toward a theory of unpleasant symptom. *Advances in Nursing Science, 17*(3), 1-13.

Levine, M.E. (1995). The rhetoric of nursing theory. *Image: Journal of Nursing Scholarship, 27*(1), 11-14.

Liehr, P., & Smith, M.J. (1999). Middle range theory: Spinning research and practice to create knowledge for the new millennium. *Advances in Nursing Science, 21*(4), 81-91.

Merton, R.K. (1967). *On theoretical sociology.* New York: Free Press.

Moody, L.E., Wilson, M.E., Smyth, K., Schwartz, R., Tittle, M., & VonCott, M.L. (1988). Analysis of a decade of nursing practice research: 1977-1986. *Nursing Research, 37*(6), 374-379.

Newman, M.A. (1984). The continuing revolution: A history of nursing science. In N.L. Chaska (Ed.), *The nursing profession: A time to speak.* New York: McGraw Hill.

Pettengill, M.M., Gillies, D.A., & Clark, C.C. (1994). Factors encouraging and discouraging the use of nursing research findings. *Image: Journal of Nursing Scholarship, 26*(2), 143-147.

Reed, P.G. (1995). A treatise on nursing knowledge development for the 21st century: Beyond postmodernism. *Advances in Nursing Science, 17*(3), 70-84.

Rizzuto, C., & Mitchell, M. (1988). Research in service settings: part I. Consortium project outcomes. *Journal of Nursing Administration, 18*(2), 32-37.

Schumacher, K.L., & Gortner, S.R. (1992). (Mis)conception and reconceptions about traditional science. *Advances in Nursing Science, 14*(4), 1-11.

Silva, M.C. (1986). Research testing nursing theories. *Advances in Nursing Science, 9*(1), 1-11.

Silva, M.C., & Sorrell, J.M. (1992). Testing of nursing theory: Critique and philosophical expansion. *Advances in Nursing Science, 14*(4), 12-23.

Titler, M.G. (1997). Research utilization: Necessity or luxury. In J.C. McCloskey & H.K. Grace (Eds.), *Current issues in nursing* (5th ed., pp. 104-117). St. Louis: Mosby.

Titler, M.G., Kleiber, C., Steelman, V., Goode, C.J., Rakel, B., Barry-Walker, J., Small, S., & Buckwalter, K. (1994). Infusing research into practice to promote quality care. *Nursing Research, 43*(5), 307-313.

Tripp-Reimer, T., Woodworth, G., McCloskey, J.C., & Bulechek, G. (1996). The dimensional structure of nursing interventions. *Nursing Research, 45,* 10-17.

Walker, P.H., & Redman, R. (1999). Theory-guided, evidence-based reflective practice. *Nursing Science Quarterly, 12*(4), 298-303.

Yura, H., & Torres, G. (1975). Today's conceptual framework within baccalaureate nursing programs. In G. Torres & H. Yura (Eds.), *Faculty-curriculum development. Part III: Conceptual frameworks, meaning and function* (pp. 17-25). New York: National League for Nursing.

Standardized Terminologies and Integrated Information Systems

Building Blocks for Transforming Data into Nursing Knowledge

SUZANNE BAKKEN, MORI COSTANTINO

The premises of this chapter are two. First, nursing theory, nursing research, and nursing practice must be related integrally in order to foster the development of nursing knowledge. Second, building blocks for the development of nursing knowledge include standardized terminologies for patient problems (e.g., nursing diagnoses, medical diagnoses, symptoms), nursing interventions, and nursing-sensitive patient outcomes as well as integrated information systems to support the acquisition, storage, transformation, and presentation of data relevant to nursing. The discussion supporting these premises is organized around three questions:

- Why have traditional nursing information systems not fostered the development of nursing knowledge?
- How can standardized terminologies and integrated information systems foster the development of nursing knowledge?
- What informatics competencies are required to complement the technological building blocks of standardized terminologies and integrated information systems?

WHY HAVE TRADITIONAL NURSING INFORMATION SYSTEMS NOT FOSTERED THE DEVELOPMENT OF NURSING KNOWLEDGE?

Although various types of nursing information systems have been in place for several decades, these systems have, for the most part, failed to foster the development of nursing knowledge. Several reasons can be posited for

this void, including the traditional role of the nursing record as a transaction log rather than an evolving repository of practice-based nursing knowledge; limited incorporation of standardized terminologies in information systems in a manner that facilitates data reuse; and application-specific rather than integrated information systems.

The Nursing Record as a Transaction Log

In his discussion of a framework for the transition from nursing records to a nursing information system. Turley (1992) notes that storage of the transaction log (what the nurse does when) is not likely to add to the understanding of the patient's condition and problems. He states,

> Alone, transaction logs do not reflect the evolution of patient status, condition resolution, or expected long-term outcomes. All those lost data represent the forfeiture of documented nursing knowledge and will critically affect the development of decision support components of any nursing information system. [Turley, 1992, p. 178]

This thought is consistent with the recommendations by the Institute of Medicine (Dick & Steen, 1991; Dick, Steen, & Detmer, 1997) reports on the computer-based patient record (CPR), which identified the documentation of the logical bases for all diagnoses or conclusions and the clinical rationale for decisions about the management of the patient's care as essential attributes of CPR systems. In addition, these attributes are critical to knowledge development in health care.

Standardized Health Care Terminologies

Standardized health care terminologies, that is, the set of terms representing a system of concepts (International Standards Organization, 1990), are necessary to reliably and validly describe, support, and analyze health care processes and outcomes (Clark & Lang, 1992). During the last several decades, development of standardized health care and nursing terminologies has been extensive (American Medical Association, 1993; Brown, O'Neil, & Price, 1998; Grobe, 1996; International Council of Nurses, 1999; Johnson, Maas, & Moorhead, 2000; Kleinbeck, 1996; Martin & Scheet, 1992; McCloskey & Bulechek, 2000; NANDA, 1999; Ozbolt, 1996; Saba, 1992; Spackman, Campbell, & Cote, 1997; Werley & Lang, 1988). Table 8-1 summarizes the content of selected terminologies related to aspects of the nursing process.

Given the obvious need for the information and the availability of multiple terminologies, one might ask, "Why are standardized terminologies not universally implemented in computer-based systems?" A number of organizations and terminology experts have proposed criteria or standards related to the suitability of terminologies for incorporation into computer-based systems (American Nurses Association, 1999; Chute, Cohn, & Campbell, 1998; Cimino, 1998). Evaluation studies of standardized terminologies against these criteria provide some answers to this question.

The evaluation criteria can be broadly conceptualized into two categories. The first category is composed of criteria that focus on the content of a terminology in relationship to the needs of a particular domain (American Nurses Association, 1999; Chute et al., 1998). These include breadth of coverage and depth of clinical detail (e.g., nursing diagnoses vs. individual symptoms; nursing interventions vs. individual tasks). In contrast, the second set of criteria (e.g., concept permanence, formal definitions) focuses on the extent to which a terminology is represented in an information system in a manner that supports computer processing for data manipulation and reuse (CEN ENV #12264, 1995; Chute et al., 1998; Cimino, 1998).

The primary focus of nursing terminology development has appropriately been on the collection and categorization of nursing concepts. Evaluations of terminologies against domain coverage criteria support several conclusions:

- Standardized nursing terminologies demonstrate broad coverage for nursing diagnoses, nursing interventions, and nursing-sensitive outcomes (Henry, Warren, Lange, & Button, 1998).
- Terminologies not specifically designed for nursing include some terms used by nurses to document problems (e.g., SNOMED International) and interventions

TABLE 8-1 Standardized Terminologies for Representing Concepts Relevant to the Nursing Domain

Terminology	Assess[1]	Diagnose	Intervene
Nursing			
Home Health Care Classification[2] (Saba, 1992)	✓	✓	✓
International Classification of Nursing Practice (International Council of Nurses, 1999)	✓	✓	✓
NANDA Taxonomy 1[2] (NANDA, 1999)		✓	
Nursing Intervention Lexicon and Taxonomy (Grobe, 1996)			✓
Nursing Interventions Classification[2] (McCloskey & Bulechek, 2000)			✓
Nursing Outcomes Classification[2] (Johnson, Maas, & Moorhead, 2000)	✓		
Nursing Minimum Data Set[2] (Werley & Lang, 1988)	✓	✓	✓
Omaha System[2] (Martin & Scheet, 1992)	✓	✓	✓
Patient Care Data Set[2] (Ozbolt, 1996)	✓	✓	✓
Perioperative Data Set[2] (Kleinbeck, 1996)	✓	✓	✓
Health Care			
International Classification of Diseases (1992)	✓	✓	
Logical Observation Identifiers Names and Codes (Huff et al., 1998)	✓		
National Health Service Clinical Terms (Brown et al., 1998)	✓	✓	✓
Physicians' Current Procedural Terminology (American Medical Association, 1993)			✓
SNOMED RT[2] (Spackman et al., 1997)	✓	✓	✓

[1]Includes assessment to generate a nursing diagnosis, goal setting, and outcome evaluation.
[2]Recognized by American Nurses Association.

(e.g., Physician's *Current Procedural Terminology* [CPT] Codes) (Griffith & Robinson, 1992; Henry, Holzemer, Randell, Hsieh, & Miller, 1997; Henry, Holzemer, Reilly, & Campbell, 1994; Lange, 1996).

- In addition to the abstract terms (e.g., nursing diagnoses and nursing interventions) predominant in standardized nursing terminologies, less abstract, i.e., more atomic, terms (e.g., symptoms and specific nursing activities) are also needed to represent nursing concepts with sufficient clinical detail (Campbell et al., 1997; Henry et al., 1994; Henry & Mead, 1997).

The findings of these evaluation studies document that the existing set of standardized terminologies provides terms for the majority of concepts required to represent nursing domain content in information systems. Additionally, recent efforts have focused on the development of terminologies that include atomic terms for nursing concepts (e.g., Patient Care Data Set [Ozbolt, 1996], International Classification of Nursing Practice [International Council of Nurses, 1999], SNOMED RT [Spackman et al., 1997]).

The second set of criteria fall primarily within the purview of informaticists, standards development organizations, and system developers rather than that of those developing standardized nursing terminologies. However, both sets of criteria are essential to achieve the goal of building nursing knowledge from data in information systems. Thus, recent collaborative efforts among these groups toward the representation of nursing concepts in a manner that maximizes the capacity for data manipulation and reuse are significant (Bakken et al., 1999; Ozbolt, 2000).

Challenge of Information Systems Integration

Systems integration is still a major challenge in most health care organizations, thereby limiting the potential of information systems to influence the quality of nursing practice and also providing a barrier to nursing knowledge development. Historically, stand-alone, application-specific information systems have constrained the relationships that can be examined among various types of data as well as the transformation processes applied to the data.

Great strides made during the last decade have the potential to decrease the technological barriers to using information systems as facilitators of knowledge development. Most significant among these are the growth of the Internet and resources available on the World Wide Web and the evolution of standards for data exchange among

systems (Hammond & Cimino, 2000). In addition, the move toward tailored (e.g., user-specific) views to a shared data repository rather than to separate information systems has decreased barriers and broadened the types of data available. In order to maximize knowledge development and use, future efforts must include enhancing the understanding of human-computer interactions at the individual user and organizational level.

HOW CAN STANDARDIZED TERMINOLOGIES AND INTEGRATED INFORMATION SYSTEMS FOSTER THE DEVELOPMENT OF NURSING KNOWLEDGE?

Framework for Design Characteristics for Nursing Information Systems

Graves and Corcoran (1989) defined nursing informatics as "a combination of computer science, information science, and nursing science designed to assist in the management and processing of nursing data, information, and knowledge to support the practice of nursing and the delivery of nursing care" (p. 3). The phenomena of interest in nursing informatics are nursing data, nursing information, and nursing knowledge. Nursing informatics involves the rules and processes that relate to symbolic representations of nursing phenomena.

The role of nursing informatics in fostering knowledge development in nursing will be discussed using the framework for design characteristics of a nursing information system provided by the National Commission on Nursing Implementation Project (NCNIP) Task Force on Nursing Information Systems (Zielstorff, Hudgings, Grobe, & The National Commission on Nursing Implementation Project [NCNIP] Task Force on Nursing Information Systems, 1993). The framework includes three categories of information required to support professional nursing practice. *Patient-specific data* are data about a particular person and may be acquired from a variety of data sources (e.g., provider observations and interventions, self-reports of functional status). *Agency-specific data* are those data relevant to the specific organization under whose auspices the health care is provided (e.g., standards of care, case mix). *Domain information and knowledge* are specific to the discipline of nursing or to health care in general (e.g., bibliographic literature, clinical practice guidelines, comparative databases). The NCNIP framework also delineates four types of information system processes that relate to the three categories of information. *Data acquisition* is the set of methods by which data become available to the information system (e.g., monitoring devices, entry of symptom data by the patient via the World Wide Web, keyboard or voice entry of data by the health care provider). *Data storage* includes the methods, programs, and structures used to organize data for subsequent use and reuse (e.g., data structures, databases). *Data transformation* or processing comprises the methods (e.g., calculation, abstraction, production rules, data mining algorithms) by which data or information is "acted upon" according to the needs of the end user. *Presentation* encompasses the forms in which information is delivered to the end user after processing. These include simple textual as well as graphic and multimedia presentations (Starren & Johnson, 2000). For example, vital signs or functional status might be best displayed as a line chart in order to examine trends over time, whereas the defining characteristics of altered oral mucous membrane, which include leukoplakia, hyperemia, and hemorrhagic gingivitis, could be presented most effectively using video images.

Transforming Data Through Standardized Terminologies and Information System Processes

The following examples illustrate the dynamic interaction among types of information and system processes.

Pressure Ulcer Management. Figure 8-1 illustrates the integration and iterative transformation of patient-specific data, agency-specific data, and domain information and knowledge using the clinical example of pressure ulcer management. Domain information and knowledge (i.e., a practice guideline) is applied to patient-specific assessment data, resulting in the generation of a "pressure ulcer risk score." The level of pressure ulcer risk score triggers agency-specific policies and protocols (e.g., ordering the appropriate type of mattress suitable to the level of risk). Multiple use of the data is illustrated by presentation formats such as lists in a patient education plan and critical path. The individual-level data can be aggregated and transformed both to refine agency-specific needs and to add to the body of domain information and knowledge related to pressure ulcer management (e.g., does care given in compliance with the practice guideline affect patient outcomes?).

Validation of Nursing Diagnoses. Probabilistic data transformation approaches have been applied to medical diagnostic reasoning for several decades, resulting in the development of medical diagnostic decision support systems (Warner et al., 1988). Nursing research and theory have generated defining characteristics and labels for nursing diagnoses (NANDA, 1999). Databases containing nursing diagnoses, predicted defining characteristics, and patient-specific data have the potential to serve as the in-

frastructure for large-scale validation studies. For instance, in her sample of 414 client assessments using the Computer Aided Research in Nursing database, Chang (1993) found a 76% positive predictive power for the presence of the defining characteristic of a problem with moving body parts and the diagnosis of self-care deficit. Rios, Delaney, Knuckeberg, and Mehmert (1991) validated the predicted defining characteristics of four nursing diagnoses related to alterations in fluid volume and identified additional defining characteristics. Wide-scale implementation of information systems containing nursing diagnoses and patient attributes will facilitate not only the validation of nursing diagnoses, but also the deployment of decision support systems that are based on empirical data rather than exclusively on predicted relationships.

Linking Diagnoses, Interventions, and Outcomes. Publications have proposed linkages among diagnoses, interventions, and outcomes (e.g., see Johnson, Maas, & Moorhead, 2000; McCloskey & Bulechek, 2000). In addition, a number of efforts are focused on implementing standardized terminologies for nursing diagnoses, interventions, and outcomes in information systems at the enterprise, national, and international level. For instance, Zingo (1997) reported on efforts to incorporate nursing terminology within a convergent medical terminology for the information systems of a large health maintenance organization. Prophet, Dorr, Gibbs, and Porcella (1997) described the incorporation of the standardized nursing languages Nursing Interventions Classification (NIC) and Nursing Outcomes Classification (NOC) for on-line care planning and documentation at the University of Iowa Hospitals and Clinics. The Omaha System has been incorporated into the clinical information system supporting the faculty practices at the University of Pennsylvania School of Nursing (Button et al., 1998). At the national level the criteria used in the information system "recognition" process by the Nursing Information and Data Set Evaluation Center of the American Nurses Association includes a standard related to terminology to document all phases of the nursing process (American Nurses Association, 1997). In Europe, efforts have centered on the Telenurse Project and its demonstrations of the utility of the International Classification of Nursing Practice (ICNP) within electronic patient records (Mortensen, 1999). At the international level, the ICNP project is making tremendous progress toward an information infrastructure to examine health care phenomena, nursing activities, and outcomes globally (International Council of Nurses, 1999).

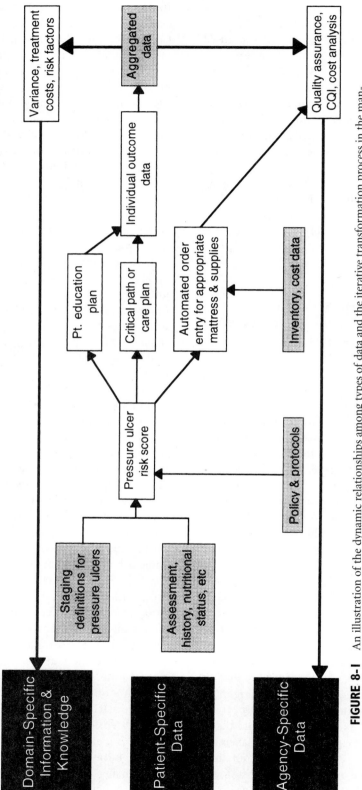

FIGURE 8-1 An illustration of the dynamic relationships among types of data and the iterative transformation process in the management of pressure ulcers.

Knowledge Discovery in Databases. As large repositories of health care data are developed, it becomes possible to apply data mining and knowledge discovery in databases (KDD) techniques in order to answer questions that were not hypothesized at the time of data collection. Similarly to the machine learning techniques applied in the artificial intelligence research of the 1980s, KDD uses pattern recognition and matching, classification or clustering schemas, and other algorithms to examine relationships in data in order to "discover" answers to the questions posed by the investigator. Recently, these techniques have been applied in several nursing informatics projects. Abbott, Quirolgico, Manchand, Canfield, and Adya (1998) examined the ability of data elements in the long-term care Minimum Data Set to predict admissions to acute care facilities. Goodwin et al. (1997) reported on an international collaborative nursing informatics research project focused on predicting adult respiratory distress syndrome risk in critically ill patients using data from clinical databases. As data of relevance to nursing become more ubiquitous, such techniques have tremendous potential for knowledge development through empirical research and theory testing.

Retrieval and Application of Heterogeneous Sources of Knowledge. In the domain of health care in general, the Unified Medical Language System, a linked collection of source terminologies developed by the National Library of Medicine, has been used to retrieve heterogeneous sources of knowledge for application in patient care settings (Humphreys, Lindberg, Schoolman, & Barnett, 1998; Lindberg, Humphreys, & McCray, 1993). MedWeaver (Detmer, Barnett, & Hersh, 1997) allows the user to move among three types of domain knowledge sources: (1) bibliographic (MedLine); (2) diagnostic decision support system (Dxplain); and (3) Web resources (CliniWeb). InfoButtons provide context-specific access to relevant information on demand at the point of care, e.g., cholesterol treatment guidelines when reporting laboratory results (Cimino, Elhanan, & Zeng, 1997). PatCIS provides the infrastructure to use patient-specific data from the clinical information system to tailor domain information and knowledge presented to patients (Cimino, 2000). Another approach to retrieval and presentation of tailored information is the Heart Care project in which a nursing assessment after coronary artery bypass graft surgery is used to create individualized Web access to a set of information resources (Brennan, Caldwell, Moore, Screenath, & Jones, 1998).

Translation of Research Protocols into Standardized Terminologies. A number of investigations have demonstrated the utility of standardized terminologies to abstract narrative records from nursing research studies (Henry et al., 1994; Parlocha & Henry, 1998). The translation of research protocols *a priori* into standardized terminologies that are also used in practice settings has the potential to expedite not only the collection of research data at the point of care but also the retrieval and application of the research findings into practice. For example, Holzemer, Henry, Portillo, and Miramontes (2000) incorporated terms from three standardized terminologies (HHCC, LOINC, and SNOMED) for structured data entry and documentation of the Client Adherence Profiling and Intervention Tailoring (CAP-IT) intervention, a nurse case manager–delivered medication adherence intervention for home care patients receiving highly active antiretroviral therapy. Nurse researchers in general, however, have yet to embrace the incorporation of standardized terminologies into research protocols.

WHAT INFORMATICS COMPETENCIES ARE REQUIRED TO COMPLEMENT THE TECHNOLOGICAL BUILDING BLOCKS OF STANDARDIZED TERMINOLOGIES AND INTEGRATED INFORMATION SYSTEMS?

Technological building blocks such as standardized terminologies and integrated information systems are necessary but not sufficient to realize the promise of utilizing information systems to facilitate the development of nursing knowledge and to link theory, research, and practice. These building blocks must be complemented by informatics competencies. The informatics competencies necessary for knowledge-intensive professions go beyond computer literacy and include the knowledge and skill to use computer-based tools to support:

- Acquisition of various types of data, information, and knowledge
- Organization of data, information, and knowledge
- Critical analysis and synthesis of data, information, and knowledge
- Application of data, information, and knowledge in the clinical decision making and care provision (including evaluation) process (personal communication, Medical Library Association, 1996).

It is essential that such competencies be incorporated into all levels of nursing education programs and into nursing practice to foster both the development and use of nursing knowledge.

SUMMARY

This chapter has described the vital role of standardized terminologies and integrated information systems as building blocks for the development of nursing knowledge. Examples have illustrated the manner in which these building blocks can facilitate the interrelationships among nursing theory, nursing research, and nursing practice. As the building blocks are broadly implemented, new questions will evolve. For example:

- How will definitions of nursing expertise evolve as sources of domain information and knowledge become more accessible at the point of care?
- What are the ways in which interventions built upon standardized terminologies and integrated information systems can and should serve as an extension of the nurse?
- Will standardized terminologies and integrated information systems assist in the delineation of a distinct body of nursing knowledge or will the boundaries of discipline-specific knowledge blur?

REFERENCES

Abbott, P.A., Quirolgico, S., Manchand, R., Canfield, K., & Adya, M. (1998). Can the US Minimum Data Set be used for predicting admissions to acute care facilities? In G. Cesnik, A.T. McCray, & J.-R. Scherrer (Eds.), *Proceedings of MedInfo* (pp. 1318-1321). Seoul, Korea: International Medical Informatics Association.

American Medical Association. (1993). *Physician's current procedural terminology.* Chicago: Author.

American Nurses Association. (1997). *NIDSEC standards and scoring guidelines.* Washington, DC: American Nurses Publishing.

American Nurses Association. (1999). *Recognition criteria for data sets, classification systems, and nomenclatures.* Report of the Committee on Nursing Practice Information Infrastructure. Washington, DC.

Bakken, S., Button, P., Hardiker, N.R., Mead, C.N., Ozbolt, J.G., & Warren, J.J. (1999). On the path toward a reference terminology for nursing concepts. In C.G. Chute (Ed.), *Proceedings of International Medical Informatics Association Working Group 6 Conference on Natural Language and Medical Concept Representation* (pp. 98-123). Phoenix: International Medical Informatics Association.

Brennan, P.F., Caldwell, B., Moore, S.M., Screenath, N., & Jones, J. (1998). Designing HeartCare: Custom computerized home care for patients recovering from CABG surgery. In C.G. Chute (Ed.), *Proceedings of the 1998 AMIA Annual Fall Symposium* (pp. 381-385). Orlando, FL: Hanley & Belfus.

Brown, P.J.B., O'Neil, M., & Price, C. (1998). Semantic definitions of disorders in Version 3 of the Read Codes. *Methods of Information in Medicine, 37*(4-5), 415-419.

Button, P., Androwich, I., Hibben, L., Kern, V., Madden, G., Marek, K., Westra, B., Zingo, C., & Mead, C.N. (1998). Challenges and issues related to implementation of nursing vocabularies in computer-based systems. *Journal of the American Medical Informatics Association, 5,* 332-334.

Campbell, J., Carpenter, P., Sneiderman, C., Cohn, S., Chute, C., & Warren, J. (1997). Phase II evaluation of clinical coding schemes: Completeness, taxonomy, mapping, definitions, and clarity. *Journal of the American Medical Informatics Association, 4*(3), 238-251.

CEN ENV 12264. (1995). *Medical informatics—Categorial structure of systems of concepts—Model for representation of semantics.* Brussels: CEN.

Chang, B.L. (1993). CARIN system: Database for Bayes' theorem applications. *Western Journal of Nursing Research, 15,* 644-648.

Chute, C.G., Cohn, S.P., & Campbell, J.R. (1998). A framework for comprehensive terminology systems in the United States: Development guidelines, criteria for selection, and public policy implications. ANSI Healthcare Informatics Standards Board Vocabulary Working Group and the Computer-based Patient Records Institute Working Group on Codes and Structures. *Journal of the American Medical Informatics Association, 5*(6), 503-510.

Cimino, J.J. (1998). Desiderata for controlled medical vocabularies in the twenty-first century. *Methods of Information in Medicine, 37*(4-5), 394-403.

Cimino, J.J. (2000). From data to knowledge through concept-oriented terminologies. *Journal of the American Medical Informatics Association.*

Cimino, J.J., Elhanan, G., & Zeng, Q. (1997). Supporting infobuttons with terminological knowledge. In D.R. Masys (Ed.), *Proceedings of the AMIA Annual Fall Symposium* (pp. 528-532). Nashville: Hanley & Belfus.

Clark, J., & Lang, N.M. (1992). Nursing's next advance: An international classification for nursing practice. *International Nursing Review, 39,* 109-112.

Detmer, W.M., Barnett, G.O., & Hersh, W.R. (1997). MedWeaver: Integrating decision support, literature searching, and Web exploration using the UMLS Metathesaurus. In D.R. Masys (Ed.), *Proceedings of the AMIA Annual Fall Symposium* (pp. 490-494). Nashville: Hanley & Belfus.

Dick, R.S., & Steen, E.B. (Eds.). (1991). *The Computer-based Patient Record: An essential technology for health care.* Washington, DC: National Academy Press.

Dick, R.S., Steen, E.B., & Detmer, D.E. (Eds.). (1997). *The Computer-based Patient Record: An essential technology for health care.* Washington, DC: National Academy Press.

Goodwin, L., Saville, J., Jasion, B., Turner, B., Prather, J., Dobousek, T., & Egger, S. (1997). A collaborative international nursing informatics research project: Predicting ARDS risk in critically ill patients. In U. Gerdin, M. Tallberg, & P. Wainwright (Eds.), *Proceedings of NI97* (pp. 247-250). Stockholm, Sweden: IOS Press.

Graves, J.R., & Corcoran, S. (1989). The study of nursing informatics. *Image: Journal of Nursing Scholarship, 21,* 227-231.

Griffith, H.M., & Robinson, K.R. (1992). Survey of the degree to which critical care nurses are performing Current Procedural Terminology-coded services. *American Journal of Critical Care, 1,* 91-98.

Grobe, S.J. (1996). The Nursing Intervention Lexicon and Taxonomy: Implications for representing nursing care data in automated records. *Holistic Nursing Practice, 11*(1), 48-63.

Hammond, W.E., & Cimino, J.J. (2000). Standards in medical informatics. In E.H. Shortliffe & L. Perreault (Eds.), *Medical infor-*

matics: Computer applications in medical care and biomedicine. New York: Springer-Verlag.

Henry, S.B., Holzemer, W.L., Randell, C., Hsieh, S.-F., & Miller, T.J. (1997). Comparison of Nursing Interventions Classification and Current Procedural Terminology codes for categorizing nursing activities. *Image, 29*(2), 133-138.

Henry, S.B., Holzemer, W.L., Reilly, C.A., & Campbell, K.E. (1994). Terms used by nurses to describe patient problems: Can SNOMED III represent nursing concepts in the patient record? *Journal of the American Medical Informatics Association, 1,* 61-74.

Henry, S.B., & Mead, C.N. (1997). Nursing classification systems: Necessary but not sufficient for representing "what nurses do" for inclusion in computer-based patient record systems. *Journal of the American Medical Informatics Association, 4*(3), 222-232.

Henry, S.B., Warren, J., Lange, L., & Button, P. (1998). A review of the major nursing vocabularies and the extent to which they meet the characteristics required for implementation in computer-based systems. *Journal of the American Medical Informatics Association, 5*(4), 321-328.

Holzemer, W.L., Henry, S., Portillo, C., & Miramontes, H. (2000). The Client Adherence Profiling-Intervention Tailoring (CAP-IT) intervention for enhancing adherence to HIV/AIDS medications: A pilot study. *Journal of the Association of Nurses in AIDS Care, 11*(1), 36-44.

Huff, S.M., Rocha, R.A., McDonald, C.J., De Moor, G.J.E., Fiers, T., Bidgood, W.D., Jr., Forrey, A.W., Francis, W.G., Tracy, W.R., Leavelle, D., Stalling, F., Griffin, B., Maloney, P., Leland, D., Charles, L., Hutchins, K., & Baeziger, J. (1998). Development of the LOINC (Logical Observation Identifier Names and Codes) Vocabulary. *Journal of the American Medical Informatics Association, 5*(3), 276-292.

Humphreys, B.L., Lindberg, D.A.B., Schoolman, H.M., & Barnett, G.O. (1998). The Unified Medical Language System: An informatics research collaboration. *Journal of the American Medical Informatics Association, 5*(1), 1-11.

International classification of disease—clinical modification, 9th revision. (1992). Salt Lake City: Med-Index.

International Council of Nurses. (1999). *ICNP Update—Beta 1 Version.* Geneva, Switzerland: Author.

International Standards Organization. (1990). *International Standard ISO 1087: Terminology—Vocabulary.* Geneva, Switzerland: Author.

Johnson, M., Maas, M., & Moorhead, S. (Eds.). (2000). *Nursing Outcomes Classification (NOC)* (2nd ed.). St. Louis: Mosby.

Kleinbeck, S.V.M. (1996). In search of perioperative nursing data elements. *AORN Journal, 63*(5), 926-931.

Lange, L. (1996). Representation of everyday clinical nursing language in UMLS and SNOMED. In J.J. Cimino (Ed.), *Proceedings of AMIA Fall Symposium* (pp. 140-144). Washington, DC: Hanley & Belfus.

Lindberg, D.A.B., Humphreys, B.L., & McCray, A.T. (1993). The Unified Medical Language System. *Methods of Information in Medicine, 32,* 282-291.

Martin, K.S., & Scheet, N.J. (1992). *The Omaha System: Applications for community health nursing.* Philadelphia: Saunders.

McCloskey, J.C., & Bulechek, G.M. (2000). *Nursing Interventions Classification* (3rd ed.). St. Louis: Mosby.

Mortensen, R.A. (Ed.). (1999). *ICNP and telematic applications for nurses in Europe: The Telenurse experience* (vol. 61). Amsterdam, Netherlands: IOS Press.

NANDA. (1999). *Nursing diagnoses: Definitions and classification 1999-2000.* Philadelphia: North American Nursing Diagnosis Association.

Ozbolt, J.G. (1996). From minimum data to maximum impact: Using clinical data to strengthen patient care. *Advanced Practice Nursing Quarterly, 1*(4), 62-69.

Ozbolt, J. (2000). Toward a reference terminology model for nursing: The 1999 Nursing Vocabulary Summit Conference. In V. Saba, R. Carr, W. Sermeus, & P. Rocha (Eds.), *Seventh International Congress on Nursing Informatics. One step beyond: The evolution of technology and nursing* (pp. 267-276). Auckland, New Zealand: Adis International.

Parlocha, P.K., & Henry, S.B. (1998). The utility of Georgetown Home Health Classification Systems for coding patient problems and nursing interventions in psychiatric home care. *Computers in Nursing, 16*(1), 45-52.

Prophet, C.M., Dorr, G.G., Gibbs, T.D., & Porcella, A.A. (1997). Implementation of standardized nursing languages (NIC, NOC) in on-line care planning and documentation. In U. Gerdin, M. Tallberg, & P. Wainwright (Eds.), *Proceedings of NI97* (pp. 395-400). Stockholm, Sweden: IOS Press.

Rios, H., Delaney, C., Knuckeberg, T., & Mehmert, P.A. (1991). Validation of defining characteristics of four nursing diagnoses using a computerized database. *Journal of Professional Nursing, 7,* 293-299.

Saba, V.K. (1992). The classification of home health care nursing: Diagnoses and interventions. *Caring Magazine, 11*(3), 50-56.

Spackman, K.A., Campbell, K.E., & Cote, R.A. (1997). SNOMED RT: A Reference Terminology for health care. In D. Masys (Ed.), *Proceedings of AMIA Annual Fall Symposium* (pp. 640-644). Nashville: Hanley & Belfus.

Starren, J., & Johnson, S.B. (2000). An object-oriented taxonomy of medical data presentations. *Journal of the American Medical Informatics Association, 7*(1), 1-137.

Turley, J.P. (1992). A framework for the transition from nursing records to a nursing information system. *Nursing Outlook, 40,* 177-181.

Warner, H.R., Haug, P.J., Lincoln, M., Warner Jr., H.R., Sorenson, D., & Fan, C. (1988). Iliad as an expert consultant to teach differential diagnosis. In R.A. Greenes (Ed.), *Proceedings of Twelfth Symposium on Computer Applications in Medical Care* (pp. 371-376). Washington, DC: IEEE Computer Society Press.

Werley, H.H., & Lang, N.M. (Eds.). (1988). *Identification of the Nursing Minimum Data Set.* New York: Springer.

Zielstorff, R.D., Hudgings, C.I., Grobe, S.J., & The National Commission on Nursing Implementation Project (NCNIP) Task Force on Nursing Information Systems. (1993). *Next-generation nursing information systems: Essential characteristics for nursing practice.* Washington, DC: American Nurses Publishing.

Zingo, C.A. (1997). Strategies and tools for creating a common nursing terminology within a large health maintenance organization. In U. Gerdin, M. Tallberg, & P. Wainwright (Eds.), *Proceedings of NI97* (pp. 27-31). Stockholm, Sweden: IOS Press.

Evidence-Based Practice

A Tool for Clinical and Managerial Decision Making

COLLEEN J. GOODE, MARY KRUGMAN

The evidence-based practice (EBP) movement continues to gain momentum in nursing, medicine, and other health care disciplines. Nurses want to base clinical and managerial decisions on the best currently available evidence to improve outcomes. When nurses subscribe to evidence-based practice, they are upholding a standard where evidence-based decisions, rather than tradition, are the drivers of practice. There is debate regarding what is valid evidence. To understand the EBP movement, nursing must be knowledgeable about its origin and the emerging views on what evidence-based practice entails.

HISTORICAL PERSPECTIVE

Research Utilization

In the mid 1970s, nurses in the United States became involved in a research utilization movement. There was a growing gap between research and practice. Although the importance of basing nursing practice, management, and education on research was discussed in the literature, there was little evidence to document that research was actively incorporated into practice. The need for the conduct of research had been established by the 1970s, but it became obvious that the need for nursing to use research in practice had not been addressed.

The Western Interstate Commission for Higher Education (WICHE) project was the first federally funded research utilization project in the United States (Krueger, 1978; Krueger, Nelson, & Wolanin, 1978). This project linked researcher and clinician to identify a nursing practice problem, retrieve and critique research related to the problem, develop a research-based plan of care, and evaluate the new research-based practice. Rogers' diffusion of innovations theory (1983), Havelock's linkage theory (1972), and Lewin's change theory (1951) provided the theoretical framework for this project. The first research utilization project published in *Nursing Research* was a product of the WICHE project. This landmark publication by Dracup and Breu (1978) used a research-based plan of care to meet the needs of grieving spouses. It is an excellent example of the research utilization process and evaluation of a research-based practice.

The Conduct and Utilization of Research in Nursing (CURN) project, led by principal investigator Dr. Joanne Horsley and director Dr. Joyce Crane, was an innovative project ahead of its time and had the greatest influence on the research utilization movement (Horsley & Crane, 1983). Rogers' diffusion of innovations theory (1983) formed the theoretical basis for this project. Their publication, *Using Research to Improve Nursing Practice: A Guide* (Horsley & Crane, 1983), is still considered the authoritative document on this subject. The CURN project synthesized current research, resulting in 10 research-based nursing protocols that have had a great impact on practice (Michigan Nurses Association, 1981-1982). For example, nurses understand the importance of a closed urinary draining system for prevention of urinary tract infections and they understand the importance of structured preoperative teaching because of the CURN protocols. In addition, the CURN project was the first to identify the correlation between organizational support and the success of implementing research utilization. The project determined that nurses were unlikely to use research in practice if they worked in an organization that placed little or no value on this activity (Horsley, Crane, & Bingle, 1978).

Other research utilization initiatives have continued to build on the work of the WICHE and CURN projects (King, Barnard, & Hoehn, 1981; Rutledge & Donaldson, 1995; Stetler, 1994; and Titler et al., 1994). The Horn Memorial Hospital projects have had a significant influence on research utilization and their educational materials are used by nursing schools and health care facilities nationally and internationally (Goode, Lovett, Hayes, & Butcher, 1987; Goode et al., 1987, 1991).

The research utilization movement had three unique problems. First, the term "research utilization" was a nursing term and other disciplines did not use this term nor understand it. This was problematic, since many practice problems require a multidisciplinary approach. Second, there was inadequate information to guide nurses regarding what type of evidence should be used when there was insufficient research or no research available. Third, the preferences of the patient were not addressed in the research utilization movement. It is possible to have a very strong research-based protocol and documentation of strong positive outcomes from its use. However, if because of cultural, religious, advance directives, or other values or beliefs the patient does not want the protocol carried out, it will not be done. Patient preferences take priority over all evidence.

Evidence-Based Practice

The EBP movement was started in England in the early 1990s. The National Health Service of the United Kingdom asserted that decisions about the provision and delivery of clinical services must be driven by evidence of clinical effectiveness and cost (National Health Service Executive, 1993, 1996). The purpose of the EBP movement in England was to provide clinically effective health care within the resources available (Coyler & Kamath, 1999). The EBP literature is dominated by medicine, to a lesser extent by nursing, and even less by other health care professions (Coyler & Kamath, 1999).

Just as the CURN project was ahead of its time, so was Dr. A. Cochrane, a British epidemiologist, when he published a book in 1972 on effectiveness and efficiency (Cochrane, 1972; Estabrooks, 1998). Twenty-one years later, in 1993, the Cochrane Collaboration was formed. This group works to prepare, maintain, and disseminate systematic research reviews, the evidence needed for health care decision making. The Cochrane library houses the Database of Systematic Reviews and the Database of Abstracts of Reviews of Effectiveness. The Cochrane Collaboration has greatly influenced the inclusion of evidence-based practice in undergraduate and postgraduate education. The Evidence-Based Medicine Working Group (1992) and the Agency for Health Care Policy and Research, which was created legislatively in 1989 to promote quality and effectiveness in health care in the United States, have built on the work of the British and have also influenced the EBP movement.

The evidence-based nursing (EBN) practice movement also began in England. The United Kingdom health care policy is grounded in evidence-based practice, and nurses in the United Kingdom have supported and participated in the development of evidence-based practice. EBN centers have been established in several countries (Ciliska & DiCenso, 1999). The United Kingdom center has been in existence the longest and has been the most productive. Most of the centers focus on developing systematic reviews of the literature for use in evidence-based decision making. The centers also conduct workshops on evidence-based practice. Challenges are faced by these centers, and these include funding sources and the need for coordination across international centers to avoid duplication of activities.

Recent contributions to furthering the development of evidence-based nursing in the United States include a publication by Stetler et al. (1998). This paper provides a definition of evidence-based nursing derived from the definition of the Evidence-Based Medicine Working Group. According to Stetler and her associates, "evidence based nursing de-emphasizes ritual, isolated and unsystematic clinical experiences, ungrounded opinions and traditions as a basis for nursing practices and stresses instead the use of research findings and as appropriate, quality improvement data or other operational and evaluation data, the consensus of recognized experts and affirmed experience to substantial practice" (Stetler et al., 1998, p. 49). Stetler and colleagues emphasize that inherent to evidence-based practice are critical thinking and research utilization competencies (Stetler et al., 1998). In the new *Evidence-Based Nursing Journal,* evidence-based nursing was defined as the incorporation of evidence from research, clinical expertise, and patient preferences into decisions about the health care of individual patients (Mulhall, 1998). Rosswurm and Larrabee (1999) have developed a model to guide nurses and other health care professionals through a systematic process leading to evidence-based practice. The authors describe applications of the model in developing an evidence-based protocol for patients with acute confusion (Rosswurm & Larrabee, 1999).

My colleagues and I (C.G.) at the University of Colorado Hospital have developed the Multidisciplinary Evidence-Based Practice Model (Goode & Piedalue, 1999).

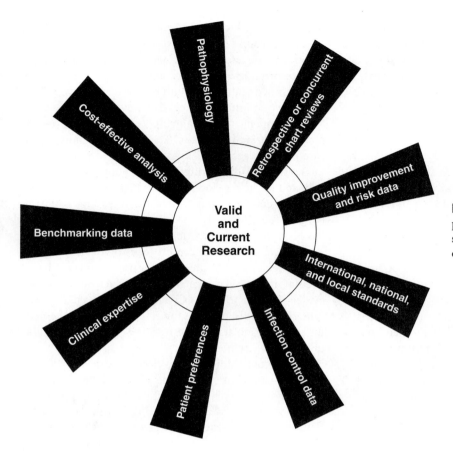

FIGURE 9-1 Evidence-Based Multidisciplinary Practice Model. Copyright University of Colorado Hospital, Denver, Colorado.

This model builds on the concepts of research utilization but includes other sources of evidence besides research (Fig. 9-1). Exploration of the evidence begins in the center or core of the model. All types of research are evaluated for their contributions to the evidence. Results from experimental, nonexperimental, and qualitative studies are synthesized to form the research base. Current, valid research is used as the basis for decision making whenever there is an adequate research base to guide practice. The nine sources of evidence attached to the research core (see Fig. 9-1) can supplement evidence obtained from synthesis of current and valid research. When research is not available to support evidence-based decision making, these sources provide the best available evidence. The selection of evidence sources will depend on the type of evidence-based project under review. For example, an evidence-based cystitis project utilized evidence from cost-effectiveness analysis, pathophysiology data, the patient's record, and infection control data to supplement the evidence from research (Goode et al., 2000). Patient preference has the power to override all other evidence sources. Providers must assure that patients are well in-

formed about the evidence so that they can make informed decisions.

Although initiatives discussed in this paper have focused on evidence-based clinical decision making, the University of Colorado Hospital model can also be used as a tool to guide managerial decision making. For example, a project on evidence-based staffing would include synthesizing current and valid research related to staffing and incorporation of other evidence sources such as benchmarking data, national staffing standards from specialty organizations, and cost-effectiveness analysis. All chief nursing officers should be able to discriminate between a good and bad research synthesis. Directors of finance should be able to locate and critique studies on health service cost-effectiveness (Gray, 1997). Both the Stetler model and the University of Colorado Hospital model contribute to furthering knowledge of evidence-based nursing practice.

WHAT CONSTITUTES EVIDENCE?

Health care providers differ regarding what constitutes "evidence" in evidence-based practice. A summary of the definitions for evidence-based practice that are in the current literature are listed in the box below. All definitions are founded on synthesis of research as the core component of evidence-based practice. Most definitions also include clinical expertise as a valid source of evidence to consider when making decisions. Some definitions strongly support patient preferences, but others do not include this evidence in the decision-making process. Stetler et al. (1998) and Goode and Piedalue (1999) include additional nonresearch sources of evidence that can be used in decision making. The models and definitions of evidence-based practice also differ regarding the type of research that can be utilized as evidence. Sackett, Rosenburg, Gray, Hayes, and Richardson (1996) have a strong emphasis on randomized controlled trials (RCT) and uphold the RCT as the gold standard. Goode and Piedalue (1999) and Stetler et al. (1998) support use of findings from research of varying designs.

FINDING THE EVIDENCE

Finding and evaluating the evidence are key steps to using EBP methods. Nurses unfamiliar with how to search for the appropriate evidence may find this process challenging. Because evidence-based methods build upon expertise nurses have already developed through evaluation of patient care data and exercising clinical decision making, acquiring the skills to carry out evidence-based decision making does not need to be intimidating.

DEFINITIONS

Evidence-Based Medicine
The conscientious, explicit and judicious use of current best evidence in making decisions about the care of individual patients. The practice of evidence based medicine means integrating individual clinical expertise with the best available external clinical evidence from systematic research (Sackett et al., 1996, p. 71).

Evidence-Based Practice, Hong Kong
The systematic interconnecting of scientifically generated evidence with the tacit knowledge of the expert practitioner to achieve a change in a particular practice for the benefit of a well-defined client/patient group (French, 1999, p. 74).

Evidence-Based Working Group
Evidence based medicine de-emphasizes intuition, unsystematic clinical experience, and pathophysiologic rational as sufficient grounds for clinical decision making and stresses the examination of evidence from clinical research (Evidence Based Working Group, 1992, p. 2420).

Evidence-Based Nursing
The incorporation of evidence from research, clinical expertise and patient preferences into decisions about the health care of individual patients (Mulhall, 1998, p. 5). Evidence-based nursing de-emphasizes ritual, isolated and unsystematic clinical experience, ungrounded opinions and traditions as a basis for nursing practices and stresses instead the use of research findings and as appropriate quality improvement data, other operational and evaluation data, the consensus of recognized experts and affirmed experience to substantiate practice (Stetler et al., 1998, p. 49).

Evidence-Based Clinical Practice
An approach to decision making in which the clinician uses the best evidence available in consultation with the patient, to decide upon the option which suits the patient best (Gray, 1997, p. 9).

Model for Clinical Decisions
Three components that bear on the management of patients' problems: clinical expertise, patient preferences for alternative forms of care, and clinical research evidence (Hayes et al., 1996, p. 2).

Multidisciplinary Evidence-Based Practice
Evidence-based practice involves the synthesis of knowledge from research; retrospective or concurrent chart review; quality improvement and risk data; international, national and local standards; infection control data; pathophysiology; cost effectiveness analysis; benchmarking data; patient preferences and clinical expertise and use of this knowledge to make patient care decisions (Goode & Piedalue, 1999).

All evidence is not of the same quality, nor is it necessarily relevant to the patient problem being examined, two important points noted by Gray (1997). Relevance of information is best determined by careful definition of the clinical problem, then by review of the University of Colorado Hospital Evidence-Based Multidisciplinary Practice Model (see Fig. 9-1) to determine the type of evidence that needs to be explored. In the past, nurses used limited sources to find evidence, often referencing only nursing journals and textbooks. Current knowledge searches may require examination of multiple types of data sources, both within the health care institution, such as medical or financial records, or by extensive computer searches. With innovations in telecommunications, distance and access are no longer barriers to a successful evidence search using the World Wide Web.

Searching for the Evidence from Research

When starting an evidence search, one should begin with the research core of the Evidence-Based Multidisciplinary Practice Model (see Fig. 9-1). Two questions should be asked when critiquing research (Gray, 1997): Is the design of the research appropriate for answering the clinical question? and How good is the quality of the research? Whether the relevant research core is within the discipline of nursing, medicine, or a related field, scientific knowledge may be examined by levels of rigor and validity. The gold standard for rigor and validity is generally regarded as research that uses the RCT (Gray, 1997; Guyatt, Sackett, & Cook, 1994; McPheeters & Lohr, 1999). This type of research, however, may not have been conducted on the problem under review, so the nurse must synthesize all types of qualitative and quantitative research available that addresses the clinical problem.

Searching for evidence usually includes the need to become familiar with how to access the major databases for health care literature. While certain sites are consistent over time, it is important to remember how quickly information technology changes. Finding information by searching databases can be complex and time consuming and may involve viewing a high volume of citations and abstracts, which quickly overwhelms the novice searcher. Classes to learn search techniques, as well as self-learning tutorials on the Web such as *A Tutorial* at http://www.lib.berkeley.edu/TeachingLib/guides/internet/findinfo.html are helpful. Web directories, search engines, and megasearch engines can be useful ways to access related databases more easily. Databases may be free, require registration, or require an institu-

tional or individual fee for service. Sources significant to evidence-based practice would include the Cochrane Library, Best Evidence, Sigma Theta Tau's *On-line Journal of Knowledge Synthesis, Evidence Based Nursing* (http://www.evidencebasednursing.com), and *Outcomes Management for Nursing Practice* at www.outcomesmanagement.com, to name a few. Nicoll's (1998) *Nurses' Guide to the Internet* is an additional resource that provides a basic overview of search methods and sources.

Searching for Evidence from Nonresearch Sources

What does a nurse do when there is no core of research to review with a particular patient problem or clinical issue? Lack of substantive research means the nurse refers back to the Evidence-Based Multidisciplinary Practice Model (see Fig. 9-1) to seek other sources of data. Each petal of the model illustrates evidence sources to be explored, and will be outlined with examples to facilitate the evidence-based search process.

Retrospective or Concurrent Patient Record Review

Nurses are familiar with patient record reviews, particularly since many health care institutions require routine audits of care to assure standards have been met. Conducting regular care audits, however, is not as extensive as reviews for evidence-based practice. Successful evidence-based record reviews include conducting a pilot of the audit tool for completeness, having several reviewers audit the same records independently to confirm interrater reliability, and selecting records by standard research methods so that the sample is representative of the clinical problem (Burns & Grove, 1998). The patient record is also a source of evidence for allergies, family history, advance directives, and other evidence that contributes to decision making.

Quality Improvement and Risk Data

Quality and risk data can provide significant information to use as evidence when evaluating a clinical problem. Although all health care institutions collect quality and risk data, not all providers collect the same information or use the same methods for data collection. It is useful to locate key individuals in the facility who are responsible for data for a particular care dimension. These persons may be in specific clinical departments, risk or quality management departments, or in an outcomes office. Relevant questions to ask are, When are the data collected (quarterly, yearly, other)? Who collects it? and What methods are used in the data collection process? These questions can help determine whether the data are reliable and can be used to support evidence-based decision making. Examples of quality or risk data are reports of patient falls, medication errors, restraint use, patient complaints, and case management variance reports.

International, National, and Local Standards

Nursing draws from rich and varied sources for standards of practice. The American Nurses Association Publication Center holds reference material for standards of practice for the profession of nursing, and can be accessed on the Web at www.nursesbooks.org. Specialty nursing organizations such as the American Association of Critical Care Nurses and the Oncology Nursing Society publish standards that can be used in evidence-based decision making. Specific specialty standards can be tracked through the specialty organization's web site. The federal government sponsors the Agency for Healthcare Research and Quality (AHRQ), which provides standards on specific clinical issues and problems for all health-related disciplines. In 1997 this agency established 12 evidence-based practice centers (EPCs) to develop reports and technology assessments on clinical topics such as sleep apnea, traumatic brain injury, and other clinical problems. Standards for pain management, pressure ulcers, and other clinical issues relevant to nurses have also been published by AHRQ. The AHRQ has a web site at http://www.ahrq.gov/, where research activities and publications can be reviewed.

National standards are also in place for provision of care by the Joint Commission on Accreditation of Healthcare Organizations (JCAHO), which surveys hospitals to ensure accreditation standards are met. The ORYX initiative of the JCAHO establishes measures for specific outcomes that trigger reporting and further review by sentinel event guidelines. Examples of these measures include neonatal mortality rates, suicide deaths, and harmful medication errors. The JCAHO Web site provides information on standards and measurement at http://www.jcaho.com. The federal government enforces specific care standards by regulations from the Health Care Finance Administration (HCFA) for those institutions receiving Medicaid and Medicare reimbursements. Information can be reviewed at http://www.hcfa.gov. Standards published by these agencies can be used in evidence-based decision making.

Infection Control

A comprehensive site for accessing evidence related to all dimensions of infection control is the Centers for Disease Control and Prevention, known as the CDC. With Web site access available at http://www.cdc.gov, the latest information on vascular access devices, line care, universal precautions, and data on a variety of clinical and infectious disease problems can be reviewed. Internal institutional infection control data are a critical component of the examination of clinical problems, and can be obtained by contacting the appropriate department. Examples of institutional data collected for the purposes of monitoring patient outcomes are nosocomial pneumonia rate for vented patients, infection rates following cesarean section, and urinary tract infection rates.

Patient Preferences

McPheeters and Lohr (1999) observe that evidence-based nursing practice includes partnering with the patient as an active participant in the decision-making process. Incorporating the patient and family in decision making offers a way to tailor care to meet religious, cultural, and other preferences. Consumers of health care have become more sophisticated about conducting their own searches for best evidence, and advocating for particular interventions or treatments based on these searches. Nurses may be in the position of helping the patient and family to assess the evidence of their own searches. HealthWeb (http://www.healthweb.org), Health on the Net (HON) at http://www.hon.ch, and Ask Jeeves (http://askjeeves.com) are examples of sources for consumer-oriented information. Ethical journals often provide rich sources of evidence related to the impact of patient preferences on outcomes of medical and nursing treatments and interventions.

Clinical Expertise

Clinical expertise is evidence drawn from incorporating knowledge of direct systematic clinical observations and the clinical judgment of the health care provider. Clinical expertise may be highlighted in protocols, pathways, and guidelines for practice, as developed through use of discipline-based literature and consensus of expert clinicians. Case studies, published in professional journals, provide a formal way of sharing clinical expertise. Evidence presented by case studies may serve to stimulate further explorations or serve as a basis for further research to validate more fully the patterns of practice or outcomes, leading to a new way of viewing patient outcomes. A new source of clinical expertise can be found in the various listservers on the World Wide Web. Numerous examples of these lists can be found in nursing, such as listserv@kentvm.kent.edu, a group for nurse researchers; listserv@lists.PSU.edu, for nursing informatics; and listserv@ulkyvm.louisville.edu, for educators. The resources now available for clinical consultations and sharing of expertise expand continuously.

Benchmarking Data

All types of patient-related data, when contributed to institution, national, or specialty organization databases, provide significant evidence regarding disease management, best practices clinically, or internal measures for improvement. National benchmarking data are collected on surgical procedures such as solid organ transplants and cesarean section rates. Benchmarking can be used for infection rates for particular patient conditions and for improvements such as monitoring the use of patient restraints. Often benchmarking data are collected, analyzed, and reported by an office of research or clinical outcomes. Health maintenance organizations also participate in benchmarking, particularly in relation to costs, services, and provider coverage. National benchmarking measurements on desired health prevention outcomes such as Pap smear rates of utilization, immunization, and mammograms, as reported by Health Employer Data Information Set (HEDIS), can contribute to evidence needed for clinical initiatives. University hospitals that belong to the University HealthSystem Consortium (UHC) provide clinical and financial data related to specific diagnoses or treatments for the UHC data bases. Hospitals are able to benchmark against the "best practices" in the UHC databases.

Cost-Effective Analysis

Finding the evidence related to cost has become an essential component of evidence-based practice methods as the costs and expenses of heath care rise and efforts are initiated to contain costs. Cost analysis may range from a simple calculation, such as the cost of a drug when implementing a particular clinical trial, to a complex analysis of the cost benefits of programs related to diabetes patient management. Cost-effective analysis takes into consideration both indirect and direct costs. In addition to evidence related to efficiency and productivity, cost-effective analysis may include episodes of care, numbers of interventions that would do more harm than good when compared with the costs of each, and beneficial versus adverse events (Gray, 1997). Another dimension to cost-effective analysis is the calculation of quality of life (pain, disability, distress) as compared with the number of years of life, examining the psychosocial as well as the medical and fiscal dimensions of outcomes (Gray, 1997). Cost-effective analysis draws upon multiple sources of evidence

to provide sufficient detail to guide direct care decisions, management of populations, and resources related to health care programs and policy decisions.

Pathophysiology

Examining fully the pathophysiology of the patient condition provides insights into management of a disease. Nurses often turn to textbooks when evaluating pathophysiology, a limiting strategy. Searching further for evidence will lead to more up-to-date sources that enrich the plan of care and help guide more informed decisions. Disease-specific Web sites contribute to expanding the nurse's knowledge, such as http://neurguide.com/, which covers all aspects of neurological diseases. The medical record, patient rounds, clinical conferences, and morbidity and mortality conferences also contribute to a more complete understanding of the patient's pathophysiology and how this evidence is used to guide best practices.

SUMMARY

The EBP movement will continue to grow in importance. Nursing *must* be an integral part of this movement. It is still unclear what the best evidence really is. There is disagreement regarding whether all types of research designs can be included in the synthesis of evidence and whether some studies should be weighted more heavily than others in the synthesis. In addition, the value and contribution of nonresearch sources of evidence to evidence-based practice must be evaluated.

Payers and policy makers have become interested in evidence-based practice because of a desire to identify costs that do not result in benefit to the patient, thereby freeing resources for other use (Goode et al., 2000). Evidence-based practice should enhance best practice and eliminate those practices that do not contribute to improved outcomes. Surveys have demonstrated that clinical decisions are often not based on the best evidence (Alspach, 1999; Gibbs, Mead, Hager, & Sweet, 1994; Institute of Medicine, 1992).

EBP frameworks such as those developed at the Baystate Medical Center (Stetler et al., 1998) and at the University of Colorado Hospital (Goode & Piedalue, 1999) must be developed and supported at other hospitals and health care agencies. Organizational support is essential for evidence-based nursing to advance in these environments. In addition, schools of nursing must continue to teach the principles for critiquing and synthesizing research. The research curriculum must expand to include the current knowledge regarding evidence-based practice.

Estabrooks (1999) reminds us that nursing is a practice discipline sanctioned by a society with expectations, and one of these expectations is that we will use the best available evidence with the intent of making outcomes better for our patients.

REFERENCES

Alspach, G. (1999). When the evidence in evidence-based practice is ignored: A time for advocacy. *Critical Care Nurse, 19*(4), 10-14.

Burns, N., & Grove S. (1998). *The Practice of Nursing Research.* Philadelphia: Saunders.

Ciliska, D., & DiCenso, A. (1999). Centres of evidence-based nursing: Directions and challenges. *Evidence-Based Nursing, 2*(4), 102-104.

Cochrane, A.L. (1972). *Effectiveness and efficiency: Random reflections on health services.* London: Nuffield Provincial Hospitals Trust.

Coyler, H., & Kamath, P. (1999). Evidence-based practice: A philosophical and political analysis: Some matters for consideration by professional practitioners. *Journal of Advanced Nursing, 29*(1), 188-193.

Dracup, K.A., & Breu, C.S. (1978). Using nursing research findings to meet the needs of grieving spouses. *Nursing Research, 27*(4), 212-216.

Estabrooks, C.A. (1999). Will evidence-based nursing practice make practice perfect. *Canadian Journal of Nursing Research, 30*(4), 273-294.

Evidence-Based Working Group. (1992). A new approach to teaching the practice of medicine. *Journal of the American Medical Association, 268*, 2420-2425.

French, P. (1999). The development of evidence-based nursing. *Journal of Advanced Nursing, 29*(1), 72-78.

Gibbs, R.S., Mead, P.B., Hager, W.D., & Sweet, R.L. (1994). A survey of practices in infection diseases by obstetricians-gynecologists. *Obstetrics and Gynecology, 83*(4), 631-636.

Goode, C.J., Butcher, L.A., Cipperley, J.A., Ekstrom, J., Gosch, B.A., Hayes, J.E., Lovett, M.K., & Wellendorf, S.A. (1987). Videotape: *Using research in clinical practice.* Ida Grove, IA: Horn Video Productions.

Goode, C.J., Butcher, L.A., Cipperley, J.A., Ekstrom, J., Gosch, B.A., Hayes, J.E., Lovett, M.K., & Wellendorf, S.A. (1991). *Research utilization: A study guide.* Ida Grove, IA: Horn Video Productions.

Goode, C.J., Lovett, M.K., Hayes, J.E., & Butcher, L.A. (1987). Use of research based knowledge in clinical practice. *Journal of Nursing Administration, 17*(12), 11-17.

Goode, C.J., & Piedalue, F. (1999). Evidence-based clinical practice. *Journal of Nursing Administration, 29*(6), 15-21.

Goode, C.J., Tanaka, D.J., Krugman, M., O'Connor, P.A., Bailey, C., Deutchman, M., & Stolpman, N.M. (2000). Outcomes from use of an evidence-based practice guideline. *Nursing Economic$, 18*(4), 202-207.

Gray, J.A.M. (1997). *Evidence based healthcare.* New York: Churchill Livingstone.

Guyatt, G.H., Sackett, D.L., & Cook, D.J. (1994). Users' guides to the medical literature: II. How to use an article about therapy or prevention B. What were the results and will they help me in caring for my patients? Evidence-Based Medicine Working Group. *Journal of the American Medical Association, 271*(1), 59-63.

Havelock, R.G. (1972). *Resource–user linkage and social problem solving.* Ann Arbor, MI: Center for Research on Utilization of Scientific Knowledge, Institute for Social Research.

Hayes, R.B., Sackett, D.L., Gray, J., Muir, A., Cook, D.J., & Guyatt, G.H. (1996). Transferring evidence from research into practice: 1. The role of clinical care research evidence in clinical decisions. *ACP Journal Club, 125*, A-14.

Horsley, J.A., & Crane, J. (1983). *Using research to improve nursing practice: A guide.* New York: Grune & Stratton.

Horsley, J.A., Crane, J., & Bingle, J.D. (1978). Research utilization as an organizational process. *Journal of Nursing Administration, 8*, 4-6.

Institute of Medicine. (1992). *Guidelines for clinical practice from development to use.* Washington, DC: National Academy Press.

King, D., Barnard, K.E., & Hoehn, R. (1981). Disseminating the results of nursing research. *Nursing Outlook, 29*(3), 164-169.

Krueger, J.C. (1978). Utilization of nursing research: The planning process. *Journal of Nursing Administration, 8*(1), 6-9.

Krueger, J.C., Nelson, A.H., & Wolanin, M.O. (1978). *Nursing research: Development, collaboration, and utilization.* Germantown, MD: Aspen.

Lewin, K. (1951). In D. Cartwright (Ed.), *Field theory in social science.* New York: Harper and Brothers.

McPheeters, M., & Lohr, K.N. (1999). Evidence-based practice and nursing: Commentary. *Outcomes Management for Nursing Practice, 3*(3), 99-101.

Michigan Nurses Association. (1981-1982). *Conduct and Utilization of Research in Nursing (CURN) project (DHEW NU00542).* New York: Grune & Stratton. Series of clinical protocols: Clean intermittent catheterization (1982); Closed urinary drainage systems (1981); Distress reduction through sensory preparation (1981); Intravenous cannula change (1981); Mutual goal setting in patient care (1982); Pain: Deliberate nursing interventions (1982); Preoperative sensory preparation to promote recovery (1981); Preventing decubitus ulcers (1981); Reducing diarrhea in tube-fed patients (1981); Structured preoperative teaching (1981).

Mulhall, A. (1998). Nursing, research and the evidence. *Evidence Based Nursing, 1*, 4-6.

National Health Service Executive. (1993). *Improving clinical effectiveness.* Leeds, UK: Author.

National Health Service Executive. (1996). *Promoting clinical effectiveness: A framework for action in and through the NHS.* Leeds, UK: Author.

Nicoll, L. (1998). *Nurses' guide to the Internet.* Philadelphia: Lippincott.

Rogers, E.M. (1983). *Diffusion of innovations* (3rd ed.). New York: Free Press.

Rosswurm, M.A., & Larrabee, J.H. (1999). A model for change to evidence-based practice. *Image: Journal of Nursing Scholarship, 31*(4), 317-322.

Rutledge, D.N., & Donaldson, N.E. (1995). Building an organizational capacity to engage in research utilization. *Journal of Nursing Administration, 25*(10), 12-16.

Sackett, D.L., Rosenburg, W.M.C., Gray, J.A.M., Hayes, R.B., & Richardson, W.S. (1996). Evidence-based medicine: What it is and what it isn't. *British Medical Journal, 312*, 71-72.

Stetler, C.B. (1994). Refinement of the Stetler/Marram model for application of research findings to practice. *Nursing Outlook, 42*(1), 15-25.

Stetler, C.B., Brunell, M., Guiliano, K.K., Morsi, D., Prince, L., & Newell-Stokes, V. (1998). Evidence-based practice and the role of nursing leadership. *Journal of Nursing Administration, 28*(7/8), 45-53.

Titler, M.G., Kleiber, C., Steelman, V., Goode, C.J., Rakel, B., Walker, J.B., Small, S., & Buckwalter, K.C. (1994). Infusing research into practice to promote quality care. *Nursing Research, 43*(5), 307-313.

Benchmarking

A Tool for Management Decision Making

SALIMA MANJI LIN, CAYCE P. TRUONG, CAROLYN SMELTZER, RUTH WILLIAMS-BRINKLEY

The new millennium brings with it empowered consumers who will demand to know more about the treatments proposed for them, their effectiveness, and the track record of the medical team offering the treatments. This will undoubtedly accelerate the demand for the standardization of health processes, despite resistance from some health care professionals and hospitals who have in the past resisted the "grading process." Moreover, governments, health purchasers, providers, and insurers will support standardization because without common platforms and benchmarks, inefficiencies and costs will continue unchecked. Benchmarking not only is an essential source of information for managers in health care organizations but also allows consumers and physicians to make personalized health decisions in a more objective manner without the wide variations that currently exist (PricewaterhouseCoopers, 1999).

STANDARDIZATION + E-BUSINESS = SPEEDY DISSEMINATION OF INFORMATION

The Internet has emerged as a new and important vehicle for accessing health care information. In fact, recent reports in several publications demonstrate that after the physician, the Internet is the second most used source by health consumers. Seventy million of the 97 million Americans who used the Internet in 1999 used it for health advice (Harris Poll, 1999). We expect that these trends will continue to grow in the year 2000. The publishing of "report cards" in health care is also becoming more prevalent on the Internet. Consumers are actively searching for information that will demonstrate to them that one provider, hospital, or health system is "better" than another. As consumers spend an increasing percentage of their disposable incomes on health care, they will become more demanding, expecting "more for less."

This phenomenon of consumerism and e-business is happening while health care costs continue to escalate. Between 1960 and 1997 the percentage of gross domestic product (GDP) spent on health care by 29 members of the Organization for Economic Cooperation and Development (OECD) nearly doubled from 3.9% to 7.6%. The United States spent the most, 13.5% in 1998. The U.S. government projects this percentage will increase to more than 16% by 2010 (Health Care Financing Administration, 1998; PricewaterhouseCoopers, 1999). In addition, medical price inflation still continues to outpace general inflation: 3.5% medical inflation compared with 2.6% general inflation in 1999 (Rate Controls, 1999).

RESPONSE TO CHANGE

The need to standardize processes and achieve a low-cost–high-quality mode of operation is no easy task. Several management tools are available to assist organizations to respond to consumerism, e-business, and standardization. However, as a health care provider, unless you know how you rank in comparison to others in your industry and unless you know how you are improving one year to the next, you may be "fixing the wrong problem." Experience from other industries shows that the most successful organizations have remained leaders through a continual process of changing and adapting to their environments. Expertise in benchmarking is one consistent feature of such leading organizations today. To meet the needs of today's sophisticated and informed health care consumer, radical changes will need to be made by providers. As with leaders in other industries, successful health care organizations increasingly rely on benchmarking to maintain a competitive advantage. Moreover, nurse executives play a critical role in benchmarking, using the results to enhance processes, provide better patient care, and communicate the need for change to top leadership.

BENCHMARKING DEFINED

Benchmarking is a tool used for the achievement of superior performance through continuous improvement. Xerox Corporation, a leader in the field of benchmarking, used the following definition: "Benchmarking is the continuous process of measuring products, services, and practices against the toughest competitors or those companies recognized as industry leaders" (Camp, 1989). Benchmarking involves establishing operating goals based on industry best-practice standards and adopting superior practices to improve one's own operations significantly.

WHAT TO BENCHMARK

It is common for line managers and administrators to view benchmarking only in terms of *performance measures*, and experience with a broad range of our clients has reflected this approach (Camp, 1995). Performance measures offer a snapshot for managers to compare their results with others in the field. However, performance measures do not offer insight into *how* another organization has achieved superior results. Thus, managers are often left with the problem of explaining a "performance gap" that is identified through comparisons of performance measures without an understanding of the *processes* that achieved the superior results. Most experts now believe that the focus of benchmarking should be on business processes, because ultimately it will be the adoption of proven practices and technologies to one's internal operations that will result in increased value to one's customers. However, performance measures are important in identifying superior performers and in estimating the magnitude of improvement necessary once superior practices have been benchmarked.

Why do health care providers typically focus less on processes than on performance measures? Performance measures are generally inexpensive, readily available, and seemingly offer a quick answer to the question, How are we doing? In addition, because providers for many years enjoyed consistent growth in the absence of serious pressures on operating margins and profitability, cost containment and productivity gains were less important than they are today. This resulted in a management orientation on budgets in which planning was done based on past performance, with allowances for inflation and

growth. In an expanding market, an internal focus was effective because any necessary cost reductions were generally minor and were executed through the budget process. Fundamental changes in operating processes were rarely required. While suitable in its day, this approach is no longer desirable because of increased competitive pressures and a volatile health care marketplace. An external focus on customers, competitors, and industry best-practice organizations, including the continual search for superior practices, is now a key to industry leadership.

TYPES OF BENCHMARKING

There are several major categories of benchmarking from which to choose, including internal benchmarking, competitive benchmarking, and functional benchmarking. *Internal benchmarking* involves comparisons among similar operations within one's own organization. With the rapid consolidation of health care providers, especially hospitals, opportunities for benchmarking with members of a system or network are increasingly available. Our experience has also shown that pursuing internal benchmarking within a multihospital health system can also be valuable. A typical example would be a health system that monitors and measures performance levels, such as nursing care hours per patient-day, in similar specialty nursing units across its hospitals over a period of time. The advantage of this method is that the underlying practices that produce the best results over time should be known to the institution. The main disadvantage of this method is that, by definition, its focus is strictly internal.

The next level of analysis, *competitive benchmarking,* assumes an external focus on best-practice competitors. In the hospital industry, it is also common for institutions to include other hospitals that are not considered direct competitors due to geography; this follows from the extensive similarities found among most hospitals throughout the country. Groups of hospitals with similar sizes, services, and patient acuity can be compiled readily from various databases, facilitating comparisons of processes across institutions.

Competitive benchmarking has several advantages over internal benchmarking, the most important of which is that it capitalizes on the significant amount of information available on the processes employed by best-practice organizations that achieve superior levels of quality, service, or productivity. Another benefit is that competitive benchmarking requires an external focus, which reduces the organization's attention on itself and increases its attention on customers. Finally, this tool provides a means to gauge how key competitors fare who use various process and performance standards.

An example of competitive benchmarking with which we are familiar involves an acute-care hospital (hospital A) that was interested in further reducing its costs without sacrificing quality or service. Having been the largest hospital and leading health provider in its local market for several years, the leadership from hospital A decided that its organization needed a comparison base that would better reflect its service mix and size. After selecting a more appropriate list of comparable facilities (expanding outside its local market), an assessment of its current performance suggested that hospital A was operating predominantly at a median level among this selected peer group. A more detailed examination revealed that hospital A's productivity was consistently lower in ancillary services. This prompted hospital A to contact an organization (hospital B) on its selected peer list that was known to have succeeded in significantly standardizing and reducing the utilization of clinical resources in ancillary services, thereby gaining efficiencies and reducing costs. Hospital A has now developed planning steps to implement clinical resource management best practices enjoyed by Hospital B.

Functional benchmarking compares the methods of one's organization with similar processes in other industries. It also offers the greatest potential rewards through the discovery of the best practices that industry has to offer. A classic example in health care is bar coding, which is used extensively to track the flow of patients and information as well as to ensure accurate medical records. Bar coding originated in the grocery industry as a mechanism to improve distribution, inventory tracking, and customer check-out. Another example of functional benchmarking is the use of practices employed by auto racing pit crews to evaluate operating room practices. When viewed from a process perspective, the objectives of pit crews and operating room teams are similar, including minimizing cycle times and effectively managing materials inventories.

These examples illustrate the importance of resisting the "not invented here" mentality that prevails in many organizations. An external focus, combined with a process orientation, provides avenues to performance improvement that would otherwise be unavailable to an organization.

BENCHMARKING PROCESS

The benchmarking process can be divided into four phases (Fig. 10-1), each of which consists of several steps. The *planning* phase involves three key steps: deciding what to benchmark, identifying whom to benchmark, and gathering data and observing best practices. In order to decide what to benchmark, it is important to have identified and prioritized key work processes. In our experience, the prioritization of processes is often enabled through the use of performance measures, which can help to identify areas of weaknesses. Identifying whom to benchmark will first require a decision as to the type of

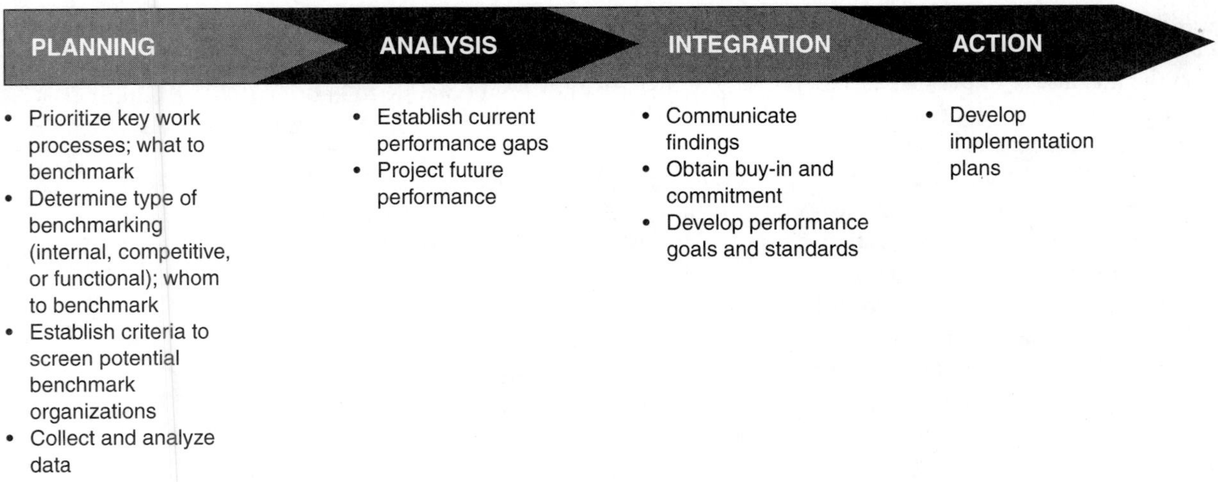

PLANNING	ANALYSIS	INTEGRATION	ACTION
• Prioritize key work processes; what to benchmark • Determine type of benchmarking (internal, competitive, or functional); whom to benchmark • Establish criteria to screen potential benchmark organizations • Collect and analyze data	• Establish current performance gaps • Project future performance	• Communicate findings • Obtain buy-in and commitment • Develop performance goals and standards	• Develop implementation plans

FIGURE 10-1   Benchmarking process.

SAMPLE SCREENING CRITERIA FOR A LARGE ACUTE-CARE HOSPITAL

- >500 beds
- Provide cardiac surgery services
- At least level II trauma center
- Case mix index >1.6
- Distribution of consumer mix
- Urban or suburban location
- Teaching versus nonteaching

---

benchmarking to be done: internal, competitive, or functional. Once this has been accomplished, it may be helpful to establish criteria in order to screen the pool of potential benchmark organizations. These criteria will vary and will be driven by the desired goals and the processes to be benchmarked. Possible criteria for a competitive benchmarking process involving a large acute-care hospital are outlined in the box above.

Gathering data involves a thorough review of relevant literature and on-line databases. In addition, industry associations and watchdog groups, securities analysts, consultants, suppliers, and the benchmark organization itself can serve as important sources of information on benchmark organizations. A proliferation of benchmarking clearinghouses has also been developed in the past few years that provide a range of services and cover a wide range of industries.

The *analysis* phase consists of estimating the current performance gap and projecting future performance. Once benchmarking organizations have been identified and data collected, analysis will help to determine how much better their best practices are than the current internal practices. Further, these data should be used to project the magnitude of performance improvement that would result from the adoption of best practices, as well as the implications for the organization.

The *integration* phase of the benchmarking results involves extensive communication of the findings to all relevant constituencies in the organization. This is a critical step to maximize buy-in and commitment from others. In addition, the findings must be translated into operational statements that describe specifically how internal practices must change in order to adopt the characteristics of best-practice organizations.

Finally, the *action* phase involves the development of detailed implementation plans for the adoption of best practices, including monitoring results and communica-

tion with key stakeholders on a consistent basis. Continual updating of benchmarks should also be done in order to keep pace with industry changes.

PERFORMANCE MEASURES

In our experience, most hospitals typically benchmark specific performance measures against other hospitals. The data needed to perform such comparisons are readily available from a number of vendors, consultants, and publicly available sources.

Performance measures can be oriented to costs, quality, or service. Historically, most benchmarking in hospitals has been done on the basis of productivity in an effort to monitor expenses. Regional and national databases to facilitate comparisons of quality and service have only recently become available; however, as consumers demand that hospitals be compared on the basis of medical care and service quality, hospitals will be evaluated increasingly against these criteria.

Most performance measures that track productivity have an input and output component. Typical inputs and outputs used in a hospital environment are provided in the box below. These inputs and outputs can be combined in a variety of ways to create performance measures used by administrators, nurse executives, and other patient care executives. Examples include salary cost per full-time equivalent (FTE), worked hours per patient-day, and total expense per discharge.

Performance measures are of great importance to leadership for two reasons. First, they provide a mechanism to evaluate the ongoing operations of an organization over time. For a manager with a broad scope of responsibility, performance measures are an efficient means

---

COMMON PERFORMANCE MEASURES IN ACUTE CARE HOSPITALS

Inputs
- Average length of stay
- Total worked hours
- Total expense
- Total salary costs
- Total supply costs

Outputs
- Full-time equivalent
- Patient-day
- Discharge

---

for tracking performance at a macro level across functions. Performance measures also provide executives with the ability to compare their organizations against others in the industry. This type of competitive benchmarking is widespread, especially in the environment of increased competition and increasing use of the Internet, which allows such comparisons to be readily accessible by the empowered consumer. However, external benchmarking based solely on performance measures is not always straightforward and usually leaves important questions unanswered.

When comparing productivity measures across institutions, both external and internal consistency are of great importance. From an external perspective, relevant comparisons require that both inputs and outputs be measured consistently in all institutions included in the benchmarking. One common issue involves the grouping of input data (e.g., salary dollars, worked hours, supply costs), which is often done by department. Due to organizational and operational differences between hospitals, the consistency of departmental groupings for inputs can vary significantly, thus affecting any resulting comparisons.

From an internal perspective, productivity measures should be consistent with the objectives of the organization and the needs of customers. For example, measuring productivity by tracking FTEs per patient-day may not be consistent with the drivers of success in some markets. In markets with a high percentage of per-case reimbursement, the organization should be focused on providing the most cost-effective care per case. In such cases, discharges may be a more appropriate output unit than patient-days. In markets in which per-diem reimbursement predominates, patient-days may be an important indicator; however, expenses are likely to be more relevant than FTEs. Customers are less concerned with a hospital's number of FTEs than with its costs. Further, while FTEs are an indicator of costs, they can be misleading. In reengineering their patient care operations, some of our clients have reduced labor expenses significantly while increasing the number of FTEs. An increasing number of hospitals are now examining productivity on an expense per discharge basis for these reasons.

In summary, hospital-specific performance measures are an extremely important tool for managing day-to-day operations. They are also valuable in identifying suitable partners to benchmark in the hospital industry. However, performance measures do not provide information on how best-practice institutions achieve superior performance. In order to understand how superior results are achieved by others and how one's own organization can

benefit from this knowledge, competitive and functional benchmarking must be done based on *processes*.

PATIENT CARE PROCESSES

Benchmarking processes provide insight into the practices of organizations that have achieved superior results and provide an excellent foundation for subsequent operations improvement and reengineering initiatives (see box, below). Our experience has shown that many hospitals desire to benchmark processes with other hospitals because of the similar nature of their operations. While perhaps limiting in terms of breakthrough potential, this type of benchmarking can offer significant potential yield along the dimensions of cost, quality, and service. One such process is the administration or provision of medications to patients. When examining the medication administration process, it is important to benchmark not only the cost of the medication itself, but also the steps involved from order inception (prescription) through procurement and administration or provision of the drug to the patient. This entire process most often occurs across at least two or more functional operating units

---

**SAMPLE PATIENT CARE PROCESSES:
ILLNESS MANAGEMENT**

Diagnosis and Treatment
Order entry
Order processing
Scheduling
Patient preparation
Treatment, medication, procedure administration
Test results reporting
Documentation

Operative Procedures
Preoperative preparation
Surgery
Postoperative care
Follow-up clinic appointment

Customer Service
Patient processing
   Admission
   Discharge
Room preparation and maintenance
Meal distribution
Pastoral care
Social work

KEY REMINDERS TO ENSURE SUCCESSFUL BENCHMARKING

1. Benchmarking is an activity that provides guidance and direction but it is not the answer. The data that are used are not perfect and, therefore, it is essential to determine what confidence level the organization is willing to accept to move forward. The higher the associated risk with a given decision, the greater the level of confidence required in the validity of the information.
2. Communicate to your staff the importance of benchmarking and how the results will be used; lack of understanding can lead to fear and an unwillingness to use the results to improve performance.
3. Ensure that the benchmarks used are relevant to organizational objectives. Benchmarking for the sake of benchmarking provides little value.
4. Go the extra step to ensure that the benchmarks used match up well with internal data; otherwise you will end up with an "apples to oranges" comparison.
5. Benchmark departments using the most applicable performance measure for the specific department, e.g., for a med/surg unit, worked hours per patient-day; for laboratory, consider worked hours per billed test.
6. In order to maximize the outcome of the benchmarking process, both external and internal data must be examined. There are various levels of aggregation and types of health care information available to leadership.
7. Before the results of benchmarking are converted into departmental targets, validation of data and benchmarks with departmental leaders is critical to their acceptance.
8. Use benchmark results to develop performance measurement indicators for ongoing monitoring and evaluation of future performance.

---

within the organization (patient care unit and pharmacy); therefore, it is essential that each step is examined and that improvements are made to the entire process, rather than just to the steps that occur in either functional unit. The gains in cost, quality, and service to customers (patients and others) are usually more significant when the boundaries of the process are defined and the work-steps evaluated across functional groups.

While benchmarking is not yet used in many health care organizations, patient care executives have begun to recognize its value within and across industries. As the health care market continues its pace of rapid change, process benchmarking will be an important tool to achieve superior performance and stay ahead of the competition.

SUMMARY

Benchmarking is one of the most important tools available to health care leadership to provide information for management decision making. In comparison to the 1990s when benchmarking was used primarily by providers to compare their performance to best practices, the start of the millennium signals an environment in which health care organizations need to communicate

their performance scorecards or "grades" to sophisticated and informed consumers. Benchmarking takes on a more prominent role as the Internet continues to be an increasingly important channel for consumers to compare and "shop" for the most efficient, consumer-friendly provider. The box above lists key reminders for organizations who decide to use benchmarking for management decision making. Among the industry leaders, benchmarking is becoming part of the organizational culture to achieve superior long-term performance. It is an ongoing process, part of the continual search for excellence.

REFERENCES

Camp, R. (1989). *Benchmarking: The search for industry best practices that lead to superior performance.* White Plains, NY: Quality Resources.

Camp, R. (1995). *Business process benchmarking: Finding and implementing best practices.* Milwaukee: ASQC Quality Press.

Harris Poll. (1999, August 5). Trends & timelines—online health: Number of users continues to grow.

Health Care Financing Administration. (1998). *National Health Expenditures: 1998 Highlights.* Washington, DC: U.S. Government Printing Office.

PricewaterhouseCoopers. (1999, November). *HealthCast 2010. Smaller world, bigger expectations.*

Rate Controls. (1999, November 30). *Health Economic Indices, 23*(11), 5.

CHAPTER 11

Use of Distance Technology for Education, Practice, and Research

JOAN E. PREDKO

As we enter a new millennium, we are just beginning to experience the effect that distance technologies or telecommunications will have on the delivery of health care and education. Sophisticated telecommunications equipment has enabled health care providers, educators, and researchers not only to view but also to interact with patients, students, and subjects located at distant sites.

Imagine yourself as an advanced practice nurse employed by a large, international, nurse-managed health center with its office in San Francisco, California. The phone rings in your home office located in Chicago, Illinois. One of your clients is calling from his home in Miami, Florida, and complains of sore throat, unproductive cough, shortness of breath, and earache. You immediately bring up his electronic health care record on your computer while instructing him to turn on his home two-way interactive video system. You are now able to control a remote camera and to receive data from an array of telemetric instruments including a thermometer, otoscope, ophthalmoscope, and stethoscope. Your client can also see you on his home monitor, and you instruct him on how to position these devices to collect and electronically send you the appropriate images and textual data. As he does this, you read the client's health history and note several complicating factors; you call up an on-line expert decision support program. It suggests checking on epidemiological data that are available on line from Florida health department databases. You can, if needed, connect with other members of your cyber health team and together formulate a diagnosis and treatment plan. On the basis of the data you have collected so far, you decide that a chest x-ray, streptococcus screen, complete blood count (CBC), and arterial blood gases are needed and, using a universal locator program, direct your client to the nearest electronic health care testing facility. Test results are made available within an hour of the client's visit. You are

sent a special alert e-mail message, and the results are transmitted directly into the patient's electronic record.

While you wait, you enter into your on-line continuing education plan that you have registered with several educational institutions and nursing organizations and note that several options have been added. You have been looking for an on-line course on advanced pharmacology for primary care practitioners, and you note that one offered by an accredited university has been found. You check out their course preview site and decide to enroll. You realize that this is the same virtual university from which your husband is completing his on-line doctoral degree using your home-based electronic study room. As you begin to ponder the growing extinction of residential universities, a news message flashes on your monitor alerting you to the results of a new study showing serious interactions of two commonly prescribed drugs. After reading the full on-line report of the study, you determine that a meeting of the cyber team is necessary and set up an on-line video meeting for later in the day to which you have invited the principal investigator of the study as well as the cyber team's clinical pharmacologist. Although this scenario is fictitious, many parts of it are being played out in multiple pilot programs around the country. Distance technology has changed and will continue to change the delivery of health care and education.

This chapter focuses on the use of distance technologies or telecommunications in nursing education, practice, and research within a broad health care framework. Remembering that the prefix "tele" means distant, it is easy to see why the following terms have entered the health care arena: telenursing, telemedicine, telepsychiatry, teleradiology, teleresearch, and telecourses. These are only a few of the terms that have been coined to represent use of technology to delivery a service that is not bound by geographical constraints. The more encompassing term *telehealth* represents the use of telecommunication devices to deliver any aspect of health care, including education, regardless of geographical location or physical limitations. Telehealth can enable us to reach people with limited or no current access to educational and health care services. It can help to eliminate the health care gap that separates the city from the rural community and developed nations from undeveloped countries.

The most successful telehealth systems employ a variety of telecommunication modalities including two-way interactive video consultations, teleradiology, and telepathology that link primary care providers in rural areas or inner-city clinics to experts in large, tertiary centers. Virtual environments for health care delivery and education have been made possible by the same advances in technology that have given us lifelike, computerized video games and military robotic medics. Virtual classrooms are here, and virtual hospitals, clinics, and operating rooms are soon to follow. It is primarily the cost that holds us back; perhaps appropriately, since virtual reality is not always the best or most cost-effective application. Consider the complexity of computer programming that is necessary to construct a three-dimensional virtual reality to simulate one clinical decision-making scenario and contrast that with the low cost and reality of actual role playing of the same scenario. The challenge in telehealth lies in maintaining or improving quality while containing costs and improving access. The use of telecommunications in each of the three areas (distance education, health care delivery, and research) will now be addressed.

DISTANCE EDUCATION

Distance education, commonly defined as education provided to students who are separated from the instructor by either time or distance, is not new. Consider the fact that correspondence courses by mail have been available since 1840, when Sir Isaac Pitman, the English inventor of shorthand, came up with the idea of delivering instruction by mail (Phillips, 1998). What *is* new is the variety of synchronous and asynchronous technologies available to deliver the education, including radio, television, audiotapes, videotapes, audioconferencing, desktop videoconferencing, room-based two-way interactive videoconferencing, satellite broadcasts, electronic mail, facsimiles, computer media (CD-ROM), and the World Wide Web. Most distance education programs now utilize a combination of audio, video, and computer technology, with the most common technologies being two-way interactive video and the Web (U.S. Human Resources and Ser-

vices Administration, Office of Advancement for Telehealth, 1999).

Some believe that all education in the future will be delivered via distance learning, as expressed by Peter Drucker, nationally renowned management consultant: "Thirty years from now the big university campuses will be relics. . . . The college won't survive as a residential institution" (cited in Lenzer & Johnson, 1997). Others believe that there are economic, demographic, and pedagogical principles (what we know about how people learn) that will ensure the survival of traditional educational institutions (Neal, 1999). Perhaps the more relevant question is not whether traditional residential campuses will perish, but how the expanding distance education market will influence them.

Joseph Coates (1996), futurist, offers these key questions:

- Should future growth in universities be more "bricks and mortar" or in telecommunication?
- Will on-campus classes be only for social purposes and for hands-on laboratories that cannot be virtualized?
- Will there be top teams of educational experts in the country teaching everyone via distance education versus every college and university teaching the same content?
- Will educational institutions cooperate and collaborate to maximize learning for students?

Additionally, Michael Moore (2000) has asked these important questions related specifically to the impact on faculty:

- When the majority of faculty become engaged in online teaching, what will be the impact on their other responsibilities such as research, service, and teaching in residential programs?
- Will new faculty be hired to do residential teaching or will this be done by adjunct faculty or perhaps graduate assistants?
- Will distance education courses replace residential courses?
- Will only a few "star" faculty take on content development and ownership roles while the majority of faculty will be supporting facilitators of that content?

It is critical that nursing engage in a debate over the answers to these questions and become involved in the decisions that will determine the future direction of higher education. There is evidence that this has begun.

The American Association of Colleges of Nursing (AACN) convened the Task Force on Distance Technology and Nursing Education, which published a white paper outlining the issues schools face when developing distance education programs and offering some recommendations (AACN, 1999). The task force members identified the potential benefits of distance technology in nursing education, which included improving the quality and access to nursing education and increased collaboration among nursing faculties in teaching, research, and practice. This white paper also identified multiple issues to be addressed in order to fully utilize technology to realize those benefits. These issues included limits on financial aid for distant students, accreditation and quality assurance for distance programs, high costs for the development of technology infrastructure, need for faculty development and student supports, limited research on the quality, cost, and efficiency of distance education programs in nursing, and legal and ethical concerns related to intellectual property, copyright, and confidentiality. The National Center for Education Statistics (U.S. Department of Education, NCES, 1999) identified some additional policy issues emerging from the support and adoption of distance education: equity of access, changes and challenges facing the role of faculty, and pressures on existing organizational structures and arrangements.

The use of technology to deliver distance learning is changing how we think of educational institutions and learning communities. In a keynote address at a multimedia conference in 1996, Diane Skiba, nursing educator and leader, summarized thoughts on our transformation from the industrial to the information age and its effect on education in this way. She felt that we are moving from:

- a teaching franchise to a learning franchise
- provider-driven to individualized learning
- teacher-focused to student-focused, e.g., from semester courses to skill sets
- time out for education to "just-in-time" education
- continuing education to perpetual learning, i.e., K-12 to K-80
- teachers as "sages on the stage" to "guides on the side"
- technology push to a learning vision pull (Skiba, 1996)

Dr. Skiba has outlined a learning vision that has been adopted by many but not all. Why might that be? Let's consider the benefits and challenges related to distance education.

Benefits of distance education to the student include increased access to higher education especially for non-traditional students, flexible scheduling of personal time, convenient location, individualized attention, less travel, and increased time to think about and respond via e-mail to questions posed by the instructor or other students. Benefits to the institution offering distance education include increased enrollment, reduced need for campus buildings, attraction of new teaching staff interested in distance education, and enhanced image of an institution perceived to be forward-thinking and technologically advanced (Matthews, 1999).

Disadvantages of distance education include high cost of course development and technology infrastructure, increased workload of faculty because it is more labor intensive to teach an on-line or interactive video class, need for ongoing staff development in the use of technology, equipment failures especially when there is limited infrastructure, need for electronic libraries, difficulty in facilitating interaction among students, decreased spontaneity, possible fraud in authenticating submission of materials, legal issues of intellectual property rights, and restrictions on financial aid available for distance learners. If these disadvantages were considered barriers, would eliminating these barriers produce successful distance education programs? There is one very important factor that needs to be considered before that question can be addressed: Are distance education programs effective?

The proverbial question of effectiveness always comes into play when new teaching strategies are implemented. The gold standard of educational quality has been the outcomes achieved with traditional classroom teaching. The results of 248 studies reviewed by T.L. Russell (1999) conducted from 1928 to 1997 demonstrate no significant differences in learning outcomes of students taught by traditional classroom methods versus distance education methods. However, greater precision in outcome measurement (most studies use course grades) is needed to determine differences in teaching methods. If one considers the true gold standard for teaching effectiveness to be one-to-one tutoring (Bloom, 1984), then use of multiple media via the Web could offer this type of individualized learning. It is possible to design a course on the Web so that each student would interact with different Web pages and assignments based on results of a pretest, an assessment of learning style preferences, and ongoing monitoring. Further study may indeed show that distance education methods are superior to traditional face-to-face classroom methods. I have had the opportunity to witness faculty using more active learning strategies in their face-to-face classrooms after first using them in the delivery of distance education classes.

Now, back to the question of producing successful distance education programs. Rather than focusing only on eliminating barriers, it is strongly suggested that a broader, more systematic approach to producing quality outcomes be used. Criteria for implementing and evaluating effective distance education programs are available from several sources including Michigan State University (1996), the Western Cooperative for Education Telecommunication Project (1999), Penn State University (1999), and the AACN White Paper (1999). In addition, lessons learned from 8 years of experience in planning, implementing, and evaluating distance teleeducation programs in nursing prompt me to offer these recommendations:

- "Custom-oriented" library and advising services for distant learners are essential.
- Adequate technical support both on and off campus is critical.
- Always have plan B when technology fails.
- Have high expectations for students and faculty; orientation is the key.
- Ensure high levels of interactivity between faculty and students and among students.
- Continuously monitor teaching and technology and make needed changes often.
- Keep focused on the instructional design and meeting student learning needs; use technology as a tool rather than allowing learning to be driven by technology.
- Provide ongoing training, support, and rewards for faculty.
- Assign a "point person" to manage the outreach efforts and keep the team focused.

Literature on distance education in nursing is growing rapidly. Billings and Bachmeier (1994) in a review of the literature on distance education in nursing from 1966 to 1992 found only 69 articles written over the 26-year period. In comparison, my search of these same databases for only a 2-year period from 1998 to 2000 located 98 articles. Many of these 98 articles focused on use of the Web for delivering the education. This is not surprising since a 1997-1998 survey by the National Center for Education Statistics (NCES) found that the Internet has become the medium of choice for most of the 1,600+ higher education institutions providing distance education (U.S. Department of Education, National Center for Education Statistics, 1999).

Currently, nursing supports and views distance education in a positive way, perhaps because it is being seen as the panacea for a number of problems, for example, an increasing national nursing shortage (practitioners and faculty), a maldistribution of health care resources in rural settings, a need for nurses to practice in underserved areas, an ever increasing need for continuing and "just-in-time" professional education in this "Information Age," and a need for increased collaboration among nursing faculties in teaching, practice, and research because of constrained resources.

USE OF DISTANCE TECHNOLOGY IN PRACTICE

Rapid changes in technological development and innovation have come at an opportune time to provide us with a set of tools for dealing with a dynamic, increasingly complex health care scene. Telecommunications has presented potential solutions to the problems of access and delivery of health care to underserved areas in rural United States and in developing countries worldwide as well as efficient delivery of professional continuing education to widely dispersed and isolated health care practitioners.

> Imagine a world where no matter who you are or where you are, you get the health care you need when you need it. A world where people living in far-flung areas need not travel hundreds of miles to get specialty care that could save their lives? A world where you will be treated in an emergency room by a nurse at your side and a physician at a distant emergency department? A world where doctors and nurses in rural America can learn about new medical practices at the touch of a computer key? (U.S. Human Resources and Services Administration, Office of Advancement for Telehealth [OAT], 1999)

These words, found on the Web site of the Office of Advancement for Telehealth (OAT), portray the "real" world for some of us, but not all of us.

Although the technologies such as videoconferencing, the Internet, store-and-forward imaging, streaming audio and video, and satellite and wireless communications already exist for use in telehealth, they are not yet readily available for our nation's rural and urban underserved peoples. "In fact, the health care industry itself lags behind other industries such as finance, insurance and education which have already integrated information systems into their daily routines. Health care analysts believe that health care is at least ten to fifteen years behind in computing" (U.S. Human Resources and Services Administration, OAT, 1999). Since its inception in May of 1998, OAT continues to focus on improving the "digital divide" between the "haves" and "have nots" in telehealth and to serve as a catalyst for the wider adoption of advanced technologies in the provision of health care services and education. In 1998 in 29 states, OAT administered 41 tele-health-telemedicine grants totaling more than $13.6 million. Approximately $5 million will be available to fund 12 to 15 new awards for fiscal year 2000. In 1999 the U.S. Human Resources and Services Administration's Bureau of Health Professions in collaboration with the OAT announced a 5-year $4 million demonstration project to help rural registered nurses earn a bachelor's degree in nursing using distance learning technologies. It is important to note that nursing is well represented in the OAT with Carole Gassert, PhD, RN, as the senior advisor for distance learning methodologies and Cathy Wasem, MN, RN, as the director of telehealth/telemedicine programs and evaluation.

As depicted in the opening scenario of this chapter, interactive home telehealth is here and growing. With the miniaturization of sophisticated health self-monitoring devices and the increasingly low cost of interactive technologies, it is likely that the home will replace providers' offices as the primary entry point into much of the health care system. Personal monitoring devices are being developed to assist in the prevention of disease through everyday use by large numbers of people. A monitor in the bathroom shower that scans for signs of melanoma, a wristwatch-like device that constantly checks pulse, respiration, and temperature, computerized eyeglasses that jog a failing memory with whispered cues, and a "smart bandage" that senses a developing infection and identifies the antibiotic needed are only some of the devices being explored by the University of Rochester's Center for Future Health (Rickey, 1999-2000). Advanced digital and compression techniques are making it possible to store vast amounts of medical information (data, voice, still images, and motion-video) on smaller and smaller chips. Electronic patient records on a card the size of a credit card can support continuity of care while assuring security, privacy, and confidentiality. Technology can bring all types of services to individuals, rather than the individual to the services. Access to services such as banking, shopping, employment, and social activities from home via the Internet and wireless videophones can support independent living for the older and disabled populations. The potential for and actual implementation of these telehealth services will clearly influence the what, when, where, and how of health care delivery as well as the education of health care professionals and clinical research agendas.

What prevents us from using the innovative telehealth technologies that will increase access and improve quality of health care services? Loeb and Puskin (1999) identified several economic, social, and technical barriers:

1. Reimbursement mechanisms do not currently support telehealth services. Medicare, the largest single third-party payer, provides limited reimbursement for tele-consultation services but no payment for telehome care services.
2. Lack of communication standards for medical devices prevents the expansion of telehealth technologies. Health care devices that do not work together or are not easily upgraded frustrate health care professionals. These care providers are reluctant to make large-scale investments in technologies today that will become outdated systems tomorrow.
3. Lack of affordable or reliable telehealth telecommunication services in some rural and inner-city communities limits access to the infrastructure necessary to support sophisticated telehealth technologies.
4. Insufficient broad-based education about home and self-care technologies and their effective utilization hinder acceptance.
5. State regulatory requirements and licensure for health care professionals currently inhibit cross-border delivery of consultative services. Within the United States, nurses and physicians are licensed within the state in which they practice. If they wish to practice in more than one state, they must receive a separate license for each state in which they practice. There is disagreement whether health care professionals need to be licensed in the state in which they reside or in the state in which the patient resides. One could assume patients are being transported electronically from their state to the consulting professional (the view of the American Telemedicine Association) or that the professional is being transported to the patient's state (the view taken by the Federation of State Medical Boards). The National Council of State Boards of Nursing (NCSBN) recommends a hybrid tool for licensure using a format similar to a driver's license, a component of mutual recognition (NCSBN, 1997). A more in-depth discussion of multistate licensure in nursing, including the mutual recognition model, can be found in the May 31, 1999, issue of the *Online Journal of Issues in Nursing* at http://www.nursingworld.org/ojin/topic9/tpc9intr.htm. Nursing is to be praised for recognizing the need to evaluate the current regulatory model that has been in place for nearly 100 years. If this licensure issue is not resolved at the state level, it invites the

federal government to consider federal licensure relative to interstate commerce regulation.

As these barriers are overcome, we can anticipate that technology will enable consumers to access a wide range of health care services from the home and that health care will move to a proactive, preventative consumer-driven model rather than the reactive, episodic, provider-driven model utilized today (Loeb & Puskin, 1999). Considering the nursing profession's focus on health promotion and disease prevention, nurses will be uniquely positioned to provide the leadership needed in this new health care delivery scene. Will we be ready?

Just as we have benefited from having guidelines to promote quality distance learning, we will benefit from guidelines for promoting quality telenursing. The American Nurses Association has produced two documents related to telehealth: The *Core Principles on Telehealth* (ANA, 1999) and *Competencies for Telehealth Technologies in Nursing* (ANA, 1999). The *Core Principles on Telehealth,* a report of the interdisciplinary telehealth standards working group, was endorsed by the ANA in 1998. It identified 12 core principles that can guide health care professionals as they determine their needs for policy development in telehealth. It was primarily written to protect clients receiving telehealth and to guard against policies being established only on the basis of commercial marketing interests. *Competencies for Telehealth Technologies in Nursing,* endorsed by the ANA in 1999, recommends 11 competencies for registered nurses using telehealth in nursing practice; it resulted from a collaboration among the ANA and specialty nursing organizations. These documents are useful guides for both practitioners and educators.

RESEARCH AND TELECOMMUNICATIONS

There are vast repositories of raw data that are more accessible to researchers because of telecommunication advances. Data warehousing and data mining are terms frequently used by researchers today. Data warehouses are for storing data, while data mining turns data into information. It is a process for discovering patterns and trends in large data sets to find useful decision-making information. These data can be analyzed and transformed into knowledge and then disseminated so that they can be used for decision making in health care planning and delivery. Computerized data entry and decision support programs have also presented a possible solution to the increasing errors in health care delivery. The electronic medical or health record is here and poses ethical dilemmas of confidentiality and privacy, as well as how best to capture and code patient and nursing data. Almost any data, e.g., medical imaging, videos of consultations, and text materials can be digitized for storage, organization, and retrieval. Comparison and analysis of universal patient records allow identification of trends and therapeutic interventions. Not only are there large data sets available, but researchers now can use telecommunications (especially the Internet and videoconferencing) to solicit subjects and collect data for their own studies. The Internet has created a global community of scholars with instant access to one another's expertise and research. Nurses can access instantly and on demand the latest research and diagnostic data from national databases and other Internet sources. Considering the fact that anyone can publish almost anything on the Web, one of our greatest challenges lies in evaluating the sources so as to attain reliable and trustworthy data.

Use of distance technologies in education and practice raises many questions in need of further research. Only a few will be listed here as samples of what is needed. Are there paradigm shifts in education and nursing practice based on the increasing use of the Internet and other telecommunications by consumers and health care professionals? How are the roles of teachers and students changed by distance education? What mix of technologies is best for which types of learning? What are the characteristics of successful, effective distant learners and teachers? What effect have copyright and intellectual property issues had on development of on-line courses? What strategies are effective in dealing with identified ethical and legal issues in distance education and telehealth? How much interaction or teacher immediacy (defined as behaviors that enhance physical and psychological closeness) is most effective and how is it achieved in distance education? How is the role of the nurse changing? Will skills such as decision making, patient education, therapeutic communication, and case management become as definitive to what a nurse does as the traditional hands-on care? Endless patient data are available and can create information overload, so which types of data are important for clinical decision making and are worth monitoring? Are there effective information systems and decision support systems to help nurses sift through the mountains of data available? Which clinical nursing services are appropriately and effectively delivered via telehealth systems versus in person? How do telehealth technologies influence the structure of the health care system and especially the delivery of nursing care (positive and negative)? How can we assure equitable distribution of home care technology? What are the economic, social, policy, and other barriers that continually emerge as the technologies in telehealth and distance education change?

Whether we are educators, clinicians, or researchers, we must take advantage of every opportunity to increase our knowledge and skills in the current and potential use of distance technologies. As we continue to share best practices and accumulate results of needed research, we will discover new paradigms and solutions for problems where telecommunications are the best tool. Policy development, regulatory reform, and legislation will certainly influence the outcome of telecommunication technologies in nursing practice, education, and research now and in the future. It is critical that nurses be involved in directing and shaping this policy and reform. The greatest technology is worthless if we are not committed to its use and willing to put forth the extra effort to make it work. On the other hand, we must be careful that technology and innovation do not become the driving forces for the delivery of education and nursing practice. Distance technologies are tools that extend our skills and help us solve problems and improve the quality and cost-effectiveness of what we do.

Nursing has come a long way since 1997 when McCloskey and Grace asked, "This is the computer age, will nursing be a part of it?" (McCloskey & Grace, 1997). Today we can answer that we not only are a *part* of it but also are the emerging leaders in the use of distance technology for education, practice, and research in health care!

REFERENCES

American Association of Colleges of Nursing. (1999). AACN White Paper: Distance technology in nursing education. Washington, DC: American Association of Colleges of Nursing. Available: http://www.aacn.nche.edu/publications/positions/whitepaper.htm.

American Nurses Association. (1999). *Core principles on telehealth.* Washington, DC: American Nurses Publishing.

American Nurses Association. (1999). *Competencies for telehealth technologies in nursing.* Washington, DC: American Nurses Publishing.

Billings, D.M., & Bachmeier, B. (1994). Teaching and learning at a distance: A review of the nursing literature. In L.R. Allen (Ed.), *Review of research in nursing education* (vol. VI, pp. 1-32). New York: National League for Nursing.

Bloom, B.S. (1984). The 2-sigma problem: The search for methods of group instruction as effective as one-to-one tutoring. *Educational Researcher, 13*(6), 4-16.

Coates, J. (1996, March). *Technology revolution: Possibilities and perils for higher education.* Keynote presentation at the annual meeting of the National University Continuing Education Association (NUCEA), Boston.

Lenzner, R., & Johnson, S.S. (1997, March 10). Seeing things as they really are. *Forbes* [Online]. Available: http://www.forbes.com/forbes/97/0310/5905122a.htm.

Loeb, J., & Puskin, D. (1999, April). *Interactive "home" telehealth: Future technologies and services.* Topical report of workshop on homecare technologies for the 21st century sponsored by Catholic University of America and Food and Drug Administration. [Online]. Available: http://www.hctr.be.cua.edu/HCTWorkshop/HCTr_A.htm.

Matthews, D. (1999). The origins of distance education and its use in the United States. *T.H.E. Journal, 27*(2), 54-67.

McCloskey, J.C., & Grace, H.K. (Eds.). (1997). *Current issues in nursing* (5th ed.). St. Louis: Mosby.

Michigan State University. (1996). *Points of distinction: A guidebook for planning and evaluating quality outreach.* [Online]. Available: http://www.msu.edu/unit/outreach/pubs/pod.pdf.

Moore, M. (2000). Editorial on technology-driven change: Where does it leave the faculty? *The American Journal of Distance Education, 14*(1), 1-6.

National Council of State Boards of Nursing. (1997, August). *Boards of nursing adopt Mutual Recognition Model.* [Online] Available: http://www.ncsbn.org/search/documents/accufacts/newsreleases/nr970825.asp.

Neal, E. (1999). Distance education—prospects and problems. *National Forum: The Phi Kappa Phi Journal, 79*(1), 40-43.

Penn State University. (1999). [Online]. Available: http://www.cde.psu.edu/DE/IDE/guiding_principles/.

Phillips, V. (1998). Virtual classroom, real education. *Nation's Business, 86*(5), 41-44.

Rickey, T. (1999-2000, Winter). Memory glasses, wristwatch monitors, and smart socks . . . here's to your health. *Rochester Review,* pp. 21-23.

Russell, T.L. (1999). *The "no significant difference" phenomenon, a comparative research annotated bibliography on technology for distance education.* Raleigh, NC: Office of Instructional Telecommunications, North Carolina State University. Available: http://cuda.teleeducation.nb.ca/nosignificantdifferences/.

Skiba, D. (1996, November). *A virtual academic village: A framework for the future.* Keynote presentation at a conference sponsored by FITNE on Discover Multimedia: Using Interactive Technology to Further Nursing and Healthcare Education, Philadelphia.

U.S. Human Resources and Services Administration, Office of Advancement for Telehealth. (1999). *Telehealth update.* [Online]. Available: http://telehealth.hrsa.gov/pubs/future.htm.

U.S. Department of Education, National Center for Education Statistics. (1999). *Distance education at postsecondary education institutions: 1997-98,* NCES 2000-013. Report prepared by Lewis, L., Snow, K., Farris, E., & Levin, D. Washington, DC: U.S. Government Printing Office. Available at http://nces.ed.gov.

Western Cooperative for Education Telecommunication Project. (1999). [Online]. Available: http://www.wiche.edu/telecom/projects/balancing/principles.htm.

Electronic Information Exchange in the Year 2010

JOANN M. ELAND

A DAY IN THE ELECTRONIC LIFE OF A NURSE ACADEMICIAN

The current generations of technical tools are finally making academic life more manageable. Early electronic mail services with only text and primitive file attachments were expanded several years ago and now include a number of useful additions including voice input and the ability to include a number of different types of file attachments. Instead of endless hours of time-consuming typing, e-mail content is either spoken directly into a microphone or typed by the computer or sent as an audio or video file attachment using a small video camera attached directly to the computer. When face-to-face communication is necessary but not physically possible, the same video camera allows video communication over thousands of miles using the Internet. Video communication is not the same as face-to-face communication, but it also does not incur the expense or difficulty associated with travel. A faculty workday begins by logging on to a computer that uses a security system that identifies the user by a scan of the retinal vessels of the eye. With the implementation of retinal scans, the electronic world is far more secure than it has ever been.

RESULTS OF A LITERATURE SEARCH

Every night the search engine software on the computer explores the international nursing and medical indexes searching for the particular keywords specified in query statements. When the search engine finds a match to the keywords, it retrieves the abstract and bibliographical information and places this information in a designated mailbox on the faculty member's computer. With the click of the mouse the software can request a full copy of an article from the publisher that will be delivered to the user's computer mailbox with a $3.00 charge billed to an electronic account. The same retrieval software will also index and store the electronic copy on the hard drive, which makes future use of it far easier than using primitive paper filing systems.

Publishers prefer electronic publishing because electronic publications are less expensive to produce, save time and valuable resources, and reach a larger market. The ability to sell individual articles has greatly increased revenue because these articles are reaching more readers via a worldwide market. Traditional paper journal subscriptions are becoming more uncommon, are costly, and arrive months out of date and thus will soon be a thing of the past because users cannot afford to purchase them. Most faculty members continue to subscribe only to specialty journals and retrieve additional references as needed. Publishers offer the added service of providing previous years' journals with their subscription rates, making article retrieval effortless.

There currently are discussions within the publishing industry that would sell on-line services on a fee-for-usage basis. For example, for $20 a month a subscriber could have unlimited access to the search engine and download 20 articles at no additional cost. If the need was greater than those 20 articles, the user could subscribe for a higher level of service. Universities are particularly interested in such services because of the escalating costs of maintaining their library collections and resources.

AN ARTICLE ACCEPTED FOR PUBLICATION

When an author finishes a manuscript for publication, it is posted on a protected area of the publisher's World Wide Web site for review. Each of the reviewers and the editor place their comments directly on the manuscript and can see each other's comments. Authors make the necessary changes, incorporating suggestions, and resubmit the manuscript electronically to the Web site, where it will be internationally indexed and made available through the publisher's Web site within 24 hours of submission. The volume of important work that the discipline of nursing is generating can finally be shared with colleagues around the world in a brief time, and the electronic indexes will allow newly published works to be accessed as quickly as they are published. It is hard to imagine that the discipline ever advanced when it took publishers 2 years to put accepted works into print and then were able to make them available to only a small number of the persons who would benefit from the knowledge.

The advent of hyperlinks within the text and bibliography of articles also has revolutionized the way scholars work. Hyperlinks are words that are linked to other words, x-rays, photographs, and audio or video files. With the click of a mouse the reader is shown on screen whatever the link is referencing. For scholars new to the field it is an opportunity to click hyperlinked text and have the *primary source* appear before their eyes. Never has scholarship been so media rich, enabling, and relevant. Historical nursing references include audio files such as the voice of Florence Nightingale and video files of many great nursing leaders including, for example, Jessie Scott! The same hypertext has a large number of photographs that further enhance the learning experience. This type of reference makes history come alive and gives a far better sense of the people and the time than words on paper ever did.

Another colleague is finishing an article on a new treatment for chronic wound healing. Annotations for the article include photographs and video clips to show *exactly* what wound characteristics justified the treatment tested in her research, as well as photographs of wound conditions for which the treatment was inappropriate. In a field of study such as wound healing, in which visual clues direct treatment alternatives, it seems archaic to suggest that such content could effectively be communicated in any other way.

INTERNET RESEARCH OPPORTUNITIES

Most cable television services have World Wide Web access as a part of their basic service, which has created an entirely new pool of research subjects. With Web-based data collection forms, it has never been easier to do this type of nursing research. Data entered into the forms are placed into a database and exported effortlessly for analysis by statistical packages. The use of the Web has had a tremendous impact on increasing sample size and diversity of the respondents and has also proved particularly helpful in acquiring larger samples from small populations of subjects such as children with cancer.

Because the data are easily exported and analyzed, researchers can analyze data during the data collection period and make necessary sample or design modifications. A colleague who is involved in an experimental design investigating a treatment protocol for neonatal pain recently made a design modification based upon an analysis of 270 subjects of a target sample of 1,500 infants. He reduced his three-group design to a two-group design because one of the experimental treatments was extremely significant in the reduction of mortality and morbidity in the sample and the other treatment arm was making no difference whatsoever. Because his data were essentially being entered into his statistical program, he could confirm his suspicion that one of his treatments was simply ineffective and was having a significant negative impact on the lives of the children in this group.

FEDERAL GRANT REVIEWS

Grants submitted for review are now completed on line, and Web cameras are used for discussion and funding determinations. Grants are distributed electronically, and reviews by the primary and secondary reviewers are posted on line by the granting agency for other members of the review panel to read. After reading the primary and secondary reviews, all members of the panel rate the proposals and participate in an on-line conference to set funding priorities. Each reviewer sees the face of every other reviewer in small windows on his or her individual computer screen. The result of reviewing grants in this manner has literally saved tons of paper, postage, travel moneys, and reviewer time.

GUEST LECTURES

Guest lectures are delivered from the office of the presenter to students around the world. A Web-based camera is used to broadcast the guest lecture to students in the class as well as to students enrolled in the course anywhere in the world via the Web. Members of the class and the professor see the face of any student who asks a question because each lecture seat is equipped with a Web camera.

Before the class, students will be involved in an on-line discussion on the topic of pain in neonates. A two-page position paper on the use of morphine around the clock for all premature infants admitted to neonatal intensive care unit will be posted on the Web for student reaction. All students in the class will be required to respond either to the position or to comments posted by other students from the class. The student responses will be summarized, and then all students will be required to write one additional response.

Students in the class will have a list of required and optional reading for the guest lecture that are all Web based and hyperlinked to other references of interest. This is a particularly useful strategy for student learning because an individual learner can easily obtain required resources 24 hours a day, 7 days a week, learn on her or his own schedule, and not be bound by conventional timelines or geographic location. Many students enrolled as distance learners live literally hundreds of miles from a health science library, and completion of the readings would virtually be impossible without electronic communication.

PROGRAM OF STUDY

Students are now able to pick and choose courses from any university in the world. Graduate students are the most frequent subscribers to the international courses because of the variety of course offerings and the ability to study with specific leaders in the field. Because the number of on-line students is limited, competition for enrollment is intense, which makes the learning environment particularly rich and diverse. A variety of teaching and learning strategies had to be developed to accommodate such a large number of learners and ensure the quality of the course work. On-line discussion of topics, group projects facilitated by the Web, bulletin boards, audio and video streaming of lectures, on-line texts and articles, and live Web camera interactions with professors had to be further developed for these strategies to provide this exceptional educational experience.

OFFICE SCHEDULE

Face-to-face meetings are still held, but when faculty members are out of town, they attend via Web camera. A laptop computer communicates to those assembled from wherever the faculty member chooses because fast Ethernet and light-based connections are as common as telephones were 10 years ago. No one minds an electronic presence on a computer screen because the input into a meeting is so critical; using technology to facilitate discussion is only a minor inconvenience.

MANUSCRIPT

In the electronic mail is a manuscript being coauthored with a Japanese colleague on children with cancer pain and their experiences with caregivers. The manuscript will compare and contrast the cultural differences in the two societies, and several photographs and video clips will be part of the published manuscript. Readers will be able to see the faces of the parents discussing this important topic and will not have to rely on words on a printed page for their impressions. Selection of what clips to use is an important part of the editing work because the instructions for authors from the journal request that there be no more than 30 minutes of video submitted for publication. Inclusion of media-rich content once again greatly enhances publication.

TEACHING RESPONSIBILITIES

A typical teaching schedule has students in two sections, including one on campus and a distance learner section. How to maintain the quality of the offerings for individuals at distant sites was once a challenge, but on-line, media-rich libraries and the newer methods of faculty and student communication have greatly eased faculty concerns. Some students attend class at the time it is delivered while others view the content using Web-based video at a time convenient for them. Originally only audio and electronic presentation software such as Power Point were used, but with the improvements in the speed of transmission it is now much easier to use video. What students like most about this type of learning is that it is available when they are available to explore the content. Many students still come to class, but if their work schedule does not permit it, if there is a snow storm, or if one of their children needs to see an advance practice nurse, they can still get the course content over the Web. As opposed to 10 years ago, the number of traditional lectures has been greatly reduced and the learners themselves are given more control over their learning.

The nature of student assignments has changed dramatically with the integration of technology. Students in the course for nursing management of the patient with pain are responsible for the maintenance of 5,000 pages on the Web related to pain management. Course assignments include updating information, addition of new information, and answering the patient's, family's, and health professional's questions on pain management. Students use a variety of on-line references to answer the questions and, when the question is too complex, refer to graduate teaching assistants or to the instructor. Because the Web site is an international resource, the assignments provide purpose and meaning for the students completing the course. Course work is not simply a course project for a grade but rather a contribution to the discipline. Participating in this course is an intense nursing-based activity, and students are required to have completed the introduction to on-line communication course before enrolling. The on-line communication course provides them with the technical tools of how to work with on-line projects, how to search the information available, and the communication skills required for the electronic age. Because all assignments are electronic, where a student resides is of no consequence.

The on-line discussions in the course are particularly interesting because of the contributions of the distance learners. The Midwest is pretty much a cultural, homogeneous melting pot, but the international students add a dimension to the course that would be unattainable by any other means. Last week nurses from Italy requested information about the use of the analgesic tramadol in epidural catheters for children. One of the students from Children's Hospital in Boston was familiar with the epidural administration of the drug, but no one else from the United States had experience with it. The ensuing discussion was a lively one that ranged from discussion of changes in practice to the fact that many innovations are started in Europe because the restrictions on research are often less stringent. In the previous week an on-line discussion focused on allowing children at the end of their lives to die in their homes. In general the consensus of the student body was that children should be allowed to die at home if it was humanly possible; however, a student in Japan countered that "death" in the home would be culturally inappropriate in Japanese society.

STUDENT TEXTBOOKS

Instead of traditional nursing textbooks, students subscribe to on-line service based on hours used per month for current media-rich references. Their on-line "texts" are full of photographs and audio and video clips and are hyperlinked to related topics. A traditional pediatric textbook explains a respiratory condition known as croup as characterized by respiratory difficulty, substernal retractions, and a "seal-like" barking sound. The current on-line Web-based resource uses the same words to describe the illness but features a video clip of the child with respiratory difficulty and substernal retractions, provides an x-ray, and allows the learner to hear the unmistakable sound of that "seal-like" barking sound. There is little question that the latter teaching tool would have a greater chance of remaining in a student's memory.

Because they are Web based, texts are available anywhere; this might be a student's home, the workplace, a hospital bedside, a client's home, or a coffee shop. On-line texts have revolutionized learning and make it available when the learner needs it, and thus learning is no longer a function of where a 10-pound "media-poor" textbook might be physically located.

VIDEO CLIPS AND SKILL ACQUISITION

Although the use of video and audio clips is useful in research-based activities, they are absolutely essential in practice-based articles and in teaching students new psychomotor skills. Students can play Web-based video clips over and over until they understand the content. There is no escaping the need to practice skills using the actual equipment in learning laboratories, but students now have access to video clips *where* they need them to learn or reinforce essential content. Such learning is particularly useful for novice learners for whom it may literally be weeks or months between learning the skill in the laboratory and completing it in the clinical setting. For the experienced nurse, clips are helpful when skills or equipment are used infrequently and a refresher is needed to ensure consistency and client safety. The use of video clips has made delivery of home care services far easier and safer because home care nurses can also pull up a clip of instructions on a treatment, a psychomotor skill, or a communication from another caregiver. Families use video clips to reinforce cares they provide including intravenous infusions, epidural catheters, or care of venous access devices. It is hard to believe that families were once expected to correctly and safely complete complex care activities with little more than one or two live demonstrations.

OFFICE HOURS

On-line office hours become a particularly interesting challenge when students live in multiple time zones around the world. Professors have found that e-mail and on-line bulletin boards answer many student questions. Using bulletin boards has drastically reduced the volume of e-mail, and what e-mail is generated is easier to reply to using the microphone to verbally answer student questions.

CONSULTATION

A traditional text-based electronic mail message from a hospice nurse anticipates the failure of an analgesic regimen and requests ideas for future implementation. The hospice nurse had begun her day by checking electronic communication that included both text and video from hospice clients, other nurses, and physicians. On a given morning messages may include routine questions such as ones surrounding physician visits or they may contain information that a crisis has occurred that requires immediate attention. Because of the placement of Web cameras in patient homes, a hospice nurse can check in with clients who have left messages. Those who are stable and doing well may only need a quick Web camera check-in, whereas others may need immediate intervention. The use of Web cameras has conquered time and distance by negating the need of getting in one's car, a bus, or the subway to travel to another location.

All hospice patients and their families are offered the opportunity to be connected to each other via an on-line caring network. The work of caring for those who are so ill remains physically and emotionally difficult, and establishment of the caregiver network has greatly eased the emotional toll such work encompasses. Family members involved in caring for hospice patients communicate fears, joys, mutual concerns, and caring to others who are involved in the same phase of life. The support these individuals generate for each other is inspiring, and many remain a part of the hospice family for a year or two after their loved one has passed away. It keeps them connected to others with similar life experiences and losses and, in my opinion, is one of the best things about this electronic age. Interestingly enough there is also a nurse caregiver on-line network as well, where hospice nurses routinely communicate with each other about the issues, cares, and concerns about being hospice nurses.

SUMMARY

Internet-based electronic information resources have revolutionized the science of nursing by virtue of the variety of the types of media resources available and the ability to access them 24 hours a day, 7 days a week. Traditional universities have truly become universities without walls, and the community of students taking advantage of this unique system of learning is spread around the world. The teaching and learning experiences of professors and students have become international in scope, and the learning environment is far from traditional.

Section Three

Changing Education

Nursing Education in Transition

JOANNE McCLOSKEY DOCHTERMAN, HELEN KENNEDY GRACE

As massive changes are occurring in the health care delivery system, nursing education must adjust to this changing environment and prepare nurses equipped to face a whole new set of challenges. Much of the history of nursing education has been tied to the need to prepare nurses to practice in hospital settings. Nurses within hospitals substituted for the family, who in earlier times had cared for the patient in home settings. Historically, preparation of nurses in diploma schools of nursing provided a ready workforce for hospitals. When this source of cheap labor "dried up" and the need for nurses to staff hospitals increased following World War II, the associate degree nursing programs provided in two-year programs continued the trend of supplying nurses to staff hospitals. This need to produce more nurses to meet the ever increasing demand has served to fuel the ongoing debate within the nursing profession regarding appropriate preparation for entry to practice. While nursing educators have engaged in this heated internal debate and have made various attempts to move basic nursing education to the baccalaureate level, other professions such as medicine have increasingly changed their focus from entry issues to those of graduate and postgraduate education. Entrance to the field of medicine is the starting point for a lifelong process of learning and maintaining professional competence. As we enter the 21st century it appears that the preoccupation of nursing educators with entry to practice is finally dissipating and shifting to a similar perspective. Preparing nurses for the changing context of practice, with ever increasing care being provided in community settings, continuing professional education to update knowledge as it develops, development of career pathways within nursing, and providing culturally competent care to an increasingly diversified population are some of the issues addressed in this section.

In the opening debate chapter, Camilleri takes a historical look at nursing and nursing education and contrasts the conflicting perspectives of nursing as a craft versus nursing as a profession. The context of hospital-based nursing has valued nursing as a craft and perceived nursing as a profession as a threat to those who exert control over the health care system. Camilleri notes that "Nursing has spawned both a strong craft culture and a strong professional culture" and that knowledge of these cultural values is important in unlocking the hold that these value systems have on the field. Dealing with the ambiguities of the future will require creative problem solving that transcends the limitations of both cultures and a more negotiable blend of elements from each of the cultures. Trends affecting nursing include increase in knowledge, use of technology, increased interdependency of the world, and finite resources. Concluding this chapter Camilleri poses a series of challenges that must be addressed by nursing education: (1) lifelong learning and mobility of the learner, (2) accessibility of education to students of all ages and ethnic backgrounds, (3) acceptance of licensure as an RN as the entrance to practice relying on continuing professional development for the professional registered nurses (PRNs), and (4) increased interdisciplinary collaboration. She challenges nursing to remain open to a diversity of ideas about nursing and to continue to engage other health care stakeholders to bring about the highest level of care most effectively.

In the first viewpoint chapter, Miller explores issues in the education of nurses that have emerged as a result of the rapidly changing methods of education. Technological advances resulting in the increased use of computer technology have made distance education—education that occurs when the student and the teacher are not in the same physical location—possible. Miller goes on to describe a wide array of teaching methods that utilize computer technology. Approaches to assuring clinical competence of nurses include objective structured clinical examinations, use of simulators, and creation of virtual reality experiences.

Expanding the scope to an international perspective, Lewis provides an extensive overview of varying approaches to international education. International students studying in U.S. universities constitute a substantial percentage of the students seeking graduate degrees. Increasingly, U.S. academic institutions are seeking to provide a broader worldview to students through study abroad programs integrated into their programs of study. While there is this increased flow of students across international boundaries the current approaches have their limitations. International students are encouraged to fit into the programs of study that have been developed from the predominant U.S. perspective with limited concern for applicability in the context from which the students have come. Study abroad programs for U.S. students are limited in terms of their in-depth exposure to another culture. As an alternative to these approaches, Lewis advocates development of an alternative approach, a truly international program. There is an urgent need to prepare nursing leaders worldwide that could be met through an integrated model for graduate nursing education. This international nursing educational program would bring together students of many nations, including those from the United States in a shared program brought together through the appropriate use of educational technology and use of an international faculty to mentor students.

Turning to the need to broaden the clinical component of nursing education, Tagliareni and Mengel address the development of interactive and contemporary curriculum models in basic nursing education. "The need is for faculty in basic nursing education to find reward and fulfillment by being with students in emerging environments of care." To do so requires moving away from traditional patterns of nursing education that focus on *what* rather than on *how* to teach and from *content* to the *process* of learning. The shift in care from acute care hospital settings to community-based practice requires a fundamental shift in focus and methodology. Faculty must join with students in a whole new world of discovery. Calling for a common ground for education and practice, the authors advocate multiple exit points (associate, baccalaureate, master's, and doctoral degrees) and a focus on population-based local health needs in a community-based health care system. The change in focus from institutions to communities requires that the issues of diversity in community settings be addressed and that a concerted effort be made to increase the diversity of the student body accordingly.

Continuing in a similar vein, Rothert and Talarczyk address the need to broaden clinical education in ad-

vanced practice nursing (APN) graduate programs. The rapidly changing health care system and the changing demographics of the population with the increased percentage of elderly and minorities have profound implications. To meet the challenges of the future, nurses must be prepared to be collaborators in practice and to participate in decision making relevant not only to practice issues but also to the context of care, particularly its business aspects. To prepare APNs for the world of practice their curricula should include experiences related to health care finance, management, and policy. Sites for clinical education should be collaborative, and clinical education should not only prepare nurses to be expert clinicians but to make appropriate use of technology as a part of practice. For nurses to be full participants in the health care system of the future, they must benchmark their practice and validate the outcomes, costs, and benefits of their interventions.

At all levels of nursing education the future requires increased attention to critical thinking. Rubenfeld and Scheffer report on their work in clarifying the concept, its critical elements, and the implications of critical thinking to altering approaches to curriculum design and process. Based on seven skills integral to critical thinking, as defined by an international panel of nursing experts, the authors suggest ways in which learning experiences can be designed to hone these skills. Use of critical thinking skills as an organizing framework would allow students to acquire knowledge in a different manner than the traditional approach of teaching content. The future requires a nurse able to draw on an ever increasing body of knowledge and use her critical thinking abilities to seek the best ways of applying this knowledge and her thinking abilities to the care of patients.

Continuing the theme of lifelong learning, Muhl describes a statewide approach developed in Wisconsin, in which all baccalaureate nursing programs contribute to making nursing education readily available to nurses in their home settings. Her description of the way in which the curriculum has been developed and the way in which collaboration has been built among institutions provides a positive example of nursing education adjusting to the changing world in which we live.

This section provides an interesting and exciting window on far-reaching shifts in nursing education that are long overdue. The themes are amazingly consistent and provide positive hope for an exciting future for nursing education.

The Century Ahead

Old Traditions and New Challenges for Nursing Education

DOROTHY D. CAMILLERI

Wherever a heterogeneous group of nurses gathers and the discussion turns to how nurses should be educated, the dialogue is likely to be spirited, with definite and opposing positions advanced. The differences of opinion among nurses, be they educators or clinicians across the broad spectrum of today's nursing positions, is both a strength and a weakness for our profession. These differences of opinion about educational patterns are hardly surprising, however, given the diversity of types and levels of practice covered by the designation "nursing" and the different paths that lead to becoming credentialed for that practice.

OUR DIVERSE PATHS: TO A GARDEN OR A WEED PATCH?

This chapter focuses on nursing and nursing education as they have developed in the United States. In the United States, nurses constitute the largest single division of health care providers and as a division are themselves quite segmented. In 1996, over two and a half million people held the registered nurse (RN) license, the credential that legally qualifies a person for the practice of professional nursing. Just over 2 million of these nurses were practicing as RNs (Health Resource and Services Administration, Division of Nursing, Notes from the National Sample Survey of Registered Nurses, March 1996.) During the first half of the 20th century most people qualifying for licensure were graduates of 3-year hospital diploma programs. Patterns have changed markedly, and today the majority of people meeting requirements graduate from 2-year associate degree programs. A growing minority graduates from generic baccalaureate programs, and a sharply shrinking minority from 3-year hospital

diploma programs. And as it becomes more commonplace to regard the baccalaureate as the minimum requirement for true professional practice, many diploma and associate degree graduates return to school to complete baccalaureate degrees. Taking 1996 student enrollments in nursing as an indication of the trends, just over 122,000 were in associate degree programs, just over 103,000 were in generic baccalaureate programs, over 12,500 were in diploma programs, and just over 48,000 licensed practical or registered nurses were in baccalaureate programs (NLN, 1997).

To further complicate matters, an additional small group of people with non-nursing degrees are entering nursing and qualifying for RN licensure through generic master's programs or even professional doctoral programs. In 1998 there were twelve generic master's programs and three professional nursing doctoral programs (Berlin & Bednash, 1999).

Nurses with the basic preparation outlined earlier are sandwiched between two additional levels of nursing staff to be found on the health care scene. On the one side are the growing numbers of nurses with graduate education who are in advanced practice roles such as nurse midwives, nurse anesthetists, administrative nurses, and nurse practitioners and clinical specialists in a variety of clinical areas. These roles are becoming more numerous and have always entailed some specialized training for the nurse to be publicly recognized as a specialist. In more recent years, a graduate degree (master's or doctoral) is the common requirement as well as certification for the role by the specialized professional nursing organization.

On the other side are licensed practical or vocational nurses, whose scope of practice is legally defined but more limited than that of the RN. In addition, most health care settings categorize all individuals in assistive roles as nursing staff. These individuals and their roles are variable, ranging from certified nurses' aides (who have some training) to relatively untrained assistive workers. The common denominator for this particular side of the sandwich is that all the work falls under the direction and supervision of the registered nurse staff. Given the many positions classified under nursing, it is possible for a patient in a health care setting to report having talked to a nurse and mean anyone from a nurse's aide to an advanced practice nurse.

The path shown in the box below is considered confusing by most and does resemble an untended foot path in a weed patch more than a cultivated garden walk. Many nurses are troubled by it. On the issue of basic licensure for professional practice, for instance, many critics argue that the wide range of educational programs at different educational levels, all purporting to prepare for professional practice, simply defies credibility. How is it possible for such different programs to produce the same ends? Some critics contend that our discipline is undermined by the claims to professional practice made by this wide array of programs. They believe that the profusion of educational backgrounds as well as the differences in roles make it highly improbable that other professionals and the public will take us seriously.

Other commentators acknowledge the educational inconsistencies but advise a more tolerant attitude about them. This group reminds us that the RN credential is a

legality with limited meaning. It is a political matter of legislation in each of the 50 states and should not be taken as evidence of equality among programs or of true professional practice. In other words, passing the examination and meeting other standards for licensure ensures a minimum standard of safe practice; it does not discriminate between higher and lower levels of ability, professionalism, or the quality of the nurse's practice.

On balance, it seems futile to bemoan the lack of one precise meaning for the term *nurse* or our profusion of titles and educational paths. This is not because there is no confusion; there *is* confusion. It is because they represent the reality of our development, the breadth of nursing roles, and the different ways that nurses are contributing to our nation's health care enterprise. We would do better to consider the factors that account for how we have evolved in concert with social circumstances and to profit from our past in order to maximize our ability to contribute in the future. There is no doubt that nursing roles and educational practices will continue to evolve, as well as health care and society in general. To choose wisely the best directions to take in nursing education during the next century, we would do well to identify some of the important traditions in our past and to examine the different ways in which nursing is connected to and influenced by the society in which it is developing. This type of assessment provides a vantage point for predicting the challenges that will shape both nursing education and health care in the century just beginning.

This chapter forwards such assessment by first looking to our past practice to identify two of the most potent traditions or cultures that have flourished, showing their fit into the larger social context of the times. It then turns to some of the challenges that can be expected in the years ahead. Some ideas about the implications of these challenges are elaborated, with differing points of view presented on a number of unresolved topics. The discussion is limited to the period of the development of modern nursing (roughly the post-Nightingale era). Although the focus of the chapter is on nursing in the United States, we trace our heritage to Nightingale and so need to take into account the forerunning developments as they occurred in Great Britain during that period.

DISCORDANT TRADITIONS

Historically, the story of modern nursing is closely tied to the story of women, with some subplots related to social class, economics, and gender. Trends or themes at odds with one another could always be identified as the story

---

EDUCATIONAL PATHS IN NURSING

Assistive Roles
Vocational school programs for licensed practical nurses
On the job training for certified nurse's assistants and
  other assistive workers

Registered Nurse Roles
Prelicensure
  Diploma
  Associate degree
  Generic baccalaureate
  Generic master's
  Professional doctorate
Postlicensure
  Baccalaureate for RNs

Advanced Practice Roles
Master's degrees in a clinical or other specialty
Doctoral degrees with emphasis on research

played out in Great Britain and the United States, and the updated version of these opposing trends sometimes seems clearly responsible for our current differences of opinion on educational practice.

The Experiment in Great Britain

Most of us are familiar in broad outline, if not in detail, with the Nightingale Fund Nursing School program. This program staffed a number of hospitals in Great Britain with nurses who were well trained in comparison with the prevailing standards of that day. Worthy of note was the social class of the recruits (genteel rather than low), their status in the hospital (pupils rather than domestics), and the focus of their loyalty and identification (to the fund rather than the hospital). These women were an experimental group who would use the skills and habits acquired through Nightingale's regimented system of training to bring about a transformation in the nursing care of hospitalized patients. Both pupil and trained nurses were responsible to the fund and were assigned to hospitals by that body. The elements of this Nightingale training had been established two years earlier by Breay, who clearly thought of the training as entailing a whole set of new principles, requiring new institutional arrangements, and yielding a new occupational identity (Williams, 1980). (I'm sure we all recognize an early "professionalizer" at work!) The Nightingale Fund program, of course, reflected the same principles as had been established by Breay. Physicians and superintendents in charge of the hospitals were happy with the advent of training because they were pleased at the upgrading or improvement in both the characters and skills of the nurses. Although the training ushered in the separation of nursing work from domestic work, the physicians and superintendents did not realize the significance of the change, nor did they recognize it as fuel for the start of a new occupation, with the potential for upsetting the status quo.

Before long, however, discordant voices were heard from the superintendent and physician group, based on their disapproval of the pupil nurses being taught theory. A medical historian wrote, "As time passed on the training of probationers became more specialized; from clinical and practical it became to a greater extent theoretical, . . . and a bad style of nurse has resulted from this false training" (Williams, 1980, p. 52). According to Williams, the physicians were willing to accept the "skilled profession" in terms of changes in the character of nurses. They were unwilling, however, to accept the changes in their status and work that did not stem directly from a medical view of what nursing should be. The viewpoint of those

in charge of the hospital was that nursing required a docile discipline, a good heart and character, and capable, well-trained hands. In their view, nursing clearly did not call for anything like independent thought or problem-solving skills.

Thus, opposing trends are to be found at this first strong push to modernize nursing, with a small group of visionary women attempting to upgrade the status of nurses and to reform nursing care for patients. The positions of the different stakeholders were based on advancing or protecting their particular interests, with opposition arising from those who believed that the nursing advances would harm their own positions. The men in control of hospitals welcomed improvements in nursing up to the point where the nurses seemed to be growing into a body with an identity and function of its own, outside the sphere of control of either the physician or superintendent. Note that the nursing care of the day *was* in need of change. Most stakeholders were in agreement on that point, though no one asked for the opinion of the previous incumbents of nursing positions. The hospital nursing positions of these women were of low status, but they had provided a sinecure of little accountability or responsibility; if the women had had the power to do so, they may well have objected to the new directions nursing was taking.

Although the nursing professionalizers did not achieve all their goals, the balance that was struck between improvements in the structure and function of nursing, without altogether capsizing the boat of conventional hospital control, allowed the course of modern nursing to unfold—never out of trouble—but unfold nonetheless. The dynamic of stakeholders advancing or protecting their own interests is most fundamental. It is as pervasive today among and within all groups as it was in Nightingale's time.

The subordinate status of women in the Victorian era and early 20th century undoubtedly contributed to these developments. Davies (1980) suggests that only such a subordinate group would accept the compromises that these nurse reformers did. She points out that only meager resources were allocated to the training of nurses and that the reform movement resulted in a minimal amount of change in the status quo. However, the nurse leaders of the day had not expected miracles. They regarded their efforts as one strand in the progress and social change of the day: promoting the wider participation of all women in society. Many in the cadre of well-educated women of respectable social class who were involved in upgrading nursing in both Great Britain and the United States were suffragists or feminists. Improving the general social order by improving the status of women was an important goal for them. For instance, responding to criticisms about nurses being taught too much, Dock, a renowned American nursing leader and suffragist of her day, said, "The thing of real importance is not that nurses be taught less, but that all women be taught more" (Melosh, 1982, p. 76).

The American Scene

American women of similar class and bent as their British sisters were greatly influenced by the Nightingale system, and this was reflected in early efforts at reform and upgrading of nursing in the United States. There was fertile ground for such upgrading, and the same conflicting themes that were apparent between the nurse reformers and the conventional sources of social control in Great Britain found expression here. In an insightful review essay on nursing history, James (1984) characterizes the social ideology held by the professionalizing segment of turn-of-the-20th-century nurses as the progressive view, one reflecting great faith in the strengthening of democracy through the education and elevation of women. Educated women and nurses would be forces for social reform and world peace. This viewpoint, James claims, infuses the history texts written by Nutting and Dock that were used for students in hospital schools in the early decades of the 20th century. The students were thereby exposed to a morally uplifting, optimistic view of the nature of nursing that was a marked contrast to the realities of their daily life.

The conditions for nurses at the time were far from ideal. There was an explosive growth in the hospital industry as all classes of people, not just the poor, began to turn to hospitals for illness care (Vogel, 1979). At the same time, social changes were propelling women into the workforce, although the working woman was not commonplace and work choices were few. A window of opportunity had opened, creating a joint niche for hospitals and women. Hospitals survived by opening their own nurse training programs as a means of staffing their institutions, and women improved their situations, acquiring a toehold on a better life through the training and discipline they acquired in these programs. Note that for many women the need to be self-supporting was their motivation, rather than the wish to improve society or upgrade the status of women.

Typically, the hospital training programs were short on curriculum, long on hours of unpaid labor benefiting the hospital, strong on discipline and subservience to au-

thority, and weak on career security for the fledgling nurse. Thus the cadre of nursing reformers of the day were injecting a note of high morale and moral purpose into the bleak nursing landscape experienced by students and trained nurses alike. Training was an apprenticeship affair, with students carrying out the work of the hospital wards under the supervision of more advanced students or the nursing superintendent. Graduates were expected to leave the hospital for private duty practice since there were few hospital positions available. Although the pattern had many positive points, service demands always took precedence over educational needs. Stewart commented:

> The big question was not how much the probationer understood about her duties but how much she could get done in a ten hour day and how fast she could learn to take a full share of the work of the hospital ward. [quoted in Davies, 1980, p. 110]

The reformers concentrated on issues such as raising standards of recruitment, allowing time for classes, and improving and standardizing the curriculum for nursing. For them, better education was the key to better health care for society and an improved status for nurses. The reformers had taken on a formidable task. James (1984) describes one group of them as "ambitious nurses [who] earned bachelor's and master's degrees at [Teachers College, Columbia] and dedicated themselves to the Sisyphean labor of upgrading the hospital training schools" (p. 571).

Loyal and Not-So-Loyal Opposition. Disagreement with their agenda for upgrading nursing came from both hospital officials and the trained nurses themselves. Those in charge of hospitals regarded the student apprenticeship training with its emphasis on submission to institutional authority as ideal. It created a disciplined if temporary workforce, and as the students graduated, new students replaced them. Because the students received little, if any, stipend, they were a relatively inexpensive source of labor. Any move to reduce the amount of service provided by students or to loosen the reins of hospital authority was, of course, objectionable.

Objections within the ranks of nursing itself had different bases. While the reformers were concerned with issues like the heavy workloads of students, their overarching concern was with the dual matter of improving health care and upgrading nursing into professional status with all that implies about such characteristics as a conceptual knowledge base, autonomy, independent judgment, and professional regulation of members. They wanted to have professional organizations to foster professional goals. They wanted nursing programs to be in educational institutions and had some success in achieving that goal, although progress was gradual until after the midpoint of the century. They wanted entering students to meet the same requirements that entering students in other programs of study were meeting. In other words, the seeds of a professional culture, first sown by Breay in Great Britain, were transplanted to this early 20th century cadre of nursing reformers in the United States. Since then, the culture of professionalism has sometimes waxed and sometimes waned, as it has been tempered by developments in the women's movement, society at large and health care, and by both support and opposition within the ranks of nurses. Professionalism is undoubtedly one of our strongest traditions.

Professionalism was not a welcome prospect to many rank-and-file or mainstream nurses who were developing their own strong tradition. This group was reasonably satisfied with the apprenticeship training they had acquired in hospital schools and with the work they now performed. They worried about being left behind should the upgrading of standards proceed as the nursing leadership wished. If academic degrees became a sine qua non for practice defined as professional, they faced the prospect of becoming second-class professionals or of being eliminated entirely. This seemed unjust to many of these nurses who considered themselves well prepared for the work of nursing.

In addition to the threat of lowered status, they had a somewhat different perspective about the work of nursing, frequently identified as the craft orientation. They took great pride in their craft, with its hands-on skills, shared standards of work and deportment, and esprit de corp. They downplayed the conceptual or theoretical and focused on the immediate conditions in their work situations. To oversimplify the differences in outlook between the professional culture and the craft culture of the rank-and-file or mainstream nurse, it can be said that the leaders and aspiring professionals "looked outward, beyond the work experience to its social context and implications. [They] . . . sought to improve nurses' positions within the medical division of labor" (Melosh, 1982, p. 5). Nursing for this group had an important cognitive aspect to it; it was to be a field of study. The rank and file, on the other hand, were absorbed in the nature, pace, requirements, and rewards of daily work. They looked inward, focusing on the immediate situation. Their concerns were on the practical, such as the conditions of work and whether the nurse had sufficient control over how it was performed. Their culture, constructed from their accumulated experiences and understandings of the workplace, guided and interpreted the tasks and social relations of work. Of value was their apprenticeship tradition, careful craft methods, practical experience, and self-control.

Melosh (1982) claims that the mainstream in nursing has always embraced the craft culture; professional ideology, though influential, was a definite minority view. Throughout every decade of this century both cultures have been much in evidence, though the issues generating the most passion for each group have varied, depending on other contextual factors of the times. Having different values the cultures have often taken divergent rather than convergent paths. Professional culture, over the years, has downplayed the apprenticeship means of learning because it was tainted with authoritarianism and illegitimate free labor and because of its neglect or even disparagement of anything conceptual. With their eyes on the broader picture, professionalizers frequently paid little attention to the actual workplace concerns and welfare of the nurse in the trenches. The craft culture for its part has tended to distrust the theoretical approach of the professionals, thinking of them as abandoning nursing skills, being too upwardly mobile, and creating an elitist class system in nursing. In the craft view, patient care deteriorates as nurses' education moves away from the bedside (Melosh, 1982). Feelings over specific proposals have run high over the years, as demonstrated by this sentence from a letter to a nursing journal, following the publication of the 1948 Brown report (which recommended a baccalaureate education for nurses):

> It's not the university graduate who knows how to give a better back rub or how to administer to the patient's comfort in countless ways, but the nurse who has been trained for it and who does not feel too far superior to carry out the everyday tasks. [Melosh, 1982, p. 68]

Lest we think such sentiments have disappeared, consider the following quote from a letter to *Nursing Spectrum* in 1999. The letter writer is canceling her subscription, saying,

> I strongly feel that you overlook and diminish the average nurse in your publication. By average, I mean those of us who practice on the front lines of health care every day. Your articles are always written by nurses with so many degrees after their names it looks like alphabet soup. . . . I have a diploma degree, although many of you may not remember what that is. I continue to give good compassionate patient

care, regardless of those nurses in their ivory towers. [*Nursing Spectrum,* 1999]

Nursing Voices as Just One Section of the Orchestra. While nursing's two cultures continue to influence the positions nurses take on educational and practice issues, they do not entirely dictate what nurses think, nor do they explain all the practices that have been adopted in education and clinical practice in nursing. And while some nurses feel that the confusion in our definition of the professional and in our pathways to practice happens because we, as a group, cannot or will not make up our minds, the facts are more complicated. It is true that nursing speaks with a chorus rather than with a single voice (Reverby, 1979), but it is also true, to continue the analogy, that our chorus is only one section of the orchestra. The panoply of events and conditions as they unfold in society add their own particular tunes and influence the outcomes. Economic factors, for instance, are potent. They have certainly played a key role in determining where and what kind of educational programs are supported, as well as in determining the degree to which we have layers of lesser prepared as well as more elaborately prepared nursing personnel. Economic factors have always played a commanding role in nurse shortages and nurse oversupplies, as reflected in the availability of jobs and the kinds of qualifications required for all types of nursing positions. It is noteworthy that the addition of lesser prepared people usually occurs at the time of shortages as a less expensive mechanism for increasing supply, and that this usually occurs over the objections of nurses with both professional and craft ideologies.

Political factors frequently interact with economics in societal decisions about nursing and nursing education, and the case of the associate degree nurse is a good example of the interplay. The position and educational program were created as a compromise that was to meet diverse goals for diverse groups. The severe post–World War II nursing shortage would be addressed because the program would attract previously untapped pools of potential recruits. These recruits would be among the influx of students entering the community college system, which was rapidly developing as a publicly supported means for extending educational opportunities to previously non-college-bound people. The control of the program (college, not hospital) and level of practitioner (technical, not professional) overcame the objections among many professional culture nursing groups, although it left many questions unanswered for other groups. The compromise acknowledged the need for different levels of practice within nursing and was part of a strategy that placed all education in educational institutions and professional practice at the baccalaureate level. The technical nurse would be under the direction of the professional nurse, a matter that would require appropriate licensing arrangements to be made by each state's board of nursing (Lynaugh, 1995) and approved by each legislature. These boards of nursing and legislatures never did, however, create that distinction in licensing (a political move, for sure) and neither did hospitals (most likely an economic move). Consequently, we have a single license for practice, with various paths to achieve it.

The influence of an interacting web of societal events on decisions about nursing would be difficult to overestimate. Starting with politics, consider the impact of wars on available workers, the need for health services for civilian and military populations, and the reorganization of male and female roles. Consider also the impact of the change in social and political ideology in this country regarding entitlements of all to health care and redressing the inequalities of treatment and entitlement based on race and ethnic issues, gender, or economics. These are just examples of factors that, while external to nursing, form a powerful context for influencing decisions that are made about nursing.

THE CHALLENGES AHEAD

Nursing has spawned both a strong craft culture and a strong professional culture. How will understanding these traditions help us to design educational patterns and policies that will be equal to the challenges ahead? Our traditional cultures have programmed us with a readiness to respond or think in certain ways. We typically do not test the waters anew each time we must react to determine what response would be a good fit for the particular situation because we believe that we already have the answer. Nurses become steeped in these cultures through the educational paths they take and through their workplace experiences. Knowledge of how the cultures evolved through the interacting web of factors that generated them enables us to take a more objective stance about them. It helps to reduce their automatic hold on our values and decision making, thus freeing us from what sometimes is the tyranny of blind adherence, to either culture. Both cultures encapsulate important insights about how nursing does, or might, fit into the emerging world of work, health care, and gender. Yet both can constrict the ability to solve problems comprehensively, taking contextual factors into account.

Perhaps the biggest challenge that we face as a group is to reform and adjust nursing education to thrive in the face of the ambiguities that lie ahead in the century just beginning. We will be challenged to develop creative problem solving that transcends the limitations of both cultures and to adopt a more negotiable blend or synthesis of elements from each one. With the hindsight we have gained from experience, we might insist on a culture that allows us to be more deliberate and self-conscious about our values and priorities, how we weigh options, and how we can address the needs of many rather than a few. The options chosen would have to meet the litmus test of improving nursing's ability to respond to society's health care needs, if we are to garner widespread support and become potent players in health care. This may require us to change our vision of the appropriate structure for nursing, from time to time, as we keep pace with social change.

LANDSCAPE OF THE 21st CENTURY

What will this 21st century be like? Without a crystal ball, certainty is elusive at best. Think of the years when the hospital was thought to remain an almost exclusive focus for nursing practice. Few people would agree with that prediction today. But caution notwithstanding, most evidence points to a high probability for certain conditions to prevail in the future, and ubiquitous change is top on the list (National Academy of Science Committee on Science, Engineering, and Public Policy, 1995). Concomitant with a rapid rate of change in knowledge and technology, the information superhighway will be immense, and knowledge itself will be a vital commodity. Technology will have an ever expanding role in business as well as in personal lives, and a global perspective on all matters will be required, as the interdependency of all communities on our planet becomes increasingly apparent. Finally, because the amount of most resources in the world is finite and the demand for resources is high from all societal sectors, we can expect a smaller share of the total resources to be allocated for either education or health care. This means we must find ways of sharing resources, rather than simply competing with others for them. Doing more with less will become a familiar refrain to those who have not become acquainted with it already.

Meeting the Challenges

The National Academy of Science committee dealing with education for engineers and scientists, in response to the increasing rates of change and technological develop-

ment expected in the 21st century, asserts that, "A world of work that has become more interdisciplinary, collaborative, and global requires that we produce young people who are more adaptable and flexible, as well as technically proficient" (National Academy of Science, 1995, p. 2). In the face of intense development and rapid obsolescence of technology, they advocate avoiding the temptation of a vocational approach to education (meaning graduate education) that results in narrowness and overspecialization. When applied to nursing and extended to also include undergraduate education, this approach calls for a sound generalist emphasis in our curricula, with attention to preparing graduates who can accommodate change with ease. The rationale is that knowledge about principles is readily transferable and will equip practitioners to face a future that is unknowable at the present time. The knowledge of principles allows the practitioners to adapt readily to technologies as they evolve rather than being constrained by technical information and proficiency that has outlived its usefulness.

The workplace is frequently unhappy with such emphasis on principles at the expense, they think, of developing skills and expertise. They point out with justification that it is skills and expertise that are needed in the workplace. However, turning novices at all levels into skilled practitioners had best be regarded as a system problem and solving it will require some creative planning and collaboration so that new graduates at all levels will continue to learn as they begin their work roles. If predictions about the future are correct, the workplace will have to adopt a continuous learning mechanism for all employees, seasoned as well as novice. The informal "picking it up in the workplace" will not suffice in an age when treatment modalities and technology change so rapidly. Educational renewal needs to be an important part of the system.

There are many additional questions that will require thoughtful responses from our nursing community if we are to rise to the broad challenges listed earlier. There may be several ways of meeting these challenges, and we need to remain open to the idea that different answers may be operationalized in different locales and should be evaluated on their own merits. Particularly from an international perspective, care should be taken so that our answers fit the requirements of the specific local situations. The following provisional list of questions is not intended to be either exhaustive or to contain what are necessarily the most important issues. All entries on this list do, however, have at least a tangential connection to the dominant cultures described in this chapter.

How can we transform our thinking about the conceptual in general and education in particular to embrace career-long learning and mobility? How can we increase the accessibility of our programs to students of all ages and ethnic backgrounds? It has been said (Day, J., as cited in Sullivan & Clinton, 1999) that by the year 2010, about 52% of the population of the United States will be composed of minorities. Surely this change in the ethnic composition of the United States population is a clarion call for facilitating the recruitment of minority students into nursing. Our success in addressing access to education issues will determine to a great extent what we will accomplish in accommodating wisely and well to change, in increasing cultural diversity within nursing, and in improving our ability to care for diverse and global populations. One other aspect of the access challenge is the matter of age and status of our students. An increasing number of students are nontraditional in terms of their ages and family and work responsibilities; they require educational programs that allow them to accommodate to such restraints. Our programs cannot be designed solely for young, full-time students with few, if any, family responsibilities.

The idea of finishing one's education is passé and had best be replaced by a career orientation at every level from nurse's aide to advanced practice nurse. This development poses a challenge to both cultures. Both cultures must recognize that old standards for judging and acquiring expertise are outmoded and that expertise is time limited. We need to come together on a new standard involving periodic renewal of knowledge and skills. Considerable change has already taken place, particularly in acute care settings, but what about career mobility from lower ranks to higher, and some of the less intense or long-term settings? A career orientation calls for looking ahead, assessing opportunities and demands of the future, and making a conscious effort to prepare for that future. The professional culture so prominent in academia and the rigidities of the workplace have been charged with setting roadblocks that make the pursuit of education difficult, and many times nursing personnel themselves have not made any effort to become prepared. Innovative programs are needed to overcome these personal and institutional roadblocks. Distance education is one such strategy; devising ways of validating experiential learning is another.

How can we provide experiential learning in our educational programs? There are many thorny issues related to this question. Most people regard it as essential for honing skills and clinical judgment. But it is time-consuming for students, preceptors, and faculty and frequently involves logistical problems. Simulated learning has been substituted with success in some instances. But without experiential learning some wonder how we will prepare graduates to exercise good clinical judgment, especially when that judgment contradicts a particular protocol.

Is it time to revisit the issue of differentiating between technical-level and professional-level practice? This has always been a divisive issue, with nurses who have less than a baccalaureate degree feeling unfairly relegated to second-class citizenship should that change come about. But if we were to succeed in engendering as a standard career-long learning for all and if service and educational institutions removed current roadblocks that nursing personnel face, maybe the issue could be viewed in a different light. Since our current licensing examinations are concerned with minimum standards for safe practice, why not keep the RN as the technical-level credential and establish a PRN for professional nursing that would have additional requirements and mechanisms for its achievement? This could be another version of the "ladder" concept already in use for distinguishing levels of clinical expertise in service settings, with the expectation that many nurses on the first or RN step would continue their professional development and qualify for the PRN. Most prognosticators expect the complexity of health care to increase, not to decrease, and it seems a given that there will be a need for different levels of nursing staff. It may well be time for service agencies to make explicit different expectations of technical-level nurses and professional-level nurses and to adjust salary levels accordingly. Added to the economic and political factors that make technical versus professional levels a difficult issue is the fact that nursing has yet to develop generally accepted measures for true professional practice.

Should we increase interdisciplinary collaboration? Collaboration and the sharing of resources (as for learning experiences) are advocated frequently as means of doing more with less (Cawley, 1993; National Academy of Science, 1995; Smith, 1995). This is not always simple, however, and is not always considered wise. Although becoming interdisciplinary is one way to break down traditional barriers between disciplines and between professionals and communities, it can also result in establishing hegemony on the part of one or another more powerful group when the power relations are not equal. It therefore requires careful attention to be given to establishing rational bases of equality among the partners and the nurturing of equality as a group norm to ensure full participation and true collaboration. This usually means relative equality of educational preparation of the collaborators and the acceptance of patients and communities as full participants in decision making.

SUMMARY

The challenges ahead for nursing and nursing education are plentiful. Although our course is far from clear, we have a wonderfully diverse supply of possible actions to pursue, and these will be tested in the decades ahead. We also have the will, optimism, and perseverance to succeed in our quest.

Because what nursing ought or needs to be depends on developments in health care delivery and other societal trends, there probably will be no such thing as a final shape to our nursing workforce or the educational system. As we examine our garden of nursing positions and the paths to them, it may still be difficult to tell the weeds from the flowers, but surely the distinctions will become clearer with the passage of time, as some are found to suit societal and health care ends more than others. The process is lengthy and requires the toleration of a few weeds until such time as their status as weeds rather than precious flowers is clear. Most new role developments in nursing have stimulated strong objection at their outset. With this thought in mind, let us remain open to a diversity of ideas about nursing roles and educational pathways and continue to engage other health care stakeholders in discussions and negotiations that will bring about the highest level of care most effectively.

REFERENCES

Berlin, L., & Bednash, G. (1999). *Enrollments and graduations in baccalaureate and graduate programs in nursing* (AACN Publication No. 98-99-1). Washington, DC: American Association of Colleges of Nursing.

Cawley, J. (1993). Physician assistants in the health care workforce. In D.K. Clawson & M. Osterweis (Eds.), *The roles of physician assistants and nurse practitioners in primary care* (pp. 21-39). Washington, DC: Association of Academic Health Centers.

Davies, C. (1980). A constant casualty: Nurse education in Britain and the USA to 1939. In C. Davies (Ed.), *Rewriting nursing history* (pp. 102-122). Totowa, NJ: Barnes and Noble.

Health Resources and Services Administration, Division of Nursing. (1996). *Notes from the national sample survey of registered nurses.* Available: http://www.hrsa.dhhs.gov/bhpr/dn/survnote.htm. (15 Oct. 1999).

James, J.W. (1984). Writing and rewriting nursing history: A review essay. *Bulletin of the History of Medicine, 58,* 568-584.

Lynaugh, J. (1995). Nursing and the W.K. Kellogg Foundation. *Nursing in Health Care, 16*(4), 174-183.

Melosh, B. (1982). *"The physician's hand": Work culture and conflict in American nursing.* Philadelphia: Temple University Press.

National Academy of Science Committee on Science, Engineering, and Public Policy. (1995). *Reshaping the graduate education of scientists and engineers.* Washington, DC: National Academy Press.

National League for Nursing Center for Research in Nursing Education and Community Health. (1997). *Nursing Data Review 1997* (Publication No. 19-7327). New York: National League for Nursing Press.

Nursing Spectrum. (1999, October). Letter to editor.

Reverby, S. (1979). The search for the hospital yardstick: Nursing and the rationalization of hospital work. In S. Reverby & D. Rosner (Eds.), *Health care in America: Essays in social history* (pp. 206-225). Philadelphia: Temple University Press.

Smith, G. (1995). Lessons learned: Challenges for the future. *Nursing in Health Care, 16*(4), 188-191.

Sullivan, E., & Clinton, J. (1999). Achieving a multicultural nursing. In E. Sullivan (Ed.), *Creating nursing's future* (pp. 317-326). St. Louis: Mosby

Vogel, M. (1979). The transformation of the American hospital, 1850-1920. In S. Reverby & D. Rosner (Eds.), *Health care in America: Essays in social history* (pp. 105-116). Philadelphia: Temple University Press.

Williams, K. (1980). From Sarah Gamp to Florence Nightingale: A critical study of hospital nursing systems from 1840 to 1897. In C. Davies (Ed.), *Rewriting nursing history* (pp. 41-75). Totowa, NJ: Barnes and Noble.

Changing Methods of Education

KAREN L. MILLER

Nursing education of the future will be one by-product of the quantum leaps occurring in telecommunications, biomedical discoveries, and computer innovations. The beginning of the 21st century finds our nursing students capable of assimilating many contemporary changes in education. They are learning in virtual classrooms, clinical simulation laboratories, interdisciplinary models, video testing situations, and self-paced programs. Nursing students are graduating from academic programs that are far from traditional. They are requesting education that combines quality with convenience and innovation. They are older, often have multiple academic degrees, and are attuned to professional opportunities for nurses in the job market. Prospective nursing students, like most students, have many career choices. Analysis of the future nursing workforce indicates that fewer young people will be available to enter nursing programs and those that do will seek flexible education and workplace options (Buerhaus, Staiger, & Auerbach, 2000). This Viewpoint chapter explores issues in the education of future nurses that have emerged as a result of rapidly changing methods of education.

The burgeoning of technological advances to deliver educational coursework is revolutionizing higher education. The combination of the personal computer with an experienced academic mind provides the ideal medium for faculty creativity. After five decades of steady improvements in curriculum, teaching methods, and degree programs, nursing educators have recognized signs of the need for faster change. Recent advances in educational technologies have prompted an array of innovative methods for distance education and classroom teaching. Distance education may be broadly defined as teaching and learning that occurs when students and teachers are not in the same physical location. Technologies currently used for distance education encompass a variety of content delivery methods, including audioconference by telephone, audiocassette tape, videotaped instruction, courier service,

electronic mail (e-mail), faxing, fixed computer media (CD-ROM and floppy disk), Internet list-servers, room-based videoconference by interactive television, desktop videoconference, and Internet-based programming (Baldwin, Bingham, & Connors, 1996).

The *virtual classroom* is one term used to describe the use of one or a combination of distance education technologies. A virtual classroom implies that no actual classroom exists, but rather the perception of a classroom exists based on student-to-student and student-to-teacher interactions via technology. The ability of faculty to use a variety of computer-based technologies to create educational programs has opened a vast array of new learning opportunities for students. Nursing faculty have developed some of the most creative interactive television and Internet-based courses available to students in any profession (American Association of Colleges of Nursing, 1999). Students at all levels of nursing education are demanding more flexibility in education. Through the combination of multiple clinical practice experiences with virtual classroom learning options, students can choose the time and place of their courses, as well as learning options suited to their individual needs.

The development of the World Wide Web for general use in the early 1990s provided a comprehensive, virtual environment for delivering text, graphics, audio, video, animation, and interactive media. The web is the infrastructure for viewing information. The Internet describes a web-based technical medium full of telecommunication lines and switches all linked together by so-called Internet protocol (Dyson, 1997). Anyone connected to the Internet through a computer has access to information available from millions of other computers and communications networks. This technical capacity makes it possible to enhance faculty and student creativity for unlimited possibilities for educational innovations.

The virtual classroom is the best way to achieve access to courses and optimal scheduling flexibility. On-line classes are asynchronous in that participation may occur at any time of day and in any place where computer and Internet access are available. Some virtual classrooms also use *desktop videoconferencing* as a way for students to meet with faculty from distant locations. Desktop video-conferencing is a synchronous educational method because it requires that students and faculty meet at the same time, although they may be at their desks in separate locations. Most virtual classroom courses existing today are similar in many ways to traditional courses. The outline, syllabus, and assignments reflect the objectives of the course. The primary difference is that most, if not all, class activities occur electronically. Required readings, projects, examinations, and papers are submitted by *electronic mail (e-mail)*. Faculty respond to student work in the same way. Faculty-student interactions via e-mail will be routine for future nursing students, regardless of whether the students are registered for virtual classroom courses. Threaded discussions, or a set of Internet-based conversations among participants, and the use of on-line bulletin boards to post these discussions are two common types of communication in the virtual classroom. Even students in traditional courses will be involved in electronic class discussions in the future. The Internet allows immediate access to nearly unlimited sources of information. Links to governmental agencies, scientific meetings, research institutions, and informational sources throughout the world can add dimensions to learning experiences never previously possible.

One key to using technology in education is for students and faculty to have access to appropriate computer equipment and technical support for these changing methods of education. Rapid integration of computer technology into everyday life for many people worldwide leaves little doubt that the virtual classroom will be available for future students seeking nursing education.

Concurrent multiple-method course presentation is familiar to many of today's nursing students. They may participate in interactive television classes, Internet-based classes, and traditional lectures and seminars all in the same course. Although there are rapidly growing numbers of completely on-line or Internet-based courses, future nursing students may be able to choose courses on the Internet from more than one school or university. It is expected that higher education will become more businesslike, with benchmarking standards for access, cost, support, outcomes, and quality (National Center for Education Statistics, 1999). A student will be able to compare courses and programs among schools based on his or her individual needs. Since some students prefer more

traditional classroom settings, courses will continue to be taught this way, although changing educational methods will allow more in-class options.

Other types of technology-based educational methods have become part of nursing programs. *Computer-assisted instruction (CAI)* modules are familiar to graduates from many schools of nursing. Using fixed computer media such as CD-ROM and floppy disks, faculty can offer specialized content in a format that students can use multiple times. Like a good textbook, a good CD-ROM program can be an inexpensive way of delivering rich, detailed cognitive content. Current technology allows for video and audio "streaming" in these programs for innovative and entertaining learning. Future use of CAI will be more interactive and integrated with Internet-based educational methods. Students will be able to use a CD-ROM as a textbook that will allow them to link to Internet sites for assignments and other sources of information on the subject under study.

Successful completion of future programs in nursing at all levels will depend on students' abilities to be self-paced and motivated to use new informational tools. Curriculum of the future will support more self-directed choices for application of knowledge to diverse clinical situations. A variety of methods are available that can help make the most of self-directed learning options. Most students are familiar with currently available on-line journals and digital reference libraries. *Knowledge hyperdocuments* and *analysis programs* are computer software tools that organize information for student use, allowing increased self-directed intellectual exploration. Hyperdocuments, also called hypermedia or "edutainment," are CD-ROMs that present snippets of text, pictures, video, and sound. These tools allow "point and click" excursions driven by the learner, rather than the teacher (Dertouzos, 1977). Analysis tools are computer programs that help students evaluate the underlying causes of phenomena in specialized areas of knowledge. These tools are designed for quantitative disciplines, such as mathematics, physics, and engineering. Health professions education emphasizes scientific inquiry as the basis for clinical practice. In the future, more sophisticated analysis of clinical data in nursing research will be possible through the use of these faster and more comprehensive analysis tools.

Today's graduate students are making the most of the multimedia capability of CD-ROM technology. An increasing number of student dissertations are being submitted electronically. This format allows films, sound recordings, and video images to be integrated into the text of a dissertation or thesis. Some universities now require electronic submission of dissertations by students, making the final product far more accessible than current requirements. A digital library has been implemented by the United Nations Educational, Scientific and Cultural Organization and the Organization of American States. The goal of this international digital library is to spotlight the literary and scientific work of scholars outside the United States. International collaboration among students and faculty will become routine and, often, required for future higher education (Leibowitz, 2000).

An interesting development from CD-ROM technology is the *digital bookbag* (Guernsey, 2000, p. 1). Instead of purchasing textbooks, course syllabi, or manuals, students may have the opportunity to acquire the entire curriculum for a course, including textbook materials, through the purchase of a single digital video disk (DVD). Creators of this technology estimate that DVDs will replace text, images, manuals, and even laboratory slides used in courses, as well as syllabi and past course materials. Since each DVD weighs only 2 ounces and can hold millions of pages and images, nursing students may find the convenience of this method appealing. It is not expected that the digital bookbag will be less expensive than traditional texts and course materials, at least in the near future.

Early evidence from studies of technology-based distance education shows that students are willing to use computer technology for all facets of their education, especially if the course content is interactive, challenging, and visually stimulating (Connors and Davies, 1999). DVD technology adds the capacity of extensive search of textbook materials by topic and digital quality of visual and sound information. Today, many publishers add a CD-ROM to their textbooks to give students enhanced versions of the printed materials. Tomorrow's students may combine their laptop computers with DVD players in order to have immediate access to all their past course materials, current course requirements and handouts, more convenient sources of information, and superior audiovisual quality.

In addition to changing methods of education that have evolved from computer technology, there are new methods for teaching clinical practice skills in the health professions. Objective structured clinical examination (OSCE) is a form of standardized evaluation of clinical skills that is an accepted method in primary care education of nurse practitioners and other advanced practice specialties. With the increased need for reliable, objective measures of professional competencies, future nursing

education will include more of this type of student evaluation. OSCE testing originated with medical student education in the late 1970s (van der Vleuten & Swanson, 1990). In response to increased need for primary care providers in the United States during the 1990s, nurse practitioner (NP) programs expanded to meet the demand for advanced practice nurses. Accurate assessment of primary care skills, including patient and family interactions, became an important requirement of NP programs, and standardized patient testing was introduced in nursing education. Today this method is widely used in medical schools to create an environment for clinical practice that is similar to real-life situations. Some schools of nursing with extensive graduate nurse practitioner and clinical specialist programs are incorporating OSCE testing as part of their complement of clinical teaching and learning methods.

Standardized patients are "actors" or persons not involved in the health professions. These persons are taught to portray patients with a variety of symptoms and conditions in a consistent, standardized manner. During interactions with these "patients," students are rated by instructors who directly observe each encounter or view videotaped student-patient interactions. Most often, the OSCE method is used to measure history taking, physical examination, diagnostic skills, laboratory utilization, patient management, and communication skills. Future nursing education will incorporate more computer and clinical information systems technology to improve OSCE evaluation methods. This method is ideally suited to improve interdisciplinary learning among nurses and other health professionals as they interact together as students with actor patients.

One of the most notable changes in education for baccalaureate students will be the methods used to teach introductory and advanced clinical skills. The clinical learning laboratory of the future will house high technology simulators and virtual reality programs for learning the many technical skills required in nursing practice. Simulators are computer-driven machines that present realistic situations in a teaching environment that appeals to the human senses and emotional status of students, in addition to cognitive abilities. Computerized simulators originated in the military and have been widely adapted for use by airline pilots, air-traffic controllers, race car drivers, and technical equipment operators. As the number of hospitalized patients declines with improvements in the management of clinical care, fewer opportunities are available for student clinical experiences. Patient care simulators are available today that provide a realistic model for anesthesia, surgery, and trauma care. These are computerized mannequins that recognize more than 200 medications, respond to painful stimuli, simulate an array of clinical symptoms, and react to physical interventions. Others are available for practicing intravenous therapy, neurological examination, and cardiopulmonary care. Nursing students and faculty can expect to see more high technology simulators as accurate substitutes for real patients in their clinical education.

Virtual reality technology presents the most promising method for enhanced nursing clinical education in the future. This method creates an environment for learning that involves the student in actual hands-on clinical situations using computer-generated tactile capabilities. Students can learn intricate clinical skills, such as suturing, invasive and laser procedures, orthopedic interventions, and ophthalmology examinations without ever picking up the real equipment or actually touching a patient. Using special devices, such as electronic gloves, computerized eyewear, or adapted flexible tubing, students can practice a virtually real clinical skill that feels and acts like the real thing. Virtual reality technology is in early stages of development. However, the opportunities to bring optimal clinical reality to the confines of the clinical learning laboratory will help students gain greater confidence at a faster pace than can currently be achieved using human subjects.

The enormous capacity of technology to improve and extend teaching and learning will add many new dimensions to nursing education. The essential challenge for faculty and students is to retain the core values of higher education while meeting growing expectations for convenient, instant communication. Students are responding positively to changing methods for education. This situation raises important concerns for faculty, both seasoned and less experienced teachers. Issues of time, access, skills, and workload impinge on faculty comfort with information technologies. University and college executives worry about the broader issues of quality, cost, student outcomes and competition among schools. The current shift in education demands that faculty and students be open to change and prepared for new opportunities. In the discipline of nursing, progress in educational methods will be the platform for the assimilation of new discoveries in biomedicine. Biotechnology, biotherapy, genomics, and next-generation pharmaceuticals are a few of the many clinical advances that future nurses will need to understand and utilize in practice. Changes in the educational environment make it possible for learner-centered teaching methods. The aim of higher education in the information age will be to help students learn to learn throughout their lives. The rapid pace of technology-based social and biomedical change will make lifelong learning imperative. It is an evolving challenge for everyone!

Educational methods of the past that have led to our collective discoveries of today incorporated the spirit of inquiry with thoughtful analysis. The fundamental objectives of higher education to improve life and to seek new knowledge will undergird future educational models. According to Judith Eaton, president of the U.S. Council for Higher Education Accreditation, "technology-based changes in educational methods will force traditional institutions to pay closer attention to the results of their educational efforts. Quality and evidence of positive outcomes for students will remain the most important factors for judging the merits of educational methods in the future" (Eaton, 1999, p. 24).

REFERENCES

American Association of Colleges of Nursing. (1999). *AACN White Paper: Distance technology in nursing education.* Washington, DC: Author.

Baldwin D., Bingham J., & Connors, H. (1996). *Teaching with technologies. Distance Education Strategies Report.* Kansas City, KS: University of Kansas Medical Center.

Buerhaus, P.I., Staiger, D.O., & Auerbach, D.I. (2000). Implications of an aging registered nurse workforce. *Journal of the American Medical Association, 283*(22), 2948-2954.

Connors, H.R., & Davies, L.L. (1999). Using technology to teach. In E.J. Sullivan (Ed.), *Creating nursing's future* (pp. 116-124). St. Louis: Mosby.

Dertouzos, M.L. (1997). *What will be: How the new world of information will change our lives* (pp. 175-189, 281). New York: Harper Collins.

Dyson, E. (1997). *Release 2.0: A design for living in the digital age.* New York: Dell Publishing Group.

Eaton, J.S. (1999, January/February). Distance education is on your doorstep. *Trusteeship,* pp. 23-27.

Guernsey, L. (2000, March 2). Bookbag of the future: Dental schools stuff 4 years' worth of manuals and books into 1 DVD. *New York Times,* p. D1.

Leibowitz, W.R. (2000, January). University of Texas says it may require digital dissertations. *Chronicle of Higher Education.* [Online]. Available: http://www.chronicle.com/free/2000/01/2000010401t.htm.

National Center for Education Statistics. (1999). Distance education at post-secondary education institutions: 1997-1998. Washington, DC: Department of Education.

van der Vleuten, C.P.M., & Swanson, D.B. (1990). Assessment of clinical skills with standardized patients: State of the art. *Teaching and Learning in Medicine, 2*(2), 58-76.

International Graduate Nursing Education

A Modest Proposal

JUDITH M. LEWIS

Countries around the world have long recognized the value of an international experience for university students and faculty. In the United States the American Council on Education (Commission on International Education, 1998) extensively addressed the need for university graduates to have "global competence." Professional nursing in the United States has highlighted the importance of preparing practitioners with global perspectives. This paper explores the origins and current status of international education and the implications for graduate nursing education. A new model that capitalizes on technology is proposed as a means of achieving greater participation in an international program without the drawbacks of existing models.

BACKGROUND

It can be argued that Europe's oldest universities were international institutions by convention, rather than intent. They began as a guild of students and evolved into a guild of scholars studying primarily in the fields of religion and medicine. Latin was the language of the academic transaction, and a cross-national student body was not unusual (Altbach & Davis, 1999). Some students wandered from country to country seeking a particular learning experience, an activity akin to exploring the Internet. Rossman (1992, p. xii) describes "the end of the twentieth century as a time comparable to the twelfth century when the rise of the university in western Europe helped enable the Renaissance." The rebirth this time is the electronic revolution and all its implications for academia worldwide.

Comparative education is sometimes used in conjunction with international education, but it is a distinct area that involves "the analysis of educational systems and problems in two or more national environments in terms of socio-political, economic, cultural, ideological, and

other contexts" (Fraser & Brickman, 1968, p. 1). Comparative education is an area of study that can be traced back to the classical period of civilization and still impacts the field of international education. Although the original intent of comparative studies was to know one's neighbors, inevitably news about what a particular university in one country was doing did positively influence the academic quality of universities in other countries (Fraser & Brickman, 1968).

Today, even though a myriad of terms may be encountered in academia, all international efforts can be grouped under one of three rubrics: movement of scholars and students; educational programs offered beyond national boundaries; and curriculum (Vestal, 1994). The motivation for such offerings includes ethnocentric, altruistic, and political purposes. Universities in the role of a receiving institution embrace an altruistic societal belief that educating foreigners contributes to a better world for all and that their own students and faculty profit from interacting with international students. The political benefits of such endeavors is expressed by Keith Geiger, Deputy Assistant Secretary for Academic Programs, U.S. State Department: "The presence of international students on our campuses brings a wealth of benefits to our country. It insures that there will be a cadre of people around the world who understand the United States in very profound ways, which in turn will lead to improved bilateral relations, enhanced business relationships, and increased cultural ties" (Jenkins, 1997).

After World War II there was a movement in the United States to promote within the country a wider interest and deeper comprehension of other societies and to create a climate of public opinion in which the actions, motives, and policies of the United States would be fairly interpreted abroad (Melby, 1961). Congress formalized a commitment to international education in 1946 by fund-

TABLE 15-1 Programs for Individuals and Institutions Encompassed by the Fulbright Program

Title	Type	Purpose
American scholar	Scholars and professionals	Lecture or conduct research abroad
Visiting scholar	Foreign scholars	Lecture or conduct research in United States
Predoctoral fellowships	American and foreign graduate students or graduating seniors	Americans study abroad; foreigners study in United States
Teacher exchange	American and foreign one-for-one exchange	Elementary, secondary, and postsecondary teachers
Hubert Humphrey fellowships	Midcareer foreign professionals	Year of study and related professional experiences
College and university affiliations	Exchange of faculty and staff	Establish linkages between U.S. universities and overseas institutions
Fulbright-Hays foreign area and language training	Individual Americans and U.S. institutions	Support research and training efforts abroad focusing on non-Western foreign languages and world area studies

Data from Council for International Exchange of Scholars, scholars@cies.iie.org.

ing the Fulbright Program (Public Law 584, the Fulbright Act) to increase mutual understanding between the people of the United States and people of other countries. Grants are awarded to American students, teachers, and scholars to study, teach, lecture, and conduct research abroad and to foreign individuals to engage in similar activities in the United States (Table 15-1).

GROWTH OF INTERNATIONAL EDUCATION

Another motivational force has emerged in recent years: academic capitalism. All major industrialized countries are seeking a share of the "international education pie," estimated to be worth $50 billion in 2010 (Schofield, 1999, p. 90). Governments, including those of Canada, Australia, and many of the 26 countries of the European Union, are pushing academia to become entrepreneurial (Green, 1997), and the international arena is a key target for income-generating activities. The United States is no different and actually "imports" or receives more students and scholars than it "exports" or sends (Table 15-2). In 1998–1999, nearly 500,000 foreign students enrolled in American colleges and universities, comprising 3% of America's higher education population and contributing approximately $13 billion annually to the U.S. economy. During the same academic year the number of foreign scholars teaching or conducting research at doctoral degree granting universities grew almost 5% over the preceding year. A related entrepreneurial endeavor capitalizes on this same population of foreign students and scholars: intensive English programs. Rubin (1997, p. A48) describes these programs as "big business" and "money-makers."

The United States exports students through study abroad programs offered by the sending universities. Through such study students have an opportunity to heighten their cultural awareness, to further develop skills in a particular foreign language, to gain additional knowledge and skill in a particular field of study, and to gain a deeper appreciation of the diversity and the oneness of the world. Although they are called exchange programs, a one-to-one exchange is unusual.

The typical American participants are traditional university students: young and unencumbered. But less than 1% of this population, estimated at 13 million in 1998, actually takes advantage of international opportunities. According to the Institute of International Education Online (2000), of those participating abroad, approximately 90% are involved in programs of a semester duration or less. Western Europe remains the destination of choice, but recently some Asian countries have grown in popularity. The largest group of participants (35%) studied in

TABLE 15-2 United States Participation in Study and Teaching Activities Abroad

	1998-1999	Prior Year Change
U.S. Exports		
Students	113,959	+15.0%
Teachers and scholars	n/a	
U.S. Imports		
Students	490,933	+ 2.0%
Teachers and scholars	70,501	+11.3%

Data from Institute of International Education Online. (2000). Available: http://www.opendoorsweb.org.

the field of social sciences and the humanities, whereas only 3% studied in a health field.

Professors as well as students are exported, exchanged, or "loaned." Visiting professorships for a semester or for a year or more are available for many of the same reasons previously identified for students. Cross-pollination is intellectually stimulating for academia. In developing countries there may be insufficient numbers of qualified teachers; visiting scholars can help "round out" a faculty or provide consultation toward planning and implementing a new program. The visiting professor benefits, colleagues and students in the receiving institution benefit, and when the professor returns home, colleagues and programs in the sending university also benefit.

Beginning in the 1920s the idea of a supranational institute of higher learning surfaced from time to time with a designation such as World University. Essentially, the proposed models involved establishing a university in a small European country that would operate under the auspices of a multinational authority. The concept was laudable, but the initiatives did not come to fruition. Petty jealousies, worry that an existing national university would be offended, and concern that such an institution would not attract top quality personnel were among the roadblocks (Zweig, 1967).

The less grandiose international models of today usually involve existing universities in two countries that have worked out an agreement for sharing of curriculum and exchange of students and professors. In 1969, however, a unique international model got underway: the United Nations University (UNU). It is headquartered in Tokyo and has no students of its own. Rather, postgraduate or young postdoctoral researchers, mainly from universities in developing countries, are accepted as participants in a UNU training course, seminar, or workshop or are selected as UNU fellows. The mission of UNU is to contribute, through research and capacity building, to efforts to resolve the pressing global problems that concern the United Nations and its member states (source: United Nations University 2000. http:www.unu.edu).

Duderstadt (2000) believes that the existing traditional higher education model is inadequate but that the entrepreneurial nature of U.S. higher education is a strength that will help it adapt to new societal demands. He proposes nine models or paradigms as a response to the demands of the 21st century (Table 15-3).

In summary, Duderstadt (2000, p. B7) concludes, "It is unlikely that any one university will assume the exact form of any one of the models. . . . But each paradigm has features that will almost certainly be part of the character of higher education in America in this century."

INTERNATIONALIZING AMERICAN NURSING EDUCATION

The literature reveals the growing value American nursing places on internationalization, including curriculum, movement of students and scholars, and, to a lesser extent, programs offered across national borders. In fact, respected educator and past president of the International Council of Nurses, Dr. Gretta Styles (1994), referred to the new millennium as the "International Century" and described the world as a classroom.

Internationalization of nursing education began in earnest with curricular efforts to address America's nondominant cultures and promote cultural competence (Lester, 1998). Some schools include immersion experiences within an American cultural group that differs from the student's heritage (St Clair & McKenry, 1999). As national borders became more porous, the preparation of culturally competent practitioners was broadened to address a wider spectrum of people, cultures, customs, idioms, and health belief systems. And, in recognition of an increasingly interconnected and interdependent world, nursing added courses or curricular threads that incorporated international health issues (Freda, 1998; Henry, 1998). Concomitantly, many universities added or increased the comparative education aspects of their liberal arts/general education courses, thus complementing the nursing major courses.

Sending Institutions

But the changing world beckoned U.S. nursing across international borders, and academic programs became more involved with the movement of students and scholars. While opportunities for American students to study abroad have increased, it can be inferred from the numerical data presented earlier that only a few of the American participants in international programs are pursuing a degree in nursing. The programs reported in the literature vary in duration, but a few weeks is more typical than an entire academic term (Goldberg & Brancato, 1998; Haloburdo & Thompson, 1998; Ross, 1998; Stevens, 1998). A faculty member arranges for the experience and usually accompanies the nursing students. Before going abroad, students prepare themselves by exploring the culture, health, education, and other relevant aspects of the host country. Because many countries do not have the same legal constraints that govern practice and education

TABLE 15-3   Nine University Models Proposed for the 21st Century

Model	Description
World University	A research university with stated international focal points. While rooted in a local culture, its students, faculty, and programs reflect international diversity. Funding would come from international as well as state and national resources.
Diverse University	A bolder, richer model open to a multiplicity of approaches and opinions while recognizing that the institution is a "uni"-versity, not a "di"-versity. The challenge is to weave together the dual objectives of unity and diversity in a way that best serves the institutional mission and society.
Creative University	Shifts focus and priority from preservation or transmission of knowledge to the creation of new knowledge. Different forms of pedagogy will be needed to nurture creativity, and alliances with other creative entities such as the entertainment industry or Madison Avenue will occur.
Divisionless University	A far less specialized and more integrated institution with a web of structures, some real and some virtual, will provide both horizontal and vertical integration among the disciplines. Just as there is blurring between basic and applied research and between science and engineering, the academic disciplines and the professions will have more intimate relationships.
Cyberspace University	A distributed learning environment where the institution is a "knowledge server" linking learners anywhere in the world to a vast information network. Learning opportunities are available to anyone, anywhere, any time.
Adult University	A research university that admits only advanced, academically and emotionally mature students directly into graduate and professional schools. Reduces costs by relieving institution of its general education and parenting roles.
Lifelong University	The institution commits itself to a lifetime of interaction with its students. It would respond to changing goals/needs of graduates. Students and graduates would network, and alumni would actively participate in academic programs.
Ubiquitous University	The institution serves as a nexus of public culture, linking myriad social systems. It is a community learning center and knowledge network available to all either with local hubs or cyberspace entities—something more creative and accessible than present university extension programs and distance education.
Laboratory University	A testing site where new models of teaching, scholarship, and service would be investigated. It would exemplify a risk-tolerant culture for students and faculty in which failure would be accepted as part of the learning process associated with ambitious goals.

Data from Duderstadt, J.J. (2000). *A university for the 21st-century.* Ann Arbor, MI: University of Michigan Press.

in the United States, it is often possible for students to provide hands-on nursing care.

Receiving Institutions

A number of nursing schools receive foreign students, but the circumstances for foreign nurses who wish to study in the United States is more complex. Because of licensure issues, most students pursue graduate (postlicensure) study. For example, Emory University offers a bachelor of science in nursing (BSN) completion program to nurses who are graduates of a Taiwanese associate degree in nursing (ADN) program (Ryan, Markowski, Ura, & Liu-Chiang, 1998). Other institutions such as the University of Texas Medical Branch School of Nursing, the University of California, and the University of Michigan, to name a few, are well known for accepting foreign nurses as students.

Concerns arise when foreign nurses study in the United States or elsewhere for long periods, especially when these nurses come from countries with long-standing needs for more nurses. Akinsola (2000) purports that

these shortages far exceed those experienced in the United States. For example, in many countries empirics (people with elementary school education who are trained on the job) provide almost all direct nursing care. Can these countries afford to lose the services of even one of their educated nurses for a year or more of study? Does the perceived benefit to the nurse and, ultimately, to his or her country and its citizens justify this practice? What are the moral, let alone legal implications if a visa "overstay" occurs and the nurse disappears into the American populace. It is not uncommon that an individual from a developing country might find the United States more attractive given the substantial differences in the standard of living, remuneration for nursing services, and the quality of the work environment. Whether the educated person remains in America legally or otherwise, a country is deprived of its human resources, a phenomenon known as "brain drain" (Glaessel-Brown, 1998; Xu, Xu, & Zhang, 1999). "One nation's healthcare gain should not be another nation's drain" (Akinsola, 2000, p. 28).

STRESS AND INTERNATIONAL STUDENTS IN NURSING

Even though universities offer a great deal of support and specialized services to international students, the cultural differences, the curricular demands, and their own expectations for academic performance all add up to a stressful learning environment regardless of the field of study. Loneliness was identified as a problem for foreign nurse students by Kayser-Jones and Abu-Saad (1982). Other researchers identified stress arising from varied academic and practice expectations (Abu-Saad & Kayser-Jones, 1981; Maroun, 1991; Shearer, 1989; Wang & Lethbridge, 1995). Julian, Keane, and Davidson (1999) discuss problems of language and cultural differences as well as a sense of isolation and vulnerability. English language proficiency is considered pivotal. And, according to Julian et al. (1999), even formal lectures include nonstandard English. The clinical setting is even more challenging, the language requirements now extend to understanding professional jargon and nonstandard abbreviations. Technical procedures, role expectations, and problem-solving skills may differ greatly from their prior experience (Julian et al., 1999). These experiences all contribute to culture shock. Klineberg (1976) discusses two other kinds of shock. "Status shock" may occur when a student who was an individual of some renown at home is treated without deference in the host country. This individual perceives a great loss of personal stature. A third condition that may be more insidious is termed "national status shock." It occurs when foreigners sense that citizens in the host country consider their country inferior and backward.

RATIONALE FOR A NEW MODEL

It is possible to say with confidence that whether it is through curriculum, movement of students and scholars, or cross-national programs, efforts to internationalize education are desirable. And, there is agreement across the profession that there is a great need for nurses with a global perspective. The reality is that few American nursing students have an experience abroad. Nursing programs are also trying new ways to extend across borders, but currently the efforts are limited. The literature reveals that traditional university nursing programs have had some success using strategies such as e-mail, desktop video conferencing, Internet, and two-way video, but problems were also identified (Kim & Vetter, 1999; Kirkpatrick & Brown, 1999; Waddell, Tronsgard, Smith, & Smith, 1999). Some of the difficulties reported may have been related to unfamiliarity with the technology, lack of infrastructure within the university, or technical support services.

For foreign nurses coming to America there are concerns related to language difficulties, brain drain, licensure and hands-on care, culture, status, or national shock, the associated financial toll to the individual or sponsoring entity, and the emotional toll of leaving family and friends for extended periods. The efforts of existing traditional universities are needed, but more can be done through a different educational model for graduate nursing education.

In the proposed model an existing or emerging Internet university develops a graduate program in nursing that is committed through curriculum and cross-national partnerships to international nursing education. By beginning anew there is no need to try to make over an existing program or delivery system. The mission and philosophy of the new school of graduate nursing as well as its program delivery strategies are dedicated to preparing nurses who are able to approach practice with a global perspective and with experience in problem solving through international networking. By housing the new school in an on-line university the necessary infrastructure and technical support are already in place; the administrators, staff, and faculty are there because of expertise and commitment to a university without borders.

The curricula for the proposed graduate programs are derived from a review of the literature and through collaboration with cross-national nurse educators and practitioners. The master's curriculum focuses on problem identification and problem solving and the options are relevant to international practice including primary health care and international health (Bajnok, 1995; Orchard & Karmaliani, 1999; Parfitt, 1999; Thorne, 1997), forensic nursing and international law (Weaver & Lynch, 1998), humanitarianism and disaster relief (Murray, 1999; Robbins, 1999), health care systems and Western-non-Western foundations of health care and science (Brown, 1988; Henry, 1998; Lindquist, 1990), and cross-national practice and international credentialing (Glaessel-Brown, 1998; Parfitt, 1999; Xu et al., 1999). Students pursue functional role preparation as collaborator, researcher, and educator. At the doctoral level the focus is on the conduct of original research that addresses an international issue or problem related to one of the areas identified above. At both the master's and doctoral level, joint research among students of different countries is encouraged.

With cross-national practice and other international issues as the foci of a university program the number of international nursing experts would grow along with a

TABLE 15-4 International University—Graduate School of Nursing

Element	Description
Faculty	A core faculty of nurse educators at International University is responsible for the overall operation of the school and academic quality control. In addition, qualified nurse educators from countries throughout the western hemisphere hold part-time appointments. All faculty members come together at regularly scheduled on-line meetings through the use of two-way video technology.
Applicants	Must be a graduate of a baccalaureate program in nursing and recognized by the country of residence as a professional nurse.
Campus	The world. Coursework, including field experience, occurs in the country of residence; anywhere the student has access to a computer with Internet capability.
Library	Comprehensive library—including e-books, full-text journals, newspapers, and other periodicals—is available on-line all day, every day.
Services	Equipment specified; all software provided on CD-ROMs. On-line and telephonic technical support. Introductory modules to orient students to library usage and to various course components. Audio and video programs available on-line and by CD-ROM. Assistance with financial aid applications is provided. Translation programs provided.
Student life	Informal student exchange, such as might take place in the campus "quad," occurs in a dedicated chat room. Mechanisms for confidential on-line voting are in place. Bidirectional events such as candidate forums, guest speakers, and other social events are presented using teleconferencing capability.
Research defense	Theses and dissertations are orally defended before faculty, students, and other members of the university at on-line forums that may be open to the community.

body of research to address and assess this emerging field and discover its theoretical foundations. Fitzpatrick (1995, p. 166) emphasizes the need for involvement in a "global nursing education research community." However, notwithstanding the global rhetoric, nursing has not significantly changed its nature to be more globally relevant (Ketefian & Redman, 1997). A graduate level school of nursing dedicated to the international arena could significantly address this need. Future nurse leaders must be well versed in the global community and be a part of effective international networks (Kim & Berry, 1998). Advanced practitioners in international nursing will play an important role in the century of the global village, providing leadership and expertise, and making sure that nursing has input into global policy making affecting nursing and the health of nations.

PROPOSED INTEGRATIVE MODEL

To illustrate the proposed model the author draws on almost 20 years of experience in distance education, including 8 years working with accomplished colleagues in a number of Latin American countries. Among them are individuals who have earned a master's or a doctoral degree in nursing from the United States, many of them Kellogg Foundation fellows. The W.K. Kellogg Foundation has also supported the development of baccalaureate and master's in nursing science traditional and distance

education programs in Latin America. Given the extent of the region, however, opportunities for graduate nursing education are limited, and no Latin country presently offers a doctorate except Brazil, where the language is Portuguese. Thus, Spanish-speaking nurses seeking a doctorate face the same challenges and stresses identified earlier for foreign nurses who are away from home and studying in a second language. For all of these reasons and because the Western hemisphere countries will become more interdependent (the North American Free Trade Agreement is just a beginning), the proposed nursing education model deliberately links the United States and Latin America.

Located in the United States, the fictional International University (IU) offers an on-line graduate nursing program to professional nurses interested in international nursing issues. Although the Western hemisphere is the initial focal area, the program delivery system is such that students anywhere in the world can earn a master's or doctoral degree without going abroad. The tuition is reasonable because of low overhead: the campus is virtual—no classrooms, dormitories, cafeterias, or bookstores—just a headquarters for administration, student services, and faculty offices and conference facilities all equipped with the latest technology. A team of technical experts train faculty and students and stand by to assist them with hardware and software problems and to maintain the main server and several backup servers. Core faculty for each of the various disciplines are responsible for academic quality control assisted by faculty members from around the world who work with IU on a part-time basis. The library is extensive and virtual. Easily accessible databases lead students to books, journals, periodicals, and other publications, with full text download capability wherever available, a great resource that is covered by the tuition. The key elements of the program are presented in Table 15-4.

THE ACADEMIC TRANSACTION

The academic transaction, a dialogue between student and teacher in which raw information is transformed into knowledge through *negotiation of meaning,* is the heart of the teaching-learning process. Mallow and Gilje (1999, p. 250) further describe the process as the "translation of information as words, phrases, symbols, and nonverbal cues, which are filtered through the context of previous life experiences so meaning is assigned and concepts make sense. Traditionally, the academic transaction occurs simultaneously with information given in the classroom. In the proposed on-line program the teacher (or a team of teachers) prepares the learning materials that are available to students at any time through unidirectional asynchronous on-line formats. The academic transaction takes place through synchronous or asynchronous bidirectional on-line formats. These formats (Table 15-5) are automatically archived in print and audio versions. The computer transcript can be retained for use as a course reference, and it can be used by the institution for documentation of outcomes and subsequent program improvement.

Threaded Discussion. Many commercial on-line course templates include threaded discussion capability. This strategy is primarily a student discussion around a topic or question posed by the professor. The professor monitors the discussion to assess the frequency and quality of each student's participation and to interject and bring the discussion back on track when things go too far afield. The discussion appears in the form of a tree structure, and multiple areas can be on the table simultaneously. Even so, it is easy to follow from both a student and teacher standpoint. Students can also agree to meet on their own for discussion purposes. For example, they may want to pose their research question, and if it is of interest to other students, they may form an interest group or secure a research partner.

Video-on-Demand. This strategy allows the student to retrieve video clips that the professor has previously prepared or selected from commercial sources. The professor can easily tape a video through a computer-mounted camera in the faculty member's office. Also, impromptu videos can be prepared quickly. By following the threaded discussions, listening to student questions, and reading papers the professor becomes aware of areas that need clarification. A presentation via video-on-demand is an efficient way to provide the information.

Chat Room. Analogous to the quad, the cafeteria, or the coffeehouse on campus, the chat room is an on-line place for students to converse informally about academic and nonacademic topics. Students can chat asynchronously or, by planning ahead, they can arrange with peers to meet in the chat room at the same time. In this way they can have a synchronous, text-based conversation on line. The professor does not grade chat room activities and does not take any official role in the discussions. Since it really is a student convenience, a professor may elect not to drop in.

On-line capabilities are under continual refinement and expansion. By the time this publication is distributed, there will be more teaching-learning technology options to consider. It is important that an institution such as IU remain on the cutting edge and maintain its commitment

TABLE 15-5 On-Line Communication Methods

On-line Method	E-Mail	Audio Conference*	Video Conference*	Threaded Discussion	Chat Room	Video on Demand
Synchronous		X	X			
Asynchronous	X			X	X	X
Text	X	X		X	X	
Audio		X	X			X
Video			X			X
Bidirectional	X	X	X	X	X	
Privacy	X					X

*Teacher can send a private print message to an individual student during the conference.

to providing a superb infrastructure and technical support services to faculty and students.

LANGUAGE REQUIREMENT

Some readers no doubt have been pondering the question: How does International University, an accredited American institution, accommodate students whose primary language is either English or Spanish? The present reality is (1) most of the professional literature is only available in English; (2) most graduates of Latin American universities speak and read some English; and (3) most American university graduates do not speak or read Spanish. In the United States the regional accrediting bodies for higher education require that entering students are native English speakers or are graduates of a high school or university where the medium of instruction was English. If this is not the case, the applicant must demonstrate proficiency in English, usually through acceptable performance on the Test of English Fluency Language (TOEFL). There are solutions, however. For example,

- *Adjunctive strategies:* Through the use of technology, faculty, interpreters, and on-line translation programs, the language barrier can be surmounted, allowing the academic transaction to take place between student and professor. Accreditors may be willing to approve a pilot program to assess the effectiveness of this cross-national strategy.
- *Twinning:* One or more Latin American universities would formally validate the entire IU nursing curriculum and award the degree. Adjunctive strategies may be employed. The agreement between IU and the affiliating university could take a variety of forms, depending on particular needs and goals of the affiliating institution. For example, a consortium of Latin American schools might join with the IU to make the most effective use of resources. This is also a strategy to build the capacity of the Latin American university; as more nurses have graduate degrees the human resource issue as a barrier to initiating a master's or even a doctoral program is lessened.

SUMMARY

The proposed model takes extensive advantage of educational technology to span national borders and focuses on developing graduates with a worldview, particular expertise in international issues, and a ready network of international colleagues. The current state of educational technology, such as that described for IU, allows a variety of teaching-learning methods to occur at a distance in an academically sound and cost-effective manner (Lewis, 2000). Any number of studies over the years have concluded that it is not the methodology but the planning and execution of the program and the quality of the academic transaction that makes the difference, no matter whether the program is traditional or nontraditional and no matter whether the program is no-tech, low-tech, or high-tech (Jevons, 1990; Russell, 1999). The proposed model begins anew, not beholden to an existing faculty or curriculum but international from day 1 in its planning, execution, and faculty mindset. It is not heretical; it capitalizes on current university practices and extends them in unique ways. And, finally, it is not intended as a replacement for existing international programs but as another means of bringing students of many nations together through appropriate use of technology.

REFERENCES

Abu-Saad, H., & Kayser-Jones, J. (1981). Foreign nursing students in the USA: Problems in their educational experiences. *Journal of Advanced Nursing, 6*, 397-403.

Akinsola, H.Y. (2000, First Quarter). Nigeria unnoticed. *Reflections on Nursing Leadership*, 27-29.

Altbach, P.G., & Davis, T.M. (1999). Global challenge and national response. In P.G. Altbach & P.M. Peterson (Eds.), *Higher education in the 21st century* (pp. 3-10). (IIE Research Report No. 29). Annapolis, MD: IIE Books.

Bajnok, I. (1995). Organizational aspects of nursing education from a global perspective. In D.M. Modly, J.J. Fitzpatrick, P. Poletti, & R. Zanotti (Eds.), *Advancing nursing education worldwide* (pp. 151-159). New York: Springer.

Brown, L.D. (1998). Exceptionalism as the rule: U.S. health policy innovation and cross-national learning. *Journal of Health, Politics, Policy and Law, 23*(1), 35-51.

Commission on International Education. (1998). *Educating for global competence: America's passport to the future.* Washington, DC: American Council on Education. ERIC 421940.

Duderstadt, J.J. (2000, February 4). A choice of transformations for the 21st-century university. *The Chronicle of Higher Education,* pp. B6-B7.

Fitzpatrick, J.J. (1995). Pathways to implementing nursing education research globally. In D.M. Modly, J.J. Fitzpatrick, P. Poletti, & R. Zanotti (Eds.), *Advancing nursing education worldwide* (pp. 163-167). New York: Springer.

Fraser, S.E., & Brickman, W.W. (1968). *A history of international and comparative education.* Scott, Foresman.

Freda, M.C. (1998). International nursing and world health: Essential knowledge for the 21st century nurse. *American Journal of Maternal-Child Nursing, 23*(6), 329-332.

Glaessel-Brown, E.E. (1998). Use of immigration policy to manage nursing shortages. *Image, 30*(4), 323-331.

Goldberg, L.K., & Brancato, V.C. (1998). International education: A United Kingdom nursing student partnership. *Nurse Educator, 23*(5), 30-34.

Green, M.F. (1997, December 19). A choice of transformations for the 21st-century university. *The Chronicle of Higher Education,* pp. B6-B7.

Haloburdo, E.P., & Thompson, M.A. (1998). A comparison of international learning experiences for baccalaureate nursing students: Developed and developing countries. *Journal of Nursing Education, 37*(1), 13-24.

Henry, B. (1998). Globalization, nursing philosophy, and nursing science. *Image, 30*(4), 302-304.

Institute of International Education Online. (2000). Available: http://www.opendoorsweb.org.

Jenkins, K. (1997). Preparing students of color for global opportunities. *Black Issues in Higher Education, 14*(19), 33-35.

Jevons, F. (1990). Blurring the boundaries: Parity and convergence in distance education. In D.R. Garrison & D. Shales (Eds.), *Education at a distance* (pp. 135-144). Malabar, FL: Robert E. Krieger.

Julian, M.A., Keane, A., & Davidson, K. (1999). Language plus for international graduate students in nursing. *Image, 31*(3), 289-295.

Kayser-Jones, J.S., & Abu-Saad, H. (1982). Loneliness: Its relationship to the educational experience of international students in the United States. *Western Journal of Nursing Research, 4*(3), 301-315.

Ketefian, S., & Redman, R. (1997). Nursing science in the global community. *Image, 29*(1), 11-15.

Kim, S., & Berry, D. (1998). Beneath the surface: Models and strategies of collaboration across countries in doctoral education. *Nursing Leadership Forum, 3*(4), 130-135.

Kim, Y.S., & Vetter, R. (1999). An international distance learning nursing course in the U.S. and Japan. *Journal of Cultural Diversity, 6*(2), 48-56.

Kirkpatrick, M.K., & Brown, S. (1999). Efficacy of an international exchange via the Internet. *Journal of Nursing Education, 38*(6), 278-283.

Klineberg, O. (1976). *International educational exchange.* Paris: Mouton.

Lester, N. (1998). Cultural competence: A musing dialogue. *American Journal of Nursing, 98*(8), 26-33.

Lewis, J. (2000). Foundations in distance education. In J. Novotny (Ed.), *Distance education in nursing* (pp. 4-22). New York: Springer.

Lindquist, G.J. (1990). Integration of international and transcultural content in nursing curricula: A process for change. *Journal of Professional Nursing, 6*(5), 272-279.

Mallow, G.E., & Gilje, F. (1999). Technology-based nursing education: Overview and call for further dialogue. *Journal of Nursing Education, 38*(6), 248-252.

Maroun, V.M. (1991). Optimizing the potential of foreign nurses in the United States—Education's role. *Journal of Professional Nursing, 7,* 74.

Melby, J.F. (1961). The rising demand for international education. In T. Sellin (Ed.), *The Annals of the American Academy of Political and Social Science, 335.* Philadelphia: The American Academy of Political and Social Science.

Murray, J.S. (1999). Pediatric nursing health care delivery plan for humanitarian missions in developing countries. *Pediatric Nursing, 25*(4), 387-394.

Orchard, C.A., & Karmaliani, R. (1999). Community development specialists in nursing for developing countries. *Image, 31*(3), 295-299.

Parfitt, B. (1999). Working across cultures: A model for practice in developing countries. *International Journal of Nursing Studies, 36*(5), 371-378.

Robbins, I. (1999). The psychological impact of working in emergencies and the role of debriefing. *Journal of Clinical Nursing, 8*(3), 263-268.

Ross, C.A. (1998). Preparing American and Nicaraguan nurses to practice home health nursing in a transcultural experience. *Home Health Care Management and Practice, 11*(1), 66-70.

Rossman, P. (1992). *The emerging worldwide electronic university: Information age global higher education.* Westport, CT: Greenwood Press.

Rubin, A.M. (1997, December 12). Intensive English programs are lucrative for universities. *The Chronicle of Higher Education,* p. A48.

Russell, T.L. (1999). *The no significant difference phenomenon: As reported in 353 research reports, summaries, and papers* (4th ed.). Raleigh, NC: North Carolina State University.

Ryan, D., Markowski, K., Ura, D., & Liu-Chiang, C. (1998). International nursing education: Challenges and strategies for success. *Journal of Professional Nursing, 14*(2), 69-77.

Schofield, J. (1999, November 15). Learning on the front lines. *Maclean's, 112*(46), 90-94.

Shearer, R.A. (1989). Teaching foreign students. *Journal of Nursing Education, 28*(9), 427-428.

St Clair, A., & McKenry, L. (1999). Preparing culturally competent practitioners. *Journal of Nursing Education, 38*(5), 228-238.

Stevens, G.L. (1998). Research briefs. Experience the culture. *Journal of Nursing Education, 37*(1), 30-33.

Styles, M.M. (1994). Empowerment: A vision for nursing. *International Nursing Review, 41*(3), 77-80.

Thorne, S. (1997). Global consciousness in nursing: An ethnographic study of nurses with an international perspective. *Journal of Nursing Education, 36*(9), 437-442.

Vestal, T.M. (1994). *International education.* Westport, CN: Praeger.

Waddell, D.L., Tronsgard, B.A., Smith, A., & Smith, G. (1999). An evaluation of international nursing education using interactive desktop video conferencing. *Computers in Nursing, 17*(4), 186-192.

Wang, R.Y., & Lethbridge, D.J. (1995). Becoming gold-plated: Chinese nursing studying abroad. *Image, 27,* 131-134.

Weaver, J.D., & Lynch, V. (1998). Forensic nursing: Unique contributions to international law. *Journal of Nursing Law, 5*(4), 23-34.

Xu, Y., Xu, Z., & Zhang, J. (1999). International credentialing and immigration of nurses: CGFNS. *Nursing Economic$, 17*(6), 325-334.

Zweig, M. (1967). *The idea of a world university.* London: Feffer & Simons.

Broadening Clinical Education in Basic Nursing Programs

M. ELAINE TAGLIARENI, ANDREA MENGEL

The process of leading a faculty group into new territory is more about not knowing than knowing. The secret is in the searching for the answers, not in the answers themselves.
— Waters (1995, p. 75)

Nurse educators face a daunting task in today's health care environment. The task to develop interactive and contemporary curriculum models is complicated by the fact that there are no clear indicators to provide direction. Nursing faculty are perplexed by broad goals established by national organizations that provide focus but do not furnish clear indications for action: Healthy People 2000 (U.S. Department of Health and Human Services, 1990, 1995); Nursing's Agenda for Health Care Reform (American Nurses Association, 1991); A Vision for Nursing Education (National League for Nursing [NLN], 1993); the Pew Health Professions Commission (Shugars, O'Neil, & Bader, 1991); and National League for Nursing Accrediting Commission (1999). In this context, nursing faculty search for right answers and prescriptive pathways. Yet, at the same time, they look for ways to cling to traditional, more certain approaches. The notion that the process of seeking new ways is more about not knowing than knowing (Waters, 1995) can create confusion and inertia.

Today, professional education in the allied health sciences is concerned with balancing the known with the unknown. All health professions have been challenged to train tomorrow's practitioners for a health care environment that is more managed, integrated, dependent on evidence for performance, and focused on better utilization of information and communication technology. In fact, this new system, with ambulatory and community-based care as its locus, is expected to place greater emphasis in psychosocial dimensions of care (O'Neil & Coffman, 1998).

The need for faculty in basic nursing education to find reward and fulfillment by being with students in emerging environments of care is the most pressing challenge facing nurse educators today. Broadening clinical education to include interdisciplinary education, the ethic of social responsibility, technology (Heller, Oros, & Durney-Crowley, 2000), and integration of population-based, primary health care as the focus of the curriculum, is imperative. A corollary and related challenge is the need for all nursing educators, particularly on the undergraduate level, to find the common ground in nursing education and practice. This common ground will build strong articulation pathways for nursing students and reveal a shared purpose for nursing: working together to improve the health status of Americans.

THE CHALLENGE TO FACULTY: MOVING AWAY FROM TRADITIONAL MODELS

Neither undergraduate nor graduate education in nursing has prepared faculty for any but the behaviorist curriculum model . . . most faculty, regardless of academic degrees, have not been prepared for the shift in thinking and interacting with students. [Bevis & Watson, 1989, pp. 111-112]

Coming to terms with new approaches to basic nursing education is not easy. It requires a posture that traditionally has not been played out in nursing education where earnest desire to embrace innovation has been counterbalanced by a tendency to retain traditional approaches. But the old ways, developed when acute care and less integrated systems provided direction for curriculum choices, no longer fully address the needs of the health care environment (Tagliareni & Sherman, 1999). The old ways create gaps in basic nursing education as preparation for future professional practice. In a fluid and rapidly changing work environment, the traditional objective driven approach, with a focus on content rather than process, does not prepare students for interactive and collaborative practice.

As Bevis and Watson (1989) suggest, nursing faculty's preparation impedes their ability to forsake institution-based curriculum strategies and shift to health promotion and disease prevention models of nursing care delivery. Nothing in the history of nursing has helped to ground faculty in a large-scale, community-based health care system where a collaborative and colearner model of teaching and learning is required. Nursing faculty first learned to be nurses in a behavioral, content-laden, measurable, structured curriculum (Bevis & Watson, 1989). Objectives for learning flowed from an orientation to what to teach rather than how to teach. Traditionally teachers were aligned to content rather than the process of learning. Nursing faculty's introduction to nursing and their allegiance to the profession occurred in a curriculum model in which it was possible to learn "all" nursing content in the basic curriculum. And nursing faculty have taught subsequent generations of nurses utilizing this same model, spending endless hours at curriculum planning meetings moving content from one semester to the other and debating the efficacy of adding or deleting content (Tagliareni & Sherman, 1999). Nursing faculty grew and developed as practitioners of nursing in an acute care, disease, and hospital-based care system. In this context, there has been little time to think about the process of learning and to align the teacher with the student as the primary way to promote learning.

It requires new thinking for faculty to move from an allegiance to cure models of intervention to ones that include community-based health promotion, disease prevention, and health restoration. It is imperative that chairs and deans in basic nursing programs create opportunities for all faculty to free themselves from traditional approaches to curriculum design that cannot and will not hold true in today's health care system and empower faculty to implement strategic curriculum change. With strong leadership and a work environment that supports and fosters experimentation, innovation will unfold.

This is not a shift that faculty in undergraduate nursing education traditionally embrace. The resulting chaos and paradoxes contrast with the comfort of certainty and right answers that derive from old lecture notes and time-honored approaches to clinical education (Tagliareni &

Sherman, 1999). Yet this is the challenge to nursing faculty today: to create collaborative, interactive education models that enhance community-based approaches to clinical learning.

BECOMING AN EXPERT NOVICE

> [S]tudents are not the only novices; any nurse entering a clinical setting where she or he has no experience with the patient population may be limited to the novice level of performance if the goals and tools of patient care are unfamiliar. [Benner, 1984, p. 21]

Moving to new practice settings and new curriculum models unsettles nursing faculty. In order for faculty to understand fully the environment of a new practice setting and take on new teacher roles, they must first become novices in that setting. Yet faculty are not complete novices in an integrated health care system, where community-based care is the cornerstone of practice. They bring expert knowledge of teaching and learning strategies to this environment and convey years of experience from acute care on curriculum decisions. Assuming the novice posture presumes that these abilities will not transfer intact and that faculty will be open to experiences in new settings, in order to learn new and different ways of knowing students and clients. During the W.K. Kellogg Community College Nursing Home Project, the term "expert novice" was developed to describe the lived experience of the faculty adapting to the unique characteristics of a new practice setting (Waters, 1991). "Being an expert novice then means being open to the differences in the practice setting in order to recognize opportunities for innovative nursing approaches to healthcare delivery. It means entering a new practice environment knowing that previous acute care models cannot be wholly transferred to the new setting" (Tagliareni & Murray, 1995, p. 367).

The community, as well as in the nursing home, requires a shift from reactive to proactive teaching and interactive caregiving. In the community, faculty must create the learning opportunities rather than react to urgent acute care needs. In the community it is essential for both faculty and students to collaborate with interdisciplinary staff and with families to understand significant health care needs. Interventions develop slowly because it takes time to listen, collaborate, and plan health care outcomes together with clients and community partners.

To faculty accustomed to reactive, fast-paced, and more structured clinical learning environments, this change can seem inefficient, cumbersome, and less than rewarding. Therefore, the move to community-based clinical settings requires that deans and chairs allow faculty time to be expert novices and develop new clinical experiences. It requires deans and chairs to support faculty during their adjustment to a proactive and collaborative teaching and practice environment.

It is our belief that with support and guidance faculty can move out of their comfort zones and embrace new approaches to teaching. What is essential is a fundamental understanding that the ways that worked in acute care do not work in a consumer-driven, integrated, health care system. The old ways do not assist faculty and students to develop skills for a community-based model of care. A fundamental change in the faculty teaching role is required in new community-based environments of care.

THE CHALLENGE TO FACULTY: FINDING COMMON GROUND

We need to focus less on the traditional meaning of the degree and more on the purpose of the basic preparation at each level. [Mengel & Donnelly, 1999]

The big challenge facing basic nursing education today is preparing RNs for emerging roles. Practice in community-based settings requires new management and technical skills and a new emphasis on health promotion and disease prevention. Traditionally these competencies have been part of baccalaureate nursing education. However, the current distribution of registered nurses by educational levels and the demographic characteristics of the registered nurse workforce should spur faculty in both associate degree and baccalaureate degree nursing programs to create complementary paths in all levels of nursing education in order to meet the health care needs of the country.

What are the implications of current demographic trends in the registered nurse population? Associate degree nursing programs graduate more registered nurses per year than baccalaureate degree programs, and the number of graduations from associate degree programs has risen faster than the number from baccalaureate degree programs. Every year approximately 60% of new registered nurse graduates are educated at the associate degree level. The last 25 years have witnessed a shift to associate degree programs as the main source of new RNs with only a relatively modest increase in the percentage of new registered nurses educated at the baccalaureate level (O'Neil & Coffman, 1998).

To adjust for this change, an updated model for basic nursing education is needed. This model would build in the strengths of the present model. This model requires a willingness by nursing faculty on both the associate degree and baccalaureate level to forgo traditional curriculum models and conventional definitions of 2-year and 4-year nursing programs. What is needed is a common ground for education and practice. This common ground would have multiple exit points (associate degree, baccalaureate, master's, and doctorate) and would focus on population-based local health needs in a community-based health care system.

Already changes are taking place. Baccalaureate nursing programs have used in-depth community assessment to determine the character of the community and the shape that care delivery should take. Associate degree educators, cognizant that many of their graduates will deliver care in the local community, are beginning to include educational experiences to heighten the students' awareness of the nature of the community and its resources (Tagliareni & Marckx, 1999).

In Philadelphia, for example, associate degree and baccalaureate nursing educators are finding complementary paths as they reinvent nursing education at both levels to meet the needs of the changing health care delivery system. At Community College of Philadelphia, associate degree nursing students in the 19130 Zip Code Project learn to develop partnerships with community-based agencies (Tagliareni & Coleman, 1999). The project focuses on extending existing primary health care services rather than on creating new services. As a result, the nursing students are developing ways to connect people with existing services. In the process, students are learning collaboration skills and extending care to those in need.

The complementary path widened in Philadelphia, spurred on by unmet health needs as well as the collegial relationships and mutual respect of nursing leaders in both associate degree and baccalaureate nursing programs. This unique collaboration is successful for two reasons. Both types of nursing programs have adopted populations in their local neighborhoods, providing an opportunity for students to learn in homes, schools, churches, and other nontraditional settings. As a result, concerns about overlapping service areas and competition for community sites have not materialized. Second, movement to neighborhood-based care has taught nursing faculty that concepts of population-based health care and research are essential in all levels of the undergraduate nursing curriculum. Rather than beginning with a model to differentiate practice and education, which traditionally has created barriers to collaboration, faculty have worked together to build coherent articulation pathways that acknowledge the skills and abilities acquired at the associate degree level. Thus, community-based care has become the common ground for strong articulation models.

Undergraduate nurse educators share the mission of designing learning activities to prepare nurses for the job market. Enhanced articulation models for nursing education can build on the strengths of the current educational system, grafting each level of education on the previous level, resulting in a more efficient and effective model. Grafting is an apt metaphor for another reason: it symbolizes a commitment to living in harmony and sharing the same space and resources as a thriving, integrated whole (Mengel & Donnelly, 1999).

It is our belief that there are complementary roles for associate degree and baccalaureate nurse educators. The move to population-based systems of care has reinforced that nursing curricula derives from practice and practice demands a workforce that is competent in population-based approaches to nursing care. Past models of conflict and competition will not address this demand. Practice today requires a new set of skills that includes community assessment, interdisciplinary management competencies, documentation for evidenced-based practice, utilization of research for care planning, and evaluation of health impact and cultural sensitivity in nontraditional community-based settings (American Association of Colleges of Nursing, 1999; National League for Nursing Accrediting Commission, 1999; O'Neil & Coffman, 1998; Tagliareni & Mengel, 1999). For nurse educators to meet the challenge of preparing registered nurses with these competencies, this skill set can and must be taught and leveled at both associate degree and baccalaureate levels of nursing education.

BASIC NURSING EDUCATION: REFINING THE MISSION

For a viable future, we must discover how to be vibrantly alive to one another, to inhabit one another's worlds . . . to be committed to the welfare of the whole. We must learn to look at health problems, indeed at world problems, not from a standpoint of how they will affect me now, but how they will affect the community as a whole now and in the future. [Bevis, 1993]

Historically, commonalities have existed in both levels of basic nursing education. Both associate degree and

baccalaureate nursing education have sought a balance between liberal and technical education. Both have seen social relevance as part of their mission. An outstanding example has been the public health efforts with immigrant populations of baccalaureate educators and the education of immigrant populations in community colleges. While social relevance remains a deeply held value in both kinds of programs, one of the most crucial issues facing nursing is the underrepresentation of minority nurses.

Today the nursing profession includes only small numbers of individuals from culturally diverse backgrounds. Though individuals from minority populations represent about 35% of the United States population, minorities comprise less than 10% of the approximately 2 million nurses currently licensed to practice. A significantly lower percentage of minority registered nurses hold a graduate degree in nursing. Minority representation in basic nursing education is equally disheartening. The percentage of minority nurses in undergraduate programs has grown to only 7% to 10% within the last 5 years (NLN, 1997; O'Neil & Coffman, 1998). It is our belief that education of a diverse workforce hinges on community colleges, which will continue to be the entry point for many ethnic minorities.

If current trends continue, the number of racial and ethnic minority students enrolled in basic nursing education programs will not be sufficient to alter significantly the racial and ethnic composition of the registered nurse workforce. Basic nursing education needs to prepare nurses who are qualified to address health issues germane to a growing minority population and provide culturally sensitive care. The enrollment and retention of nursing students from minority backgrounds is a critical issue in nursing education.

These enrollment data are particularly worrisome when viewed in the context of changing demographics of the American population and the increased health care needs of vulnerable minority populations. Urban and rural poor Americans, historically underserved, have been the primary beneficiaries of public health initiatives and public health nursing. Their lack of access to health care continues to be a considerable problem that needs to be addressed by all levels of nursing education.

With an ethnically diverse workforce, nursing will be better able to provide culturally sensitive health care. This should enhance nurses' ability to collaborate with individuals and communities when delivering population-based care. The current and continuing emphasis on cost-effective care, the nursing care needs of home care clients, aggregates with specific health risks, and the undeserved present challenges as urgent as addressing the primary care needs of the general population (Mengel & Sherman, 1997).

In some ways, debate about whether an associate or baccalaureate degree is the right educational preparation for nursing's mission to serve the public is an artifact of the late 20th century. The new health care system demands a nurse who can prove effectiveness of both cost and quality through evidence-based practice. Now is the time for nursing to consolidate its place in a rapidly changing system by supporting multiple entry and exit points for nursing education while integrating community-based approaches across all levels of basic education.

FUTURE IMPLICATIONS

As nurses, we are magnetically attracted to certainty. There are surely good explanations for our discomfort with ambiguity, both historical and sociological, but continuing to act as though there is always or almost always one right answer handicaps us now more than ever. [Waters, 1995, p. 75]

Changes in the health care system are changing basic nursing education and nursing practice. Negotiating these changes and strengthening nursing's position in the reordered health care system will test nurse educators' cohesion and flexibility. As nurse educators from both associate degree and baccalaureate degree nursing programs fully embrace a common ground in a community-based health care system, basic nursing education will begin to define a new vision for action. It is imperative that nurse educators find ways to develop faculty commitment to a collective vision that calls for a greater sense of collaboration and to a curriculum that is responsive to changes in health care.

Waters' discovery that the key to faculty development and curriculum reform is found in the searching for answers, not in the answers themselves (Waters, 1995) provides a framework for faculty action in an emerging health care system. There is no magic formula for curriculum reform; no one design will fit all nursing programs uniformly. The challenges of an ambiguous, uncertain health care future cannot be addressed with rigidity. Nor can these challenges be addressed with standardized or traditional approaches to undergraduate nursing education. Faculty who are creative, agile, innovative, and willing to accept community-based care as the common ground will lead the way.

In a recent editorial, Dr. Helen Grace of the W.K. Kellogg Foundation asked nursing to champion the educa-

tional diversity (multiple entry points) of the profession. She cautioned nursing leaders that the biggest political risks for nursing were the divisions within nursing itself. Dr. Grace concluded by asking nursing to speak with one voice on the complex educational structure of nursing education. "If nursing unites, celebrating its diversity by demonstrating the role that nurses, from all educational levels, play in improving the health of the people, the future is promising. If the divisions continue, nursing's seat at the table will continue to be in jeopardy" (Grace, 1998, p. 3). If the divisions continue and if undergraduate nursing faculty continue to hold on to traditional, time-honored approaches to curriculum development and clinical education, they will miss the opportunity to recast, revitalize, and restructure for the future of nursing.

REFERENCES

American Association of Colleges of Nursing. (1999). *Essential clinical resources for nursing's academic mission.* Washington, DC: Author.

American Nurses Association. (1991). *Nursing's agenda for health care reform.* Kansas City, MO: Author.

Benner, P. (1984). *From novice to expert.* Menlo Park, CA: Addison-Wesley.

Bevis, E.O. (1993). All in all, it was a pretty good funeral. *Journal of Nursing Education, 32*(3), 101-105.

Bevis, E.O., & Watson, J. (1989). *Toward a caring curriculum: A new pedagogy for nursing.* New York: National League for Nursing Press.

Grace, H. (1998). Missed opportunities, use and abuse of private philanthropic resources by nursing. *Nursing and Health Care Perspectives, 19*, 3.

Heller, V.R., Oros, M.T., & Durney-Crowley, J. (2000). Ten trends to watch. *Nursing and Health Care Perspectives, 21*(11), 7-15.

Mengel, A., & Donnelly, G. (1999). Associate degree and baccalaureate degree nursing education, finding complementary paths in a population-focused health care system. In M.E. Tagliareni & B. Marckx (Eds.), *Teaching in the community, preparing nurses for the 21st century* (pp. 95-101). Boston: Jones and Bartlett.

Mengel, A., & Sherman, S. (1997). Access to higher education for all Americans—the role of associate degree nursing. In V. Ferguson (Ed.), *Educating the 21st century nurse* (pp. 109-118). New York: National League for Nursing Press.

National League for Nursing. (1993). *A vision for nursing education.* New York: Author.

National League for Nursing. (1997). *NLN nursing data book.* New York: Author.

National League for Nursing Accrediting Commission. (1999). *Interpretive guidelines for standards and criteria.* New York: Author.

O'Neil, E., & Coffman, J. (Eds.) (1998). *Strategies for the future of nursing.* San Francisco: Jossey-Bass.

Shugars, D., O'Neil, E., & Bader, J. (1991). *Healthy America: Practitioners for 2005, an agenda for U.S. health professional schools.* Durham, NC: Pew Health Professions Commission.

Tagliareni, M.E., & Coleman, I. (1999). Associate degree nursing students assess neighborhood health care. In M.E. Tagliareni & B.B. Marckx (Eds.), *Teaching in the community, preparing nurses for the 21st century* (pp. 210-223). Boston: Jones and Bartlett.

Tagliareni, M.E., & Marckx, B.B. (Eds.). (1999). *Teaching in the community, preparing nurses for the 21st century.* Boston: Jones and Bartlett.

Tagliareni, M.E., & Mengel, A. (1999). Nursing competencies in community settings, results of a community-based DACUM activity. In M.E. Tagliareni & B.B. Marckx (Eds.), *Teaching in the community, preparing nurses for the 21st century* (pp. 51-64). Boston: Jones and Bartlett.

Tagliareni, M.E., & Murray, J. (1995). Community focused experiences in the ADN curriculum. *Journal of Nursing Education, 43*(8), 366-371.

Tagliareni, M.E., & Sherman, S. (1999). When ambiguity replaces certainty, new faculty roles in community settings. In M.E. Tagliareni & B.B. Marckx (Eds.), *Teaching in the community, preparing nurses for the 21st century* (pp. 20-34). Boston: Jones and Bartlett.

U.S. Department of Health and Human Services. (1990). *Healthy people 2000: National health promotion and disease prevention objectives.* Washington, DC: U.S. Government Printing Office.

U.S. Department of Health and Human Services. (1995, Fall). Healthy people 2000—a mid-decade review. *Prevention Report,* 1-60.

Waters, V. (1991). *Teaching gerontology.* New York: National League for Nursing Press.

Waters, V. (1995). *The narrative enlarging.* New York: National League for Nursing Press.

Broadening Clinical Education in APN Graduate Education Programs

MARILYN L. ROTHERT, GERALDINE J. TALARCZYK

Nursing education has the task of preparing the next generation of nurses to practice successfully in a rapidly changing health care system. The expectations and opportunities new graduates will face are difficult to predict at the time of the students' entry into a nursing program. As the roles, competencies, and practice sites change, so too must the education. This chapter focuses on the clinical education component of programs for advanced practice nurses (APN). Factors including population demographics, competencies identified by the profession for APN curricula, and the relationship between the health care systems and nursing education have a major impact on the future of nursing education for APNs.

BACKGROUND

Changing demographics influence health care priorities as well as nursing practice. By 2020 more than 20% of the population will be 65 years of age or older, with the fastest growing group those over 85 (Heller, Oros, & Durney-Crowley, 2000). The country's aging population is requiring more health care resources, which is adding to the growing shortage of nurses, particularly APNs (American Association of Colleges of Nursing [AACN], 1999).

Population diversity is also impacting nursing and practice. Gary, Sigsby, and Campbell (1998) note that workplace leaders of the future must be able to manage unity in diversity. They argue that cultural diversity should be a key element in all components of nursing. The 1996 U.S. Census Bureau predicts that by 2010 the percentage of Hispanics will exceed the percentage of blacks. After 2050 Hispanics are predicted to comprise more than 25% of the population, and blacks, Asians, and American Indians will comprise 24% (U.S. Department of Commerce, 1997). These population characteristics will require the ability of nurses and other health profes-sionals to understand the risk variance, unique lifestyle, and diets across populations, as well as the communication skills needed to understand the multiethnic, multicultural patient mix for whom they will care (Katz, 1999).

A number of guidelines have been developed that give direction to the overall curricula for APN educational programs. For example, the AACN published *The Essentials of Master's Education for Advanced Practice Nursing* in 1996. This document presents a graduate core curriculum that addresses major content areas but is less specific about the description of clinical experiences for APN nursing curricula. It directs the reader to advanced practice nursing specialty organizations and accrediting bodies for the defined number and types of clinical experiences required for specific educational programs.

The National Organization of Nurse Practitioner Faculties (NONPF) Curriculum Guidelines Task Force (1995) has established guidelines for educational programs for nurse practitioners. These guidelines are organized into domains that represent practice competencies. The content included in the NONPF document is nearly identical to the AACN guidelines, although different in organizational format. It addresses recommendations for required number of clinical hours, faculty and preceptor qualifications, and contractual agreements but offers little detail regarding the characteristics of clinical learning experiences. Specialty organizations have also developed curriculum guidelines for their unique groups.

Other guidelines have been developed related to essential competencies for practice in managed care. These often are directed at physician education but are similar to those cited earlier, with increased emphasis on such areas as evidence-based practice, population-based medicine, continuous quality improvement, teamwork and coordination of care, and economics of health care (Council on Graduate Medical Education, 1997).

Recently a study was reported that determined the extent to which nurse practitioner (NP) educational programs are addressing the curricular topics related to practice competencies recommended in the AACN and NONPF documents as well as those recommended by the Pew Health Professions Commission in 1995 (Bellack, Graber, O'Neil, Musham, & Lancaster, 1999). Program Directors were asked to rate curricular topics by ideal emphasis and current emphasis. The topics that evidenced the greatest discrepancy between ideal and current were information systems, health care economics and financing, environmental health, and case management. In addition, Hall and Stevens (1995) emphasized the need for core courses about community health in all graduate nursing programs regardless of specialty and role. They argue that nurses must look not only at individual health behaviors and responses to health problems but must also focus on larger community-based conditions that affect health and illness.

Since nursing is a practice profession, nursing education must rely on a collaborative relationship with the health care system to acquire teaching and learning sites for students. The dynamics of the health care delivery system, especially its financing, are threatening the conventional means of access to clinical practice sites and are requiring a rethinking of how nurse educators facilitate clinical learning and experiences. The magnitude of the issue was identified in a survey of AACN members in 1998 in which 84% of the respondents indicated their programs were experiencing problems related to a decline in number of or a difficulty in placing students at clinical sites. Most frequently cited barriers were a shortage of new available sites, sites not accepting a large enough number of students, difficulties in recruiting or retaining preceptors, potential preceptors already fully committed to other professional responsibilities, competition for access to clinical facilities with other schools of nursing and other health professional schools (Task Force on Essential Clinical Resources for Nursing's Academic Mission, 1999).

Increasingly clinical institutions have little or no vested interest in the educational enterprise. Contrasted with other fields, the health care industry has focused attention primarily on the funding, development, and advancement of medicine to the exclusion of most other health professions. With the pressures from managed care for increased productivity coupled with declining financial resources, there is an increasing expectation of some clinicians and agencies to be compensated for educational effort, funds nursing programs do not currently

have. One contributing factor to the inequitable distribution of moneys may be the failure of nursing education to include clinical staff and agencies in the planning and implementation of nursing education programs. This results in a lack of buy-in and access to industry financial support for educational programs. This is in contrast to other professional schools, such as colleges of medicine and business, who partner with their respective industries. Lack of involvement by clinical nursing staff in the educational process may also stem from failure of nursing to create a professional culture that embraces the mentoring and instruction of future members of the profession. To date, neither nursing education nor practice has advocated for the formation of partnerships.

According to the AACN 1998 Institutional Database, 113 of 568 institutions reported having a nursing center administered or owned by the school of nursing. These nursing centers represent a dramatic shift away from dependence of nursing education on outside clinical agencies. Nursing centers provide not only needed clinical services, frequently in underserved areas, but also rich opportunities for both faculty and student practice and research. The financial impact of a nursing center on the school is variable and is dependent on external sources of funding, contracts with third-party payers, and patient resources.

These background characteristics require institutions of graduate nursing education to reassess traditional clinical education for APNs, including curricular content, sites for clinical education, instructional strategies, and financing. Discussion and recommendations are addressed below.

REDEFINING CLINICAL EXPERIENCE

Recommendation: The clinical experience for NP students should include exposure to health care finance, management, and policy and application of concepts related to evidence-based practice, decision making, ethics, and cultural competence.

No longer is health care delivered by practitioners with a sole focus on the health care needs of a single patient and the family. Today's practice takes place in a complex network of health care systems within the context of political, social, and financial agendas that directly affect the APN's practice. Cost-effective health care is a major focus of funding and health care agencies.

In the education of APNs it is essential that students gain the skills and knowledge necessary to practice within this environment and learn strategies to apply this knowledge in clinical practice. This suggests that a part of the clinical experience be a rotation in areas such as risk management, claims, practice management, and billing. APN students need to gain experience with practice report cards reflecting benchmarks of practice. In addition, APN students need to understand the relationship between health care policy and practice and to learn skills and gain experience in strategies designed to influence policy.

Patient care is the focus of clinical education, and this too has added dimensions that are important to the functioning of an APN. The education of an APN must include experiences in application of concepts of evidence-based practice, decision making, ethics, and cultural competence.

Evidence-based practice involves integrating clinical expertise with the best available external clinical evidence drawn from research (Sackett, Haynes, Guyatt, & Tugwell, 1991). The core content drawn from epidemiology and economics is relatively new to nursing. The broader term of clinical decision making includes concepts drawn from social psychology and cognitive processes (e.g., bounded rationality, heuristics, and biases), foundational knowledge from the study of ethics, and a basic understanding of statistics and the decision analysis model based on Bayes theorem.

APNs function in a health care setting that requires rapid decision making. The magnitude of information available is enormous, yet prediction is uncertain and the knowledge available is almost always incomplete. APNs require a set of skills to identify the key information for the patient problem and to understand the notion of probability and the change in probability of a disease or outcome based on new information. To understand their own and patient decision-making processes and behaviors, they need to know human limitations to cognitive processing and the limitations of human information processing that can lead to inappropriate shortcuts and biases in the decision-making process.

In addition, APNs need to have skills and knowledge to support patients in making wise choices about their health. There is a growing supply of decision supports for patients and providers that can assist them in making informed decisions (Bernstein et al., 1998; Michie, Smith, McClennan, & Marteau, 1997; O'Connor et al., 1998; Rothert et al., 1997). Clinical education should include knowledge of and experience in the use of decision supports and the ethical decisions related to health care. For example, if an informed patient chooses, after reviewing all information, to refuse recommended therapeutics that constitute the standard of practice, the APN must know

the ethical, legal, and political issues related to the situation to best support the patient and maintain integrity of practice. These components of clinical decision making should be integrated into the practice setting in an applied rather than conceptual way.

To be prepared to care for all the people of this country, APNs must have knowledge of other cultures at a level that enables them to respect the differences and understand patients in the context of their culture. This requires more than textbook definitions and conceptual discussions. It requires experience with other cultures, preceptoring and mentoring by caregivers with other cultural backgrounds, and language skills where appropriate. An international experience in which a student can be immersed in another culture for a period of time may become an important part of the curriculum. While this may not be a possibility for all at the present time, course objectives can require skills and a minimum knowledge base. Clinical experiences can be acquired among local populations and through student and faculty exchanges with nursing programs involved with diverse populations.

SITES FOR CLINICAL EDUCATION

Recommendation: Instead of health professions competing for clinical education sites, collaborative sites should be developed where students in medicine, nursing, and other professions learn together, define their roles and their differences, and develop strategies to work as a team.

Both medicine and nursing have identified issues in locating sites for clinical education. As clinical care has moved from hospitals to primary care sites in the community, clinical education sites have become smaller and are competing for revenues. Clinical sites have indicated increasing reluctance to accommodate students unless they are reimbursed for the "lost revenue" associated with educating students (Bellack & O'Neil, 2000). Medical education is, by any definition, better funded than nursing education, and the ability to pay preceptors at clinical sites is more of an option for medicine than nursing. It is also extremely difficult to have interdisciplinary education without interdisciplinary practices, and such practices are difficult to find. So, on the face of it, the argument that there should be collaboration among health professions related to clinical education may seem naïve and self-serving.

However, putting aside the argument of cost, there are strong reasons why interdisciplinary education should continue to be pursued. In 1997 the AACN called for the health care industry to scrutinize costs and maximize efficiency by shifting from an environment of competition to one of collaboration (AACN, 1997). Interdisciplinary education is necessary for interdisciplinary practice and visa versa. The AACN and others have differentiated the terms *multidisciplinary* and *interdisciplinary*. Multidisciplinary efforts involve several professions working in parallel and often with separate goals; interdisciplinary education coordinates health care and other fields in collaborations that include joint planning, decision making, and responsibility. The latter is clearly the needed focus of clinical education.

Foundations have identified interdisciplinary education as a critical need and invested in developing such programs. For example, seven community-focused projects were funded in 1992 by the W.K. Kellogg Foundation to increase the number of primary care providers by establishing academic primary care centers where students could be educated in primary care with an interdisciplinary approach. While the outcomes were impressive, so too were the challenges identified during these projects in bringing together community and multiple health professional schools, usually including medicine, nursing, and others. The Robert Wood Johnson Foundation is currently funding initiatives identified as Partnerships for Quality Education (PQE). The newest effort asserts that a key element in the new practice environment is the ability to provide seamless coordination of care that can best be achieved by teams of people working together. It is noted that for primary care practitioners to work effectively in teams, they must train in teams. This concept led the most recent phase of educational grants to address building team and collaborative practice among APNs and physicians (Moore, 1998).

Collaboration in clinical education requires the active support of the clinical setting. Creative solutions are needed, and Bellack and O'Neil (2000) challenge us by asking, "Can partnerships with managed care organizations be created in a way to enlarge the learning space, number of faculty, and clinical learning experiences of students while maintaining quality of the educational program?" Hospitals are rapidly developing into health networks that include a variety of settings for clinical education related to primary care and tertiary care services. Clinical sites in health care networks would be logical places for collaborative education. However, the professions will be required to provide data regarding the benefit of such arrangements to the health care system.

Health care centers owned and operated by nursing should take their place in the list of sites for collaborative health professions clinical education. Centers run by nurses may have collaborative arrangements with medicine that include arrangements for physician services with faculties of medicine to support patient care. This arrangement can provide a strong basis for collaboration in education. The centers must, however, be established on solid business principles so that the management and business aspect can be a realistic experience for students. Most frequently, nurse-managed centers focus on underserved populations and are built financially on grants, college funds, and other soft money sources rather than relying on revenue generated from practice. Use of nonrecurring funds to support recurring costs does not provide a realistic setting to teach health care finance.

For interdisciplinary education to occur, there must be strategies to address appropriate content as well as location for clinical education. The skills needed for collaboration such as negotiation and team building are not frequently found in current curricula (AACN, 1997). It would seem logical that interdisciplinary approaches need to be taught experientially, placing the burden on clinical education to bring together multiple disciplines. If we can bring together medical and nursing students to learn together, debate issues related to role, and pool their thinking in the care of patients, we may achieve the goal of interdisciplinary approaches to health care. Content of mutual concern such as finance and the business of health care, ethics, and the role of technology could be taught across professions.

INSTRUCTIONAL STRATEGIES

Recommendation: Clinical education should incorporate the various technological methods needed in practice.

Technology is becoming imbedded in the practice of APNs in a variety of ways. Communication with patients can take place through e-mail, web, and fax. Telehealth options allow for video images of patients from their homes as well as patient data among providers at distant sites. Medical records are increasingly computerized providing accessibility from various locations. The APN must become comfortable with the technology to incorporate strategies that enhance the care of the patient.

Technology has also revamped the information flow in health care. Patients can access information from the Internet, information that may or may not be consistent with standards of practice. Decision aids are increasingly available to assist patients in understanding and making wise choices regarding their health. Decision supports are also available to providers in a variety of formats. Palm-held computers hold current information that the APN can access regarding guidelines for a specific condition, medication options, and differential diagnoses given a specific symptom complex. Specific programs are available on CD-ROM or other formats to address complex areas such as the management of menopause. Clinical information is available on the Web from journals, research sites, and associations focused on specific disease entities.

With the avalanche of information, the APN must be able to navigate and evaluate the resources to provide effective, efficient care. The clinical educational experience must provide the foundation by integrating the technological resources into the student experience. This is necessary to build the skills that enable APNs to continually increase their professional knowledge and draw on technology for decision support in their practice.

FINANCING OF CLINICAL EDUCATION

Recommendation: Nursing needs to benchmark the need, cost, and contributions of APN education to inform the graduate medical education (GME) debates and build new partnerships with community settings.

In recent years there has been growing recognition of the need for primary care practitioners, both physicians and APNs, because of managed care and inadequate access for patients. Primary care takes place predominately in the ambulatory setting. Ambulatory settings are finding it difficult to accommodate health professional students citing issues such as clinical productivity, cost, and space (Boex et al., 1998).

Although a large portion of hospital-based GME costs are reimbursed by Medicare ($6.3 billion for 1996), essentially no such funds are directed to pay the costs of ambulatory care training. Nursing, with the exception of diploma programs, has generally not shared in the GME dollars and has few options to obtain sustained funding for APN education. The need for and investment in medical education is clearly recognized; the need for investing in nurse practitioner education has not been clearly recognized.

Gold (1999) notes that a major impediment to reimbursement is the lack of understanding of the costs of training and the tradeoff between clinical productivity and educational productivity of faculty. To understand the costs, it is necessary to measure clinical productivity of the trainee, which depends on educational level.

The literature identifies little data on the costs of nursing training in the ambulatory setting. When asking for increased funding for health professions education, the Bureau of Health Professions is challenged to present evidence-based hard data to support requests for level or increased funding for nurse education. Also, the Office of Management and Budget seeks data proving the market does not assure an adequate supply of nurses to justify requests for additional funding for nurse education (Spencer, 1999).

This raises questions about nursing that we are ill prepared to answer. Nursing frequently cites that the graduate APN student functions on the student's own license and, therefore, can be more productive than medical students. However, the benchmarks used for productivity do not always capture the nursing practice. Gold (1999) states that the professions of faculty and trainees affect the cost equation since nonphysician faculty as a rule do not command the high level of reimbursement that physicians do, and nonphysician trainees are not usually capable of residents' high level of clinical productivity.

Two concepts are missing from this argument. The first is reassessment of the variable productivity currently measured only by time and quantity. Nursing must add variables such as patient outcomes, number of return visits and hospitalizations to capture fully the productivity of APNs. These variables not only reflect quality of care but also cost containment in capitated models.

Secondly, nursing must collect data around need and impact of clinical education on primary care sites. We must accurately define productivity and cost implications on primary care settings serving as clinical sites. This assessment must include individual provider by profession, case mix, and quantity and quality of outcome redefined to include patient status. Work such as that of Mundinger (2000) provides a framework for the task facing nursing to identify the data needed to garner the resources required for APN education.

These issues are critical to nursing education. The serious issue of funding cited frequently in medical literature in relation to GME impacts the future of APN education. If primary care providers receive payment for serving as preceptors to medical and other health professional students, nursing may well lose their sites for clinical education unless new revenue streams can be identified.

SUMMARY

In summary, APN clinical education is facing critical issues as well as opportunities. After reviewing key constructs related to changing demographics, current guidelines, and status of collaborative relationships, a series of recommendations are proposed:

1. The clinical experience for NP students should include exposure to health care finance, management, and policy and application of concepts related to evidence-based practice, decision making, ethics, and cultural competence.
2. Instead of health professions competing for sites for clinical education, collaborative sites should be developed where students in medicine, nursing, and other professions learn together, define their roles and their differences, and develop strategies to work as a team.
3. Clinical education should incorporate the various technological methods needed in practice.
4. Nursing needs to benchmark the need, cost, and contributions of APN education to inform the GME debates and build new partnerships with community settings

These recommendations do not require a linear sequence of experiences but can be organized to fit within the time frame allocated to clinical education in most APN programs. It must be acknowledged that clinical education must continue to change as the health care needs and systems change. The goal is to position the student to learn within the system so that the changes are immediately experienced by the student.

One other note is essential. As the new skills and knowledge are identified for students, they must also be learned by faculty. This requires strategies to support faculty development and developing sites for faculty practice. The skills and knowledge required in practice is changing at a rate that requires nursing education to be positioned within the system to prepare the APNs of tomorrow.

REFERENCES

American Association of Colleges of Nursing. (1996). *The essentials of master's education for advanced practice nursing.* Washington, DC: Author.

American Association of Colleges of Nursing. (1997, July). Once rare, interdisciplinary training gains ground. *AACN Issues Bulletin,* Washington, DC: Author.

American Association of Colleges of Nursing. (1999, April). Faculty shortages intensify nation's nursing deficit. *AACN Issues Bulletin,* Washington, DC: Author.

Bellack, J.P., Graber, D.R., O'Neil, E.H., Musham, C., & Lancaster, C. (1999). Curriculum trends in nurse practitioner programs: Current and ideal. *Journal of Professional Nursing, 15*(1), 15-27.

Bellack, J.P., & O'Neil, E.H. (2000). Recreating nursing practice for a new century: Recommendations and implications of the Pew Health Professions Commission's final report. *Nursing and Health Care Perspectives, 21*(1), 14-21.

Bernstein, S.J., Skarupski, K.A., Grayson, C.E., Starling, M.R., Bates, E.R., & Eagle, K.A. (1998). A randomized controlled trial of information-giving to patients referred for coronary angiography: Effects on outcomes of care. *Health Expectations, 1,* 50-61.

Boex, J.R., Blacklow, R., Boll, A., Fishman, L., Gamliel, S., Garg, M., Gilchrist, V., Hogan, A., Meservey, P., Pearson, S., Politzer, R., & Veloski, J. (1998). Understanding the costs of ambulatory care training. *Academic Medicine, 73*(9), 943-947.

Council on Graduate Medical Education. (1997). *Resource paper: Preparing learners for practice in a managed care environment.* Washington, DC: U.S. Department of Health and Human Services, Public Health Service, Health Resources and Services Administration, Bureau of Health Professions.

Gary, F.A., Sigsby, L.M., & Campbell, D. (1998). Preparing for the 21st century: Diversity in nursing education, research, and practice. *Journal of Professional Nursing, 14*(5), 272-279.

Gold, M. (1999). The changing US health care system: Challenges for responsible public policy. *The Milbank Quarterly, 77*(1), 3-37.

Hall, J.M., & Stevens, P.E. (1995). The future of graduate education in nursing: Scholarship, the health of communities, and health care reform. *Journal of Professional Nursing, 11*(6), 332-338.

Heller, B.R., Oros, M.T., & Durney-Crowley, J. (2000). The future of nursing education: Ten trends to watch. *Nursing and Health Care Perspectives, 21*(1), 9-13.

Katz, L.B. (1999, January). Growing Hispanic population poses major health care implications. *Health Policy Bulletin.* Lansing, MI: Public Sector Consultants, Inc.

Michie, S., Smith, D., McClennan, A., & Marteau, T.M. (1997). Patient decision making: An evaluation of two different methods of presenting information about a screening test. *British Journal of Health Psychology, 2,* 317-326.

Moore, G.T. (1998). Preparing for change. *The Q Connection: A Newsletter Published by Partnerships for Quality Education, 6,* 1.

Mundinger, M.O., Lane, R.L., Lenz, E.R., et al. (2000). Primary care outcomes in patients treated by nurse practitioners or physicians. *Journal of the American Medical Association, 283*(1), 59-68.

National Organization of Nurse Practitioner Faculties Curriculum Guidelines Task Force. (1995). *Advanced nursing practice: Curriculum guidelines and program standards for nurse practitioner education.* Washington, DC: Author.

O'Connor, A.M., Tugwell, P., Wells, G.A., Ehnslie, T., Jolly, E., Hollingworth, G., et al. (1998). Randomized trial of a portable, self-administered decision aid for postmenopausal women considering long-term preventive hormone therapy. *Medical Decision Making, 18,* 295-303.

Rothert, M.L., Holmes-Rovner, M., Rovner, D., Kroll, J., Breer, L., Talarczyk, G., Schmitt, N., Padonu, G., & Wills, C. (1997). An educational intervention as decision support for menopausal women. *Research in Nursing Health, 20,* 377-387.

Sackett, D.L., Haynes, R.B., Guyatt, G.H., & Tugwell, P. (1991). *Clinical epidemiology: A basic science for clinical medicine* (2nd ed.). Boston: Little, Brown and Company.

Spencer, S. (Ed.). (1999). Slants & trends. *Legislative Network for Nurses, 16*(9), 67.

Task Force on Essential Clinical Resources for Nursing's Academic Mission. (1999). *Essential clinical resources for nursing's academic mission.* Washington, DC: American Association of Colleges of Nursing.

U.S. Department of Commerce. (1997). The Hispanic population in the United States: March 1996 (update). *Current Population Reports* (US Census Bureau Report P20-502). Washington, DC: Census Bureau.

Critical Thinking

What Is It and How Do We Teach It?

M. GAIE RUBENFELD, BARBARA K. SCHEFFER

While critical thinking has been on parade as the sine qua non of nursing for the past decade, as a profession we are still diversified—and at times mystified—in our conceptions of just what critical thinking is and is not. To date nurses and nurse educators have borrowed definitions of critical thinking from outside the profession, the most recent being those of the American Philosophical Association (Facione, 1990) and Paul (1992). Our teaching of critical thinking is as diversified as the multiple definitions that are used. Nursing literature is full of suggestions for teaching approaches (e.g., Baker, 1996; Dowd & Davidhizer, 1999; Perciful & Nester, 1996; Thompson & Rebeschi, 1999; Weis & Guyton-Simmons, 1998). Much of the focus on teaching critical thinking has been spurred on by the mandates from accrediting bodies to teach and evaluate nursing students' critical thinking abilities. Unfortunately, because nursing has not committed itself to a nursing-specific definition of critical thinking, what and how we teach may not have the best grounding in critical thinking in nursing. An even more serious issue is the use of standardized and/or nonstandardized test scores that purport to represent critical thinking of students. Because the existing standardized tests for measuring critical thinking are not based on nursing conceptualizations of critical thinking, what is being tested may not indicate who will or will not be a good critically thinking nurse in practice.

We hope some light will be shed on the subject of defining critical thinking in nursing with a recently completed descriptive research study (Scheffer & Rubenfeld, 2000). Between 1995 and 1998, the authors conducted a Delphi study to develop a consensus statement on critical thinking in nursing. An international panel of 55 expert nurses from nursing practice, education and research participated in five rounds of questions and answers that resulted in a consensus statement, a list of 10 habits of the mind and seven skills for critical thinking in nursing and definitions of those habits and skills. Habits of the mind are affective dispositions toward critical thinking, and skills are those cognitive tasks used to think critically. The consensus statement is:

> Critical thinking in nursing is an essential component of professional accountability and quality nursing care. Critical thinkers in nursing exhibit these habits of the mind: confidence, contextual perspective, creativity, flexibility, inquisitiveness, intellectual integrity, intuition, open-mindedness, perseverance, and reflection. Critical thinkers in nursing practice the cognitive skills of analyzing, applying standards, discriminating, information seeking, logical reasoning, predicting and transforming knowledge. [Scheffer & Rubenfeld, 2000]

While this statement has not been widely disseminated yet, it is tempting to conjecture about its impact on the profession and, specifically, on nursing education, which have not heretofore had a discipline-specific description of critical thinking. Although there are certainly similarities between this statement and others found in the critical thinking literature, there are also significant differences. Specifically, expert nurses think that creativity, intuition, and a contextual perspective are important habits of the mind necessary for critically thinking nurses. Among the skills, transforming knowledge and predicting stand out as unique to nursing's definition of critical thinking.

Huge implications for teaching accompany the acceptance of this consensus statement. In this chapter we will present each habit of the mind and skill along with the definitions of those terms as agreed on by the Delphi study panel. (See boxes on pp. 126 and 129.) Then we will discuss the implications for teaching those components of critical thinking to nursing students. The habits and skills are arranged in alphabetical order because the Delphi participants elected not to attempt consensus on prioritizing them at this time.

Before addressing each habit and skill, it is important to clarify two points. First, it is becoming apparent that some of our existing teaching methods may actually prevent nursing students from developing critical thinking. We will offer some suggestions to counter this situation. Second, although we artificially separate the components of critical thinking, it is extremely important to appreciate that, in reality, the components work together. They are in synergy with each other.

The first habit of the mind (see the box below) is confidence, defined as "assurance of one's reasoning abilities." This is a tough habit to develop in novices who feel inadequate and believe they can do nothing right at first. Confidence in their critical thinking skills has been found to be low in nursing students (Colucciello, 1999; Haffer & Raingruber, 1998). Nursing's tradition of academic ter-

---

CRITICAL THINKING IN NURSING HABITS OF THE MIND

Confidence: assurance of one's reasoning abilities

Contextual Perspective: considerate of the whole situation, including relationships, background and environment, relevant to some happening

Creativity: intellectual inventiveness used to generate, discover, or restructure ideas; imagining alternatives

Flexibility: capacity to adapt, accommodate, modify, or change thoughts, ideas, and behaviors

Inquisitiveness: an eagerness to know by seeking knowledge and understanding through observation and thoughtful questioning in order to explore possibilities and alternatives

Intellectual Integrity: seeking the truth through sincere, honest processes, even if the results are contrary to one's assumptions and beliefs

Intuition: insightful sense of knowing without conscious use of reason

Open-mindedness: a viewpoint characterized by being receptive to divergent views and sensitive to one's biases

Perseverance: pursuit of a course with determination to overcome obstacles

Reflection: contemplation on a subject, especially one's assumptions and thinking for the purposes of deeper understanding and self-evaluation

Data from Scheffer, B.K., & Rubenfeld, M.G. (2000). A consensus statement on critical thinking in nursing. *Journal of Nursing Education, 39,* 352-359.

---

rorism, under the guise of teaching and learning principles, has done much to promote this lack of self-confidence. In spite of proponents of humanistic nursing education (Ironside, 1999a, 1999b; Middlemiss & Van Neste-Kenny, 1994; Bevis & Watson, 1989; Watson, 1999), some teaching methods have not changed much since Florence Nightingale was in the business! Nursing students are led to believe they cannot make mistakes, that "only perfect practice is permissible in clinical areas" (Watson, 1999, p. 37). In such anxiety-producing situations students' brains regress to what Hart (1983) called reptilian (survival) levels of function. Anxiety prevents them from accessing their higher order thinking skills to retrieve even their basic knowledge. Classic oppressed group behavior that has plagued our female-dominant profession is too often what students see among nurse educators and practicing nurses (Jewell, 1994). No wonder students have no self-confidence! Nursing faculty can no longer teach as they themselves were taught—with fear tactics—and expect students to learn to think critically. Learning must become a safe partnership process between educator and student. This is no easy feat; however, it is imperative that we break the bonds of oppressive behavior that have squelched nursing's potential for years.

The second habit of the mind identified by the Delphi panel, contextual perspective, means "being considerate of the whole situation, including relationships, background and environment, relevant to some happening." That context is what makes nursing so nonlinear, muddy, and challenging to teach. Nursing students, particularly those in early adulthood, tend to be linear thinkers when they start out (Benner, 1984; Rambur, 1999); they are used to memorizing content given to them in lock-step lectures and readings. Helping them to become relativistic thinkers is no small endeavor. One of nursing's great ironies is that we preach the importance of the context but evaluate learning through context-free multiple choice tests. Even state board exams are set up this way. There is little room for the "but what if" style of thinking when students are expected to produce the one "correct," noncontextual answer that will be the basis of their grades. One way to overcome this in a classroom situation is to allow and encourage students to challenge test answers, to show how alternative answers could be just as valid or better. Situational, application-style questions on exams increase students' contextual perspective to some degree, but there is still emphasis on the one "right" answer. Evaluating students' contextual perspective is probably best done in clinical situations where the context is real or in computer simulations using "nonsterilized" case studies.

Creativity is one habit of the mind that is unique to nursing's definition of critical thinking as compared to those of other disciplines. Yet, Daly (1998) proposed that the generation of new ideas (creativity) is a necessary component of the problem-solving process used in critical thinking in general. It was defined in our study as "intellectual inventiveness used to generate, discover, or restructure ideas; imagining alternatives." We believe that nursing is one of the most creative professions. For example, consider the student nurse who was able to engage a resistive adolescent on the psychiatric unit by challenging her to walk backwards with the student through the hallways. How much do faculty promote this kind of creativity in students? Is the student rewarded for creativity or chided for not maintaining "norms"? Watson (1999) saw it this way: "Despite nursing faculty rhetoric about nurses being autonomous professionals . . . faculty . . . usually reward obedience and conformity rather than assertiveness, questioning and difference. Such authoritarian approaches stifle the creative, inquisitive, risk-taking behaviors necessary for a mature health profession" (p. 37). Do we stifle creativity by giving students boxes into which they must confine their thinking? Mind mapping, or concept mapping, is one approach that gets away from thinking in boxes (Beitz, 1998; Daley, Shaw, Balistrieri, Glasenapp, & Piacentine, 1999; Rooda, 1994; Rubenfeld & Scheffer, 1999). Students are encouraged to record their unique thinking paths in learning situations. In clinical situations, for example, students can be coached to articulate and follow their personal thinking journeys as they work with patients.

"Flexibility—the capacity to adapt, accommodate, modify or change thoughts, ideas and behaviors"—is certainly important in the ebbs and tides of nursing's muddy waters. It is difficult for nursing students to be flexible, especially if, as novices, they have just learned the "right" path. Beginning students have a limited repertoire of approaches with which to achieve flexibility. Flexibility is best learned through role-modeling by faculty who are comfortable thinking aloud as situations change around them. Faculty who can address student questions during a class and still stay on task exemplify classroom flexibility. Those who can maintain calm approaches as patient situations change drastically provide excellent examples of flexibility in practice. The nurse educator who says to the student, "Hmm, this doesn't look like it's going to work. Let's rethink what and how *we* need to do this," is modeling flexibility, thinking, and partnership in learning.

Inquisitiveness, that wonderful characteristic of 3-year-olds, somehow gets snuffed out early in the student's educational journey that begins in grade school. The Delphi panel of experts defined this habit as "an eagerness to know by seeking knowledge and understanding through observation and thoughtful questioning in order to explore possibilities and alternatives." This habit has also been identified in most other disciplines' descriptions of critical thinking. Colucciello (1999), using the California Critical Thinking Dispositions Inventory, found inquisitiveness scores to be low in her sample of nursing students. Students who have managed to hang on to their natural curiosity and bring it to their learning of nursing are a joy to most teachers. On the other hand, trying to reinstill that characteristic in those who have lost it is a huge challenge. Certainly the biggest deterrent to inquisitiveness is when a teacher responds by saying, "That's a stupid question." "You should know that; you had that last year," while not as blunt, is a comparable comment. The student who does not want to be revealed as having forgotten something may stop asking questions. Faculty nonverbal behavior, voice tone, raised eyebrows, or frowns send even stronger messages than words. Rewarding the process of learning or the questioning as being equal to the outcome of learning is one approach that works. Instead of only grading end products, faculty can also grade students' questions. Mind maps, especially when they are shared among groups of students, are one way to promote that questioning. Questions asked by students during their thinking journeys can be as important as the answers. When students hear faculty exclaiming, "Great question!" they soon learn that questioning is a good thing.

"Intellectual integrity is seeking the truth through sincere, honest processes, even if the results are contrary to one's assumptions and beliefs." This habit is similar to what Facione (1990) called "truthseeking" and was one of the stronger traits found in Colucciello's samples of BSN students (1999). In nursing, it is intellectual integrity that will keep a nurse away from premature closure during conclusion making and will remind the nurse to verify those conclusions. Many students, used to being "spoon-fed" information, need to learn how to question what they read, to critique more openly. Because students often choose one tried-and-true path to knowledge, they need help to recognize that there are multiple ways of knowing and discovering information (Rambur, 1999; Stein, Corte, Colling, & Whall, 1998). Unfortunately for some students, these multiple paths to knowledge reveal the ambiguity of many health care issues. To work through that ambiguity, they must persevere in their quest to find the best "truth" in the situation. Taking time to explore various perspectives on complex issues is a helpful exercise. Consider the concept of family for example; it may be defined biologically, legally, sociologically, ethically, etc. Asking students to define family, therefore, can be a lesson in intellectual integrity.

"Intuition, the insightful sense of knowing without conscious use of reason," is not surprisingly a habit of the mind for nurse critical thinkers. It is not, however, acknowledged as a part of conceptualizations of critical thinking in other disciplines. In recent years, intuition has received "sanction" through descriptive nursing research (Benner, 1984; Benner, Tanner, & Chesla, 1996). Prior to that time, it was suspect in nursing, for some a subjective, "woman" thing that should not be promoted in the credible, positivistic world of science-based nursing. Talk to any practicing nurse, however, and you will soon hear that intuitive responses are an essential part of the repertoire of everyday nursing decision making. Intuition, because it develops with experience, is difficult to teach to beginners. Faculty can help students pay attention to how mature nurses use intuition every day and encourage them to pay attention to their own beginning "gut reactions." Guiding students to describe their thinking processes will help them become aware of the intuitive parts of their thinking. Those descriptions come with reflection, which is the 10th habit of the mind to be described later. A simple intuition-promoting activity is to ask students to describe their first responses to a situation and to reward them for not self-censoring their responses to such a question. Following up with, Why do you think that was your first reaction? can promote reflection on intuitive responses. Students can be helped to acknowledge their growing intuition in nursing and learn how to validate it before acting on it. They can also develop nursing intuition by reflecting on how they use intuition in other parts of their lives.

The eighth habit of the mind is "open-mindedness—a viewpoint characterized by being receptive to divergent views and sensitive to one's biases." That attitude of openness has been the gold standard for approaches to diverse patient needs throughout nursing's history. We say that we value open-mindedness. We are seeing more and more emphasis through courses and content on multicultural perspectives. On the other hand, we don't see students being encouraged to challenge faculty viewpoints, nor do we consistently encourage debate within our faculty ranks. Faculty cannot hold themselves up as infallible and all-knowing, not in today's complex world. We must look at our self-confidence and question if it can withstand student challenges and challenges from other faculty as well. Critical thinking is nurtured by open debate with our students and our peers.

"Perseverance—pursuit of a course with determination to overcome obstacles"—has implications for clinical teaching. Do faculty promote perseverance or do they hinder it if students don't perform appropriately on the first try? Within the time constraints of clinical teaching it is far too easy to give students the answers or show them where to find answers, without supporting their efforts to slog through various options until they overcome obstacles and make a path through the chaos. How should faculty promote perseverance? Obviously, there is a high risk of frustrating students with assignments that become complex hunting trips. A happy medium will have to be found between allowing for perseverance and necessary efficiency. Faculty must also give students credit for the process of hunting and not just for the end product of the hunt.

Reflection is the final habit of the mind identified by the nursing Delphi panel. It was defined as "contemplation upon a subject, especially one's assumptions and thinking for the purposes of deeper understanding and self-evaluation." Like confidence, inquisitiveness, intellectual integrity, and open-mindedness, reflection seems to be a universally accepted characteristic of critical thinkers across disciplines. It is often referred to as metacognition. Reflection was the cornerstone of Schon's seminal work *The Reflective Practitioner* (1983), as well as the subject of many other texts (Brookfield, 1995; Osterman & Kottkamp, 1993). Yet, reflection does not happen automatically, nor is it easy to do. Sure, students can relate what they think about, but they often do not have an adequate vocabulary to describe how they think. They can be helped in this task by written guides such as the Critical Thinking Inventory (Rubenfeld & Scheffer, 1999) or Brookfield's (1995) four lenses to achieve reflection. Reflection takes time and energy; faculty must take care that they do not expect students to have immediate insights into their thinking and their behaviors. Detailed self-reflection must be valued and rewarded so students will develop this as a habit.

In summary, the critical thinking habits of the mind can be promoted through teaching methods that focus on the process as well as on the outcomes of learning. With beginning definitions of these habits, there is an increased probability that both faculty and students can operationalize these habits.

The seven critical thinking skills identified by the international panel of nurse experts (see the box on page 129) also have some similarities to critical thinking skills

---

CRITICAL THINKING IN NURSING SKILLS

Analyzing: separating or breaking a whole into parts to discover their nature, function, and relationships

Applying Standards: judging according to established personal, professional, or social rules or criteria

Discriminating: recognizing differences and similarities among things or situations and distinguishing carefully as to category or rank

Information Seeking: searching for evidence, facts, or knowledge by identifying relevant sources and gathering objective, subjective, historical, and current data from those sources

Logical Reasoning: drawing inferences or conclusions that are supported in or justified by evidence

Predicting: envisioning a plan and its consequences

Transforming Knowledge: changing or converting the condition, nature, form, or function of concepts among contexts

---

Data from Scheffer, B.K., & Rubenfeld, M.G. (2000). A consensus statement on critical thinking in nursing. *Journal of Nursing Education, 39,* 352-359.

---

in other disciplines. However, some skills emerged that are specific to nursing. Just as faculty can promote critical thinking habits of the mind, so too they can help students develop the skills. Care must be taken, however, that the skills are not taught outside the context of the habits of the mind. If faculty try to teach skills rigidly, as entities unto themselves, students will have difficulty learning the skill, and their companion and complementary habits can be squashed as well.

The first skill identified by the nurse experts in the Delphi study—analyzing—seems to be fairly universal to conceptualizations of critical thinking across disciplines. "Analyzing is separating or breaking a whole into parts to discover their nature, function and relationships." At face value, this skill seems to be in conflict with the contextual perspective habit of the mind, but effective analysis must also be seen in context. For example, each component of a community (police department, health department, citizenry) can be separated and assessed as individual entities, but they must also be examined in context as they relate to each other and the community as a whole. Although the breaking apart is artificial, it is a necessary task to better understand the role of the pieces. Unfortunately, there are no rules about how far or in what ways something must be broken down to best understand the issue at hand; it is a highly individualized skill. Take for example, an IV drug calculation. There are a variety of ways to break down that process to achieve the accurate drug administration. Some ways make sense to some students and no sense to others. A great teaching challenge is to help students find their own method of breaking things down so that the analysis process can be both meaningful and produce accurate results. Analyzing for some requires keeping the overall picture in mind for the parts to make sense; for others, analyzing requires focusing on the individual pieces without worrying about the bigger picture. For faculty who have long practiced a personal analytical approach, allowing for, trying to understand, and valuing the analytical approaches of students or peers takes open-mindedness and self-confidence.

The second skill, applying standards, defined as "judging according to established personal, professional, or social rules or criteria," is, perhaps, unique to nursing's definition because nursing is an applied science in the health care field. This skill must constantly be balanced with creativity. There are certain things that just *have* to be done in nursing—period. Patient rights, for example, cannot ever be ignored; nurses cannot restrain patients without absolute safety justifications. A nursing challenge is to define clearly just what those standards are and to consider if they confine or stimulate thinking possibilities. Take, for example, the perceived "standard" that nurses must have a physician's order to perform certain nursing interventions. That perception has stifled many a critical thinking opportunity. If a diabetic patient starts to act strangely, believe it or not, there are nurses who think they cannot check a glucose level via a finger stick without a doctor's order. This, of course, virtually eliminates the possibility that the nurse can collect adequate information to make a reasoned decision. Faculty must help students understand the fuzzy perimeters of nursing and medical practice and how Nurse Practice Acts and institutional rules can and should be operationalized. Case situations that reflect muddy reality are always helpful for such learning. Discussions of what nurses can or cannot do are especially helpful to beginning level students who come into the profession having formed their opinions of nursing from the media, which often depict nurses in confined roles and the nursing profession as ancillary to medicine.

Discriminating is another skill necessary for critical thinking in nursing as well as in other fields. It is defined as "recognizing differences and similarities among things or situations and distinguishing carefully as to category or rank." This skill is vital to clustering patient data so that all possible conclusions can be considered. Students need help distinguishing crucial pieces of information from those with less importance. Consider the thinking involved in making a decision about timing the administration of ferrous sulfate, for example. Drug books state that it is absorbed better without food but that at the same time it can cause gastrointestinal (GI) upset on an empty stomach. The beginning nursing student has no frame of reference to know that avoiding the GI upset is more important, that it is better to give the drug with meals and risk the less-important loss of absorption. It becomes a matter of probabilities. From our perspective, that lack of knowledge about relative importance is one of the most frequent frustrations expressed by students. Faculty need to emphasize constantly the discriminatory aspects of information to help students make distinctions. Guidelines for setting priorities are helpful, but experience and critical thinking, not books, provide the best guidelines.

Information seeking, the next skill, is the "searching for evidence, facts or knowledge by identifying relevant sources and gathering objective, subjective, historical and current data from those sources." This skill may seem so obvious that it could be overlooked in its importance to critical thinking. But the appropriate depth of information-seeking must be identified. Students learn the basic skill of collecting information from patients, families, and others in health assessment courses. To achieve more depth, students need to learn alternatives to gathering information, for example, with patients who are noncommunicative. Perhaps even more necessary is helping students learn how to dig for information and to appreciate that no one person, book, or computer search has all the answers. Rambur (1999) argued that we must "help students reconceptualize themselves as seekers of information" (p. 272). This skill, of course, is closely tied with the habits of perseverance, creativity, and intellectual integrity.

The fifth skill, logical reasoning, defined as "drawing inferences or conclusions that are supported in or justified by evidence," is often misconstrued as encompassing the whole of critical thinking. Granted it is important, but only in context with the other critical thinking skills and habits. Helping students to describe their logical reasoning to the point of a conclusion will help them see that there must be supporting evidence for their conclusions. Such learning helps students consider the power of their biases as well. We have developed one exercise we call Bertha's Body, which is helpful in examining the logical reasoning behind conclusions. Bertha, 5 feet, 2 inches, and 150 pounds, wears baggy sweat pants to her clinic appointment. Based only on that information, beginning students are asked to describe their initial hunches about Bertha. Some conclude she is depressed about her weight or self-conscious about her looks. When asked to support their conclusions with evidence, they see that the conclusions are completely based on societal or personal biases and not on evidence. When other possibilities are pointed out (e.g., Bertha is pregnant; she has just come from a gym workout, where she is a weight-lifter), students begin to recognize the impact of biases and the need for evidence-based conclusion making.

Predicting, defined by the Delphi panel as "envisioning a plan and its consequences," is unique to nursing's definition of critical thinking skills and also gets overlooked as a skill that beginning students must start to learn. Because of the complexity of nursing, faculty often reduce problem solving to a linear process as a way to teach it to novices. When students make decisions about the best nursing diagnosis for a particular cluster of data, they will be more discriminating if their developing skills in prediction are prompted. They can be encouraged to look beyond the diagnostic label to what they will do to implement care for their first choice of a nursing diagnosis. For example, a patient is crying over the death of her husband a month earlier. Most novice students jump to the language-matched nursing diagnosis of dysfunctional grieving. Students who are encouraged to think forward to their nursing interventions for that diagnosis soon realize that they would not encourage that patient to stop crying, that the grief is not dysfunctional, and so on. Without that predictive thinking, the student may waste time and energy going through a linear version of the nursing process trying to force ineffective interventions to fit the selected nursing diagnosis. Nurse educators can help students develop their skills of predicting by nurturing students to ask themselves consistently, What will happen if . . .?

The seventh skill, transforming knowledge—"changing or converting the condition, nature, form or function of concepts among contexts"—is a most valuable skill in nursing as a practice discipline and applied science. This is perhaps the skill most crucial to students applying classroom-learned knowledge to clinical situations. To the frustration of many faculty, students do not automatically recognize the importance of assessing peripheral circulation in diabetics just because they had a lecture on the complications of diabetes. Students need help in seeing how that situation is similar to what was discussed in class, or transforming that knowledge to the clinical situation. In the "old school" approach to nursing, it was thought that faculty could teach all the vital health care and nursing content to students. We know today that this is impossible. Health care and nursing have become much too complex; the sheer volume of content is so huge, it is unthinkable that it can be taught. We propose countering that reality with the skill of transforming knowledge; we must teach students how to find and transfer the information rather than simply parroting back facts on an examination.

In summary, as a result of the Delphi study, the nursing profession, including nurse educators, has consensus on descriptions of critical thinking habits of the mind and skills that are unique to nursing. The hours and hours of critical thinking contributed by the international panel of nurse experts has broadened our perspective of critical thinking in nursing. According to their consensus, nursing has several components that are unique to nursing—creativity, intuition, contextual perspective, predicting, and transforming knowledge—in addition to the other habits of the minds and skills that have similarities with descriptions found in other disciplines.

Accepting this new, consensus-based, nursing-specific description of critical thinking may add fuel to the fire for a paradigm shift emerging in nursing and particularly in nursing education. For the last several decades the profession's primary research focus has been on developing a scientific knowledge base or, as we now call it, evidence-based practice. Although the majority of that knowledge has come from a logical positivist model, alternative ways of knowing through qualitative methods have begun to contribute their share to evidence-based practice and are the foundation of this paradigm shift (Daly, 1998).

It is time to take the next step, to acknowledge that we can never teach all the expansive knowledge base of nursing. We must now focus a significant portion of our teaching on nurturing and enhancing students' critical thinking processes so they can seek and use ever-changing knowledge in the most effective and efficient ways.

Now, it would be ludicrous to think we can give up teaching knowledge and focus all energy on teaching the processes of critical thinking. One cannot learn critical thinking in a vacuum. But it is paramount that nurse educators embrace the teaching of critical thinking with at least as much vigor as they now teach nursing knowledge.

It has been said that knowledge is power. We believe that critical thinking abilities operationalize that power. It is the synthesis of nursing knowledge and critical thinking that will be identified as the hallmarks of nursing expertise. Nurse educators have a key role in nurturing this synthesis. We encourage dialogue, debate, and further research to continue the journey.

REFERENCES

Baker, C.R. (1996). Reflective learning: A teaching strategy for critical thinking. *Journal of Nursing Education, 35*(1), 19-22.

Beitz, J.M. (1998). Concept mapping. Navigating the learning process. *Nurse Educator, 23*(5), 35-41.

Benner, P. (1984). *From novice to expert: Power and excellence in nursing practice.* Menlo Park, CA: Addison-Wesley.

Benner, P., Tanner, C.A., & Chesla, C.A. (1996). *Expertise in nursing practice: Caring, clinical judgment, and ethics.* New York: Springer.

Bevis, E.O., & Watson, J. (1989). *Toward a caring curriculum: A new pedagogy for nursing.* New York: National League for Nursing.

Brookfield, S. (1995). *Becoming a critically reflective teacher.* San Francisco: Jossey-Bass.

Colucciello, M.L. (1999). Relationships between critical thinking dispositions and learning styles. *Journal of Professional Nursing, 15,* 294-301.

Daly, W.M. (1998). Critical thinking as an outcome of nursing education, what is it? Why is it important to nursing practice? *Journal of Advanced Nursing, 28*(2), 323-331.

Daley, B.J., Shaw, C.R., Balistrieri, T., Glasenapp, K., & Piacentine, L. (1999). Concept maps: A strategy to teach and evaluate critical thinking. *Journal of Nursing Education, 38*(1), 42-47.

Dowd, S.B., & Davidhizer, R. (1999). Using case studies to teach clinical problem solving. *Nurse Educator, 24*(5), 42-46.

Facione, P.A. (1990). *Critical thinking: A statement of expert consensus for purposes of educational assessment and instruction.* The Delphi Report: Research findings and recommendations of the American Philosophical Association, ERIC Doc. No. ED315-423.

Haffer, A.G., & Raingruber, B.J. (1998). Discovering confidence in clinical reasoning and critical thinking development in baccalaureate nursing students. *Journal of Nursing Education, 37*(2), 61-70.

Hart, L.A. (1983). *Human brain and human learning.* New York: Longman.

Ironside, P.M. (1999a). Thinking in nursing education: Part I, A student's experience learning to think. *Nursing and Health Care Perspectives, 20,* 238-242.

Ironside, P.M. (1999b). Thinking in nursing education: Part II, A teacher's experience. *Nursing and Health Care Perspectives, 20*(5), 243-247.

Jewell, M.L. (1994). Partnership in learning: Education as liberation. *Nursing and Health Care, 15,* 360-364.

Middlemiss, M.A., & Van Neste-Kenny, J. (1994). Curriculum revolution: Reflective minds and empowering relationships. *Nursing and Health Care, 15,* 350-353.

Osterman, K.F., & Kottkamp, R.B. (1993). *Reflective practice for educators: Improving schooling through professional development.* Newbury Park, CA: Corwin Press.

Paul, R. (1992). *Critical thinking: What every person needs to survive in a rapidly changing world* (rev. 2nd ed.). Santa Rosa, CA: Foundation for Critical Thinking.

Perciful, E.G., & Nester, P.A. (1996). The effect of an innovative critical thinking method on nursing students' knowledge and critical thinking skills. *Journal of Nursing Education, 35*(1), 23-28.

Rambur, B. (1999). Fostering evidence-based practice in nursing education. *Journal of Professional Nursing, 15,* 270-274.

Rooda, L.A. (1994). Effects of mind mapping on student achievement in a nursing research course. *Nurse Educator, 19*(6), 25-27.

Rubenfeld, M.G., & Scheffer, B.K. (1999). *Critical thinking in nursing: An interactive approach* (2nd ed.). Philadelphia: Lippincott, Williams & Wilkins.

Scheffer, B.K., & Rubenfeld, M.G. (2000). A consensus statement on critical thinking in nursing. *Journal of Nursing Education, 39*, 352-359.

Schon, D.A. (1983). *The reflective practitioner: How professionals think in action.* New York: Basic Books.

Stein, K.F., Corte, C., Dolling, K.B., & Whall, A. (1998). A theoretical analysis of Carper's ways of knowing using a model of social cognition. *Scholarly Inquiry for Nursing Practice, 12*(1), 43-60.

Thompson, C., & Rebeschi, L.M. (1999). Critical thinking skills of baccalaureate nursing students at program entry and exit. *Nursing and Health Care Perspectives, 20*, 248-252.

Watson, J. (1999). *Postmodern nursing and beyond.* New York: Churchill Livingstone.

Weis, P.A., & Guyton-Simmons, J. (1998). A computer simulation for teaching critical thinking skills. *Nurse Educator, 23*(2), 30-33.

CHAPTER 19

Collaborative Institutional Approaches to Nursing Education

V. JANE MUHL

Registered nurses (RNs) are often geographically bound and unable to relocate to an area in which there is an educational institution that offers a baccalaureate degree in nursing. This is especially true for RNs living in remote rural areas. Educational institutions often lack resources to provide learning opportunities for adult learners unable to travel to campus. Collaborative institutional approaches may provide opportunities that single institutions do not have the resources to offer independently.

In 1992 the five University of Wisconsin degree granting institutions that offer a baccalaureate degree in nursing collaborated with the University of Wisconsin Extension to discuss a method of providing baccalaureate education that was more accessible to RNs throughout the state. The result of this effort is the Collaborative Nursing Program (CNP), a program using distance education modalities and the combined resources of the five nursing programs. The goal of the program is to provide a high-quality education that is flexible so that Wisconsin nurses may pursue their baccalaureate degree without having to relocate or travel great distances to a campus.

This chapter will discuss the process used for the development of the CNP. It will identify the key collaborative participants, the elements of the Facilitation Process Model used in the development of the program, a description of the characteristics of the CNP, and the positive aspects associated with the CNP.

BACKGROUND

Wisconsin is a large, rural, midwestern state covering over 54,000 square miles. In the Wisconsin system of higher education, of the thirteen 4-year institutions, only five offer baccalaureate nursing programs. These five institutions include an urban university, a land-grant research university, and three regional comprehensive universities. One of

the regional comprehensive universities offers a baccalaureate completion program only, while each of the others offer basic nursing education through graduate education. While part of a state system, each institution contributes to the state's vision but maintains its own unique mission, including regional and nursing accreditation.

Faculty in the nursing programs recognized that because of the geographic location of the institutions, educational opportunities were limited for many of the RNs, especially those in the northern sector of the state. In addition, the deans of the nursing programs identified that resource limitations prioritized the focus of the programs on the needs of students who could come to campus. The demand for off-campus instruction, however, continued.

EDUCATIONAL NEEDS STUDY

To determine the extent of the need for baccalaureate education completion opportunities, a survey of RNs was conducted in 1993. At that time there were just over 46,000 licensed RNs in the state. The total population was geographically stratified into four strata based on zip code. A sample of 1,500 individuals was drawn and surveyed. The survey determined that over 60% of the nurses in the state did not have a baccalaureate degree in nursing. Of the nurses who indicated that they were thinking of continuing their education in the next 5 years, 86% responded positively to the idea of obtaining the courses through distance education technology. Further, 67% stated that a degree completion program delivered entirely by distance education technology would be either very or somewhat attractive to them. From the stratified sampling process, it was extrapolated that nearly 9,000 RNs were interested in baccalaureate education.

Conclusions of the study indicated that it was essential to make opportunities for degree completion available to

RNs close to work or home and at a reasonable cost. This could be accomplished only through a collaborative effort of the five institutions, using distance education technologies.

COLLABORATIVE PARTICIPANTS

The University of Wisconsin Board of Regents had a vision for the 21st century. They identified that bringing student-centered learning environments to the citizens of the state by removing time and place as barriers to learning and by using technologies that would expand the traditional walls of the campus should be a priority (The University of Wisconsin System Board of Regents, 1996). This set the educational climate for change and innovation.

The deans of the five nursing programs reported that, independently, they could not address the need of RNs across the state for baccalaureate completion. The University of Wisconsin Extension, a nondegree granting entity of the UW-System, offered to provide the leadership and personnel to facilitate the collaborative process among the five institutions.

The development of the CNP resulted from the combined energies of a university system interested in serving the educational needs of all of its citizens, without regard to time and place, to the dedication of the deans and faculty of the five institutions with nursing programs who were willing to risk entering into a collaborative approach to address the needs of RNs across the state, and to the insight of the personnel of the UW-Extension to provide an opportunity to facilitate a statewide collaborative effort.

FACILITATION PROCESS MODEL

The process used in the development of the CNP will be described in the context of a Facilitation Model, which was developed and applied to this institutional collaborative effort by M. Offerman (1997), UW-Extension Dean of Continuing Education. The process was facilitated by an external and objective team, who were joined by a faculty "champion." For this situation, the facilitation team members were not nurses, had no vested interest in any of the existing nursing programs, and were not employed by any of the nursing schools. They were, however, informed about collaboration, knowledgeable about nursing education, and able to engage with the planning group. The faculty "champion" was a known and highly regarded leader in the nursing education community. Even though she was from one of the University of Wisconsin Schools of Nursing, she was

trusted and embraced by colleagues across the state as one of the nursing leaders in the state.

The Process Model consists of the following elements: (1) agreement to collaborate, (2) faculty control, (3) curriculum focus, (4) iterative planning, (5) attention to student needs, (6) structured curriculum planning, and (7) assertive conflict management. These elements will be described and the related actions identified.

ELEMENTS OF THE FACILITATION MODEL
Agreement to Collaborate

The faculty champion and members of the facilitation team made visits to all five schools, asking them to enter into discussions for the purpose of determining whether a collaborative effort might assist in addressing the needs of RNs seeking a baccalaureate degree, using distance technology as the methodology for delivery. Schools were assured that their participation was voluntary, that they could withdraw from the discussions at any time, that faculty were to be actively involved, and that decisions needed to be embraced by all. Each dean of the five nursing schools agreed to participate. In addition, the facilitators obtained the support of the vice-chancellor of each of the institutions, as well as the Wisconsin system administration. This was done so that policies could be changed, if need be, to support the collaborative effort and address existing barriers.

Faculty Control

The initial joint meeting brought together one or two faculty from each of the five nursing programs. The facilitators structured the meeting to allow faculty an opportunity to express concerns about a collaborative endeavor, to determine the operational ground rules, and to outline the expectations and responsibilities of the faculty. By engaging faculty early in the process, it was felt that there would be a greater willingness to support an effort in which they had participated in its development stage.

Curriculum Focus

While each of the institutions had their own baccalaureate completion curriculum, it was agreed to engage in an exercise early in the process to develop an "ideal curriculum." Since the committee meetings were facilitated by persons without vested interests in any one program and included one or two faculty from each of the participating institutions, each school could contribute to the evolving common nursing curriculum. In addition, by initially focusing on the curriculum, the potential logistical barriers did not surface or interfere with the development of the curriculum.

Iterative Planning

Committee members were asked to take information, ideas, and concerns back to their home institutions, where they would, in turn, receive support and input to share with the committee. Because one of the ground rules stated that decisions and issues could be revisited, all faculty had an opportunity for input at every juncture.

Attend to (Focus on) Student Needs

The vision of the curriculum was to attend to the needs of the adult employed learner, who had many roles and responsibilities and who was living at a distance from the campuses. During the curricular development process, the logistics of addressing the specific student needs were discussed.

Structured Curriculum Planning

Curricular planning considerations focused on the adult learner's needs, content needed to meet those needs, and the essential elements of an RN to baccalaureate nursing curriculum. With representatives from each of the five institutions, the essential elements of the curriculum were identified. This included five core courses in nursing, upper-level nursing electives, clinical experiences, and a capstone nursing course. This upper-division nursing curriculum would contain approximately 30 credits.

Further decisions about the curriculum included that nurses with an associate degree in nursing (ADN) could transfer up to 60 credits of prior learning. The additional credits needed to obtain the baccalaureate degree would be institution specific and include the general education and nursing support courses unique to each institution (approximately 30 to 38 additional credits).

Once the curriculum was determined, the collaborative effort focused on developing common courses across the five institutions to offer the advanced nursing component content. Faculty groups with representatives from each institution developed the outlines and basic syllabi for the core courses. These five core courses included health assessment (including decision making based on data analysis), theoretical foundations of nursing practice, leadership/management (including change agent or multidisciplinary care issues), nursing research, and community health nursing (including health promotion, families and groups, community-based practice).

Courses were approved on each campus through the nursing program's and institution's approval process.

Each institution took responsibility for developing and delivering at least one of the core courses and one elective. Initially, each of the courses was developed to be delivered in a synchronous format to sites throughout the state. Over 30 sites were identified and contracted with for technology support. The distance education technologies identified for delivery of the courses included the following synchronous site to site modalities:

Audiographics: Combines audio teleconferencing with computer graphics. Students use a computer to view prepared graphics and a desktop microphone to communicate with the instructor.

Interactive videoconferencing (compressed video): Students and instructors are linked through live audio and video.

Telecourses: Broadcast on Wisconsin Public Television.

Conference call service: Connects students and instructor through audioconference lines.

As the program has developed and with the assistance of grants, the courses are also being developed for on-line (Internet) delivery.

Assertive Conflict Management

The facilitation team was charged with managing the entire process, from objective facilitation of the agreement to collaborate, through the design and development of the curriculum, through the implementation of the program, including confronting conflict. This included making explicit the ground rules, which involved putting all the issues on the table and then addressing them. It focused on respect for all persons and ideas. It provided that all ideas would be heard and that all decisions could be revisited. It also identified that the outcome of the process needed to be a win-win situation for all. This last concept was especially vital to the one comprehensive institution whose only nursing program was a baccalaureate completion program.

CHARACTERISTICS OF THE CNP

The CNP was implemented in spring 1996. It is a multiple institution collaborative effort to deliver a baccalaureate nursing degree by distance education technologies and the combined resources of the five nursing programs. The CNP began using synchronous technologies but is now expanding into the asynchronous, Web-based format.

During the visioning and development process, the logistical considerations were deferred so that they would not emerge as barriers. However, before the program could be implemented, they were addressed. The facilitation team worked with faculty, a steering committee that provided oversight to all components, an administrative committee that made decisions about cost of technology support and tuition issues, and the deans and administrators of each of the institutions. The following further describe how the program functions:

- Each institution maintains its own unique baccalaureate degree rather than offering a common degree.
- Each institution participates in developing and offering portions of a shared nursing curriculum.
- The home institution concept evolved to implement the program, so that students choose one of the five institutions to be their designated home institution, from which they receive their degree. The home institution provides the advising, financial aid, registration, and specified degree requirements. In most cases, students select the institution that is the closest to where they live or work.
- Students register and take courses through the home institution, although faculty from one of the other institutions might provide the instruction.
- A central coordinating body was identified to maintain a central database of class rosters and demographic information. It also coordinates the site assignments and rotation of courses.
- Tuition and fees are the same across the institutions, to maintain a level playing field.

POSITIVE ASPECTS

Kuramoto (1999) identifies positive aspects of being involved in this multiinstitutional collaborative effort. These include a reduced sense of competition among the institutions since marketing, tuition costs, and the curriculum have previously been agreed upon. In addition, sharing the teaching load by all five institutions reduces the duplication of efforts to deliver the program on a statewide basis. The central administrative office coordinates the collection of student information and scheduling of the courses. Further, instructional technology support for faculty and students has been positive. Increased communication among the five schools of nursing has resulted.

However, perhaps the most positive aspect of the collaborative effort is that RNs throughout the state now have access to a baccalaureate degree in nursing without having to relocate or travel great distances to a campus through the application of distance education. These opportunities are expanding with the redesign of the synchronously delivered courses into delivery over the Internet. It is providing educational opportunities for RNs that any one institution was unable to offer independently.

REFERENCES

Kuramoto, A.M. (1999). The challenges and rewards of institutional collaboration in distance education. *Journal for Nurses in Staff Development, 15*(6), 236-240.

Offerman, M.J. (1997). Collaborative degree programs: A facilitational model. *Continuing Higher Education Review, 61,* 28-55.

The University of Wisconsin System Board of Regents. (1996). *A study of the UW System in the 21st century.* Wisconsin: Author.

Section Four

Changing Practice

A Nurse Is Not a Nurse Is Not a Nurse

JOANNE McCLOSKEY DOCHTERMAN, HELEN KENNEDY GRACE

Following a form that we began in the 5th edition, the changes and issues in practice are presented in this section by specialty area. Although all nurses share certain perspectives and experiences, the chapters in this section reflect that nurses working in different specialties have a wide range of skills and are faced with different issues. Communicating these differences with each other helps us all to understand the vast profession that we share. Space limitations prevent us from including all the specialties; we have selected for inclusion those areas of practice that reflect most nurses and may be of most interest to nursing students. The last chapter is about a recent, but rapidly growing, trend that affects nurses in all specialties, the use of alternative therapies.

The debate chapter by Joel is about home care and related issues and questions that are developing as this arena of care delivery assumes more importance. Joel demonstrates that, slowly, home care is moving to a functional social model suitable to the needs of some, but not all, consumers. Joel begins her chapter by relating the history of home care in the United States. Although nursing has traditionally dominated the home care scene, things are changing. Individual consumers of home care want more say, but home care is dictated by public policy and overall public preference. The definition and philosophy of home care are being challenged by new consumer groups such as the disabled. Joel addresses many questions: To what extent should providers and consumers be able to exercise choice in the selection of a setting for care? Does the consumer have the right to choose home care regardless of cost, or only as the least costly option? Joel frames the debate statement as to whether the recipients of in-home services should have increased autonomy and responsibility in making decisions about their care. On the pro side is a strong consumer lobby complicated by the need to make policy decisions about reimbursement. On the con side are the opinions of providers, especially physicians, who are returning to home care driven by economics and need, and the issues related to supervision of assistive personnel. The debate is only beginning. Joel's chapter helps us to understand the current situation as the issues continue to emerge and take shape. This is a well-written, informative chapter that should be read by all nurses.

The viewpoint chapters are in alphabetical order by specialty, with the first being that of ambulatory nursing. According to Androwich and Haas, despite the growing workforce, the role of the ambulatory nurse remains undefined. What exactly is ambulatory nursing and what do ambulatory nurses do? Ambulatory care occurs in multiple settings, including outpatient departments, physician offices and group practices, health maintenance organizations, and nurse-managed centers. Furthermore, each setting may have a different model or philosophy of health care. The authors discuss several issues related to ambulatory care: the diversity of practice settings, inadequate documentation, need to incorporate technology and evidence-based practice precepts, educational preparation, delegation and supervision, the rapid pace of care, preparation for telephone communication, need for multistate licensure, and the difficulty of maintaining a common culture across various settings. Despite the issues, they believe there are a number of opportunities and many rewards for nurses in this specialty.

The specialty of emergency nursing is discussed by Rice, Abel, and Smith. This is a specialty in which the patient volume and complexity has increased rapidly in the past few years. The issues for nurses in this specialty include a shortage of well-prepared nurses, working with unlicensed caregivers, increasing exposure to unknown infectious diseases and hazardous materials, increasing patient acuity, the addition of observation units, the high risk of violence, the movement to contracted services, and the need for data management skills. The authors also overview the numerous credentials and certifications these nurses are required to have, the use of advance practice nurses in the emergency department, and the opportunities for expanded roles. A new role is the emergency services case manager. Legislative changes frequently have an impact on the role and responsibilities of the emergency department nurse. The emergency department nurse manager must be prepared to work with various physician groups. The authors conclude with an overview of the role of the Emergency Nurses Association in the popular television show called "ER."

Some specialties focus on setting, others on the age of the population. People older than 65 comprise 12% of the U.S. population but account for more than 33% of the country's health care expenditures. While the aging population is growing rapidly, the number of nurses specializing in gerontology remains small. In their chapter, Zwygart-Stauffacher and Rantz provide an overview of the issues related to the care of our aging population. Increasingly, the elderly are using services across the continuum, and new roles for caregivers are emerging as a result. The authors point out that within the new reimbursement systems, gerontological nurses must often assume tough gatekeeping functions about what services will be provided. They discuss the role of the gerontological clinical specialist compared with that of the gerontological nurse practitioner. Qualifications of faculty, adequacy of associate degree programs to prepare nurses to work in nursing homes, the need for specialty gerontological content in master's practitioner programs, and the need for more research are discussed. In this chapter the authors wrestle with many of the issues related to this specialty that will be helpful to others working in the area.

Another specialty that includes care of a number of elderly as well as other age groups is hospice care, the topic of the next chapter. Poleto begins her chapter with a historical overview of hospice care in the United States. The first hospice in the United States was established in New Haven, Connecticut, in 1974. During the 1980s and 1990s, hospice programs sprang up all across the United States. There are currently over 3,000 hospice programs in the United States; in 1983 hospice care became available under Medicare for those with a life expectancy of 6 months or less. The author discusses the need to make an early referral for care and the advantages to the patient and family. She discusses the barriers to early referral and to use of hospice care in general. This is a good overview of a specialty area of practice that all nurses should be informed about.

Medical-surgical nursing is the subject of the next chapter. The new name for this specialty is adult health nursing. It involves care of the adult patient and occurs in many settings. According to Fetter and Grindel, the change in the title of the specialty recognizes the broadened role and responsibilities. In the past, the medical-surgical nurse worked only with hospitalized acute patients, but today's adult health nurse cares for adults across the care continuum. The multiple changes in hospitals related to economic pressures and changing technologies, as well as an aging patient population that requires new and different services, have challenged this nursing workforce to maintain quality. Job stress has also increased. The authors overview the changes and issues related to the care of the adult patient. The challenges are many. Practicing adult health nurses need to retool to meet the demands. Fetter and Grindel outline the competencies needed by adult health nurses and the roles that must be assumed by adult health specialty organizations. There is much that needs to be done if the nation's adults are to be well cared for.

Nursing's newest specialty is parish nursing, begun in 1984 and recognized by the American Nurses Association as a specialized area of practice in 1997. In her chapter, Solari-Twadell defines parish nursing as the combination of ministry and nursing. The nursing role component is health promotion and disease prevention. The author covers the controversy as to whether the specialty should be more closely aligned with nursing, seen by some nurses and clergy as tinkering with the integration of faith and health in the life of the church. Other issues include the development of a standardized curriculum, the need for role clarity, the development of certification for the specialty, and the financing of the role. Some parish nurses are paid, others are not. In some congregations the existence of parish nursing is seen as one nurse's contribution to the congregation. But this approach has little permanency. Solari-Twadell wants the role of the parish nurse to be fully integrated into the congregation, to have the nurse be a visible member of the ministerial team. The final issue discussed is the need for documentation of services rendered. The author discusses some recent efforts to accomplish this using the standardized languages of North American Nursing Diagnoses Association (NANDA), Nursing Interventions Classification (NIC), and Nursing Outcomes Classification (NOC).

The specialty of perinatal nursing is discussed next by Simpson. Perinatal nurses care for mothers and babies during pregnancy, labor, birth, and the postpartum and newborn period. Few health care events are more joyous than attendance at the birth of a healthy baby. Given that this is a normal event in the lives of most women, a reader might think that the specialty would have few issues. Quite the opposite. The changes in the health care delivery system that favor the financial bottom line and convenience have resulted in several challenges for those practicing in this specialty. Simpson does an excellent job of presenting several issues: the continued medicalization of labor and birth, increased use of technology for healthy women, the ongoing conflict between usual practice versus evidence-based care, errors by health care providers, increasing nurse/patient ratios, the proliferation of convenience as the foundation for care, lack of education about the impact of the convenience philosophy among childbearing women, and the forces challenging nurse midwives as providers. Even though a pregnant woman plans and prepares for a low-tech childbirth, she often agrees during labor to interventions that are unnecessary and have the potential for injury. The use of drugs to artificially stimulate labor contractions has increased 110% since 1989. This and other practices in many perinatal units are done more for convenience, for both the provider and patient, rather than allowing the normal process of birth to occur. Unfortunately, adverse outcomes happen related to these convenient practices. Simpson urges perinatal nurses to be advocates for pregnant women and give them the necessary information they need to make the important decisions during labor and birth. This is a stimulating chapter that is a must read for anyone interested in this area of practice.

Perioperative nursing, a specialty that is currently under siege, is the topic of the next chapter. Beyea addresses the issues in perioperative nursing related to the many changes in surgery. For example, more older adults with more co-morbidities are undergoing surgery; more surgery is done in ambulatory care and office settings with minimally invasive technologies; enhanced imaging devices and robotic technologies have improved the diagnosis and treatment of numerous conditions; there are mandates for more equipment and supplies that protect health care workers. These changes and others have challenged the traditional roles of nurses in operating rooms. Surgical technologists have replaced nurses in the traditional scrub role and are lobbying to take on the roles of circulating, first assisting, and supervision in operating rooms. A new role of registered nurse first assistant whereby nurses with master's degrees who are an integral part of a surgeon's practice provide preoperative and postoperative assessment and management has emerged. The perioperative nurse role in the ambulatory setting is highly diversified. Other new roles such as gene therapy nurse are emerging. The recent name change of the spe-

cialty organization from Association of Operating Room Nurses to Association of PeriOperative Registered Nurses reflects many of the changes in the specialty. One of the most serious nursing shortages is in this specialty. The author worries that unless there are effective ways of recruiting students and nurses to the surgical setting, this specialty nursing practice may approach extinction.

Psychiatric nursing is the subject of the next chapter by Stuart, who begins by listing several areas of vulnerability that nurses in this specialty face: fewer nurses are attracted to the specialty; psychiatric nurses are often viewed as expensive workers who can be replaced; there are few outcome studies that document the nature and effectiveness of care delivered by psychiatric nurses; and graduate nursing programs have less course work in psychiatric illness. Stuart overviews the changes that have occurred in five areas: role, activities, models of care, treatment settings, and evidence-based practice. She first reviews the history of psychiatric nursing and how the role has evolved since the emergence of the specialty in the 1950s. Next she lists psychiatric practice activities in three groups: direct care, communication, and management. She says that communication and management activities need to be better integrated in the current role of the psychiatric nurse. In the area of model of care she outlines four stages of treatment and overviews the goal, assessment, intervention, and outcome for each. This is a helpful model as hospital length of stay continues to decline and much of psychiatric treatment is now in community-based settings. She then discusses the expansion of mental health treatment settings and the challenges and opportunities provided by the change. Finally, she urges psychiatric nurses to articulate the nature of their care and collect data on the outcomes that they achieve. This is an informative chapter about a specialty that is undergoing a number of changes and is challenged to respond or else.

The last chapter in this section is not about a particular specialty but about a trend that affects nurses in all specialties. Eliopoulos discusses the growing and extensive use of complementary and alternative therapies, defined as practices outside the dominant system of managing health and disease taught in American medical schools. Although the rest of the world has long used these therapies, their use is relatively new in the United States. The Office of Alternative Medicine was established only in 1992 at the National Institutes of Health and became freestanding in 1998 as the National Center for Complementary and Alternative Medicine. Eliopoulos discusses the factors that contribute to the rapid growth of complementary and alternative therapies in the United States. She states that the introduction of these new therapies offers nurses an opportunity to reclaim the role of healer. New opportunities for nurses in the areas of aromatherapy, herbal medicine, homeopathy, acupuncture, therapeutic touch, guided imagery, massage therapy, and others are emerging. Nurses can use these therapies to enhance traditional care or to establish private practices. Challenges are also emerging, including the risk that physicians will seek the gatekeeper role to the use of these therapies, licensure issues, and safe use of the therapies. Eliopoulos urges nurses and nursing to find a strong voice that will help integrate these therapies with traditional medicine.

As the chapters in this section demonstrate, nurses in all specialties are challenged to keep up with many health care system changes. As we attempt to streamline our care to save unnecessary steps and cost, we must also continue to provide enough time to attend to the tasks of caring for people. Nurses need to be vocal about the services that must be retained to ensure safety and quality. We also need to help others to see that nurses are not interchangeable. The nursing profession is large and composed of a vast array of individuals with differing skills and knowledge. We need to acknowledge our similarities and differences as we move forward amid the turmoil of overwhelming change.

Moving the Care

From Hospital to Home, from Nurses to Whom?

LUCILLE A. JOEL

The trend toward community-based services, or more correctly alternatives to institutional settings, was set into motion by the growing demand for health care in the face of economic pressures to curtail escalating costs. Demographics had become our destiny with rapidly growing numbers of the aged, disabled, and chronically ill; family caregivers were less readily available; and technological advancement made the movement of sophisticated medical diagnostics and therapeutics out of the hospital possible. The initial presumption was that community-based services would be less costly.

Home care has been both an active participant and passive respondent in this transition. Home care has been aggressive in the use of telecommunications to extend their capability (Kinsella, 1998), developing community-based primary care programs for special populations, conceptualizing the community as client to tailor personal care service to a geographical area (Glick, 1999). Home care has always thrived on creativity and ingenuity. In turn, home care has been shaped and reshaped by the fortunes of government funding and internal competition. The result was two dominant home care markets, the post-acutely ill, and the disabled and chronically ill with varying degrees of restorative potential.

THE CONTEXT OF CARE IN THE NEW MILLENNIUM

Senge (1990) tells us that success depends on tracking the patterns of social trends so that we may be strategically positioned to create our own preferred future. This statement is not an oxymoron but truth that is so basic as to be frightening. These trends are set in motion by the society and are not debatable (assuming that they are interpreted correctly), yet they are broad enough so stewards of the society can be creative in their response. The challenge is to rise above self-interest, the temptation to protect our field of work, and natural caution about change. Once we have faced our own biases, the world looks more logical, if not more acceptable.

The American public is intrigued by high technology, specialization, freedom of choice, and fierce individualism. Applying these qualities, many would best define our ethic toward health as, "A basic package of services for everyone, but the guarantee that those who have the resources can obtain more for themselves and their own." In contrast, countries with more socialized systems would say, "The greatest good for the most people." This interpretation may answer a lot of questions about why we act as we do.

Many among us expect health to be a personal responsibility. Because most of us have a minor amount of serious illness in our lives, this makes good sense. On the other hand, the progress of medical science has created a cohort of the frail and vulnerable who continue to have primary health care needs, but those needs take on a new meaning. The frail elderly, disabled and chronically ill, persons with acquired immunodeficiency syndrome (AIDS), and low-birth-weight babies are all among those whose health becomes a public concern and creates serious liabilities should it be ignored. Homelessness, poverty, the absence of family, and environmental pollution are also by-products of industrial and scientific progress, complicating the picture more and generating more need for personal health services.

The financial burden of health care has become substantial for Americans. They continue the search for efficiencies that will allow them to honor a commitment to the needy, yet maintain some control over the total number of dollars spent. Americans are neither proud nor complacent about the fact that 14% of the population have no guaranteed access to health care, and an equal number have inadequate provisions.

The search to produce access has begged the question of a defined standard in health care but focused almost irrationally on cost. Hospitals were targeted as the major offender, given their association with high-tech and aggressive and defensive diagnostics and therapeutics. Rather then searching for programmatic options that promise a better use of resources, the years since 1982 (beginning of the Medicare hospital prospective payment system) have held a flurry of public policy activities with the obvious goal of preserving the status quo in the health care industry to whatever extent possible. Antics included reducing reimbursement for services to the poor so far below cost that few providers would care for them, increasing the co-payments and deductibles under Medicare to the extent that seniors pay more out-of-pocket than before the program was established, and cross-subsidizing public entitlement programs and the medically indigent through private sector payers, which practice has since been declared illegal in many states. Over the years, generations of statistical equations have been developed (diagnosis-related groups [DRGs], Current Procedural Terminology, resource-based relative value scales, resource utilization groups [RUGs], medical data system, medical data system 2, medical data system +, Outcome and Assessment Information Set [OASIS]) with the ultimate goal of controlling cost through prediction of resource use on an episode of illness or encounter basis. Each of these case mix methods has been gamed by the industry. We continue to pursue technical solutions to political problems. Some of the most hopeful programmatic redesigns have surfaced from private sector: home respite services to ease caregiver burden, case management, a focus on self-care, sensitivity to consumer preference, and seamless programs that provide consumers with access to all services through a single point of entry.

Despite final defeat in the fall of 1994, the Health Security Act of 1993 served as a wake-up call for the public conscience. It included many of the programs that have since offered some response to public discontent. Clear distinctions between levels of care are becoming common: intensivist, critical care, acute, subacute, skilled, intermediate, custodial, ambulatory, nursing homes, home care. Assisted living programs with a broad range of on-site and in-home services are popular but are still rarely an option through public entitlements. The bill proposed movement away from the medical model and toward functional ability as a major indicator for defining the need for home care services. Broader definitions of home and community care included companion and chore services. In its vision the Healthy Security Act of 1993 was

often brilliant but in its process is politically naive (Joel, 1995).

THE HOME CARE INDUSTRY

A definable sequence of events over the past 35 years has shaped modern home care and generated the dilemmas this segment of the industry faces today. Titles 18 and 19 of the Social Security Act created Medicare and Medicaid. It was within those entitlements that home care was recognized as reimbursable but not at first mandatory. Subsequent legislation in 1971 made home health services mandatory as a covered benefit under these programs and in 1972 expanded service to the disabled and to end-stage renal disease patients in 1978. Elimination of the prior hospitalization requirement and a more flexible redefinition of the term "homebound" followed over time and brought home care into its own. The Medicare hospital prospective payment system (PPS) of 1982 heightened the use of this segment of the industry. Incentives were offered to hospitals for the early discharge of patients. Referral to home care was the natural consequence.

There currently are more than 20,000 organizations providing in-home services to 8 million individuals in the United States. In 1998, there were 9,655 Medicare-certified home care agencies, 2,287 Medicare-certified hospices, and more than 8,000 agencies that offered a variety of services but did not participate in Medicare. The 1998 statistics offer the first departure from home care's consistent pattern of growth over the past 30 years. The reader is referred to Table 20-1, showing a decrease of almost 800 agencies in 1 year (National Association for Home Care, 1999).

Home care organizations also vary in their structures, sponsorship, and auspices. The major types of agencies are the Visiting Nurse Associations (VNAs) (freestanding nonprofit), public agencies (governmental), hospital-based (operating unit of a hospital), and proprietary agencies (freestanding, for-profit). Proprietary and hospital-based agencies showed the most growth until 1998, when all of the traditional agency types showed a decline. Home care agencies depend on governmental funding, with more than 65% of revenue coming from Medicare (38.7%) and Medicaid (27.2%) in 1996 (National Association for Home Care, 1999). Consequently the Balanced Budget Act of 1997 (BBA) had serious implications for this sector of the health care industry. The BBA rules and regulations designated 1994 as the base year for rate setting, turning back the clock to a period when cost-consciousness was less common among home health agen-

TABLE 20-1 Number of Medicare-Certified Home Care Agencies, by Auspice, for Selected Years, 1967-1998

	Freestanding Agencies						Facility-based Agencies			
Year	VNA	COMB	PUB	PROP	PNP	OTH	HOSP	REHAB	SNF	Total
1967	549	93	939	0	0	39	133	0	0	1,753
1975	525	46	1,228	47	0	109	273	9	5	2,242
1980	515	63	1,260	186	484	40	359	8	9	2,924
1985	514	59	1,205	1,943	832	4	1,277	20	129	5,983
1990	474	47	985	1,884	710	0	1,486	8	101	5,695
1991	476	41	941	1,970	701	0	1,537	9	105	5,780
1992	530	52	1,083	1,962	637	28	1,623	3	86	6,004
1993	594	46	1,196	2,146	558	41	1,809	1	106	6,497
1994	586	45	1,146	2,892	597	48	2,081	3	123	7,521
1995	575	40	1,182	3,951	667	65	2,470	4	166	9,120
1996	576	34	1,177	4,658	695	58	2,634	4	191	10,027
1997	553	33	1,149	5,024	715	65	2,698	3	204	10,444
1998*	508	32	1,131	4,418	678	66	2,631	3	188	9,655

*Data for 1998 were obtained on September 30. Actual FY counts are expected to differ.

VNA: Visiting Nurse Associations are freestanding, voluntary, nonprofit organizations governed by a board of directors and usually financed by tax-deductible contributions as well as by earnings.

COMB: Combination agencies are combined government and voluntary agencies. These agencies are sometimes included with counts for VNAs.

PUB: Public agencies are government agencies operated by a state, county, city, or other unit of local government having a major responsibility for preventing disease and for community health education.

PROP: Proprietary agencies are freestanding, for-profit home care agencies.

PNP: Private not-for-profit agencies are freestanding and privately developed, governed, and owned nonprofit home care agencies. These agencies were not counted separately prior to 1980.

OTH: Other freestanding agencies that do not fit one of the categories for freestanding agencies listed above.

HOSP: Hospital-based agencies are operating units or departments of a hospital. Agencies that have working arrangements with a hospital, or perhaps are even owned by a hospital but operated as separate entities, are classified as freestanding agencies under one of the categories listed above.

REHAB: Refers to agencies based in rehabilitation facilities.

SNF: Refers to agencies based in skilled nursing facilities.

From Health Care Financing Administration (HCFA), Office of the Actuary, National Health Statistics Group, Center for Information Systems, Health Standards and Quality Bureau.

cies. Meanwhile, those agencies that had begun to monitor costs and institute efficiencies early on were penalized for their good business practices. This entire regulatory scene limits the profitability of home care and creates a situation in which care is given to public entitlement recipients at a price less than cost. The most severe effects of the BBA will fall on the sickest and highest cost patients, in fact forcing them to opt for higher cost skilled nursing facilities or hospital care (Benner, 1998; Mackin & Forester, 1999). And the future bodes no better circumstances as home care moves into PPS based on the OASIS case mix method. In many ways the best hope for the industry is PPS with its capitated rates. Medicare and Medicaid are also moving decisively into managed care, which builds on the same concept. Rather than being labeled as a negative, such arrangements provide the opportunity to distance home care from the medical model and into the mode of personal assistance to normalize life. Services recognized in this model, provided through integrated systems, and financially bundled within the managed care package hold the best promise for quality of life (Landi et al., 1999). Economic survival and quality of life can only peacefully coexist where providers have the freedom to be creative in partnership with the recipient of services, new technologies are called into play to improve the human condition, and atypical support systems are encouraged when they contribute to the desired outcomes.

Despite a great dependency on public dollars, those dollars have not been extensive. In 1999, home health services, including hospice, accounted for a projected 7.6% of Medicare dollars spent, and 9% of total Medicaid dollars in 1996, the last year for which data are available. The number of Medicaid home care recipients has continued to steadily increase through 1997, whereas Medicare numbers show a decline in the same period (National Association for Home Care, 1999). This shuffling can be traced to the BBA, which placed new restrictions on home care payments to purposely reduce growth of home care services for the Medicare population (ANA House of Delegates, 1998). By 1998, it is estimated that 90% of home care agencies had costs that exceeded revenue by 32% for services to Medicaid recipients. VNAs and hospital-based agencies were the most dependent on government funds, with 80% of their revenues coming from this source. In comparison, only 55% of the revenue of for-profits come from public entitlements (National Association for Home Care, 1999). These figures are important and allow us to make some predictions about the future of home care. Medicare serves clients with episodic problems in the form of skilled nursing needs or potential for some return to self-care through rehabilitative efforts. If the Medicare home care market continues to decline, long-term patients will dominate to a greater degree than currently observed. VNAs and hospital-based agencies will face critical economic times. Medicare recipients will be directed into skilled nursing and subacute care facilities.

The caregivers in home care are both formal and informal. Unpaid help, especially family members, are the backbone of home care in the United States. Because the Bureau of Labor Statistics (BLS) and the Health Care Financing Administration (HCFA) count workers in different ways, much of our data is imprecise. However, the general nature of the workforce and the inevitable problems are clear. The largest number of workers are home care aides and registered nurses. In 1998, total home care employment declined by 7.2% (National Association for Home Care, 1999). The profile of the home health aide is remarkably consistent. Studies describe a middle-aged female, disproportionately minority workforce with low education, low pay, and a high degree of part-time employment. There is no consistent rule for the education of home health aides comparable with the federal standard that exists for nursing assistants in skilled nursing facilities. Once more highly paid than in hospital nursing, this is not the current case for registered nurses in home care. But nurses have always expressed particular satisfaction with the high degree of professional autonomy in home care practice.

The case for home care is often based on arguments of cost-effectiveness. The hospital per diem charge or subacute or skilled nursing daily rate is compared with the charge for a home visit. This logic is specious, given the fact that these are not comparable services. There have been, however, specific clinical situations that have been carefully and inclusively analyzed and found to be particularly suited to home care. These include low-birth-weight babies, ventilator-dependent adults, oxygen-dependent chil-dren, chemotherapy in children, intravenous antibiotics for osteomyelitis and cellulitis, congestive heart failure, and psychiatric care, to name a few (National Association for Home Care, 1999). In these situations, there were either significant dollar savings by moving treatment to the home, or more expensive institutional care was shortened or readmissions averted when home care was provided.

THE ISSUES

The issues in home care do not stand alone but are immensely affected by other aspects of the health care industry and consumer choice.

Whether movement of health care services into the community is a response to the declining use of hospitals or primarily is due to other factors, it is a trend that seems irreversible. The hospital length of stay (LOS) continues to decrease but at a slower pace: 1996 (5.5 days), 1997 (5.3), 1998 (5.3). Even when hospital-based subacute care is factored into the calculations, we only see a modest increase in the length of stay and a continuing pattern of decline: 1996 (6.2), 1997 (6.1), 1998 (6.0) (Interview: Roger Cero, New Jersey Hospital Association, Princeton, NJ, February 11, 2000).

Community-based service, in the form of home care and health promotion, has a long and proud tradition. They are not newcomers but took on new significance with social pressure to curtail cost and favor those service settings that are less expensive. Some of our original presumptions have proved to be naïve. Where medical intensity is great or functional ability is so seriously compromised as to require continuous care, home care can be costly. Subacute care has appeared to fill some of these gaps. At the other end of the spectrum, the less needy have chosen assisted living, which does not always eliminate the presence of home care. With these new levels of care as options, the arguments for personal choice and humane and compassionate care are gaining in prominence. Home care is best suited to reinforce and complement the care provided by family, friends, and community resources. It can be the optimum venue for the preservation of dignity and independence. The home continues to be the best place to maintain control over your own care.

Confusion over roles and responsibilities will be part of any transition from medical to social model. New patterns of accountability and authority are not only inevitable but necessary to do the most with the least for the most needy. And this seems to be the manner in which public policy is reshaping this segment of the industry.

There will be questions about who has the right to authorize services; where are the quality controls, and how will quality be defined; and who is responsible for the practice of nonprofessionals who provide 80% of the hands-on care? Note that this percentage will increase if more skilled nursing patients choose subacute options in hospitals and nursing homes. Most especially, the supervisory issues around home health aides have become public and frightening.

Nursing has long dominated the home care scene. The roots of many of our most illustrious leaders can be traced to home care. This has often been touted as the setting that provides the best showcase for our practice: autonomy, equality, respect. The pioneering home care agencies were nurse managed and nurse controlled and built on a social model that went far beyond the diagnosis and treatment of illness. Can this tradition be recaptured and sustained as home care responds to governmental policy and public preference.

The "wild card" in the equation continues to be the consumer, or just as often consumer advocates. Consumerism has become militant, and the reaction is no longer new or unexpected. Recipients of care have become uncomfortable with deferring to professionals. The historic practice of "protecting the public from themselves" has been seriously called into question as consumers have access to more information. Direct access to diagnostics and therapeutics is growing. Consumer satisfaction and dissatisfaction as expressed to insurers, particularly in managed care plans, are a driving determinant in who does what and which providers and facilities will be included in a network. The good will of plan members is necessary if they are to continue their subscriptions. Medicaid is moving rapidly toward managed care through state waiver programs; Medicare is moving at a slower, but deliberate, pace.

Chiefly deriving from consumers and their advocates, a broad definition of home care is becoming popular and receiving much favor in managed care plans, where functional ability and quality of life can be addressed with more latitude. Case management is a natural complement to this "social" approach, monitoring abuses and educating the recipient of care to the pros and cons of choices. In 1993, the President's recommendations to the Congress for long-term care entitlements included personal assistance for persons with functional impairment where they live, where they recreate, where they work, and where they do business. The intent was to normalize life through personal assistance suited to the preference of the individual (The White House Domestic Policy Coun-

cil, 1993). The extreme application of this principle to nursing homes could involve separating personal care and nursing services from nontherapeutic and hotel services so the clients or their agents, usually the family, may choose what suits them best, thereby controlling resources . . . the ultimate weapon. It suffices to know that this broader vision of home care and in-home services exists, has been proposed for public policy, and enjoys growing support.

Issues of Control

As the home and community become the prevailing sites for care, the control of the medical establishment declines, and this includes nurses. Some may say that consumer demand for more control was the catalyst in this reformation and not its by-product. Consumer allegations of forced dependence on entering the health care system and frequent distrust of provider professionals should have been an anticipated consequence of specialization and high technology. As the personal relationship between the provider and patient began to erode, the vulnerable easily came to feel victimized.

The position of the consumer is further strengthened by the growing trend to have public entitlement recipients (Medicare, Medicaid, Civilian Health and Medical Program of the Uniformed Services [CHAMPUS]) use their resources to "buy" into a managed care plan of their choice. Currently, this ability to choose is compromised when managed care plans are specifically designed for the poor, and choice is often limited to providers and facilities that can not attract a middle class or private payer client base. State law frequently requires that plan subscribers must include a mix of Medicaid and non-Medicaid recipients.

Discussion inevitably leads to issues of "turf protection," and the public patience has worn thin on this topic. A medicalized system has concentrated services in settings in which the balance of power weighs in the direction of the industry and provider professionals. Public dissatisfaction with this paradigm was slow coming, but long building. The issue is who defines the nature and context of services? The Agency for Health Care Research and Quality (formerly Agency for Health Care Policy and Research), the Patients' Bill of Rights, advance final directives, and the Patient Protection Bill are all examples of public policy intended to guarantee the ability of consumers to make their own informed choices. The dramatic growth of the complementary health market is another consumer strategy to avoid medicalization. Although the migration to home care was primarily motivated by cost, what it will be is based on public preference.

The frail and chronically ill have been the major recipients of home care, and they have frequently been poor. Today they are joined by those in a recuperative mode, who are in a position to demand more and different services, having access to more personal resources: private insurance, workplace benefits. There is also the addition of younger disabled persons who object to both the terms home and care, because of the connotations that have become associated with them in this society. They prefer to reserve the term *care* for relationships of intimacy and affection and note that assistive services should not be limited to the home in the usual sense of the word. Rather, services that allow you to maintain a home in the community should help you to live and to flourish wherever that may be. Rather than promoting a "caring in place" philosophy, services should follow you from the home to places where you can be productive, recreate, socialize, or do your business such as it is. Advocates of the disabled, this often younger and more militant constituency, contend that the recipient of services should be able to select those in an assistive capacity to them and decide whether family is an option. This is contrary to the traditional view that bases the authorization of services on the potential for rehabilitation or the need for skilled nursing as determined by professionals. The expanded definition of "homebound" was a breakthrough, but rigid interpretation still prevails. More latitude has been observed in state-funded or Medicaid waiver programs in which personal assistance and functional impairment are the priority. This has also been the response in programs created to substitute for nursing home confinement.

The ability of home care personnel to provide some rather technically complex care and the frequency and immediacy of supervision, if any, are controversial issues. Many arguments for the increased use of nonprofessional personnel hinge on the ability of the disabled to direct their own care, thereby maintaining control. One such situation is the creation of a category of worker called the home care medication aide. It has been proposed that the medication aide should only be able to help cognitively intact home care patients who are able to recognize their medications and understand their use and side effects. Other controversy focuses on the delegation of specific activities by the professional, notably the nurse. In Oregon, non-nurses may "perform nursing functions if they have been taught by a nurse on a patient-specific and procedure-specific basis."

THE DEBATE

Statement: Recipients of in-home services should have increased autonomy, flexibility, and commensurate responsibility in making determinations about their care.

Pro

The medical model is increasingly out of step with the restructuring delivery system. Primary health care, integrated systems, and community-based services all begin to move us toward a new paradigm that values self-care, personal responsibility, prudence in resource use, and increased commitment to the common good as the true test of community. The frail elderly, one major market for in-home services, are most concerned with functionality and their perception of their own health than they are with illness. Illness only becomes a priority when it gets in the way of living. The Clinton administration's 1993 report on health care reform recommended eligibility for assisted living arrangements and home health services based on measurable functional impairments as opposed to medically defined problems and a shift to personal, client-directed care with the standard being that the persons providing service, to the extent possible, be selected, trained, supervised, and evaluated by the recipient (The White House Domestic Policy Council, 1993).

Realistically, a fence may have to be put around the liberties and choices allowed within the context of home care, especially where public dollars are used. A cap on the total amount of funding available in a preestablished period is one approach. Caution would have to be taken that the spirit of flexibility and choice is not violated by inadequate funding. Withholding funding is a common back-door strategy to reach your goal without the unpleasant policy decisions that would be required with a more forthright approach. Examples abound, but two should suffice, given their familiarity to the reader. Few, if any, restrictions are placed on the services provided to Medicaid recipients. However, the fees paid to the provider are so low that few accept these patients. Abortions are legal, but the poor are denied the public dollars to access the procedure.

The tough policy decisions to allow the consumer to retain maximum control will be slow in coming. The first challenge requires the honesty to separate the control and funding aspects. Although only a finite number of dollars may be available to an individual, allowing decisions about the use of those dollars could honor the spirit of consumer choice. Allowing flexibility may lead to some creative options. Pooling resources in a setting such as a group residential home may pay for more services and consequently more freedom, for the more acutely ill or those recovering from acute illness, fluid movement between levels of care including, but not limited to the home, all within a predetermined spending cap. This could be accomplished through managed care plans with the proper policies and benefit structure. In many ways, this is the broader application of the "true" hospice concept. These decisions are most comfortably made by the consumer if they are supported by case management, at best independent case management. A case manager engaged by the payer could be subject to conflict of interest, the need to hold a job versus acting as an advocate for the client.

Con

Consumer militancy and the growing political influence of both the elderly and younger disabled persons has led to a gradual restructuring of home care to distance it from the mainstream of health care, broaden the definition of home care and in-home assistance, and increase consumer's right to engage and dismiss services.

A first wave of consumerism predated the dramatic onslaught of acute and subacute clinical situations into the home. With the appearance of this new clinical population in the home, more justification appeared for medicalization. Physicians who once abandoned home practice are returning to that setting, some out of economic motivation and others as a response to consumer need. The federal government has approved Medicare reimbursement to physicians for their supervision of the medical regimen in home care based on the observation that much of home care has become so medically dependent that close supervision is not only justified but also necessary.

Putting aside the very apparent medical needs in home care, there remain the chronically ill, frail, and disabled. These populations have traditionally used significant amounts of nonprofessional and assistive services in the home. Surveys indicate that home health agencies rely on part-time, temporary workers and have been assigning heavier case loads with resultant alienation of the workforce. A high turnover rate is common among home health aides and can lead to a lack of reliability and inconsistency of services. Observable quality of care problems follow, such as incomplete work, inadequate skills even for simple activities, failure to carry out orders, client injury or abuse, exploitation of the client, theft, absenteeism, and on and on. Given the frequency of such incidents and the basic vulnerability of many home care

recipients, closer professional controls can be justified. There is little state-to-state consistency in maintaining records on disciplinary actions, requiring criminal background checks, or imposing any standard for training or competency testing.

Despite the outcry for consumer empowerment, the American public has always found comfort in the medical establishment and the assurance that professionals would act in their best interest. There is a clear distinction in home care between those situations in which medical necessity drives the use of resources and others in which functional ability and basic services to compensate for functional deficits are needed. It was just such a distinction that differentiated Medicare and Medicaid, episodic versus continuing care. Whether these distinctions should be perpetuated and how they should, if at all, be recognized in the process of authorizing services for the public is a serious question, more rooted in philosophy than financial expedience.

BEYOND DEBATE

Home care, not unlike other segments of the health care industry, is in a struggle over "consumer control and choice," the definitions to describe it, the public policy to allow it, the dollars to fund it, the economic models to distribute those dollars, and the provider systems to actually make it happen. And this observation forces many issues:

- What are the appropriate criteria for maintaining a patient in the home, putting aside economic motivation?
- To what extent should providers and consumers be able to exercise choice in the selection of a setting for care?
- How appropriate is the medical model to the home care population?
- How much direct consumer access to providers and services should exist?
- If home care is a cost-efficient proxy for the hospital or nursing home, how is the break-even point identified and what happens once it is reached?
- Does the consumer have the option to choose home care regardless of cost or only as the less costly option?
- Who is responsible for the supervision of volunteers in the home, including family members if they undertake medical or nursing activities?
- Are family members supervised or are they the supervisors?
- To what extent can activities be delegated?

- The expanded use of volunteers and family caregivers raises questions of caregiver burden and new categories of reimbursable services, either through dollars paid or tax credits allowed.
- The many relatively unskilled in-home services create a market for home care workers. When and to what extent does nursing supervise these workers?
- And this list is not exhaustive.

CONCLUSION

The dispute over turf ownership in home care or any sector of health care pits the consumer against the government and their agents, the industry, and the professions. Slowly over time home care and in-home services are moving to a functional-social model that is more suitable to the needs of some; whereas a large constituency of the acutely ill have a real need for continuing medical expertise in the home and are confronted with decisions beyond the capability of most lay people. The challenge will be to see the distinctions and accommodate them. This was the original premise for the division between the Medicare and Medicaid populations. So, there may be something we can learn from past practice, including when past practice has outlived its usefulness.

REFERENCES

American Nurses Association House of Delegates. (1998). *Home health care payment systems.* Washington, DC: Author.

Benner, M. (1998). The Medicare interim payment system's impact on home health services. *Home Care Provider, 3*(3), 169-170.

Glick, D.F. (1999). Advanced practice community health nursing in community nursing centers: A holistic approach to the community as client. *Holistic Nursing Practice, 3*(4), 19-27.

Joel, L.A. (1995). Health care reform: Getting it right this time. *American Journal of Nursing, 95*(1), 7.

Kinsella, A. (1998). Home telecommunication services: Their role in home care today. *Home Care Management, 2*(5), 17-22.

Landi, F., Gambassi, G., Pola, R., Tabaccanti, S., Cavinato, T., Carbonin, P.U., & Bernabei, R. (1999). Impact of integrated home care services on hospital use. *Journal of the American Geriatric Society, 47*(12), 1430-1434.

Mackin, A.L., & Forester, T.M. (1999). Home health at the crossroads. *Caring, 18*(9), 12-13, 15.

National Association for Home Care. *Basic statistics about home care 1999.* Available: http://www.nahc.org/consumer/hcstats.html.

Senge, P. (1990). *The fifth discipline.* New York: Doubleday.

The White House Domestic Policy Council. (1993). *The President's health security plan.* New York: Times Books.

Ambulatory Care Nursing

Challenges for the 21st Century

IDA M. ANDROWICH, SHEILA A. HAAS

The ambulatory care setting offers numerous opportunities for nurses to practice in a variety of roles. Of the nearly 200,000 registered nurses (RNs) identified as employed in ambulatory care settings, approximately 18% are managers, 52% are staff nurses, 11% are nurse practitioners, 4% are clinical specialists, and the rest are in roles such as clinician, researcher/consultant, instructor, certified nurse anesthetist, or other (U.S. Department of Health and Human Services, Division of Nursing, National Sample Survey of Registered Nurses, March 1996).

Statistics at the national level demonstrate an increase from 1.7 million to nearly 1.9 million health care workers employed in ambulatory care in the years from 1997 to 2000 (http://www.stat-usa.gov). It is difficult to get exact figures for nursing because of the tremendous growth in primary care settings. Thus, given the size, growth, and importance of the field, defining the practice would appear straightforward. This is not the case. In fact, Stavins (1993) claims that the most difficult challenge facing ambulatory nursing is "defining our role." This chapter will focus on the definitional aspects of the ambulatory care nursing role and identify and discuss several of the issues facing nurses in this practice field.

DEFINING AMBULATORY CARE NURSING

Verran is credited with an early interest in delineation and definition of ambulatory care nursing. In her seminal study (1981) she used a Delphi method and ambulatory nurses' expert opinions to delineate seven "responsibility areas" in the ambulatory nurse role. Other researchers have continued this effort (Haas & Hackbarth, 1995a; Hackbarth, Haas, Kavanagh, & Vlasses, 1995; Hastings & Muir-Nash, 1989; Hooks, Dewitz-Arnold, & Westbrook, 1980; Joseph, 1990; Parrinello & Witzel, 1990; Pinkney-Atkinson & Robertson, 1993).

In the American Academy of Ambulatory Care Nursing's (AAACN) *Administration and Practice Standards* (1993), ambulatory care nursing is operationally defined as "nursing practice in an ambulatory care setting. Nursing care provided to patients with institutional episodes of care of less than 24 hours" (p. 19). Although this definition delineates nursing practice by the environment in which the nurse practices and the amount of time the nurse spends with a patient, it is not useful in capturing essential characteristics and role elements.

This need to depict ambulatory nursing as it is today for practicing nurses, other health care providers, policy makers, and the public led the American Nurses Association (ANA) and the AAACN to establish a joint task force to write a monograph on ambulatory care nursing: *Ambulatory Care Nursing: The Future Is Now.* As part of this charge, the task force developed a conceptual definition of ambulatory care nursing. In the absence of a rich and recent literature from which to cull the universal characteristics of ambulatory care nursing, members of the task force were asked to assemble focus groups in their ambulatory care organizations. Each focus group responded to the question: "What are the universal characteristics of ambulatory care nursing?" (AAACN/ANA Task Force, 1997). Commonly occurring themes in the reports assisted the task force in the evolution of a conceptual definition of ambulatory care nursing.

Using the ANA's Social Policy Statement (1995) as a foundation, the task force developed the following definition:

Professional ambulatory care nursing includes those clinical, management, educational, and research activities provided by registered nurses for and with individuals who seek care for health-related problems or concerns or seek assistance with health maintenance and/or health promotion. These individuals engage predominantly in self-care and self-managed health activities or receive care from family and significant others outside an institutional setting.

Ambulatory care nursing services are episodic, less than 24 hours in duration, and occur as a single encounter or a series of encounters over days, weeks, months, or years. Ambulatory nurse-patient encounters take place in health care facilities as well as in community-based settings, including schools, workplaces or homes.

They occur as personal visits or as encounters using the telephone and other communication devices. Ambulatory care nursing services focus on cost-effective ways to maximize wellness; prevent illness, disability, and disease; minimize symptoms of acute minor ailments; and support patients in the management of chronic disease to effect more positive health states throughout the life span up to and including a peaceful death. [AAACN, 1997, pp. 13-14]

The AAACN is "the association of professional nurses who identify ambulatory care nursing as essential to the continuum of high quality, cost-effective patient care." The Mission of the AAACN is to advance the art and science of ambulatory nursing (AAACN, 2000). The AAACN was established in 1978 by a group of nursing directors and supervisors in ambulatory care who recognized the need for well-prepared nurse administrators in the expanding arena of ambulatory care. The AAACN was originally named the American Academy of Ambulatory Nursing Administration (AAANA), and the name was changed in 1993 to reflect the organization's commitment to development of all nurses working in ambulatory care. As part of this commitment the AAACN publishes and updates standards for ambulatory care nursing.

The fifth edition of the *Ambulatory Care Nursing Administration and Practice Standards* (2000, p. 6) reflects five core ambulatory care nursing values:

1. Shared responsibility among patients, families, and other members of the health care team in all phases of the episode of care.
2. Education to enable patients and families to understand and make informed decisions.
3. Continuity of care.
4. Excellence in care that balances patient needs, cost-effectiveness, outcomes, and appropriate resource utilization.
5. The opportunity to serve as patient advocate.

The nine *Ambulatory Care Nursing Administration and Practice Standards* (2000) are designed to "promote effective management of increasingly complex ambulatory care nursing roles and responsibilities in a changing health care environment which requires not only expanded clinical and administrative skills but methods to

evaluate the quality, appropriateness and effectiveness of services" (p. 4). The standards are designed to be used in conjunction with specialty practice nursing organization standards such as those promulgated by the American Nurses Association. They address issues such as the structure and organization of ambulatory care nursing, staffing, competency of nursing staff, nursing practice, continuity of care, ethics and patient rights, environment, research, and quality management. Each standard includes a rationale for the standard and criteria by which to measure the contribution of nursing. The AAACN standards are presented as recommendations and are intended to be adapted to fit many diverse ambulatory care settings. Because ambulatory care practice is ever expanding and changing, the AAACN is committed to revising, updating, and promulgating its standards.

CURRENT ISSUES IN AMBULATORY CARE NURSING

Along with the need for definitional clarity, there are also several issues or concerns relating to the ambulatory care environment. These include (1) the diversity of practice in ambulatory care settings, including the use of varied conceptual models of health and evolving issues with costs of ambulatory care for the individual patient, (2) inadequate documentation of nursing practice leading to limited understanding of ambulatory nursing practice, (3) the need to incorporate technology and evidence-based practice precepts into the delivery of care, (4) the limited number of nurses with baccalaureate or advanced academic preparation, (5) the increased need for delegation and supervision of unlicensed assistive personnel, (6) the rapid pace of ambulatory patient encounters, (7) the expectations placed on the nurse related to telephone communication, (8) the need to negotiate within multiple organizational cultures, and (9) the need for multistate licensure for professional nurses.

Diversity in Practice

There is marked diversity in the types of settings in which ambulatory care is delivered. Among the major private sector ambulatory care settings are university hospital outpatient departments, community hospital outpatient departments, physician group practices, health maintenance organizations (HMOs), physician offices, and nurse-managed centers. Ambulatory care settings that are publicly funded include community health clinics, Indian Health Service, and Community, Migrant Worker Health Centers. Within each of these distinct settings, the philosophy of care and the model of care delivery may have a different model of health as a foundation. Smith (1981) defines four such models of health: the clinical model, the role-performance model, the adaptive model, and the eudaimonistic model that could be operative in a given setting.

It is not surprising that the clinical model, or medical model, is frequently the driving force in physician group practices and even in university hospital ambulatory care and community hospital ambulatory care. However, it is somewhat surprising that it predominates in many HMOs (Haas, Hackbarth, Kavanagh, & Vlasses, 1995). HMOs, by definition, should be more focused on health promotion and disease prevention.

Diversity in types of settings, models of health, and the consequent models of care delivery is an issue for nursing when nurses who work in a setting find that they have difficulties working under the prevailing model and philosophy. Furthermore, they may have difficulty identifying this lack of congruence in values as the root of the problem. They will say "I want to have time to do health promotion with my clients, yet I have so much paperwork and clerical work that I just can't get to it." Or, "I want to work with the vast array of patient and family problems, but all I have time for is their physical ailments." Or, "I want to work as a colleague with the physicians and really get into health promotion." Operative in each of these situations is a clinical model of health driving the practice model; consequently, the scheduling of patient visits and the provider's time is dictated by this view of health.

Solutions to this issue involve educating nurses about the many and various types of ambulatory care settings, educating nurses and physicians about multiple models of health with their practice implications, and enhancing the care provider's ability to diagnose operative models of health in different settings. The optimal outcome would be health care professionals who will choose a practice setting for employment where there is a good fit between their professional goals and the mission, philosophy, model of health, and care delivery model of the organization. If there is not a good fit, at least the professional enters the organization with an understanding and awareness of the model currently operating and, if needed, the wherewithal to initiate change.

With the movement of complex infusion therapies for infectious disease, oncology, and cardiac patients into ambulatory care settings, questions are now being raised and studies done on the cost-effectiveness (Liptak, Burns, Davidson, & McAnarney, 1998; Tice, Poretz, Cook, Zinner, & Strauss, 1998) of these treatments for the array of patients receiving them and the incidental costs of ambulatory care for patients and their caregivers. Ambulatory nurses as patient advocates must be aware of such costs for patients and work with community agencies making referrals where possible for transportation to and from ambulatory sites and scheduling therapy in such a way that it is feasible for patients to comply with the therapeutic regimen.

Inadequate Documentation of Practice

The nature of ambulatory practice, with its relatively rapid pace for patient encounters, high patient volume, and scheduled time constraints, does not contribute to comprehensive documentation of nursing care. The use of the Nursing Minimum Data Set (NMDS) (Werley & Lang, 1988) in ambulatory practice is limited (Androwich & Stoupa, 1994). With no documentation trail, paper or electronic, justifying the value of nursing is problematic, and the care rendered by nurses becomes invisible. At a research conference held by the AAACN (Androwich & Phillips, 1992) several documentation concerns were identified. These included limited use of the elements of the NMDS in practice settings, documentation systems designed primarily for physicians, no classification scheme for interventions or outcomes, and limited use of the problem list. When nursing interventions are documented, the assessment data leading to the individual nursing judgment is omitted, and any link to patient outcome is unknown. In addition, there are no generally accepted methods of measuring productivity, nursing intensity, or patient acuity in the ambulatory setting, nor have we defined the concept of *episode of care* in a manner that could link visits within an episode of care to determine the effectiveness of specific interventions in achieving outcomes. Documentation needs to be captured in an automated patient record to link encounters in a meaningful, retrievable manner.

In 1992 the Nursing Interventions Classification (NIC) was published (McCloskey & Bulechek, 1992). To prepare to implement NIC in an ambulatory field test site, an assessment survey, modeled after a similar national survey used by the Iowa Research Team (Bulechek, McCloskey, Denehey, & Titler, 1994) asking about the interventions used in practice, was distributed to professional nursing staff ($n = 197$) at that ambulatory site. This survey was designed to elicit the frequency of use of each of the 336 nursing interventions in the taxonomy. Respondents were asked to identify the frequency of use of each of the interventions based on a 5-point Likert scale, ranging from *"rarely or never"* to *"many times a day."*

The response rate for the ambulatory survey was 64%, yielding 126 completed surveys from each of 12 service areas in the outpatient center. Table 21-1 lists the top 30 interventions by frequency of use in ambulatory care across all 12 settings.

The use of standardized language systems, such as NIC for interventions, is an important step toward implementing a nursing minimum data set in ambulatory care and is necessary to allow collection and aggregation of data across ambulatory care sites. When documentation of care is inaccurate or incomplete, the value of having professional nurses rather than less "expensive" staff

TABLE 21-1 Frequency of Use of NIC Interventions in Ambulatory Care (Top 30, *n* = 126)

Intervention	Rarely or Never	Many Times Daily
	Rating (%)	
Active Listening	10.32	76.19
Vital Signs Monitoring	15.32	60.48
Infection Control	17.60	57.60
Body Mechanics Promotion	30.16	50.79
Emotional Support	17.46	47.62
Health Screening	24.59	42.62
Specimen Management	22.40	41.60
Teaching: Prescribed Medication	16.80	40.80
Communication Enhancement	16.80	39.20
Infection Protection	27.64	39.02
Medication Management	19.05	38.89
Presence	18.40	38.40
Teaching: Disease Process	18.55	37.10
Humor	24.00	36.80
Touch	28.00	36.80
Teaching: Individual	24.19	36.29
Teaching: Procedure/treatment	21.77	33.06
Medication Administration	33.60	32.00
Medication Administration: Parenteral	31.75	31.75
Energy Management	38.40	31.20
Technology Management	41.13	29.84
Preparatory Sensory Information	30.08	28.46
Environmental Management: Safety	32.26	28.23
Fall Prevention	36.80	26.40
Anxiety Reduction	24.80	25.60
Risk Identification	36.00	25.60
Medication Administration: Oral	34.40	25.60
Decision-Making Support	20.63	25.40
Transport	41.13	25.00
Environmental Management: Comfort	39.20	24.00

practicing in ambulatory settings becomes difficult to justify.

Another major issue with documentation involves the inability to link visits into meaningful units in which goals are set over time periods that vary. For example, many of the nursing interventions that are identified for a pregnant woman occur over the duration of the pregnancy and into the postpartum period. When the single visit is documented, but not linked to related visits, there is an inability to demonstrate an effective outcome related to nursing care. As we move to increasingly automated documentation in ambulatory care, we will need to determine the best method to conceptually examine and capture an entire episode of care.

Need to Incorporate Technology and Evidence-based Practice Precepts

We are surrounded with an overwhelming increase in our technological capabilities: Web-based information retrieval and storage, telehealth delivery modes for patient education, and clinical decision support systems that automate care processes. Teich and Wrinn (2000) describe systems in which results review, electronic records, referral processing, secure messaging, order entry for prescriptions, and tests and decision support in the form of alerts—all using a Web-based portal—are possible. The development and use of these systems will likely have an impact on the role elements of the nurse in ambulatory care settings. With many of the coordination of care activities that would normally "belong" to the RN becoming automated, how will the ambulatory care RN of the 21st century reshape her role? Kerfoot (2000) identifies a technical intelligence quotient (TIQ) as a survival skill for the new millennium. She defines TIQ as not merely being aware of how a specific technology works but as understanding the relationships among the technology, the users, and the affected systems and how they all interact to produce outcomes.

This brings us to a discussion of evidence-based medicine or nursing. The standard definition of (EBM) (or EBN) is "the conscientious, explicit and judicious use of the current best evidence in making decisions about the care of individual patients" (Sackett, Rosenberg, Gray, Haynes, & Richardson, 1996). The goal of EBM is to provide rigorous answers for "simple" questions. If I am a patient, what is my "best" care option? If I am a provider, how am I doing? How am I doing compared with others? Inside the system? Outside the system? For the profession, how can we improve what we are doing? We know that measures of quality require accurate, timely, relevant data. Consequently we need information on health outcomes, clinical outcomes, consequences of care, utilization data, and processes of care.

Educational Preparation

Significant numbers of nurses currently working in ambulatory care have many years of nursing and ambulatory care experience; however, many also have less than baccalaureate preparation as their highest level of nursing education (Hackbarth et al., 1995). With expansion of ambulatory nursing roles, there are increasing expectations that ambulatory nurses coordinate care within the health care network and the community. Yet nurses without baccalaureate preparation have not had formal coursework or clinical experiences with community health nursing. Adding to this problem is the fact that significant numbers of currently practicing ambulatory care nurses do not belong to any professional nursing organizations (Haas & Hackbarth, 1995a). Therefore, continuing education through programs, newsletters, and collegial information sharing is less available to ambulatory nurses who are not members of professional organizations.

The issue of basic nursing preparation and continuing education for nurses practicing ambulatory care presents a challenge. Yet without ongoing education, it is becoming increasingly difficult for the non-master's-prepared nurse to compete with persons with a master's in business administration for management positions in the ambulatory setting. Creative mechanisms are needed to provide incentives for nurses to enhance their formal educational preparation and to keep current with regional and national practice issues and trends. Clinical ladders or professional nursing advancement programs offer mechanisms that provide both incentives and rewards for nurses who seek educational opportunities to enhance their practice. Distance learning through videoconferencing or on-line computer coursework offers opportunities for formal for-credit coursework and continuing education. Learning through distance education formats provides accessibility and flexibility for nurses no matter the size or location of their practice environment. The challenge is to get sufficient credible distance learning programming prepared in a timely fashion. The need for more bachelor of science in nursing (BSN) nurses to work in ambulatory care organizations has been identified, yet there is currently no way to provide entrée to employment of new BSN graduates in ambulatory care.

Ambulatory care organizations might be more willing to hire new nurse graduates if they were educated to practice in ambulatory care. For example, BSN students should have parallel ambulatory care clinical experiences. Students should spend as much time caring for pediatric, obstetric, mental health, and elderly clients in ambulatory settings as they do in hospital settings.

Delegation and Supervision

Nonlicensed assistive workers have traditionally been used in ambulatory care settings. As in inpatient settings, there is a push in ambulatory care to maximize the use of assistive personnel. There is even a movement to remove all professional nurses from some ambulatory care organizations on the basis of the misinformed assumption that "nursing care" in ambulatory settings is strictly technical care and can be provided by technicians at a lower cost.

There are patient care delivery roles for both assistive personnel and professional nurses in ambulatory care. Assistive personnel should be doing lower level nursing activities, ones that do not require discretionary judgment or critical thinking. Nurses working in ambulatory care want to delegate many activities that fall under the dimensions of enabling operations and technical procedures (Haas & Hackbarth, 1995a). Delegation of these dimensions would allow the professional nurse time for higher level activities in dimensions such as teaching, care coordination, and community outreach. Nurses working in ambulatory care also need time both to delegate and to supervise assistive personnel. Currently there are no empirical data to give direction as to the optimal number of assistive personnel that one nurse can supervise in the ambulatory setting. Many nurses working today grew up under primary nursing in hospitals. They have little experience with delegation and supervision of assistive workers, and many have mistaken notions about how assistive workers are "working on their license." Consequently they are reluctant to delegate to them for fear of what may happen not only to the patient but also to their license and livelihood.

As more assistive workers are incorporated in delivery models in ambulatory care organizations, nurses will need to be educated regarding delegation and supervision, and evaluation studies will be necessary to identify optimal staffing ratios, including optimal spans of control. Haas and Gold (1997) recommend effective supervision strategies:

1. Know your assistive workers, role expectations for them, and their level of competency (in ambulatory care there is marked confusion or blurring of scopes of practice between licensed practical nurses [LPNs], nursing assistants [NAs], and medical assistants [MAs]).

2. Allocate time for supervision, rounding, and evaluating care delivery.
3. Develop open communication channels.
4. Adhere to patient care and work performance standards.
5. Give timely feedback, positive and negative, and make time for sharing improvement strategies.

A need also exists for nursing intensity indexes and systems in ambulatory care so that client demands for nursing care can be tracked and appropriate staffing can be planned and budgeted (Haas & Hackbarth, 1995b; Hastings, 1992; Verran, 1986). Caveats to consider regarding assistive workers are that assistive workers are more costly than professional nurses when there is insufficient work to occupy their time for an entire shift. When assistive workers are in a delivery model, a significant portion of professional nursing time will be consumed in delegation and supervision; thus, when the bulk of the care needs are higher level care, it may be more cost-effective to hire a nurse who can do all care and who does not require supervision. For example, there will be more activities that can be assigned to assistive workers in high-volume clinics such as general surgery or ophthalmology and perhaps less work for assistive workers in an oncology clinic, where chemotherapy is being given and emotional support, care planning, and education needs are many.

Rapid Pace of Care

The high volume of patients with which the nurse must interact affords limited time for each patient. This means that the nurse must make rapid assessments, plan nursing care, and execute that plan in quick order. This leads to a continuing tension between the available time in an encounter and the ideal time needed for a complete nursing assessment. It is difficult for the nurse to be the patient's advocate if there is no time to spend in understanding what the patient's needs, values, and preferences are.

Continuity of care, the extent to which the same provider is seen during a sequence of encounters, has been given attention with the number of physician providers seen as a determinant of quality of primary care (Spooner, 1994). If we believe that nursing care can have an impact on patient outcomes in ambulatory practice, it is necessary to develop models of care delivery to ensure similar continuity. Dickey (1998) recommends visit planning in ambulatory care. "The primary purpose of visit planning is to improve recognition, and ultimately treatment of patients' major health needs regardless of when or how the patient present" (Dickey, 1998, p. 89). Steps in visit planning include (1) 24 to 48 hours before seeing a patient, an experienced ambulatory care nurse (a) previews the chart, (b) updates the problem list, and (c) makes a preliminary visit plan; (2) during the visit the nurse (a) obtains a clear, concise understanding of the reasons for the visit and (b) develops a final visit plan based on the patient's needs; (3) throughout the process the nurse (a) manages the patient flow and (b) serves as a patient advocate; (4) exit visit planning occurs at the conclusion of the providers portion of the visit (Dickey, 1998). In the exit interview the nurse has the opportunity to go over the visit with the patient, assessing learning needs and correcting any misapprehensions the patient may have with respect to future therapeutic plans, medications, or educational needs (Phillips, personal communication, 1994).

Frequently, nurses in ambulatory care are used primarily to leverage the physician's practice, and little value is placed on the dimensions of the nursing role or the nursing interventions themselves. A number of differentiated nursing practice models can be used to address this (Hermann, 1993; Schroeder, Trehearne, & Ward, 2000). In the model described by Hermann, nursing practice is diversified to incorporate RNs with differing educational preparation and practice experience. There are three levels of nursing: the staff RN (usually associate degree or diploma prepared), who typically supervises unlicensed personnel, provides basic triage patient education, and administers medications; the RN II (BSN), who functions with a broader, yet still limited scope; and the clinical nurse specialist–nurse practitioner.

Telephone Nursing Practice (TNP)

The phone communication dimension (Haas & Hackbarth, 1995a; Hackbarth et al., 1995) of the ambulatory nurse role is an aspect of the role that is unique to ambulatory nursing practice. It is also a role dimension about which ambulatory nurses have concerns. Some of these concerns are related to the amount of education that they receive regarding phone communication, particularly phone triage and phone advice, both of which have a high liability risk potential. Assessment of the client over the phone requires a high level of assessment, including the ability to identify nuances in each situation, well-developed communication and decision-making skills, and proficiency in documentation. Nurses in ambulatory settings need to collaborate with physicians and other members of the health care team in establishing protocols that include health promotion and disease prevention, as well as treatments for symptoms. Finally, nurses need to learn that all phone communication must be documented appropriately. The AAACN has developed and promulgated *The AAACN Telephone Nursing Practice Administration and Practice Standards* (1997) and in 2000 will offer a revision to these standards and a Telephone Nursing Practice Verification Program, which is a continuing education offering that provides didactic content and skills development opportunities to prepare ambulatory nurses to do telephone nursing practice. Haas and Androwich (1999) used the Nursing Interventions Classification (NIC) to enhance understanding of the breadth and depth of nursing practice by means of communication devices. They proposed four telephone interventions to reflect the complexity of TNP. These are Telephone Consultation, Telephone Follow-Up, Surveillance: Telephone, and Triage: Telephone. These telephone interventions can be used to educate nurses regarding telephone practice and to evaluate performance of telephone practice nurses. Because advanced knowledge and skills are required for TNP, development of a certification examination in TNP is in process.

Demand management is a term given to a method of care delivery and a marketing initiative. Once used predominantly by managed care organizations, it is now common in many types of ambulatory care organizations. Kastens (1998) defines demand management as "the provision of health information to consumer, creating an educated and empowered member who accesses and participates in medical decisions to assure that the right kind of care is provided at the right time" (p. 321). Kastens maintains that demand management is essential for managing the well population, as well as acute or chronically ill patients. Demand management centers include nurse triage and advice and physician referral. Many demand management centers use established protocols for nurse triage and advice.

Need for Multistate Licensure

As telephone nursing practice became more and more prevalent, it became obvious that there were potential violations of state nurse practice acts by nurses who were consulting, providing surveillance, triaging, or following up with patients who reside across state lines if the nurse is not licensed to practice nursing in the state where the patient is residing. The AAACN developed a position statement regarding multistate licensure in an effort to inform nurses of the risks to their license and took this position statement to the National Federation of Specialty Nursing Organizations, so that those organizations could have the opportunity to endorse it if they so wished and begin to educate their members as to the risks (Haas, 2000).

The current licensure system does not address issues that have come about as a result of health care restructuring, technology advances, and increasing consumerism: (1) increases in multistate and national health care systems, (2) movement toward community-based care, (3) increases in managed care, use of telephone triage, and telephone consultation, (4) increases in use of automated monitoring of patients and telehealth modalities in the delivery of care, and (5) growing expectations by consumers of inclusion in health care decision making (Haas & Hutcherson, 1999). Legal authority for practice is a concern for any professional nurse who provides care for clients in a state in which the nurse is not currently licensed, such as nurses working in integrated delivery systems, nurses working in tertiary referral health care systems, telephone practice nurses, flight nurses, and nursing faculty. Current state licensure laws do not adequately address whether states have authority to regulate practice of a nurse who is physically located in another state. The mutual recognition model of nurse licensure would allow a nurse to have one license (in his or her state of residency) and practice in other states as long as the individual acknowledges that he or she is subject to each state's practice laws and discipline. Under mutual recognition, practice across state lines would be allowed, whether physical or electronic, unless the nurse is under discipline or a monitoring agreement that restricts practice across state lines. To achieve mutual recognition, each state would have to enter into an interstate compact that allows nurses to practice in more than one state (NCSBN, 1999). According to the NCSBN (1999), *Black's Law Dictionary* defines an interstate compact as "an agreement between two or more states established for the purpose of remedying a particular problem of multistate concern." An interstate compact supersedes state laws and may be amended by all party states agreeing and then changing individual state laws (NCSBN, 1999).

The National Council of State Boards of Nursing (NCSBN) believes that the Mutual Recognition Model of Nurse Licensure enacted through the interstate compact is the preferred regulatory model because it (1) maintains a state-based regulatory system, (2) can be implemented incrementally on a state-by-state mode, (3) can be implemented without uniform requirements for licensure in each state, (4) meets demands of integrated delivery systems, (5) meets the challenges of technological advances in telehealth, and (6) meets the public's need for access to nursing care. The benefits of the interstate compact include (1) enhancing nurses' mobility, (2) maintaining a state-based system of licensure and discipline, (3) does not change practice laws in each state and allows each state nurse practice act to maintain the authority to regulate nursing practice in the individual state, (4) deals only with licensure issues, and (5) expands consumer access to qualified nurses (Williamson, 1998).

By 2000, 12 states had adopted the interstate compact. Legislation is pending in other states. The interstate compact requires that nurses obtain only one license in the state of residency (domicile, IRS tax status), that nurses agree to abide by the state practice act in their home state and states where clients are resident at the time care is provided, and that if an incident occurs, both the "home state" and "remote state" can take disciplinary action and the compact will enable exchange of investigative information. Advantages of the one license concept include reduced barriers to interstate practice for nurses, cost-effectiveness and simplicity for the licensee, unduplicated listing of licensed nurses (we would have accurate national data on the nursing population), improved tracking for disciplinary purposes, and increased interstate commerce.

Some nursing organizations have concerns about mutual recognition and the interstate compact; the issues include lack of uniform requirements for licensure in each state; confidentiality and information sharing, particularly in terms of discipline issues (however, less than 1% of all licensed registered and practical nurses experience final disciplinary actions in a given year [NCSBN, 1999]); the potential for the compact to facilitate strike breaking; limited access by nurses to laws, rules, and other practice-related information in states where the nurse is not a resident; and licensure linked to state of residence and the need for a separate compact and time line for advanced practice nurses. In the latter, there is so much variability between states in the scope of practice for advanced practice nurses that a separate compact is being devised for their practice.

Challenges with the interstate compact begin with informing all nurses of the need for and benefits of, as well as the time line for enactment of, the interstate compact. Current information is available on the National Council of State Boards of Nursing Web site: http://www.ncsbn.org. The National Federation of Specialty Nursing Organizations (NFSNO) and the American Organization of Nurse Executives also have information on multistate licensure as does the American Academy of Ambulatory Care Nurses: http://www.inurse.com.

Promulgation of Organizational Culture and Collaborative Practice across Settings in a Network

As more acquisitions and mergers occur, health care networks will encompass multiple health care organizations and agencies. Conceivably, networks will include several different types of ambulatory care agencies. For example, an academic health center may have in its network one or more HMOs, a university hospital outpatient center, a community hospital outpatient center, and two or more physician group practices. Ambulatory patients will move between these settings. Patients may receive primary care in an HMO or physician group practice or the community hospital outpatient center and then be referred to the university hospital outpatient center for consultation with specialists. Referrals may be made from the university hospital outpatient center back to the original primary care referral source. Ambulatory care nurses working in each of these agencies will need excellent negotiation skills, and, furthermore, they will need to be expert at assessing the cultures in each of the agencies with which they interact. A "seamless system of care" demands that each agency's culture and requisite practices not impede a patient's progress. At this time we are but neophytes in understanding organization culture. The survival of evolving health care networks will depend on management and blending of multiple organizational cultures.

SUMMARY

Although concerns and challenges abound in the rapidly evolving world of ambulatory care nursing, they also provide multiple opportunities for nursing. Experienced ambulatory care nurses say that they would work in no other field of nursing. The opportunities to provide primary health care and build long-term relationships with patients, families, and health care colleagues are but a few of the rewards of working in ambulatory care nursing.

REFERENCES

American Academy of Ambulatory Care Nursing Standards Revision Task Force. (1993). *Ambulatory care nursing administration and practice standards.* Pitman, NJ: Jannetti.

American Academy of Ambulatory Care Nursing Standards Revision Task Force. (2000). *Ambulatory care nursing administration and practice standards.* Pitman, NJ: Jannetti.

American Academy of Ambulatory Care Nursing Telephone Practice Standards Task Force. (1997). *Telephone nursing practice administration and practice standards.* Pitman, NJ: Jannetti.

ANA/AAACN Task Force. (1997). *Ambulatory care nursing: The future is now.* Washington, DC: ANA.

ANA. (1995). *Social policy statement.* Washington, DC: Author.

Androwich, I., & Phillips, K. (Eds.). (1992). *The use of the minimum data set in ambulatory nursing.* American Academy of Ambulatory Care Administration. Pitman, NJ: Jannetti.

Androwich, I., & Stoupa, R. (1994). Count what counts: The nurse manager's role in automating data. *Seminars for Nurse Managers, 2*(2), 85-91.

Bulechek, G.M., McCloskey, J.C., Titler, M.G., & Denehey, J.A. (1994). Report on the NIC project: Nursing interventions used in practice. *American Journal of Nursing, 94*(10), 59-62.

Dickey, L. (1998). Outpatient visit planning: Turning episodic care into comprehensive care. *Nursing Economic$, 16*(2), 88-90.

Haas, S. (2000). Update on multi-state licensure. *Viewpoint, 22*(1), 3-4.

Haas, S., & Androwich, I. (1999). Telephone consultation. In G. Bulechek & J. McCloskey (Eds.), *Nursing interventions: Effective nursing treatments.* Philadelphia: Saunders.

Haas, S., & Gold, C. (1997). Supervision of unlicensed assistive workers in ambulatory care. *Nursing Economic$, 15*(2), 57-59.

Haas, S., & Hackbarth, D. (1995a). Dimensions of the staff nurse role in ambulatory care: Part III—Using research data to design new models of nursing care delivery. *Nursing Economic$, 13*(3), 230-241.

Haas, S., & Hackbarth, D. (1995b). Dimensions of the staff nurse role in ambulatory care: Part IV—Use of research data to develop nursing intensity measures, standards, clinical ladders, and quality improvement programs. *Nursing Economic$, 13*(5), 285-294.

Haas, S., Hackbarth, D., Kavanagh, J., & Vlasses, F. (1995). Dimensions of the staff nurse role in ambulatory care: Part II—Comparison of role dimensions in four ambulatory settings. *Nursing Economic$, 13*(3), 152-165.

Haas, S., & Hutcherson, C. (1999). *Multi-state licensure: It's coming faster than we thought possible.* Nursing Shortage Conference, September 19, 1999. Fort Lauderdale, FL: The Forum on Healthcare Leadership.

Hackbarth, D., Haas, S., Kavanagh, J., & Vlasses, F. (1995). Dimensions of the staff nurse role in ambulatory care: Part I—Methodology and analysis of data on current staff nurse practice. *Nursing Economic$, 13*(2), 89-98.

Hastings, C. (1992). Classification issues in ambulatory care nursing. *Journal of Ambulatory Care Management, 10*(3), 50-64.

Hastings, C. (1997).The changing multidisciplinary team. *Nursing Economic$, 15*(2), 106-108.

Hastings, C., & Muir-Nash, J. (1989). Validation of a taxonomy of ambulatory nursing practice. *Nursing Economic$, 7,* 142-149.

Hermann, C.E. (1993). Diversified nursing practice in ambulatory care. *Nursing Economic$, 11*(3), 176-179.

Hooks, M., Dewitz-Arnold, D., & Westbrook, L. (1980). The role of the professional nurse in the ambulatory care setting. *Nursing Administration Quarterly, 4*(4), 12-17.

Joseph, A. (1990). Ambulatory care: An objective assessment. *Journal of Nursing Administration, 20*(11), 18-24.

Kastens, J. (1998). Integrated care management: Aligning medical care center and nurse triage services. *Nursing Economic$, 16*(6), 320-322, 329.

Kerfoot, K. (2000). TIQ (technical IQ)—A survival skill for the new millennium. *Nursing Economic$, 18*(1), 29-31.

Liptak, G., Burns, C., Davidson, P., & McAnarney, E. (1998). Effects of providing comprehensive ambulatory services to children with chronic conditions. *Archives of Pediatric and Adolescent Medicine, 152*(10), 1003-1008.

McCloskey, J.C., & Bulechek, G.M. (Eds.). (1992). *Nursing Interventions Classification.* St. Louis: Mosby–Year Book.

National Council of State Boards of Nursing. (1999). Available: http://www.ncsbn.org.

Parrinello, K., & Witzel, P. (1990). Analysis of ambulatory nursing practice. *Nursing Economic$, 8*(6), 322-328.

Pinkney-Atkinson, V., & Robertson, B. (1993). Ambulatory nursing: The handmaiden/specialist dichotomy. *Journal of Nursing Administration, 23*(9), 50-57.

Sackett, D.L., Rosenberg, W.M.C., Gray, J.A.M., Haynes, R.B., & Richardson, W.S. (1996). Evidence-based medicine: What it is and what it isn't. *British Journal of Medicine (BMJ), 312,* 71-72.

Schroeder, C., Trehearne, B.B., & Ward, D. (2000). Expanded role of nursing in ambulatory managed care, Part I: Literature, role development, and justification. *Nursing Economic$, 18*(1), 14-19.

Smith, J. (1981). The idea of health: A philosophical inquiry. *Advances in Nursing Science, 3*(3), 43-50.

Spooner, S.A. (1994). Incorporating temporal and clinical reasoning in a new measure of continuity of care. *Proceedings of the Annual Symposium on Computer Applications in Medical Care* (pp. 716-721). American Medical Informatics Association. Philadelphia: Hanley & Belfus.

Stavins, M. (1993). Ambulatory nursing: Facing the future. *Journal of Ambulatory Care Management, 16*(4), 67-71.

Teich, J., & Wrinn, M. (2000). Clinical decision support systems come of age. *MD Computing, 17*(1), 43-46.

Tice, A., Poretz, D., Cook, F., Zinner, D., & Strauss, M. (1998). Medicare coverage of outpatient ambulatory intravenous antibiotic therapy: A program that pays for itself. *Clinical Infectious Diseases, 27*(6), 1415-1421.

Verran, J. (1981). Delineation of ambulatory care nursing practice. *Journal of Ambulatory Care Management, 4*(2), 1-13.

Verran, J.A. (1986). Patient classification in ambulatory care. *Nursing Economic$, 4*(5), 247-251.

Werley, H.H., & Lang, N.M. (Eds.). (1988). *Identification of the nursing minimum data set.* New York: Springer.

Williamson, S.H. (1998). Moving toward multistate licensure: Proposal revamps current system. *AAACN Viewpoint, 20*(5), 1, 16-17.

Current Issues in Emergency Nursing 2000

MARILYN L. RICE, CYNTHIA J. ABEL, DEBORAH SMITH

More than 99 million patient visits were made to emergency departments (EDs) annually in the United States at the end of the twentieth century (American Hospital Association [AHA], 2000). This large volume of ED visits is a result of the frequent, chaotic, and complex changes in the health care industry and society. An aging population, increased outpatient procedures, difficult access to primary care services, managed care bureaucracy, and the consumer's expectation for convenient, expedient, friendly care have all contributed to this rise in emergency department visits. The spectrum of patient illness, injury, and acuity presented to EDs on a daily basis ranges from nonurgent to emergent in nature and spans all possible medical, surgical, and social conditions. This multitude of patient complaints challenges nurses practicing in this setting to achieve competencies and skills for an infinite variety of medical problems and social situations.

The increasing volume and complexity of emergency clientele has had an impact on emergency services. At the same time, health care delivery systems are transitioning to a more integrated model of care, and legislators are introducing initiatives intended to protect the public's access to health care services. These changes in health care delivery and medical legislative efforts, combined with institutional initiatives for efficiency and economy, have required emergency nurses and administrators to confront difficult issues and develop creative solutions.

These issues and solutions have also created new and unique opportunities for professional practice in emergency nursing. As the volume of emergency visits increases, the demand for nurses in this specialty rises proportionately. Today, the total number of nurses practicing in emergency care settings in the United States is estimated to be as high as 90,000 professional registered nurses (RNs). More than 25% of these nurses, or approximately 24,000 emergency nurses, are members of the Emergency Nurses Association (ENA), the professional association for emergency nurses.

The ENA offers emergency nurses from all over the country and the world the opportunity for education in their clinical specialty, development of leadership and management skills, collegial relationships, and professional growth. ENA's annual meetings, scientific assemblies, products, and services have been produced by emergency nurses who volunteer as members of the board of directors or as members of one of the standing committees or vision councils. In addition, the Emergency Nurses Foundation, established in 1992, affords emergency nurses new opportunities for funding of scientific studies and advanced education.

ENA leaders continually struggle with the issue of meeting and maintaining the needs of current members, while attracting and mentoring new members. The ENA, like other professional organizations, has experienced a slight decrease in membership for a variety of professional and personal reasons. Emergency nurses, like other professionals, work more hours with greater demands and fewer resources, have less free time, and have much less employer support for professional activities. More frequently the profession's newer emergency nurses tend to ask, What can the organization do for me? rather than What can I contribute to my profession and specialty?

PRACTICE ISSUES

Increasing Acuity

Because the volume of emergency visits tripled over the last 30 years, a single-bay "emergency room" has evolved into a large, multisuite ED with state-of-the-art critical care equipment designed to care for increasingly more acutely ill patients. Advances in technology, along with episodic or chronic shortages of critical care beds or critical care nurses, can have an impact on the time that critically ill patients stay in the emergency department. In some instances, EDs today might hold critically ill patients for extended periods of time, possibly hours to days waiting for critical care inpatient beds to open or critical care nurses to staff them. However, 1998 data from ENA's national survey show that the national averages did not require patients to stay excessively long in the ED. In 1,417 EDs, 92% were able to discharge the patient, categorized as urgent, to another area within 5 hours. Only one ED, or 0.1%, held any emergent patient for longer than 24 hours (ENA, 1999a).

Triage

The increasing volume and mixed acuity of patients seen in the ED has resulted in the development and refinement of nurse triage systems. Triage nurses sort, prioritize, and control the flow of patients, as well as initiate minor interventions. Triage is actually one of the highest skills associated with emergency nursing and requires a high level of critical thinking and decision making. Triage nurses are faced with multiple challenges related to patient mix, patient rights, federal legislation, and managed care requirements. A successful triage system relies on well-educated, highly skilled, and experienced emergency nurses.

Standards of Care

As emergency patient acuity and length of stay have increased, so has the expectation in standard of care. A Joint Commission on Accreditation of Health Care Organizations (JCAHO) accredited hospital must ensure that ED standards reflect the current standards of practice. These standards must apply across the continuum whether the patient is cared for in the ED or critical care unit. Expectations for nursing assessment, analysis, evaluation of care, and documentation of that care are greater than ever before.

Emergency nurses today must be prepared to manage ever more complex procedures and equipment. Invasive monitoring devices, balloon pumps, pulse oximetry, and end tidal CO_2 monitoring are but a few of the advanced procedures and equipment found in today's ED.

This increasing acuity, along with higher standards of care, and the episodic and unpredictable nature of patient arrivals and length of stay present challenges to ED administrators attempting to meet the nursing needs of these patients while remaining fiscally responsible. Current ED managers must adjust staffing and skill mix on an hour-to-hour and day-to-day basis to meet the needs of the changing mix of ED patients.

Practice Setting

Emergency nursing practice is not limited to the hospital ED. Alternative practice settings include sites from prehospital care to urgent care clinics. Emergency nurses can be found practicing in helicopters, fixed-wing aircraft, ambulances, fast tracks, observation units, chest pain centers, after-hours clinics, occupational health clinics, poison control centers, and the traditional ED. Many emergency nurses have blended their experience into more nontraditional roles, such as health care and medical legal consulting, information system experts, sales, and even architecture. The practice of emergency nursing in an alternative setting offers both excitement and challenge. However, the emergency nurse must maintain competency in emergency care and in concepts more specific to those unique environments. As an example, an emergency nurse working in a prehospital setting must be familiar with scene safety, extrication, and immobilization. Flight nurses must be knowledgeable about the effects of altitude on patients, crew, and equipment.

Practice in an alternative setting also requires emergency nurses to be aware of issues related to role and scope of practice. Some of these issues are addressed in individual state or federal legislation, and practice may vary from state to state. Practice in an alternative setting may cross state lines and even international borders. Emergency nurses must be aware of these practice differences and act accordingly.

Changing Roles in Emergency Care

Many of the changes in health care and the emergency setting have provided new opportunities for emergency nurses to develop new roles and skills. Roles have expanded to include experiences in management, education, advanced practice, collaboration of care, and research. The emergency services case manager is a relatively new role developed to coordinate the services of the multiple departments and agencies involved in meeting the needs of emergency patients. As more and more patients access the hospital through the ED, clinical paths and practice guidelines have been redesigned to include the emergency phase of patient care.

Numbers of nonlicensed assistive personnel used in the hospital and EDs grew steadily in the 1980s and continues to grow as hospitals attempt to meet the increasing demand for health services, yet reduce costs. Titles used to delineate nonlicensed providers in the emergency setting include patient care technicians, multiskilled workers, orderlies, care partners, clinical associates, and patient care assistants.

The use of nonlicensed personnel in EDs was originally limited to tasks such as patient transport, stocking rooms, passing meal trays, and making beds or stretchers. Currently, nonlicensed assistive personnel may be used for additional tasks, such as measuring vital signs, procedural assistance, Foley catheter insertion, nasogastric tube insertion, dressing changes, respiratory treatments, 12-lead electrocardiogram performance, dysrhythmia recognition, and phlebotomy (Beardsley & Hatler, 1994). The expansion of the role of the nonlicensed assistive personnel in the ED requires that emergency nurses be prepared to delegate, supervise, and establish competency of these caregivers. It has been argued that this supervisory role requires leadership skill beyond what is taught in some nursing programs. The use of nonlicensed assistive personnel is not expected to decrease in light of the current specialty nurse shortage and aging of the nurse workforce.

Advance Practice Nurses

The newest advance practice nursing role used in the emergency care setting is that of the nurse practitioner. During the 1970s, emergency nurse practitioner programs opened for nurses with curricula similar to the current physician assistant programs. Graduate level education was not a requirement. It is estimated that approximately 200 emergency nurses completed such programs before the federal funding was discontinued in the 1980s.

Curry estimated in 1994 that only 1% of all nurse practitioners were practicing in EDs. Since that time, nurse practitioner programs have flourished to meet the increased demand for midlevel providers. Family nurse practitioners (FNPs), adult nurse practitioners (ANPs), pediatric nurse practitioners (PNPs), and, since 1994, emergency nurse practitioners (ENPs) have been employed in EDs in an attempt to meet the demand for emergency health care services.

FNPs used in the ED have traditionally been limited to caring for the nonurgent or fast-track emergency patients. ENPs, however, on graduation are educated to care for the emergent, urgent, and nonurgent patient population. Their practice sites might include a tertiary hospital ED, flight program, urgent care setting, or a rural, underserved ED.

Issues that have developed with the increase in numbers and variety of nurse practitioners moving into emergency care include the question of certification, third-party reimbursement, and autonomy of practice. The resolution of these issues varies from state to state. Nationally, the Board of Certification for Emergency

Nursing (BCEN) is exploring the potential for the development of an advance practice certification for ENPs. At present, ENPs must obtain certification through the American Nurses' Association critical nurse practitioner examination, the family nurse practitioner examination, or the adult nurse practitioner examination. ENA has published the "Scope of practice for the nurse practitioner in the emergency care setting" (ENA, 1999b).

Credentialing

One of the realities of emergency nursing is that an unusually high number of credentials and certifications are expected of nurses practicing in this specialty. Certification in the specialty of emergency nursing is granted by the BCEN. Established in 1980, the certified emergency nurse (CEN) credential is currently held by more than 25,000 practitioners. Prerequisites for the examination are 2 years of experience in emergency nursing care. The CEN's purpose is to validate the specialized body of knowledge unique to emergency nursing. The evaluation of this knowledge at the competency level by the CEN examination contributes to quality of care by validating that a defined body of emergency nursing knowledge has been demonstrated. The CEN has gained greater recognition internationally, with the first CEN examination offered in 1995 in Australia and New Zealand. For emergency nurses in the specialty of flight nursing, the certified flight registered nurse (CFRN) examination has been available since 1993.

In addition to the CEN, basic life support (BLS) and advanced cardiac life support (ACLS) standards are expected for practicing emergency nurses (ENA, 1999c). Emergency nurses caring for trauma patients may also be expected to achieve and maintain the trauma nurse core course provider (TNCC) verification, the trauma nurse specialist (TNS) certification, or the ENA comprehensive advanced trauma nursing course (CATN). Nurses working in EDs caring for pediatric patients may be expected to achieve and maintain the pediatric advanced life support (PALS) provider certification or the emergency nursing pediatric course (ENPC) verification. In states that require emergency nurses to supervise prehospital care, the mobile intensive care nurse (MICN) or emergency communication registered nurse (ECRN) certification may be required. In hospitals with burn centers the advanced burn life support (ABLS) credential is recommended.

Achievement and maintenance of these credentials requires commitment, time, and money investment, which is reimbursed by hospitals at lower and lower rates. As resources dwindle, ED administrators are challenged to attract, maintain, and reward a highly credentialed group of nurses. In more and more hospitals, emergency nurses must decide to use personal time and funds to achieve, or maintain, these credentials.

MANAGEMENT ISSUES IN EMERGENCY CARE

As health care organizations have eliminated layers of management, ED administrators, managers, and even staff members have found themselves accountable for a broader scope of responsibility. The nurse manager role has evolved from single department supervisor to multi-department facilitator, mentor, advisor, and coach. The ED nurse manager of today must be able to interface with all hospital departments and outside agencies and community services (Bailey, 1991). ED staff are expected to assume previous managerial duties, which might include scheduling, policy and procedure development, and quality improvement.

Contract Management

Five years ago, more than 50% of the approximately 5,200 hospital EDs in this country contracted with services for managing their business (Greene, 1994). The traditional emergency physician practice management company provided capital, managed care, and physician practice expertise while achieving economies of scale in return for a percentage of revenues of management fees. It was also speculated that nurses would eventually become part of the contract groups, thus allowing the group to provide all physician and nursing services. During the past 5 years, however, emergency physician contract groups have experienced mergers, acquisitions, and buyouts, resulting in fewer, but larger contract groups. As health care organizations began buying out physician practices, many physicians, including emergency physicians, became hospital employees. Health care organizations have realized the incredible costs associated with physician employees and, increasingly, are re-evaluating and eliminating this business relationship. As a result and as an alternative to joining the larger practice groups, emergency physicians are again forming emergency practice groups for single hospitals and smaller health care systems. More emergency advanced practice nurses have become partners in all groups.

Some hospitals are entering into joint ventures with these companies to ensure a piece of the capitation dollar or steady referral stream (Jaklevik, 1995). The emergency nurse manager, who generally is a hospital employee, must be prepared to work with, and frequently manage, these various-sized physician groups. Nurse entrepreneurs may find opportunities by venturing within these groups, and perhaps nurse-owned and nurse-managed practice management companies will become a reality. At the least, nurse managers must understand how these contracts function and the financial impact changes in the department make on these contracts.

Managed Care and Reimbursement

Managed care and ensuing changes related to the ambulatory payment classifications (APC) are the greatest financial challenges faced by emergency nurses today (Lee, 1994; Shaeffer, 2000). Managed care contracting, utilization review, new product and service development, and innovative pricing strategies are just a few of the elements the emergency administrator must include in any plans to compete in a managed care marketplace (Donker, 1992). Even in communities where managed care has had little impact, these strategies can be used to help provide the delivery of cost-efficient emergency health care.

The Health Care Financing Administration (HCFA) has proposed using APCs as the method of reimbursement for hospitals for providing emergency and other outpatient services to Medicare beneficiaries. APCs are a prospective payment system in which the hospital shares in the risk of providing care to patients in a concept similar to the diagnosis-related groups used for inpatient payments. Under the APC fee schedule, listed services and procedures are each paid at a predetermined rate. The system makes little allowance for variations in acuity. For example, a simple laceration requiring three sutures will be reimbursed at the same amount as a larger more extensive laceration requiring layers of closure. Implementation of this system took place in July 2000. The financial impact of this change will be significant for most EDs (Shaeffer, 2000). More than ever before, better cooperation will be required among the emergency service and other hospital departments.

Informatics

The expression "we're drowning in information but starved for knowledge" represents the need for automation of ED data (MacLean, 1995). The efficient processing of these data into systems useful in the management of emergency services is not perfect. ED data management capabilities include registration, automated triage, and patient flow monitoring. Clinical uses include reference information retrieval, drug dosage calculations, patient history profiling, medical record management, trauma registries, point-of-service billing, hospital-to-hospital linkages, and automated patient discharge instructions (Matson, 1992). A 1998 database survey conducted by the ENA indicated that in more than 25% of EDs, 76% use computers for registration. Order entry occurs in 63% of those EDs, and charge capture is done in 33% of those facilities (ENA, 1999a).

Voice-activated report dictation, patient assessment and treatment information, on-line consultation by means of teleconferencing, and voice recognition documentation are becoming realities. The ability to use databases and spreadsheets to improve management and performance is a necessity for emergency managers and administrators.

Results of multiple year and multiple ED strategic research projects are beginning to emerge. After identification of serious system problems that have an impact on emergency patient care, best practices are emerging and will continue to be studied. Benchmarking and patient satisfaction tools continue to serve as important monitors of care.

RISKS ASSOCIATED WITH THE PRACTICE OF EMERGENCY CARE

The very characteristics of emergency care that attract nurses to this specialty are the same characteristics that place nurses practicing in this environment at physical and emotional risk. Emergency nursing is described as dynamic, fast paced, ever changing, never boring, "adrenalin pumping," "blood and guts," and "you never know what's going to walk or be carried through the door next." The potential exposure to infectious diseases, hazardous materials, and violence are a daily part of the emergency care climate.

Violence in Emergency Care

A response of more than 1,400 ED nurse managers to a 1994 ENA survey revealed that violence within the ED is a frequent, if not daily, occurrence in many EDs (ENA, 1997). Data from a 1998 ENA National Emergency Department survey indicate that 42% of EDs surveyed had experienced an increase in violence-related visits (ENA, 1997).

Violence in the emergency care setting can be precipitated by a number of factors: ED overcrowding, easy hospital access through the ED, the family and friends of patients in a crisis situation, family and friends of victims of gang violence, long wait times, and the availability of controlled substances and other drugs. A study performed by the California Emergency Nurses Association (Keep & Glibert, 1992) of five metropolitan areas revealed that of 103 hospitals surveyed, 58% reported injuries by staff members, visitors, or patients as a result of violence. The most common weapons used were guns and knives.

Information from the ENA workplace violence survey has been used extensively for legislative action at state levels to protect health care workers from violence. Strategies that are being promoted as a deterrent against violence or the consequences of violence include such things as education of emergency staff to recognize hostile situations and practice skills for defusing or dealing with violence. Use of trained security personnel and environmental controls, which serve as a deterrent against violence, is also being promoted.

Infectious Disease

The increased incidence of human immunodeficiency virus (HIV), hepatitis B, hepatitis C, tuberculosis, and the threatened use of biological weapons of mass destruction put emergency personnel on the front line of exposure to infectious diseases. Patients with these diseases may not be able to communicate or even realize that they have these diseases. It is imperative that emergency personnel, particularly those charged with triage responsibilities, be able to quickly identify a suspicious set of symptoms or pattern of illness and be knowledgeable about disease transmission, treatment, and use of appropriate personal protective equipment.

According to a 1995 ED database survey, approximately 33% of the 2,224 ED physical plants were built during the last 10 years. However, from 1970 and 1984, the greatest number, or 40% of EDs surveyed, were constructed. Between 1995 and 1997, 41% anticipated either remodeling or new construction, and 40% did not plan on ED physical changes (ENA, 1996). Facility design and renovation of emergency care areas requires structural, functional, and strategic planning. In addition to providing current and future patient care, education, service, and research, these environments should minimize exposure to a variety of agents and materials.

EDs must include sufficient and strategically located negative pressure rooms. State-of-the-art supplies and equipment designed to provide protection for health care personnel should be standard in emergency settings. Such equipment might include the latest version of needleless intravenous systems, safe needle disposal devices, and the usual personal protective equipment, nonpermeable gowns, gloves, and masks.

Hazardous Materials

Emergency care personnel are often the first to receive and care for the victims of hazardous materials exposure.

These patients may or may not have been decontaminated before arrival and can present risk to emergency personnel, other patients, and visitors. Therefore, it is essential that emergency nurses participate in continuing education, both didactic and drills, regarding the identification and management of hazardous materials. EDs should be designed to support isolation and decontamination of patients who have been exposed to hazardous materials, while protecting health care workers, patients, and visitors from contamination.

TRAUMA AND INJURY PREVENTION

Traumatic injury is the leading cause of death in the first four decades of life. Each year more than 150,000 Americans die, and approximately 80,000 are permanently disabled as a result of injury (National Safety Council, 1998). Each year approximately 2.6 million people are hospitalized for injuries and about 37.2 million people are treated in hospital EDs for injury. The economic impact of these fatal and nonfatal injuries exceeded $478 billion in 1997. In addition, traumatic injury typically involves children and young adults and therefore results in the loss of more productive work years than other diseases.

Clear evidence exists that optimal outcomes for injured patients are best obtained in an organized system for trauma care. A regional trauma system consists of hospitals, personnel, and public service agencies that have a planned response for caring for injured patients. This plan integrates all aspects of care from the time of the injury through the rehabilitative phases.

Optimal trauma care requires that costly equipment and experienced personnel must be immediately available in EDs, operating suites, and critical care areas 24 hours per day. A priority system must often be developed to determine access to support services, such as radiology and laboratory facilities, as well as operating rooms and critical care beds. Trauma care services must often coexist or compete with other key services, such as cardiovascular services, offered by a facility.

Because of the costs and requirements associated with the provision of trauma care, some regions of the United States experienced the closure of many trauma centers in the late 1980s and early 1990s. The problems associated with the cost of trauma resources and poor reimbursement are being partially addressed on the federal and state level through the introduction of legislation supporting the development of regional trauma systems and providing a base for uncompensated care.

The most recent piece of federal legislation that addresses this issue is the Trauma Care Systems Planning and Development Act of 1990. This Act was an amendment to the Public Health Service Act (Public Law 101-590), which allows for $60 million of support through grants and technical assistance for trauma system development on a state level. Currently, not every state has initiated a statewide program for trauma system development.

Emergency and trauma care professionals are challenged to continue to pursue a system of trauma care, which ensures the highest quality of care for injured patients by managing programs efficiently in a cost-effective manner while maintaining excellent outcomes. Trauma care providers must constantly work to maintain the skill and knowledge required to provide the best possible care for injured patients.

Injury Prevention

Perhaps the most cost-effective method of managing the impact of trauma and injury is implementation of injury prevention strategies. Legislation, enforcement, technology, and education are all strategies used in the fight for injury prevention. Mandatory seatbelt laws, child-passenger restraint laws, laws requiring motorcyclists to wear helmets, and laws that prohibit drunk driving are all examples of legislation and enforcement strategies. Shatterproof glass, head restraints, seatbelts, and airbags are examples of technology that has reduced injury and saved lives. The ENA's Institute for Injury Prevention are emergency nurses who are active volunteers who conduct injury prevention activities and educate the public. Education is thought to reduce preventable injuries and death by increasing awareness and promoting healthy lifestyles.

Professional emergency nurses, as well as professional associations, today find themselves in a strategic position to place pressure on manufacturers to market safety aspects of products and to create safer products. Nurses can support national organizations that focus on promoting safety, such as Mothers Against Drunk Driving (MADD) and the National Safe Kids Campaign. Who better than the emergency nurses who deal with the direct results of trauma every workday to spread the message for injury prevention?

LEGISLATIVE ISSUES
Access to Care

The increased number of people covered by managed care insurance providers in the United States, many of which require precertification for emergency treatment, has presented a dilemma for emergency care personnel. Both the Consolidated Omnibus Budget Reconciliation Act (COBRA) of 1985 and the Emergency Medical Treatment and Active Labor Act (EMTALA) of 1994 were congressional responses to address public concerns related to access, denial of care, and inappropriate patient transfers. This legislation requires that hospitals receiving Medicare funds evaluate all patients presenting to a hospital for care to determine whether an emergency condition exists. Such a condition, if found, requires the hospital to provide immediate and stabilizing care within its capability before transfer is considered (Niersbach, 1999; Southard, 1989).

Because a patient cannot be questioned about financial information before the medical screening examination, an increasing number of EDs have implemented nurse triage systems, provided treatment to all patients who presented to the ED, and obtained financial information after treatment. If the managed care plan would not authorize ED treatment after the fact, patients were then "stuck with the bill." The ethics and difficulties presented to both patients and emergency care providers have resulted in a joint effort by emergency physicians and nurses to work with their legislators for solutions.

A bill entitled Access to Emergency Medical Services Act of 1995 was introduced into Congress in 1995. This legislative initiative, developed in cooperation with the American College of Emergency Physicians (ACEP) and supported, in concept, by the ENA Board of Directors, established a uniform "prudent layperson" definition of an emergency medical condition and enacted it for all health plans, including Medicare and Medicaid (ENA, 1995). The national standard of prudent layperson definition of an emergency is that "patients who present to the emergency department should have their treatment covered by insurance based on the initial symptoms, not the final diagnosis, and no prior authorization of services should be required." Passage of the bill by Congress is being urged to require the prudent layperson standard for health care consumers, advocating for the Access to Emergency Medical Services Act of 1999.

Although Congress approved the prudent layperson standard for Medicare and Medicaid, millions of Americans are not covered by the prudent layperson standard. Preauthorization continues to be required by health plans for hospital services, including the EDs in many states.

Legislative issues that remain of high priority to emergency nurses include issues related to the scope of emergency nursing practice and advanced practice, the welfare of emergency care workers, bans on the sale of assault weapons, monitoring child health issues, the prevention of domestic violence and the treatment of domestic violence victims, support for vehicle passenger safety measures, drunk-driving legislation, and legislation that addresses other means of injury prevention and funding of trauma and emergency care.

MEDIA REPRESENTATION OF EMERGENCY NURSING

The number one rated television program since 1994, NBC's *ER*, gave emergency nurses the unique opportunity to have an impact on the image portrayed of emergency nurses to the general public. Producers and writers of the program took an early opportunity to work with emergency nurses across the country to develop an authentic and accurate portrayal of emergency nursing and ED operations. After the first five episodes, the roles of emergency nurse actors strengthened on the program. Members of the cast portraying nurses attended the ENA annual meeting and scientific assembly in 1994 and 1995 to meet and network with practicing emergency nurses. A positive relationship between the producers, writers, actors, and the emergency nurses has continued (Rice, 1996).

In 1994, Julianna Margulies won the coveted Best Female Actor Emmy for her role as *ER*'s emergency nurse manager, Carol Hathaway. *ER* has been honored with numerous prestigious awards from peers, the Hollywood media industry, and emergency and health care organizations. In many acceptance awards by actors and other representatives of the show, emergency nurses are specifically cited and given tremendous thanks.

On a weekly basis, *ER* reinforces strong favorable impressions of emergency nursing. The program and cast members from the program have been used to help promote the message of injury and violence prevention. What has been learned from emergency nursing's involvement with the media is that a powerful message of education and prevention can be sent out to the public through the media, and nursing can have an impact on how the image of nursing is portrayed.

REFERENCES

American Hospital Association. (2000). *Hospital statistics 1998.* Chicago: Health Forum.

Bailey, M.M. (1991, September). What the future holds for E.D. nursing. *Nursing, 91*, 84-89.

Beardsley, S., & Hatler, C. (1994). Nonlicensed, multiskilled workers in the emergency department. *Journal of Emergency Nursing, 20*(5), 377-382.

Donker, R.B. (1992). Managed care. In T.A. Matson & P. McNamara (Eds.), *The hospital emergency department: A guide to operational excellence* (pp. 115-124). Chicago: American Hospital Publishing, Inc.

Emergency Nurses Association. (1995, July 27). *Federal legislative report.* Park Ridge, IL: Author.

Emergency Nurses Association. (1996). *1995 National Emergency Department Database.* Park Ridge, IL: Author.

Emergency Nurses Association. (1997). *ENA position statement on violence in the emergency care setting.* Park Ridge, IL: Author.

Emergency Nurses Association. (1998). *ENA position statement on domestic violence.* Park Ridge, IL: Author.

Emergency Nurses Association. (1999a). *1998 ENA National Emergency Department Database.* Des Plaines, IL: Author.

Emergency Nurses Association. (1999b). *Scope of emergency nursing practice.* Des Plaines, IL: Author.

Emergency Nurses Association. (1999c). *Standards of emergency nursing practice.* Des Plaines, IL: Author.

Greene, J. (1994, January 31). Contracts are catching on. *Modern Healthcare, 24,* 29-34.

Jaklevik, M.C. (2000, January 3). Back to basics for docs. *Modern Healthcare, 30,* 30.

Keep, N., & Glibert, P. (1992). California Emergency Nurses Association informal survey of violence in California emergency departments. *Journal of Emergency Nursing, 18*(5), 433-439.

Lee, M. (1994). Emergency nursing at the crossroads. *American Journal of Nursing, 18*(5), 433-439.

MacLean, S.L. (1995). The ENA national emergency department database. *ENA Management Update, 2*(3), 5.

Matson, T.A. (1992). Information systems. In T.A. Matson & P. McNamara (Eds.), *The hospital emergency department: A guide to operational excellence* (pp. 115-124). Chicago: American Hospital Publishing, Inc.

National Safety Council. (1998). *Accident facts.* Itasca, IL: Author.

Niersbach, C. (1999). Managers forum: EMTLA. *Journal of Emergency Nursing, 25*(6), 541-542.

Rice, M.L. (1996). ER nurses fight stereotype: A win for all nurses. *Revolution: The Journal of Nurse Empowerment, 6*(1), 77-81.

Shaeffer, C. (2000). Ambulatory payment classifications. *Journal of Emergency Nursing, 26*(1), 20-23.

Southard, P. (1989). COBRA legislation: Complying with ED provisions. *Journal of Emergency Nursing, 15*(1), 23-25.

SUGGESTED READINGS

Bayley, E.W., & Turcke, S.A. *A comprehensive curriculum for trauma nursing* (2nd ed.). Chicago: Roadrunner Press.

Centers for Disease Control and Prevention. (1999). Fact sheet on dating violence. *International Journal of Trauma Nursing, 5*(4).

Curry, J.L. (1992). Oil on troubled waters: Unlicensed assistive personnel in the emergency department. One hospital's experience. *Journal of Emergency Nursing, 18*(5), 428-431.

Curry, J.L. (1994). Nurse practitioners in the emergency department. *Journal of Emergency Nursing, 20*(3), 207-212.

Emergency Nurses Association. (1997). *ENA position statement on advanced practice in emergency nursing.* Park Ridge, IL: Author.

Emergency Nurses Association. (1997). *ENA position statement on autonomous emergency nursing.* Park Ridge, IL: Author.

Emergency Nurses Association. (1997). *ENA position statement on the enhanced 9-1-1 system.* Park Ridge, IL: Author.

Emergency Nurses Association. (1997). *ENA position statement on healthcare worker protection act.* Park Ridge, IL: Author.

Emergency Nurses Association. (1997). *ENA position statement on hospital and emergency overcrowding.* Park Ridge, IL: Author.

Emergency Nurses Association. (1997). *ENA position statement on latex allergies.* Park Ridge, IL: Author.

Emergency Nurses Association. (1997). *Position statement on observation/holding areas.* Park Ridge, IL: Author.

Emergency Nurses Association. (1997). *ENA position statement on bloodbourne infectious disease.* Park Ridge, IL: Author.

Emergency Nurses Association. (1997). *ENA position statement on the care of the pediatric patient during interfacility transport.* Park Ridge, IL: Author.

Emergency Nurses Association. (1997). *ENA position statement on children's gun violence prevention act.* Park Ridge, IL: Author.

Emergency Nurses Association. (1997). *ENA position statement on educational recommendations for nurses providing pediatric emergency care.* Park Ridge, IL: Author.

Emergency Nurses Association. (1997; addendum, 1998). *ENA position statement on staffing and productivity in the emergency care setting.* Park Ridge, IL: Author.

Emergency Nurses Association. (1997). *ENA position statement on specialty certification in emergency nursing.* Park Ridge, IL: Author.

Emergency Nurses Association. (1997). *ENA position statement on the use of non-registered nurse (non-RN) care givers in emergency care.* Park Ridge, IL: Author.

Emergency Nurses Association. (1998). *ENA position statement on access to health care.* Park Ridge, IL: Author.

Emergency Nurses Association. (1998). *ENA position statement on conscious sedation.* Park Ridge, IL: Author.

Emergency Nurses Association. (1998). *ENA position statement on family presence during invasive procedures and/or resuscitation.* Park Ridge, IL: Author.

Emergency Nurses Association. (1998). *ENA position statement on hazardous material exposure.* Park Ridge, IL: Author.

Emergency Nurses Association. (1998). *ENA position statement on injury prevention.* Park Ridge, IL: Author.

Emergency Nurses Association. (1998). *ENA position statement on interfacility transport of the critically ill or injured patient.* Park Ridge, IL: Author.

Emergency Nurses Association. (1998). *ENA position statement on domestic violence.* Park Ridge, IL: Author.

Emergency Nurses Association. (1998). *ENA position statement on the role of delegation by the emergency nurse clinical practice settings.* Park Ridge, IL: Author.

Emergency Nurses Association. (1998). *ENA position statement on the role of the registered nurse in the prehospital care environment.* Park Ridge, IL: Author.

Emergency Nurses Association. (1998). *ENA position statement on the treatment of sexual assault survivors.* Park Ridge, IL: Author.

Emergency Nurses Association. (1998). *ENA position statement on tuberculosis exposure in the emergency department.* Park Ridge, IL: Author.

Emergency Nurses Association. (1999). *Emergency nursing core curriculum* (5th ed.). Philadelphia: Saunders.

Emergency Nurses Association. (1999). *ENA position statement on health care worker needlestick and sharps injury prevention act.* Park Ridge, IL: Author.

Emergency Nurses Association. (1999). *ENA policy statement on minimal trauma nursing education recommendations.* Park Ridge, IL: Author.

Emergency Nurses Association. (1999). *Position statement on OSHA hazardous information bulletin on latex gloves.* Park Ridge, IL: Author.

Emergency Nurses Association. (1999). *ENA position statement on bill of rights act.* Park Ridge, IL: Author.

Emergency Nurses Association. (1999). *Scope of practice for the nurse practitioner in the emergency care setting.* Des Plaines, IL: Author.

Evans, S.S. (1991). Delegation: What do we fear? [Editorial]. *Heart Lung, 20,* 17A-20A.

Geraci, E.B., & Geraci, T.A. (1994). An observational study of the emergency triage nursing role in a managed care facility. *Journal of Emergency Nursing, 20*(3), 189-194.

Gibbs, H., & Duncan Ross, A. (1996). *The medicine of ER, or how we almost die* (pp. 21-28). New York: Basic Books.

Joint Commission on Accreditation of Healthcare Organizations. (1999). *2000 hospital accreditation standards.* Oak Brook Terrace, IL: Author.

Lenehan, G.P. (1999). ED short staffing: It is time to take a hard look at a growing problem and strategies such as standard nurse-patient ratios. *Journal of Emergency Nursing, 25*(2), 77-78.

MacLean, S.L., Bayley, E.W., Cole, F.L., Bernardo, L., Lenaghan, P., & Manton, A. (1999). The LUNAR project: A description of the population of individuals who seek health care at emergency departments. *Journal of Emergency Nursing, 25*(4), 269-282.

McKay, J.I. (1999). The emergency department of the future—The challenge is in changing how we operate. *Journal of Emergency Nursing, 25*(6), 480-488.

Pouroy, J. (1995). *Behind the scenes at ER* (pp. 121-124). New York: Ballantine Books.

Purnell, L. (1993). A survey of the qualifications, special training and levels of personnel working in emergency department triage. *Journal of Nursing Staff Development, 9*(5), 223-226.

Southard, P. (1994). Trauma in a reformed health care environment. *Journal of Emergency Nursing, 20*(5), 422-423.

Recent Changes and Current Issues in Gerontological Nursing

MARY ZWYGART-STAUFFACHER, MARILYN J. RANTZ

For more than 30 years there has been an awareness of the aging of America and that there would be an explosion of older adults in America. The beginning of the new millennium finds us facing this aging explosion with increased knowledge about the aging process and needed care for the elderly, yet only a limited number of adequately prepared professional nurses is available to address the needs. The time is here, the time is now, and the elderly population projections for the 21st century are staggering. Cost implications for caring for the elderly are equally staggering. Costs are associated with not only vast increases in numbers of elderly but in the complexity of the multiple chronic diseases and acute exacerbations that occur. Although people older than 65 comprise approximately 12% of the population, they account for more than one third of the country's personal health care expenditures (U.S. Special Committee on Aging, 1991). As the older population grows, so will be their use of services. In 1990, about 1.5 million impaired people older than age 65 used some type of community service at least once. By the year 2020, 2.4 million impaired older people will use community services (U.S. Special Committee on Aging, 1991). To understand the scope of the costs of these services, in 1992, more than $60 billion were spent on long-term care and home and community care for the elderly (Cohen, Kumar, McGuire, & Wallack, 1992). This compares with the substantial increase of cost of these services by 1996, when $125.5 billion was spent on nursing home and home health care for the elderly (Health Care Financing Administration [HCFA], 1996; Levit et al., 1997). In addition, Medicare's Hospital Insurance and Supplementary Medical Insurance program financed $203.1 billion in spending for health care of the aged and disabled, bringing the total spent on those older than 65 years of age to $326.6 billion (Levit et al., 1997). Considering the costs and needs for services for older people to-

day and in the future, one must ask, Do we have the nursing work force to address the needs of the gerontological clients? Can today's work force adjust to work effectively in our changing delivery systems? How can we better prepare the gerontological nursing work force of tomorrow? These are major issues confronting gerontological nursing today.

CHANGING DELIVERY SYSTEMS

Older adults are using services across the continuum of care; they no longer depend on hospitalizations, which are coupled with ongoing supervision from their primary care physician to manage their chronic conditions. Older adults are using a multitude of community-based home care and social services, subacute care, and long-term care services delivered in multiple sites (Vladeck, Miller, & Clauser, 1993). New roles are emerging as nurses assist seniors to navigate the continuum of care. The nurse becomes the person who helps them navigate those uncertain waters as they try to use services from multiple settings across multiple agencies funded from a variety of sources (Ebersole & Hess, 1998). New nursing roles are not without dilemmas. Gerontological nurses must now make decisions that are not only client focused but also economic focused. Seldom before have nurses played such integral roles in the allocation of resources. Nurses in the past cared for seniors without concern for cost implications. Today, as nurses assume case management or care coordination roles, cost must be considered. Subsequently, nurses must make tough decisions about allocation of resources for the client. It is a new era for gerontological nurses. We must be aware of what services cost and help seniors make wise cost-effective choices, while assuring they receive the service they need. Yet, gerontological nurses, like other health care providers, are dually challenged because they may not identify needs consistent with those of their clients (Zwygart-Stauffacher, Lindquist, & Savik, 2000).

As seniors use a variety of services across the continuum of care, funding of services by means of managed care contracts becomes a tremendous challenge for gerontological nursing. When funded through managed care contracts, services must be provided within a capitated budget. This means there is a set fee for *all* services that people will use, and nurses must assume gate-keeping functions and make tough decisions about which type of services seniors will receive. Capitation is a very different approach than the fee-for-service approach, in which costs of services are totaled and billed at the end. Because managed care is fully implemented for Medicare recipients, limits on acute care utilization and hospitalization will become apparent. No longer will seniors with multiple chronic illnesses primarily use multiple hospitalizations for the management of their illnesses. As much as possible, they will be managed on an outpatient basis, and some tough decisions will have to be made about when to stop treatment. Subsequently, the elderly that will be seen in the acute care setting will be most complex with multiple-system disorders or illnesses requiring a tremendous depth and breadth of knowledge for care of that older adult. The nurse in the community will be part of a health care team that will be making some tough decisions to not hospitalize some very sick people with complex illnesses and allow them to die at home, in a nursing home, or in a subacute unit.

ADVANCED PRACTICE NURSE IN GERONTOLOGICAL NURSING

With the evolution of managed care and complex care delivery systems the gerontological nurse prepared at the graduate level is being viewed as the appropriate provider or coordinator of care services. Therefore, an increase in the number of individuals prepared with graduate degrees in gerontological nursing is required. Historically, the advanced practice gerontological nurse is a master's-prepared individual with a clinical specialization in gerontological nursing.

In the 1970s there were only a few programs at the master's level preparing gerontological nurse practitioners; this was not embraced by the nursing community until the mid to late 1980s. There are now two advanced clinical practice roles in which gerontological specialization developed: the gerontological clinical nurse specialist and the gerontological nurse practitioner. Yet even

with the expansion of two graduate preparation options, the numbers of individuals prepared with gerontological nursing specialization have not been realized. Although the number of certified gerontological nurse practitioners has risen from 1,570 in 1993 (American Nurses Credentialing Center [ANCC], 1994) to 3,240 by January of 2000 (ANCC, personal communication, 2000) with an additional 847 nurses certified as gerontological clinical nurse specialists, this is not even half as many certified as pediatric nurse practitioners, which is in excess of 10,000 (National Certification Board of Pediatric Nurse Practitioners and Nurses, personal communication, 2000).

There is support in the literature that these two roles (nurse practitioner and clinical nurse specialist) will merge, and a single advanced practice gerontological nurse preparation will emerge in the near future (Fulmer & Mezey, 1994; Schuren, 1996). Although there are similarities in the role, there are also differences that have had little discussion within all the nursing communities (Page & Arena, 1994). At issue is whether one individual can be prepared who can integrate the competencies of both these roles when minimal research has been conducted to compare these roles (Fenton & Brykczynski, 1993; Lyons, 1996). These roles have traditionally been setting-specific, with the nurse practitioner as the provider of ambulatory and primary care services and the clinical specialist providing services to special patient populations in long-term care and acute care settings and staff education or development. If a blending of these roles can occur, the resulting issue becomes: Can we prepare clinically competent people in a blended role who can successfully meet the demands of the role expectations across settings? Nurse practitioners have been prepared with a variety of primary care skills that have been specifically targeted to develop skills to direct primary care of older adults. That has not been the case for clinical nurse specialists. They have received information and education targeted to managing nursing problems older adults present, not assuming responsibility for directing with the client the management of their health alteration. These are two distinct role functions.

Historically, the individuals who have merged both these role functions have done so with a clinical nurse specialist master's degree followed with a post-master's specialization for nurse practitioner. How to configure both the merged curriculum and the specialized focus is at issue. Another key issue is whether family nurse practitioners or adult nurse practitioners will be viewed as having the knowledge and experience necessary to work with the elderly in their health care management. Technically, individuals prepared as family or adult nurse practitioners were allowed to sit for the ANCC certification as gerontological nurse practitioners (GNP) until 1996, when the ANCC instituted the policy that allowed only individuals who have been prepared in a gerontological nurse practitioner program to sit for the GNP examination. No longer is the crossover from family and adult to gerontological allowed. Given the complexity of gerontological clients and the complexity of the knowledge base that is required for successfully managing the role functions of the gerontological nurse practitioner, it is clear that formal gerontological education needs to be the foundation for gerontological certification and clinical practice.

An additional issue related to preparing individuals at the advanced practice level is the need to restructure curricula in academic institutions in light of cost containment. There is a trend to minimize specialization content in an effort to try to include more students in all courses. These cost-containment efforts are likely to have an impact on specialized courses, such as specialized gerontological courses. It is likely that the cost-containment efforts will delete those courses as options for students, because it is more costly and time consuming to arrange both specialized didactic and clinical components. It is presumed by some that one can obtain the knowledge that is necessary for delivering gerontological care by simply completing clinical practica with older adults without specialized didactic content within the graduate program. This is a disturbing trend.

Assuming that broad didactic courses, such as a general primary care management course applied across the lifespan, and clinical experience with older people is adequate for preparation as an advanced practice gerontological nurse is a disservice to both students *and* clients. Students need both didactic and well-planned clinical experiences with theoretical content specific to the gerontological population. Specialty courses should be available for further specialization. Haight and Stewart (1994) describe geropsychiatric specialty courses for graduate nursing education. In light of the scope of clinical problems and the frequency with which nurses are confronted with mental health and behavior problems of older adults, such specialty courses are appropriate and needed. Students also need an understanding of cost of care delivery. We can no longer afford to teach students how that care should be delivered without an understanding of what that care will cost.

Aside from the content issues of what should be taught, qualifications of the faculty are at issue. A report of the planning committee for the White House Conference on Aging revealed that an alarming 40% of the nursing faculty teaching in graduate level gerontological nursing programs have *no* formal gerontological preparation. Three fourths (77%) of all clinical preceptors and instructors in all programs in nursing have no formal preparation working with the elderly (Dye, 1992). Mezey (1995) has advised that failure to produce adequate number of faculty to teach gerontology has adversely affected the care of the elderly. How can gerontological advanced practice nurses be prepared by faculty without gerontological preparation?

UNDERGRADUATE NURSING EDUCATION

On the basis of our experience, we concur with Fulmer and Mezey (1994) that traditionally, basic nursing programs have included very little geriatric nursing content and that most faculty lack preparation in geriatric nursing. If they do have course work in geriatric nursing, the faculty lack preparation in geriatric nursing to be qualified to teach those courses (National League for Nursing, 1991). Yurchuck and Brower (1994) reported that only 12% of undergraduate faculty have specific gerontological preparation. Minimal progress has been seen since these initial reports. Rosenfeld, Bottrell, Fulmer, and Mezey (1999) examined the geriatric content in the baccalaureate curriculum of 80% of university programs in 1997. Of the respondent nursing programs, only 40% reported at least one full-time faculty member American Nurses Association or ANCC certified in geriatrics. (ANCC is the only body certifying gerontological nurses.) Twenty percent of the part-time faculty was reported to be certified. How can a school of nursing hope to achieve the standard proposed by Rosenfeld et al. "that the nursing community assure that every nurse graduating from a baccalaureate nursing program have a defined level of competency." When one considers the approach to undergraduate nursing education, it is clear that nurse educators would not be put in the position of teaching pediatric or obstetric nursing without preparation in those fields. Why have we allowed nurse educators to teach gerontological nursing without a knowledge base or practice base for their instruction? Because of the sheer numbers of older adults using the health care delivery system and the complexity of the clinical problems that they present, it is imperative that faculty be prepared clinically and theoretically to teach these courses. Simply having "taken care of elders" is not sufficient preparation.

Sister Rose Therese Bahr (1994) said it so well:

What's wrong? Despite the amount of money made available for post-doctoral study, few faculty are taking advantage of the opportunity to upgrade their knowledge in gerontological nursing. I would hazard a guess that the attitude problems of students not wishing to choose gerontological nursing as a career starts with the faculty who also have an attitude problem. To be based in reality means that all of us are on the continuum of aging. All persons will get old unless a traumatic event occurs that ends life much earlier. What are faculty afraid of that they shy away from content and clinical experience that evolves around the care of the aged? [p. 38]

Issues surrounding undergraduate nursing education must include grappling with the problem of associate degree education. Most of the registered nurses working in nursing homes are prepared at the associate degree level. Many associate degree curricula do contain content concerning gerontological nursing; however, most do *not* contain a specialized gerontological nursing course. These curricula also lack content and practica in nursing leadership and advanced health assessment. How can nurses prepared at this level be expected to assume a supervisory level position or coordinate comprehensive assessments as are required in nursing homes and hospitals across the nation.

The Institute of Medicine (1986) has recommended that "Nursing homes should place their highest priority on recruitment, retention, and support of adequate numbers of professional nurses who are trained in gerontology and geriatrics to insure an adequate number and appropriate mix of professional and non-professional nursing personnel to meet the needs of all types of residents in each facility." However, many nursing homes have received waivers from even the Omnibus Budget Reconciliation Act's (OBRA) minimal increases in staffing standards (Francese & Mohler, 1994). These homes claim shortages of registered nurses and inadequate reimbursement to pay their salaries are the reasons that they cannot meet the staffing standards. Nursing must become involved to correct these delivery system problems. What creative strategies will nurse administrators conceive to address the shortage of adequate staffing during the present workforce issues that are facing the United States at this time.

In addition, nursing must deal with the issue of how much preparation a student can receive in a 2-year program to be able to deal with complex problems of elderly in nursing homes and other settings. However, it must be acknowledged that one of the major providers of nursing services in nursing homes is the licensed practical nurse prepared with even less formal education.

Home care is an exploding source of services for seniors. Most nurses working in the home care arena are prepared at the associate degree level. Traditionally, public health or community-based services were to be provided by the baccalaureate-prepared nurse, but this is no longer the case. We have nurses going into homes, a most complex environment to care for people with complex clinical problems, with minimum formal nursing education and frequently coupled with limited experience. At some point nursing must address this issue and establish the baseline for professional gerontological nursing and general nursing practice at the baccalaureate level. Education aside, nursing assistants and homemakers with little or no formal nursing preparation are delivering many in-home services to seniors.

CURRENT CLINICAL AND SYSTEMS ISSUES

To identify the current and changing clinical and systems issues of gerontological nursing discussed in gerontological literature, the journals listed in the box below for the years 1992 to 1995 and subsequently 1995 to 1998 were analyzed using qualitative methods (Zwygart-Stauffacher, Bowman, & Rantz, 2000). The trends in order of frequency of publication are identified for these two time periods in the box on page 172.

When comparing the trends in the gerontological nursing literature from 1992 to 1995 and 1995 to 1998 with trends identified from a 1980 to 1990 literature review for

---

**JOURNALS REVIEWED
1992-1995 AND 1995-1998**

Journal of Gerontological Nursing
Geriatric Nursing
The Gerontologist
Journal of the American Geriatrics Society
Journals of Gerontology
Journal of Long-Term Care Administration
IMAGE: The Journal of Nursing Scholarship
Nursing Research
Research in Nursing and Health
Nursing Outlook

TRENDS IN GERONTOLOGICAL RESEARCH LITERATURE*

Identified in 1992-1995

Clinical Issues
Reminiscence
Restraints
   Problems associated with
   Efforts to reduce use
Disruptive or aggressive behavior
   Nursing strategies to manage
Wandering
Functional status
   Maintaining function
   Measurement of functional status
   Using functional status to predict illness
Activities of daily living
Elderly response to hospitalization
Use of life sustaining or life-saving procedures
Tube feedings
   Positive and negative aspects of use
   Ethical dilemmas of use
Relocation stress
Urinary incontinence
Failure to thrive
Substance abuse
Depression
Alzheimer's
Elder abuse
Wellness promotion

Systems Issues
Dementia special care units
   Resource use
   Regulation of
   Effectiveness of
Subacute units
Discharge from acute care settings
Family caregiving
   Collaboration between facilities and families
   Stress associated with
Community-based services
   Continuum of care
   Financing
   Gaps in home health coverage
Life-care community developments
Advanced directives and self-determination
Delaying nursing home placement
Financing long-term care
Staffing issues in nursing homes
   Use of nurse practitioners and clinical nurse specialists
   Retention of staff and training issue

Minimum data set for nursing homes
   Validation of and research using
Health care reform
Financing acute care

Identified in 1995-1998

Clinical Issues
Assessment Issues
Wellness
   Promotion and
   Disease prevention
Alzheimer's
Functional status
Urinary incontinence and other issues
Disruptive or aggressive behavior
   Nursing strategies to manage
Restraints
   Problems associated with
   Efforts to reduce use
Activities of daily living
Falls
Depression
Relocation stress
Sustaining or saving life
Wandering
Elder abuse

Systems Issues
Family caregiving
   Collaboration between facilities
   Stress associated with
Community-based services
Staffing issues
Dementia special care units
   Resource use
   Effectiveness of
Discharge from acute care settings
Self-determination
Financing long-term care
Financing acute care
Minimum data set
Subacute units
Health care reform
Life-care community developments
Delaying nursing home placement

*In order of frequency of publication.

a report to the Institute of Medicine (Lang, Kraegel, Rantz, & Krejci, 1990), one sees some new issues have surfaced. Although during the early 1990s the emergence of dementia special care units and subacute units was paramount with controversy surrounding these special care programs and units, this was less of an issue by the late 1990s. Some have seen these units as options for long-term care agencies to improve their financial position, whereas others are concerned if the agencies can provide the level of clinical expertise that these more acutely ill elderly need. The Minimum Data Set (MDS) assessment instrument mandated for use in all nursing homes in 1990 is a new issue at the turn of the 1990s, although its use and usefulness were being addressed by the end of the century. Controversy continues to surround the MDS instrument and the data that are collected. Some are concerned about pursuing research activities using MDS data, raising concerns about validity and reliability. Others are concerned about how regulators will interpret aggregated assessment information from MDS data, how payment mechanisms may be designed using the data, and how comparisons will be made across agencies. In the later 1990s, issues surrounding assessment, wellness, and functional status were more frequently represented in the gerontological literature. Possibly, this is a result of the emergence of advanced practice roles and the use of this provider in all settings, but particularly the nursing home setting.

In the early 1990s there was a marked increase in the number of studies related to advance directives and the use of life-sustaining procedures. It may be that the Patient Self-Determination Act of 1991 is raising these issues for discussion, or perhaps public debate surrounding health care reform and costs of services are bringing these issues forward. Elder abuse in the current survey is more clearly represented in the nursing gerontological literature. It is likely that this is related to increased public and professional awareness of the problem and attention by nurse researchers. The issues of restraints and behavioral issues were more prominent at the end of the century, possibly related to the effect of OBRA 87 and new HCFA and Joint Commission on the Accreditation of Healthcare Organizations (JCAHO) guidelines for restraint use for clients in nursing homes and hospitals.

The development of community-based services across the continuum of care is also a recent phenomena in the nursing literature, as well as the development of life-care communities for older adults. These services are considered by many authors to be significant trends for the future of gerontological care delivery. Other trends for the future identified in the literature are delivery of acute care services in long-term care facilities and an increased emphasis on research about care delivery and care needs of older adults. These trends could hold much promise for improving the quality of care and quality of life of long-term care residents.

WHERE GERONTOLOGICAL NURSING NEEDS TO GO NEXT

With the complexity and diversity of clinical problems it is clear that gerontological nursing education must be enhanced so that nurses working with older adults are educationally prepared to deal with their complex problems. In addition, nurses need to be prepared to deal with the complex systems issues that permeate the complicated delivery systems that older persons must traverse. Gerontological nursing education must prepare professionals to not only deal with these complex issues but also to shape the future of care delivery for older adults.

We must have nurse researchers who have gerontological nursing experience to guide research that is relevant and clearly addresses the issues of older adults. Gerontological nurse researchers who are grounded in clinical experience with older adults can direct relevant research that truly adds to improving the quality of care that older adults receive or improve the education that nurses receive for gerontological nursing. In addition, nurse researchers who are out of touch with the realities of clinical service systems are not prepared to ask relevant questions that will make significant differences for older adults. With shrinking research dollars and increased competition for resources for research activity, the true relevance of the topic under investigation and the impact it will have on clinical practice and patient outcomes must be clear. Researchers who are formally educated and experienced in the care of the elderly are crucial to the future of gerontological nursing.

It is important that we recruit individuals into gerontological nursing practice who have a true commitment to the elderly and the services that they need. Gerontological services are in a growing market with growing opportunities. As with any expanding market, it is not always clear whether people are motivated to choose gerontological nursing because they are truly interested in caring for older adults or whether job and economic security are the prime motivators. This motivation can clearly affect the outcome of care and the individualization of the care provision.

Nurses who have a gerontological commitment need to embrace this time of health care reform and configure systems of care, determine what appropriate care outcomes will be, and pursue building those service delivery systems. It is time for gerontological nurses to design the future, not react to someone else's designs. It is time for gerontological nurses to designate what the critical outcomes of gerontological nursing should be and design a path to achieve the outcomes. "In view of the projections of dramatically increasing elders in the next century, gerontological nursing will hold a critical position in the health of the nation and the world" (Southern Council on Collegiate Education for Nursing, 1995).

REFERENCES

American Nurses Credentialing Center. (1994). *Credentialing catalog.* ANA.

Bahr, R.T. (1994). Response to "Issues facing faculty in long-term care." In E.L. Middy (Ed.), *Mechanisms of quality in long-term care: Education* (pp. 37-41). New York: National League for Nursing Press.

Cohen, M.A., Kumar, N., McGuire, T., & Wallack, S.S. (1992). Financing long-term care: A practical mix of public and private. *Journal of Health Politics, Policy, and Law, 17*(3), 403-423.

Dye, C.A. (1992). *Education and training. Report of the White House Conference on Aging Planning Committee.* Washington, DC: U.S. Government Printing Office.

Ebersole, P., & Hess, P. (1998). *Toward healthy aging.* St. Louis: Mosby.

Fenton, M., & Brykczynski, K. (1993). Qualitative distinctions and similarities in practice of clinical nurse specialist and nurse practitioners. *Journal of Professional Nursing, 9*(6), 313-326.

Francese, T., & Mohler, M. (1994). Long-term care nurse staffing requirements: Has OBRA really helped? *Geriatric Nursing, 15*(3), 139-141.

Fulmer, T., & Mezey, M. (1994). Contemporary geriatric nursing. In W.R. Hazard et al. (Eds.), *Principles of geriatric medicine and gerontology* (3rd ed., pp. 249-258). New York: McGraw-Hill.

Haight, B.K., & Stuart, G. (1994). Answering need: Gero psychiatric nursing course development. *Journal of Gerontological Nursing, 20*(12), 12-18.

Health Care Financing Administration. (1996). Baltimore, MD: Bureau of Data Management & Strategy, Office of Health Care Information Systems.

Institute of Medicine Committee on Nursing Home Regulations. (1986). *Improving the quality of care in nursing homes.* Washington, DC: National Academy Press.

Lang, N.M., Kraegel, J.M., Rantz, M.J., & Krejci, J.W. (1990). *Quality of care for older people in America.* Kansas City, MO: American Nurses Association.

Levit, K.R., Lazenby, H.C., Braden, B.R., Cowan, C.A., Sensenig, A.I., McDonnel, P.A., Miller, J.M., Won, D.K., Martin, A.B., Sivarajan, L., Donham, C.S., Long, A.M., & Stewart, M.W. (1997). National health expenditures. *Health Care Review, 19*(1), 161-200.

Lyons, B.L. (1996, June 16). Meeting societal needs for the CNS competencies: Why the CNS and NP roles should not be blended in master degree programs. *Online Journal of Issues in Nursing,* pp. 1-6.

Mezey, M.D. (1995). Why good ideas have not gone far enough: Improving gerontological nursing education. In T. Fulmer & M. Matzo (Eds.), *Strengthening gerontological nursing education* (pp. 3-19). New York: Springer.

Page, N., & Arena, D. (1994). Rethinking the merger of the clinical nurse specialist and the nurse practitioner. *Image, Journal of Nursing Scholarship, 26*(4), 315-318.

National League for Nursing. (1991). *Gerontology in the nursing curriculum.* New York: Author.

Rosenfeld, P., Bottrell, M., Fulmer, T., & Mezey, M. (1999). Gerontological nursing content in baccalaureate nursing programs: Findings from a national survey. *Journal of Professional Nursing, 15*(2), 84-94.

Schuren, A.W. (1996). The blended role of the clinical nurse specialists and the nurse practitioner. In A.B. Hanrick, J.A. Spross, & C.M. Hanson (Eds.), *Advanced nursing practice: An integrative approach.* Philadelphia: Saunders.

Southern Council on Collegiate Education for Nursing. (1995). Gerontological nursing issues and demands beyond the year 2005. *Journal of Gerontological Nursing, 21*(6), 6-9.

U.S. Senate Special Committee on Aging. (1991). *Aging America: Trends and projections* (DHS # [FCoA] 91-28001). Washington, DC: U.S. Department of Health and Human Services.

Vladeck, B.C, Miller, N.A., & Clauser, S.V. (1993). The changing face of long-term care. *Health Care Financing Review, 14*(4), 5-23.

Yurchuck, E., & Brower, H. (1994). Faculty preparation for gerontological nursing. *The Journal of Gerontological Nursing, 20*(1), 17-24.

Zwygart-Stauffacher, M., Bowman, A., & Rantz, M. (2000). A critical review of gerontological nursing research: Where we have been and where we are going. (In review)

Zwygart-Stauffacher, M., Lindquist, R., & Savik, K. (2000). Development of health care delivery systems that are sensitive to the needs of stroke survivors and their caregivers. *Nursing Administration Quarterly, 24*(3), 33-42.

CHAPTER 24

Hospice Care

Underutilized and Misunderstood

MOLLY A. POLETO

The tongues of dying men enforce attention like deep harmony.
—William Shakespeare, *Julius Caesar*

For most of human history, medicine could do little to cure disease, prevent death from accident, or treat infections and plagues. Living to be an elder was unusual and considered good fortune. The 20th century has witnessed tremendous advances in public health and medical and nursing care, in which antibiotics, infection control, and vaccines account for a dramatic decrease in morbidity and mortality. In addition, advances in surgery, trauma care, and the pharmaceutical and technical management of diseases have lengthened the average lifespan. People now live long enough to have chronic diseases develop, where they once succumbed to death quickly and often at a young age.

In the United States, death at home in the care of the family has been widely superseded by an institutional and technological process of dying. By the 1950s, it was not uncommon for a chronically or terminally ill patient to be hospitalized for weeks, even months. Withholding diagnosis and prognosis was common, and individuals frequently died in a facility alone, frightened, and uncomfortable. Critics and reformers argued that medical technology obscured humanistic compassion for dying people and those close to them (Field & Cassel, 1977). Advances in 20th century medicine did little to address the medical, emotional, and social needs of the dying.

HISTORICAL PERSPECTIVE

Beginning in 1935, interest began to grow in the psychosocial aspects of dying and bereavement. In the late 1950s and 1960s nurses and physicians began to dialogue and publish their observations and concerns about how

people were dying. The institutionalization of the ill and dying resulted in isolation, poor management of physical symptoms, and left families to grieve unprepared and isolated.

Cicely Saunders, a young physician previously trained as a nurse and social worker, worked with dying patients in England from 1957 to 1967. Dr. Saunders studied pain control in cancer patients and pioneered the practice of prescribing opioid analgesia "around the clock" versus "as needed" on the premise that when pain exists throughout the day and night, analgesia should be given correspondingly (Hospice Education Institute, 1998).

In 1962, Harriet Goetz, a registered nurse, noted in her article focusing on a different approach to the care of the dying, "Once we know that the patient is aware of impending death, we can bring to him sympathetic, forthright friendship. We can be open to him, not denying the truth or pretending we don't know" (Goetz, 1962, p. 61). These practices were then quite controversial because patients were often not told their diagnosis and prognosis. Goetz also suggested such therapies as the use of atropine to relieve terminal secretions and environmental adjustments, such as soft lighting in the patient's room, to render comfort. Both concepts would later be integrated into components of hospice care.

In 1964, John Hinton, a psychiatrist from England, published a study on the care of dying patients. He compared the physical discomforts, mental state, and personal history of 102 patients dying in a hospital to a group of patients on the same ward with serious but nonfatal illnesses (Hinton, 1964). The results were alarming and troubling. The physical discomfort of the dying was disturbingly greater than that of the control patients. For the dying the intensity and amount of suffering more than doubled in the last 2 weeks of life. Nausea and vomiting were sufficiently alleviated in 63% of the dying patients; however, dyspnea was only alleviated in 18% of those studied. In measuring emotional distress, a significant degree of depression occurred in 46% of the dying compared with 10% among patients with nonfatal illnesses. In addition, Hinton looked at the correlation between emotion and physical symptoms. He found that 71% of patients with dyspnea experienced anxiety, whereas only 30% had anxiety when they did not have dyspnea. He also found that twice as many parents of school-aged children were anxious compared with those without dependents. Hinton attempted to open communication between the physician and patient by noting "It has also shown to those who believe the fatal prognosis should never be revealed to the patient that there is cause to reconsider their opinion as some have found it beneficial to speak more openly to the dying and their families" (Hinton, 1964, p. 204). Hinton's findings and recommendations helped to begin early movement toward quality care of the dying.

In 1966, Jeanne Quint, a nurse-sociologist, published an article about two types of situations as reported by nurses that were common and very troublesome: patients who do not know their diagnosis and patients whose behavior does not conform to expectations (Quint, 1966). The nurses reported extreme discomfort when dealing with uninformed patients because conversations could never venture into the "forbidden" topics that surround diagnosis and prognosis. The nurses' efforts to avoid these discussions resulted in tension and ineffective communication with their patients. Quint believed that dying was a social and a biological experience and urged health care providers to consider seriously the consequences for patients who are not informed.

Quint also discussed nurses' responses to patients who progressed through their fatal illness in ways that were not peaceful or "cooperative." Nurses' behaviors such as avoidance and making judgments about patients led to less than optimum nursing care.

In 1967, St. Christopher's Hospice in London was founded by Dr. Saunders and emphasized a multidisciplinary approach to the care of the dying (Beresford, 1993). St. Christopher's Hospice, an inpatient facility, was homelike and offered soft lighting, flowered wallpaper, and linens from home and an open kitchen stocked with refreshments. Twenty-four-hour visitation and the welcoming of pets made the environment as close to home as possible.

In 1969 the publication of Elizabeth Kübler-Ross's book *On Death and Dying* became a sentinel event in the care of the dying (Kübler-Ross, 1969). Kübler-Ross, an English physician, brought death out of the closet by reporting her conversations with dying patients. Ross was a storyteller and through her stories brought the lives of the dying and their families into the living rooms of the reader. Areas formerly forbidden or, at best, underaddressed by the medical society were presented openly and honestly. Her patients discussed where and how they wanted to live until they died, where they wished to die, personal and family fears and worries, and how much pain medication they preferred.

Five stages of dying were presented by Kübler-Ross: denial, anger, bargaining, depression, and acceptance. Medical caregivers and academia accepted these stages; *On Death and Dying* became required reading, a cornerstone for education for many nurses, social workers, and chaplains in training. Most professionals currently agree that patients may not progress through these stages in the exact order as described in 1969. The stages, however, remain a foundation for caregivers in understanding the challenges and needs, as well as the beauty and potential growth, that may be experienced by people in the process of dying.

The first hospice in the United States opened in 1974 in New Haven, Connecticut (originally named New Haven Hospice), where hospice home care was offered first and inpatient care soon followed (Hospice Nurses Association, 1997). The Connecticut Hospice became a model for new hospice programs as word about the hospice philosophy and care spread across the nation. Hospitals created discreet inpatient hospice units where staffs were trained in hospice philosophy and care, and the atmosphere was designed to soothe and comfort all who entered. Hospice home care became, and remains, the most prevalent level of care because the opportunity to die in one's own home is usually desired.

During the 1980s and 1990s, hospice programs sprang up across the United States. In the year 2000, major urban and most rural communities have access to hospice care. As of 1999, 3,100 operational or planned hospice programs existed in the 50 states, the District of Columbia, Puerto Rico, and Guam. An estimated 540,000 patients were served by hospices in the United States in 1998 (National Hospice Organization, 1999). In 1989, nursing home legislation allowed hospices to offer services in nursing home facilities.

With the passing of the 1990 Patient Self-Determination Act, statutes were introduced requiring informed consent and communication about patient decision making by all health care providers (Omnibus Budget Reconciliation Act, 1990). Informed decision making was considered an important step toward patient autonomy and the opportunity to determine the direction and intensity of one's health care.

To learn how advance directives affected patient choice surrounding their care and to study care of seriously ill hospitalized patients, a large and comprehensive study funded by the Robert Wood Johnson Foundation was performed. The Study to Understand Prognosis and Preferences for Outcomes and Risks of Treatments (SUPPORT) was conducted in two phases (Connors et al., 1995). The study of 4,301 patients was designed to examine outcomes and clinical decision making for seriously ill hospitalized patients. Phase I (primarily observation) documented shortcomings in communication, frequency of aggressive care, and the characteristics of a hospital death. Only 47% of physicians knew when their patients preferred to avoid cardiopulmonary resuscitation (CPR), and for 50% of conscious patients who died in the hospital, family members reported moderate to severe pain at least half the time. Phase II, an intervention study, focused on those areas identified in phase I as the most concerning. Physicians in the intervention group (phase II) received estimates for the likelihood for their patients' survival every day up to 6 months for their patients and outcomes of CPR and functional disability 2 months after CPR. In addition, a specially trained nurse had multiple contacts with the patient, family, physician, and hospital staff to elicit preferences, improve understanding of outcomes, focus on pain management, and facilitate effective communication regarding advance directives and communication across the medical team and patient and family. SUPPORT investigators hypothesized that accurate predication of risk for death, counseling about patient and family preferences, and team communication would result in improved outcomes in end of life care for this population of patients.

The results bewildered end-of-life care specialists. In phase II there was no improvement in the timing or incidence of do not resuscitate (DNR) orders or physicians' knowledge of patients' preferences, no decrease in the number of intensive care unit days spent for the dying, and no change in the level of reported pain. It was concluded that societal commitment and more proactive and forceful measures may be needed to improve the experience of seriously ill and dying patients. Since the SUPPORT study, several national and international groups have formed to study ways to improve care of the dying. However,

SUPPORT investigators and other leaders in end-of-life care all agree that although hospice care remains the "cadillac" of programs for the terminally ill, it remains underused, surrounded by myths and misinformation.

HOSPICE CARE DEFINED

Hospice is a program of specialized care for patients with terminal illness that provides interdisciplinary services in multiple settings; universally in the home and hospital, and many in nursing homes and residences. The physical, spiritual, psychological, and social aspects of the patients and their families are incorporated into the hospice plan of care, in which the *patient and family* is the unit of care because they guide the direction and intensity of care. The interdisciplinary team (IDT) consists of a nurse, physician, chaplain, social worker, home health aide, and volunteer. Physical, speech, and occupational therapy and a dietician are included when warranted. Respite care for the family during the illness and bereavement care for the year that follows the death are standard in hospice care.

Hospice focuses on the dignity, autonomy, and comfort of the patient and admits patients of all ages, including children. Hospice professionals teach caregivers about care of the patient and assess and respond to concerns to ease both physical and existential suffering. All terminal diseases qualify for hospice care such as end-stage diseases of the heart, lung, liver, and kidney, amyotrophic lateral sclerosis (ALS), stroke, dementia, cancer, and acquired immunodeficiency syndrome (AIDS).

Most hospice patients die at home (in 1995, 77% of hospice patients died in their own home) (National Hospice Organization, 1999). When providing services in a facility, the IDT regularly travels to coordinate the care of hospice patients by support for and education of facility staff and assuring physical comforts for the patient and family (i.e., comprehensive pain management, nourishment for patient around the clock, and an overnight place for family to rest) and providing 24-hour availability for questions and concerns. Prisons, foster homes, shelters, and assisted living facilities represent other institutions that have arranged contracts with hospice. The fundamental components of hospice care are delivered to all patients and their families (in a facility, the staff may be regarded as "family"), regardless of their location. This includes 24-hour availability of a registered nurse for guidance and visits, expert pain and symptom management, the provision of medications, medical supplies, and equipment needed for comfort, chaplain and social worker intervention, volunteers, and bereavement care for a year after the death.

MEDICARE HOSPICE BENEFIT

On November 1, 1983, hospice care became available under Medicare. The beneficiary is eligible for coverage of hospice services when the primary physician and the hospice medical director certify that the patient has a life expectancy of 6 months or less (Christakis & Ecsarce, 1996). Hospice providers are required to deliver comprehensive services to the patient and family, which include such unique provisions as respite care, bereavement care for 1 year after the death, continuity of care (the patient and family plan of care transfers when moving between home and facility care), and a certain percentage of hours provided by volunteers is mandatory. The benefit authorizes 210 days of care. The hospice medical director may approve care beyond the original time allotted if the patient lives longer than the 6-month expectation and remains terminally ill. The hospice Medicare benefit was a new and innovative model to deliver services; however, it currently remains underused by the medical and lay community.

A comparison of the Medicare home health and Medicare hospice benefits demonstrates the differences in services and the clear advantages of the hospice benefit for the patient with a life-limiting illness (Table 24-1). Communication between home health and hospice is crucial to ensure movement of eligible patients between the programs as deemed appropriate.

"END OF LIFE" (EOL) CARE VERSUS "BRINK OF DEATH" CARE

To experience the full benefits of hospice care, patients must be enrolled as early as medically appropriate. A timely hospice referral ensures the patient and family will be offered the full range of services with adequate time and assistance to address issues at the close of life. Unfortunately, hospice providers across the nation experience referrals so late in the process, they often have time to provide only the very essentials of care, such as pain relief and a visit at the time of death, with a sketchy and hasty bereavement plan. As a result of late referrals, "end-of-life" care becomes "brink-of-death" care, clearly missing the established goal of hospice.

The hospice nurse is often performing a physical and psychospiritual assessment on a weak, uncomfortable, and often semiresponsive patient. There is often inadequate or no time for social work or chaplain care, and the volunteer may be left out of the picture, a true loss for the patient and family. After death (often hours or a few days subsequent to admission), the family is left to deal with the aftereffects of the delayed admission. They have endured months of worry, uncertainty, and witnessing their loved one uncomfortable and often not in the physical location in which the patient wished to die.

Patients deserve to have their physical symptoms well managed, be eased of financial burdens of medical care during the terminal phase, have their fears and concerns addressed, and be assured that practical yet important is-

TABLE 24-1   Major Differences Between Home Health and Hospice Benefits

Home Health Medicare Benefit	Hospice Medicare Benefit
Requires skilled need	No skilled need required
Patient must be homebound	Patient not required to be homebound
May require copayment for durable medical equipment and supplies	No copayment for durable medical equipment and supplies
Patient is responsible for prescriptions	Medications related to the terminal illness are provided by hospice
Nursing visit requires physician order, schedule fixed per medical treatment plan	Physician order not required for nursing visits; visit schedule determined by interdisciplinary team
Reimbursement is based on services and supplies provided, per patient, per visit, or per beneficiary	Reimbursement at approximately $90 per day regardless of services or supplies provided (inpatient rates vary)
Patient must meet skilled care requirements	Patient must be deemed terminally ill by physicians (considered to have prognosis of 6 months or less)
No respite care is provided for family	Short-term inpatient care is available, including respite care
No continuous (24-h) home care	Continuous (24-h) home care available on short-term basis

Adapted from Wright, P.M. (1999). Expanding the role of the home health nurse: Recognizing the hospice eligible patient. *Journal of Hospice and Palliative Nursing, 1,* 139. Copyright 1999 by Nursecom Inc.

TABLE 24-2 Outcomes of a Timely Referral versus a Late Referral as Experienced by the Patient and Family

Timely Hospice Referral (Months Before Death)	Late Hospice Referral (Weeks, Even Hours, Before Death)
Management of Symptoms Early management; avoids severe symptoms; avoids "crisis" management	Symptoms severe and complex by now; "crisis" management common
Patient Participation or Autonomy Increased autonomy; patient participates	Less autonomy; function and alertness of patient decreased
Caregiver Needs Early identification of needs before exhaustion and stress occur	Caregiver discouraged, tired; "I can't go on like this."
Tasks of Life Closure (Financial, Housing, Psychological and Emotional Adjustment, Dependent Children, and More) Time to prepare family for future loss; time to say "good bye"	Not possible to fully assess and counsel; planning last minute; crisis
Existential Suffering Addressed early, relationship essential for quality spiritual care; healing and reconciliation possible	Often profound by now; patient often too ill to participate Healing and reconciliation difficult
Bereavement (1 Year After Death) Less complicated; issues are addressed before death; patient may participate	More complicated; unaddressed issues can worsen after death
Caregiver Satisfaction Higher lever of fulfillment; able to receive support over time	Lower level of fulfillment; not ample time to receive guidance or instruction

sues are dealt with, such as a guardianship for dependent children and financial or legal affairs. *Caregivers deserve* to have their worries heard, their loved one comfortable and at peace, assistance with the burden of providing care, time for closure (to say "goodbye"), and their bereavement needs anticipated and coordinated. To consent to or decline hospice care is a decision each patient and family will make, but only when given an opportunity to decide. When individuals are not provided information about hospice, they progress through a crucial phase in life without this option when deciding their destiny.

A patient recovering from a stroke is automatically referred for rehabilitation services and prenatal care is a standard referral for a pregnant woman, both individuals being availed the coordination of medical and social needs in anticipation of future problems and rewards. Why do some medical providers, particularly physicians and nurses, overlook comprehensive and compassionate care that hospice offers when there are clearly benefits for all involved? To avoid, delay, or obstruct discussion about hospice *early in the terminal phase* is medically unwise and unethical and should be considered malpractice, especially when the patient and family are suffering or when suffering is anticipated (Table 24-2).

BARRIERS TO HOSPICE CARE

Barriers to hospice include the physician or nurse who delays or refuses to refer to hospice, inadequate prognosis criteria needed to accurately estimate survival time, hospice providers who impose strict or burdensome admission requirements, a culture that avoids death, and myths and misunderstandings that surround hospice care.

The *physician* is sometimes considered the "gatekeeper" of hospice care. Although some physicians have a deep commitment to quality care of the dying and refer patients at the appropriate time, many still see death as the enemy, as a sign of their failure as a doctor. They may avoid or delay discussion with the patient or family and often fail to even broach the subject at all. Physicians also consider the 6-month prognosis requirement restricting and may be reluctant to refer to hospice for fear that they will be held responsible if the patient exceeds the prognosis. Although hospice programs carry the burden to justify longer stay patients (patients receiving hospice services longer than 210 days), physicians remain skeptical and in dislike of the restrictive time frame.

In the ideal physician-patient relationship the "hospice talk" comes after a number of conversations during the patient's illness, in which earlier discussions about treatments and the patient preferences and concerns occurred. On the contrary, when the physician-patient relationship is new or lacking depth and trust, the physician is challenged to enter a conversation that is complex and emotionally charged. The patient's greatest concerns and preferences for care will be difficult to ascertain in this setting.

Accurate prognostication would lend tremendous aide in the timing of the hospice referral. In the early days of hospice the predominant diagnosis was cancer; therefore estimating survival time for patients was fairly uncomplicated because it was based on the natural progression of the malignancy. The ability to predict the estimated lifespan for an individual with congestive heart failure (CHF) or chronic obstructive lung disease (COPD), however, is far more problematic. The trajectory of these diseases in their late stages has many highs and lows in relation to the patient's functional status, severity of symptoms, and possible medical treatments that can result in remission, however brief it may be. A patient with CHF may have multiple hospitalizations for exacerbations of their disease with reasonable quality of life in between.

In response to this dilemma the National Hospice Organization (NHO) published *Medical Guidelines for Determining Prognosis in Selected Non-Cancer Diseases* (Stuart et al., 1996). Originally published in 1995 and edited in 1996, the guide incorporates objective assessment scales (e.g., Karnofsky Performance Status), frequency of emergency department visits, laboratory and radiological findings, and the percent of weight loss to predict patient survival time. The diseases included in this guide are heart disease, pulmonary disease, dementia, human immunodeficiency virus (HIV), liver and renal disease, stroke, coma, and ALS.

Although these guiding principles and other guidelines with similar intent aided the process of survival estimation, research indicates that currently available criteria for predicting 6-month survival with seriously ill patients are not helpful with COPD, CHF, or end-stage liver disease (ESLD) (Fox et al., 1999). Fox et al. concluded that it is not necessarily the use of objective criteria that is flawed in predicting survival but rather that the events around the disease process are difficult to predict with reasonable accuracy. Because it is impossible to predict prognosis with 100% certainty, many physicians often avoid considering hospice for their patients (Slomski, 1995). The dilemma to accurately predict prognosis remains; further research is clearly indicated.

Currently some hospice providers have what might be considered *strict admission criteria* that may hinder the ease with which the referral and admission occur. As a result of stringent review by the federal regulatory bodies, some hospice providers will not approve an admission until requested laboratory and/or radiological reports are received from medical providers. This requirement can be problematic for the medical provider, often resulting in resentment and frustration by the very source that requested hospice for their patient.

Some hospice programs have adjusted their evaluation and admission processes to ease the work for the referral source. This has improved relations between agencies, thereby lengthening the time that patients receive hospice care. When the community provider of end-of-life care strives to make intake and admission procedures uncomplicated, the patient and family ultimately benefit by timely and appropriate care.

"Americans are more afraid of how they will die in today's health care system than they are of death itself" (Executive Summary, 1997, p. 1). This quote was taken from an executive summary in a report by American Health Decisions, where it was concluded that people fear reaching the end of their lives connected to machines and prefer a natural death in familiar surroundings with loved ones. Important to note was that although Americans consider planning for their death and dying important, they remain uncomfortable with the topic and resist or avoid taking action. *One can conclude that even when the primary physician and nurse fully support hospice and the hospice provider in the community is easily accessible, the patient may often be the "barrier" to hospice care at the end of his or her life.*

The last barrier to hospice care for discussion may be the area best addressed by hospices alone. These include the *myths and misunderstandings* that surround hospice. *Myths* about hospice include the following: hospice is only for cancer patients, only for the elderly, not covered by insurance companies, just for Catholics (many grassroots programs originated in Catholic institutions), is only for the last few days or weeks of life, only available in the hospitals, not for persons with IVs or treatments, and requires a DNR order and a responsible caregiver. All of these statements are untrue. It is the responsibility of the hospice provider to inform their communities through education, support, and collaboration with community agencies caring for prehospice clients. Although resources for community education and marketing funds may be restricted for many programs, hospices are morally obligated to ensure accurate information is conveyed and reinforced.

SUMMARY

Society must prepare for death as well as it prepares for birth. When an expectant mother learns of her pregnancy, she quickly receives information and advice regarding her medical care, as well as emotional support and social assistance. Nature allows her 9 months for her and her family to plan for the practical, economic, social, and psychological impact of the new baby. Information about parenting, financial assistance to those in need, and good prenatal medical care focus on one common goal, a "good birth." This same level of care must be made readily available for the individual with a terminal illness. Months of medical, financial, and social adjustments for the future are essential for a "good death."

Nurses are called to research and develop systems, educate communities, and provide care that is available to all with serious illnesses. The vulnerable, scared, and frail can find comfort, companionship, and expert care with the help of hospice.

> Of all the wonders that I yet have heard,
> It seems to me most strange that man should fear;
> Seeing that death, a necessary end,
> Will come when it will come.
>
> —William Shakespeare, *King Richard II*

REFERENCES

Beresford, L. (1993). *The hospice handbook*. Boston: Little, Brown.

Christakis, N.A., & Escarce, J.J. (1996). Survival of Medicare patients after enrollment in hospice programs. *The New England Journal of Medicine, 335*, 172-178.

Connors, A.F., Dawson, N.V., Desbiens, N.A., Fulkerson, W.J., Goldman, L., & Knaus, W.A. (1995). A controlled trial to improve care for seriously ill hospitalized patients. *Journal of the American Medical Association, 274*, 1591-1598.

Executive Summary. (1997). The quest to die with dignity: An analysis of Americans' values, opinions and attitudes concerning end-of-life care. *A Report by American Health Decisions.*

Field, M.J., & Cassel, C.K. (Eds.). (1997). *Approaching death: Improving care at the end of life*. Washington, DC: National Academy Press.

Fox, E., Landrum-McNiff, K., Zhong, Z., Dawson, N.V., Wu, A.W., & Lynn, J. (1999). Evaluation of prognostic criteria for determining hospice eligibility in patients with advanced lung, heart, or liver disease. *Journal of the American Medical Association, 282*, 1638-1645.

Goetz, H. (1962). Needed: A new approach to care of the dying. *RN, 25*, 61-62.

Hinton, J.M. (1964). Problems in the care of the dying. *The Journal of Chronic Diseases, 17*, 201-205.

Hospice Education Institute. (1998). *A short history of hospice and palliative care*. New Haven, CT: Author.

Hospice Nurses Association. (1997). *The hospice nurses study guide: A preparation for the CRNH candidate* (2nd ed.). Pittsburgh: Author.

Kübler-Ross, E. (1969). *On death and dying*. New York: Macmillan.

National Hospice Organization. (1999). *Hospice fact sheet*. Arlington, VA: Author.

Omnibus Budget Reconciliation Act of 1990. (OBRA-90), Pub L 101-508.

Quint, J.C. (1996). Obstacles to helping the dying. *American Journal of Nursing, 96*, 1568-1571.

Slomski, A.J. (1995, September 25). Doctors' misconceptions about hospice care. *Medical Economic$, 72*(18), 72-88.

Stuart, B., Alexander, C., Arenella, C., Connor, S., Herbst, L., & Jones, D. (1996). *Medical guidelines for determining prognosis in selected non-cancer diseases*. Arlington, VA: National Hospice Organization.

Recent Changes and Current Issues in Adult Health/Medical-Surgical Nursing Practice

MARILYN S. FETTER, CECELIA GATSON GRINDEL

Numerous, complex, and interrelated forces are causing dramatic changes in the delivery of health care services, and adult health nurses are facing increasing challenges as they work to provide quality, cost-effective, accessible patient care. New care delivery systems challenge all nurses. However, the traditional focus of medical-surgical nurses' practice, hospitalized acutely ill patients, has undergone a paradigm shift (Barnum & Kerfoot, 1995). Medical-surgical nurses must now identify themselves as adult health nurses and broaden their focus, roles, and responsibilities to the care of adults across the care continuum (Academy of Medical-Surgical Nurses [AMSN], 2000; Fetter & Grindel, 1997; Mc-Closkey & Grace, 1997). In the past decade, intense pressure to reduce health care spending has resulted in numerous changes in health care practices, organizations, and finances. Insurers and other payers have shifted incentives from cost-plus reimbursement for delivered services to individuals to prospective, capitated payments for sets of negotiated services to select populations (Jacobs, 1998). As a result, hospitals and care providers have been forced to develop not only more cost-effective ways to deliver traditional services, such as inpatient hospitalization care, but also innovative approaches to promote well-being and reduce customer demand for more costly programs (American Organization of Nurse Executives [AONE], 1999). Working with increasingly strict financial targets, hospitals and other providers have engaged in numerous efforts to cut costs and service utilization. Managed care, mergers, and the formation of health care networks are among the alternatives implemented in attempts to deliver more cost-effective health care.

Economic pressures, as well as advancing technologies, have shortened hospital lengths of stay, and thus increased acuity levels. These changes have resulted in greater reliance on outpatient settings and demand for skilled home care. Concomitantly, home care agencies are experiencing intense economic pressures, as new regulations now tightly restrict reimbursable patient care visits (Waggoner, 1999). There are numerous reports in the lay and professional literature of patients and families struggling to provide and pay for needed care (Appleby, 1999; Miller, 1999). Socially, these demands are occurring as increasing numbers of Americans reach middle and old age, when health care and family care giving needs increase (U.S. Census Bureau, 1996). The widening diversity of the population in terms of culture, language, religion, socioeconomic status, and literacy further challenges health care organizations and adult health nurses (Sullivan & Clinton, 1999). Politically, rampant consumer complaints, coupled with existing economic threats to Medicare and Medicaid, and rising numbers of uninsured and underinsured persons have driven legislators to regulate patients' rights care delivery components, such as length of stay and mandatory coverage for specific treatments. Among adult health nurses, there is alarm about the lack of coordinated and comprehensive concern for adult patients' well-being, regardless of their insurance or payor status (Gothberg, 1999). Technological and other scientific advances are improving the prevention, diagnosis, and treatment of many acute and chronic illnesses. However, implementing these innovations fairly, safely, and cost-effectively is straining providers, insurers, and delivery systems (Institute of Medicine, 1996). Many nurses believe that the delivery of quality nursing care is threatened by these multiple stressors and nursing work force issues (Miller, 1999; Miller & Fry, 1999). Understanding these factors and their effects on patients and families challenges nurses to provide the leadership to implement strategies that will improve clinical care and outcomes of adults (Joint Commission on Accreditation of Health Care Organizations [JCAHO], 1997).

CHANGING CONSUMER POPULATIONS AND NEEDS

The U.S. population is aging and requiring more, different, and new health services. As life expectancy increases, American demographics shift (U.S. Census Bureau, 1996). In 1995, 33.6 million Americans were 65 years of age and older. By 2010 this number is expected to climb to more than 40 million persons, representing more than 13% of the total population. As the "baby-boomers" age, the number of "old" and "old-old" is increasing and expected to reach 4.6 million by the end of this decade. Most older adults remain in the community, with only 1.3% of persons 65 to 74 years of age and 6% of individuals between the ages of 75 and 84 living in long-term care facilities (American Association of Retired Persons [AARP], 1993). Although Americans are healthier than ever before, significant chronic health problems such as hypertension and other cardiovascular disease, diabetes mellitus, musculoskeletal disorders, visual and hearing impairments, and dementia are likely to develop as they age (National Center for Health Statistics, 1997a). They often receive numerous medications, recover more slowly from episodes of illness and surgical procedures, and require more assistance from family and health care providers (Fetter & Grindel, 1997).

Changes in the American population suggest that much of the health care dollar will be spent in efforts to prevent and manage chronic illness. Preventing the onset of and controlling health conditions are major goals in managing care and costs (Brownson et al., 1997; Institute of Medicine, 1996). Implementing strategies to promote positive health behaviors such as optimal nutrition and moderate the effects of controllable or so-called lifestyle factors such as tobacco, alcohol and other drugs, and violence are significant tasks for health providers (Brown, 1999; Lantz et al., 1998). Maximizing the efficiency of health care demands that, in each encounter with the health system, patients receive a wide range of preventive services, including information about how to navigate the system and negotiate for needed services and reimbursement.

When acute clinical problems arise, consumers want quick and effective health care services. Payors want patients to use services appropriately. However, limited access to care continues to be an issue. The number of working poor is growing, and these individuals are five times more likely than other Americans to lack health insurance from any source (Seccombe & Amey, 1995; U.S. Census Bureau, 1997). In 1997 the poverty rate of children (19.9 %) exceeded that of all other Americans (National Center for Health Statistics, 1997b). Thus a new generation is reaching adulthood with compromised health status. In addition, many Americans who have some degree of health insurance are underinsured, and as many as 40% of these persons lack the coverage to pay for catastrophic and other illnesses (Short & Banthin, 1995).

Over the past few years, federal and state governments have been working with HMOs and other insurers to shift Medicare clients into managed care programs for the delivery of services. In several states, insurers are failing to renew contracts for these health care services for Medicare clients (Appleby, 1999). The Health Care Financing Administration (HCFA) reported that 90 insurers will end service in 329 counties, pulling out of the HMO programs that give seniors and the disabled an alternative to regular Medicare. Thus meeting the nation's health care needs continues to plague health care providers, legislators, insurers, and consumers.

CHANGES IN HEALTH CARE SYSTEMS

Currently, adults are hospitalized as a last resort when medical management, particularly pharmaceutical interventions, fails to produce positive clinical outcomes. New hospital systems have developed to accommodate more acutely ill patients, shortened lengths of stay, and the increasing reliance on outpatient settings for surgery and diagnostic procedures (Fralic, 1999). With decreasing revenues from payors, hospitals have engaged in numerous strategies to cut costs (Barnum & Kerfoot, 1995). Mergers, downsizing, redesigned care processes, and new staffing patterns have been introduced. Mega-mergers have created health care networks that offer extensive health care services under the umbrella of the parent organization. These networks have been designed to use economies of scale to reduce administrative costs; increase purchasing power for drugs, equipment, and supplies; and increase their market share by offering discounts to employers. The aim of these organizations is to develop a seamless, interwoven, and cost-effective network of health care services, but many are struggling to achieve this goal.

Although the effects of changing demographics and cost containment have affected all health care organizations, the most dramatic implications of these forces have been experienced by hospitals. Rising numbers of acutely ill patients require intense nursing care, yet daily turnover of patient beds disrupts this care. Rapid cycle rounds of patient admissions, discharges, and transfers add to the workload of nurses charged with the often unrealistic goal of providing holistic patient care to very sick patients (Valentine, 1997). In an effort to reduce nursing labor costs, many institutions have elected to change staffing patterns by replacing registered nurses with unlicensed aides. Because research has documented that care by registered nurses results in better patient outcomes (American Nurses Association [ANA], 1997), this strategy, implemented as patient acuity continues to increase, raises serious concerns about the quality of care being delivered to the nation's sickest adults. Nurses and other providers have articulated their concerns about unsafe patient care conditions and inadequate patient access to services (Miller, 1999). In the ANA study, 78% of the nurses surveyed stated that managed care had decreased the quality of care for persons who are ill, and 85% reported less time available to care for patients.

Patients discharged from acute care settings are going home much sicker than ever before. Initially, home care agencies expanded to manage the flood of patient referrals. Soon thereafter reimbursement for home visits was limited. As a result, many patients are released from nursing follow-up before their clinical condition warrants or before family members are ready to independently handle the patients' care (Waggoner, 1999). These experiences have challenged patients, families, and health care providers to ensure that optimal outcomes will result even if health care support is withdrawn early in the trajectory of healing (Boland & Sims, 1996).

In addition to leaving home care patients at high risk for complications requiring rehospitalization, capitation on patient visits has resulted in severe financial crises for some home care agencies. The General Accounting Office (GAO) reported that since October 1997, 760 home care agencies had closed nationwide. The National Association for Home Care (NAHC) (1998), stating that the GAO underestimated the number of agency closures under the Interim Payment System, indicated that the number of closures was double that reported. Furthermore the NAHC emphasized that the extent of patient access problems that resulted from these closures was not well documented but considered problematic.

Limitation of reimbursable visits highlights the need for measuring and managing patient outcomes. Variables such as rehospitalization, complication rates, and patient and family satisfaction must also be included in evalua-

tion data so that the total picture of outcomes can be viewed. Measurement of clinical outcomes documents the degree to which patient needs are being met, yet outcomes measurement places additional burden on home care nurses who are required to collect patient data using the HCFA Outcome and Assessment Information Set (OASIS) instrument (HCFA, 1999). For example, completion of each OASIS data set takes 30 to 90 minutes, depending on the patient's condition. However, this additional time for data collection and documentation is not reimbursed by insurers or the federal government (Waggoner, 1999).

Consumers and health care providers are voicing major concerns about the deteriorating quality of health care. As access to care became more complicated with the advent of managed care (Taylor, Beauregard, & Vistnes, 1995), consumers have become increasingly dissatisfied as reflected by declining patient satisfaction scores and consumer demands for legislative controls on the delivery of health care services. These legislative initiatives threaten to undermine the basic economic incentives and gains achievable under managed care (Wilensky, 1997).

Dissatisfaction with health care delivery is a nationwide problem. Nurses caring for adults report frustration in their ability to care comprehensively for patients. Despite the fact that preventing illness and promoting health are two important maxims of managed care that are purported to enable cost savings, nurses are challenged to implement these strategies because of constrained resources and inadequate research knowledge about which programs work. The diffusion of adult consumers across health care settings and plans has retarded the emergence of a unified voice expressing patient, family, and providers' concerns (AMSN, 2000). However, nurses caring for adults report the need and desire to advocate for their patients' welfare and demand accessible programs that deliver care at acceptable levels of quality and cost-effectiveness.

Practice Changes

Changes in health systems have created difficult work environments for adult health nurses and threaten these organization's abilities to recruit and retain competent professionals (AONE, 1999). Nurses are dealing with increasingly demanding workloads, complaints by patients and families, and employers' added expectations to collect and manage data, supervise unlicensed staff, and work within severely restricted budgets (Barnum & Kerfoot, 1995). Charged with upholding quality of care, many nurses see deteriorating care conditions. The problem is most serious on understaffed adult hospital units, often filled with acutely ill older adults with numerous complex health problems.

Working conditions that cause concern for patient safety and quality patient care, along with hospital census reductions, have resulted in many nurses leaving staff and unit management positions in hospitals (Fralic, 1999). This exodus of experienced nurses occurs as the nursing workforce ages and approaches retirement (Miller, 1999). In 1996 the average age of the registered nurse (RN) was 44 years, up from 40 years of age in 1988. Only 9% of RNs were younger than 30 years of age in 1996. It is expected that a high percentage of nurses will retire over the next 10 to 15 years. This profile of the RN added to the fact that staff turnover in acute care facilities reached an all-time high of 15% in 1998 (Miller, 1999) has set the stage for nurse shortages.

Nurse shortages are occurring across the country. A 1998 study of 178 hospitals reported 81% of the hospitals indicated that they have or anticipate a shortage of nursing middle managers, RNs, licensed vocational nurses, and unlicensed nursing assistants (Hay Group, 1998). The seeds of the current shortage were planted in the mid-1990s when hospitals changed staffing mix, replacing some RNs with unlicensed assistive personnel (Miller, 1999). These downsizing strategies may have been a quick fix for cost containment; however, these lower paid, lower skilled personnel were not prepared to care for acutely ill patients. The remaining RNs picked up the slack in patient care. As the workload and job stress increased, nurse morale and job satisfaction decreased. Widespread burnout has resulted, and many nurses are seeking jobs outside the hospital walls, often outside of nursing (Gothberg, 1999; Valentine, 1997).

Nursing shortages have been a part of the past, but the current shortage is unique because of the shortage of nurses with competence, skills, and experience (AONE, 1999). Enrollment in bachelor's degree programs has declined over the last few years (Malone & Marullo, 1997). In many states the number of applicants for the state RN examination has decreased. New graduate nurses require supervision by competent staff as they gain needed experience. This training period puts more demands on experienced staff and takes time away from caring for very sick patients. The shortage of nurses is not limited to hospital settings in large cities. Rural areas have reported a continuous shortage of RNs (Miller, 1999).

The complexity of adult care and the intricate nature of health care networks require that nurses are well prepared to attend to multiple patient and family needs while managing scientifically and technologically advanced care within large, complicated systems. Numerous skills are necessary to ensure quality, cost-effective nursing care (Christman, 1998). The complexity of today's patients and care environments requires an ever-expanding knowledge base (see box, below). Nurses must be able to provide skilled care to hospitalized, acutely ill adults, and simultaneously incorporate health promotion and disease prevention strategies into clinical care (American Association of Colleges of Nursing [AACN], 1997; AMSN, 2000; Valentine, 1997). The rapid pace of knowledge development in basic and clinical health sciences offers the potential for significant reductions in mortality and morbidity. Nurses must keep abreast of emerging practice standards and guidelines, pharmaceutical and product innovations, and genetic and other scientific advances altering entire practice specialties (Brown, 1999).

The diversity of patients and staff, family needs, and diminishing resources further challenge nurses skills in communication, problem solving, delegation, supervision, and advocacy (Sullivan & Clinton, 1999). Current and future nurses must have the management and leadership skills to direct teams caring for adults across a wide variety of settings and the wellness-illness continuum. The complexity of the health care environment demands that future nurses also possess additional skills and knowledge in such areas as case management, resource management, delegation, computer competency, data

---

ADULT HEALTH NURSING PROFESSIONAL EDUCATION NEEDS

- Cutting-edge nursing information
- Scientific advances in such areas as technologies, genetics, pharmacology, and epidemiology
- Managerial and organizational concepts
- Measuring and managing outcomes
- Evidence-based practice
- World health and international outreach
- Legal, ethical, and economic issues
- Patient and family advocacy
- Infection prevention and control
- Gerontology
- Mental health issues and treatment
- Collaboration with other health care providers
- Cultural diversity and competence
- Foreign language skills
- Computer technologies and skills
- Career and financial planning

management, outcomes measurement, organizations and systems, health care economics, and legislation. Demonstrating that interventions improve patient outcomes is essential for health care organizations and nursing departments (Miller & Fry, 1999). The demand for measuring and managing patient outcomes highlights the need for nurses who are competent in data management, outcomes measurement, and research utilization (JCAHO, 1997). Documenting the effectiveness of changes in the delivery of health care services ensures that these new models enhance patient care and consumer satisfaction (Carey, Garrett, & Jackson, 1995; Hofer et al., 1999; Jollis & Romano, 1998; Romano, Rainwater, & Antonius, 1999; Rudy et al., 1995).

Along with the entire nursing profession, adult health nursing is facing perhaps its greatest challenges in history. In making the transition in title from medical-surgical to adult health nursing, the specialty recognizes a broadly expanded domain of roles, responsibilities, accountability, and professionalism (AMSN, 2000). As professionals, adult health nurses must remain committed to patient care and lifelong learning despite major role strain. These values set the stage for nursing care that is "on the cutting edge." An energetic, talented, and capable cadre of individuals must be recruited into the adult health nursing practice. These newest nurses will be older and more diverse than previous nursing cohorts and will have taken a variety of educational pathways into the profession. They will require nurturing, mentoring, and educational and professional development to meet the demands of current and future patients. Nurses caring for adult populations are challenged to use the latest medical, technological, and pharmaceutical advances to provide patients with quality care. Their knowledge must be applicable across a wide range of ages and clinical conditions. Furthermore, to advance adult health status, they must take an active role in developing prevention initiatives designed to address targeted health goals for specific populations (Fetter & Grindel, 1997). Adult health nursing's specialty organizations must provide the leadership to accomplish these goals.

Implications for Adult Health Nurses

Assuring quality health care for the American public is the responsibility of consumers, health care providers, insurers, health care systems, and legislators. Although many of the recent changes in the delivery of health care are or have the potential to be positive, adult health nurses are faced with many challenges. Recently, a major adult health nursing specialty organization articulated expectations for nursing professionals and organizations.

According to the Academy of Medical-Surgical Nursing (AMSN, 2000),

> Expert nurses caring for adult populations must:
> - Be on "the cutting edge" of practice through continuous professional development
> - Provide quality patient care that is sensitive to the physical, psychological, cultural, and socioeconomic needs of individuals, families, groups, and communities
> - Participate in outcomes measurement and program evaluation to assure quality care
> - Be politically active regarding issues that affect the health and well-being of the American public
> - Use their knowledge of health economics to influence health resource allocations for the good of the American public
> - Test interventions that support healthier lifestyles for U.S. citizens
> - Demonstrate proficiency at patient care management through coordination of care, referrals, and resource utilization
> - Demonstrate expert communication skills with consumers, patients, families, professional colleagues, and the media

Adult health nursing specialty organizations must share in the profession's responsibility to influence the delivery of health care (Wakefield, 1999). They must:

- Advocate for patients and their families in local, state, and national discussions about health care legislation and initiatives
- Recruit talented and committed persons into the specialty
- Monitor the collection and dissemination of data regarding patient outcomes
- Give direction for documenting the effectiveness of nursing interventions in patient care
- Work to ensure that the workplace is an environment that ensures patient safety and quality nursing care

Nursing's major professional organizations challenge nursing education programs to provide nursing students with real work experience before employment in health care agencies (AACN, 1997; ANA, 1997; AONE, 1999). Some special concerns are related to adult health nursing. These nursing education programs must:

- Provide a strong clinical foundation that students can apply to the care of adults and their families across settings
- Implement strategies that foster clinical decision making and critical thinking

- Strengthen content in organizations and systems, cultural diversity, health care economics, political activism, and computer competency
- Focus research content on research utilization, outcomes measurement, and program evaluation

Providing accessible, cost-effective health care requires committed, dedicated, knowledgeable nursing professionals who will advocate for patients' and families' well-being and interests. Changes in patient populations, care delivery settings, technologies, and resources are challenging nurses to provide quality patient care. At the same time, concerns about future nurse shortages and recruitment are coming to the public's attention. The nursing professional and specialty organizations can and must play a significant role in ensuring a future nursing workforce that is capable of fulfilling its patient responsibilities. Adult nursing specialty organizations must take the lead in developing initiatives that advocate for quality clinical care for patient populations, ensure maximum accessibility for basic services, and promote cost-effective care delivery without compromising patients' rights and dignity. To achieve these goals, these specialty organizations must advocate for their current and future nurse constituents, who need support in their ongoing efforts to develop and maintain expert clinical and professional skills.

To serve adult health patients and their families in this era of fast-paced changes, the specialty of adult health nursing and its members must evolve and grow. The expanded diversity and complexity of patient populations and practice will continue. Practicing adult health nurses must retool to meet clinical and organizational demands. Adult health nursing organizations must work together to support their members' broader and more comprehensive roles and opportunities. They must promote excellence in patient care by nurturing their members' knowledge, professional development, and leadership. The health care of the nation's adults depends on it.

REFERENCES

Academy of Medical Surgical Nursing. (2000). *"Project Tomorrow"* *draft report.* Pitman, NJ: Author.

American Association of Colleges of Nursing. (1997). *Executive summary. A vision of baccalaureate and graduate nursing education.* Washington, DC: Author.

American Association of Retired Persons. (1993). *A profile of older Americans.* Washington, DC: Author.

American Nurses Association. (1997). *Implementing nursing's report card: A study of RN staffing, length of stay, and patient outcomes.* Washington, DC: Author.

American Organization of Nurse Executives. (1999). *Executive summary: Nursing staffing survey.* Chicago: Author.

Appleby, J. (1999, July 29). Why are insurers dropping Medicare HMO? *USA Today,* p. A1.

Barnum, B.S., & Kerfoot, K. (1995). *The nurse as executive.* Gaithersburg, MD: Aspen.

Boland, S.L., & Sims, S. (1996). Family care giving at home. *Image, 28,* 55-58.

Brown, P.A. (1999). Nutrition and cancer. *MedSurg Nursing: The Journal of Adult Health, 8,* 333-345.

Brownson, R.C., Newschaffer, C.J., & Ali-Abarghoui, F. (1997). Policy research for disease prevention: Challenges and practical recommendations. *American Journal of Public Health, 87,* 735.

Carey, T.S., Garrett, J., & Jackson, A. (1995). The outcomes and costs of care for acute low back pain among patients seen by primary care practitioners, chiropractors, and orthopedic surgeons. *New England Journal of Medicine, 333,* 913-917.

Christman, L. (1998). The future: A challenge for nurses and nursing. In G. Deloughery (Ed.), *Issues and trends in nursing.* St. Louis: Mosby.

Fetter, M.S., & Grindel, C.G. (1997). Recent changes and current issues in medical-surgical nursing practice. In J.C. McCloskey & H.K. Grace (Eds.), *Current issues in nursing* (5th ed.). St. Louis: Mosby.

Fralic, M. (1999). Planning for tomorrow's health care system. In E.S. Sullivan (Ed.), *Creating nursing's future.* St. Louis: Mosby.

Gothberg, S. (1999). In pursuit of safe staffing. *Med-Surg Nursing: The Journal of Adult Health, 8,* 329.

Hay Group, Inc. (1998). *1998 Nursing shortage study: Preliminary report.* Philadelphia: Author.

Health Care Financing Administration. (1999). *Federal Register: Rules and Regulations, 64*(15), 3764-3784.

Hofer, T.P., Hayward, R.A., Greenfield, S., Wagner, E.H., Caplan, S.H., & Manning, W.G. (1999). The unreliability of individual physician "report cards" for assessing the costs and quality of care of a chronic disease [see comments]. *Journal of the American Medical Association, 281*(22), 2098-2105.

Institute of Medicine. (1996). *Primary care: America's health in a new era.* Washington, DC: National Academy Press.

Jacobs, P. (1998). The economics of health care. In G. Deloughery (Ed.), *Issues and trends in nursing.* St. Louis: Mosby.

Joint Commission on Accreditation of Healthcare Organizations. (1997). *Nursing practice and outcomes measurement.* St. Louis: Mosby.

Jollis, J.G., & Romano, P.S. (1998). Pennsylvania's focus on heart attack: Grading the scorecard. *New England Journal of Medicine, 338*(14), 983-987.

Lantz, P.M., House, J.S., Lepkowski, J.M., Williams, D.R., Mero, R.P., & Chen, J. (1998). Socioeconomic factors, health behaviors, and mortality results from a nationally representative prospective study of U.S. adults. *Journal of American Medical Association, 279*(21), 1703-1708.

Malone, B., & Marullo, G. (1997). *Workforce trends among U.S. registered nurses.* Report for the International Council of Nurses ICN Workforce Forum, Stockholm, Sweden. Available: www.ana.org/readroom/usworker.htm.

McCloskey, J.C., & Grace, H.K. (1997). A nurse is not a nurse is not a nurse. In J.C. McCloskey & H.K. Grace (Eds.), *Current issues in nursing* (5th ed.). St. Louis: Mosby.

Miller, A. (1999, August 1). Nurse alert: Caring touch compromised by shortages, burnout. *The Atlanta Journal-Constitution,* pp. A1, 10.

Miller, K.L., & Fry, S.C. (1999). Practice of the future. In E.S. Sullivan (Ed.), *Creating nursing's future.* St. Louis: Mosby.

National Association for Home Care. (1998). Official state data reveal more than doubling of home health care closures (News release: October 2, 1998). Available: www.nahc.org/NAHC/NewsInfo/98nr/hcdoubling.html.

National Center for Health Statistics. (1997a). *Healthy people 2000 review.* Hyattsville, MD: U.S. Public Health Service.

National Center for Health Statistics. (1997b). *America's children: Key indicators of well-being.* Available: www.cdc.gov/nchswww/default.htm.

Romano, P.S., Rainwater, J.A., & Antonius, D. (1999). Grading the graders: How hospitals in California and New York perceive and interpret their report cards. *Medical Care, 37,* 3295-3305.

Rudy, E.B., Daly, B.J., Douglas, S., Montenegro, H.D., Song, R., & Dyer, M.A. (1995). Patient outcomes for the chronically critically ill: Special care unit versus intensive care unit. *Nursing Research, 44*(6), 324-331.

Seccombe, K., & Amey, C. (1995). Playing by the rules and losing: Health insurance and the working poor. *Journal of Health and Social Behavior, 36,* 168-181.

Short, P.F., & Banthin, J.S. (1995). New estimates of the underinsured. *Journal of the American Medical Association, 274,* 1302-1306.

Sullivan, E.S., & Clinton, J.F. (1999). Achieving a multicultural nursing profession. In E.S. Sullivan (Ed.), *Creating nursing's future.* St. Louis: Mosby.

Taylor, A.K., Beauregard, K.M., & Vistnes, J.P. (1995). Who belongs to HMOs: A comparison of fee-for-service versus HMO enrollees. *Medical Care Research and Review, 52*(3), 389-408.

U.S. Census Bureau. (1996). *Population projections of the United States by age, sex, race, and Hispanic origin (1995-2050).* Washington, DC: Author. Available: http://www.census.gov/population/projections/nation/hh-fam/table6n.txt.

U.S. Census Bureau. (1997). *Press briefing on 1997 income and poverty estimates.* Washington, DC: Author. Available: www.uscb.gov/hhes/income/income97/prs98asc.html.

Valentine, N. (1997). Nursing's new world—A guide for taking professional responsibility to make healthcare better in the next century. In V.D. Ferguson (Ed.), *Educating the 21st century nurse.* New York: NLN Press.

Waggoner, M.G. (1999). OASIS: Measuring outcomes in home care. *Med-Surg Nursing: The Journal of Adult Health, 8,* 214-215.

Wakefield, M. (1999). Nursing's future in health care policy. In E.S. Sullivan (Ed.), *Creating nursing's future.* St. Louis: Mosby.

Wilensky, H. (1997). Social science and the public agenda: Reflections on the relation of knowledge to policy in the United States and abroad. *Journal of Health, Politics, Policy, and Law, 22,* 1241.

CHAPTER 26

Recent Changes and Current Issues in Parish Nursing

ANN SOLARI-TWADELL

It was 1984 when Reverend Granger Westberg, a Lutheran clergyman, approached Lutheran General Hospital, Advocate Health Care, about piloting an innovative nursing role to be called "parish nursing" (Holst, 1987). Sixteen years later the parish nurse ministry can be found across the United States, in most religious denominations, and internationally in such countries as Canada and Australia (Olson, Clark, & Simington, 1999; Van Loon, 1999).

Parish nursing is one form of health ministry that can be found in a congregation. The congregation is a term that means "an assembly of people whose beliefs about God combine with a common identity, a shared history, regular worship and common values to effect personal and social transformation" (Anderson, 1990, p. 265). A health ministry that is integral to the life of a congregation can be a catalyst for change. For example, congregations can reshape the understanding of health as being more than the absence of disease providing a more comprehensive view of health (Foege, 1990).

Parish nursing is a health promotion, disease-prevention role based on the care of the whole person and encompassing seven functions. These functions are integrator of faith and health, health educator, personal health counselor, referral agent, trainer of volunteers, developer of support groups, and health advocate. This nursing role does not embrace the medical model of care or invasive practices such as blood drawing, medical treatments, or maintenance of intravenous products. It is a professional model of health ministry that uses a registered professional nurse (Solari-Twadell, 1999). The focus of the practice is the faith community and its ministry (McDermott & Burke, 1993).

RECENT CHANGES IN PARISH NURSING
Designation as a Specialty Practice

The American Nurses Association identified parish nursing as a specialized area of practice in 1997. This altered the impression of parish nursing from that of being an innovative "grass roots" nursing practice model to a recognized nursing practice with a specialized body of knowledge and a particular skill set. This designation of a specialty practice came more than 10 years after the establishment of this nursing role in many congregations. It is a clear statement of the profession of nursing that this role is not only a ministry within a congregation but a form of nursing practice. It requires that those nurses functioning in the parish nurse role in a congregation need to be practicing within the parameters of the nurse practice act of the state in which they are providing services, as well as the guidelines for ministry of the denomination they are serving.

Some nurses and clergy are concerned with the vested interest of this professional nursing organization in parish nursing. It is perceived as a possible secularization and tinkering with the integration of this nursing ministry of faith and health into the life of the church. This kind of interest rather than being seen as strengthening the role of the parish nurse is viewed as opening the door to external requirements for the nurse along with meddling into that which is of the church (Smith, 2000).

Development of an Endorsed Standardized Curriculum for the Preparation of Parish Nursing

The International Parish Nurse Resource Center identified in the early 1990s more than 60 different curricula that claimed to offer some level of preparation in parish nursing. The review of these curricula resulted in the identification of the diversity in content. This raised concern as to the consistency with which nurses were being prepared to enter the practice of parish nursing. Given this diversity in preparation, the International Parish Nurse Resource Center in partnership with Loyola University of Chicago and Marquette University in Milwaukee initiated a 3-year project that resulted in a standardized endorsed curriculum for the preparation of parish nurses and parish nurse coordinators (McDermott, Solari-Twadell, & Matheus, 1998). The dissemination of these curricula includes an orientation for the parish nurse education program coordinator to the particular differences in preparing a parish nurse to practice health ministry in a congregational setting. To date there are 43 sites in the United States using these standardized curricula. These sites have prepared more than 2,000 parish nurses and parish nurse coordinators. In 1997 when the curricula were completed, it was agreed that the content would need review and revision in 3 years. That process is currently underway with the revisions anticipated to be complete by July 2000. The creation of these standardized curricula support a consistent preparation for those beginning a parish nurse practice.

Publishing of a Scope and Standards for Parish Nursing Practice

The American Nurses Association continued their investment in parish nursing with the publication of the "Scope and Standards of Parish Nursing Practice" (ANA, 1998). The Health Ministries Association initiated the development of the material for this document. The content of this booklet lays out the competent level of care and professional performance expected of a parish nurse (ANA, 1998). For many parish nurses this document was welcomed because it further substantiated the credibility of the parish nurse role. For others it represented deconstruction of not only the medical model but the secular compromising of the congregational ministry known as parish nursing (Smith, 2000).

A concern for the specialty practice of parish nursing following the availability of the scope and standards document is not only the dissemination of the document. It is important that there is a level of understanding by those that are practicing in the parish nurse role as to the importance of the integration of the standards into their day-to-day practice of the parish nurse. The purposes of the standards are to protect the integrity of this ministry that is a specialty practice within the profession of nursing. This can only be done if those that are practicing in the role understand the importance of this document, evalu-

ate their present parish nurse practice, and make changes to comply with the scope and standards for parish nursing as published by the American Nurses Association.

CURRENT ISSUES IN PARISH NURSING
Role Clarity

Is any nurse who works in the setting of a congregation a parish nurse? What makes a nurse a parish nurse? The congregation is a location in the community. Practicing nursing in this community site known as a congregation is not the only qualification for a nurse to be called a parish nurse. Nurse practitioners may have a clinic in a congregation and thus also are practicing in this setting. They are not parish nurses. They are nurse practitioners. Nurse case managers may use a congregation as a site for following up on clients. This is not parish nursing. This is nursing case management. These are but a few examples that reflect the presence of different nursing roles practicing in the setting of the congregation.

Particular parameters differentiate the parish nurse role from other nursing practices found in the location of the congregation. The following are some questions that can clarify the presence of a parish nurse in a congregation:

- Is the nurse a registered professional nurse?
- Has the nurse completed a basic preparation course in parish nursing?
- Is the nurse considered part of the ministerial staff of the congregation?
- Does the nurse have the potential to actualize the seven functions of the parish nurse role?
- Is the focus of the nurses' practice that of whole person health promotion and disease prevention with an emphasis on spiritual care?
- Does the nurse participate in some ongoing process of theological reflection that nurtures the pastoral dimensions of the parish nurse role?

It is important that there be role clarity as this role is introduced into the life of a congregation. If there is a blurring of the role, it will only cause confusion for the clergy, church members, and other health professionals. Role confusion also has the potential to compromise the integrity of the parish nurse practice and diffuse the focus of parish nursing practice.

Development of a Certification Process for Parish Nurses

A professional certification process in nursing is one means for a member of a specialty practice to substantiate a level of expertise and competency in that nursing role. By engaging in the process of certification, the nurse seeks a credential that will communicate to the public a particular level of knowledge of the specialty practice. Once a specialty practice has developed a scope statement and standards of practice, the next step is the construction of a certification process.

There is presently a requirement that the nurse be prepared at the baccalaureate level to participate in a certification process. As parish nursing seeks to develop such a certification process for parish nursing, there arises several concerns. Are there sufficient numbers of parish nurses this early in the development of the specialty prepared at the baccalaureate level? Another major consideration is the financial investment in becoming certified in the specialty. The question of finances is a real one when some parish nurses are not being paid for the time they are committing to the parish nurse role in their congregations.

Some parish nurses are serving as parish nurses in denominations that have a process for qualifying individuals to assume ministry roles in the congregation. Because parish nursing is seen as a form of health ministry, nurses are participating in these denominational ministerial processes to receive endorsement by a particular church hierarchy. Because the parish nurse role is both ministry and nursing practice, not just one or the other, this will be a major consideration in the development of a certification for this parish nursing. The nursing certification will be addressed by the nursing certifying body, and the religious dimension of practicing ministry would be the responsibility of the denomination. It remains to be seen whether a dual process of this nature will be too costly, time intensive, and rigorous for the parish nurse. The requirements could have the capability of deterring nurses to follow their call to this ministry of parish nursing practice. A certifying process that considers the uniqueness of this ministry of parish nursing practice will be a challenge in design—one worth the effort if it offers the two worlds of nursing and religion a long-awaited reconciliation.

Financing of the Parish Nurse Role

The original organizational framework for parish nursing that was developed through the efforts of Reverend Granger Westberg and Lutheran General Hospital required a 20-hour-a-week, paid position. The employer was the hospital with a contract that detailed the specific congregation(s) the nurse was to serve. The salary was to be paid by the congregation with the benefits and liability of the nurse to be covered by the hospital (Solari-Twadell

& Westberg, 1991). Today there are many such organizational arrangements that mimic this original design to financially support the parish nurse role. However, today, with more and more concern regarding the reimbursement for health care services and the shrinking margin of health care institutions, this model of financing the parish nurse is being challenged.

Early in the parish nurse movement the word spread about parish nursing with excitement and possibility. Without much understanding of the role or how to begin this health ministry nurses, clergy, and lay people became creative in developing new and different organizing frameworks for this ministry. Many, however, included no financial remuneration for the nurse. For some religious denominations this is in keeping with religious traditions that see ministry as a gift of "time and talent." So although some see the parish nurse position as having more credibility when the nurse is paid, other belief systems do not see it is necessary to pay the nurse or may even believe that payment for ministry is contrary to beliefs and traditions.

The other factor that enters into the consideration for payment of the services of the parish nurse is the nature of the role. This is a health promotion, disease prevention nursing role. Health promotion programming has never been funded adequately in the health system of the United States. Funding for programs of this nature are frequently underwritten by foundations and grant writing. This kind of funding is time limited and eventually will need to be identified if the program is to sustain long-term financial support.

The idea that the services provided by the parish nurse should be considered for reimbursement through an HMO or other health insurance mechanism raises some concern. Would the nature of the parish nurse role be compromised by documentation for reimbursement? Would this kind of financing for services create further problems with the congregation being seen as a health clinic versus a health place in the community? Does this mode of financing compromise the very nature of the congregation, its ministry, and independence?

Integration

So that parish nursing may continue as a viable contributor to the transformation of health care, it must be integrated—integrated both into the life of the congregation served and the overall health care system in the United States. At this point in the history and development of parish nursing as a specialty practice, this is a tremendous challenge.

The existence of parish nursing in some congregations is perceived as an individual contribution on the part of a nurse to the membership of the congregation. If that particular nurse would leave the congregation, the ministry would disappear. This is not the intention of this ministry. The plan for parish nursing from the beginning was that it would be integrated into the life of the congregation. The most visible manifestation of this ideology is that the nurse is an integral part of the ministerial team in the congregation (Holstrom, 1999). In other words the parish nurse on a day-to-day basis is privileged with information regarding individuals, program development, worship development, and special liturgical events. In this way health and wholeness is woven into everything that is occurring within the congregation's life. This level of involvement requires pastoral leadership that understands and therefore facilitates an integration of this health ministry into everything that is part of the life of the congregation.

Integration of parish nursing into the continuum of care of the health care system is no less challenging. This is based on the congregation being valued as a partner in the formation of the health of individuals in society. It requires new thinking and relationships in which the acute care provider or financial reimbursement system is not seen as the only source of health care services. This requires the consumer to be the driver of not only where their health care dollar will be spent but how much of it will be spent on prevention of illness and how much on acute care of illness. Clearly as a society, the consumers in the United States are not at this level of understanding or investment, but over the last 5 to 7 years there has clearly been a move in that direction. Consumers in the United States are paying more out of their pocket for alternative means of health care. This has a close kinship with or may be a preparation for demanding more say in the expending of their health care dollar in the future.

Documentation of the Practice

Early in the development of the parish nurse movement the documentation of the services rendered was insufficient. For some nurses going into this practice it actually meant an opportunity to abandon this professional responsibility! The setting of the congregation does not require documentation of services rendered by any other staff member. So in some settings the concept of documentation of services rendered by the nurse was debated or not accepted well by the pastoral leadership. Today this responsibility of the parish nurse is more clearly understood and clarified as a necessity in the standards of practice for

parish nursing. However, the requirements for documentation in the standards do not adequately address the system that should be used. This is leaving the system of documentation up to the nurse, and the result is a variety of formats and systems for parish nurse documentation.

Recently there has been a system of parish nurse documentation developed that is based on the use of standardized nursing languages (Burkhart, 1997). The use of the North American Nursing Diagnosis Association (NANDA) (1999) and the Nursing Interventions Classification (NIC) (McCloskey & Bulechek, 2000) standardized nursing languages brings with it the ability to cross specialties within nursing and create a common understanding of the contribution of each nursing specialty. This has the capability of forming a linkage across the various sites in the continuum of health care services. The use of standardized nursing languages has presented additional work for those within parish nursing. Initially, there was no adequate language to describe the interventions of the parish nurse. This has resulted in the parish nurses expanding the standardized language so that particularly the phenomena of spiritual care could be adequately documented. The expansion of the standardized nursing languages in the area of spiritual care will not only enhance the practice of the parish nurse but also any nurse in any practice arena who is interested in caring for the spiritual dimension of the client served.

Identification of Outcomes

There has been a growing interest over the last 7 years as to what the health outcomes are related to the presence of a parish nurse. The stories told by those practicing in the parish nurse role are impressive as to how the parish nurse is making a difference in the life of not only members of the congregation, but the life of the congregation. There has been no consistent method for reporting the outcomes of parish nursing practice, however. Data that are most useful for a health care system evaluating their investment in parish nursing are numerical. Numbers, although not able to tell the full story, can give a quick overall evaluation.

Again, the importance of using a standardized language as part of the system for documenting parish nurse outcomes is important. Therefore the use of the Nursing Outcomes Classification (NOC) (Johnson, Maas, & Moorhead, 2000) will be important. Use of this standardized language will offer the same benefit of NANDA and NIC terminology in furthering communication across specialties of nursing within the continuum of care. At present there is a research study through the University of Iowa that will support the NOC system's validity and reliability. Parish nurses are participating in this study. This participation not only will contribute to nursing as a whole but also will include outcomes pertinent to the practice of the parish nurse. This will ensure that within time there will be a system of documenting parish nurse outcomes that will be useful not only to the parish nurse but also to those nurses providing spiritual care across the continuum of care.

SUMMARY

Many who pioneered the role of the parish nurse are stunned at what has occurred over the last 15 years. The possibilities and opportunities for the contribution that this specialty practice will make to the well-being of individuals and communities is not clear at this time. In some instances, for some nurses in the role, for many pastors providing leadership to congregations, and for both congregations and health care institutions making a financial investment it is still very much a journey of faith and trust. One thing is for sure, if we are going to have a different outcome to the problems in our health care system, we have to apply different methods. Parish nursing offers this opportunity.

REFERENCES

American Nurses Association. (1998). *Scope and standards of parish nursing practice.* Washington, DC: Author.

Anderson, H. (1990). The congregation as a healing resource. In D. Browning, T. Jobe, & I. Evison (Eds.), *Religious and ethical factors in psychiatric practice* (pp. 264-278). Chicago: Nelson Hall in association with the Park Ridge Center for Health, Faith and Ethics.

Burkhart, L. (1997, spring/summer). Nursing standardized languages to promote professionalism. *Perspective in Parish Nursing Practice,* 1, 3-11.

Foege, W. (1990). The vision of the possible: What churches can do. *Second Opinion, 13,* 36-42.

Holst, L. (1987). The parish nurse. *Chronicle of Pastoral Care, 7*(1), 13-17.

Holstrom, S. (1999). Perspectives on a suburban parish nursing practice. In P.A. Solari-Twadell & M.A. McDermott, *Parish nursing: Promoting whole person health within faith communities* (pp. 67-75). Thousand Oaks, CA: Sage.

Johnson, M., Maas, M., & Moorhead, S. (Eds.). (2000). *Nursing outcomes classification (NOC)* (2nd ed.). St. Louis: Mosby.

McCloskey, J.C., & Bulechek, G.M. (Eds.). (2000). *Nursing interventions classification (NIC)* (3rd ed.). St. Louis: Mosby.

McDermott, M.A., & Burke, J. (1993). When the population is a congregation: The emerging role of the parish nurse. *Journal of Community Health Nursing, 10*(3), 179-190.

McDermott, M.A., Solari-Twadell, A., & Matheus, R. (1998, January). Promoting quality education for the parish nurse and parish nurse coordinator. *Nursing Health Care Perspectives,* 4-7.

North American Nursing Diagnosis Association. (1999). *Nursing diagnoses: Definitions and classification 1999-2000.* Philadelphia: Author.

Olson, J.K., Clark, M.B., & Simington, J.A. (1999). The Canadian experience. In P.A. Solari-Twadell & M.A. McDermott, *Parish nursing: Promoting whole person health within faith communities* (pp. 277-285). Thousand Oaks, CA: Sage.

Smith, S.D. (2000, winter). Parish nursing: A call to integrity. *Journal of Christian Nursing,* 18-20.

Solari-Twadell, P.A. (1999). The emerging practice of parish nursing. In P.A. Solari-Twadell & M.A. McDermott, *Parish nursing: Promoting whole person health within faith communities* (pp. 3-24). Thousand Oaks, CA: Sage.

Solari-Twadell, A., & Westberg, G. (1991, September). Body, mind and soul: The parish nurse offers physical, emotional and spiritual care. *Health Progress,* 24-28.

Van Loon, A.M. (1999). The Australian concept of faith community. In P.A. Solari-Twadell & M.A. McDermott, *Parish nursing: Promoting whole person health within faith communities* (pp. 287-297). Thousand Oaks, CA: Sage.

CHAPTER 27

Recent Changes and Current Issues in Perinatal Nursing

KATHLEEN RICE SIMPSON

Every day in the United States approximately 11,000 babies are born to women in more than 6,000 hospitals that provide perinatal services (Martin, Smith, Mathews, & Ventura, 1999). These mothers and babies are cared for during pregnancy, labor, birth, and the postpartum period by perinatal nurses dedicated to providing a safe and therapeutic environment to promote the best possible outcomes for their patients. Few professional experiences are more rewarding than attendance at the birth of a healthy newborn and sharing the joy with the new mother and her family (Simpson & Chez, 2001). Perinatal nursing offers the best of all specialty areas of professional nursing practice and includes the prenatal course, obstetrical triage, and labor, birth, perioperative, postanesthesia, postpartum, and newborn care. Perinatal nurses caring for women with high-risk pregnancies and preterm infants use medical-surgical and critical care nursing knowledge and skills. No other specialty in nursing offers a wider range of activities and opportunities to make a difference in the lives of women, newborns, and their families. The focus of perinatal nursing is on making families and creating our future (Simpson & Chez, 2001). Although approximately 4% of registered nurses in the United States are men (Geolot, 1999), perinatal nursing remains predominantly a specialty of nurses who are women. This woman-to-woman connection is powerful for both perinatal nurses and patients.

As a specialty we face many challenges; some are specific to perinatal care, and others we share with nursing in general. These challenges are related in part to recent changes in health care delivery systems that seem to favor the financial bottom line and convenience over practices that promote patient safety and to the socialization of women to childbearing. Current issues of importance that require assertive actions by perinatal nurses if sig-

nificant changes are to occur are the continued medicalization of labor and birth, increased use of technology for healthy women, the ongoing conflict between "the way we've always done it" versus evidence-based care, errors by health care providers that contribute to maternal-fetal injuries, increasing nurse/patient ratios, the proliferation of convenience as the foundation for care during labor and birth, lack of education about the impact of this convenience philosophy among childbearing women, and the forces challenging nurse midwives as the primary care providers for healthy women. Each of these issues will be discussed in the context of why we are in this situation and what can be done to make significant changes.

THE MEDICALIZATION OF LABOR AND BIRTH

Unlike other nursing specialties, perinatal nurses care for women during a healthy, natural life event. Labor and birth are natural physiological processes. Most women do well with support and selected minimal intervention (Simpson & Knox, 1999). Yet many women in the United States give birth in a high-technology, low-touch environment with electronic devices monitoring every physiological parameter possible (Simpson, 1999). Even when an unmedicated, low-technology childbirth is planned and prepared for extensively, many women who are vulnerable during labor and birth find themselves agreeing to interventions that clearly are unnecessary and have the potential for iatrogenic injuries (Knox, Simpson, & Garite, 1999). When birth occurs in a hospital, there is a tendency to view the process as a medical event. In this setting birth is controlled and managed; arbitrary time frames rule what is a natural process. Despite a substantial body of evidence to suggest this is not the best approach, if labor is not proceeding according to the "labor curve," interventions are routinely used to hasten the process. For example, amniotic membranes are frequently artificially ruptured to speed labor, which causes a significant increase in umbilical cord compression evidenced by variable fetal heart rate decelerations. The use of drugs to artificially stimulate labor contractions has increased 110% since 1989, the first year these data were collected (Martin et al., 1999). Most women in the United States labor in bed, eliminating the normal physiological advantages of an upright maternal position. If the second stage of labor does not proceed within outdated time frames, vacuum extractors using between 400 and 600 mm Hg of pressure are applied to the fetal head to hasten birth. The U.S. Food and Drug Administration (FDA) has issued warnings to health care providers about risk of fetal injuries with this device (FDA, 1998); however, the procedure is at an all-time high (Martin et al., 1999). Although an extensive body of research suggests otherwise, most women in the United States have an episiotomy immediately before birth (Martin et al., 1999). This unnecessary procedure is painful, delays recovery, and increases risk of urinary and fecal incontinence for women later in life (Renfrew, Hannah, Albers, & Floyd, 1998). Many hospitals in the United States have strict visitor policies based on crowd-control principles that disregard the desires of women to have those she wishes attend birth.

This medicalization of childbirth continues for many reasons. Hospitals have invested millions in high technology related to the birthing process. That technology, once in place, becomes the part of the routine for caring for women during labor and birth. There was hope that this technology would reduce the incidence of cerebral palsy; however, despite continuous electronic fetal monitoring (EFM) during labor as the routine in U.S. hospitals since the late 1970s, the incidence of cerebral palsy remains the same as it was before the introduction of this device. There was hope that EFM would be a factor in reducing professional liability for health care providers and institutions; however, "bad baby" cases have instead increased over the years. Conflicts in interpreting the data from EFM has now become a major part of lawsuits alleging perinatal malpractice. Problems with interrater and intrarater reliability related to EFM are reality in everyday clinical practice. Thus it is no surprise that experts disagree when asked to offer testimony for the defense and plaintiffs. Another significant reason for the continued medicalization of childbirth is that perinatal care is provided primarily by physicians (Martin et al., 1999), who are educated and trained to monitor and intervene, rather than nurse midwives who believe less is more when it comes to interventions for childbearing women. Nurse midwives believe in and support the inherent power of women to give birth naturally and with selected interventions as needed. Unfortunately, only 7% of births in the United States are attended by nurse midwives (Martin et al., 1999). Financial and philosophical reasons prohibit or inhibit certified nurse midwives (CNMs) from getting privileges to attend births in many hospitals. In some areas of the country there are more obstetricians-gynecologists than are needed to support the target population. Thus there is an effort to prevent CNMs from effectively entering the market. Healthy women at low risk for complications during pregnancy can be managed by CNMs and have been shown to have similar clinical outcomes and lower costs of care (Brown & Grimes, 1993). Increased access to CNMs by this healthy patient population would help to reverse the current trend in making birth a medical event.

INCREASED USE OF TECHNOLOGY

Some argue that the lack of one-to-one nursing care in the United States for women in labor has led to electronic monitors providing much of the maternal-fetal assessment data during labor and birth. It is just as likely that the increased use of technology has contributed to the perception by health care administrators that one-to-one nursing care during labor is no longer needed. The latest monitors allow electronic assessment of multiple physiological variables that are displayed on a central screen at nurses' stations. In this type of setting, nurses have less need to personally interact with the woman in labor. Consider the following scenario: a healthy woman at term agrees to an induction of labor, which leads to epidural anesthesia, slow progress of labor and attachment of the following nine intervention and monitoring devices: a main intravenous line and additional line with oxytocin, internal fetal scalp electrode, intrauterine pressure catheter, epidural catheter, automatic blood pressure device, cardiac monitor, pulse oximeter, and Foley catheter (Simpson, 1999). It is interesting to note that none of these devices or interventions are recommended by the professional associations that promulgate guidelines and standards of care for women in labor such as the Association of Women's Health, Obstetric and Neonatal Nurses (AWHONN), the American College of Nurse Midwives (ACNM), the American College of Obstetricians (ACOG), or the American Society of Anesthesiologists (ASA), yet they are the routine in many labor and birth units in the United States (Simpson, 1999).

THE "WAY WE'VE ALWAYS DONE IT" VERSUS EVIDENCE-BASED PERINATAL CARE

The lack of integration of evidence-based care for healthy pregnant women contributes to high-technology labor and birth becoming the norm. Perinatal nurses only can be advocates for healthy childbearing women when they have knowledge of current standards and guidelines from their professional associations (Simpson & Knox, 1999). Many nurses are unaware of their specialty nursing organization. Of those who are aware, few are members. Although there are 2.5 million registered nurses in the United States, AWHONN has approximately 23,000 members. Undoubtedly there are many more perinatal nurses in the United States. In addition to the awareness of and adherence to professional guidelines and standards of care, perinatal nurses must have knowledge about all areas of their specialty practice. The ability to search computer databases for pertinent literature and critically evaluate the combined weight of what is known about each intervention is requisite for perinatal nurses in the advocacy role who want to provide safe and effective care (Gennaro & Lewis, 2000). Perinatal nurses must be aware of the body of evidence to suggest that routine interventions during labor and birth lead to iatrogenic injuries (Knox, Simpson, & Garite, 1999). They must be willing to work collaboratively with physician colleagues to make evidence-based perinatal care a reality (Simpson, 1999).

Commitment to practice based on evidence and standards is an ongoing process and may require substantial changes and more professional energy than the usual methods of implementing and evaluating changes in patient care, but it is well worth the additional effort (Simpson & Knox, 1999). Discussions about clinical practice that are based on evidence and standards of care rather than hierarchical relationships, personal preferences, and old routines can be helpful in setting the stage for real collaboration. For the perinatal nurse to have an equal voice in these discussions about clinical practices, efforts must be made to keep abreast of current evidence and evolving trends that have the potential to enhance maternal-fetal outcomes (Simpson & Knox, 2001). However, to be able to critically evaluate the evidence that is available and present credible recommendations, nurses need knowledge of the research process and skills in critiquing research studies. Unfortunately, according to the latest data, 59% of registered nurses (RNs) in the United States today do not hold a 4-year college degree (Geolot, 1999). Without the education about the research process that is provided during baccalaureate education, it is difficult for nurses to bring a similar level of understanding and evaluation of the evidence under consideration to a clinical discussion with physician colleagues. The wide disparity in education between nurses and physicians is one of the contributing factors to the lack of equal partnership in developing and implementing evidence-based clinical interventions. An equal voice in clinical discussions must be the voice of one who has been educated in an institution of higher learning in a manner similar to other members of the health care team (Simpson & Knox, 2001). The lack of college education among the majority of practicing nurses is one of the most significant barriers to enhancing the professional status of nurses and contributes to the present hierarchical relationships between nurses and physicians. Nurses have been debating this issue for too long. The time is now to set a date for requiring the baccalaureate degree as the criteria for entry into professional nursing practice. Grandfather in the current nurses and move forward united in providing consumers with care they deserve, delivered by professionals that have been adequately educated to provide that care (Gennaro & Lewis, 2000). Only with additional education will nurses be able to fully participate in processes that promote evidence-based care for mothers and babies.

ERRORS BY HEALTH CARE PROVIDERS THAT RESULT IN MATERNAL-FETAL INJURIES

Even though use of multiple interventions and sophisticated technologies to monitor maternal-fetal status has become the norm, these techniques and machines have not decreased risk of maternal-fetal injuries. This is a serious issue facing perinatal nurses today. Along with emergency departments and perioperative services, perinatal units account for most of the claims of patient injuries and death (Simpson, 2000). The release of the report from the Institute of Medicine *To Err is Human: Building a Safer Health System* late in 1999 highlighted what risk managers and perinatal care providers already knew: errors by health care providers are an unfortunate common occurrence during inpatient stays (Kohn, Corrigan, & Donaldson, 1999). Forty-two percent of all Americans are aware of at least one medical error either through personal involvement or an experience of a relative or friend (National Patient Safety Foundation [NPSF], 1999). According to NPSF (1999) there are approximately 3 million errors per year in the inpatient setting, costing an estimated $200 billion dollars annually. An error occurs during 17% of all inpatient admissions; fortunately, only 4% result in an adverse outcome (NPSF,

1999). An adverse outcome is generally defined as an injury caused by treatment. A preventable adverse outcome for a mother or baby can be tragic, with long-term and even fatal consequences in some cases. Between 44,000 and 98,000 patients die every year in hospitals because of errors by health care providers, more than due to traffic accidents, breast cancer, and human immunodeficiency virus, making these types of deaths the fourth leading cause of death in the United States (Kohn et al., 1999). These deaths include mothers and babies. Many of these patient injuries related to human error are preventable. Fetal and neonatal injuries are more common than maternal injuries. Five common recurring clinical problems account for most fetal and neonatal injuries (Knox, Simpson, & Garite, 1999):

1. Inability to recognize or appropriately respond to both antepartum and intrapartum fetal compromise
2. Inability to effect a timely cesarean birth (30 minutes from decision to incision) when indicated by fetal or maternal condition
3. Inability to appropriately resuscitate a depressed baby
4. Inappropriate use of oxytocin or misoprostol, leading to uterine hyperstimulation, uterine rupture, and fetal compromise or death
5. Inappropriate use of forceps, vacuum, or fundal pressure, leading to fetal trauma or preventable shoulder dystocia

Most errors are not the result of individual recklessness or incompetence but rather from flaws in the system (Kohn et al., 1999). We are a decade behind other high-risk industries in attending to basic safety (Simpson, 2000). For example, in the airline industry and in nuclear power plants, safety is the number one priority, ranking above production (Knox et al., 1999). Their motto is "Safety First." To create a culture of safety, systems must be designed that are geared toward preventing, detecting, and minimizing the likelihood of error, rather than attaching blame to individuals (Kohn et al., 1999). Perinatal providers must look to other industries in which safety is the number one priority for solutions to promote the best possible maternal-fetal outcomes. Perinatal unit operations and health care provider relationships must be reexamined in the context of implementing a system designed for maternal-fetal safety (Simpson, 2000).

NURSE/PATIENT RATIOS

The increasing nurse/patient ratio during labor and birth is a major barrier to quality perinatal care. When the nurse has more patients than can be adequately cared for, there is a constant priority setting and elimination process that contributes to shortcuts and only the most basic care (Knox, Kelley, Simpson, Carrier, & Berry, 1999). Unfortunately, for some nurses the basics may be high-tech interventions and documentation, while supportive care in labor is considered a luxury. As costs of care have accelerated, perinatal units have suffered staffing cuts. The increased use of technology to monitor maternal-fetal status during labor, the high rate of epidural anesthesia, and the fact that most women and fetuses are healthy have contributed to the ability of institutions providing perinatal care to "get away with" using less nurses in perinatal services (Knox, Simpson, & Garite, 1999). A multicenter randomized clinical trial is currently underway in the United States and Canada to evaluate the impact of one-to-one nursing care during labor and birth when compared with routine care. These nurse researchers are studying an important issue for perinatal nurses. It is hoped that results will demonstrate that one-to-one nursing care does have a significant positive effect on maternal-newborn outcomes. More rigorously designed clinical research projects are needed to evaluate and quantify the importance of continuous nursing care during labor and birth.

PROLIFERATION OF CONVENIENCE AS THE FOUNDATION FOR LABOR AND BIRTH

Artificial induction of labor is at the highest level in the United States since these data began being collected from birth certificates in 1989 (Martin et al., 1999). The incidence of labor induction is most likely much higher than reported, because of inaccuracy issues with data retrieved from birth certificates. Multiple factors influence the decision to induce labor (Simpson & Poole, 1998a). Clearly not all indications are clinical or are in the best interests of mothers and babies. Increasingly, convenience has become a significant factor in artificial induction of labor. This is a complex issue that involves all participating parties, the pregnant woman, her family, the obstetrician or CNM, the institution, and the perinatal nurse (Simpson & Poole, 1998a). In 1995, ACOG included "psychosocial indications" as an accepted reason for induction. Previously ACOG's position had been that induction of labor solely for convenience was not recommended (ACOG, 1991). The most likely reason for this change was that routine practices were not consistent with published standards, exposing physicians to liability risks if adverse outcomes resulted from artificial labor induction. The controversial issue is: Who benefits more from this convenience approach to labor induction? Women agree to or choose induction of labor for many reasons. For some women, advance planning and prior arrangements can provide reassurance and a sense of control over an otherwise unpredictable process (Simpson & Poole, 1998b). Additional factors such as child care for other children, availability of the labor support person or father of the baby, choice of attending physician on call, avoidance of holidays, maternity leave constraints, and even a federal income tax deduction in the preferred year can enter into the pregnant woman's decision to agree to or request an elective induction of labor (Simpson & Poole, 1998b). If pregnant women are fully informed about the indications for induction, risks and benefits of the proposed method, and possible alternative approaches as recommended by ACOG (1999), the woman's choice should be honored if there are appropriate resources available to safely induce labor. However, many discussions between women and their physician before induction fall short of meeting these criteria. An all-too-common occurrence during admission of a pregnant woman for induction is the realization by the nurse that the woman did not request an induction of labor and is unaware of the indications, potential risks, and alternative approaches. Although not well documented in the literature or discussed openly in professional forums, a scheduled induction of labor offers some real convenience advantages to the physician and CNM (Simpson & Poole, 1998b). Scheduling several women for an induction of labor on the same day starting early in the morning allows patient management to be done concurrently and increases the likelihood that most women will give birth by the end of the day (Simpson & Poole, 1998b). When physicians and CNMs schedule inductions routinely, the risk of women's going into spontaneous labor and giving birth at a time that is inconvenient is avoided. As the number of patients who have scheduled inductions increase, the number of physician and CNM phone calls and trips to the hospital in the middle of the night and on weekends is likely to decrease (Simpson & Poole, 1998b).

Another example of provider convenience is shortening the second stage of an otherwise normal labor by application of forceps or a vacuum extractor and cutting an episiotomy. Perinatal nurses can help to avoid the temptation by physicians to shorten the second stage when there are no maternal-fetal indications by calling physicians at appropriate times when birth is imminent, so they are not delayed in the hospital when they have an office full of pregnant women waiting to be seen. This re-

quires knowledge of the labor process and keen assessment skills. All interventions for convenience involve some risk of an adverse outcome. Unfortunately the current culture in many perinatal units supports routine practices for convenience rather than patience and allowing the normal process and progress of birth to occur. In this situation, routine practices for convenience continue until the inevitable adverse outcome occurs.

Another way to understand how practices that involve risk can come to be favored over patience and patient safety is provided by Vaughn (1996) in her analysis of the *Challenger* disaster. She found that professional standards of any work group will degrade slowly and incrementally over time. Vaughn (1996) termed this progressive degradation in safe practice *the normalization of deviance.* Operational systems and clinical practices that are known to be risky continue because the risk is continually redefined in the context of injuries that do not occur (Vaughn, 1996). This phenomena of human behavior is especially prevalent when the chances of the risk occurring are small. Most mothers and babies are healthy, so care involving increased risk does not usually result in patient injury (Knox et al., 1999). As time goes on, practice becomes increasingly less safe because "they get away with it." Perinatal practices that involve convenience for health care providers should be evaluated in terms of risks and benefits for mothers and babies. Women should be fully informed that practices or interventions being considered are for convenience, and they should be allowed to make a decision about whether to proceed. Avoiding risk of the normalization of deviance in any perinatal setting is a significant challenge for perinatal nurses, but one that can be met if the goal of the best possible outcomes for mothers and babies is ranked higher in priority than convenience. This will require physicians and nurses coming to consensus that patient safety is the number one priority and that some may be inconvenienced waiting for nature to take its course.

LACK OF KNOWLEDGE AMONG CHILDBEARING WOMEN ABOUT THE IMPACT OF PHILOSOPHY OF CONVENIENCE

There has never been more information about pregnancy and birth available than there is today for childbearing women. A visit to the local bookstore will reveal aisles of books on all sorts of related topics. More than 3,000 Internet sites are devoted to pregnancy and childbirth. Yet many pregnant women seem to be uninformed about the implications of artificial induction of labor, epidural anesthesia, assisted instrumental vaginal birth, and elective cesarean birth on the eventual outcomes of pregnancy. It is the rare woman admitted for an elective induction of labor who is able to accurately articulate the risks involved. Most women are not actively involved in the decision to use forceps or a vacuum to shorten the second stage of labor or are informed about the risks of the procedure versus waiting for the fetus to descend spontaneously. Few women question the need for an episiotomy when the procedure is imminent. Women put their trust in their health care providers. Trust is a good thing, but not blind trust. A fully informed woman is a partner in the decision-making process. However, even women who are fully informed agree to things they had planned to avoid when they are vulnerable during the process of labor and birth. Perinatal nurses, as advocates for pregnant women, need to make sure that women have the necessary information to make important decisions during labor and birth. Unfortunately this advocacy can be seen by some as interfering with the physician-patient relationship. One way to increase the likelihood that women who are informed and have made choices actually realize care based on those choices is the implementation of a birth plan listing available options that can be completed by women during the prenatal period and made part of the medical record. The perinatal nurse can then review requests and appropriateness on the basis of the individual clinical situation on admission for childbirth. The content of prepared childbirth classes should include an objective review of the risks and benefits of commonly used interventions during labor and birth, and this information should be reinforced by nurses who care for women during the intrapartum period.

SUMMARY

Many issues in perinatal care could benefit from the collective efforts of all perinatal nurses to improve the way we routinely care for childbearing women. Much of what we do in perinatal care is based on myths, rituals, and "the way we've always done it" (Simpson & Knox, 1999). Those who are invested in the old ways will resist attempts for significant change. The best hope for change is a firm commitment to providing care based on the combined weight of available evidence. This commitment involves perinatal nurses making an effort to become educated about how to critique these data and apply the evidence to everyday clinical practice. Knowledge is power. This power is within all perinatal nurses who arm themselves with the skills required to have clinical discus-

sions with physician colleagues based on evidence and thus become true partners in determining the best practices for routine perinatal care.

REFERENCES

American College of Obstetricians and Gynecologists. (1991). *Induction of labor.* Technical Bulletin No. 157. Washington, DC: Author.

American College of Obstetricians and Gynecologists. (1995). *Induction of labor.* Technical Bulletin No. 217. Washington, DC: Author.

American College of Obstetricians and Gynecologists. (1999). *Induction of labor.* Practice Bulletin No. 10. Washington, DC: Author.

Brown, S.A., & Grimes, D.E. (1993). *A meta-analysis of process of care, clinical outcomes, and cost-effectiveness of nurses in primary care roles: Nurse practitioners and certified nurse midwives.* Washington, DC: American Nurses Association.

Food and Drug Administration. (1998). *FDA Public health advisory: Need for caution when using vacuum assisted delivery devices.* Washington, DC: Author.

Gennaro, S., & Lewis, J. (2000). Is the BSN as the criteria for entry in professional nursing practice still worthwhile and realistic? *MCN The American Journal of Maternal Child Nursing, 25*(2), 62-63.

Geolot, D. (1999). *Nursing workforce characteristics.* Presented at the Tri-Council Meeting, May 3, Washington, DC.

Knox, G.E., Kelley, M., Simpson, K.R., Carrier, L., & Berry, D. (1999). Downsizing, re-engineering and patient safety: Numbers, newness and resultant risk. *Journal of Healthcare Risk Management, 19*(4), 18-25.

Knox, G.E., Simpson, K.R., & Garite, T.J. (1999). High reliability perinatal units: An approach to the prevention of patient injury and medical malpractice claims. *Journal of Healthcare Risk Management, 19*(2), 27-35.

Kohn, L., Corrigan, J., & Donaldson, M. (Eds.) and the Committee on Quality of Health Care in America, Institute of Medicine. (1999). *To err is human: Building a safer health system.* Washington, DC: National Academy of Sciences Press.

Martin, J.A., Smith, B.L., Mathews, T.J., & Ventura, S.J. (1999). Births and deaths: Preliminary data for 1998. *National Vital Statistics Report, 47*(25), 1-38.

National Patient Safety Foundation. (1999). *Finding cures for medical error.* Chicago: Author.

Renfrew, M.J., Hannah, W., Albers, L., & Floyd, E. (1998). Factors that minimize trauma to the genital tract in childbirth: A systematic review. *Birth: Issues in Perinatal Care, 25*(3), 143-160.

Simpson, K.R. (1999). Routine care during labor and birth: Is this really how we want to practice perinatal nursing or are we ready to advocate for childbearing women and insist on evidence-based care? *Mother Baby Journal, 4*(4), 5-7.

Simpson, K.R. (2000). Creating a culture of safety: A shared responsibility. *MCN The American Journal of Maternal Child Nursing, 25*(2), 61.

Simpson, K.R., & Chez, B.F. (2001). Professional and legal issues. In K.R. Simpson & P.A. Creehan (Eds.), *AWHONN's perinatal nursing* (2nd ed., pp. 23-55). Philadelphia: Lippincott Williams & Wilkins.

Simpson, K.R., & Knox, G.E. (1999). Strategies for developing an evidence-based approach to perinatal care. *MCN The American Journal of Maternal Child Nursing, 24*(3), 122-132.

Simpson, K.R., & Knox, G.E. (2001). Perinatal teamwork: Turning rhetoric into reality. In K.R. Simpson & P.A. Creehan (Eds.), *AWHONN's perinatal nursing* (2nd ed., pp. 57-71). Philadelphia: Lippincott Williams & Wilkins.

Simpson, K.R., & Poole, J.H. (1998a). *Cervical ripening, induction and augmentation of labor.* AWHONN Practice Symposium. Washington, DC: AWHONN.

Simpson, K.R., & Poole, J.H. (1998b). Labor induction & augmentation: Knowing when and how to assist women in labor. *AWHONN Lifelines, 2*(6), 39-42.

Vaughn, D. (1996). *The Challenger launch decision: Risky technology, culture and deviance at NASA.* Chicago: University of Chicago Press.

CHAPTER 28

Recent Changes and Current Issues in Perioperative Nursing

SUZANNE CUSHMAN BEYEA

Perioperative nurses face a number of challenges as we move into the next decade. Changes in the health care delivery system, advances in technology, and increases in the cost of care are occurring at an accelerated pace, creating many new opportunities. Concurrently, the traditional role of the registered nurse in the operating room is being threatened. It is anticipated that these changes will affect nursing practice, leading to role diversification and ultimately the emergence of new positions and responsibilities for perioperative nurses in a variety of clinical settings.

Powerful economic, social, political, environmental, and technological forces are contributing to these dynamic changes in surgical settings across the United States (Seifert, 2000). These forces are complex, diversified, and often interrelated. A few examples include:

- Health care costs currently consume 13% to 14% of the gross national product (Rundle, 1999).
- Managed care has failed to address the problem of ever increasing health care costs. It is estimated that more than 40 million Americans lack health insurance.
- In greater numbers than ever before, older adults with many more comorbidities are undergoing surgery and account for increased health care costs and longer lengths of stay.
- In an unprecedented manner, health care consumers are demanding quality care and are increasingly active participants in their health care decisions.
- Changes in the ethnic, racial, cultural, and spiritual or religious diversity of society require cultural sensitivity toward patients and coworkers. Health care workers need to better understand how various cultural beliefs and values influence health care practices.
- Changes in regulatory and legislative mandates designed to improve the quality of care require health care

institutions and providers to continually evaluate and improve care.
- Federal mandates related to the computerized patient record will result in the automation of some or all of the patient data collected in health care facilities.
- Work-related illnesses and injuries such as latex allergy and needlestick and sharp injuries have led to changes in equipment and supplies and mandates about protecting health care workers.
- Enhanced imaging devices have and will continue to improve the diagnosis and treatment of and surgery for numerous health conditions.
- Innovations such as minimally invasive surgery, virtual reality technology, and artificial intelligence have begun to transform surgical technique and will lead to greater precision, less tissue injury, and improved patient outcomes.
- Developments related to genetics and pharmaceuticals will change the way health care conditions are evaluated and treated.

These forces work in synergy and contribute to role changes in perioperative nursing practice. The survival of perioperative nursing will largely depend on whether nurses within this specialty become active participants in the development of new roles and pursue these opportunities. Recent changes and current issues in perioperative nursing will be addressed by exploring the changes within the health care system and the resultant nursing practice issues.

CHANGES IN THE SURGICAL DELIVERY SYSTEM AND SETTING

Since the mid-19th century, surgery has been primarily hospital-based. Before that time, surgery was performed on kitchen tables, in makeshift operating rooms, and any place the patient was located. Transitioning surgery to operating rooms within hospitals led to marked improvements in surgical techniques and health outcomes. Along with these improvements came increased costs due to the personnel, equipment, supplies, and technological breakthroughs needed to achieve these outcomes. During this era, nurses in the operating room assumed the roles of scrub and circulating nurse and practiced within the four walls of the surgical suite.

By the 1980s, the trend of moving surgery from the hospital to ambulatory settings had begun. Estimates suggest that approximately 20% of surgeries were being performed outside of the traditional hospital operating room at this time (Maksud & Moody, 1997). Ambulatory surgical centers were established in an effort to decrease costs and create an efficient process for both patient and staff members. Changes in reimbursement, the shift to minimally invasive surgical techniques, cost containment efforts, and high levels of patient and staff satisfaction further contributed to the expansion of ambulatory surgical settings.

In hospitals the role of the nurse continued to be limited to the operating room suite. Surgical technologists were gradually replacing nurses in the traditional scrub nurse role. The registered professional nurse retained the role of circulator, and in some clinical situations there were limited efforts to extend that role to preoperative visits and teaching. Meanwhile, the role of the perioperative nurse in the ambulatory setting became highly diversified. Perioperative nurses in ambulatory settings assumed responsibility for the care of the patient throughout the entire perioperative period, from preadmission to discharge. In fact, some ambulatory-based perioperative nurses made discharge follow-up calls or visits.

The trend toward performing surgery in ambulatory settings continues at a steady rate. According to current projections, 70% or more of all surgeries or minimally invasive procedures will be performed outside of hospital operating rooms (Maksud & Mooney, 1997). In addition to the growth in ambulatory procedures, office-based surgery is emerging as the latest trend in surgery. It is anticipated that as more procedures are performed in office settings, the number of surgeries performed in both hospital and ambulatory settings will decrease. These changes in clinical settings will continue to drive significant changes in the traditional role of the operating room nurse.

These trends became apparent recently when the premier organization for perioperative nurses changed its name from the Association of Operating Room Nurses to the Association of periOperative Registered Nurses (AORN). This name change was intended to better represent the various roles of the surgical nurse, rather than describe the place where their practice had traditionally been confined. The name change recognized the diversification of perioperative nursing roles during the past two decades and acknowledged the role diversity within the association's membership.

Role Diversification

Perhaps the most dramatic changes in surgical nursing during the past two decades are the movement of the registered nurse away from the scrub role and out of the confines of the four walls of the operating room. In many surgical settings, today's perioperative nurse is concerned with the patient's entire surgical experience from preadmission to discharge. No longer is the nurse's single focus the intraoperative period. The development of surgical technology programs in hospitals and in technical colleges has lead to an increased availability of ancillary personnel who are assuming the scrub role. Acceptance of the surgical technologist in this role occurred quickly, partly because of the decreased availability of qualified surgical nurses and the lower costs associated with unlicensed personnel in this role.

Concurrent to the trend of surgical technologists replacing scrub nurses, the role of the registered nurse first assistant (RNFA) emerged. Nurses performing in this role have the requisite education, skills, knowledge, and judgment to assist a surgeon during surgery. Nurses with advance practice credentials and designation have further expanded the first assistant role. After obtaining a master's degree, many RNFAs have assumed the role of nurse practitioner, providing preoperative and postoperative assessment and management. As midlevel providers, nurses with these qualifications are an integral part of a surgeon's practice, have hospital privileges, and provide ongoing and follow-up care for their patients.

Other perioperative nursing roles include case manager, educator, clinical specialist, consultant, and patient care coordinator. Some of these roles are recent innovations or reflect an expansion of existing roles and responsibilities. Perioperative nurse case managers are used in acute care settings, office practices, and by insurance companies. Implementation of this role includes helping patients access surgical care, obtain second or third opinions, coordinate care, and obtain presurgical authorization for reimbursement purposes. With shorter hospital stays, more outpatient surgery, and greater numbers of older adults undergoing surgery, there are continually increasing needs for coordination of home care services. Perioperative nurse case managers or patient care coordinators are often in the best position to develop and implement a plan of care that best meets the patient's needs.

With the increasingly complex technological aspects of intraoperative care, there has been a resurgence of the role of clinical specialist and nurse educator within the operating room. Nurses assuming these roles are often responsible for the design, implementation, and evaluation of perioperative education programs for staff, patients, and families, inservice education, and orientation programs for members of the surgical team. Clinical specialists and educators often serve as clinical resource people to staff and assist with clinical research and continuous quality improvement efforts, while supporting the day-to-day operations of a surgical department.

Many perioperative nurses with extensive surgical experience choose roles as consultants for companies that provide health care services or manufacture perioperative supplies and equipment. Nurses working as consultants may implement new clinical programs, provide consultation or interim management services, market new products and services, provide education related to new products or equipment, and contribute to product development teams. Roles such as these often require extensive travel to various health care facilities and medical exhibits. With additional specialized education and training, perioperative nurses are developing roles of the nurse business manager, laser safety officer, biomedical engineer, or informatics specialist. In these roles, nurses provide clinical support services in the role of consultant. Some potential future roles for nurse consultants in the operating room will emerge with advances in tissue engineering, telecommunications, robotics, and virtual reality.

Threats to Traditional Nursing Roles

As these various new or diversified positions have emerged and as the surgical technologist replaces the scrub nurse, there are ongoing threats to the registered nurse in the circulating role. A significant threat emerged in December 1997 when the Health Care Financing Administration (HCFA) proposed a rule change that would allow hospitals and ambulatory surgery centers reimbursed by Medicare and Medicaid to determine their own staffing patterns for surgical services. This proposed rule would replace prescriptive rules that currently state that a physician, osteopathic physician, or registered nurse must supervise an operating room. To date, no final decisions on this proposed rule change have been made, and ongoing debate continues related to this controversial change (Romig, 2000).

Also threatening the role of the registered nurse (RN) in the operating room is the Association of Surgical Technologists' national legislative and regulatory initiatives to expand the role of the surgical technologist from scrubbing to circulating, first assisting, and supervision in operating rooms. As surgical technologists pursue expanded roles, their national organization has identified strategies in every state to remove surgical technologists from nursing authority and place them under the state medical authority. Typical of these efforts is a proposed regulation in 1999 of a new "intraoperative assistant" position under the physician assistant and specialist assistant statute in New York State (Romig, 2000).

Threats from outside the nursing profession are real and appear to have gained momentum as agencies use unlicensed assistive personnel as part of their cost-savings programs. Health care facilities have adopted the concept of multiskilled health care workers, many of whom have limited training and experience. In some surgical departments, one RN may supervise two or more operating rooms. As surgery moves to less regulated areas such as physician offices, the trend of using unlicensed personnel and not having an RN circulator appears to be somewhat more pervasive. These trends may be even further confounded by the fact that there is a national shortage of nurses and increasing competition to recruit perioperative nurses.

The Hay Group (1999) reported that in a survey of 178 hospitals conducted during the spring of 1998, 81% of respondent hospitals reported a shortage of nursing managers, RNs, licensed practical nurses, or unlicensed assistants. The survey results reported in the *Nebraska Nurse* indicated that the most serious shortages were for RNs in critical care, the operating room, medical-surgical, and obstetrics. The most likely reason given for the shortage was an insufficient supply of experienced nurses. With the existing shortage, the aging nursing workforce, diminished student enrollments, and fewer opportunities for students to have educational opportunities in perioperative settings, it is anticipated that the shortage of perioperative nurses will continue to increase in the next decade.

The roles and responsibilities of the perioperative nurse in the acute care setting are extremely complex and changing at an unprecedented rate. Depending on the clinical setting, nurses who circulate and take on-call hours may need to be cross-trained to every specialty in the operating room so that they can provide safe, competent care. The challenge of maintaining the requisite skills and expertise can be overwhelming in light of the technological advances and changes in surgical techniques in all specialties. Perioperative nurses question their ability to provide an acceptable standard of care if they have limited experience in a specific specialty.

The burden of maintaining scheduled hours and taking "on-call hours" can be stressful and potentially disruptive to a nurse's personal and family life. With the increased number of RN vacancies in many surgical departments, remaining staff members share the workload by working extra or overtime hours. Inherent workplace health and safety issues such as latex allergies, smoke plume evacuation, and sharp and needlestick injuries are of growing concern to many perioperative nurses. The demands of the highly technological, fast-paced environment of the inpatient operating room, complicated by the ever-shrinking number of qualified nurses, makes jobs outside of the hospital or in less stressful roles attractive.

Changes in Surgical Interventions

Certainly the current health care environment and threats to the RN role make it apparent that it will not continue to be business as usual in the operating room for the perioperative nurse. Advances in medical and surgical diagnostic technique and interventional approaches promise to even further confound the future. Breakthroughs in medical and scientific knowledge may remarkably change the way we conceptualize health problems and diagnosis. New imaging techniques, simulation, minimally invasive surgery, interventionist techniques, and robotics are expected to revolutionize surgical care.

For example, computed tomography scans, magnetic resonance imaging, and software can create three-dimensional views and support microscope-assisted guided interventions and image-guided minimally invasive brain surgery. Virtual reality technology provides surgeons with many new learning opportunities and promises to enhance surgical technique. Minimally invasive techniques, such as laparoscopic video-assisted cholecystectomies, have and will continue to influence surgical technique for all major surgeries. A recent development is the use of laparoscopic procedures for individuals donating a kidney and minimally invasive techniques for cardiopulmonary bypass surgery.

Perhaps the most dramatic change is that many surgical procedures are being replaced by nonsurgical and noninvasive interventions. For example, angioplasty is done instead of coronary artery bypass surgery or vascu-lar surgery. New innovations such as GammaKnife and CyberKnife are promising sophisticated radiological advances. CyberKnife enables physicians to target brain tumors with a precise dose of radiation and minimize the effects of radiation on healthy tissue. These technologies offer great promise for the treatment of tumors in other parts of the body. Robotic technologies are fast becoming an integral part of the surgical team; advances include voice-controlled robotic arms that enable visualization and computer- and image-controlled robots that actually perform surgery (Popolow, 1999). Others predict that in the future, microscopic miniature robots or nanobots will be inserted in a patient's bloodstream and be used to repair tissue and cells (Merkle, 1996). Some even predict that what we think of as traditional surgery will eventually become obsolete. See the box on page 205.

All of these advances in surgical technique, equipment, and instrumentation will require an ever-increasing number of technology-proficient and skilled nurses. Nurses will assume roles to support these technologies so that these advances can be effectively integrated into clinical practice. Within the surgical department, it is most often the RN who has the requisite education, training, and resultant proficiency to operate or provide support for a specific technology. Surgical departments will be increasingly challenged to identify qualified and competent caregivers while staying on or ahead of the technology curve to provide state-of-the-art clinical services. Another significant challenge will be affording these emerging technologies.

Financial Pressures

In the 1990s, managed care resulted in capitation for services and reduced reimbursement rates and payments. In this decade, both the Balanced Budget Act of 1997 and the Ambulatory Payment Classification will markedly change health care financing as agencies face further reductions or changes in their existing payment structures. Neither of these legislative initiatives has been fully implemented, and their full effects have not been fully delineated or experienced.

For example, it is predicted that the ambulatory payment classification system, a prospective payment system, will drive significant changes in outpatient health care, the magnitude of which may be equivalent to the changes observed in acute care hospitals when the diagnosis-related groups system was implemented in the early 1980s. The Balanced Budget Act enacts some of the most significant changes to both the Medicare and Medicaid programs since their inception. Other changes, including the

PERIOPERATIVE NURSING PRACTICE: ISSUES, CHALLENGES, AND OPPORTUNITIES

Economic
Spiraling costs of health care
Balanced Budget Act of 1997
Implementation of Ambulatory Patient Classification system
Costs related to the development and implementation of new technologies
Downsizing and program consolidation
Capitation and managed care
Costs of benefits for health care workers
Reuse of single use devices

Political (Legislative)
Role of registered nurse in surgical settings
Role of surgical technologists in the operating room
Third-party reimbursement for registered nurse first assistants
Supervision of and delegation to unlicensed assistive personnel
Patient and personnel health and safety (latex allergy, needlestick injuries, smoke plume evacuation, patient bill of rights)
Computerized patient record

Environmental
Workplace safety and health (latex allergy, injuries, workplace violence, smoke plume evacuation, potential exposure to HIV infection or resistant strains of pathogens)
Nursing shortage
Globalization of health care
Trend toward patient-directed care

Social
Aging population
More than 40 million Americans uninsured
Trend toward complementary medicine and holistic health approaches
Increased emphasis on wellness and disease prevention
Multicultural aspects of society and health care
Demand for quality, cost-effective health care

Technological
The Internet as a pathway to access health care, services, education, and information
Breakthroughs in imaging, 3-D technology, artificial intelligence, robotics, informatics, and virtual reality
The Human Genome Project
Bioengineering of pharmaceutical products

reduction of hospital payments for inpatient capital and graduate medical education and revising physician fee schedules, promise to further affect the current structure of health care and its financing in the United States.

Financial issues specific to perioperative settings are occurring in synergy with these legislative initiatives. The increasing costs of labor, equipment, and supplies constantly challenge perioperative managers. The costs of acquiring new technologies such as virtual reality, robotics, and artificial intelligence, along with advances in genetics and pharmaceuticals, will transform health care and surgery.

It is likely that certain facilities will be able to afford the latest technologies and innovations, limiting their availability. Kaiser (2000) suggests that in the future, certain facilities will emerge as freestanding diagnostic centers, whereas others will become specialized surgical, intervention, and treatment centers. The desire for high-quality outcomes and low costs will also drive the market. Even now, health care insurers are bargaining to obtain the most cost-effective care and will pay travel costs for patients who are referred to a specialized referral center.

Development in surgical services information systems will help perioperative managers better understand how resources are used and expended in surgical settings, calculate productivity, enhance efficiencies, integrate services, reduce delays and down time, and develop activity-based costing systems. As Medicare, Medicaid, and other insurers implement incentives for a healthy lifestyle, the numbers of surgeries related to cancer, heart disease, and trauma may fall at a steady rate. This trend, along with projections about gene therapy, pharmaceuticals, and nonsurgical interventions may drastically change the traditional surgical setting. Instead of increasing the number of operating rooms and needing more perioperative nurses, the need for certain hospitals and operating rooms may be reduced or eliminated. Traditional operating room nurses may see their role totally eradicated.

But that does not signal the death knell for the perioperative nurse. New roles will be developed such as the gene therapy nurse or minimally invasive interventions nurse. Other perioperative nurses may develop skills and provide wellness or complementary therapy care. Competition for these new roles may come from nurses who previously worked in intensive care and other acute care units. Roles for professional nurses may completely disappear if the computerized patient record does not include the contributions of nurses and their care to patient outcomes. The need to incorporate a standardized nursing language into computerized documentation has never been more apparent. Without an ability to demonstrate the effectiveness of nursing care, professional nurses will be replaced by unlicensed personnel, first in highly technical areas like the operating room and critical care units and perhaps eventually in all clinical settings.

Perioperative nurses face numerous challenges within the next decade. The number of proficient RNs willing to work in surgical settings will continue to shrink as many older nurses choose retirement or leave for other opportunities. Unless there are effective ways of recruiting students and nurses to the operating room and other surgical settings, our specialty practice may approach extinction.

Using valid and reliable data, perioperative nurses need to demonstrate their contributions to quality care in surgical settings through outcomes management. Currently there is little research to support the regulatory staffing standards requiring the presence of RNs in the operating room. Surgical technologists are well positioned from an organizational perspective to assume new roles and responsibilities. If legislative initiatives create opportunities for role changes, the economics of health care could result in the elimination of the traditional RN role.

Within the next 20 years the health care system in this country will probably be a totally reinvented industry. The human genome project and technological innovations have only just begun to suggest how our understanding of health, illness, and medical-surgical treatment will radically change the future. Perioperative nurses must stay alert and remain well positioned to address the economic, social, political, environmental, and technological forces at work in surgical settings. If the role of the nurse in the operating room is eliminated, it may be a forewarning to the profession of nursing. There has never been a more critical time to examine and validate the contributions of nurses to quality patient care and positive patient outcomes regardless of the setting or specialty.

REFERENCES

Hay Group. (1999). 1998 report on nursing shortage study. *Nebraska Nurse, 32*(2), 17.

Kaiser, L.R. (2000). Looking forward to the new century. *Surgical Services Management, 6*(1), 12-17.

Maksud, D.P., & Mooney, K.M. (1997). Trends in ambulatory surgery. *Plastic Surgical Nursing, 17*(2), 80-81.

Merkle, R.C. (1996). Nanotechnology and medicine. *Advances in Anti-Aging Medicine, 1,* 277-286. Available: http://www.zyvex.com/nanotech/nanotechAndMedicine.html.

Popolow, G. (1999). How robotics is transforming the OR. *Surgical Services Management, 5*(12), 35-39.

Romig, C. (2000). Legislative update. *Surgical Services Management, 6*(1), 49-52.

Rundle, R.L. (1999, August 9). The outlook: Can managed care manage costs? *The Wall Street Journal,* p. A1.

Seifert, P.C. (2000). Leaving the nineties behind. *Surgical Services Management, 6*(1), 18-22.

Recent Changes and Current Issues in Psychiatric Nursing

GAIL W. STUART

The contemporary practice of psychiatric nursing is challenged by both issues internal to nursing and changes in the external health care environment. Externally, managed behavioral health care dominates the treatment of mental illness. The federal Balanced Budget Act of 1997 has led to the further restriction of mental health services, and the struggle for parity of coverage for physical and mental illness continues. At present, parity has been enacted at the national level and by many states across the country. Advances in genetics and neurobiology abound, and the field is moving quickly to a paradigm of evidence-based practice. Finally, in 1999 the Surgeon General released a Report on Mental Health (U.S. Department of Health and Human Services, 1999) containing the following messages:

- Mental health is fundamental to health.
- Mental disorders are real health conditions.
- The efficacy of mental health treatments is well documented.
- A range of treatments exists for most mental disorders.

There are more than 82,000 registered nurses working in mental health organizations in the United States, and more than 17,000 of them have graduate degrees (Manderscheid & Henderson, 1999). Internally, psychiatric nurses have to face the question of whether they are vulnerable to becoming extinct and replaced by others, or whether they are viewed as valuable, competent clinicians who can function in a world of changing mental health care needs, processes, priorities, and structures. Areas of vulnerability are many:

- Fewer nurses are attracted to the specialty of psychiatric nursing.
- The amount of content devoted to understanding psychiatric illnesses and working with psychiatric patients in nursing educational programs has decreased steadily over the past decade and is almost nonexistent in some curricula.
- The biopsychosocial skills and expertise of psychiatric nurses are often poorly delineated and underused in many mental health care systems.
- Psychiatric nurses are frequently viewed as expensive mental health care providers who can be replaced by two or more less costly personnel.
- There are increasing threats to nursing autonomy as state boards of nursing and other regulatory bodies delimit master's-prepared psychiatric nurses to practicing in the "extended" role requiring the full supervision of physicians.
- There are relatively few outcome studies that document the nature, extent, and effectiveness of care delivered by psychiatric nurses.
- Psychiatric nurses continue to struggle to be perceived as revenue producers and to receive direct reimbursement from third-party payers for the services they provide.
- Role differentiation for psychiatric nurses based on education and experience is often lacking in the position descriptions, job responsibilities, and reward systems of the organizations in which they practice.
- The specialty is struggling with the education and certification of advanced practice psychiatric-mental health nurses in clinical nurse specialist, nurse practitioner, and combined roles. Graduate programs in psychiatric nursing are moving away from the preparation of clinical nurse specialists and toward that of nurse practitioners who often have significantly less course work related to the diagnosis and treatment of psychiatric illnesses.
- Advanced practice registered nurses–psychiatric mental health (APRNs–PMH) are underused in managed care and primary care delivery systems.

These issues must be addressed if psychiatric nursing is to continue to develop as a specialty area. Nurses need to continue to move into the continuum of care and clearly articulate their skills, functions, and abilities. They must also demonstrate their cost-effectiveness and establish differentiated levels of practice based on education, experience, and credentials (Stuart, Worley, Morris, & Bevilacqua, 2000). Other survival skills needed by psychiatric nurses in the future include management of negative emotionality, achievement of collegial unity, understanding the nature of transitions, revising career trajectories, and marketing themselves (Thomas, 1999). Such strategies will position psychiatric nurses as visible, interdependent, central, and collaborating professionals who have much to offer a reformed health care system.

Recent changes and current issues are occurring in five discrete areas of psychiatric nursing practice: (1) role, (2) activities, (3) models of care, (4) treatment settings, and (5) evidence-based practice. Each of these will be explored on the basis of historical perspectives, recent developments, and future challenges in the field.

PSYCHIATRIC NURSING ROLE

The decades of the 1950s and 1960s are fondly remembered by psychiatric nurses because they mark the emergence of the identity of the specialty. It was an exciting and stimulating time, and the early psychiatric nursing leaders who contributed to this identity formation, Peplau (1952, 1962, 1978), Crawford, Gregg (1954), Tudor (1952), and Mellow (1968) will forever remain larger than life for their early contributions to the emerging specialty area. The challenges they faced were to identify and describe the roles and functions for psychiatric nursing specialty practice and to disseminate them widely within the broader community of nurses.

The challenges for psychiatric nurses in the 1970s and 1980s were somewhat different. During these years nurses worked to define the nature and focus of nursing as a practice discipline and examined aspects of both the art and science of nursing. Psychiatric nurses worked parallel to the overall nursing profession and moved psychiatric nursing into the mainstream of nursing practice by helping elaborate psychosocial concepts, thus further defining the caring and holistic dimensions of professional nursing practice.

Psychiatric nurses in the 1990s faced a new challenge—that of integrating the rapidly expanding bases of psychobiology, the neurosciences, psychopharmacology, and psychotherapy into the holistic biopsychosocial prac-

tice of psychiatric nursing (Abraham, Fox, & Cohen, 1992; Babich & Tolbert, 1992; Hays, 1995; McEnany, 1991; Pothier, Stuart, Puskar, & Babich, 1990). Advances in understanding the interrelationships of biology, brain, behavior, emotion, and cognition offered new opportunities for psychiatric nurses. In addition, the taxonomy used to categorize and diagnose mental illnesses was becoming increasingly precise and more interdisciplinary. A final issue to emerge was the importance of sociocultural factors in psychiatric care. Psychiatric nurses saw the need to become realigned with care and caring, which represent the art of psychiatric nursing and give balance to the science and high technology of current mental health care practices (McBride, 1996). These changes led to the revised *Scope and Standards of Psychiatric-Mental Health Clinical Nursing Practice* (American Nurses Association, 2000).

The task for psychiatric nurses today and in the years ahead is to evolve beyond the formative work in the field and enact psychiatric nursing roles and functions on the basis of current realities (Flaskerud & Wuerker, 1999; Haber & Billings, 1995; Lanza, 1997a, 1997b; Shea, Pelletier, Poster, Stuart, & Verhey, 1999). For example, the nurse-patient relationship as first described by Peplau (1952) has grown in complexity from its original historical elements. It needs to be reconceptualized in a health care environment in which there is greater consumer responsibility and a broader context of clinician accountability. The concept of the nurse-patient relationship has thus evolved into that of the nurse-patient partnership, which incorporates new dimensions of the professional psychiatric nursing role (Fig. 29-1).

Enacting the nurse-patient partnership requires expanding the traditional roles of the nurse to include the elements of clinical competence, patient-family advocacy,

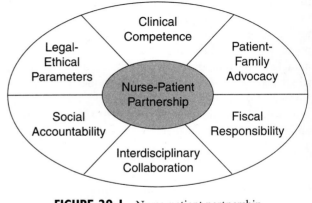

FIGURE 29-1 Nurse-patient partnership.

fiscal responsibility, interdisciplinary collaboration, social accountability, and legal-ethical obligations (Stuart, 2001a). No longer can psychiatric nurses focus exclusively on bedside care and the immediacy of patient needs. Rather, they must broaden the context of their care and the responsibility and understanding they bring to the caregiving situation. Thus, the current practice of psychiatric nursing requires greater sensitivity to the social environment and active advocacy for the diverse needs of patients and families of the mentally ill (Clement, 1997; Geller, Brown, Fisher, Grudzinskas, & Manning, 1998; Mohr, 1997). It also mandates thoughtful consideration of complex legal and ethical dilemmas that arise from a health care system that is embracing the efficiencies of managed care, which often disadvantages and discriminates against those with psychiatric illness (Dee, van Servellen, & Brecht, 1998; Fletcher, 1998; Goldman, 1999; Gregory, 1998). New models of delivering mental health care require greater skill in interdisciplinary collaboration built on the psychiatric nurse's clinical competence and professional self-assertion (Akhavain, Amaral, Murphy, & Uehlinger, 1999; McCloskey & Maas, 1998) and balanced by a clear understanding and respect for the cost indices and financial aspects of psychiatric care in general and psychiatric nursing care in particular (Baradell, 1994; Mohr, 1998; Olfson, Sing, & Schlesinger, 1999). Each of these elements must permeate to a greater degree the education, research, and clinical components of the current state of psychiatric nursing.

PSYCHIATRIC NURSING ACTIVITIES

There are three domains of contemporary psychiatric nursing practice: direct care, communication, and management activities. Within these overlapping domains, the teaching, coordinating, delegating, and collaborating functions of the psychiatric nursing role are expressed. Often the communication and management domains of practice are overlooked, minimized, or discounted when discussing psychiatric nursing. However, these integrating activities are critically important and time-consuming aspects of the psychiatric nurse's role. They are also valuable in a reformed health care system that places great emphasis on efficient patient assessment, triage, and management. Thus, they are critical aspects of contemporary psychiatric nursing practice.

It is important for psychiatric nurses to be able to further delineate the various activities they engage in within each of these domains. The range of specific activities that can be enacted by a psychiatric nurse in each area are listed in the box on page 210 (Stuart, 2001a). Although not all psychiatric nurses participate in all of these activities, they do reflect the current nature and scope of competent caring by psychiatric nurses. In addition, psychiatric nurses:

- Make biopsychosocial health assessments that are culturally sensitive
- Design and implement treatment plans for patients and families with complex health problems and comorbid medical conditions
- Engage in case management activities, such as organizing, accessing, negotiating, coordinating, and integrating services and benefits for individuals and families
- Provide a "health care map" for individuals, families, and groups to guide them to community resources for mental health, including the most appropriate providers, agencies, technologies, and social systems
- Promote and maintain mental health and manage the effects of mental illness through teaching and counseling
- Provide care for the physically ill with psychological problems and the psychiatrically ill with physical problems
- Manage and coordinate systems of care integrating the needs of patients, families, staff, and regulators

Finally, psychiatric nurses must be able to articulate both the general and the specific aspects of their practice to patients, families, other professionals, administrators, and legislators. When such skills and competencies are identified, psychiatric nurses will be able to ensure their appropriate role utilization, adequate compensation for the nursing care provided, and the most efficient use of scarce human resources in the delivery of quality mental health care. Health care reform, patient and family needs, scientific developments, economic realities, and societal expectations are the forces that will shape the future roles and activities of psychiatric nurses.

PSYCHIATRIC NURSING MODEL OF CARE

As a result of rising health care costs, changing reimbursement trends, and problems with accessibility of care, there has been a reformulation of the model of care for psychiatric illness in this country. Fifteen years ago, most psychiatric care was provided in hospital units, where the average length of stay for acute inpatient treatment was about 25 days, compared with 19 days in 1991 and 10 days in 1995. Not surprisingly, most psychiatric nurses were employed by inpatient facilities. Now, however, most inpatient psychiatric settings have an average

PSYCHIATRIC NURSING ACTIVITIES

Direct Care Activities
Activity therapy
Advocacy
Aftercare follow-up
Behavioral treatments
Case consultation
Case management
Cognitive treatments
Community assessment
Community-based care
Community education
Complementary interventions
Compliance counseling
Counseling
Crisis intervention
Discharge planning
Environmental change
Environmental safety
Family interventions
Group work
Health maintenance
Health promotion
Health teaching
High-risk assessment
Holistic interventions
Home health care
Individual counseling
Informed consent acquisition
Intake screening and evaluation
Interpreting diagnostic and laboratory
   tests
Medication administration
Medication management
Mental health promotion
Mental illness prevention
Milieu therapy
Nutritional counseling

Ordering diagnostic and laboratory
   tests
Parent education
Patient triage
Physical assessment
Physiological treatments
Play therapy
Prescription of medications
Promotion of self-care activities
Provision of environmental safety
Psychiatric rehabilitation
Psychobiological interventions
Psychoeducation
Psychosocial assessment
Psychotherapy
Rehabilitation counseling
Relapse prevention
Research implementation
Social action
Social skills training
Somatic treatments
Stress management
Supporting social systems
Telehealth

Communication Activities
Clinical case conferences
Developing treatment plans
Documentation of care
Forensic testimony
Interagency liaison
Peer review
Preparing reports
Professional nurse networking
Staff meetings
Transcribing orders

Treatment team meetings
Verbal reports of care

Management Activities
Budgeting and resource allocation
Clinical supervision
Collaboration
Committee participation
Community action
Consultation/liaison
Contract negotiation
Coordination of services
Delegation of assignments
Grant writing
Marketing and public relations
Mediation and conflict resolution
Mentorship
Needs assessment and forecasting
Organizational governance
Outcomes management
Performance evaluations
Policy and procedure development
Practice guidelines formulation
Professional presentations
Program evaluation
Program planning
Publications
Quality improvement activities
Recruitment and retention activities
Regulatory agency activities
Risk management
Software development
Staff scheduling
Staff and student education
Strategic planning
Unit governance
Utilization review

From Stuart, G., & Laraia, M. (1998). *Stuart and Sundeen's principles and practice of psychiatric nursing* (6th ed.). St. Louis: Mosby.

length of stay of 7 days, and inpatient crisis stabilization programs involve only a 2- or 3-day length of stay. These changes stimulated reciprocal changes in the goals, assessments, interventions, and expected outcomes of psychiatric care. Mental health providers, including psychiatric nurses, have reevaluated the models of care they use on the basis of the patient's treatment stage, setting, and resources.

One current psychiatric nursing model of care identifies four treatment stages: (1) crisis, (2) acute, (3) maintenance, and (4) health promotion (Stuart, 2001b). These stages reflect the range of the adaptive-maladaptive continuum of coping responses and suggest a distinct set of psychiatric nursing activities. For each stage, the psychiatric nurse identifies the treatment goal, focus of the nursing assessment, nature of the nursing interventions, and expected outcome of nursing care (Fig. 29-2).

In the *crisis stage of treatment* the nursing goal is the stabilization of the patient; the nursing assessment focuses on risk factors that threaten the patient's health and well-being; the nursing intervention is directed toward managing the environment to provide safety; and the expected outcome of nursing care is that no harm will come to the patient or others.

In the *acute stage of treatment* the nursing goal is for the patient's illness to be placed in remission; the nursing assessment is focused on the patient's symptoms and maladaptive coping responses; the nursing intervention is directed toward treatment planning with the patient and

the modeling and teaching of adaptive responses; and the expected outcome of nursing care is symptom relief.

In the *maintenance stage of treatment* the nursing goal is the complete recovery of the patient; the nursing assessment is focused on the patient's functional status; the nursing intervention is directed toward reinforcing the patient's adaptive coping responses and patient advocacy;

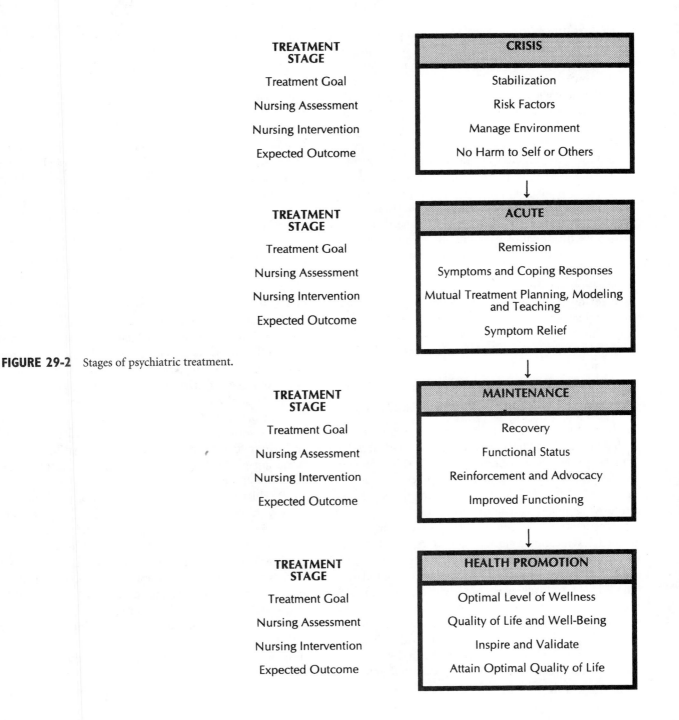

FIGURE 29-2   Stages of psychiatric treatment.

and the expected outcome of nursing care is improved patient functioning.

In the *health promotion stage of treatment* the nursing goal is for the patient to achieve the optimal level of wellness; the nursing assessment is focused on the patient's quality of life and well-being; the nursing intervention is directed toward inspiring and validating the patient; and the expected outcome of nursing care is that the patient will attain the optimal quality of life.

These treatment stages have often been overlooked in traditional psychiatric nursing practice, which did not value or reimburse maintenance or health promotion activities. With health care reform and the emergence of managed mental health care, however, activities related to these stages are becoming essential aspects of the contemporary psychiatric nursing role.

This model of care also helps to determine how the psychiatric nurse functions in each setting. For example, in previous years most psychiatrically ill patients entered the psychiatric hospital in the acute treatment stage and were able to stay in the hospital until the goal of symptom remission was attained. This created the need for comprehensive treatment plans with long-term interventions for recovery. Today, however, most patients are admitted to inpatient units in the crisis treatment stage and have stabilization as their treatment goal, thus mandating very different nursing interventions and expected outcomes. The psychiatric care goals of symptom remission and recovery are now most often pursued in community-based settings, requiring new skills and competencies of psychiatric nurses.

PSYCHIATRIC NURSING TREATMENT SETTINGS

Traditional practice settings for psychiatric nurses have included psychiatric hospitals, community mental health centers, psychiatric units in the general hospital, residential treatment facilities, and private practice. More recently, alternative treatment settings throughout the continuum of mental health care have emerged for psychiatric nurses. Specifically, hospitals are being transformed into integrated clinical systems that provide inpatient care, partial hospitalization or day treatment, residential care, home care, and outpatient or ambulatory care (Fig. 29-3). Psychiatric nurses who continue to work within inpatient units have seen the goals, processes, and structures of care change drastically, reflective of the new models of psychiatric nursing care described earlier (Delaney, Ulsafer-Van Lanen, Pitula, & Johnson, 1995; Maree, in press; McGihon, 1994). Nurses who staff inpatient

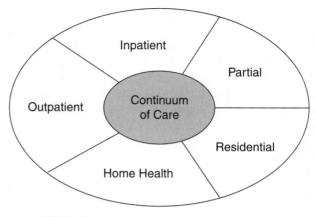

FIGURE 29-3   Continuum of mental health care.

units no longer have their responsibilities limited to activities delivered exclusively in the hospital setting. Rather, they are likely to be flexibly assigned on a daily basis to other settings in the continuum of mental health care on the basis of fluctuating patient census and organizational need.

Community-based treatment settings have expanded to include foster care or group homes, hospices, visiting nurse associations, emergency departments, nursing homes, shelters, primary care clinics, schools, prisons, industrial settings, homes, managed care facilities, and health maintenance organizations. Psychiatric nurses are moving into the domain of primary care and are working with other nurses and physicians to diagnose and treat psychiatric illness in patients with somatic complaints. Cardiovascular, gynecological, respiratory, gastrointestinal, and family practice settings are appropriate for assessing patients for anxiety, depression, and substance abuse disorders. As health care initiatives continue to move into schools and other community settings, psychiatric nurses are assuming leadership roles in providing expertise through consultation and evaluation.

Psychiatric nurses are well suited to provide comprehensive health care to patients in both psychiatric settings and primary care environments. In particular, advanced practice psychiatric nurses acting as consultants to nonpsychiatric providers in hospital-based or outpatient clinics are in a unique position to assess and triage these patients on the basis of the immediacy of their needs. Early assessment and triage can minimize the length of time between psychiatric referral and intervention. By identifying patients in crisis and intervening in a timely fashion, they may reduce failed appointments and enhance the efficacy of treatment.

Psychiatric nurses also provide medical and medication management for selected groups of patients in collaborative practices. For example, patients who are having difficulty being stabilized on their medications or who have co-morbid medical illnesses are seen in a psychiatric nursing clinic in which nurses and physicians collaborate to provide high-quality patient care. Psychiatric nurses who obtain prescriptive authority can further expand the services they provide and deliver cost-effective psychiatric care to communities that do not have access to a psychiatrist.

This widened range of settings maximizes the psychiatric nurse's potential contribution to the delivery of mental health care. The specific role the nurse assumes in any one of these psychiatric treatment settings, however, depends on a number of factors including the:

- Legal parameters of practice as defined by one's state's nurse practice act
- Clinical competence of the nurse as a consequence of education, experience, and certification in psychiatric nursing
- Philosophy, mission, values, goals, and organizational structure of the treatment setting
- Needs of the consumers of mental health services
- Number of available staff and the services they are able to provide
- Consensus reached by the mental health care providers who work together regarding their respective roles, responsibilities, and accountabilities
- Resources and revenues available to offset the cost of care needed and provided

The new opportunities for psychiatric nursing practice that are emerging throughout the continuum of mental health care are exciting for the specialty. They allow psychiatric nurses to demonstrate their flexibility, accountability, and self-direction as they move forward into these expanding areas of practice. They also require that psychiatric nurses be proactive in articulating their skills and activities and demonstrate their expertise in designing interventions, planning programs, implementing treatment strategies, managing staff, and collaborating with other health care providers in a variety of traditional and non-traditional treatment settings. Perhaps most important, the expansion of mental health treatment settings is providing psychiatric nurses with the opportunity to implement primary, secondary, and tertiary prevention functions from a holistic, biopsychosocial perspective, thus expanding their base of practice to better meet the mental health needs of individuals, families, groups, and communities.

PSYCHIATRIC NURSING EVIDENCE-BASED PRACTICE

A final aspect of current psychiatric nursing is the emphasis being placed on evidence-based practice. This includes the identification, description, measurement, and use of data pertaining to the efficacy and effectiveness of the care provided by psychiatric nurses (Newell & Gournay, 2000; Rosswurm & Larrabee, 1999; Stetler et al., 1998). This is the greatest area of challenge for the specialty that has found it difficult to articulate the nature and outcomes of psychiatric nursing care (Barrell, Merwin, & Poster, 1997; Merwin & Mauck, 1995; Poster, Dee, & Randell, 1997). This has created problems in justifying the need for psychiatric nurses in various treatment settings and in giving psychiatric nurses the recognition and compensation they deserve on the basis of their actual and potential contributions to the mental health delivery system.

Evidence-based care and clinical effectiveness emphasize the importance of clinical practice, which when delivered to patients, is effective in achieving expected health outcomes. Psychiatric nurses must be sensitive to the issues of cost and quality and support their practice with data from outcome studies that reflect clinical, functional, satisfaction, and financial indicators. This is the essence of evidence-based psychiatric nursing practice. The use of measurement or rating scales must be viewed as an essential part of psychiatric nursing practice, and nurses would benefit greatly from mastering the technology that supports this process. Nurses need to research the impact of their activities and control the data set related to nursing outcomes. Finally, nurses need to know how to access, interpret, and use findings from efficacy and effectiveness outcome research (Stuart, 1999).

Outcome data for psychiatric nurses can include health status, functional status, quality of life, the presence or absence of illness, type of coping responses, and satisfaction with treatment. Outcome evaluation can focus on a psychiatric clinical condition, a nursing intervention, or the caregiving process (Faulkner & Gray, 2000). The outcomes that need continued examination by psychiatric nurses fall into four categories:

- Clinical outcomes—the patient's treatment response
- Functional outcomes—the maintenance or improvement in the patient's biopsychosocial functioning
- Perceptual outcomes—the patient's and family's satisfaction with the response to treatment, caregiving process, and health care providers

• Financial outcomes—costs and resources used to achieve the treatment response

Specific indicators related to each of these categories are presented in the box below (Stuart, 2001c).

Outcome data documenting the quality, cost, and effectiveness of psychiatric nursing practice are perhaps the most important issue on the psychiatric nursing agenda. More work is needed in this area, and studies must be able to stand up to the scientific review of the broader community of mental health professionals, regulators, and payors by being methodologically sound, empirically

---

CATEGORIES OF OUTCOME INDICATORS

Clinical Outcome Indicators
High-risk behaviors
Symptomatology
Coping responses
Relapse
Recurrence
Readmission
Number of treatment episodes
Medical complications
Incidence reports
Mortality

Functional Outcome Indicators
Functional status
Social interaction
Activities of daily living
Occupational abilities
Quality of life
Family relationships
Housing arrangement

Satisfaction Outcome Indicators
Patient and Family Satisfaction with:
    Outcomes
    Providers
    Delivery system
    Caregiving process
    Organization

Financial Outcome Indicators
Cost per treatment episode
Revenue per treatment episode
Length of inpatient stay
Use of health-care resources
Costs related to disability

From Stuart, G., & Laraia, M. (1998). *Stuart and Sundeen's principles and practice of psychiatric nursing* (6th ed.). St. Louis: Mosby.

---

grounded, and replicated across the continuum of psychiatric treatment settings (National Advisory Mental Health Council's Clinical Treatment and Services Research Workgroup, 1999). The results of this work can then be used to provide a shared knowledge base, formulate practice guidelines, provide data on clinical course, and better manage mental health care and the way in which it is delivered in this country.

Finally, the need to implement evidence-based practice and to critically evaluate the outcomes of psychiatric nursing care is a task for each psychiatric nurse regardless of role, activity, model of care, or treatment setting. Psychiatric nurse clinicians, educators, administrators, and researchers all must assume responsibility for answering the question that is likely to determine the future of psychiatric nursing. What difference does psychiatric nurse caring make? Only a clear and credible answer to this question will position psychiatric nurses as central, visible, competent, interdependent, and collaborating professionals who have much to offer a reformed health care system.

REFERENCES

Abraham, I., Fox, J., & Cohen, B. (1992). Integrating the bio into the biopsychosocial: Understanding and treating biological phenomena in psychiatric-mental health nursing. *Archives of Psychiatric Nursing, 6,* 296.

Akhavain, P., Amaral, D., Murphy, M., & Uehlinger, K. (1999). Collaborative practice: A nursing perspective of the psychiatric interdisciplinary treatment team. *Holistic Nursing Practice, 13*(2), 1-11.

American Nurses Association. (2000). *Scope and standard of psychiatric-mental health clinical nursing practice.* Washington, DC: Author.

Babich, K., & Tolbert, R. (1992). What is biological psychiatry? How will the trend toward biological psychiatry affect the future of the psychiatric mental health nurse? *Journal of Psychosocial Nursing and Mental Health Services, 30,* 33.

Baradell, J.G. (1994). Cost-effectiveness and quality of care provided by clinical nurse specialists. *Journal of Psychosocial Nursing, 32*(3), 21-24.

Barrell, L., Merwin, E., & Poster, E. (1997). Patient outcomes used by advanced practice psychiatric nurses to evaluate effectiveness of practice. *Archives of Psychiatric Nursing, 11*(4), 184-197.

Clement, J. (1997). Managed care and recovery: Opportunities and challenges for psychiatric nursing. *Archives of Psychiatric Nursing, 11*(5), 231-237.

Dee, V., van Servellen, G., & Brecht, M. (1998). Managed behavioral health care patients and their nursing care problems, level of functioning, and impairment on discharge. *Journal of the American Psychiatric Nurses Association, 4*(2), 57-66.

Delaney, K., Ulsafer-Van Lanen, J., Pitula, C.R., & Johnson, M.E. (1995). Seven days and counting: How inpatient nurses might adjust their practice to brief hospitalization. *Journal of Psychosocial Nursing, 33*(8), 36-40.

Faulkner & Gray. (2000). *2000 Behavioral outcomes & guidelines sourcebook.* New York: Author.

Flaskerud, J., & Wuerker, A. (1999). Mental health nursing in the 21st century. *Issues in Mental Health Nursing, 20*(1), 5-17.

Fletcher, J. (1998). Mental health nurses: Guardians of ethics in managed care. *Journal of Psychosocial Nursing, 36*(7), 34-37.

Geller, J., Brown, J., Fisher, W., Grudzinskas, A., & Manning, T. (1998). A national survey of "consumer empowerment" at the state level. *Psychiatric Services, 49*(4), 498-503.

Goldman, H. (1999). The obligation of mental health services to the least well off. *Psychiatric Services, 50*(5), 659-663.

Gregg, D. (1954). The psychiatric nurse's role. *American Journal of Nursing, 54,* 210-212.

Gregory, R. (1998). Ethics and practice in the helping sector: Common myths. *Administration and Policy in Mental Health, 25*(5), 555-559.

Haber, J., & Billings, C. (1995). Primary mental health care: A model for psychiatric-mental health nursing. *Journal of the American Psychiatric Nurses Association, 1*(5), 154-163.

Hayes, A. (1995). Psychiatric nursing: What does biology have to do with it? *Archives of Psychiatric Nursing, 9*(4), 216-224.

Lanza, M. (1997a). Power and leadership in psychiatric nursing: Directions for the next century, part I. *Perspectives in Psychiatric Care, 33*(1): 5-13.

Lanza, M. (1997b). Power and leadership in psychiatric nursing: Directions for the next century, part II. *Perspectives in Psychiatric Care, 33*(2): 5-9.

Manderscheid, R., & Henderson, M. (Eds.). (1999). *Mental health United States, 1998.* Washington, DC: Department of Health and Human Services, Center for Mental Health Services.

Maree, E. (2001). Hospital based psychiatric nursing care. In G. Stuart & M. Laraia (Eds.), *Principles and practice of psychiatric nursing* (7th ed.). St. Louis: Mosby.

McBride, A. (1996). Psychiatric-mental health nursing in the twenty-first century. In A. McBride & J. Austin (Eds.), *Psychiatric-mental health nursing: Integrating the behavioral and biological sciences.* Philadelphia: Saunders.

McCloskey, J., & Maas, M. (1998). Interdisciplinary team: The nursing perspective is essential. *Nursing Outlook, 46*(4), 157-163.

McEnany, G. (1991). Psychobiology and psychiatric nursing: A philosophical matrix. *Archives of Psychiatric Nursing, 5,* 255.

McGihon, N.N. (1994). Health care reform: Clinical implications for inpatient psychiatric nursing. *Journal of Psychosocial Nursing, 32*(11), 31-33.

Mellow, J. (1968). Nursing therapy. *American Journal of Nursing, 68,* 2365.

Merwin, E., & Mauck, A. (1995). Psychiatric nursing outcome research: The state of the science. *Archives of Psychiatric Nursing, 9*(6), 311-331.

Mohr, W. (1997). Outcomes of corporate greed. *Image: The Journal of Nursing Scholarship, 29*(1), 39-45.

Mohr, W. (1998). Managed care and mental health services: How we got to where we are now. *Journal of the American Psychiatric Nurses Association, 4*(5), 153-161.

National Advisory Mental Health Council's Clinical Treatment and Services Research Workgroup. (1999). *Bridging science and service.* Rockville, MD: National Institutes of Health, National Institute of Mental Health.

Newell, R., & Gournay, K. (2000). *Mental health nursing: An evidence-based approach.* London: Churchill Livingstone.

Olfson, M., Sing, M., & Schlesinger, H. (1999). Mental health/medical care cost offsets: Opportunities for managed care. *Health Affairs, 18*(2), 79-90.

Peplau, H. (1952). *Interpersonal relations in nursing.* New York: GP Putnam's Sons.

Peplau, H. (1962). Interpersonal techniques: The crux of psychiatric nursing. *American Journal of Nursing, 63,* 53.

Peplau, H. (1978). Psychiatric nursing: Role of nurses and psychiatric nurses. *International Nursing Review, 25,* 41.

Poster, E., Dee, V., & Randell, B. (1997). The Johnson behavioral systems model as a framework for patient outcome evaluation. *Journal of the American Psychiatric Nurses Association, 3*(3), 73-80.

Pothier, P., Stuart, G., Puskar, K., & Babich, K. (1990). Dilemmas and directions for psychiatric nursing in the 1990s. *Archives of Psychiatric Nursing, 4,* 284.

Rosswurm, M., & Larrabee, J. (1999). A model for change to evidence-based practice. *Image: The Journal of Nursing Scholarship, 31*(4), 317-322.

Shea, C., Pelletier, L., Poster, E., Stuart, G., & Verhey, M. (1999). *Advanced practice nursing in psychiatric and mental health care.* St. Louis: Mosby.

Stetler, C., Brunell, M., Giuliano, K., Morsi, D., Prince, L., & Newell-Stokes, V. (1998). Evidence-based practice and the role of nursing leadership. *Journal of Nursing Administration, 28*(7/8), 45-53.

Stuart, G. (1999). Mental health services research. In C. Shea, L. Pelletier, E. Poster, G. Stuart, & M. Verhey (Eds.), *Advanced practice nursing in psychiatric and mental health care.* St. Louis: Mosby.

Stuart, G. (2001a). Roles and functions of psychiatric nurses: Competent caring. In G. Stuart & M. Laraia (Eds.), *Principles and practice of psychiatric nursing* (7th ed.). St. Louis: Mosby.

Stuart, G. (2001b). A stress adaptation model of psychiatric nursing care. In G. Stuart & M. Laraia (Eds.), *Principles and practice of psychiatric nursing* (7th ed.). St. Louis: Mosby.

Stuart, G. (2001c). Evidence-based psychiatric nursing practice. In G. Stuart & M. Laraia (Eds.), *Principles and practice of psychiatric nursing* (7th ed.). St. Louis: Mosby.

Stuart, G., Worley, N., Morris, J., & Bevilacqua, J. (2000). Role utilization of nurses in public psychiatry. *Administration and Policy in Mental Health, 27*(6), 423-441.

Thomas, S. (1999). Surrounded by banana peels: Is psychiatric nursing slipping? *Journal of the American Psychiatric Nurses Association, 5*(3), 88-96.

Tudor, G. (1952). Sociopsychiatric nursing approach to intervention in a problem of mutual withdrawal on a mental hospital ward. *Psychiatry, 15,* 193.

U.S. Department of Health and Human Services. (1999). *Mental health: A report of the surgeon general.* Rockville, MD: Substance Abuse and Mental Health Services Administration, Center for Mental Health Services, National Institutes of Health, National Institute of Mental Health.

Alternative and Complementary Therapies

An Overview and Issues

CHARLOTTE ELIOPOULOS

Be it the woman using ginger to control morning sickness, a senior citizen group who wants to reduce the risk of falls by establishing a daily tai chi routine, or the surgical patient who asks for therapeutic touch to be performed postoperatively to speed the elimination of anesthesia, clients in virtually all practice settings are challenging nurses with the use of complementary and alternative medicine (CAM).

More than 40% of all Americans are using CAM, and most of these individuals are doing so without the knowledge or advice of their health care provider (Eisenberg et al., 1998). Consumers are demonstrating their support of new CAM modalities not only philosophically but also financially, spending as much for these therapies as they do for all out-of-pocket physician expenditures (Eisenberg et al., 1998). The consumer-driven growth of CAM poses interesting possibilities for nurses if they are ready to meet the challenge. A proactive approach is essential to promoting quality in the use of new modalities and ensuring a strong role for nursing in the integration of CAM into conventional practice settings.

GROWTH OF CAM

By definition, CAM consists of practices outside of the dominant system for managing health and disease that have not been taught in American medical schools or practiced in U.S. hospitals (Eisenberg et al., 1998). Although nearly 90% of the world population uses what we consider CAM as their primary source of medical care and were doing so for centuries before America was discovered, CAM is relatively new to the United States (see box, p. 217, top). It was just in 1992 that the National Institutes of Health (NIH) established the Office of Alternative Medicine (OAM) for the purpose of evaluating the growing use of CAM. The OAM became a freestanding center within NIH in 1998 and was renamed the National Center for Complementary and Alternative Medicine (NCCAM). NCCAM has categorized CAM into seven fields of practice (see box, p. 217, bottom):

- Mind-body (biobehavioral) interventions
- Alternative (nonbiomedical) systems of healing
- Manual healing methods
- Pharmacological and biological treatments
- Herbal medicine
- Bioelectromagnetic applications
- Diet, nutrition, and lifestyle changes

Many factors are responsible for the increasing use of CAM, not the least of which is consumers' dissatisfaction with the experience of using conventional medicine. During the same period in which conventional care has become characterized by skyrocketing costs, abbreviated hospital stays, and 5-minute impersonal office visits, CAM practitioners have created practices in which the consumer is treated with a holistic, nonrushed approach in an appealing environment (i.e., pleasant scents, sights, and sounds versus the cold sterility of the usual conventional practice setting).

In addition to being a "feel good" experience, CAM has proven to be effective in treating many conditions without the side effects or risks of medications and other conventional treatments. Today's increasingly well-informed, health-conscious consumers desire interventions that can promote wellness and stimulate the body's own healing capabilities, rather than merely treat symptoms. They appreciate an active role in their health care and to be empowered to affect their own health status.

The baby boomers have played a role in the popularity of CAM. This generation, like no other, has demonstrated

FACTS ABOUT THE USE OF COMPLEMENTARY AND ALTERNATIVE MEDICINE IN THE UNITED STATES

- More than 40% of Americans use alternative therapies.
- The most common users of alternative therapies are white women aged 35-49 years, college educated, and with annual incomes greater than $50,000.
- Alternative therapies are used most often for chronic conditions, including back problems, anxiety, depression, and headaches.
- Less than 40% of persons using alternative therapies disclose this information to their physicians.
- Nearly 60% of services provided by alternative medicine practitioners are paid entirely out-of-pocket.
- Annual out-of-pocket expenditures for alternative therapies exceeded expenditures for all U.S. hospitalizations.
- An estimated 15 million adults (18.4% of all prescription users) took prescription drugs concurrently with herbal remedies or high-dose vitamins or both.

Data from Eisenberg, D.M., Davis, R.B., Ettner, S.L., Appel, S., Wilkey, S., Van Rompay, M., & Kessler, R.C. (1998). Trends in alternative medicine use in the United States, 1990-1997: Results of a follow-up national survey. *Journal of the American Medical Association, 280,* 1569-1575.

EXAMPLES OF ALTERNATIVE AND COMPLEMENTARY THERAPIES

Mind-Body or Biobehavioral Interventions
Aromatherapy
Art therapy
Biofeedback
Dance therapy
Hypnosis
Imagery
Meditation
Music therapy
Prayer
Relaxation
Self-help support groups
T'ai chi
Yoga

Alternative Systems of Healing/Nonbiomedical Systems
Acupuncture
Anthroposophic
Ayurvedic medicine
Community-based health care practices (e.g., Native American, shamans)
Environmental medicine
Homeopathy
Naturopathy
Traditional Oriental medicine

Diet, Nutrition, and Lifestyle Modifications
Cultural diets (e.g., Native American, macrobiotic, Mediterranean)
Diet modification regimens
Supplemental therapies (e.g., amino acids, vitamins, minerals, enzymes)

Manual Healing Methods
Chiropractic
Energy work (e.g., healing touch, polarity, Qigong, Reiki, therapeutic touch)
Massage and related techniques (e.g., manual lymph drainage, Alexander technique, Feldenkrais method, pressure point therapies, Trager psychophysical integration)

Herbal Medicine
European
Latin American
Native American
Oriental

Pharmacological and Biological Treatments
Antineoplastics
Bee venom
Cartilage products
Ethylenediamine tetraacetic acid (EDTA) chelation therapy
Hoxsey method
Ozone therapy

Bioelectromagnetic Applications
Electroacupuncture
Neuromagnetic stimulation
Transcranial electrostimulation

an interest in diet, exercise, and other health-promoting measures and is unwilling to accept disease and disability as expected outcomes of aging. They desire that which is natural, appreciate the mind-body connection, and have heightened sensitivity to their spiritual dimensions. Unlike previous generations who showed a blind obedience to the medical establishment, baby boomers have challenged authority and redefined professional-client relationships. Natural, holistic therapies that empower and actively engage individuals in activities to promote health and well-being are well received by this group.

NURSING AND CAM

Nurses historically have been identified as healers; this was the foundation on which the profession was built. As the profession grew, there was a legitimate need for nursing to become more science based, and it did so rather successfully. But we must now question whether the pendulum has swung too far in the direction of science and technology. In many settings, nurses can recite a patient's laboratory results, yet know nothing of that patient's unique life story; provide a treatment to the patient, yet have their minds and hearts elsewhere; sense that the patient could benefit from their presence, yet retreat to the desk to satisfy documentation requirements.

CAM offers an exciting arena for nurses to reclaim their role as healers. The basic principles that are woven through CAM are consistent with nursing's views of health and healing (Eliopoulos, 1999):

The body has the ability to heal itself. Florence Nightingale promoted this principle when she wrote that medicine and surgery can remove obstructions, but nature alone cures (Nightingale, 1859). Nursing has long assisted individuals in getting their bodies and minds in optimal states for healing to occur.

Health and healing are related to a harmony of mind, body, and spirit. Long before CAM was recognized in the United States or the term *holistic* was commonly used, nursing attended to the needs of the whole person. Whole person care is the thread woven through the nursing process.

Basic, good health practices build the foundation for healing. In most practice settings, nurses are the primary discipline responsible for assessing and planning for all aspects—physical, emotional, socioeconomic, spiritual—of the individual. It is nursing who educates, counsels, and coaches individuals in diet, exercise, safe medication use, lifestyle modifications, and other practices that promote good health.

Healing practices are individualized. Learning about the uniqueness of each patient through comprehensive assessment, and planning and implementing care that is tai-

lored to fit the patient are basic nursing standards of practice that foster individualized care.

Clients are responsible for their own healing. The promotion of self-care and maximum independence are highly valued foundations of nursing practice.

As can be seen, the principles embraced in CAM are consistent with those long advanced by nursing. These basic principles of healing that guide CAM offer nursing an opportunity to highlight nurses' historical and special role as healers in this new arena.

CAM offers nurses the potential for innovative practice models. Increasing numbers of nurses are obtaining training in aromatherapy, herbal medicine, homeopathy, acupuncture, acupressure, therapeutic touch, guided imagery, massage therapy, and other modalities. Advanced preparation or certification in a specific modality can enable nurses to offer a wider range of services to clients in traditional care settings, as witnessed when a nurse in a primary care setting helps an individual correct incontinence with the use of biofeedback or when a nurse in an intensive care unit assists a patient in controlling pain with the use of therapeutic touch and guided imagery. These new skills also can enable nurses to establish private practices in which clients contract directly with nurses for specific therapies (e.g., therapeutic touch, stress reduction classes), wellness counseling, coaching for effective living with a chronic condition, or guidance in the integration of CAM and conventional therapies.

CHALLENGES

Exciting new opportunities within the realm of CAM can be accompanied by new problems for nurses to address. Although many of the interventions used within CAM are healing modalities that nurses are competent to independently practice, there is the risk that physicians will seek a gatekeeper role that requires that CAM therapies be ordered and managed through them. The medical model is the paradigm in which physicians have been socialized, thus it is understandable that they would gravitate toward a physician-led and physician-controlled approach to CAM. Furthermore, it is understandable that the health care system would support a physician-led model for reimbursement of CAM services (i.e., CAM therapies would require a physician's order to qualify for reimbursement). The implications could be that a qualified nurse in a conventional practice setting would be restricted from doing therapeutic touch, recommending an herbal alternative, or performing acupuncture—or obtaining reimbursement for these activities—without a physician's order. Because most CAM therapies are not medical procedures, the wisdom of a physician-directed paradigm is questionable.

Rather than a physician-directed paradigm, nurses could be working in settings that are directed by non-physician CAM practitioners. For example, a healing center that offers the services of an acupuncturist, a homeopath, and a hypnotherapist may employ a nurse. Confusion may arise related to delegation, direction, and supervision of the nurse. Strong role models of nursing will be needed to work in collaboration with CAM practitioners without allowing them to determine nursing practice or delegate inappropriately to nurses.

Licensure issues could develop for nurses who practice CAM. The area of massage therapy exemplifies the potential complications that could arise. How much of a massage can a nurse perform in caregiving before it becomes a therapeutic massage requiring licensure as a massage therapist? Would a nurse who is a licensed massage therapist and works exclusively doing massage therapy meet a state's practice requirements to maintain a nursing license? These questions already are surfacing in various states and are likely to be compounded as nurses increasingly practice CAM modalities.

Nurses may need to assume leadership in helping consumers use CAM safely. As mentioned earlier, most consumers are using CAM without the knowledge of their conventional practitioners. Many consumers are influenced and make decisions regarding their use of CAM by advertising claims and testimonials. They may see a television commercial describing an herbal preparation that can "melt pounds away" or have a neighbor who is a distributor for a magnet company advise them of the benefits of magnets for pain control. Consumers could be tempted to self-diagnosis and seek CAM remedies without the benefit of a comprehensive evaluation, thereby delaying the diagnosis and treatment of medical conditions; they also could use CAM therapies that could prove harmful to them, as could happen with herb-drug interactions. A strong advocacy role by nurses will be essential to protecting consumers in this new arena.

Nurses need to play an important role in developing the new paradigm that emerges as CAM therapies become more accepted and used in the conventional health care system. CAM, although widely used in holistic practices, does not equate to holistic care. Substituting a medical technology with a CAM modality without identifying the interrelationships and factors affecting the bio-psycho-social-spiritual dimensions of the person is not holistic care. Rather, it is a continuation of a fragmented system of health care delivery using a different set of treatment modalities. Nursing must be a strong voice in promoting a holistic model that integrates the best from CAM and conventional medicine.

REFERENCES

Eisenberg, D.M., Davis, R.B., Ettner, S.L., Appel, S., Wilkey, S., Van Rompay, M., & Kessler, R.C. (1998). Trends in alternative medicine use in the United States, 1990-1997: Results of a follow-up national survey. *Journal of the American Medical Association, 280*, 1569-1575.

Eliopoulos, C. (1999). *Integrating alternative and conventional therapies: Holistic care of chronic conditions* (pp. 76-77). St Louis: Mosby.

Nightingale, F. (1859). *Notes on nursing*. London: Harrison and Sons.

Section Five

Quality Improvement

Preserving Quality in an Era of Cost Control

JOANNE McCLOSKEY DOCHTERMAN, HELEN KENNEDY GRACE

In this time of continued transition in health care with intense pressure to control costs, maintaining quality of care becomes a major concern. In the past, incentives have focused on doing more rather than less in a system where payment was based on the services provided. Under managed care the incentives have been reversed so that minimalist care could easily become the norm. Within a system in which funding is based upon capitation and income to a practice is based on an average cost per enrolled member, the challenges to deliver quality care and also to make a profit are often at odds with one another. Costs can be controlled by limiting the number of diagnostic tests and procedures, by limiting the amount of time spent talking to patients, by denying care to patients with prior chronic conditions that would be costly to treat, and by limiting the amount of time patients spend in hospitals for treatment. In this era of cost control, minority groups and the poor are particularly vulnerable.

These intense pressures to control costs create both a formidable challenge and an opportunity structure for nursing. Nurses can play important roles in managed care systems in providing and coordinating cost-effective and preventive health care. In institutional settings, quality nursing care has been shown to be effective in reducing expensive complications such as infections and conditions arising from drug reactions. Nurses have particular expertise in extending care outside of institutional settings through home health, hospice, and long-term care. While nurses have unique strengths to offer in this era of cost control, there are intense pressures upon nurses to cut corners as an immediate "fix" and to sacrifice the long-term gains to be achieved through quality care. A major challenge is to document carefully the effects of quality nursing care, including the associated costs, so that nurses can have a positive impact upon the entire health care system. The challenge of "selling quality nursing care" is particularly great in this era of "business man-

agers" who view health care as a commodity and consider the costs from a short-term perspective. The challenge to nursing is to retain its "rootedness" in clinical care while serving as an effective spokesperson in the business aspects of patient care. This section provides an interesting overview of the issues related to maintaining standards at different points in the health care system, including nursing education and practice.

In the opening debate chapter, Stahl frames the debate in terms of the balance of maintaining quality of care while preserving a solid "bottom line." She notes that many health maintenance organizations (HMOs) are managing by pulling out of Medicare and Medicaid contracts that pay less for the care of the poor than do other insurers. Stahl notes that "managed care" is not managed and that the system is "fragmented, uncoordinated, poorly organized, and unmeasured." She advocates a change in orientation from disease treatment to health promotion, a capitation system built around patient contacts, the use of innovative approaches to the delivery of care, and a focus upon service. She notes the tendency to deal with problems in the short term through such measures as cutting staff and reducing professionals, particularly registered nurses. Specific approaches to improving quality while maintaining cost control would be to make better use of information technology such as comprehensive health care profiles of patients that follow the patient through the system, and consumer empowerment. There is a need to develop common ground for the measurement of quality. Physicians and patients tend to see quality on an individual basis, whereas HMOs measure quality on the basis of disease groups and cost of care. There is a need to develop objective measures that include the interpersonal aspects of care and amenities. Report cards that grade such things as access and service, effectiveness in keeping people healthy, appropriateness of treatment, and follow-up might be one approach in bridging the individual versus the group orientation. Clinical decision support criteria and "think and action" panels that encourage working together to solve problems would be desirable rather than the current adversarial relations.

In the first viewpoint of this section, Dean-Baar raises the question of "Standards and Guidelines: Have They Made Any Difference?" The model for standards and guidelines for professional nursing practice was designed for the purpose of creating a unifying framework that could be used to evaluate the quality of nursing in a variety of settings. "Standards are commonly interpreted from a legal perspective as being written documents that are intended to be applied rigidly and to be followed in virtually all cases. . . . Guidelines are recommendations for patient management and may include a range of interventions. The intent of guidelines is to describe alternatives and to assist in decision making." Practice guidelines are being developed throughout the health care system. Noting that many of the interventions commonly used have no basis in published scientific research, Dean-Baar advocates that practice be grounded in valid research and that standards and practices built from this base improve the quality of patient care. The importance of consistency across areas of nursing and of speaking with one voice would be facilitated through the use of unifying standards and guidelines.

Another approach, the use of clinical pathways, is advocated by Kyzer. This entails the use of multidisciplinary plans for patient care that sequence interventions and clinical outcomes on a timeline. Bringing together the multidisciplinary team to develop the clinical pathway and continually monitoring the progress of care are important parts of the process. Results from a variety of settings using the clinical pathways as a methodology indicate positive improvements in the quality of care provided.

In this era of cost control the interest in measuring the outcomes of care has greatly increased. Titler addresses this issue, pointing to the need to measure outcomes at multiple levels: patient, unit, department, organization, or health care system levels. Stressing the importance of linkages between the processes of care and the outcomes, she notes that many outcome measures focus solely on medical care, ignoring the contributions of nursing care. In outcome management programs she stresses the importance of clearly delineating the purpose and of using a conceptual model of the salient factors in producing specific outcomes and in selecting and defining the outcomes to be measured. In validating the contributions of nursing to specific outcomes, it is of particular importance to consider the processes and context of patient care. A successful outcome management program requires careful atten-

tion to data collection and management and requires sufficient resources. Once data are collected and analyzed, the importance of presenting information to relevant groups so that the information can be used for improvement of quality of care is stressed. The author cautions about the translation of outcomes into revised policies and procedures without the "buy in" and involvement of the nurses in changing the processes of care.

Noting the current trend toward "customer satisfaction" as a supreme goal, Zimmerman urges caution against over-reliance on these measures. Most customer satisfaction scales address issues easily measured while not addressing the more complex dimensions. Health care is not an objective "measurable" product, and in most instances, the patient is not the one filling out the form. In addition, sometimes what the customer wants is not the desired treatment. For example, parents who bring a child to the doctor because they have a cold might want the doctor to prescribe antibiotics. Although the parents might be satisfied should the doctor do so, it would not be appropriate treatment. Inappropriate use of "customer satisfaction" measures frequently leads to finding "someone to blame," and in most instances this would be someone from nursing. While resisting customer satisfaction as the measure of care, nurses could profit from training in principles of "customer service."

Turning to nursing licensure as another facet of maintaining quality of care, Dorsey addresses the process of nurse licensure. Traditionally, licensure has been a matter of state laws that govern the licensure process. While preserving licensure as a state prerogative, the changes in health care require greater flexibility. The interstate practice of nursing is now necessary. Until recently, law required that a nurse be licensed in the state in which care is being provided. But frequently nurses live in one state and provide care in another. Also, nurses may provide care in home settings that are in different states, or provide care through the Internet that is delivered to multiple sites. One way of managing licensure while maintaining states rights is through the use of multistate compacts. Such a compact is in place involving five states. A mutual recognition model allows nurses to practice in different states if the state recognizes the license of another as valid in their state. While some groups, such as the American Nurses Association, oppose such an approach because of its impact on collective bargaining, others view this as a positive change, the first change in licensure in 100 years.

In the concluding chapter to this section, Welton and Nieves-Khouw address performance evaluation as a means of measuring clinical competence. Tracing the history of competency testing, the authors then address its application to nursing. "Nursing competence is the application of knowledge and skills related to caring, critical thinking, communication and clinical intervention expected for the nurse's practice role within the context of the public health, welfare, and safety." The authors then go on to describe the complexities of selecting a model, of testing for competency, and the discrepancies that might exist between written competency testing and actual clinical practice.

Ironically, as the pressures for increasingly cost-effective care increase, the need for measuring the quality of care and the competence of caregivers becomes increasingly important. Like a kaleidoscope, different players in the drama of health care see quality from differing perspectives. The challenge for nursing is to be able to speak to the effects of nursing on care outcomes in such a way that within this ever-changing field the contributions of nursing can be readily identified.

Can Quality of Care Be Maintained in a Managed Care System?

DULCELINA ALBANO STAHL

Three major trends in the health care arena that constitute the crux of whether quality of care can be maintained in a managed care system are (1) the transitional changes occurring in various types of health plans and in the health care delivery system, (2) information technology, and (3) consumer empowerment. Amidst these trends are critical issues that must be thoroughly explored and understood in order to ascertain whether or not quality of care can be maintained in a managed care system.

TRANSITIONAL CHANGES IN HEALTH PLANS

According to the 1999 Annual Employer Health Benefits Survey conducted by the Kaiser Family Foundation and the Health Research and Educational Trust, health maintenance organizations (HMOs) now provide 28% of health coverage for employees while traditional indemnity insurance provides only 9%, a dramatic drop from the 73% the latter provided 9 years ago. Meanwhile, preferred provider organizations (PPOs) have become the most popular type of health plan offered to employees, accounting for coverage to 38% of all workers. Notwithstanding the high numbers of PPOs and HMOs, managed care organizations (MCOs) are in a transitional flux. MCOs are beset by Wall Street expectations, consumerism, legislative and political pressures, and litigation.

A major dilemma facing MCOs is how to balance solid bottom-line financial performance and the provision of consistent, high-quality health care. On January 15, 1999, Donna Shalala, Secretary of the Department of Health and Human Services (HHS), unveiled the new risk adjustment program initially contained in the Balanced Budget Act (BBA) of 1997 as a way to pay health plans more fairly and "reduce incentives for plans to enroll only healthier [Medicare] beneficiaries." HMOs continue to oppose this risk adjustment because this would reduce payments to them by about $11 billion over the reductions already mandated by the BBA of 1997. Many HMOs pulled out of their Medicare risk contract with the Health Care Financing Administration (HCFA) as a result of the decreased reimbursement under the BBA of 1997. Consequently, many elderly patients were left without coverage as they sought to enroll in other health plans that might or might not offer a Medicare-risk contract.

To curb this trend of HMOs opting not to provide coverage for Medicare recipients—a trend detrimental to the HCFA's goal of reducing the skyrocketing costs of providing health care services to the elderly—the HCFA agreed to phase in the implementation of the new risk adjustment program for health plans commencing in 1999.

The public at large has been critical of the MCOs' stance on this risk-adjustment issue. The arguments that have been leveled against HMOs in this regard are:

1. HMO executives are being paid millions of dollars, far above what other business executives receive (e.g., 1997 compensation for Wilson Taylor, chairman and CEO of CIGNA, $12.5 million; for William McGuire, CEO of United HealthCare, $8.6 million; for James Stewart, executive vice president of CIGNA, $7.3 million), and therefore a reduction in their salaries and bonuses would make up for these organizations' risk-adjustment loss of revenue.

2. Many HMOs have enrolled mostly healthy seniors who have not used services through the years, and yet the HCFA has been paying the HMOs rates that were based on risks of utilization. Therefore the HCFA deemed that the new risk-adjustment was justified.

Although HMOs do not offer any counter-argument, there are serious implications on the maintenance of quality of care if HMOs continue to pull out of the

Medicare-risk contract with the HCFA. One of the benefits that Medicare-risk contracts usually provide is discounts on medications. Seniors tend to have higher utilization of medications because of chronic and debilitating conditions. Without discounts on medications, they may not be able to afford the drugs they need. Data indicate that today seniors who are not in HMOs pay two times more for drugs than those with HMO coverage. Many seniors who are not enrolled in HMOs and who are receiving brand name drugs for chronic conditions even go outside the United States to purchase their drugs solely to save money. For example, the ulcer drug Prilosec has a U.S. retail price of $116.52 for a 1-month supply. This same quantity of Prilosec costs $55.10 in Canada and $32.10 in Mexico. In 1995, those who had drug supplemental coverage paid an average of $600 per year for outpatient medications. Ten percent of Medicare beneficiaries pay more than $1,500 per year for medications. Because medications are critical in maintaining the health status of many seniors, a continued trend of HMOs to pull out of their Medicare risk contract with the HCFA would seriously affect the maintenance of quality care for these seniors.

Some MCO experts are raising issues regarding the direction and goal of managed care companies. For instance, David Lawrence, M.D., Chief Executive Officer of Kaiser Foundation Health Plans and Kaiser Foundation Hospital, recently commented that most of what we call "managed care" is not that at all. He contends that the delivery of care is "fragmented, uncoordinated, poorly organized, and unmeasured. It is not systematic, thereby making quality improvement and safety management difficult, if not impossible" (Troy, 1999). He then proposes that health care delivery be organized through health care teams, that there should be performance tracking, and that the determination of improved performance be based on measured outcomes.

One can argue that Lawrence is wrong in his contention. After all, is it not true that currently there are many integrated delivery systems (IDS) whose goal is to improve efficiency and effectiveness of care delivery and ultimately improve quality of care? Although the answer to this question is in the affirmative, Lawrence *is* right in proposing that there should be performance tracking and performance improvement based on measured outcomes. Unfortunately, measurable outcomes of an IDS's effects on maintaining quality of care are not readily discernible to consumers and the public at large.

J.D. Kleinke, an independent medical economist, states that "managed care companies must move from being claims-based insurance companies to become organizations that are proactively involved in managing people's health care and wellness" (Troy, 1999). Many HMOs would contend that they are *already* doing a great deal of proactive health promotion and education. For example, recognizing that as of 1996 nearly 23 million women aged 50 years and older have or were at risk for developing osteoporosis and that this figure is anticipated to increase to 35 million by 2015, many health plans are using a range of interventions with pharmacists, including educational programs and screening to reduce the risk of developing the disease and incidence of fractures (osteoporosis is the primary cause of 1.5 million fractures in the United States). Thus Kleinke has no grounds for his statement. Nevertheless the truth of the matter is that MCOs can do more than they are currently doing. In fact, there are still some who are just beginning to address this issue. If MCOs continue to promote wellness and illness prevention, then quality of care can be maintained and enhanced.

Some experts advocate for contact capitation. Under this arrangement, physicians are reimbursed a fixed fee as in capitation but only for the patients they actually treat. This also holds true for specialists. In effect, physicians are paid a fixed amount per referral, which is intended to pay for an episode of care, that is, all associated costs for a specified time. Thus the HMO retains the risk for the number of referrals (Fine, 1999). If this trend continues in managed care, then quality of care can be maintained and improved as consumers gain better access to specialists for their specific health care needs without the need of obtaining a referral and approval from their respective primary care physician.

Today, MCOs offer many of the benefit options specified in patients' rights bills. Nationally, two thirds of workers (67%) enrolled in HMOs can designate an obstetrician-gynecologist (OB-GYN) as their primary care physician, up substantially from only 49% in 1998. One fourth of HMO members with a chronic condition (25%), compared with 22% in 1998, can select a specialist as their primary physician. Many health plans also dropped preexisting condition exclusion clauses in their contracts in response to legal requirements and market demands (Wechsler, 1999a). These changes have improved the quality of care services provided, especially for those having chronic conditions. Patients can access specialists directly and have continuity of care treatment and management rather than being bounced back and forth between the primary care physician and the specialist.

Other transitional trends occurring in MCOs include innovative approaches to health care delivery models.

Two of these are the targeted service delivery and cross-service management. The former focuses on understanding the needs of the enrollee in the workplace, in the community, or at home. Response to the needs of the individual patient or community served rather than focusing on high cost providers and inefficient use of services as a means of controlling costs in order to shore up bottom-line performance is being advocated by MCO experts as the future of managed care. Continuation of this trend will eliminate the issue of denial of services for economic reasons, thereby ensuring quality of care.

Under a cross-service management approach, patient-focused care or service-focused care is the goal. This entails "coordination of care at various levels to streamline access to health care services, support a cost-accounting system that permits more accurate pricing of the costs of services provided, improve quality of services, and ultimately the satisfaction of clients and providers" (Grazier, 1999). The coordination of services would also prevent unnecessary duplication of tests and procedures performed at various health care delivery sites: emergency department, outpatient, inpatient, subacute care, home care, and long-term care. Patients benefit from being spared the pain, inconvenience, or side effects of repeated procedures and tests.

On the litigation front, several MCOs have been sued. In the case of Goodrich vs. Aetna the plaintiff was awarded $116 million, the largest verdict against an MCO ever given by the courts. The case is interesting because it involved denial of care based on the justification that the treatment was "experimental," and yet there was nothing mentioned in the health plan's handbook regarding experimental treatment (Robbins, 1999).

Another case that did not even involve serious injury or death but was just the contention of a "bad faith" breach of fiduciary responsibility was that of Karen Johnson, who sued Humana and was awarded $13 million. Johnson had carcinoma in situ of the cervix. Her physician recommended a hysterectomy, which would have cost Humana thousands of dollars. Only a cervical conization was approved and performed, which cost only several hundred dollars. Consequently, Johnson's lawyer argued in the court that the cure rate for her cancer with this procedure was not as great as with a hysterectomy.

MCOs tend to recoup losses from incurred litigation costs by increasing fees charged to its enrollees and by reducing reimbursements to contracted providers in future contract negotiations. To what extent a consumer is willing to pay higher costs of health care will determine the breadth of his or her benefit coverage. The only alternative for those who cannot afford increased fees may be to sign up with an HMO that offers only basic coverage. Thus, if more sophisticated treatment and procedures are needed, these individuals may not then seek health care services. In such a case, quality of care cannot be maintained. In another scenario, those who are enrolled in a PPO may also not seek health care services if the out-of-pocket costs are dramatically increased. Similarly, their quality of care cannot be maintained.

TRANSITIONAL CHANGES IN HEALTH CARE DELIVERY

Although many health care providers have used managed care as the rationale for downsizing, reengineering, and changing their delivery models, the extant literature reveals that the profits of hospitals and medical centers are much better than anticipated. It could be argued that this phenomenon is the result of improved systems, increased productivity, and improved efficiencies required to survive and thrive under a managed care system. On the other hand, the counter-argument could be that this resulted from the dramatic budget reductions gained by decreasing the registered nurse staff and replacing them with patient care technicians—the doing more with less philosophy—and changing the role expectations and job descriptions of staff.

The Balanced Budget Act of 1997 threw yet another curve ball at health care providers. The objective of the BBA is to reduce Medicare outlays by $115.1 billion between fiscal years 1998 and 2002 and reduce federal Medicaid outlays by $10.1 billion. To achieve this, the BBA will reduce Medicare's rates of increase in payments to hospitals by more than $40 billion, with $17.1 billion reductions in the hospital prospective payment system update factor alone. Physician payments will be reduced by $5.3 billion, managed care plan payments by $21.8 billion, home health agency payments by $16.2 billion, and skilled nursing facility payments by $9.5 billion. However, more than $23 billion of new spending money is provided to states to fund expansion of children's health care insurance coverage (Deloitte & Touche, 1997).

As a result of the implementation of the BBA, many teaching hospitals and skilled nursing facilities have experienced financial difficulties. In 1999, many health care associations and the American Medical Association have lobbied for legislation to be passed to restore some funding to alleviate the serious financial dilemma that health care providers have been experiencing. Congress finally passed legislation to restore some funding. Although health care providers felt some relief, they still contend that the substantial reductions in Medicare payments will pose a threat to their ability to provide quality care to the patients they serve. Thus a critical and legitimate question to ask while health care providers continue to carry out their transitional strategies for delivering health care services is, Can quality of care be maintained under the BBA of 1997?

The registered nurse shortage is definitely creating serious issues of quality of care in acute care settings. In long-term care, the shortage of qualified nursing assistants also is dramatically affecting facilities' ability to care for the elderly. Consequently, with the increased scrutiny of skilled nursing facilities by the Office of the Inspector General (OIG) and state regulatory agencies, many facilities have been fined thousands of dollars or were closed because of violations, particularly those related to quality of care issues. In effect, the crisis in health care providers' ability to provide quality care has significant implications in maintaining quality of care in a managed care system.

INFORMATION TECHNOLOGY

Today MCOs have data systems that can have a tremendous impact on the quality of health care services delivered. Computerized records, centralized treatment protocols, community-based assessments, disease management protocols, and service utilization data offer a wealth of information that has dramatic implications for maintaining the quality of services provided. Unfortunately, these data have not been shared with health care providers by MCOs. Yet it is clear that increased availability of such information from MCOs to providers and enrollees can improve the quality of care.

Conversely, many health care providers also have their own data systems that contain enormous amounts of information that, if utilized, could significantly improve the quality of services provided to their consumers. For instance, a patient's comprehensive health care profile that can be accessed immediately on line in case of an emergency could prove to be the difference in being able to save a life or preventing serious complications.

Patient care advocates argue that patients' rights to privacy supersede the benefits of sharing clinical information between MCOs and providers. The 1996 Health Insurance Portability Act required the Department of Health and Human Services (HHS) to issue rules to protect unauthorized use of electronic medical records if Congress failed to enact legislation dealing with the problem by August 21, 1999. Consequently in early November 1999 the HHS issued a proposed rule that basically limits the release of private health information without a patient's consent. It requires health plans to inform patients regarding how their medical information is used and to whom it is disclosed. Moreover, patients gain the right to see and correct their own records. This HHS proposal was open for comment until February 17, 2000. The over 40,000 comments received are currently being reviewed while Congress continues to prepare legislation to protect the privacy of health information for all Americans. There are several problems with this proposed rule.

First, while the HHS contends that it will cost $3.8 billion to implement the proposal over 5 years, the managed care industry estimates it will cost more than $40 billion. Second, the HHS will hold health plans legally responsible for compliance by their contracted entities—hospitals, pharmacists, physicians, consultants, and data processing firms. Penalties for unintentional disclosure are fairly low, but intentional disclosure can mean a $50,000 fine and imprisonment. MCOs argue that being held legally responsible for their contracted entities is unfair and will be very costly; MCOs will have to revise all their contracts to include provisions relative to the responsibilities of their contracted entities to minimize their risk exposure to the HCFA fines and penalties. Third, physicians and patient advocates believe that the rule is too lax because it allows health plans to disclose medical information for too many purposes without individual consent. Fourth, the rule does not preempt state laws, which means that the federal rule will have to be adhered to along with 51 other rules from the states and the District of Columbia (Wechsler, 1999b).

It is apparent that this privacy rule does not address the issue of maintaining and improving the quality of care through sharing of clinical data between MCOs and providers. Yet, as previously mentioned, there is a need for MCOs to share their wealth of information with providers for quality of care purposes. Until this issue is resolved, unnecessary duplication of services will continue, the outcomes of various disease management protocols that improve quality of care will remain within the domains of only those who have the data rather than with the public at large, and disease prevention and health promotion will continue to be just topics for more educational seminars or perhaps even e-commerce business for the entrepreneurial individual.

CONSUMER EMPOWERMENT

Consumerism has definitely paved the way for the transitional changes that have occurred and continue to occur in MCOs. Yet there are major issues that this trend has not addressed that definitely affect the quality of services provided in a managed care arena. These issues include, but are not limited to, lack of common definition of quality, failure to utilize report cards of health plans, employers' persistent narrow focus on costs and other minimal criteria in deciding which health plans to offer their employees, and failure to harness consumer empowerment to influence the quality of services provided.

COMMON GROUNDS FOR DEFINING QUALITY OF CARE

Emily Rhinehart, vice president of AIG Consultants, Inc., in Atlanta, has made cogent, provocative observations regarding health care quality. She contends that health care quality is still in the eyes of the beholder, irrespective of how MCOs or providers try to define what quality service is. She further observes that there seems to be a disparity between the focus of MCOs and that of the press. While the press focuses on individual cases, particularly those who have experienced denial of needed services, MCOs focus on "attempting to measure the quality of care for populations, age groups and other homogeneous groups based on diagnoses. They are not focused on one member at a time" (Rhinehart, 1998). Then the question becomes, who should really be ensuring that an individual consumer receives quality services? Rhinehart suggests that individual providers must oversee the quality of services provided to their patients.

It may be argued that Rhinehart's view is too myopic and very subjective. Clearly, there are now objective measurements for quality of care, such as health care outcomes. For instance, the rate of nosocomial infection in the hospital setting is a very important objective measurement of how well the hospital staff are adhering to infection control guidelines and universal precautions. A low rate of nosocomial infections means a lower incidence of complications from admitting diagnosis to surgical intervention, thereby maintaining quality of care. On the other hand, there are anecdotal notes that indicate instances wherein patients measured the quality of the care they received by how they felt about the nurse who took care of them, even if that nurse may have committed an error in administering medications.

More than two decades ago, Shortell already recognized the importance of what he termed the transactional aspect of quality in physician referral behavior. He contended that physician referral behavior was a "system of rewards, costs, and outcomes perceived by physicians in referring patients to one another" (Shortell, 1972). In effect, a patient was referred by a physician to another physician specialist who not only had technical competence but also had positive treatment outcomes. Moreover, Shortell also observed that clear communication between the consultant and referring physician can affect the quality and continuity of care received.

In a group model HMO the HMO contracts directly with a medical group consisting of physicians who are paid a certain amount of money per HMO member per month regardless of whether the members use any services. The physician group is then responsible for providing health care services to the HMO members. This is referred to as capitation. There is financial incentive to control utilization of services; there may even be instances of underutilization because the less the utilization, the more the money saved for the physician group at the end of the year (Stahl, 1997).

While Shortell commends the value of physician referrals based on technical competence and treatment outcomes in promoting quality of care, the primary care physician of a group model HMO who is financially motivated may elect to handle cases himself or herself instead of referring patients to a specialist who has more technical competence. When this happens, maintaining quality of care for the patient is at risk.

Other experts on what constitutes quality services, such as A. Donabedian, have advocated models of defining common grounds for determining quality services in terms of specific criteria and parameters. Three criteria common to these models are technical services, interpersonal aspects of care, and amenities. Each of these criteria has specific parameters to determine quality of care (Donabedian, 1980).

In terms of technical services, the parameters include availability of latest equipment needed, the qualifications and expertise of the staff, accuracy of diagnoses, appropriateness of treatment, practice guidelines, effectiveness of treatment, morbidity, mortality rates, and increase or decrease in the patient's functional status. These parameters obviously have an impact on the issue of whether quality of care can be provided in a managed care system, not necessarily as a result of the type of managed care contract but rather as the direct result of the technical capabilities of the provider. For example, misdiagnosis of an HMO patient who is admitted for inpatient care can adversely affect the person's health. There is documented evidence that misdiagnosis does occur in health care settings.

If a particular provider, such as a hospital, does not have practice guidelines for its physician, nursing, and allied health professionals to ensure quality of care provided for specific cases, then an MCO patient may be deprived of the quality care that he or she deserves. Although large teaching hospitals and medical centers do have practice guidelines, there are still many providers, such as community-based private hospitals, that are still in the developmental stage of their practice guidelines. Delays in providing treatment can also occur in settings in which the latest equipment and other resources, such as a physician specialist, are not available. Consequently, an MCO patient may have to be transferred to another hospital for care, thereby disrupting the continuity of care that the patient deserves.

The second criterion used to determine quality of care is that of interpersonal aspects of care. Shortell and others contend that the roles and expectations of the health care professionals and allied staff, their sensitivity and compassion in service delivery, their honesty and integrity in the treatment of patients, their compliance with regulatory and ethical standards, and their spirituality are critical parameters for ensuring quality of care.

With the transitional changes occurring in the health care delivery system today, complicated by the BBA of 1997 and the shortage of nursing staff, overworked registered nurses may not be able to exercise compassion and sensitivity for their patients. In the long-term care industry, the high turnover of staff has been exacerbated by the relentless efforts of the OIG in enforcing the Omnibus Budget Reconciliation Act (OBRA) regulations through continued closer inspections of skilled nursing providers and facilities. High turnover is no longer just a phenomenon of nursing assistants. It is also true for administrators, directors of nursing, and other department heads. Many have become frustrated because they must spend more time on paperwork documentation, as required by the prospective payment system, than on actual patient care. Moreover, these persons also have felt that working in a skilled nursing facility is no longer worthwhile because they find that their compensation is generally lower than that of other service jobs.

The third criterion for quality of care determination is that of amenities. This includes the ambiance of the care site, the appearance of the staff, a sound environment that is conducive to health care recovery from illness, efficiency and effectiveness of care delivery, and patient and family satisfaction.

The above-mentioned common grounds for determining quality of care are akin to the performance standards of the National Committee on Quality Assurance's (NCQA) Health Plan Employer Data and Information Set (HEDIS), used to accredit health plans. These include member satisfaction, access, preventive care, health promotion, and wellness.

In its second annual State of Managed Care Quality report, the NCQA reported the overall satisfaction of enrollees with their health plans in 1998 at 55.7%. In terms of access to care, the rates were 82.2% for not having a problem with delays in medical care as a patient waited for health plan approval, 81.2% in not having a problem getting referral to a specialist, and 85.3% in not having a problem receiving care that the patient and his or her physician believed was necessary. These results indicate that quality of care can be maintained in a managed care system.

REPORT CARDS OF HEALTH PLANS

In 1999 the NCQA revamped its accreditation process and adopted a new report card system that consumers can use to compare various measures of quality in managed care plans. The categories used for rating health plans are based on the Foundation for Accountability's Consumer Information Framework (FACCT) and are weighted: access and service (40%), qualified providers (20%), living with illness (15%), staying healthy (15%), and getting better (10%).

The new NCQA report card for consumers will carry the accreditation status of each health plan (excellent, commendable, accredited, provisional, or denied) and its respective scores in the above-mentioned categories. The objective is to enable consumers to identify which health plan is providing superior service as opposed to those providing only average service. This report will be made available free on NCQA's web site (www.ncqa.com), for employer distribution, and to the media.

To further determine whether quality of care can be maintained in a managed care system, it is important to take a closer look at the factors included in each of the categories being measured for each health plan.

Access and service entails not only access to services but also provider skill, communication, coordination of care, and follow-up. MCOs require that physicians are credentialed when they contract with the MCO to ensure that physicians have the technical skills needed to practice their area of specialization and that they adhere to the ethical standards of their profession. Similarly, hospitals and other providers are required to have accreditation from recognized accrediting bodies such as the Joint Commission on Accreditation of Health Care Organizations (JCAHO), because accreditation provides some degree of assurance that the provider skills, coordination of care, follow-up of care, and communication of the provider's mission and goals to the entire staff and the strategies of achieving these are in place. Accreditation by JCAHO and credentialing of physicians provide assurances for the quality of care delivered.

With respect to staying healthy, the measures used are preventive care, risk reduction, and education to promote wellness and prevention of illness. There are many health plans that offer innovative programs in these areas. In 1995, Health Partners, a Minneapolis HMO, offered on-line access to the plan's data on their quality reports and provider directories through computer modem or diskette given to their members. In effect, members could then make an informed decision in choosing a provider that would not only meet their needs but also provide quality services (Atlantic Information Services, Inc., 1995). At Access Health in Broomfield, Colorado, members are given literature about their conditions, and patients at high risk receive periodic telephone calls from registered nurses who counsel, monitor, and refer them to providers, if needed. According to Rufus Scott Howe, a family nurse practitioner and vice president of population care management at Access Health, one such program for asthma patients helped the Blue Cross & Blue Shield of Massachusetts reduce emergency department visits by 90% and inpatient admission by 59% (Hoechst-Marion Roussel, 1999).

Providing appropriate treatment and follow-up after an illness are the measures for the "getting better" category. Once a patient is discharged from the acute care setting, follow-up care at home or as an outpatient is essential. More importantly, providing support through a nurse-staffed call center to handle any questions the patient has does make a difference in health care outcomes and thus maintenance of quality care. The Healthwise Communities Project in Boise, Idaho, funded by the Robert Wood Johnson Foundation, has achieved exceptional results from its nurse-staffed call center that handled about 25,000 calls and set up 52 information stations with reference books and a database of health information and decision guidance. According to estimates by researchers at the Oregon Health Sciences University, the savings from the project were from $7.5 million to $21.5 million over 22 months by forestalling unnecessary doctor and emergency department visits.

In terms of living with illness, the factors measured are reducing symptoms, avoiding complications, and maximizing quality of life for people with chronic illness. These measures are critical in maintaining quality of care

for seniors. In a managed care system, Medicare-risk HMOs offer seniors discounts on medications. This feature enhances the patient's compliance with his or her medication regimen because he or she does not have to worry so much about incurring too much cost for medications. Increased compliance with medication regimen not only prevents complications but also maximizes the quality of life for the person with chronic illness.

In the final category on changing needs, the focus is on providing the care a patient needs when his or her functional abilities change dramatically. In a managed care system, providing care after a dramatic change in functional abilities can be facilitated in an HMO model wherein the patient can be admitted immediately for care at 100% coverage in an acute care setting. This is one of the advantages of an HMO: eliminating financial concerns relative to inpatient costs.

On the other hand, one can argue that an HMO model at times presents some hurdles in accessing emergency and urgent care because of the requirement to obtain approval by the primary care physician to avoid out-of-pocket costs for emergency or urgent care services received. Consequently the patient is subjected to unnecessary anxiety and stress that are not conducive to maintaining quality of care.

Notwithstanding the values of MCOs' report cards, a survey conducted by KPMG Peat Marwick in 1977 of 1,502 firms with 200 or more employees and its 1996 survey of 1,151 firms revealed that only 1% of employers provide data on health plan quality to their employees. Moreover, only 11% of employers who offer HMOs to their employees contend that NCQA's accreditation quality measurements were important to them when making decisions about which health plans to offer their employees. Additionally, only 5% admit that HEDIS performance measures were important when selecting health plans.

The employers' failure to utilize report cards of health plans and their persistent narrow focus on costs and other minimal criteria in deciding which health plan to choose for their employees is a serious public policy issue if quality of care is to be maintained in a managed care system. Although the majority of the largest and most influential employers are already utilizing accreditation and HEDIS to guide their decisions, says Margaret O'Kane, NCQA president, the NCQA is working hard to educate other employers on the availability of report cards to help them select quality health plans for their employees.

Employers are in a position to harness consumer empowerment to pave the way for maintaining and improving quality of care in a managed care environment. These employers need to fully utilize the report cards to influence the health plans in providing benefits that better meet their employees' needs.

STRATEGIES FOR CHANGE

The debate on whether or not quality of care can be maintained in a managed care system will continue in this millennium unless strategies for change are developed and implemented by both MCOs and health care providers. The tension between MCOs and health care providers has been going on for over a decade since the introduction of managed care. Providers argue that they have lost control of clinical decision making and that MCOs are not making decisions based on patient need but on their desire to save money. On the other hand, MCOs counter that providers such as physicians sometimes provide unnecessary treatments or recommend additional diagnostic procedures that are costly when less expensive alternative courses of treatment could achieve the same results.

The rationale for the above tension lies in divergent perceived goals between MCOs and providers. Providers view their goal as providing the best medical care possible for their patients without paying much attention to costs. On the other hand, the goal of MCOs is to make providers more efficient and eliminate excesses.

Essential strategies to change these perceived divergent goals are to maintain and improve quality of care in a managed care system. Because managed care is here to stay irrespective of its transitions, it behooves providers and MCOs to work together to develop and implement strategies that would be mutually beneficial for both and would be a win-win situation for the patient, provider, and MCO.

Lynanne Balleli, MD, MBA, director of clinical services at InterQual, Marlborough, Massachusetts, offers one strategy: the use of a clinical decision–support criterion in both hard copy and software formats. This criterion help providers match appropriate treatments to demonstrated patient need by outlining a particular sequence of interventions recommended for diagnosing and treating a clinical problem (Balleli, 1999). For example, the criterion would validate when reasonable nonspecialist diagnostic steps and therapeutic interventions have been unsuccessful and that referral to a specialist is needed. Moreover, the criterion also specifies instances wherein early management by a specialist is the best course of action. The bottom line is that the most efficient delivery method is to provide the most appropriate care at the beginning of the treatment process. By so doing, unnecessary complications and additional costs are avoided, overutilization and underutilization of services are prevented, and quality of care is ascertained.

The clinical decision–support criteria, says Balleli, should be developed by an outside organization so that the biases of the clinicians and any possible financial and personal incentives are avoided. The key to achieving this strategy is to elicit the buy-in of the physicians on the principle that such criteria are based on medical research and on consensus among generalists, specialists, academics, and community-based clinicians and are thus reflective of the latest medical best practices with supporting evidence of successful outcomes.

Another strategy is for large teaching hospitals and academia to spearhead the establishment of a "think and action panel" to create a bill for Congress to enact on the use of an MCO and provider information database not just to maintain quality of care but more importantly to improve quality of care in a managed care system. This "think and action panel" should have representation from consumers, ethicists, physicians, nurses, allied health professionals, lawyers, the HCFA, information technology experts, MCOs, legislators, financial consultants, hospitals, and home health care, subacute care, rehabilitation care, and long-term care providers. The likelihood of achieving this strategy is high when there is a wide representation of those who would be directly and indirectly affected by such legislation.

The road to success in maintaining quality of care in a managed care system is not a straight one. There are several intersections that have to be crossed and navigated. Notwithstanding, there is a compass that can point in the right direction, namely, a cooperative and collaborative team of MCOs and providers (managed care provider team [MPT]) having the same agenda and working together toward a common goal: quality care delivered in the most cost-effective way. The strategies for change can pave the way for this new MPT's unified approach to maintaining and promoting quality of care in the future.

REFERENCES

Atlantic Information Services, Inc. (1995, February 27). *Managed Care Week*, p. 3.

Balleli, L. (1999, March). Criteria help to bridge the gap between providers and MCOs. *Managed Healthcare*, pp. 62-63.

Hoechst-Marion Roussel. (1999). The state of health care in America. *Business & Health* (special issue).

Deloitte & Touche. (1997). The Balanced Budget Act of 1997. Public Law 105-33.

Donabedian, A. (1980). Explorations in quality assessment and monitoring. In *The definition of quality and approaches to its assessment.* Ann Arbor, MI: Health Administration Press.

Fine, A. (1999, March). Specialists fall under capitation's umbrella. *Managed Healthcare,* pp. 50-52.

Grazier, K. (1999). The future of managed care. *Healthcare Management, 44*(6), 423-426.

Rhinehart, E. (1998, October). Health care quality still is in the eyes of the beholder. *Managed Healthcare,* p. 18.

Robbins, D. (1999, March). Legal cases associated with payment issues spawn big-dollar verdicts. *Managed Healthcare,* pp. 13-17.

Shortell, S.M. (1972). *A model of physician referral behavior: A test of exchange theory in medical practice.* Chicago: Center for Health Administration Studies, University of Chicago.

Troy, T. (1999, October). Managed care's keenest thinkers. *Managed Healthcare,* pp. 30-35.

Wechsler, J. (1999a, March). HMOs continue to oppose risk adjustment. *Managed Healthcare,* p. 17.

Wechsler, J. (1999b, December). Privacy standards tricky for HMOs. *Managed Healthcare,* p. 14.

CHAPTER 32

Standards and Guidelines

Have They Made Any Difference?

SUSAN L. DEAN-BAAR

It has been a decade since the American Nurses Association, in conjunction with more than 30 specialty nursing organizations, developed a framework designed to bring unity to the development and promulgation of professional nursing standards. Has the framework developed in 1991 (American Nurses Association, 1991a) achieved the potential that was hoped for? What is the impact of this framework on current nursing practice? Are professional standards influencing the definition and provision of quality nursing care? Standards can be categorized into three groups related to the source from which they come: (1) professional nursing association standards, (2) institution-specific agencies, and (3) regulatory agencies (Smith & Popovich, 1993). This chapter discusses professional nursing association standards and the framework developed by the American Nurses Association and specialty nursing organizations. Schroeder (1991) provides a comprehensive review of other approaches to standards in nursing.

HISTORY OF PROFESSIONAL NURSING STANDARDS

A component of the American Nurses Association's (ANA) core mission is its responsibility for defining nursing, establishing the scope of nursing practice, and for setting standards of nursing practice. In 1952, the ANA established functions, standards, and qualification committees that serve as the roots of today's current standards of practice.

In 1973, ANA's Congress for Nursing Practice published the generic *Standards of Nursing Practice*. These were based on the nursing process and provided a systematic approach to nursing practice in any setting and in any specialty area. Over the next 15 years there were numerous standards documents published both by the ANA

and by other specialty nursing organizations. Definitions of standards developed by professional nursing organizations ranged from setting a baseline for practice or minimum expectations to setting a goal for practice or level of excellence. In addition to the various definitions there were also multiple approaches to the structure and format of standards. Many used a structure, process, and outcome format that reflected the ANA model for quality assurance (ANA, 1975).

An analysis of standards published by the ANA between 1973 and 1989 found that standards related to areas other than the nursing process were being included (McGuffin & Mariani, 1990). These additional standards included the areas of theory, organizations, continuity of care, collaboration, professional development and continuing education, quality assurance and peer review, research, community systems, and ethics. There was considerable repetition among these standards and apparent confusion between the concepts of professional development and continuing education and quality assurance and peer review. McGuffin and Mariani also found that at least four specialty areas had published criteria for selected nursing diagnoses in the specialty area. The authors recommended that those aspects of practice that consistently appear in or affect practice be shared among areas of nursing to avoid duplication and that agreement be reached on the broad category headings. In addition, they concluded that clarification and consistency were needed in several areas, including how the categories of professional practice and professional performance standards are defined, and whether standards indicate a minimum or maximum level of practice.

The diversity of definitions and frameworks for standards during this time resulted in a fragmented approach and confusion over the purpose of standards for nursing practice. In 1988, the ANA began a process of reevaluating the nature and purpose of standards of nursing practice because of the concerns that had been raised during this evolution of standards of professional practice. These concerns included the inability to use standards to evaluate the effectiveness of care, the lack of consistency in the process used to develop professional standards, the proliferation of standards of nursing practice, and the wide range in the intent, format, and scope of standards. The divergent and numerous approaches used in establishing standards limited their usefulness for nurses, other health care providers, payers, policy makers, and consumers when applied to a variety of activities such as clinical decision making and quality activities. As a result of other activities within the health care arena, including some of the activities being performed by the Agency for Health Care Policy and Research, the body of work on evaluating the nature and purpose of standards was expanded to include the purpose and format of guidelines for practice (ANA, 1991a).

The development of the framework for nursing practice standards and guidelines that resulted from this evaluation began with a critical analysis of the environment internal and external to nursing. This included discussion representing the perspectives of nurses in a variety of practice roles and settings, with input from numerous specialty groups, state nurses' associations, and ANA structural units. This process and the framework that resulted were substantially different from previous standards work done by the ANA.

The standards published in 1991 reflected the first revision of professional nursing standards in 18 years (ANA, 1991b). They were published with a commitment to establish a collaborative process for a more timely review and revision every 5 years. As a result, the standards were reviewed and minor revisions were made (ANA, 1997).

MODEL FOR PROFESSIONAL NURSING STANDARDS AND GUIDELINES

The model for standards and guidelines for practice was designed with the purpose of creating a unifying framework that could be used to evaluate the quality of nursing in a variety of practice settings. The combined model for standards of nursing practice and practice guidelines is designed to provide direction for nursing practice, a means to evaluate practice, and a way in which the profession can describe what its accountability is to the public. Each of these is important to building a foundation to assure quality.

Standards

Within the model, standards and guidelines primarily differ in their scope and intent. The purpose of standards is to provide broad direction for the overall practice of nursing, including the provision of care and professional role activities. Standards are authoritative statements that describe a level of care or performance common to the profession of nursing by which the quality of nursing practice can be judged (ANA, 1997). Standards reflect the values of the profession and further explicate the definition of professional practice. Standards of clinical nursing practice are divided into two categories—standards of care and standards of professional performance. The intent of standards of care is to describe an acceptable level of client or patient care; the intent of standards of professional performance is to describe an acceptable level of behavior in the professional nurse's role.

Standards of care describe a competent level of care as demonstrated by the nursing process involving assessment, diagnosis, outcome identification, planning, implementation, and evaluation. Standards of professional performance describe a competent level of behavior in the professional role including activities related to quality of care, performance appraisal, education, collegiality, ethics, collaboration, research, and resource utilization (ANA, 1997).

STANDARDS OF CLINICAL NURSING PRACTICE

Standards of Care
- I. Assessment
- II. Diagnosis
- III. Outcome Identification
- IV. Planning
- V. Implementation
- VI. Evaluation

Standards of Professional Performance
- I. Quality of Care
- II. Performance Appraisal
- III. Education
- IV. Collegiality
- V. Ethics
- VI. Collaboration
- VII. Research
- VIII. Resource Utilization

Data from American Nurses Association. (1997). *Standards of clinical nursing practice* (2nd ed.). Kearneysville, WV: American Nurses Publishing.

These definitions of standards clearly delineate the role of standards as setting a competent level of care or performance. This is a significant change that was first noted in the 1991 standards and marked a significant departure from previous standards that were designed to describe excellence and were not intended to define minimum levels of nursing care or legal parameters for measuring the quality of care. Each of the standards of nursing practice includes criteria that will allow them to be measured. These criteria are relevant, measurable indicators of the standard. The framework was developed with the belief that standards are anticipated to remain relatively stable over time but that the criteria may change over time because of advancements in knowledge and technology.

This model for standards deletes the use of the structure, process, and outcome format frequently used in the past. The deletion of this format does not negate the importance of structure, process, and outcome attributes in evaluating quality of care (Donabedian, 1988). *Structure* attributes are those related to the setting in which the care occurs. What had previously been labeled as structure criteria are more appropriate as separate standards related to the administrative domain. *Process* reflects what is done in giving and receiving care and thus in this framework is reflected both in the standards and within guidelines. *Outcomes* reflect the effects of care and are patient/client-focused. Outcomes are more appropriately included as part of guidelines for practice.

The framework was intended to be a model for development of standards of clinical practice for specialty areas of practice. Differentiation among specialty areas of practice could be accomplished by developing criteria that reflected the common level of performance for nurses practicing in a given specialty area for each of the standards. The specialty area standards of practice would be congruent with the intent, format, and scope of the general standards of clinical nursing practice. Thus, the standards would not change, but the criteria will change to reflect the specialty area of practice, in essence creating standards of practice for that specialty area. As specialty areas of practice are revising standards, this approach is being used. The specialty areas of community health, dermatology, gerontology, home health, otorhinolaryngology, oncology, psychiatric-mental health, public health, rehabilitation, respiratory, and school health nursing are among those that have adopted the ANA model for the development of standards of practice.

Although many specialty groups have adopted this model, it has not been universally adopted. The American Society of Plastic and Reconstructive Surgical Nurses (Hackett, 1997) have used some of the components of the framework, such as differentiating between standards of care and standards of professional performance, using similar terms to describe each standard, and adapting the definitions found in the ANA standards. However, different language is used to describe each standard, and rather than use criteria for each standard they have developed an outcome statement that seems to include many of the criteria found for similar standards in the ANA standards. The Intravenous Nurses Society is an example of a specialty area in nursing that uses a different approach to standards of practice (Intravenous Nurses Society, 1998). The standards include 84 areas of practice and establish guidelines for competence in each of those areas. This approach is more consistent with the past requirements of the Joint Commission on Accreditation of Healthcare Organizations for identification of standards for high-frequency or high-risk areas of practice.

If specialty areas of practice develop standards using different definitions, intents, or formats, the strength of the model's application in providing a framework by which to evaluate the quality of nursing across settings and areas is weakened. Communication between nurses and others is also complicated by the different meanings associated with standards of professional nursing practice.

One area in which the model has expanded is into the area of advanced practice. The first advanced practice standards using the framework were published for the acute care nurse practitioner (ANA & American Association of Critical-Care Nurses, 1995). In 1996 the ANA completed a collaborative effort with specialty nursing organizations with the publication of advanced practice standards that followed the same framework and approach used for the generalist standards of practice (ANA, 1996). In addition to setting standards for the acute care nurse practitioner, this model has been used to describe the practice of advanced practice nurses in rehabilitation.

Guidelines

In contrast to standards the purpose of guidelines is to describe a process of patient/client care management that has the potential of improving the quality of clinical and consumer decision making. The goal of guidelines is to describe a recommended course of action to address a specific nursing diagnosis, clinical condition, or the needs of a particular patient/client population. Guidelines guide practice by providing linkages among diagnoses, treatments, and outcomes and describing available alternatives.

This approach to guidelines has similarities with previous work done within nursing and has in the past also been referred to as "standards." This is most commonly reflected in the standardized care plan approach to planning and providing nursing care. Both approaches attempted to describe a course of action to address a specific need or diagnosis. Both approaches also have the potential to reduce variation in clinical practice.

However, there are some significant differences in the approaches. One of the major differences is in the change in terminology from standards to guidelines. Standards in health care are commonly interpreted from a legal perspective as being written documents that are intended to be applied rigidly and to be followed in virtually all cases. Exceptions to following a standard would be rare and difficult to justify. In addition, standards are considered to be the foundation for safe health provider practices and not following these standards would indicate unsafe and incompetent practice. Guidelines are recommendations for patient management and may include a range of interventions or strategies, and as such, would not meet the characteristics just described. Another difference is the intent of guidelines to describe alternatives and to assist in decision making. One of the difficulties frequently encountered in practice is the inability to use standardized care plans because of the individual characteristics of the patient or client situation. Standardized plans of care do not account for the complexity and comorbidity frequently present in individuals. The intent of guidelines is to identify those circumstances when it is known that the guideline would need modification in either interventions or expected outcomes or when the guideline would not be appropriate.

Guidelines convert science-based knowledge into clinical action in a form accessible to practitioners. They reflect knowledge generated through research or professional consensus by practitioners regarding preferred interventions for a particular problem or select group of patients/clients. Guidelines have the potential for decreasing variability in practice by providing nurses and other providers with a synthesis of published information that can decrease the amount of professional uncertainty that occurs in making diagnosis and treatment decisions.

The development of guidelines is occurring in many arenas. The Agency for Health Care Policy and Research (AHCPR and renamed the Agency for Healthcare Research and Quality [AHRQ] in 1999) devoted considerable resources to developing 19 multidisciplinary guidelines. All of the guidelines developed by AHCPR included at least one nurse as a member of the panel developing the guideline. Several guidelines released by AHCPR focused on clinical conditions where nursing makes a significant contribution to the care and outcomes of individuals experiencing those problems (e.g., acute pain management, cancer pain management, prediction and prevention of pressure ulcers, treatment of pressure ulcers, and incontinence). AHRQ is no longer coordinating the development of guidelines. Its role in evidence-based practice was redefined to keep relevant information in the public domain, serve as an impartial, neutral broker, encourage multidisciplinary input to all projects, advocate for patient perspectives and needs, and protect special populations. It now has three major components, Evidence-Based Practice Centers, an on-line National Guideline Clearinghouse (http://www.guideline.gov), and a program of product research and evaluation.

To assist nursing specialty groups and other nursing groups, the ANA published a manual describing a process that could be used in the development of clinical practice guidelines (Marek, 1995). As nursing groups become involved in the development of guidelines, the following issues should be considered in choosing a topic for guideline development: nursing's contribution to the care of the client; variation in nursing interventions and outcomes; impact of the clinical condition on the client's physical, psychological, and social functioning; costs of caring for the client with the clinical condition and variation in those costs; high incidence or prevalence of the clinical condition; and extent of the research base. Once these questions have been answered, the scope of the guideline must be identified and the client/patient population, care settings, assessment criteria, interventions, outcomes, and the intended audience for the guideline must be defined.

In the development of practice guidelines, certain characteristics should be taken into consideration to maximize their usefulness. First, they should be reasonable in view of the state of the art. Interventions and outcomes described within a practice guideline should be possible and not developed in a way that makes them unreasonable to implement or achieve. They should be comprehensible or able to be understood by nurses, other health care providers, and consumers. They must be measurable or able to be evaluated, and they must be validated by research or professional consensus. The process for reviewing and updating guidelines will need to be a dynamic one so that guidelines can reflect changes in knowledge and technological capabilities.

From the early stages in the discussion of how professional nursing organizations should be involved in guideline development, the course has not been as clear and consistent as it has been with the development of standards. It is clear that the development of guidelines by professional nursing organizations would take considerable organizational resources.

Nursing organizations have actively participated in the development of multidisciplinary guidelines coordinated by other organizations. An example of this is the participation by the American Association of Spinal Cord Injury Nurses and the Association of Rehabilitation Nurses in the development of guidelines focusing on the treatment of autonomic dysreflexia (Consortium for Spinal Cord Medicine, 1997a) and prevention of thromboembolism (Consortium for Spinal Cord Medicine, 1997b) in individuals with a spinal cord injury. These guidelines were developed by the Consortium for Spinal Cord Medicine that includes representation from 17 organizations representing the interdisciplinary treatment team. These guidelines would meet the criteria described above.

Many professional nursing organizations are involved with a variety of projects and initiatives to promote and encourage evidence-based practice. More than 30 organizations, many of them nursing organizations, have joined together to create and sponsor The Best Practice Network (http://www.best4health.org). This network is devoted to providing a mechanism to encourage and recognize the development and use of best practices. To date, despite the continuing focus on evidence-based practice, no professional nursing organization has completed the development of a guideline that would meet the definition and characteristics described. The Association of Rehabilitation Nurses has begun work on a guideline that will focus on management of bowel elimination problems. This is in contrast to the expectations at the time the model for professional nursing standards and guidelines was developed. Organizational representatives that participated in the development of the model were very encouraging in their assessment that collaborative development of practice guidelines was a realistic goal. Perhaps part of the reason that guidelines have not been developed by professional nursing organizations is the realization by all groups involved that it is a complex, expensive process if it is to be done well. The U.S. General Accounting Office (1991) reported that in a review of 35 medical specialty societies it was found that guideline development generally took from 1 to 3 years and that costs ranged from $5,000 to $130,000 per guideline and did not reflect the volunteer time of members to develop the guideline.

It has also become clear that most health care practices have no basis in published scientific research. It has been suggested that this may be true of 80% to 90% of common practices (James, 1995). The use of published scientific research is a cornerstone of well-developed guidelines. This may be another reason why the development of guidelines by professional nursing organizations is not occurring.

The new model developed collaboratively by the ANA and more than 30 specialty nursing organizations makes clear distinctions between standards and guidelines for practice. These distinctions in intent and definition are important in determining the appropriate use of standards and guidelines. However, they are both equally important in evaluating nursing practice and the quality of care provided. Standards of clinical nursing practice provide a framework to evaluate the individual professional nurse's overall performance. Guidelines provide a means to evaluate the quality of nursing care provided to a specific patient or patient population. Components of the standards of care should be embedded within guidelines. Within a guideline should be information about assessment, diagnosis, outcome identification, planning, implementation, and evaluation of that specific diagnosis or clinical condition.

USE OF STANDARDS AND GUIDELINES IN PRACTICE

Standards of nursing practice and practice guidelines can serve as the basis for many activities within nursing (Dean-Baar, 1993; Taylor, 1994). Nationally published guidelines and standards can be used in the development of agency-specific documents. Guidelines can serve as the basis for the development of agency-specific policies and procedures. They are being used to develop clinical pathways (Brandt, 1994; Duncan & Otto, 1995). Guidelines also can be used to promote patient/client participation in health care decision making by clarifying health care choices (including choice of practitioner) and their consequences for the patient/client.

The standards of clinical nursing practice are being used to develop job descriptions and performance appraisal systems that support quality professional practice. In those agencies with clinical or career ladders the standards can serve as the framework for the initial stage of the ladder, with additional stages reflecting increased expectations for practice.

The components of standards embedded in guidelines can be used in conjunction with the Nursing Minimum Data Set (Werley & Lang, 1988) to develop database systems that can provide valuable information on the quality of nursing care. They also could be used to serve as the basis for including relevant nursing information in large database systems such as the Health Care Finance Administration. The inclusion of elements in databases that reflect nursing's contributions to patient/client care can make it clearer that nursing should be included in discussions of cost and payment for providing health care services.

Perhaps the most important area where standards and guidelines are used is in the area of quality improvement. Standards and guidelines can be used to develop institution-, agency-, or unit-based quality programs that demonstrate that the organization is delivering safe, effective, and appropriate care. Written, meaningful standards and guidelines are essential to developing quality improvement programs. They can serve as the basis for quality improvement systems by identifying important aspects of performance or care within either the standards or a specific guideline. These aspects can be used to identify indicators of quality nursing care that are then monitored. The AHCPR has described how to translate clinical practice guidelines into evaluation tools and how to use those tools to evaluate the quality of care provided (AHCPR, 1995a, 1995b). The data collected can be used to improve the quality of care provided.

In the area of evaluating nursing's performance in relation to professional standards, organizations can use the standards of practice and the criteria for each standard to develop their own indicators and make decisions about how and what data should be collected to determine the degree to which the standard is being met. Because of the framework's ability to include general and specialty areas of practice, an institution or agency could utilize the same approach as the framework in developing its program. This approach provides for many possibilities and includes the ability to evaluate practice not only within an agency but also across agencies.

If nursing uses the standards of clinical practice and practice guidelines to develop quality improvement programs, the potential of being able to demonstrate clearly the contribution of nursing in providing quality care within that setting would be considerable. As health care becomes increasingly competitive, information on quality becomes even more valuable than in the past.

THE FUTURE OF STANDARDS IN NURSING

It has been almost a decade since the nursing profession adopted a new framework for standards of practice and almost 30 years since the first standards of professional

practice were published. A review of recent literature reveals that the profession has not universally adopted the framework. There is also scant discussion in the literature about the use and role of professional standards in shaping professional practice. Perhaps it is time to reconsider the conceptual base that has been used to describe professional practice in the current framework. The development of the current framework in the early 1990s does seem to have addressed some of the concerns that were raised about the usefulness of standards to describe professional practice. The lack of discussion in the literature might suggest, however, that the standards are still not seen as relevant and useful in describing professional nursing practice.

The framework for standards of professional nursing practice continues to be based on the use of the nursing process. The debate about the usefulness of this approach appears to be gathering momentum. Pesut and Herman (1999) argue that the development of clinical reasoning in nursing has evolved to a point that new models of reasoning are necessary. The development of classification systems to describe the advances in nursing diagnosis, nursing interventions, and nursing-sensitive patient outcomes are all indications of the need for a new model of clinical reasoning. One major purpose of standards of professional practice is to describe the overarching process that nurses use in their practice. The science of our discipline may be leading us to a new understanding of the process we use in our practice. The developing knowledge about the process we use may result in the need to change the conceptual basis of our professional standards.

SUMMARY

Standards of clinical nursing practice and guidelines for practice have been considered essential to professional nursing practice. They are one mechanism that we use to describe and define the scope of professional nursing practice. Standards and guidelines can make a difference but not if the profession continues to be inconsistent in their development, definition, and use. As the standards of clinical nursing practice are implemented and work continues on the development and implementation of practice guidelines, we must create ways to translate this work in a manner that will assist in articulating the contributions of professional nursing practice to the health and well-being of patients and clients.

It appears that the benefits of a framework for standards and guidelines that was developed collaboratively among professional nursing organizations have not been as great as had been hoped for. It does become clearer every day, however, that the ability to speak with one voice about the role of standards and guidelines in describing our practice and our contributions to the outcomes of patients and clients is essential. The future ability to have a common definition of "standard" and "guideline" that can be fully embraced and used may require the profession to reexamine the underlying conceptual framework. Engaging in this discussion may help to articulate clearly the critical role that nursing plays in the planning and delivering of quality, appropriate, and effective health care.

REFERENCES

Agency for Health Care Policy and Research. (1995a). *Using clinical practice guidelines to evaluate quality of care* (Vol. 1: Issue). AHCPR Publication No. 95-0045. Rockville, MD: Author.

Agency for Health Care Policy and Research. (1995b). *Using clinical practice guidelines to evaluate quality of care* (Vol. 2: Methodology). AHCPR Publication No. 95-0046. Rockville, MD: Author.

American Nurses Association. (1975). *A plan for implementation of standards of nursing practice.* Kansas City: Author.

American Nurses Association. (1991a). Task force on nursing practice standards and guidelines: Working paper. *Journal of Nursing Care Quality, 5*(3), 1-17.

American Nurses Association. (1991b). *Standards of clinical nursing practice.* Washington, DC: Author.

American Nurses Association. (1996). *Scope and standards of advanced practice registered nursing.* Washington, DC: Author.

American Nurses Association. (1997). *Standards of clinical nursing practice* (2nd ed.). Kearneysville, WV: American Nurses Publishing.

American Nurses Association & American Association of Critical-Care Nurses. (1995). *Standards of clinical practice and scope of practice for the acute care nurse practitioner.* Washington, DC: American Nurses Association.

Brandt, M. (1994). Clinical practice guidelines and critical paths—roadmaps to quality, cost-effective care (Part II). *Journal of American Health Information Management Association, 65*(2), 54-57.

Consortium for Spinal Cord Medicine. (1997a). *Acute management of autonomic dysreflexia: Adults with spinal cord injury presenting to health-care facilities.* Washington, DC: Paralyzed Veterans of America.

Consortium for Spinal Cord Medicine. (1997b). *Prevention of thromboembolism in spinal cord injury.* Washington, DC: Paralyzed Veterans of America.

Dean-Baar, S. (1993). Application of the new ANA framework for nursing practice standards and guidelines. *Journal of Nursing Care Quality, 8*(1), 33-42.

Donabedian, A. (1988). The quality of care: How can it be assessed? *Journal of the American Medical Association, 260*(12), 1743-1748.

Duncan, S.K., & Otto, S.E. (1995). Implementing guidelines for acute pain management. *Nursing Management, 26*(5), 40-47.

Hackett, P. (1997). Standards of clinical practice for plastic surgical nursing. *Plastic Surgical Nursing, 17*(1), 23-25, 29-32.

Intravenous Nurses Society. (1998). Intravenous nursing: Standards of practice. *Journal of Intravenous Nursing, 21*(15), S1-S91.

James, B.C. (1995). Implementing practice guidelines through clinical quality improvement. In N.O. Graham (Ed.), *Quality in health care: Theory, application, and evolution* (pp. 157-187). Gaithersburg, MD: Aspen.

Marek, K. (1995). *Manual to develop guidelines.* Washington, DC: American Nurses Association.

McGuffin, B., & Mariani, M. (1990). Clinical nursing standards: Toward a synthesis. *Journal of Nursing Quality Assurance, 4*(3), 35-45.

Pesut, D.J., & Herman, J. (1999). *Clinical reasoning: The art and science of critical and creative thinking.* Albany, NY: Delmar.

Schroeder, P. (1991). *Approaches to nursing standards.* Gaithersburg, MD: Aspen.

Smith, T.C., & Popovich, J.M. (1993). Health care standards: The interstitial matter of quality programs. *Journal of Nursing Care Quality, 8*(1), 1-11.

Taylor, J.W. (1994). *Implementation of nursing practice standards and guidelines.* Washington, DC: American Nurses Association.

U.S. General Accounting Office. (1991). *Practice guidelines—The experience of medical specialty societies* (Publication PEMD-91-11). Washington, DC: Author.

Werley, H., & Lang, N. (Eds.). (1988). *Identification of the nursing minimum data set.* New York: Springer.

The Use of Clinical Pathways

Do They Improve Quality?

SUSAN PARK KYZER

The concept of clinical pathways has been evolving over the past decade. Very appropriate to the title of this viewpoint chapter, the idea for clinical pathways was born out of a concern for quality of care (Zander, 1991b). Although the concept has been used successfully for cost containment, clinical pathways would not have achieved the robust health they enjoy today had they not also held the key to maintaining quality. Economic necessity has forced everyone involved in health care to become cost-conscious. However, the heart of health care must not be moved from its focus on quality of care for the patient and family.

In 1983 one of the most dramatic changes in modern health care occurred with the enactment of the diagnosis-related group (DRG) legislation. Faced with the first external control of care delivery, the Nursing Department of the New England Medical Center determined to "address the demand to incorporate patient-centered, quality nursing care within the context of DRG's, length of stay and cost-effectiveness" (Zander, 1985). The clinical systems that evolved from that determination—case management plans, critical pathways, and then fully developed clinical pathway systems—require that three questions be answered. These questions aim for the root of providing quality health care: (1) What work is required to get patients within certain case types to desired outcomes? (2) What is the best way to produce these outcomes? (3) Who is accountable for the results? (Zander & McGill, 1994). These basic questions are as relevant today as they were in 1983.

DEFINITIONS

A *clinical pathway* is a multidisciplinary plan for patient care that sequences interventions and clinical outcomes on a timeline (Zander, 1991a). Clinical pathways are developed for homogeneous patient populations and are uniquely different from traditional care plans in the following ways:

• Clinical pathways are multidisciplinary, and therefore truly represent patient care plans rather than nursing care plans.

• A multidisciplinary team is formed to author the clinical pathway; therefore, care is planned in an interrelated, more comprehensive fashion and reflects the care as experienced by the patient rather than by each discipline's separate focus.

• The interventions are planned on a timeline, thereby providing shift-to-shift and day-to-day continuity and coordination of the activities needed to move the patient toward desired outcomes.

• Anticipated clinical outcomes statements at key points on the timeline assist clinicians in evaluating the clinical progress of patients (even if "This is my first day back" or "I was pulled and don't usually work with this kind of patient"), thereby focusing the caregiving team on patient outcomes of care rather than on task completion only.

• Clinical pathways are written for the environment in which the work is done by a team of expert clinicians who will be using them, thereby creating a plan of care that uniquely reflects the resources and working patterns that exist in that delivery setting.

Quality of care has been defined by a working group of the Institute of Medicine as "the degree to which health services for individuals and populations increase the likelihood of desired health outcomes and are consistent with current professional knowledge" (Mitchell, 1993). Traditionally, quality has been measured by negatives such as morbidity and mortality, unexpected returns to surgery, nosocomial infections, iatrogenic complications, and readmission rates. This level of measurement "in essence, quantifies what went wrong in patient care" (Nash, 1993). However, the absence of "something going wrong," while important, does not necessarily equate to quality care. The focus is now shifting to more positive quality measures such as "survival, clinical condition-specific endpoints, health status (physiological, psychological and emotional health), functional status, general well-being and satisfaction with care" (Mitchell, 1993). Increased consistency, continuity, and coordination of care as well as interdisciplinary collaboration are factors underlying improved quality for patients and families. Based on the previous definitions of a clinical pathway and quality of care the view expressed here is that quality of care can be improved by the development and use of clinical pathways.

IMPROVING QUALITY OF CARE

Quality of care can be improved at each step in the process of developing and implementing a clinical pathway for a specific population of patients: during the initial process of clinical pathway development, as the clinical pathway content is written, as clinicians use the pathway to guide patient care, and as data generated from use of the pathway are reviewed and evaluated and changes made to further improve care. There are many specific examples of improved quality that have occurred in various settings in relation to each of these steps.

Quality of care is often improved during the initial process of clinical pathway development. One of the first steps in writing a clinical pathway is bringing together a team of expert clinicians who are involved in caring for a specific patient population (i.e., case-type). This in itself is an exciting event because it is often the first time all of the people involved in caring for these patients are able to sit down together to talk about all of the aspects of that care. This team meeting provides a structure and a time for examining system issues and problems from a patient outcome focus. Caregivers get to know one another and understand each others' disciplines better, think of ways to smooth out communications and coordination of care, and begin to form cooperative and collaborative relationships, thereby enabling them to work toward the same outcomes.

On an orthopedic unit, for example, nurses routinely required patients with total hip replacements to sit up for lunch after their morning physical therapy. During the clinical pathway development meeting it came to light

that frequently the afternoon physical therapy session accomplished little as a result of patient fatigue. After some discussion, the unit nursing staff changed their routine and began allowing patients to rest after the morning session. Patients were then able to take better advantage of their afternoon physical therapy sessions. Instead of nursing and physical therapy attempting to obtain a certain level of patient activity individually, they became aware of each others' routines and developed a plan that would best assist the patients in reaching their desired clinical outcomes.

Quality of care can be improved as the content of the clinical pathway is written. These improvements may include better sequencing and timing of interventions, care that is based on current professional knowledge, care that is planned from a patient focus, and better coordination and continuity of care from setting to setting. Following are examples of these improvements.

In planning care for patients with elective total hip replacement the clinical outcome desired was early ambulation in order to prevent deep vein thrombosis, pneumonia, and urinary tract infection. In discussing how soon patients could be expected to ambulate, one problem identified by the physical therapist was the difficulty in teaching patients with postoperative pain to use a walker. It was decided that a physical therapist would see these patients for walker training prior to surgery when this new skill could be mastered without the added distraction of postoperative pain. The altered sequence of events involving a physical therapy consult prior to rather than after surgery resulted in earlier ambulation for this group of patients.

In another group of patients, digoxin levels were drawn routinely at 6 a.m., medication administered at 9 a.m., and reports from morning blood draws posted at 10 a.m., resulting in a day's delay in adjusting medication dosages. When unit staff and laboratory personnel realized that their respective routines were not really focused on the patients, adjustments in timing were made so that results were posted and dosages adjusted prior to the administration of morning medications.

During a team meeting to develop a clinical pathway for cesarean section, a discussion took place regarding the appropriate prophylactic intravenous antibiotic to use. The physicians at the meeting agreed that research would support the use of any one of several first-generation antibiotics, and were quite surprised when the pharmacist reported that many of their colleagues were routinely using third-generation antibiotics for this purpose, contrary to published recommendations. Using the clinical pathway process, the hospital was able to standardize a more appropriate treatment choice among the physicians.

In another example, after establishing a preadmission testing program for elective hip replacement patients, the clinical pathway team examined the provision of care from the patient's perspective. They realized that patients (who usually were experiencing pain on walking already) were being required to go to seven different departments, some of them quite distant from one another, to complete the preadmission program. Further changes were made so that patients could remain in one location to complete all testing. This decreased the average time a patient spent at the preadmission visit from several hours to about 1 hour. Patient and family satisfaction increased dramatically.

The Hospital Association of New York State has developed a model that "extends beyond the acute-care hospital stay in both directions. They (the pathways) begin with pre-admission and continue through post-discharge" (Causey, 1992). The entire episode is included, resulting in well-coordinated continuity of care.

These examples illustrate simple changes that are not difficult to make once the problems have been identified but obviously improve quality of care. The process of getting clinicians together to discuss the kind of continual quality care they would like to deliver produces these kinds of changes. Interdisciplinary collaboration is increased as clinicians get to know one another, begin to appreciate each other's viewpoints, and work together with patient outcomes as the primary focus. Not only is formal collaboration increased (e.g., in team meetings and interdisciplinary rounds) but informal collaboration is also increased, on the phone, at the bedside, and in day-to-day activities. According to Lord, "For pathways to become truly meaningful, you need to define and design the process for the continuum of care—beginning with the patient's entry into the health care system, not just the component that's delivered in the hospital" (Lumsdon & Hagland, 1993). More and more hospitals, physician offices, outpatient settings, and home care agencies are joining together to do just that—plan care from a patient's perspective so that desired outcomes can be identified, achieved, and measured for the entire episode of care across the continuum.

Quality of care is improved as clinicians use the pathway to provide continuity of plan. Creative staffing patterns, more part-time workers, flexible staffing, float pool and agency staff use, and increased use of contract staff for therapies all contribute to the loss of continuity of caregiver; and therefore it is extremely important to maximize continuity of care planning. A clinical pathway provides continuity of plan from shift to shift and from day to day even as caregivers change (Flynn & Kilgallen, 1993). Having a tool that displays the patient's progress visually and states key outcomes to evaluate greatly assists caregivers. When a patient has not met the intermediate outcomes for a particular time interval, caregivers are alerted to look for corrective actions that can help the patient continue to make progress. As a result, care is more proactive and problems are recognized earlier. Details of care that might sometimes be missed or forgotten appear on the clinical pathway to serve as a "cueing mechanism" for staff. Care is complex, and varies from patient to patient; if the essential components of care are not blueprinted they may be forgotten or not done on time. As a result, patient outcomes may be jeopardized (Campbell, 1992).

For example, a dietitian might say, "The drug-food interactions are done before I arrive!" Tasks like this no longer "fall through the cracks" as accountabilities are clarified and the clinical pathway structures the total care. Another problem with regard to the timing of administration of intravenous prophylactic antibiotics prior to surgery was eliminated by listing the time frame and the person (position) responsible for administration of the medication on the pathway. This clarified who was accountable for this procedure and provided the means to track success in meeting the specified time frame.

Another example is that of a patient who is on "post-op day 3" of a total hip clinical pathway. The anticipated intermediate outcome is "Ambulates with assistance 10 feet," but the patient is unable to accomplish this outcome. Prior to having the clinical pathway, staff would not have been particularly focused on evaluating ambulation at this point, but because this has been identified as a key outcome the nurse and physical therapist will discuss the situation and try to determine the reason. Is the patient's inability to walk a result of excessive pain? Is the problem nausea or weakness? What about the hematocrit? Depending on the situation and the answer to these and other questions the caregivers will decide whether there are any corrective actions that can be taken or whether there is a need to involve other members of the health care team. Noting the patient's lack of progression and early intervention promote accomplishing the desired outcomes.

Quality of care is improved as clinicians review data generated by aggregating variance from the clinical pathway over a period of time. The clinical pathway represents the pattern of care and the desire patient outcomes. By measuring how care actually progresses against what is planned, both process and outcome are evaluated. Looking at achievement of outcomes for groups of patients over a period of time can reveal where the plan is working and where improvements can be made.

For example, a clinical pathway for bowel resection has as a postoperative outcome of "Bowel sounds present." A quarterly aggregation and analysis of data from this pathway showed that a number of patients did not achieve the stated outcome during the appropriate time interval and experienced ileus. Further investigation revealed that preoperative bowel preparations were being started too late in the day and therefore were not finished completely. An adjustment of routines and attention to starting and completing the bowel preparations appropriately resulted in a decreased incidence of ileus during the next quarter for bowel resection patients. In another example,

> When statistical analysis found that patients with dysphagia were prone to develop pneumonia, changes were instituted: "Now the nurse assesses the patient's gag reflex and swallowing on admission. If dysphagia is suspected, the patient is made NPO, and the physician and other team members are notified." . . . The new protocol for dysphagia has reduced complications and length of stay. [Luquire, 1994]

When data are generated in a systematic, ongoing fashion, evaluated, and changes made based on that data, improvement efforts are more likely to be directed at real rather than spurious issues. A clinical pathway and its associated measurement data provide a logical, methodical approach to quality improvement that is specific to patient populations and is supported by clinicians who really understand the problems.

RESULTS OF CLINICAL PATHWAYS WITH REGARD TO TRADITIONAL QUALITY MEASURES

Traditional quality measures of mortality, morbidity, readmission rates, complication rates, and patient satisfaction, while not the whole story, certainly cannot be overlooked. Here are some examples of the results of established clinical pathway systems.

• In a study done at the Toronto Hospital in Ontario, elderly patients with a fractured hip who were managed with a clinical pathway (CareMap) statistically had a significantly better outcome at 6 months and fewer postoperative complications, and a greater number of the patients returned home within 14 days of admission (Ogilvie-Harris, Botsford, & Hawker, 1993).

• Patients having coronary artery bypass graft surgery without cardiac catheterization at Scripps Memorial Hos-

pital in La Jolla, California, spend less time on average in the intensive care unit and are extubated sooner, improvements that have in turn reduced the incidence of nosocomial pneumonia (Andersson, 1993).

• At Barnes Hospital in St. Louis, Missouri, using the Thoracotomy CarePath®, pulmonary complications such as atelectasis, pneumonia, and respiratory failure were reduced by 50% (Weilitz & Potter, 1993).

• With regard to the chemotherapy CarePath® at Barnes Hospital, "improved communication between the hospital's outpatient cancer center, the pharmacy, and the nursing divisions resulted in chemotherapy drugs arriving on the nursing unit near the time of the patient's admission rather than several hours later. As a result, the hospital achieved greater efficiency in delivering patient care and improved physician and patient satisfaction" (Weilitz & Potter, 1993).

• The conclusion from a study done by Vanderbilt University Medical Center in Nashville, Tennessee, and St. Thomas Hospital on the use of clinical pathways with cerebral revascularization patients states, "The dual approach of case management (clinical pathways) and selective use of the ICU promotes quality patient care, conserves financial resources without adversely affecting morbidity or mortality rates, enhances physician/nurse collaboration, and improves patient satisfaction" (Hoyle et al., 1994).

• At Scripps Memorial Hospital, monitoring of mortality, morbidity, and readmission rates has shown no deterioration in quality outcomes using CareTrac® (Trubo, 1993).

• Using clinical pathways at St. Luke's Episcopal Hospital in Houston, Texas, the readmission rate for neuroscience patients dropped from 5% to 1% (Luquire, 1994).

These are but a few of the published outcomes of the use of clinical pathways. Although much has been written about the use of clinical pathways to reduce length of stay and provide some measure of cost containment, this chapter has focused solely on quality improvement. It is quite evident that the development and use of clinical pathways can be a major quality strategy and that pathways are possibly the most powerful tool health care providers have to maintain and improve quality of care.

REFERENCES

Andersson, D. (1993). Scripps health: Quality planning for clinical processes of care. *The Quality Letter, 5*(8), 2-4.

Campbell, A., & Lakier, N. (1992). Process intervention—applying TQM to clinical care. *Healthcare Forum Journal, 35*(4), 81-83.

Causey, W. (1992). Clinical pathways seen as opportunity to integrate traditional QA with CQI. *Quality Improvement/Total Quality Management, 2*(4), 49-64.

Flynn, A., & Kilgallen, M. (1993). Case management: A multidisciplinary approach to the evaluation of cost and quality standards. *Journal of Nursing Care Quality, 8*(1), 4.

Hoyle, R., Jenkins, M., Edwards, W., Edwards, W., Martin, R., & Mulherin, J. (1994). Case management in cerebral revascularization. *Journal of Vascular Surgery, 20*(3), 396-401.

Lumsdon, K., & Hagland, M. (1993). Mapping care. *Hospitals & Health Networks, 67*(20), 34-40.

Luquire, R. (1994). Focusing on outcomes. *RN, 57*(5), 57-60.

Mitchell, P. (1993). Perspectives on outcome-oriented care systems. *Nursing Administration Quarterly, 17*(3), 4.

Nash, D. (1993). The state of the outcomes/guidelines movement. *Decisions in Imaging Economics,* 11-17.

Ogilvie-Harris, D., Botsford, D., & Hawker, R. (1993). Elderly patients with hip fractures: Improved outcome with the use of CareMaps with high-quality medical and nursing protocols. *Journal of Orthopaedic Trauma, 7*(5), 428-437.

Trubo, R. (1993). If this is cookbook medicine, you may like it. *Medical Economics, 70*(5), 69-82.

Weilitz, P., & Potter, P. (1993). A managed care system: Financial and clinical evaluation. *Journal of Nursing Administration, 23*(11), 51-57.

Zander, K. (1985). Defining nursing . . . roots and wings. *Definition, 1,* 2.

Zander, K. (1991a). CareMaps: The core of cost/quality care. *The New Definition, 6*(3).

Zander, K. (1991b). Critical pathways. In M. Mellum & M. Sinoris (Eds.), *Total quality management* (pp. 305-314). Chicago: American Hospital Association Publishing, Inc.

Zander, K., & McGill, R. (1994). Critical and anticipated recovery paths: Only the beginning. *Nursing Management, 25*(8), 34.

Outcomes Management for Quality Improvement

MARITA G. TITLER

The capacity to consistently analyze the outcomes of care is a critical element in management of health care organizations. Attention to outcomes management has increased as competition for services escalates. As health care organizations respond to cost pressures, the need to demonstrate to various audiences the delivery of high quality care is essential. Thus, health care systems are placing more emphasis on outcomes management as a key driving force in developing market strategies, developing new services, refining existing services, and allocating resources (Howell, 1999). Despite the resources dedicated to outcomes management, it is still difficult to describe empirically to administrators and policy makers the contributions of nursing practice to patient outcomes.

OVERVIEW OF OUTCOMES MANAGEMENT

Outcomes management includes the selection and assessment of patient outcomes and use of these data for improvement of patient care at the individual, unit, department, organization, or health care system level. Outcomes management is multidimensional as individual practitioners want to know that their care makes a difference, accrediting bodies want evidence of quality of care provided for the interest groups they represent, payers want to know what they are getting for the money spent, patients and families want to make informed choices regarding treatment options and provider services, and health care organizations want to benchmark their performance with others (Hill, 1999). Thus, outcomes management requires linkages between the processes of care (e.g., medical treatments, nursing treatments, treatments by other health care professionals) and the outcomes achieved. Although outcomes are the end results of treatments, the setting in which the treatments are delivered and the demographic and clinical characteristics of the

patient, such as age and comorbidity, also influence outcomes (Kane, 1997a).

Numerous publications address outcomes management including the selection and measurement of outcomes, analysis of outcome data, translating analyzed data into information for decision making, disseminating the information to appropriate administrators and clinical staff, and using the outcome information for quality improvement (Aiken, Sochalski, & Lake, 1997; Havens & Aiken, 1999; Kane, 1997c; Kirchhoff & Rakel, 1999; Lamb-Havard, 1997; Lepper & Titler, 1999; Mandelblatt et al., 1996; Mark, Salyer, & Geddes, 1997; Mitchell, Shannon, Cain, & Hegyvary, 1996; Nadzam & Nelson, 1997; Peters, Cowley, & Standiford, 1999; Schalock, 1995; Scott, Sochalski, & Aiken, 1999; Stonestreet & Prevost, 1997; Strickland, 1997; Titler et al., 1999; Titler & Reiter, 1994). Although it is beyond the scope of this chapter to address all issues inherent in outcomes management, several important steps are discussed when outcomes management is used as a method of quality improvement. These steps are an iterative process and are used to explicate the following viewpoint:

Many outcomes management initiatives focus on medical treatments with little attention to nursing care. Physicians document services rendered and patient outcomes through use of standardized coding schemas without detailing the contributions of treatments of other health care providers such as nurses. Nursing treatments are not accounted for in these coding schemas and thus are difficult to incorporate into outcomes management programs. This is peculiar, since much of health care is nursing care. Thus, the contributions of nursing care to patient outcomes remain essentially invisible and empirically unaccounted for in outcomes management initiatives. Until a standardized nursing language is used to document nursing treatments, nurses' ability to empirically describe the contributions of nursing care to specific patient outcomes will be limited.

DELINEATE THE PURPOSE

The first step in outcomes management is to be clear about the purpose and questions being addressed by the outcomes initiative. For example, the purpose may be to measure and manage outcomes from an organizational perspective, which necessitates selecting outcomes that are applicable across settings, sites of care, and patient populations. In contrast, the purpose may be to manage outcomes for a specific type of patient population such as those treated for heart failure or diabetes. Using outcomes wisely to manage care requires being clear about the question that is being asked and the factors that are likely to influence the answer (Kane, 1997a). Questions to think about in defining the purpose are:

- What is the major question being addressed by the outcomes initiative? Is the purpose to address and improve systems of care from an organizational perspective? Is the purpose to improve care processes for a specific high volume patient population? Is the purpose to evaluate and modify care delivered to individual patients? These questions focus on addressing the level of analysis for which the outcome is assessed: individual, nursing care unit, patient population, organization, or provider of service.
- What processes of care are the focus? How will the data be used to improve processes of care? These questions address what health care treatments will be the focus of the outcomes management initiative. The processes of care may focus on medical treatments, nursing treatments, treatments by other health care providers, or clinical programs of care such as a phase II cardiac rehabilitation program.
- Who will use the outcomes management report(s): nurses, physicians, administrators, nurse managers, case managers, third party payers?
- How will the outcomes management initiative be integrated into the quality improvement process? Does a specific outcomes management initiative replace or complement existing quality improvement initiatives?

Answering the above questions helps to solidify the major purpose of the outcomes management initiative and the context for defining and collecting the outcomes. For example, if the purposes of the initiative are to monitor a core set of organizational outcomes for decreasing cost and length of stay and increasing the market share of the health care system, the types of outcomes measured may include variables such as patient satisfaction, mortality, cost per case or unit of service, nosocomial infec-

tion rates, and adverse events such as falls, pressure ulcers, and medication errors. In comparison, an outcomes management initiative for patients with heart failure may include factors such as health status, satisfaction with the heart center services, symptoms of angina and dyspnea, and biophysical indicators such as cardiac output.

Outcomes management programs that focus solely on organizational performance run the risk of omitting outcomes that are sensitive to nursing care, making it difficult to identify the processes of care responsible for achieving the outcomes. Therefore, it is my viewpoint that outcomes management programs that focus on organizational performance must be supplemented with outcomes initiatives that are patient population specific or nursing treatment specific or that focus on care in a specific nursing unit in order to provide useful data for making improvements in practice.

The purpose and questions asked in outcomes management initiatives are traditionally driven by a medical model because electronic data sources are available that have standardized physician coding schemas for medical diagnoses and medical treatments. It is easy to determine the high-volume patient groups cared for in any organization by asking for an analysis of the medical record abstract database delineating high-volume diagnosis-related groups (DRGs) and high-volume *International Classification of Diseases, Ninth Revision (ICD-9)* diagnostic codes. If nursing care were documented electronically using standardized nursing language, such as the Nursing Interventions Classification System (McCloskey & Bulechek, 2000), outcomes management initiatives could focus on high-volume or high-cost nursing treatments. It would then be possible to determine the most frequently used nursing treatments by age, by patient care unit, and by patient group. A high-volume nursing treatment could then be the focus of an outcomes management initiative. For example, vital signs monitoring is an intervention frequently performed by nursing staff in the acute care setting. It is not well understood that the frequency of vital signs monitoring should be dictated by how critical the patient's condition is. Nurses could be performing this intervention too frequently on patients who do not require the intervention and not frequently enough on others who may benefit from earlier detection of an adverse physiological sequelae. An outcomes management initiative focused on vital signs monitoring and related patient outcomes within a patient population such as heart failure, or within a specific nursing care unit, may provide more meaningful data for improving nursing care delivery. Perhaps consumers, payers, and administrators would be better served if outcomes management programs selected high-volume or high-cost nursing treatments as a focus for outcomes management initiatives. Similarly, use of standardized nursing treatment language would capture the nursing treatments, as well as medical treatments used with specific patient populations, thereby making it possible to describe the contributions of nursing treatments to patient outcomes.

Use of nursing treatments to guide outcomes management would also prove useful in deciphering the meaning of organizational outcomes that are sensitive to nursing treatments. For example, if organizational outcomes data demonstrate a higher than desired rate of falls, the electronic patient record could be accessed to determine if those who fell received the fall-prevention intervention and the types of patients who received the fall-prevention intervention who did not fall. This would provide a focus for an outcomes initiative that (1) determines those at risk for falls and (2) implementing the fall-prevention intervention for those at risk.

Similarly, outcomes management initiatives that focus on patient populations, such as those with heart failure, could address questions such as (1) What nursing treatments account for the variation in outcomes? (2) What are the most frequently used nursing treatments in patients with heart failure? and (3) Are evidence-based nursing practices for heart failure patients being used in the delivery of care? It would be interesting to determine, for example, the amount of variation in length of stay that is accounted for by nursing treatments compared with medical treatments.

USE A CONCEPTUAL MODEL

In the development of an outcomes management initiative the purpose and question(s) to be addressed will provide guidance in conceptualizing the initiative. This necessitates developing a clear model of the factors believed to be salient and their relationship to the outcomes of interest (Kane, 1997a; Strickland, 1997). Some factors will play a direct role and other factors influence processes of care and subsequent outcomes indirectly. Each of the factors needs to be captured and defined. Setting forth a conceptual model provides a mechanism for thinking about what factors are most important in addressing the purpose and questions to be addressed by the outcomes management initiative. The conceptual model also provides the basis for the analysis plan (Kane, 1997a, 1997b). Figure 34-1 is an example of a conceptual model devel-

oped for decreasing costs and improving care of heart failure patients treated in the acute care setting.

Many outcomes management initiatives are interdisciplinary in nature. In the development of a conceptual model it is imperative to explicate the nursing care process components in the model. This includes outcomes that are sensitive to nursing practices as well as nursing diagnoses and nursing treatments. Contextual variables amenable to nursing management practices also need to be explicated. However, the lesser availability of these nursing variables may make them more difficult to capture than medical variables, which routinely are included in electronic data repositories. Perhaps time and resources should be allocated to routine collection of critical nursing process variables (e.g., nursing treatments) and contextual variables in electronic data repositories for ready inclusion in outcomes management initiatives.

SELECT AND DEFINE THE OUTCOMES

The next step is to select and define the outcomes to be measured. The conceptual model guides the selection of the aspects of health to be measured (Maciejewski, 1997). Several typologies of outcomes are available for use as a guide:

- Patient-, provider-, or payer-specific outcomes (Kleinpell, 1997)
- The Clinical Value Compass consisting of four major parts: (1) functional status, risk status, and well-being, (2) cost and resource utilization, (3) satisfaction with health care and perceived benefit, and (4) clinical outcomes such as mortality and symptoms (Nelson, Mohr, Batalden, & Plume, 1996)
- The Consumer Assessments of Health Plans Study (CAHPS) (McCormick, Cummings, & Kovner, 1997)
- Oryx indicators set forth by the Joint Commission for Accreditation of Healthcare Organizations
- The Health Plan Employer Data and Information Set (HEDIS) (McCormick et al., 1997)
- American Nurses Association (ANA) Nursing Report Card patient-focused outcome indicators (ANA, 1995)
- The Nursing Outcomes Classification (Johnson, Maas, & Moorhead, 2000)
- The 15 categories of outcomes set forth by Lang and Marek (1990)

Outcomes are generic or condition specific. Generic outcomes are comprehensive measures that assess overall effects of treatments on health status. Mortality, morbidity, and utilization are traditional generic outcomes but

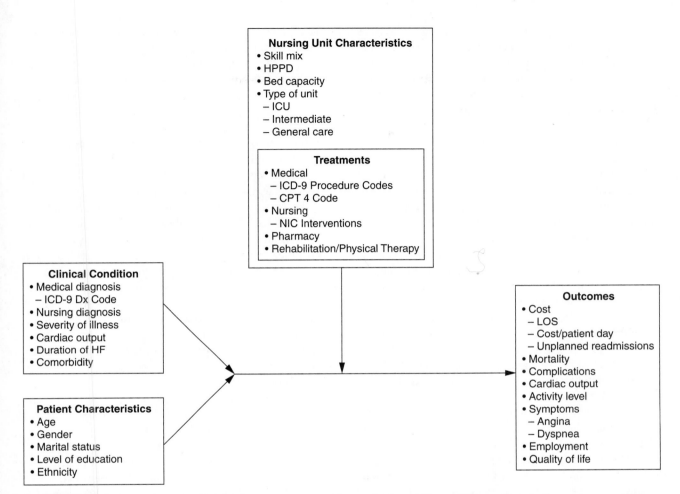

FIGURE 34-1 A conceptual model for decreasing costs and improving care of heart failure patients in the acute care setting.

are limited by comprehensiveness. Absence of mortality, for example, says little about the health of the population (Maciejewski, 1997). Health-related quality of life (HRQOL) is a generic outcome of different domains of health that are affected by disease and treatment. Several multidimensional and unidimensional HRQOL measures are available. Examples of generic, multidimensional HRQOL instruments include the Sickness Impact Profile, the 36-item Short-Form Health Survey, the Nottingham Health Profile, and the Quality of Well-Being Scale (Maciejewski, 1997; Spilker, 1996). Examples of generic, unidimensional HRQOL instruments include the RAND Social Health Battery, the Barthel Index of ADLs, and the Zung Self-Rating Depression Scale (Maciejewski, 1997; Spilker, 1996).

Condition-specific outcomes focus on aspects of health that reflect the status of a given medical condition and are likely to be sensitive to subtle changes in health

(Spilker, 1996; Titler & Reiter, 1994). These measures are designed to detect changes in the most important domains of a specific condition, such as changes in dyspnea intensity for people with chronic lung disease. There are essentially two types of condition-specific measures: (1) clinical measures that are primarily signs, symptoms, and test results and (2) experiential measures that capture the effect of the disease or problem on the individual (e.g., functioning) (Atherly, 1997). Examples of condition-specific outcome measures for heart failure include heart murmur (sign), angina (symptom), cardiac output (test), and ability of the individual to climb a flight of steps (function). Condition-specific outcomes are designed to detect small treatment effects whereas generic outcomes are designed to measure broad facets of health in several domains such as social, emotional, physical, and cognitive functioning; and overall well-being (Atherly, 1997; Maciejewski, 1997).

An essential component of outcomes management is defining the outcome domains, both conceptually and operationally. A conceptual definition uses words to depict the meaning of the domain. For example, if social functioning is an outcome of interest, it is important to define this term in relation to the outcomes management initiative. Social functioning can encompass any or all of the following: role functioning, involvement in the community, closeness of interpersonal relationships, and coping. Definitions of outcome domains should follow and be congruent with the purpose, questions to be answered, and conceptual model of the outcomes management initiative. The outcome instrument or test operationalizes the outcome measure. In choosing an instrument, reliability, validity, and sensitivity to change must be considered (Frytak, 1997; Kirchhoff & Rakel, 1999; Spilker, 1996; Strickland, 1997). Particular caution is warranted in selection of self-report measures to assure that the questions in the instrument reflect the conceptual definition of the outcome. Lastly, selection of outcome measures for outcomes management initiatives must consider the practicality of the measures selected. This includes length, readability, and cultural sensitivity (Kirchhoff & Rakel, 1999).

Selection and definition of outcomes should be done with the treatment in mind. When the outcomes management initiative includes nursing treatments, care should be taken to select outcomes that are sensitive to these treatments. In general, outcomes that are likely to pick up small treatment effects should be included as well as more global measures that permit comparisons of outcomes across different patient populations. An outcomes typology that is sensitive to nursing care, such as the Nursing Outcomes Classification (Johnson et al., 2000) or the ANA Report Card Indicators (ANA, 1995) are helpful in guiding selection of outcomes sensitive to nursing practices.

PROCESSES OF CARE

There are usually several different types of health care providers in a setting in which outcomes initiatives are planned. It is essential that the treatments be delineated for a particular outcomes initiative if the data are going to be used for improving care processes. Critical elements to consider are the type of treatment, both medical treatments and nursing treatments, the dose of the treatment (e.g., frequency, medication dosage), and the provider of the treatment (e.g., specialty physician, generalist physician, advanced practice nurse, staff nurse, educator)

(Hebert, 1997). It is my viewpoint that more attention is needed in the planning phase of outcomes management initiatives to delineate this component of the conceptual model and to operationalize it. Knowing the data source for the treatment components, how these data will be collected, and the timing of the treatment in relation to the outcomes is critical for a successful program.

Both medical and nursing treatments should be accounted for in outcome initiatives. Because physicians document services rendered through use of standardized coding schemas, it is easier and more convenient to detail medical treatments. Nursing treatments are not accounted for in these physician-dominated coding schemas and thus are more difficult to incorporate into outcomes management programs. For example, medical treatments for heart failure patients can be acquired using the *ICD-9* procedure codes and the *Current Procedural Terminology (CPT)*-4 codes. However, patient teaching regarding self-care is a nursing treatment not included in the medical records abstract electronic data repository, and thus may be overlooked as a critical nursing intervention that explains variation in outcomes of heart failure patients.

A review of 257 quality of care databased articles demonstrated that only 17 of the 257 articles addressed linkages between processes of nursing care by staff nurses and patient outcomes; a majority of the studies evaluated linkages between organizational context and patient outcomes (Lee, Chang, Pearson, Kahn, & Rubenstein, 1999). Although six studies demonstrated that nursing care processes affect patient outcomes, significant gaps were found in the extent to which nursing treatments used in daily practice were empirically evaluated in relation to outcomes. The gaps included (1) the relationship between monitoring interventions and patient outcomes and (2) the use of common nursing interventions, with most common interventions not being studied at all. Gaps in linking nursing treatments and patient outcomes for performance improvement are likely to continue until nurses electronically document nursing treatments using standardized language such as the Nursing Interventions Classification (McCloskey & Bulechek, 2000). Evaluating outcomes without linkages to nursing treatments provides little guidance for improving quality of care.

CONTEXT OF CARE

Studies on the organizational context of health care underscore the importance of contextual variables on patient outcomes (Aiken et al., 1997; Blegen, Goode, &

Reed, 1998; Mark et al., 1997; Mitchell et al., 1996; Sochalski & Aiken, 1999; Sovie, 1994). For example, studies have demonstrated that unit and organizational characteristics such as nurse staffing influence patient outcomes. Thus, it is important to consider during the planning phase organizational and nursing service variables that may indirectly impact patient outcomes. These may include staffing ratios, demand for nursing care hours per patient-day of nursing services, and nursing staff vacancy and turnover rates.

Changes in patient outcomes cannot, however, be linked directly to staffing ratios or other organizational variables because the nursing care planned and delivered is virtually unknown. Until health care organizations require use of standardized nursing language for documentation of nursing care in computerized patient records, outcomes management initiatives may focus on performance improvement actions (increasing staffing) that are not cost-effective for the health care system. It is only with the use of standardized languages for nursing treatments and documentation of those treatments in electronic data sources that we will be able to understand the relationship between organizational variables such as staffing ratios, nursing treatments ordered, and nursing treatments omitted because of insufficient staff skill or staff time to carry out particular nursing treatments.

DATA COLLECTION AND MANAGEMENT

The reality of an outcomes management initiative is brought to light when staff consider (1) how and when the chosen outcomes will be collected, (2) the data source for each outcome, (3) the number and types of patients to be included, and (4) who will be responsible for assuring that data are collected and managed in a database structure that promotes use of the data for decision making. Resources allocated to undertake the outcomes management initiative affect decisions made about methods of data collection and management. Writing a data collection and management plan with specific protocols is essential to determine if the overall conceptual model and purpose need to be modified. It is my experience that this step in the process of outcomes management often results in modifications of the overall plan. For example, incorporating self-report outcome measures into clinical practice may result in missing data or missing groups of patients that affect the overall outcomes analysis and may not be realistic. Capturing self-reported outcomes, depending on the length of the questionnaire, may require an employee dedicated to this part of the outcomes man-

agement initiative. If resources are not available for a dedicated employee, and integration of the outcome measure into clinical practice results in missing data or loss of a considerable number of patients, that particular outcome may need to be dropped or another outcome substituted as a proxy measure. Data sources for the treatment component must also be considered. For many nursing treatments, this requires concurrent or retrospective abstraction of the medical record, a costly data collection process. In contrast, physician treatments can be acquired electronically from the medical record abstract. The utilization of the electronic patient record with inclusion of nursing treatments that use standardized language will make acquisition of nursing treatment data more available in the future.

In developing a data collection and management plan, one should consider using existing data repositories that may be available in the organization. For example, patient characteristics and length of stay data are available from the UB92 and may be accessed from medical records personnel. Similarly, the institution's risk program may have adverse event and infection data that are available for use. When existing data repositories are used, it is important to know how the data were collected, the definitions of the outcome indicators, and the categorizations used in the data repository (Kirchhoff & Rakel, 1999).

Decisions about timing for measurement of the outcomes selected for a particular initiative is an essential component of data collection (Hebert, 1997; Kirchhoff & Rakel, 1999; Strickland, 1997). One must specify the points in time when each outcome will be measured (e.g., baseline, upon admission to an acute care unit, upon discharge from an acute care unit, and 6 weeks following discharge from an acute care unit). Selection of these time points must be matched carefully to when a treatment is most likely to have a measurable effect. This requires defining the episode of care that will be the focus of the outcomes management initiative. The episode of care may be an acute care hospitalization, it may be from the onset of a particular condition and continue throughout the trajectory of illness, it may be during a certain phase of a chronic condition (e.g., exacerbation of a chronic condition), or it may be from the immediate presurgical encounter through the post-surgery acute and ambulatory care services. Thus, timing for collection of each outcome measure requires that boundaries be set around the health services rendered and that the time for short- and long-term effects of treatment be delineated. The decision regarding the best time points for data collection is best made based on a thorough understanding of the health care condition and the expected points of impact of the treatment or program of focus for a particular outcomes management initiative. Treatments are matched to the stage and phase of the condition; measurement time points are matched to when the treatment is most likely to have a measurable effect; and outcomes are selected for each measurement time point that is most likely to have been changed by the treatment (Strickland, 1997). Carefully documenting when the treatment was administered and systematically measuring appropriate baseline, intermediate, and long-term outcomes are crucial to establishing relationships between treatments and outcomes (Strickland, 1997). Certain outcomes will need to be collected at several points in time, with respect to the treatment, to detect changes in the outcome over time.

Data should be managed in a database capable of handling extensive amounts of data. Data should be entered as soon as they are collected, attention given to duplicate data entry, and data verification performed to detect data entry errors. A data dictionary is essential to manage the data and assure data quality. Lastly, procedures for merging of data sets from various data repositories must be developed and adhered to. Policies that address data security and confidentiality must also be in place.

DATA ANALYSIS AND TRANSFORMING DATA INTO INFORMATION

Multiple sources are available to guide the reader in data analysis techniques (Carey & Lloyd, 1995; Kane, 1997b). Outcomes management staff should seek consultation with statistical personnel while planning the outcomes initiative and during data analysis and interpretation. When possible, outcomes management teams should include statisticians with expertise in analysis of complex data sets.

The goal of data analysis and transforming data into information is to identify processes of care that contribute to desired outcomes and to identify areas for performance improvements. Thus, the purpose, questions, and conceptual model should guide the data analysis plan. Consideration should be given to use of appropriate statistical techniques such as multiple regression modeling, multivariate analyses, and the use of risk adjustment (Kane, 1997b). Quality control techniques, such as run charts and statistical control limits, are useful to identify common and special causes of variation over time. These techniques are helpful in separating processes that are stable and that can be systematically improved from those that are affected by special causes such as equipment failure or changes in staffing level, for which efforts are needed to control the processes before system improvements in care can be made (Carey & Lloyd, 1995; Kirchhoff & Rakel, 1999).

An issue to consider is how the data will be categorized and presented. For example, will data be grouped by patient population, provider, or patient care unit? The priorities of the audience are often an important consideration in making these decisions. If current organizational structures for decision making are clinical departments, the data are best presented by groups of patients served by staff in those departments. If product or service line structures exist and are the foundation for performance improvements, data can be analyzed and presented according to a particular service line. Similarly, it may be a comparison of two or more medical treatments or nursing treatments that serves as the grouping variable for analyses (Kirchhoff & Rakel, 1999).

Writing the outcomes management report is guided by the audience who will be using it. The narrative report should be brief with data displays appended (Lepper & Titler, 1999). Important areas to consider are (1) the purpose and questions to be addressed, (2) the conceptual model, (3) variables (outcome, process, and contextual variables) addressed by the data along with data definitions, data source, and timing for collection of each variable, (4) methods of data analysis, (5) interpretation of data and findings, and (6) possible recommendations for performance improvements. The report serves as a stimulus for discussion by the users of the report. Data analysis and reporting is an iterative process and one should expect that the users might request further analysis of certain areas of interest. It is important to include in the report positive findings as well as areas for improvement.

The report should be presented to existing groups such as staff meetings or interdisciplinary quality improvement meetings. A short 20-minute presentation will facilitate beginning discussions by staff on areas for performance improvements.

IMPROVING PERFORMANCE

The essence of outcomes management is improving care delivery and patient outcomes. The treatments included in the outcomes management initiative need to be specific enough to provide some direction for what evidence-based changes in practice may be warranted. This component of outcomes management is one of the most difficult components of any initiative because it requires changes in practice for performance improvement. Changes in practice cannot be dictated but must come from the providers of care. For example, writing a policy that every heart failure patient will have a comprehensive discharge plan of care does not translate into practice behaviors of clinicians. Thus, changes in practice and development of the associated policies and procedures must come from the staff and be facilitated by the person in charge of the outcomes management initiative.

One pitfall of outcomes management initiatives is to continue to measure, measure, measure without putting resources and time into changing performance in areas that offer an opportunity for improvement. This is a waste of valuable resources if the initiative does not move beyond measurement to management.

SUMMARY

Nurses provide organizational leadership for outcomes management yet empirical data delineating the contributions of nursing care to the outcomes is limited. It is my viewpoint that these limitations come from (1) a focus on organizational outcomes rather than outcomes for specific patient populations, (2) lack of attention to developing outcomes initiatives that focus on nursing treatments, or (3) limited use of standardized nursing language in the computerized patient record. It is proposed that more outcomes management should focus on a specified nursing treatment such as outcomes management of discharge planning. The outcomes initiative should be intervention focused, with the selection of the outcomes closely related to the intervention. This would result in better data for management of the process of nursing care, which is the overall goal of outcomes management. Outcomes measurement is simple, but care can only be managed if one is clear about the treatments or care processes that are the focus of the outcomes management initiatives.

REFERENCES

Aiken, L.H., Sochalski, J., & Lake, E.T. (1997). Studying outcomes of organizational change in health services. *Medical Care 35*(11 Suppl), NS6-18.

American Nurses Association. (1995). *Nursing report card for acute care settings.* Washington, DC: Author.

Atherly, A. (1997). Condition-specific measures. In R.L. Kane (Ed.), *Understanding health care outcomes research* (pp. 53-66). Gaithersburg, MD: Aspen.

Blegen, M.A., Goode, C.J., & Reed, J. (1998). Nurse staffing and patient outcomes. *Nursing Research, 47*(1), 43-50.

Carey, R.G., & Lloyd, R.C. (1995). *Measuring quality improvement in healthcare: A guide to statistical process control applications.* New York: Quality Resources.

Frytak, J. (1997). Measurement. In R.L. Kane (Ed.), *Understanding health care outcomes research* (pp. 93-125). Gaithersburg, MD: Aspen.

Havens, D.S., & Aiken, L.H. (1999). Shaping systems to promote desired outcomes. The magnet hospital model. *Journal of Nursing Administration, 29*(2), 14-20.

Hebert, P. (1997). Treatment. In R.L. Kane (Ed.), *Understanding health care outcomes research* (pp. 93-125). Gaithersburg, MD: Aspen.

Hill, M. (1999). Outcomes measurement requires nursing to shift to outcome-based practice. *Nursing Administration Quarterly, 24*(1), 1-16.

Howell, R.E. (1999). On the scene: University of Iowa Hospitals and Clinics: Outcomes management. Perspective from the CEO. *Nursing Administration Quarterly, 24*(1), 61-62.

Johnson, M., Maas, M., & Moorhead, S. (2000). *Nursing outcomes classification (NOC)* (2nd ed.). St. Louis: Mosby.

Kane, R.L. (1997a). Approaching the outcomes question. In R.L. Kane (Ed.), *Understanding health care outcomes research* (pp. 1-15). Gaithersburg, MD: Aspen.

Kane, R.L. (1997b). Miscellaneous observations about outcomes research: Practical advice. In R.L. Kane (Ed.), *Understanding health care outcomes research* (pp. 1-15). Gaithersburg, MD: Aspen.

Kane, R.L. (1997c). *Understanding health care outcomes research.* Gaithersburg, MD: Aspen.

Kirchhoff, K.T., & Rakel, B.A. (1999). Outcomes evaluation. In M.A. Mateo & K.T. Kirchhoff (Eds.), *Using and conducting nursing research in the clinical setting* (2nd ed., pp. 76-89). Philadelphia: Saunders.

Kleinpell, R.M. (1997). Whose outcomes: Patients, providers or payers? *Nursing Clinics of North America, 32*(3), 513-520.

Lamb-Havard, J. (1997). Nurses at the bedside: Influencing outcomes. *Nursing Clinics of North America, 32*(3), 495-512.

Lang, N.M., & Marek, K.D. (1990). The classification of patient outcomes. *Journal of Professional Nursing, 6,* 153-163.

Lee, J.L., Chang, B.L., Pearson, M.L., Kahn, K.L., & Rubenstein, L.V. (1999). Does what nurses do affect clinical outcomes for hospital patients? A review of the literature. *Health Services Research, 34*(5 [Part 1]), 1011-1032.

Lepper, H.S., & Titler, M.G. (1999). Program evaluation. In M.A. Mateo & K.T. Kirchhoff (Eds.), *Using and conducting nursing research in the clinical setting* (2nd ed., pp. 90-104). Philadelphia: Saunders.

Maciejewski, M. (1997). Generic measures. In R.L. Kane (Ed.), *Understanding health care outcomes research* (pp. 19-52). Gaithersburg, MD: Aspen.

Mandelblatt, J.S., Fryback, D.G., Weinstein, M.C., Russel, L.B., Gold, M.R., & Hadorn, D.C. (1996). Assessing the effectiveness of health interventions. In M.R. Gold, J.E. Siegel, L.B. Russel, & M.C. Weinstein (Eds.), *Cost-effectiveness in health and medicine* (pp. 135-175). New York: Oxford University Press.

Mark, B.A., Salyer, J., & Geddes, N. (1997). Outcomes research. Clues to quality and organizational effectiveness? *Nursing Clinics of North America, 32*(3), 589-601.

McCloskey, J.C., & Bulechek, G.M. (2000). *Nursing interventions classification (NIC)* (3rd ed.). St. Louis: Mosby.

McCormick, K.A., Cummings, M.A., & Kovner, C. (1997). The role of the Agency for Health Care Policy and Research in improving outcomes of care. *Nursing Clinics of North America, 32*(3), 521-542.

Mitchell, P., Shannon, S.E., Cain, K.C., & Hegyvary, S.T. (1996). Critical care outcomes: Linking structures, processes, and organizational and clinical outcomes. *American Journal of Critical Care, 5*(5), 353-363.

Nadzam, D.M., & Nelson, M. (1997). The benefits of continuous performance measurement. *Nursing Clinics of North America, 32*(3), 543-559.

Nelson, E.C., Mohr, J.J., Batalden, P.B., & Plume, S.K. (1996). Improving health care. Part 1: The clinical value compass. *Journal on Quality Improvement, 22*(4), 243-258.

Peters, C., Cowley, M., & Standiford, L. (1999). The process of outcomes management in an acute care facility. *Nursing Administration Quarterly, 24*(1), 75-89.

Schalock, R.L. (1995). Outcome-based evaluation. New York: Plenum Press.

Scott, J.G., Sochalski, J., & Aiken, L. (1999). Review of magnet hospitals research: Findings and implications for professional nursing practice. *Journal of Nursing Administration, 29*(1), 9-19.

Sochalski, J., & Aiken, L.H. (1999). Accounting for variation in hospital outcomes: A cross-national study. *Health Affairs, 18*(3), 256-259.

Sovie, M.D. (1994). Nurse manager: A key role in clinical outcomes. *Nursing Management, 25*(3), 30-34.

Spilker, B. (1996). *Quality of life and pharmacoeconomics in clinical trials* (2nd ed.). Philadelphia: Lippincott-Raven.

Stonestreet, J.S., & Prevost, S.S. (1997). A focused strategic plan for outcomes evaluation. *Nursing Clinics of North America, 32*(3), 615-631.

Strickland, O.L. (1997). Challenges in measuring patient outcomes. *Nursing Clinics of North America, 32*(3), 495-512.

Titler, M.G., McCloskey, J.M. (Eds.), Ryan, J., Reiter, R.C., Rakel, B.A., Dreher, M., Berg, M.S., Greiner, J., Schlapkohl, M., Kraus, V.L., Johlin, F.C., Jensen, G.V., Mutnick, A.H., Szymusiak-Mutnick, B.A., Leo, K.C., Davenport, K.D., Shafer, M.E., & Howell, R.E. (1999). On the scene: University of Iowa Hospitals and Clinics: Outcomes management. *Nursing Administration Quarterly, 24*(1), 31-65.

Titler, M.G., & Reiter, R.C. (1994). Outcomes measurement in clinical practice. *MEDSURG Nursing, 3*(5), 395-398.

CHAPTER 35

The Problems with Health Care Customer Satisfaction Surveys

POLLY GERBER ZIMMERMANN

One organization recently adopted the following mission statement: "We will do whatever it takes to make the customer happy." Many nurses believe that, officially or not, this is the credo of their health care institutions.

The customer satisfaction bandwagon, rampant in the business world throughout the 1990s, has now been joined by health care. Fortunately the days when health care personnel could have an attitude of "just be grateful that we are here" are gone. In the search to improve both humanistic caring and profitability, however, many have allowed the pendulum to swing too far. They have adopted a misguided *excessive* and *exclusive* focus on customer satisfaction as the measurement of quality patient care. Making customer satisfaction the supreme goal has major inherent flaws, particularly when used in the health care arena for "patient" customers.

FLAWED CUSTOMER SATISFACTION CONCEPTS

The concepts of measuring customer satisfaction, even in the most appropriate applications, have difficulties. Quality expert Jarrett Rosenberg (1996) lists some common myths about achieving customer satisfaction:

Myth 1: Customer satisfaction is objective and straightforward.

Accurately finding out whether customers are satisfied is a perplexing, multidimensional task. Determining customers' attitudes takes experimentation, including looking at the customers' patterns.

One common problem is that surveyed respondents feel compelled to give an answer regardless of whether they have a strong opinion or even enough information to form one. And, unfortunately, the data from a poorly designed survey looks as valid as the data from a well-designed source (Sherman, 1998).

Myth 2: Customer satisfaction is easily measured.

Customer satisfaction is a complex attitude that includes whether the customers' experiences match their expectations. In other words, low expectations will be satisfied with a substandard performance, but attentive service will not please someone with unrealistic presumptions. Keep in mind that television portrayals include plenty of available staff, space, and time for everyone's needs.

Satisfaction is also influenced by facts that are not directly related to the current experiences, such as an institution's general reputation. Solution Point Research company's database revealed satisfaction varied based on the size of the emergency department: the larger the emergency department, the less satisfied the patients (Zimmermann, 1997a).

Quality expert Terry G. Vavra (1997) suggests that customer satisfaction surveys can actually *create* dissatisfied customers. Surveys imply promises to customers about the organization's interest in and responsiveness to their complaints. The customers feel skeptical when there are no improvements. Yet most providers report that the majority of complaints about their institution's acute health care focus on the bill and the waiting time, some of the poorly accepted intrinsic parts of care.

This is particularly true in an era of cost containment limits with a concurrent increase in patient volume and acuity. For instance, the nation's emergency departments are now handling 100 million patients, with an admission rate that rose from 12% to 20% during a time in which the number of departments have decreased from 5,000 to 4,600 (Eisenberg, 2000).

Myth 3: Customer satisfaction is accurately and precisely measured.

The "objective" numbers lull people into this common misperception. But attitudes vary, both among people from time to time and in the same people at different times.

Most rating scales contain a response bias. People opt for the middle rating or one of the extremes for the majority of the items rather than an accurate distinction between each aspect. The *mean* rating traditionally used for interpretation is really not that helpful.

Survey results will also be influenced by methodology, such as distribution (Zimmermann, 1998). Any personal contact creates more favorable responses. One emergency department had an unexpected dramatic drop in its ratings when its survey company changed from personal phone interviews to random mailings (Zimmermann & Pierce, 1999).

As some quality experts put it, standardized tests of customer perception are an oxymoron. Customer satisfaction, by its very nature, involves individual minds, behavior, responses, and attitudes (Jeffries & Sells, 2000).

Myth 4: Customer satisfaction is quickly and easily changed.

Unless experiences are significantly below or above expectations, it takes time to build a shift in customer satisfaction. It is a lagging indicator rather than an accurate reflection of current experiences. Continuous quality improvement, rather than a heroic-effort mentality, builds satisfaction and the usually desired result, *repeat* customers.

This raises another issue, though, since many health care settings by design are intended to be episodic. The best care may actually be accomplished by *preventing* the customer patients' return.

Myth 5: It is obvious who the customer is.

Every organization has distinct different groups of consumers and it is important to identify which groups are dissatisfied. Traditionally health care satisfaction surveys lump all customers into one group (e.g., patients), which is a narrow perspective. Other customers, such as managed care networks, physicians, and internal customers, are just as important.

In the end, some quality experts recommend that the health care industry stop using standardized customer satisfaction surveys. These cost-effective, "one-size-fits-all" instruments can actually place an organization at a competitive disadvantage. The reason is that a standardized survey is likely to include dimensions that this specific group of customers may not deem important or to miss entirely the dimensions driving this group's overall satisfaction. The risk for inappropriate survey content increases when users are geographically dispersed. In the end, there is a gap in which incorrect decisions were made

in response to perceptions from inaccurate generic surveys. In other words, the survey fits none (Jeffries & Sells, 2000).

HEALTH CARE CUSTOMER SATISFACTION FLAWS

The problem in applying customer satisfaction surveys to health care is further complicated because health care is not an objective, measurable "product," as in manufacturing or sales. A retail customer legitimately discerns whether the purchased toaster fulfills the promised performance of safe, quick, darkening of bread.

But customer satisfaction is more nebulous in the "healing" of a physical complaint, where biological, psychological, and environmental components are involved. It does not consider other factors, such as up to a 30% to 50% patient noncompliance with the treatment regimen in chronic conditions.

The distinction between customer satisfaction and value further clarifies this issue. Customers value a service, not as an end in itself, but because the service delivers the desired consequence. Customer satisfaction is then the customer's feeling about the value that was received (Stahl, Barnes, Gardial, Parr, & Woodruff, 1999).

It becomes difficult to make patient customers happy in our quick-fix society when they do not get instantaneous service and relief. Quality health care service, without a cure, is not always valued.

Overall, the excessive emphasis on customer satisfaction surveys in health care has flaws because these surveys

1. Tap only a limited group of customers
2. Survey people with impaired recollection
3. Do not often meet research criteria for application of results
4. Are heavily influenced by factors outside the health care interaction
5. Focus exclusively on individuals in a system
6. Assume that the health care customer always correctly identifies good care

Who is Filling Out Health Care Customer Satisfaction Surveys?

The obvious assumption is "patients," but the actual respondents are a more restrictive group than that. Although care is given to everyone, only alert, competent, English-speaking, younger (with good sensory ability), literate patients tend to actually complete surveys. Yet it is the delirious, elderly individual who requires a translator for an obscure language who requires the most nursing effort, caring, and interventions.

Hospice services share that the family, not the patient who is very ill or who has died, often completes their surveys. The *patient* was satisfied, but the *family* is not because the hoped-for outcome of their loved one's improved health was not met. Somehow, there was never enough done.

More than that, I believe that the stress of their health care needs results in foolish behavior by some. How else do you explain the man who literally threatened to kill the emergency department (ED) triage nurse if she did not immediately obtain a physician for his wife who had a gastric ulcer? Or the individual with a sprained ankle in the emergency department who stated, "I don't care; I was here first!" when informed there would be a delay because another patient was *dying* in cardiac arrest.

Coping with patients' inappropriate behaviors is part of the nurse's job. But what is bothersome is that with customer satisfaction surveys the "foolish" opinions of some disgruntled patients are now legitimized by their anonymous survey results being averaged in the totals.

The Patient's Impressions of the Experience Are Often Not Accurate

It is true that our perception becomes our reality. But when patients already feel incapacitated in some way, a problem that might normally be perceived as minute now becomes significant. One hospitalized elderly woman declared that "they don't give good care here." Her specific complaints were lack of dessert on her (diabetic) dinner tray, bruising from a blood draw (from her elderly, anti-coagulated, fragile veins), and the fact that she had to ask for her prn analgesic (because she takes it automatically at home). She could not recall that staff *had* explained the rationales to her.

Unlike other purchasing decisions that most consumers enjoy or at least feel in control of, health care service "purchases" are often made at a time of stress and vulnerability. Most emergency departments report a higher rate of complaints about the night shift. It makes sense that the patients' fatigue and inconvenience would account for the higher rate rather than some nation-wide incompetence of all night shifts.

Elderly persons comprise 20% of the U.S. population and a higher percentage of the total health care consumers. In the United States, it is estimated that 10% of individuals age 65 and older and nearly 50% of individuals age 85 or older have Alzheimer's disease, which always

affects the memory. It should not be unexpected that there may be some inaccurate recollections of the health care experience when these individuals complete their mailed survey several weeks later.

Are We Meeting Survey Validity?

Research criteria demand a return rate of 60% or more for survey validity (Polit & Hungler, 1995). Yet many health care institutions drive their customer satisfaction programs on return rates of less than 10%. Managers have been fired for failing to improve their ratings on the basis of a 6% survey return rate. Although every person is important, the extremes are overly represented at that level of sampling.

This approach then promotes a mentality that drives caregiving decisions toward those most likely to fill out a survey. One study found a 34% discrepancy between the ED patients' perception of their need for immediate care compared with the physician researcher's opinion, based on the presenting complaint (American Hospital Association, 1995). It has to be a temptation to allow an impatient business person with a minor laceration to see the physician before a quiet, elderly nursing home resident with a fever if you know your job is on the line.

Factors Outside the Experience Itself

There is a basic assumption that these sick, stressed patients are fair and accurate in the judgment of their health care experience. Yet one emergency department found that the major issue in the patients' write-in comments, either positive or negative, was their male nurses. On further analysis they found that middle-aged women almost exclusively made these comments, either as the patient or a family member. Does this not raise suspicions that other social or cultural issues are involved, outside of the actual care rendered?

In the same vein, another emergency department experienced a significant drop in their satisfaction ratings during their department's remodeling. It is reasonable to assume that environmental factors such as noise, dirt, or inconvenience were having an influence rather than a change in the level of provided nursing care and concern (Zimmermann, 1998).

Why not use a solution proven to improve satisfaction ratings if you really want that: increase the RN composition in the staffing skill mix. One study found that the percentage of hours of care delivery by RNs was inversely related to the unit rates of patient complaints (Blegen, Goode, & Reed, 1993). In another study, analyzing ANA's

10 quality indicators, the patients' perception of satisfaction with their care increased as the percentage of RNs in the nursing staff increased (Moore, Lynn, McMillen, & Evans, 1999).

Seeking an Individual to Blame

These customer satisfaction surveys focus on specific individuals within a system. The patient is often asked more than 40 questions about the specific personal behaviors of registration, admission, laboratory, nursing, physicians, and so on. Were the nurses concerned about not discharging you too soon? Was your blood drawn with skill (i.e., quickly, little pain)? Did the ED nurse treat you with the proper urgency?

There is no public outcry to scrutinize nursing. In fact, 92% of those polled trust the health care information provided by RNs, almost the same rate as that of physicians (93%) (Sigma Theta Tau International, 1999). Almost three quarters of Americans surveyed rated nurses' honesty and ethics as either "high" or "very high," placing them higher than any other profession with respect to these virtues (ANA, 2000).

Of course, some individual health care staff members can be rude, and that behavior must be dealt with. But who is blamed if a system problem causes an ED delay for an available inpatient bed or no additional pillows are available from the linen supply? Usually it is the people in front of the patient at that point who get the blame, even though there is probably nothing this particular staff can immediately change for a different result. Edward Deming's premise of avoiding individual blame and focusing on process and systems is still true. It is time to move beyond the idea that "if we only had nicer nurses" who would "work harder," the problems would be solved.

The Customer Can Judge Good Care

Any underlying premise behind these customer satisfaction surveys is that health care consumers know what is best for their needs. Do they? Are we doing them a favor to let them believe that they do? Although today's consumer is often more sophisticated and informed, health care providers undergo years of education and training to become more than a vending dispenser for the requested health care purchase.

LACK OF UNIVERSAL ACCEPTANCE

If customer satisfaction is such a gold standard of quality care, why do not all health care providers and institutions use surveys? Some revere them; others do not use them at all. Everyone adheres to other accepted universal standards, such as morbidity and mortality rates or outcome indicators.

Consider what are the outcomes in our current emphasis on pleasing the patient. Bauchner, Pelton, and Klein (1999) reported that almost all pediatricians had parents request an antibiotic that was not indicated during the past month; 40% had it happen 10 or more times. Despite our era of increasing bacterial resistance to antibiotics, one third of the pediatricians admitted they occasionally (or more frequently) comply with these requests. This is in spite of 78% believing that parent education would be the most effective way to reduce inappropriate requests for antibiotics.

Grossman, Keen, Singer, and Asher (1995) found that 65% of surveyed pediatric residents believed a low-grade fever was a good defense mechanism that should not be treated. However, 44% of them indicate that they do provide antipyretics in these cases to "satisfy the parents." What happened to being patient advocates that ultimately do what is best for the patients, even if it is not well received?

SATISFACTION NEEDED TO SUCCEED AS A BUSINESS?

A common argument for health care customer satisfaction surveys is that hospitals are businesses; businesses need satisfied customers to succeed. But that is a simplistic solution. Solovy (1998) reports that consumers overwhelmingly state that they think quality information is useful about health care plans (87%), doctors (86%), and hospitals (83%). But only about a third actually use that information to make a decision in choosing a health care plan (34%), a doctor (35%), or a hospital (30%).

Data to prove a link of profitability with customer satisfaction are sparse. Nelson et al. (1992) studied whether patient perceptions of quality care relate to a hospital's financial performance. They found a 17% to 27% attributable variation in financial measures. However, the two dimensions of hospital quality that made an independent, statistically significant contribution were the billing services and discharge.

The surprise finding was that the dimensions usually thought most important for hospital quality care—nursing service and key features of daily care including the exchange of information—were *not* significantly related to any measure of profitability. The researchers concluded that there is no guarantee that better perceived quality on the patients' part will produce a stronger financial bottom line.

CUSTOMER SERVICE TRAINING

I am not opposed to teaching nursing staff a few tricks of the service industry that can help manipulate patients' perceptions. In that way patients can appreciate the quality care they are actually being given. It does need to be clearly identified, however, that this focus is an adjunct *accessory* to nursing, not the main object of it.

Herzlinger (1997) found that patients judge ED staff by their service (not professional) skills 85% of the time. Yet rarely is any service training provided to staff. Dr. Thom A. Mayer relates INOVA Fairfax Hospital's experience. They instituted formal customer satisfaction training for all staff, including physicians. As a result, their ED complaints decreased by more than 70% while their patient compliments increased by more than 100% (Mayer, Cates, Masorovich, & Royalty, 1998).

Some of the techniques they teach include (Mayer & Zimmermann, 1999):

1. *Use "scripted" phrases to communicate caring.*
   It is difficult to create spontaneously just the right phrase for each encounter. Some phrases that seem to naturally reassure patients are "I'm sorry this happened to you"; "We'll take good care of your husband (wife, etc.)"; or "We do this kind of thing all the time and we are good at it."
2. *Restate the patients' complaints or comments in their exact terms.*
   This common therapeutic technique of reflecting allows the patient to feel "heard." They may not get what they want, but at least they feel you understood their need.
3. *Negotiate expectation with provided knowledge.*
   Help patients realistically shape their expectations by giving them appropriate limited amounts of control. For instance, inform them of the usual, reasonable amount of waiting time so they do not feel forgotten.
4. *Give generous time estimates.*
   One study found that ED patients were more satisfied if they were seen by the physician sooner than the initial estimated time than if they were given a shorter estimated time but were seen after that time estimate had elapsed. And this difference occurred despite both groups' actually being treated in the same amount of time.
5. *Navigate transitions.*
   Use language and processes to help communicate to the patient that the care is being passed on when transitioning care to a new person. This can include men-

tioning the incoming "capable staff" to the patient prior to a shift change or introducing them during walking rounds.
6. *Sit down when you talk with the patient.*
   A person will perceive that you are in the room three times longer than you are if you sit instead of stand. Keep your speech slow and frequently use their name. Rapidly spoken comments made while walking out of the room are often perceived as being abrupt and rude.

Other institutions have instituted system changes that have improved patient satisfaction. Some add amenities such as a "greeter," valet parking, improved signage, a volunteer-staffed coffee cart, or TV sets in ED patient care areas. Others improve treatment processes, such as faster digital x-rays, expanded triage protocols, bedside registration, or discharge nurses (Zimmermann, 1997a, in press; Zimmermann & Pierce, 1999).

EFFECT ON NURSING STAFF

Overall, I am most concerned about the effect all this "pleasing the customer" mentality has on health care providers themselves. The overwhelming majority went into health care to help people, realizing that sometimes it is a thankless job. But now, like eager puppy dogs seeking an approving pat on the head, the focus is to get satisfied patients. No health care provider advocates customer *dis*satisfaction, but it seems that the tail is now wagging the dog (Zimmermann, 1997b).

Nurses do have professional standards and motivation. We are the ones with the expertise and ability. I am not perfect, but I am a *professional* nurse who *does* care. Yet my nursing credibility in this regard is vulnerable to patient customer satisfaction survey results.

PATIENT CARE VERSUS CUSTOMER SATISFACTION

In fact, there is evidence that people want health care providers managing their care rather than being the shopping consumers. Preliminary findings from one Chicago suburban hospital were that more than 90% preferred to be called "patients" (rather than "customers" or "clients"). And this preference held true in the emergency department, same-day surgery unit, and the physician's office (Bernard Heilicser, personal communication, January 14, 2000).

In the end, I believe that the whole customer satisfaction concept in health care is actually *degrading* to nursing. *Customers* receive a requested *commodity* for a *price.* I obtain the book I want if I have the money. *Nursing,* on the other hand, often gives *more* than what is sought after, often *without* compensation.

• The frightened new teenage mother wants medication for her infant. The nurses also provide emotional support, teaching, and a thorough assessment of potential problems.

• The woman vaguely answers the routine assessment questions when seeking care for her injury. The perceptive nurse skillfully screens for domestic violence and intervenes with preventive measures.

• The young woman with undiagnosed abdominal pain angrily demands food and analgesics. The empathetic nurse maintains conditions for diagnostic and treatment integrity but provides alternative comfort measures.

• A heat crisis strikes the community. The nurse forgoes her lunch break to continue to manage care for the overwhelming number of patients, including the uninsured.

These are examples of *quality* health care, and ultimately that *is* what everyone wants. These are examples of *patient* care and *that* is what nursing does.

REFERENCES

American Hospital Association. (1995). *Hospital Health Network, 69,* 20.

American Nurses Association. (2000). High public esteem for nurses. *American Journal of Nursing, 100*(1), 21.

Bauchner, H., Pelton, S.I., & Klein, J.O. (1999, February). Parents, physicians, and antibiotic use. *Pediatrics, 103,* 395-401.

Blegen, M.A., Goode, C.J., & Reed, L. (1998). Nurse staffing and patient outcomes. *Nursing Research, 47*(1), 43-50.

Eisenberg, D. (2000, January 31). Critical condition. *Time,* pp. 52-54.

Grossman, D., Keen, M.F., Singer, M., & Asher, M. (1995). Current nursing practices in fever management. *Medsurg Nursing, 4*(3), 193-197.

Herzlinger, R. (1997). *Market-driven healthcare.* New York: The Free Press.

Jeffries, R.D., & Sells, P.R. (2000). Customer satisfaction measurement instruments. In healthcare does one size fit none? *Quality Progress, 33*(2), 118-123.

Mayer, T.A., Cates R.J., Masorovich, M.J., & Royalty, D. (1998). Emergency department patient satisfaction: Customer service training improves patient satisfaction and rating in physician and nurse skill. *Journal of Health Care Management, 43,* 427-441.

Mayer, T.M., & Zimmermann, P.G. (1999). ED customer satisfaction survival skills: One hospital's experience. *Journal of Emergency Nursing, 25*(3), 187-191.

Moore, K., Lynn, M.R., McMillen, B.J., & Evans, S. (1999). Implementation of the ANA report card. *Journal of Nursing Administration, 29*(6), 48-54.

Nelson, E.C., Rust, R.T., Zahorik, A., Rose, R.L., Batalden, P., & Siemanski, B.A. (1992, December). Do patient perceptions of quality relate to hospital financial performance? *Journal of Health Care Marketing, 12*(4), 6-13.

Polit, D.F., & Hungler, B.P. (1995). *Nursing research: Principles and methods* (p. 288). Philadelphia: Lippincott.

Rosenberg, J. (1996). Five myths of customer satisfaction. *Quality Progress, 29*(12), 57-60.

Sherman, B. (1998, March). How non-profits can benefit from marketing research. *Association Forum, 28*(2), 22-23.

Sigma Theta Tau International. (1999). New poll shows public concern about health care. *Reflections, 31*(2), 39.

Solovy, A. (1998, March 20). Trendspotting. *Hospitals & Health Networks, 72*(6), 60.

Stahl, M.J., Barnes, W.K., Gardial, S.F., Parr, W.C., & Woodruff, R.B. (1999). Customer value analysis helps hone strategy. *Quality Progress, 32*(4), 53-58.

Vavra, T.G. (1997). Is your satisfaction survey creating dissatisfied customers? *Quality Progress, 30*(12), 51-56.

Zimmermann, P.G. (1997a, October). Manager's ask and answer: What can be done to enhance customer satisfaction? *Journal of Emergency Nursing, 23*(5), 470-475.

Zimmermann, P.G. (1997b, December). Guest editorial: Customer service run amok. *Journal of Emergency Nursing, 23*(6), 514-515.

Zimmermann, P.G. (1998). Manager's ask and answer: How do you measure customer satisfaction? *Journal of Emergency Nursing, 24*(3), 269-271.

Zimmermann, P.G. (2000, December). Manager's forum: Customer satisfaction. *Journal of Emergency Nursing, 26*(6).

Zimmermann, P.G., & Pierce, B. (1999). Manager's forum: Customer satisfaction. *Journal of Emergency Nursing, 25*(1), 48-49.

Licensure in Nursing

Old vs. New Approaches

DONNA M. DORSEY

North Carolina passed the first nurse practice act in 1903, and by 1923 all states had adopted a nurse practice act. The practice acts were state based and built on a foundation that requires a nurse to be licensed in each state where the nurse practices. For nearly 100 years these practice acts have served nursing regulation well. This single-state licensing model provided for public protection while maintaining each individual state's authority to regulate the practice of nursing. But in today's world of rapid communication, Internet, and mobility, single-state licensing creates barriers to the practice of nursing and to full access to nursing care.

The interstate practice of nursing has increased at a rapid rate, altering the way nursing is practiced. Technology, the growth of large multistate health care systems, and the mobility of nurses are just some of the factors that have made the single-state licensure system appear as a barrier to the practice of nursing. Pressure on state boards of nursing has been increasing to change the regulatory model of licensure in order to better respond to the changing health care system. Nurses complain that licensure from one state to another takes too long. Employers cannot make full use of the workforce because of the time and expense of obtaining licensure in every state in which the nurse is working. Confusion exists regarding the requirements for licensure when the nurse is physically located in one state and is providing care to a patient in another state. Nursing regulators agreed that a change was needed.

In 1994, the National Council of State Boards of Nursing, a nonprofit organization composed of boards of nursing, began research into models of regulation that would eliminate the perceived barriers of the single-state licensure system. Following a great deal of research and evaluation, the mutual recognition model was chosen as the best approach to the regulatory needs of nursing to-

day. The mutual recognition model of nursing licensure is similar to the driver's license model. Nurses must maintain a license in their state of residence and are authorized to practice on a multistate privilege in any other state that has passed the interstate compact. An interstate compact is an agreement between two or more states established for the purpose of remedying a particular problem of multistate concern (Black, 1983, p. 421). In the case of nurse licensure, the compact resolves the barriers created by the single-state license, creates mechanisms for cooperation and information sharing regarding the licensure of nurses, and maintains the right of the state to regulate nurses.

On January 1, 2000, a new phase in nursing licensure was initiated by five boards of nursing—Maryland, Texas Board of Registered Nursing, Texas Board of Licensed Vocational Nursing, Utah, and Wisconsin—when each of the states implemented the mutual recognition model of licensure. Utah passed the legislation in 1998, with the other states following in 1999. All had agreed that implementation would not occur before January 1, 2000, to provide adequate time for development of regulations and policies. The decision of these states to become the pioneers was based on their belief in the need for change and that the mutual recognition model was the right direction for nursing regulation.

NEED FOR A CHANGE

Confusion and concern about compliance with licensure have increased with the advent of new practice modalities and technologies. A patient is released from a hospital in Maryland and returns home to Tennessee. The nurse in Maryland calls the patient to assess his progress toward recovery and provides directions for further care. Another nurse uses closed circuit television to provide nursing care to a patient in another state. It is midnight and a patient calls his managed care organization using a toll-free number. The nurse who answers is in another state, assesses the patient's complaint, and provides direction for care. None of these nurses are licensed in the state where the patient is located and are unknowingly placing themselves at risk for practicing nursing without a license. Most state boards of nursing have determined that the nurse must be licensed in the state where care is provided. Yet the majority of nurses are unclear about the licensing requirement when functioning in these nontraditional roles. Technology has erased the geographical barriers to providing nursing care but the licensing laws have remained geographically based.

In the Executive Summary of the Telemedicine Report to Congress (1997), single-state licensure was identified as a barrier. The report stated that:

> Telemedicine offers the potential to provide health services across vast distances to underserved areas. However, even though telemedicine knows no boundaries, health professionals must be licensed and regulated at the state level. Therefore, issues relating to cross-state licensure are perceived to be potential barriers to the expansion of telemedicine. [p. 4]

The report also concluded that the federal government does have the authority to set licensing standards for the practice of telemedicine. Although licensure is a state-based authority under the state's police powers, the report found that, "the Supremacy Clause of the Constitution mandates that even state regulation designed to protect vital state interests must give way to paramount Federal legislation" (p. 4). For nursing regulators the concept of federal intervention in licensing was unsuitable. Creating a separate federal license for telemedicine had the potential to make regulation of nursing practice more difficult and confusing.

A study contracted by the National Council of State Boards of Nursing provided further evidence that the current licensing system needed change. TVG Inc. (1997) conducted qualitative structured interviews with 40 key decision makers and senior executives in managed care organizations, demand management companies, and large university health centers. The overall goal of the study was to gain additional knowledge on the current and future extent of interstate practice of nurses. Of particular interest was the respondents' attitude regarding the current licensing system.

> The participants see the current system of licensure as unwieldy, archaic, and out of touch with the direction that the marketplace is moving. The general feeling is that the growth areas of healthcare are non-traditional areas such as tele-medicine, demand management, outcome measurement, and disease management. While the respondents perceive that nurses are "naturals" for filling positions in these areas, they do not necessarily believe that they are exclusively nursing roles. Consequently, they noted that a complicated licensure system, such as currently exists, if it were strictly enforced (that is, if any nurse engaged in these areas is forced to be licensed in any state in which she/he may have come in contact with clients) the demand for nurses would fall. Many respondents noted that they would simply seek out other healthcare professionals, or train other professionals, to fill such positions. [TVG, Inc., p. 9]

The respondents felt that a driver's license model would be preferable to the current licensure system. A coordinated national system was also suggested as a method to eliminate the ability of a nurse with disciplinary action on the license in one state from working in another state on a valid license (p. 9).

In a nationwide survey of a random sample of 3,000 registered nurses and 3,000 licensed practical/vocational nurses, the nurses reported that the problematic aspect of licensure was related to the endorsement process. The costs and time of obtaining the verifications of licensure for the state of original licensure and for other states where licensed, as well as turnaround time in the new state, were viewed as unreasonable (National Council of State Boards of Nursing, 1997, p. 3). In addition, anecdotal information from nurses confirms that the endorsement process is frustrating and causes a great deal of stress, particularly when time is limited. In an informal survey with 658 responses, four out of five nurses said the current system was in need of change (p. 2). These surveys also verified the perception that more nurses are working in multiple states.

It is apparent that new modes of practice, the advent of technology, and the increase in practice across state lines have created challenges for nursing regulators. Pressure to expedite licensure, increased confusion regarding the need for licensure when practicing via modalities that cross state lines, and the increased mobility of nurses have made the single-state license restrictive. The ease of movement among states has also made the disciplinary role of boards of nursing more difficult. One can even question the effectiveness of the single-state licensure system to carry out its role in public protection.

SELECTING THE OPTIMAL MODEL

The mutual recognition model was not chosen without careful and through research. There were several criteria that were important in selecting a model. Any new model had to preserve the state-based authority for regulation of nursing. A national model was not an option. The model had to allow for seamless practice across state lines along with an open system of information exchange among boards of nursing. Cost was also a consideration. Most important was that a new model had to provide for public protection by assuring competent nurses providing care in the most effective manner to meet the patient's needs (National Council of State Boards of Nursing, 1998, p. 7).

A task force composed of members of boards of nursing evaluated nearly a dozen different models for multistate regulation. Five were selected for in-depth analysis, with two approaches emerging as possible solutions—fast endorsement and mutual recognition. The analysis of each model included the impact on stakeholders such as nurses, employers, boards of nursing, and consumers. Fast endorsement was an appealing option to many boards. But it did not solve one large problem: a nurse would still need to be licensed in all states where the nurse practiced. The risks of practicing in a state without licensure would remain an issue, especially if the nurse did not have a clear understanding that the activities being performed, such as telephone triage, were considered nursing by the state board.

At the same time, a panel of legal experts composed of boards of nursing attorneys and other legal consultants reviewed the issue of multistate practice and its impact on current state laws and regulations. The panel recommended a mutual recognition model similar to the driver's license model. In the report to the Delegate Assembly of the National Council of State Boards of Nursing (1997) the rationale for the recommendation of the legal panel was outlined as follows:

- mutual recognition is the closest model to the existing system;
- mutual recognition reflects the legal concept of Full Faith and Credit between U.S. jurisdictions;
- mutual recognition could be implemented incrementally;
- work could proceed on multiple fronts: some states could move forward immediately, based on interpretations of current law, while other states could move forward creating a pathway by either interstate compact or legislative change; and
- implementation could begin with uniform requirements, although boards might agree to move toward a goal of uniform requirements. [p. 7]

An interstate compact was recommended as the preferred method of implementation. States are accustomed to interstate compacts and their implementation. The compact defines areas of cooperation among states, such as jurisdiction, information sharing, discipline, and administration, while at the same time, it maintains the state-based authority for the regulation of nursing.

The task force found that the mutual recognition model resolved the problem of requiring verification from state to state. Because the state agrees to recognize other state's license standards, there is no need for licensure in each state. The model also allows a state to retain its authority for interpretation of the nursing practice. Given the recommendation of the panel of legal experts and the research findings, the task force recommended to the 1997 Delegate Assembly of the National Council of State Boards of Nursing that the mutual recognition model be endorsed by the delegates. The delegate assembly is a body composed of two representatives of each state's board of nursing. These delegates voted to endorse the mutual recognition model. In addition, it was decided to implement the model using an interstate compact.

THE MUTUAL RECOGNITION MODEL

Implementing mutual recognition is a voluntary process. The state legislature must adopt the interstate compact for a state to participate in mutual recognition. Although titles of the compacts and format may differ from state to state, the compacts are identical in substance. The compact details the conditions of participation, the relationship with other states in the compact, and the requirements that the nurse must meet to hold a multistate privilege. Once a state joins the compact, a compact administrator is appointed. In most cases the compact administrator is the executive officer of the board of nursing. The administrators form a compact administrators' group with the responsibility to implement the compact and deal with issues related to the implementation. The administrators develop policies and procedures to carry out the provision of the compact. They are also responsible for handling any disputes related to implementation.

Fundamental to the compact is the requirement that licensure is based on the state of residence. In order for a nurse to obtain a multistate privilege, the nurse must be a resident of a state that has passed the compact and be licensed in that state. The nurse may not hold a nursing license in any other compact state, but may practice in any compact state without obtaining additional licensure. The nurse is expected to abide by the laws and regulations of the state where the nurse is working. Should the nurse change permanent residence and move to another compact state, the nurse must obtain a license in the new state and relinquish the license from the previous state. It is easy to understand how the model works, if one thinks of the driver's license model. An individual obtains a driver's license in the state where the individual lives. One can drive throughout the country without getting another license, must abide by the law of the state where the individual is driving, and must obtain a new license when one changes residence.

Until all states have joined the compact, a nurse will still need licenses in noncompact states even if the nurse is living in a compact state. For example, the nurse living in state A, a compact state, but practicing in state B, a noncompact state, must have a license in state B to practice in state B. The multistate privilege does not extend to state B since the state has not joined the compact. On the other hand, a nurse living in a noncompact state but licensed and working in a compact state does not have a multistate privilege because the nurse does not live in the compact state. Residence remains the determining factor in obtaining a multistate privilege to practice nursing.

To facilitate the multistate practice a coordinated licensure information system is required to enable tracking of nurses and enhance coordination among the boards of nursing. The system contains both licensure and disciplinary data as submitted by the boards of nursing. The public, which includes employers, may query the system rather than contacting an individual board for information regarding license status. The compact also requires that a board of nursing report disciplinary actions to the system immediately.

A nurse who violates the nurse practice act in a state is subject to discipline by the board of nursing in that state. The process does not change under mutual recognition. Should a nurse violate the law while practicing in a state under the multistate privilege, that state may take action against the privilege. The complaint is reported to the board in the state where the violation occurred, as is done under the single-state license system. Once the board initiates an investigation of the complaint, the board flags the nurse on the coordinated database. The action the compact state takes when a nurse is working in the state under the multistate privilege is against the privilege. In the single-state system the nurse would have a license in the state, and the action would be against the license. But there is no difference in the action. A board can require a nurse to cease and desist practicing in the state, which equates to revoking the license. A nurse can be reprimanded, fined, or placed on probation when working on a privilege. One difference in the single-state licensure system occurs when

the license is revoked by the state of residence. Since the nurse can only hold a license in the state of residence, the revocation would mean that the nurse could not practice in any compact state. Under the single-state system, a revocation in the state of licensure does not automatically cause revocation in other states where the nurse is licensed. Each state must take action. The compact provides the advantage that each state will no longer need to take disciplinary action if the state of residence has taken action. This eliminates the problem of disciplined nurses practicing undetected in other states.

Advanced practice nurses do not have a multistate privilege under the compact. Unlike the requirements for licensure of registered nurses and licensed practical nurses, in which the difference in standards is small, standards for licensure or certification of advanced practice nurses vary widely. Many states require collaborative agreements with physicians licensed in the state as part of the licensure or certification process. At this time, it would be extremely difficult to overcome the state differences. Attempts to expand the practice of advanced practice nurses or delete restrictive requirements have met with failure in state legislatures. The boards of nursing continue to work on resolving this problem. The ultimate goal is for advanced practice nurses to have full access to mutual recognition licensure. In the interim, the advanced practice nurse will be able to exercise the multistate privilege on the basic license and then obtain advanced practice licensure or certification on a state-by-state basis.

THE ISSUES

As with any change, there are those who believe mutual recognition is not the right direction for nursing regulation. But they are wrong. The major areas of concern voiced by the opponents of mutual recognition are licensure in the state of residence, lack of uniform requirements, discipline, costs, confidentiality of information, lack of knowledge of state laws, and strike breaking (National Council of State Boards of Nursing, 1999, p. 1). All of the issues have been extensively researched and debated. The language in the interstate compact has been carefully crafted to address issues that were identified. During the legislative process the legislators heard the opponents but were satisfied that mutual recognition and the interstate compact did not place nurses at risk and provided for public protection. In fact, many legislators could not understand why the model was so long in coming. From a policy perspective, legislators saw the change as "making a great deal of sense."

Perhaps the most contentious issue has been the linking of licensure to the state of residence rather than to the traditional state of practice. The choice between state of residence and state of practice was not a legal issue but rather an administrative issue. After careful consideration of both options, the state of practice was rejected as too complicated. Today it is not unusual to find nurses working for a number of different employers, crossing state borders in the course of their work or providing care via telehealth. How does a nurse working in more than one state choose the state of practice? How does the nurse who is not employed in nursing determine the state of practice? The difficulty in determining the state of practice when a nurse is practicing in multiple states would be too confusing for both nurses and the boards of nursing. Using the state of residence as the link for licensure allows for consistent licensing procedures, reduces the administrative burden, and provides for public protection.

Lack of uniform requirements was another issue debated. The fear has been that licensure will be reduced to the lowest common denominator. This is not the case. The core requirements for licensure have been relatively consistent for a very long time. All states use the national licensing examination and have similar educational requirements. Nurses have always been able to move with relative ease from state to state. In the last 20 years, core requirements have become more alike than different. The areas of major difference in licensure requirements are in continuing education, background checks, and prelicensure education programs. The boards continue to work to close the differences.

Concern has been expressed that mutual recognition will place the nurse at greater risk of discipline by multiple states. Taking disciplinary action against a nurse who has violated the laws of the state is a basic component of public protection. Mutual recognition will provide for better coordination among boards of nursing with regard to investigation and disciplinary actions. Boards of nursing have long communicated actions to one another and laws have allowed the other states where the nurse is licensed to take similar action. As under the single-state licensure system, mutual recognition does not require a board to take action because another state has done so. Each board makes the decision based on the board's state laws. Opponents feel that nurses are at a disadvantage should the state of licensure revoke the nurse's license because that nurse could not work in any other state. Even in the single-state license system, a nurse whose license is revoked in one state usually has the license revoked in other states where the nurse is licensed. Mutual recognition prevents the nurse from falling through the cracks in the system and practicing in a state that is unaware that the license has been revoked in another state. The interstate compact allows boards to communicate information at an earlier stage of the complaint process, which also affords greater public protection.

Both nurses and boards of nursing have expressed concerns about the costs. Revenue from renewals of licensure and endorsement will be reduced, since individuals not living in the state will not need licenses in that state. Most jurisdictions believe an increase in fees will be necessary to replace lost revenues. Any fee increase is unpopular with nurses. But one must also consider the value added. No longer will nurses need to hold licenses from multiple states or be required to obtain endorsement when working in another state. Even with an increase in fees, these fees are likely to remain the lowest of almost all regulated professions.

One cannot open a newspaper today and not see concerns raised about the confidentiality of information. The idea of a single coordinated licensure system with access available to the public, employers, and boards of nursing causes a great deal of apprehension. Any system must meet stringent security requirements, with confidentiality meticulously maintained. Each state's public information laws govern what can be released to the public. Boards of nursing will have the same kind of access to information as they have under the single-state licensure system, but can retrieve the information from a single source, allowing for better coordination. Boards that have entered into the compact have access to significant investigative data. The system only provides a flag that the information is available from the board doing the investigation. The risks to confidentiality are no greater than the risks within each state's database.

The compact grants a multistate privilege to nurses to practice in other states provided that the nurses abide by the laws and regulations of the state where they are practicing. How is the nurse supposed to know what the laws and regulations are in a state? This situation is not unique to mutual recognition licensure. It is the nurse's professional responsibility to know and understand the laws and regulations wherever the nurse practices. It is the nurse's responsibility to contact the board of nursing and request a copy of the practice act and regulations. Lack of knowledge of the laws and regulations is not an impediment to mutual recognition.

Concern has been raised that the hard-fought collective bargaining agreements could be compromised under the mutual recognition model. Strike-breaking activities were the major concern. Mutual recognition allows the nurse to move easily from one state to another. Since the nurse does not have to obtain a license, the nurse can come into the state and work immediately. Even under the single-state licensure system, nurses can move quickly into a state to work. Most states created temporary licenses to allow a nurse to work until permanent licensure was obtained. The interstate compact was never intended to impact adversely on collective bargaining. In fact, to assure that there is no unintentioned outcome from the compact, most states have included language in their laws to the effect that the compact does not supersede any state labor laws.

The American Nurses Association has been the most vocal opponent to the mutual recognition model. Even so, a number of state nursing associations have agreed to support the state boards of nursing in their efforts to pass the interstate compact. The state associations and the boards of nursing have agreed to carry out a 5-year evaluation of the implementation of mutual recognition and make any necessary modifications. No licensing system will be without challenges, but careful and thoughtful consideration of issues will allow for a continuing system that provides public protection without placing the nurse at risk.

THE BENEFITS

Mutual recognition offers many benefits. Nurses can move freely from state to state without obtaining a license in each state. When a nurse calls a patient at home to check on the patient's condition, uses a fax to send instructions to a patient, or assesses a patient via closed-circuit television, there will no longer be a risk for practicing nursing without a license when the practice crosses state lines. The frustrations experienced in obtaining licensure in a variety of states will no longer be an issue. Renewal of licensure will also be easier, since there will only be one license to renew instead of several. Mutual recognition also allows nurses to take advantage of new opportunities such as telehealth without worrying about licensure.

Public protection will be enhanced. Greater coordination and communication among boards of nursing means better assurance of safe nursing practice. It will be more difficult for a nurse who violates the laws to move from state to state undetected. Disciplinary actions will take place in a more expeditious manner while at the same time assuring that due process protections are not violated.

Health care institutions will find a more flexible nursing workforce. Those health care institutions that have hesitated to move into telehealth activities or other activities that would take nurses across state lines for fear of violating licensing laws can move forward. Verification of licensure would be enhanced by a single coordinated data base.

Access to nursing care will also be enhanced, especially in rural areas. The barrier created by the single-state licensing system will be eliminated. Consumers can choose a nurse to provide care regardless of state boundaries. Nurses can more easily manage patient care without regard to the mobility of their patients, therefore ensuring continuity of care.

Finally, the mutual recognition system resolves the federal government concern regarding access to cost-efficient care in rural areas and underserved populations by removing some of the licensure impediments. The barrier of licensure to telemedicine as described in the Telemedicine Report (1997) is no longer applicable to nursing and removes the threat of federal regulation of nursing.

Clearly, the time has arrived for mutual recognition. The need and benefits outweigh any of the issues. Those issues identified are not reason enough to delay or discard the model. Change is always difficult. In the case of nursing licensure, it is made more difficult because mutual recognition is the first major change to the structure of licensure in 100 years. If nursing regulation does not meet the needs of the health care system, others will be found to provide the care. There will be no winners. Nursing, the public, and employers will lose. With mutual recognition, nursing as well as the public will reap the benefits of a licensure regulation system designed for the 21st century.

REFERENCES

Black, H.C. (1983). *Black's law dictionary* (abridged 5th ed., p. 421). St Paul, MN: West Publishing Co.

Department of Commerce. (1997). Telemedicine Report to Congress, Executive Summary [On line]. Available: http://www.ntia.doc.gov/reports/telemed/execsum.htm.

National Council of State Boards of Nursing. (1997, August). Report of the Multistate Regulation Task Force. *Business Book.* Chicago: Author.

National Council of State Boards of Nursing. (1998, January). *Why is the National Council considering mutual recognition as a new model for nurse licensure?* Chicago: Author.

National Council of State Boards of Nursing. (1999, June). Response to ANA House of Delegates regarding concerns about mutual recognition and the interstate compact [On line]. Available: http://www.ncsbn.org/files/mutual/ana990609.asp.

TVG, Inc. (1997, February). *The interstate practice of nursing: An assessment of current practices in the healthcare industry.* Ft. Washington, PA: Author.

Performance Evaluation
Measuring Clinical Competencies

ROBERT H. WELTON, FE NIEVES-KHOUW

The concept of competencies began in the early 1970s when the U.S. State Department turned to David McClelland (1993) and his associates for help in selecting junior foreign service information officers who represent America in foreign countries. The critical part of the foreign service officers' job is to get as many people as possible to like the United States and support U.S. policies. The state department had traditionally selected foreign service officers with a foreign service officer examination. According to McClelland (1973), traditional aptitude or knowledge-based tests did not predict on-the-job success; plus these tests also tended to discriminate against minorities and candidates from less privileged backgrounds. If traditional aptitude testing does not predict job performance, then what does?

McClelland and his associates attempted to identify factors that could accomplish two objectives. One objective was to identify factors that could predict successful job performance, and second, they wanted these factors not biased by a candidate's race, sex, or socioeconomic status. They used behavioral event interviews with foreign service officer superstars, those officers who had demonstrated superior performance, to determine which factors were accurate predictors of success on the job. They compared this superior group to average and poor performers to identify characteristics that differed between the two groups, that is, behaviors generally shown by superior performers and not shown by average performers.

These success-predicting factors were not personality traits, nor were they skills in the traditional sense. Instead, they presented as sets of behaviors combined with skills, knowledge, and personal attributes. Furthermore, these factors or "competencies" were definable, observable, and measurable. Eventually, the competency characteristics that differentiated superior from average information officers were grouped into three categories (McClelland, 1993):

1. *Cross-cultural interpersonal sensitivity* or the ability to hear what people from a foreign culture are really saying or meaning and to predict how they will react
2. *Positive expectations of others* or a strong belief in the underlying dignity and worth of others different from oneself and the ability to maintain this positive outlook under stress
3. *Speed in learning political networks* or the ability to figure out quickly who influences whom and what each person's political interests are

Given the increasing cultural diversity of today's patient populations coupled with the need for nurses to advocate for patients in an increasingly regulated environment, all three of these competencies are essential to effective nursing practice regardless of the setting. Yet we rarely see or hear of them in competency discussions. These omissions are most probably due to the consistently narrow focus on competencies in the work settings as clinical skills not inclusive of critical thinking or collaborative work, which are critical elements for practice.

Since 1973 when McClelland published the psychological foundations for competencies in "Testing for Competence Rather than Intelligence," competencies have been widely applied across occupations and professions in multiple disciples and industries.

COMPETENCIES IN HEALTH CARE

Competencies in health care have attracted considerable attention over the past two decades because they are thought to represent a way to identify caregiver characteristics that can predict or contribute to successful job performance and ultimately positive patient outcomes.

267

Competency development in health care typically refers to education and training of staff to improve job performance and care outcomes (Kelly, 1992). The primary distinction between traditional approaches to instruction and competency-based instruction is in the emphasis of the educational program: traditional instruction emphasizes what a learner should *know*, while competency-based education emphasizes what a learner should be able *to do* to indicate competency for the task, skill, or role (Alspach, 1995). The emphasis in competency is on task performance and not on acquiring knowledge; knowledge acquisition is demonstrated as it applies to performance in a clinical area (Abruzzese, 1996). The focus of competency-based programs is the result, that is, the ability of new staff to do their job.

ANATOMY OF A COMPETENCY

The ability of staff to do their job is a clear and simple definition in the real world of work, but there is no consensus on this or other definitions of competence or competency. Definitions vary from "just enough to get the job done" to the inclusion of deep innate qualities that are hard to identify or measure. Table 37-1 shows the diverse range in some of these competency definitions.

Despite all these varying definitions, there does seem to be consensus on the model of Dorothy del Bueno and associates of the dimensions of competence as the integration of critical thinking skills, technical skills, and interpersonal skills (del Bueno, Griffin, Burke, & Foley, 1990). This model, shown in Figure 37-1, presents these three overlapping dimensions in the context of a given work setting. And, the box on page 269 shows examples of skills or behaviors in each of these three dimensions. When evaluating performance in the real world of work, what one sees most often is emphasis placed on staff's attaining only the clinical and technical skills, with little effort directed to developing and evaluating the skills in the other two dimensions of critical thinking and interpersonal skills.

Alspach (1995a) identified several major elements in a well-designed competency-based approach to education that distinguishes it from traditional approaches to instruction. According to Alspach, a competency-based approach is:

- Derived from and for a specific role and practice setting
- Organized around and contributes to an overall competency-based curriculum
- Based on real-world performance requirements
- Derived from and validated by practitioners
- Practice and performance based
- Structured by competency statements and performance criteria
- Learner centered
- Flexible in terms of instructional strategies used

TABLE 37-1   Competency Definitions

Author and Date	Competency Definition
Alspach, 1995b	The distinction between competence and competency lies in (a) that competence implies a person's potential capability to perform, and the term competency emphasizes a person's actual performance in a real-life situation, and (b) that competency is determined in relation to employer-defined standards of practice specific to an organizational role and setting
Benner, 1982	The ability to perform a task with desirable outcomes under the varied circumstances of the real world
Butler, 1978	The ability to meet or surpass prevailing standards of adequacy for a particular activity.
del Bueno et al., 1990	The effective application of knowledge and skill in the work setting
Gatz et al., 1982	In relation to community workers and the older residents to whom they provide services, it is the ability to perceive multiple options to dilemmas, to recognize available resources and to use them, with a result of decreased feelings of powerlessness
Guinon, 1991	Underlying characteristics of people and indicated ways of behaving or thinking, generalizing across situations, and enduring for a reasonably long period
Kelly, 1998	A person's actual performance in his or her specific job function or specified task
Spencer & Spencer, 1993	Underlying characteristics of an individual that are causally related to criterion-referenced effective or superior performance in a job or situation
National Council of State Boards of Nursing, 1996	The application of knowledge and the interpersonal, decision-making, and psychomotor skills expected for the nurse's practice role, within the context of public health, welfare, and safety
Pollack, 1981	Whatever is required to get something done

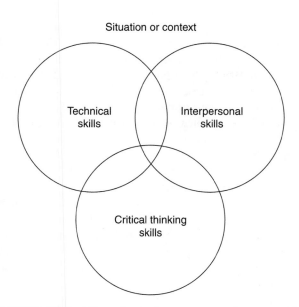

Situation or context

Technical skills

Interpersonal skills

Critical thinking skills

FIGURE 37-1 Dimensions of competent performance. (del Bueno, D.J., Weeks, L., & Brown-Steward, P. [1987]. Dimensions of competent performance. *Nursing Economic$, 5*[1], p. 23. Reprinted with permission of the publisher, Jannetti Publications, Inc., East Holly Avenue, Box 56, Pitman, NJ 08071-0056; Phone [856] 256-2300; FAX [856] 589-7463. [For a sample issue of the journal, contact the publisher.])

• Shared expectations with learners and allows for remedial instruction as necessary

COMPETENCIES FAIL TO DIFFERENTIATE EXPECTATIONS BASED ON PREPARATION

Graduates of baccalaureate degree, associate degree, and hospital-based diploma nursing programs all take the same licensing examination, which is designed to ensure safe practice. Using the same licensing examination fails to recognize the broad range of functions in nursing and the potential for improving the quality of care given, if different roles and responsibilities were identified. Realistic statements regarding the competencies of each level or category of nursing education are necessary so that each category of graduate can be used effectively and efficiently (Ellis & Hartley, 1998). No such differentiated competencies based on basic preparation for practice exist on a nationally recognized scope. The Midwest Alliance in Nursing (Primm, 1986), the Healing Web Group of six midwestern and western states (Ellis & Hartley, 1998), the Sioux Falls, South Dakota, experience (Modern Hospitals, 1994), and the Colorado experiment (Ellis & Hartley, 1998) are examples of some local and regional work to-

ward describing competencies of graduates from different types of nursing programs. However, to date, few of these projects have yielded widespread implementation.

WHY BOTHER TO USE THEM?

Competencies in the training, development, and assessment of nurses and other health care workers have been used since the 1970s. The real driver for competencies in nursing began in 1991 when the Joint Commission on Accreditation of Healthcare Organizations (JCAHO) started to require hospitals to prove that its workers had the ability to meet the performance expectations stated in their job descriptions (2000). In 1993, these requirements were extended to all hospital staff except physicians. Since 1991, all health care organizations have been working to develop, deploy, maintain, and update their competency programs to comply with JCAHO's ever evolving mandates on competency assessments while ensuring some relevancy to the real work world of daily practice.

EXAMPLES OF SKILLS IN THE THREE DIMENSIONS OF COMPETENCY

Clinical and Technical Skills
Cognitive skills
Knowledge
Psychomotor skills

Critical Thinking Skills
Problem-solving
Time management
Priority setting
Planning
Ethics
Resource allocation
Fiscal responsibilities
Clinical reasoning
Change management

Interpersonal Skills
Communications
Customer service
Conflict management
Delegating
Team facilitation
Collaborating
Directing
Articulating
Understanding diversity
Team building

Included in these standards are requirements for orientation, ongoing in-service and education, and an assessment of the ongoing learning needs of staff to ensure that the organization supports growth in its work force's ability to carry out their job responsibilities. JCAHO especially focused on the health care staff's ability to adapt care to the age of the patient and to adequately perform new procedures and techniques or operate new technology or equipment. Before these regulations, the use of competencies in hospitals was limited to "cutting edge" practices in which units used competency-based orientation to train new staff and introduce them to the skills required to care proficiently for specific patient populations. The introduction of JCAHO competency standards made this approach mandatory.

COMPETENCIES IN NURSING

Competency in nursing is not a new concept but an evolving response to shifts in practice patterns. Licensure proves minimum competency in that it demonstrates that an individual has learned the theories and standards of nursing practice. In addition, many state boards of nursing require continuing education for license renewal. With existing licensure and continuing education, why require health care agencies to develop a systematic approach to document and prove that their workers are able to meet the expectations of their role? What value does this requirement add? It is inevitable that concerns about minimum requirements to ensure safe care of patients surface as health care systems are redesigned and business factors drive patient care decisions. In essence, use of competency models in health care is a tangible way to hold organizations accountable for clearly articulating success factors in the work environment and for recruiting employees that match these descriptions. This requirement also holds the industry clearly responsible for providing training that will ensure that personnel are able to meet job expectations.

The result presumably is the achievement of the goals and objectives of the agency: good patient care. Unfortunately, when nursing competency programs are developed as a response to regulatory standards, they aim to meet *minimum* requirements and leave out other essential components of patient care: teamwork, system facilitation, timeliness, and responsiveness. The byproduct of a competency approach aimed at complying with minimum standards is a competency program that consists of skill checklists summarizing interventions that nurses usually provide. This type of competency program does not develop high performers. Instead, it accepts satisfactory but mediocre practice. It also is not useful in performance management, recognition, merit determination, or development of high performers because it does not include performance expectations of clinical "superstars."

The nurse's role in intensive care units is unique because in ICUs the nurse is the only member of the health care team who remains at the patient's bedside 24 hours a day. Through observations, continuous surveillance, and the use of complex technologies, nurses collect comprehensive data and are usually the first providers to detect subtle changes in the patient's condition. Nurses interpret data and make decisions about what information is useful, what is not, and when to call the physician. Based on their data analysis, nurses make either independent or collaborative decisions about treatments and plans of care. These unique nursing contributions to cardiac intensive care are summarized in the box below. Nurses in other acute care settings share some of these same characteristics; however, few hospitals include these essential characteristics in developing their competency models. Why? Probably because these characteristics take time, usually longer than any probationary period, and practice to develop. Thus these "competencies" are rarely seen in writing in an orientation plan for new staff. Yet these qualities are what distinguish "superstars," and they are the qualities we all would want in the nurses caring for our family members or ourselves.

CHARACTERISTICS UNIQUE TO CRITICAL CARE NURSING PRACTICE

- Maintains focus on the patient as an individual amid multiple technologies
- Uses data from multiple simultaneous sources associated with one or a few critically ill patients
- Rapidly assimilates and prioritizes information
- Rapidly intervenes because of limited patient tolerance for delay
- Identifies signs of subtle changes in a patient's condition, which can be achieved only through continuous and intensive monitoring
- Frequently communicates with other members of the health care team about the rapidly changing condition of the critically ill patient to update the patient's plan of care

From American Association of Critical Care Nurses. (1992). *Critical care in the nursing curriculum: Selecting and integrating essential content, AACN* (p. 7). Aliso Viejo, CA: Author.

TOO MANY CONFUSING DEFINITIONS AND MODELS

Initial difficulties in competency development arise from lack of consensus about what competency means and what dimensions it includes. Table 37-1 provides some definitions from the gurus. However, McGuire, Stanhope, and Weisenbeck (1998) offer a more useful definition that goes beyond minimum standards. According to these authors, nursing competence is the application of knowledge and skills related to caring, critical thinking, communication, and clinical intervention expected for the nurse's practice role within the context of the public's health, welfare, and safety. McGuire et al. (1998) also describe standards consistent with this definition as including:

- Application of knowledge
- Demonstration of responsibility
- Restriction or accommodation of practice if unable to perform full scope of nursing practice
- Responsibility for nursing competency assessment

In contrast, investigators in non-health-care industries, such as Mirabile (1997), introduce the concept that competence is associated with high performance on the job, not merely doing the job. This definition includes motives, beliefs and values and core competencies focused on what the organization does best, not what the organization does most. Parry (1998) states that competencies are closely intertwined with but should not be confused with skills and personality traits. Competencies include skills as learning points, and personality traits such as creativity, independence, decisiveness, and initiative influence the way one uses his or her competencies. Both Parry (1998) and Mc-

Clelland (1973) agree that measures of competence should be designed to reflect changes in what the individual has learned. It is expected that experience and opportunities to perform tasks increase one's competence.

There is significant disagreement regarding the role of a caregiver's values in competency development. Spencer and Spencer (1993) describe the Iceberg Model in which skills and knowledge are surface competencies that are easy and less costly to develop, observe, and measure, while motive and trait competencies, though harder and more costly to develop and measure, are ultimately more predictive of performance outcomes (Fig. 37-2).

The American Compensation Association (1996) takes the position that the primary goal of competencies is to "raise the bar" in performance and not merely to establish baseline performance. Used this way, competencies have applications in recruitment, placement, promotion, training and development, performance management, and ultimately help the organization gain a competitive edge.

SELECTING A COMPETENCY MODEL

Lack of consensus in defining competence, competency, and its component parts influences decisions hospitals make about the competency model they will adapt. Building a competency model is the first step in competency development, and it should:

- Identify outcomes to be achieved through the competency program
- Describe tools to elicit and classify those outcomes
- Include a format for describing competency requirements

FIGURE 37-2 The Iceberg Model. (From Spencer, L.M., & Spencer, S.M. [1993]. *Competence at work.* New York: John Wiley & Sons. Copyright 1993. Reprinted with permission of John Wiley & Sons, Inc.)

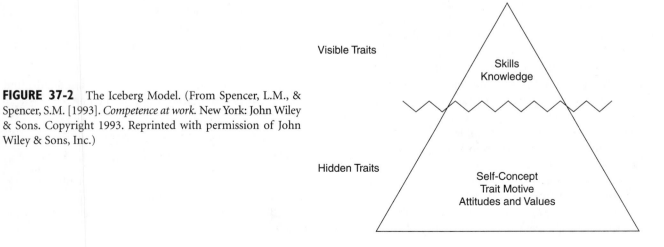

- List specific competency requirements and give each competency a basic definition and behavioral criteria to describe expected performance levels
- Be based on real work priorities
- Be developed by the people who need and use the competencies

As mentioned earlier, the general inclination in competency development and assessment is to focus on clinical skills at the exclusion of the outcomes that are important to the organization. Primary focus on patient care interventions is essential, but this focus is shortsighted, superficial, and does not allow the individual to understand the total context in which patient care has to be delivered.

One of the most difficult and controversial issues to address in building a competency model is how to prioritize what is important. The Nursing Interventions Classification (NIC) offers a useful structure to select interventions relevant to the daily nursing practice. As it is skills driven, the NIC describes critical activities for each nursing intervention that are observable, measurable, and derived from the real world. It even includes expectations around cultural competency, which is frequently missing in other frameworks. The NIC can be used to identify all nursing activities or to decide the priority of the few competencies central to practice.

Another approach to prioritizing competencies is to categorize competencies according to practice risk and opportunity or volume for the practice of selected interventions. Some organizations choose to have a competency model that includes only those competencies that are high risk–high volume, high risk–low volume, or only those competencies that are just high volume. In addition, some hospitals standardize competencies across most, if not all practice areas. Others identify core (i.e., common to all practitioners regardless of setting) competencies and allow each patient care unit to add unit-specialty competencies to the core. Still others opt to buy ready-made competencies from consulting agencies or other hospitals and adapt these to their facilities and cultures. Using ready-made competencies is risky because they may not be relevant to practice and performance norms in their new setting. While all these approaches to competency modeling are feasible and, in some cases, valid, they do not include important dimensions of patient care that will guarantee quality patient care. Patient care is not delivered in a vacuum. Patient care includes the patient, the family, and the system in which patient care is delivered. Competencies that ignore these dimensions measure the beginning competence of a neophyte,

but they do not promote the development of more experienced nurses.

Dimensions that are excluded in competencies that are focused primarily on nursing interventions are those competencies that help humanize the caregiving environment and demystify caregiving processes. Nurses have a central role in facilitating the smooth delivery of care by the multidisciplinary team. It is imperative in the nurse's clinical success that she or he become a broker and advocate for the patient and support the patient and his or her family as they negotiate a confusing system at a time of crisis. Patients in a research study by Gerteis et al. (1993) eloquently described these dimensions of patient care. They include:

- Respect for patient's values, preferences and expressed needs including preserving the patient's dignity and privacy and involvement in decision making.
- Coordination of care, which refers to integration of the care delivered by different disciplines that comprise the clinical team.
- Information, communication, and education that respect the patient's preference for the level of detail on clinical information, status, or prognoses as well as keeping the patient informed about the process of care.
- Physical comfort that goes beyond pain management to assistance with activities of daily living and providing for a personal and comfortable hospital environment.
- Emotional support and alleviation of fear and anxiety, including interventions sensitive to the crisis that acute or chronic illness creates in the patient's relationships, occupation, and finances.
- Involvement of family and friends that recognizes that family members are partners in patient care and can offer substantial support to the patient's recovery and facilitate important decision making.
- Transitions, which address the patient's specific anxieties about the appropriate information, and support needed to continue his or her successful recovery after discharge.

Critics of existing competency models frequently find these important dimensions of care missing.

WRITING COMPETENCIES: OBSESSIVE-COMPULSIVE OR GENERAL STATEMENT

Competency writers vary in how they describe expectations. These variations can influence how performance is evaluated. Some developers write in great detail while others offer general descriptions of desired behaviors.

Which is best? This decision determines the time and energy required or available to build the competency model and its application to people and jobs. Generic competencies are more universal and will remain stable over time, while skill- or detail-oriented competencies are specific to situations and require frequent changes over time. Mirabile (1997) asks a fundamental question, What do you want to be able to do as a result of the competency model? He identifies the following advantages and disadvantages to using detail in generating competency models:

The more detail you create:

- The longer it will take to build the model
- The more money it will require
- The more you restrict the range of acceptable performance
- The more you inhibit creative, alternative ways to achieve the same outcome
- The less you can compare information across jobs or people
- The less you can generalize the results
- The faster the information becomes obsolete

But with a detailed model:

- It is easier to communicate expected outcomes
- Performance management can become specific
- The more you can differentiate between performance levels and between people

Nurses tend to like marching orders and are more comfortable with specific and concrete descriptions of behavioral expectations. Specific and concrete expectations also simplify performance evaluation. Maintenance of this type of competency modeling consumes time, money, and energy, and it requires close monitoring so appropriate updates are identified and written as needed. A real danger is confusing competencies with policies and procedures so that a competency is written to accompany any new clinical standard. This confusion can lead to competencies that are too detailed, lengthy, and costly to deploy realistically and maintain in today's practice environment. In our experience at a large, East Coast, university-affiliated medical center where we choose not to use a detailed model, our efforts still took over 3 years to fully develop and deploy, and the cost estimate exceeded $85,000.

COMPETENCY ASSESSMENT SHOULD FOCUS ON WHAT A STAFF PERSON ACTUALLY DOES

Preceptors for new staff can use a variety of competency assessment methods, such as a posttest and quizzes, case studies, simulations, peer review, self-report, and observations to assess competencies. However, the merit of each method varies. The continuums of competency assessment methods with their degrees of reliability of validly assessing clinical competency are shown in Figure 37-3.

According to Alspach (1995b), when a competency-based approach to orientation is used, preceptors and managers should adjust competency assessment methods and verification to ensure reliable and valid evaluation of actual clinical performance. Her recommendations (1995) for modifications in competency evaluation include:

- *Decrease reliance on written tests* because being knowledgeable in an area is not equivalent to being clinically competent in that area.
- *Increased reliance on simulations* affords a more valid and reliable assessment because it requires the staff person to actually perform as expected rather than show that he or she is knowledgeable about a skill.
- *Maximize reliance on clinical observations,* which are the most valid and reliable means of evaluating if a new nurse can perform in actual patient care situations.

Unfortunately, direct observation of actual clinical performance is seen as time-consuming and expensive, especially in the prevailing heavily regulated work environment. Front-line staff are frequently asked to use less reliable, "fast and quick" assessment methods to save time and money.

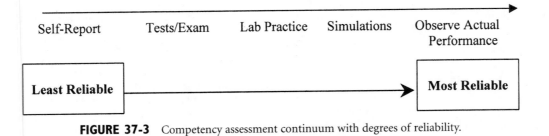

FIGURE 37-3 Competency assessment continuum with degrees of reliability.

ASSESSING THE EFFECTIVENESS OF COMPETENCY PROGRAMS

In the end, any competency program has to deliver outcomes to justify the resources provided to build it. The primary question is whether the competency program achieved or delivered the outcomes the organization wanted from it. The easiest outcome to deliver is compliance with regulatory standards. No measure of effectiveness has to be developed other than a tracking system in the human resources (HR) department to demonstrate that each worker's competencies have been assessed and documented and that there is a process for continually reviewing the same set of competencies. Hospitals often have HR policies that require that competencies central to practice be assessed by the end of orientation or prior to termination of probation.

JCAHO site surveyors prefer that competencies be observed in daily practice. This preference is a double-edged sword. On one hand, observation in daily practice is the best proof that a competency is executed as expected by the employee. On the other hand, this revalidation method is the easiest to fake. Less than conscientious assessors can easily sign off on a competency, especially if the assessors do not see the merits of the competency program and consider it an academic exercise mandated just to fulfill a regulatory requirement. The effectiveness of this competency approach is difficult to measure beyond the results that a tracking mechanism can offer.

When competencies are tied to organizational outcomes and are written to reflect critical success factors to achieve organizational goals, measures of effectiveness can include:

- Whether the competency program effectively communicated its core values to its employees
- Whether employee performance increased because the competency program "raised the bar"
- Whether the competency program aided the organization in gaining a competitive edge
- Whether teamwork and cross-functional collaborations critical to achieving goals have improved
- Whether the competency program addressed and closed gaps between low, acceptable, and high performers

SUMMARY

This discussion of competencies and their influence on performance evaluation has identified several critical issues in competency development, deployment, and assessment that must be clarified if competencies are to be useful to fully develop staff and their performance evaluation. These issues are:

- Narrow focus on skills and not inclusive of critical thinking or collaboration.
- Many models have gaps and omissions such as cultural competency.
- Used as band-aids for gaps or deficient in operational processes.
- Difficult to find an all-inclusive and comprehensive organizing framework (e.g., medical diagnoses, nursing diagnoses, or body organ systems).
- Front-line staff want them to be very prescriptive and detailed.
- Distinction among competencies, policies, and procedures are sometime unclear.
- Seen as having little value by many experienced front-line staff who may fail to fully integrate them into unit-based orientations.
- Very costly and time-consuming to develop and deploy.
- Multiple measurement methods can be unreliable or invalid.
- Difficulties in evaluating competencies in temporary staff.
- Merging performance evaluation with competency assessment frequently ensures only *readiness* to perform against established standards, and not actual performance in daily practice after orientation.
- Seen as valuable to novices but useless to expert practitioners, as they frequently do not "raise the bar" for their performance.

REFERENCES

Abruzzese, R.S. (1996). *Nursing staff development: Strategies for success* (2nd ed., p. 267). St. Louis: Mosby.

Alspach, J.G. (1995a). *The educational process in nursing staff development* (p. 162). St. Louis: Mosby.

Alspach, J.G. (1995b). *Designing competency assessment programs: A handbook for nursing and health-related professionals* (p. 14). National Nursing Staff Development Organization.

American Compensation Association. (1996). *Raising the bar: Using competencies to enhance employee performance.* Scottsdale, AZ: American Compensation Association.

Benner, P. (1982). Issues in competency based testing. *Nursing Outlook, 30*(5), 303-309.

Butler, F.C. (1978). The concept of competence: An operational definition. *Educational Technology, 7,* 7-18.

del Bueno, D.J., Griffin, L.R., Burke, S.M., & Foley, M.A. (1990). The clinical teacher: A critical link to competence development. *Journal of Nursing Staff Development, 6*(3), 135-138.

Ellis, J.E., & Hartley, C.L. (1998). *Nursing in today's world: Challenges, issues and trends* (p. 213). Philadelphia: Lippincott.

Gatz, M., Barbarin, O., Tyler, F., Mitchell, R., Moran, J., Wirzbicki, P., Crawford, J., & Engelman, A. (1982). Enhancement of individual and community competence: The older adult as community worker. *American Journal of Community Psychology, 10*(3), 291-303.

Gerteis, M., Edgman-Levitan, S., Daley, J., & Delbanco, T.L. (Eds.). (1993). *Through the patient's eyes.* San Francisco: Jossey-Bass.

Guinon, R.M. (1991). Personnel assessment, selection and placement. In M.D. Dunnettte & L.M. Hougs (Eds.), *Handbook of industrial and organizational psychology* (p. 335). Palo Alto, CA: Consulting Psychologist Press.

Kelly, K.J. (1998). *Clinical and nursing staff development: Current competence and future focus* (2nd ed., p. 240). Philadelphia: Lippincott.

McClelland, D.C. (1973). Testing for competence rather than intelligence. *American Psychologists, 28,* 1-14.

McClelland, D.C. (1993). Introduction. In L.M. Spencer & S.M. Spencer (Eds.), *Competence at work* (pp. 3-7). New York: John Wiley & Sons.

McGuire, C.A., Stanhope, M., & Weisenbeck, S.M. (1998). Nursing competence—an evolving regulatory issue in Kentucky. *Nursing Administrative Quarterly, 23*(1), 24-28.

Mirabile, R.J. (1997, August). Everything you wanted to know about competency modeling. *Training and Development,* pp. 73-77.

Modern Hospitals. (1994). 100 Top U.S. hospitals—Bench-marks for success. *Modern Hospitals, 24*(3), 8, 14.

National Council of State Boards of Nursing. (1996). *Definitions of competence and standards for competence.* Chicago: National Council of State Boards of Nursing.

Parry, S.B. (1998, June). Just what is a competency? (And why should you care?) *Training,* pp. 58-64.

Pollack, M.B. (1981, January/February). Speaking of competencies. *Health Education,* pp. 9-13.

Primm, P.L. (1986, May-June). Entry into practice: Competency statements for BSNs and ADNs. *Nursing Outlook, 34*(3), 135-137.

Spencer, L.M., & Spencer, S.M. (1993). *Competence at work.* New York: John Wiley & Sons.

Section Six

Governance

Challenges to Nursing Leadership in a Changing Nursing Practice World

JOANNE McCLOSKEY DOCHTERMAN, HELEN KENNEDY GRACE

The structures in which nursing has been practiced through the years have sometimes been a constraint to the ability of professional nurses to govern their own practice. In the changing terrain of health care at the turn of the millennium the entire field is shifting, offering unusual challenges for nursing to play a more prominent role in governance issues. The pressures for cost control push nursing leaders to be experts not only in the domain of quality of patient care but also in the economic underpinnings of the field. Use of less costly personnel to provide patient care has emerged through the years as one way of addressing cost problems. While, on the one hand, we see nursing being somewhat diminished in some aspects in institutional settings, in areas outside of hospital nursing we see the role of nursing expanding and becoming progressively more independent. Increasingly, the dichotomy between nursing education and nursing practice is narrowing. As nursing educational programs become more involved in the provision of services, the lines between funding for educational programs and funding for service become blurred. As nursing moves toward more independence, governance models for nursing centers and community-based practices are beginning to emerge. One of the hallmarks of a profession is that of being able to govern one's domain. In nursing this has always been in question with boundary problems an issue vis-à-vis medicine and institutional controls within hospital settings. This section provides a wonderful overview of the complexities of nursing and its governance in a changing health care environment.

The opening debate posed by Zimmermann addresses the question of the use of unlicensed assistive personnel (UAP): Do they erode the quality of care or make more appropriate use of professionally prepared nurses? Some argue that UAP are a necessary part of cost control. The average wage for a professional nurse is 144% higher than that for a UAP. However, this figure does not take into account fringe benefits, which are the same as for professionals, the costs of training, the lack of stability of the staff, and the costs of supervision. Zimmermann argues that there is a need to determine the skill mix necessary to provide quality care. Nurses need to know what can be delegated and what cannot. In concluding the chapter, Zimmermann takes us back to Florence Nightingale's admonition to "do the sick no harm." "Fulfilling that axiom includes more than our own individual practice. It involves making strategic and tactical choices based on all the relevant issues for the number and composition of staffing that best meets the patients' needs."

In this era of profound change, Kerfoot addresses the complex challenges faced by nurse leaders. Cataclysmic changes in the reimbursement systems place enormous pressures on nurse leaders who are trying to assure quality of care while working with management to achieve viable cost-effective services. The challenges will be even more complex in the years ahead. The breaking of the genetic codes that will make genetic interventions possible, the explosion in information technology, and the changes that are accelerated in the delivery of health care are pointed to as presenting particular challenges to nursing leadership. Of particular concern are the ethical issues that will be raised and the need for nursing to weigh interventions that will now be possible. At the same time as these scientific advances are occurring, the health care marketplace is mandating that services become much more personalized. Self-management of care, customizing of services, greater accountability to patients and their families, and the need for synergistic caregiving teams push nursing leadership to become innovative in changing practice. Kerfoot concludes this chapter by advocating for the creation of "sanctuaries of caring and healing."

In today's changing health care terrain nurses are moving beyond traditional leadership roles to broader governance roles. Malone addresses the challenges faced by nurses who move into and hold nonnursing leadership positions. One of the major obstacles is that of the ambivalence of nursing related to power. Becoming a leader in shaping health care requires the use of power. Characteristics of successful leaders include vision and risk taking along with the ability to manage boundaries, empower others, and mentor followers. Pointing out the numbers of nurses who have moved into nonnursing leadership positions Malone speaks to the challenges of being an effective leader and the ambivalence of nursing in supporting these leaders.

New structures in linking nurses in academic settings with those in community-based practice have provided opportunities for nurses to play key leadership roles in shaping these practice settings. The next three chapters address these issues. Meservey notes that we currently do not have a health care system but rather a medical intervention system. To be an effective leader in shaping health care systems for the future nurse leaders need to first have a clear vision of what such a system would involve. The author envisions a health care system as more integrated, more managed, more evidence based, more ambulatory, and dependent on information systems technology. The education of health professionals and health services research must respond to the challenge of reshaping such a system. To create such a system, there needs to be a change in the orientation of health care as a system developed for providers to one that is centered on the community; the focus of practice must be on prevention. And the research should be community based. Meservey then describes a model developed in Boston where health professions' educational programs have joined with the community to create a health careers academy. Leadership by nurses with a new vision has been key in creating this new multidisciplinary health systems model.

The changing face of health care delivery provides new opportunities for nursing centers. Lundeen notes that most of the efforts of health care reform are merely tinkering with the edges and argues that nursing centers have the potential to provide a viable alternative system of primary health care delivery. Noting the lack of progress in meeting the goals for *Healthy People 2000* in particular categories, Lundeen argues that nursing centers as a recognized part of a health care delivery system have the potential to address these problem areas. Nursing centers differ from traditional medical models in their emphasis

on prevention and coordination across the continuum of care. For nursing centers to position themselves to reach their full potential as part of a comprehensive system of health care, collaboration with other providers and documenting patient care outcomes are essential. Lundeen concludes, "As nurses, we should celebrate our proud history, claim credit for the work we are doing in our dynamic present, and proclaim in a multitude of ways that nursing centers have met and will continue to meet the call for innovation in a challenging future."

The theme of developing community-education linkages continues with the article authored by Belcher describing interdisciplinary service-learning partnership developed between five Indianapolis public schools and nursing, education, and social work programs of the university. The author notes that the challenge for faculty is to prepare professionals who are comfortable with the changing landscape of practice and equipped to address the challenges of the future. As part of creating this interdisciplinary educational program within the university, six courses have been developed: (1) communications and collaboration; (2) cultural competency; (3) public policy and public awareness; (4) development and coordination of family, school, and community research; (5) reflective practice; and (6) leadership. By having a vision for an altered future, nursing has provided important leadership to an innovative program that enriches the health and education of young people in the public schools while providing professionals of the future with a program uniquely designed to equip them for a changing environment of practice.

Shifting back to more traditional governance roles, Maas and Specht address the complex issues related to shared governance models in nursing. One of the hallmarks of a profession is self-governance of practice. Nursing in institutional settings has predominantly been governed by the institution rather than by the profession, in contrast to medicine, which has been practiced in institutional settings but governs the practice by the profession itself. The authors note that interest in self-governance in nursing fluctuates with the ebb and flow of nurse shortages. At times of shortage, self-governance becomes more predominant. Some of the issues that complicate self-governance are the lack of clearly defined criteria for self-governance, the mixed motives in instituting such systems, and disagreements about how self-governance models should be implemented. Nurses need to accommodate two systems: those of the organization and those of the profession. Noting that there is considerable confusion about participation in decision making and shared governance, the authors advocate that nurses participate in shared governance for the whole system, not of nursing as a part of the system. Noting that there is considerable room for pseudoshared governance models, these models sometimes may serve as an opiate for nursing rather than true participation. The authors conclude that there are top-down and bottom-up approaches that have been employed but that the unit approach is most desirable because of the buy-in of nurses to this model and their true participation.

The nursing leadership roles of the future will undoubtedly be more challenging than those of the past. The revolutions in the scientific realm, the explosion of information, and the movement of care from institutional to home and community settings coupled with the ever present concerns for cost control place nursing leadership in a most interesting position. How nurses rise to the challenge will likely determine how far nursing will travel from being a pawn in the game of health care to controlling its own destiny.

CHAPTER 38

The Increasing Use of Unlicensed Assistive Personnel (UAP)

The Erosion and Devotion of Nursing

POLLY GERBER ZIMMERMANN

Unlicensed assistive personnel (UAP) within health care constitutes a sizable presence. The term now comprises at least 50 different job titles of workers who are not highly skilled or otherwise credentialed. That lack is the distinguishing factor because some states do not license certain highly prepared positions, such as a respiratory care practitioner or surgical technologists, even though individuals in those roles have obtained national credentials (Carroll, 1998).

The American Nurses Association (1992a) defines UAP as "unlicensed individuals who are trained to function in an assistive role to the registered professional nurse in the provision of patient/client activities as delegated by and under the supervision of the registered professional nurse." Professional nursing organizations' position statements allow a place for such an assistive role, in both direct nursing and indirect nonnursing patient care activities, provided the RN determines, delegates, and oversees the process (American Nurses Association [ANA], 1992a; Emergency Nurses Association, 1997; Tri-Council for Nursing, 1995).

Is the increasing use of these assistive personnel necessary? Does the increasing use of this role promote efficient patient care and enhance nursing's professionalization? The answer must consider cost, quality of care, utilization, and the potential standardization of the role.

BACKGROUND

The nursing shortage in World War II created team nursing, a sharp demarcation of routine tasks under a skill mix ratio of 70% auxiliary workers and 30% registered nurses (RNs). In the 1970s and 1980s, however, primary care by RNs with undivided responsibility dominated. This change was attributed both to the administration's interest in nurses' abilities for increased productivity and to the professionalization of nursing (Brannon, 1990). UAP were used mainly in the 1980s because there was a shortage of nurses.

As health care costs were rising, many hospitals embraced reengineering in the early 1990s. This fundamental rethinking of processes often included hiring less skilled, cheaper auxiliary workers as a way to cut labor expenses, a cost that typically consumes 55% of the budget (American Hospital Association [AHA], 1996-1997). The use of UAP in the 1990s grew out of a cost-cutting focus. Currently 97% of hospitals employ UAP (Merker, Cerda, & Blank, 1991) with the skill mix at 69% RN nationwide (Huntington, 1995).

FINANCIAL ISSUES

UAP Are a Necessary Part of Cost Controls

Hospitals are under growing pressure to control their spending. This is due, among other things, to significant Medicare and Medicaid payment shortfalls, price competition, and managed care (Buerhaus, 1995; Eisenberg, 2000; Smith & Panting, 1995).

Nursing labor represents 23% of the hospital workforce. It is the single largest labor cost for hospitals (AHA, 1996-1997), making up nearly half the hospital's total budget (Davis, 1994). The average wage for an RN is 144% higher than that of UAP (Anders, 1995).

There are only so many health care dollars. If we hold out for the all-RN Cadillac model of care delivery, the result will be fewer resources to serve all the population's health care needs.

Increasing the Use of UAP Is Not an Essential Aspect of Cost Control

Looking only at the wage expense is too narrow of a perspective. Hiring and benefit costs (which typically run about 30%) are the same for all categories of workers (Rubach, 1995). However, with UAP use, there are now additional training and supervision expenses (Burda, 1994).

Overtime use often rises to compensate because RNs cover more patients for nursing functions (Manuel & Alster, 1994). A 1996 survey by the *American Journal of Nursing* found 67.5% of RNs reported increased patient loads and 35.8% said they were spending more time supervising UAP (Shindul-Rothschild, Berry, & Long-Middleton, 1996).

Productivity varies between the two types of workers. One study found that UAP have 40% downtime while the RNs only have 12% (Curry, 1992). Gardner (1991) found costs were actually reduced when care was given by primary nursing as compared to a team nursing structure.

Concentrating only on labor expenses mistakenly misses other larger health care cost drivers. They include the costs of physician residency training programs (Japsen, 1994); malpractice (Curran, 1994); administration (Woodhandler, Himmelstein, & Lewortin, 1993); overuse of technology (Prescott, 1993); critical care misuse (Smith & Panting, 1995); drugs (Kapinos, 1994); and increasing capital expenditures (U.S. Government Accounting Office, 1992).

One emergency department attempted to increase productivity by adjusting the skill mix to a higher technician percentage. Only higher-level trained personnel, such as emergency medical technicians and paramedics, were hired into the structured technician role. Although there was improved morale, the department's man-hours per patient actually went up, and the profit margin decreased. These results were attributed to the high mobility of the technician population, which then required constant training, and the high patient acuity, which required more advanced assessments and skills (Jones, 1999).

Overall, analysts believe it is unknown whether reengineering, with its labor changes, actually improves financial margins in the long run. So far, there have been mixed results (Carroll, 1998). While it has helped those hospitals in the top 75th percentile, those in the lower 25th percentile continued to lose money after reengineering (Serb, 1998).

QUALITY OF CARE ISSUES

The process of determining the exact effect of varying the total number and ratio in the skill mix of RNs is not so easy as it first seems. Early studies often showed an unambiguous relationship because many factors that affect morbidity outcomes were not considered. Some of these include care from other disciplines, the severity and complexity of the patient's condition, other characteristics of the patient (e.g., elderly, immunosuppressed), and the work environment (Blegen, Goode, & Reed, 1998).

Many question if the generic outcome of patient morbidity per se is the best criteria to judge the effects of nursing. Currently the focus is shifting toward preventable complications, such as pressure sores, infections, pneumonia, urinary tract infections (UTIs), medication errors, patient falls, and patient complaints (Blegen et al., 1998).

Two other distinctions are increasingly considered. One is the unit variance in patient acuity, such as the difference between an intensive care unit and a rehabilitation unit, rather than using hospital's cumulative results. The other is to separate out the RN hours involved in direct patient care from the institution's total RN hours, which include other roles, such as administration (Blegen et al., 1998).

Increasing UAP Use Does Not Affect the Quality of Care

A 1999 survey of hospital-based RNs found that 59% felt UAP added to, with only 18% indicating they detracted from, quality of patient care (Ventura, 1999). One consulting firm claims that their research involving 117 hospitals found that reconfiguring jobs improved mortality rates and had no effect on patient morbidity (Elias, 1995).

Nurses need to stop alarming the public about quality of health care in hospitals. The credibility of the industry and the profession suffers when staffing debates about staffing take place in the public arena.

The Institute of Medicine (IOM) Committee on the Adequacy of Nurse Staffing concluded in 1996 that there was no evidence of massive nationwide hospital RN staff reductions or of support for the opinion that changing nurse staffing patterns had adversely affected the quality of care. The report called for more research on the definitive effects of structural measures, such as specific staffing ratios (Wunderlich, Sloan, & Davis, 1996).

Increasing UAP Use Does Negatively Impact Quality

Decreases in RN staffing have coincided with a rise in hospital errors, infection rates, and readmissions. The November 1999 IOM report identified that mistakes in diagnosis and medication, failure to apply critical preventive precautions, and other preventable errors occur far more frequently than was previously thought and that many are related to staffing (Kennedy, 2000d).

There is a growing body of studies that show that a higher ratio of RNs to non-RNs improves the patient care outcomes. Even more specifically, the studies are beginning to more precisely indicate that it is the RN hours of care per patient per day that may be among the most meaningful figures to consider in the evaluation of the quality of patient care.

- Lower mortality rates were related to several factors, including a higher RN skill mix (Hartz et al., 1989).
- An extensive study comparing team nursing and primary care nursing models demonstrated that quality was better and that costs were reduced with primary care (Gardner, 1991).
- Thirteen studies have found that patient morbidity and mortality are adversely affected by changing the total number of RNs on staff and the RN component in the skill mix (Aiken & Lake, 1992; Prescott, 1993).
- In a study of downsizing of 281 hospitals, those with across-the-board staffing cuts of 7.5% or more and those with 3.35 or fewer full-time-equivalents (FTEs) per adjusted occupied bed had higher mortality levels (Murphy, 1993).
- For "magnet hospitals," a statistically significant result was that the higher the nurse staffing, the lower the mortality rate (Aiken, Smith, & Lake, 1994).
- The percentage of hours of care delivery by RNs and the RN skill mix were inversely related to the unit rates of medication errors, decubiti, and patient complaints (Blegen et al., 1998).
- An inverse relationship was found between RNs providing care and postsurgical complications of urinary tract infections, pneumonia, and thrombosis (Kovner & Gergen, 1998).
- In a study that looked at the effects of staffing in 80% of the nation's acute care hospitals, Bond, Raehl, Pitterle, and Franke (1999) found that as the number of RNs per occupied hospital bed increases, mortality rate decreases. This study, completed by three pharmacists and a biostatistician, also found that as the numbers of licensed practical nurses and hospital administrators increases, mortality rate increases.
- Using the 10 ANA quality indicators for nursing care in acute care institutions, the single most consistent and significant predictor was the percentage of RNs in the nursing staff caring for patients. As the percentage of RNs increased, so did patients' perceptions of satisfac-

tion with care, pain management, education, and overall care. The higher nurse staffing per acuity-adjusted day was highly correlated with shorter lengths of stay and a significant inverse relationship to preventable conditions: pressure sores, pneumonia, postoperative infections, and urinary tract infections (ANA, 1997; Moore, Lynn, McMillen, & Evans, 1999).
- A study from the Agency for Healthcare Research and Quality (AHRQ, formerly AHCPR) reported that one additional hour of RN care cuts a patient's risk of pneumonia by 8% and the chance of urinary tract infection by nearly 10% (Kennedy, 2000c).

Subjective opinions concur. In one survey, 87% of the surveyed RNs responded that the use of UAP had not improved the quality of care (Shindul-Rothschild et al., 1996). Nearly four out of five RNs surveyed in 1999 said managed care had decreased the quality of care to patients who are sick, and 69% pointed to inadequate staffing as their greatest concern. Physicians also support the increased use of RNs to ensure quality of care (Gordon & Baer, 1994).

The public also agrees. Focus groups across the United States cited concerns with the competency of caregivers, finding that the key indicator for quality of care was the RNs (AHA, 1997). In another study, 75% of public consumers said that a reduction in the number of RNs providing patient care in hospitals lowers quality (Princeton Research Survey Associate, 1996).

In addition, health care workers themselves can be placed at risk by staff changes. A study by the Minnesota Nurses Association found a 65.2% increase in the number of injuries and illnesses in RNs during the same time that RN positions were reduced by 9.2% (Shogren, Calkins, & Wilburn, 1996).

UTILIZATION CONSIDERATIONS

Many indicate that the UAP is a reality here to stay in health care. The question is really not "if" but "how" to best manage their use. Currently 80% of the RNs in acute care institutions and 98% of RNs working long-term care facilities are involved in some capacity with the assignment, delegation, and supervision of UAP in the delivery of nursing care (Blegen, Gardner, & McCloskey, 1992).

Supplement or Replace RNs

UAP Supplement Nursing. The UAP debate is really a turf issue. Protesting RNs are just being insecure and overprotective. Nursing needs to consider *effective* use of their time. RNs spend up to 70% of their time doing the work of other departments and lesser trained individuals instead of fully applying their higher-level skills and abilities (Manuel & Alster, 1994; Mills & Tilbury, 1995; Prescott, Phillips, Ryan, & Thompson, 1991).

One 1999 study found that 71% of the responding RNs said that UAP do provide the extra hands they need to get the work done, and 59% said UAP add to the quality of patient care (Ventura, 1999). In one program that used nursing students as RN extenders, the RNs spent 8% more time on assessment, teaching, and family support (Davis, 1994).

Besides, there is a nursing shortage. The Bureau of Health Professions predicts a shortage of 729,000 bachelor-prepared nurses by the year 2010 (Curtin, 1999). Lengthened recruitment times for RNs are increasingly being reported (Sloane, 1999).

This current nursing shortage is attributed to:

1. A growing demand: the Bureau of Labor Statistics predicts the job market for RNs will grow 23% by the year 2006.
2. Retirement of "graying" RNs: about half the RN workforce will reach retirement in the next 15 years.
3. Lower nursing program enrollments and older nursing students: the average age of the new graduate nurse is 31 years.
4. An aging population resulting in higher hospital census and acuity.
5. A robust economy with increased opportunities within and outside nursing (Curtin, 1999; Silvestri, 1997; Sloane, 1999).

These causes will not be quickly resolved. Nursing has to accept that UAP are essential to getting the work done.

UAP Positions Do Replace Current RN Positions. One survey found that RN respondents reported a reduction in the numbers of RNs providing direct patient care within the preceding year (60.2%) and the hiring of UAP to provide direct care previously provided by RNs (41.9%) (Shindul-Rothschild et al., 1996). The *RN* magazine survey of hospital-based RNs found that the nurses reported that their hospitals are hiring more UAP (39%) and cross-training personnel from other departments (33%) to handle tasks formerly performed by nurses (Ventura, 1999).

The supervision necessary with UAP consumes RN time that could be spent more productively with the patient. In two studies, a third of surveyed RNs said they were spending more time supervising UAP (Shindul-Rothschild et al., 1996; Ventura 1999).

Nursing has a unique role in health care that cannot be passed to others. The number of patient contacts is not the same as what is accomplished when a contact occurs, such as adherence to infection control protocols or ongoing assessment. The shortage does not negate the need for individuals with the necessary professional competencies.

The nursing profession must take a proactive role to fortify its ranks. Pay, bonuses, benefits, and management features (e.g., clinical ladders, shared governance, flexible hours) are traditionally successful means used to attract and retain nurses.

Additional nontraditional methods of recruitment will be needed in the future. These can include aggressive promotion of nursing as a career among younger people, adjusting the workplace to make it more receptive to retaining the older nurse, establishing internships and more extensive on-the-job training opportunities, and immigration.

UAP Percentage in the Skill Mix: What Percent Is the Most Effective?

Sovie (1995) recommends at least a 70% RN staff for medical-surgical units and an 80% RN staff for intensive and intermediate care units. Jones (1999) found that the most productivity occurred in the studied hospital's emergency department, even at peak times, when the RN staffing level was at least 71% to 72%. Blegen et al. (1998) found that the benefit from increasing RNs in the staff ratio was verified up to a staff mix of 87.5% RN (ANA, 1999).

Legislature: Are Mandatory Legislated Patient-Staff Ratios the Answer?

Some suggest the government should regulate staffing to protect the public's health. In 1999, California enacted the nation's first law mandating minimum nurse-patient staffing ratios for all acute care and psychiatric hospital units by the year 2002. The California Nurses Association claims the law was needed because hospitals would try to circumvent the current legislated ICU ratios by prematurely transferring patients to other units (Rockey, 2000).

Others raise concerns that once the patient-staff ratios are named, there will be a reluctance to adjust them when needed. The fear is that the minimum ratio will become the staff ceiling. Unit staffing should be flexible and adjusted according to (1) the skill and knowledge level of the nursing staff, (2) the accessibility of the ancillary service personnel, (3) the practice behaviors of physicians, (4) patient acuity, (5) the complexity and intensity of the care, and (6) the work environment (ANA, 1999; Buerhaus, 1997; Lamkin & Sleven, 1991; Rockey, 2000). For instance, many emergency departments find it necessary to increase staff numbers after enlarging the area, even if the census stays the same (Zimmermann, 2000). Many are adapting a "wait and see" attitude before advocating this course of action in other states.

THE NEED FOR UAP ROLE STANDARDIZATION

A common concern for all is that the UAP role lacks universal definition. There are no standards; each hospital defines their UAP's hiring, training, and scope of practice. In one study of hospitals, only 20% required a high school diploma; 26% preferred previous clinical bedside experience; and 29% preferred certification as a nursing assistant (Barter, McLaughlin, & Thomas, 1994). Another found that 70% did not require UAP to have a high school diploma or to be a certified nurse's aide (CNA) (Barter & Furmidge, 1994).

Huston (1996) lists requirements considered essential for any increased control in the use of UAP. They include that the UAP have standardized (1) titles and job descriptions, (2) training and orientation, (3) supervision, (4) periodic verification of competency, and (5) UAP evaluation by and accountability to the RN evaluation.

Training

There are established regulations of 75 hours of theory and practice, with examination, for CNAs who work in long-term care. But there is no federal or community standards for the training of the more broadly defined UAP, usually used in acute care with higher acuity patients.

UAP tend to have a high turnover rate. Employers tend to be reluctant to invest training monies where there is often no long-term benefit. Barter et al. (1994) found that 88% of surveyed hospitals provide newly hired UAP with less than 40 hours of classroom instruction. In Ventura's (1999) survey the RNs reported that 55% of their hospitals gave UAP three weeks or less of job training (Ventura, 1999). Another survey found that 59% of hospitals offered less than 20 hours of classroom orientation and 41% provided less than 40 hours of on-the-job training (Barter & Furmidge, 1994). Overall, about half the surveyed nurses felt UAP did not receive an adequate amount of training (Ventura, 1999).

It is interesting to compare this amount of training to work with a vulnerable population with Royal Carribean's standard for their stable, healthy customers. They provide an average of 92 hours of training to *each* crew member on their *Voyager* cruise ship (Fishman, 2000).

RN Delegation Skill

Improving RN Delegation Skills Is the Answer. Most RNs, especially those who entered the practice in the 1980s, don't know how to effectively delegate to UAP. The ANA (1992b) calls for all RN program curricula to "include content on supervision, delegation, assignment and legal aspects regarding nursing's utilization of assistive personnel." Jung, Pearcey, and Phillips (1994) found that educating RNs about leadership resulted in an increased amount of work being delegated while maintaining patient satisfaction, nurse job satisfaction, and the quality of nursing care.

RN Delegation Training Is Not a Significant Component. Even after training, many RNs still lack the skill and comfort level for supervising UAP (Abts, Hofer, & Leafgreen, 1994; Jung et al., 1994). Some attribute this, in part, to the fact that delegation increases the liability of the RN. But others give it a broader explanation.

Team nursing's ingrained difficulty is the frequent blurring or informal violations of the assigned distinct task delineations and responsibilities as a result of the ever changing nature of patient needs and interactions. On-the-spot decisions, requiring a depth of knowledge and trained critical thinking, are made at the bedside during "routine" care (Brannon, 1990). Many RNs feel frustration at being responsible for care they don't even witness or at being required to delegate what they are not comfortable delegating, but what their employer insists they must.

The sponsors of the California patient ratio law also included a prohibition against using unlicensed, minimally trained personnel to perform procedures normally done by nurses. These tasks included medication administration, venipuncture, intravenous therapy, parenteral or tube feedings, invasive procedures (including insertion of nasogastric tubes, catheters, or tracheal suctioning), patient assessment or education, and postdischarge care (Kennedy, 2000a).

Legitimization

Some suggest a more integrated, multiskilled, versatile assistive health care worker as the answer to the current inefficient and duplicative allied health roles (Pew Health Professions Commission, 1995). However, there was universal nursing alignment against the American Medical Association's proposed solution of the new Registered Care Technologist (RCT), an assistive position for nursing care that would be supervised by physicians.

Regulation, certification, or licensure for UAP by nursing have all been considered possibilities. In the end the

ANA (1993) decided to assume the least restrictive regulation role possible that would still maintain public safety. A key reason for this position is the belief that regulation would "legitimize" the UAP role. This could result in making UAP an "official" occupation and fuel potential growth (ANA, 1996).

WHAT IS NURSING?

An additional aspect that must be included in the debate is identifying what nursing is. Is it a list of tasks that can be prioritized, delegated, and supervised? Or is it an embodied art and skill that incorporates the whole of patient care knowledge, assessment, prioritization, and discernment into something bigger than the sum of its parts? Nurses, as a whole, do not usually clearly answer this question for themselves, let alone for the public.

Some emphasize nursing needs to focus on leadership rather than on hands-on caregiving. Nursing must begin to direct the future rather than maintain the status quo in caregiving. Shamian (2000) believes the restructuring and downsizing of health services in the 1990s unfortunately dismantled nursing leadership and diminished nursing influence at the decision-making table.

Others stress that nursing is a hands-on profession. Its essence goes beyond a performance of skills and prioritization of isolated tasks ordered by physicians. It is assessing and meeting the ever changing needs of the whole patient. A UAP can physically count a pulse. An "expert" nurse, however, also assesses circulation, perfusion, hydration, skin integrity, overall physical state, and the patient's emotions during the act. The nurse might even throw in some teaching.

Nursing often takes the profession's inherent complexity for granted because it is so familiar to them. A visit to any Nursing 101 class quickly illustrated just how much must be taught and experienced for an individual to be socialized into an RN-level caregiver. For instance, one beginning student had to ask whether to first give the breakfast tray or the bath to the diabetic patient. Another novice student decided not to give oxygen to the patient with emphysema because "his breathing isn't too bad."

One way for nursing to decide on and deal assertively with the UAP issue is to join forces through their professional organizations. Yet membership numbers remain paltry. Only 10% of nurses belong to the ANA, whereas 38% of physicians belong to the American Medical Association. Memberships are also low in specialty nursing organizations. For instance, within emergency care, about 33% of emergency nurses belong to the Emergency Nurses Association, whereas 67% of emergency department physicians in clinical practice belong to the American College of Emergency Physicians.

SUMMARY

If UAP are a fact of nursing's life, then nursing needs to monitor and control that fact. Everyone agrees that there is a need for ongoing research and for nursing to manage the UAP role. Now more than ever nurses are in a position to help shape the preferred future of human care. Nursing needs to review and raise standards continually in order to respond to our evolving world (Jones, 2000).

Patients implicitly count on the nurse to be their advocate. They trust nurses for health care information (92%), the same as they trust physicians (93%) (Sigma Theta Tau, 1999). And three fourths of Americans rated nurses' honesty and ethics as either "high" or "very high," placing them above any other profession (Kennedy, 2000b).

It is time to consider the full implications of Florence Nightingale's (1859) admonition to "do the sick no harm." Fulfilling that axiom includes more than our own individual practice. It involves making strategic and tactical choices, based on all the relevant issues, for the number and composition of staffing that best meets the patients' needs.

REFERENCES

Abts, S., Hofer, M., & Leafgreen, P.K. (1994). Redesigning care delivery: A modular system. *Nurse Manager, 25*(2), 40-46.

Aiken, L., & Lake, E. (1992, December). *Summary of empirical literature on the relationship between nursing skill mix or RN-to-patient ratio and hospital mortality.* Philadelphia: University of Pennsylvania, Center for Health Services and Policy Research, School of Nursing.

Aiken, L.H., Smith, H.L., & Lake, E.T. (1994). Lower Medicare mortality among a set of hospitals known for good nursing care. *Medical Care, 32*(8), 771-787.

American Hospital Association. (1996-1997). *Hospital statistics.* Chicago: Author.

American Hospital Association. (1997). *Reality check: Public perception of health care and hospital.* Chicago: Author.

American Nurses Association. (1992a). *Position statement on registered nurse utilization of unlicensed assistive personnel.* Washington, DC: Author.

American Nurses Association. (1992b). *Statement on registered nurse education relating to the utilization of unlicensed assistive personnel.* Washington, DC: Author.

American Nurses Association. (1993). *Monitoring and regulating unlicensed assistive personnel.* Washington, DC: Author.

American Nurses Association. (1996). *Registered professional nurses & unlicensed assistive personnel.* Washington DC: Author.

American Nurses Association. (1997). *Implementing nursing's report card: A study of RN staffing, length of stay and patient outcomes.* Washington, DC: Author.

American Nurses Association. (1999). *Principles for nurse staffing.* Washington, DC: Author.

Anders, G. (1995, February 10). Hospitals' RX for high costs: Fewer nurses, more aides. *The Wall Street Journal,* pp. B1, B4.

Barter, M., McLaughlin, F.E., & Thomas, S.A. (1994). Use of unlicensed assistive personnel by hospitals. *Nurse Economic$, 12*(2), 82-87.

Barter, M., & Furmidge, M. (1994). Unlicensed assistive personnel. Issues related to delegation and supervision. *Journal of Nursing Administration, 24*(4), 36-40.

Blegen, M.A., Gardner, D.L., & McCloskey, J.C. (1992). Who helps you with your work? *American Journal of Nursing, 92*(1), 26-31.

Blegen, M.A., Goode, C.J., & Reed, L. (1998). Nursing staffing and patient outcomes. *Nursing Research, 47*(1), 43-50.

Bond, C.A., Raehl, C.L., Pitterle, M.E., & Franke, T. (1999). Health care professional staffing, hospital characteristics, and hospital mortality rates. *Pharmacotherapy, 19*(2), 130-138.

Brannon, R. (1990). The reorganization of the nursing labor process: From team to primary nursing. *International Journal of Health Services, 20*(3), 511-524.

Buerhaus, P.I. (1995). Economics and reform: Forces affecting nurse staffing. *Nursing Policy Forum, 1*(2), 9-14.

Buerhaus, P.I. (1997). What is the harm in imposing mandatory hospital nurse staffing regulations? *Nursing Economic$, 15*(2), 66-72.

Burda, D. (1994, August 8). A profit by any other name would still give hospitals fits. *Modern Healthcare, 24*(32), 115-134.

Carroll, P. (1998). Buyer beware? *Subacute Care Today, 1*(5), 24-28.

Curran, C. (1994). Work redesign: The key to true health care reform. In J.C. McCloskey & H.K. Grace (Eds.), *Current issues in nursing* (4th ed.). St. Louis: Mosby.

Curry, J. (1992). Bridge over troubled waters: ED nurses share strategies regarding use of prehospital care providers in the emergency department. *Journal of Emergency Nursing, 18*(6), 30A-35A.

Curtin, L. (1999, October). A crisis in the making: Key facts. *Curtin Calls, 1*(10), 15.

Davis, B. (1994). Effective utilization of a scarce resource: RNs. *Nursing Management, 25*(2), 78-80.

Eisenberg, D. (2000, January 21). Critical condition. *Time, 155*(4), 52-54.

Elias, M. (1995, January 1). Caregiving is shifting from RNs to aides. *USA Today,* pp. 1D, 2D.

Emergency Nurses Association. (1997). *Position statement: The use of non-registered nurses (non-RN) caregivers in emergency care.* Des Plaines, IL: Author.

Fishman, C. (2000, March). Fantastic voyage. *Fast Company,* Issue #32, 170-200.

Gardner, K. (1991). A summary of findings of a five-year comparison study of primary and team nursing. *Nursing Research, 40*(2), 113-117.

Gordon, S., & Baer, E.D. (1994, December 6). Fewer nurses to answer the buzzer. *The New York Times,* p. A23.

Hartz, A.J., Krakauer, H., Kuhn, E.M., Young, M., Jacobsen, S.J., Gay, G., Muenz, L., Katzoff, M., Bailey, R.C., & Rimm, A.A. (1989). Hospital characteristics and mortality rates. *New England Journal of Medicine, 321,* 1720-1725.

Huntington, J.A. (1995). Restructuring: Safety, quality and cost. Staff nurses' view. *Nursing Policy Forum, 1*(2), 16, 19, 38.

Huston, C.L. (1996). Unlicensed assistive personnel: A solution to dwindling healthcare resources or the precursor to the apocalypse of registered nursing? *Nursing Outlook, 44*(2), 67-73.

Japsen, B. (1994). Teaching hospitals face hard lessons. *Modern Healthcare, 24*(6), 36-40.

Jones, C. (1999). Staffing standards. In P.G. Zimmermann & B. Pierce (Eds.), Manager's Forum. *Journal of Emergency Nursing, 25*(3), 221-223.

Jones, D. (2000). What matters most in nursing's future: Future standards. *Reflections on Nursing Leadership, 26*(1), 36.

Jung, F.D., Pearcey, L.G., & Phillips, J.L. (1994). Evaluation of a program to improve nursing assistant use. *Journal of Nursing Administration, 24*(3), 42-47.

Kapinos, T. (1994, July 13). When aides replace RNs at the bedside. *The Chicago Tribune, NursingNews,* p. 3.

Kennedy, M.S. (2000a). News: California nurses win landmark victory. *American Journal of Nursing, 100*(1), 20.

Kennedy, M.S. (2000b). News: High public esteem for nurses. *American Journal of Nursing, 100*(1), 21.

Kennedy, M.S. (2000c). News: Study shows link between nursing care and improved patient health and safety. *American Journal of Nursing, 100*(2), 21.

Kennedy, M.S. (2000d). News: A medical error wake-up call. *American Journal of Nursing, 100*(2), 21.

Kovner, C., & Gergen, P.J. (1998). Nurse staffing levels and adverse events following surgery in US hospitals. *Image: Journal of Nursing Scholarship, 30*(4), 315-321.

Lamkin, L.R., & Sleven, M. (1991). Staffing standards: Why not? A report from the ONS administration committee. *Oncology Nursing Forum, 18*(7), 1241-1243.

Manuel, P., & Alster, K. (1994). Unlicensed personnel no cure for an ailing health care system. *Nursing & Health Care, 15*(1), 18-21.

Merker, L.R., Cerda, F., & Blank, M. (1991). *1990 utilization of nurse extenders.* Chicago: American Hospital Association.

Mills, M.E., & Tilbury, M.S. (1995). Restructuring: Safety, quality and cost. Nursing administration's perspective. *Nursing Policy Forum, 1*(2), 17-19.

Moore, K., Lynn, M.R., McMillen, B.J., & Evans, S. (1999). Implementation of the ANA report card. *Journal of Nursing Administration, 29*(6), 48-54.

Murphy, E.C. Ltd. (1993). *Cost-driven downsizing in hospitals: Implications for mortality.* Amherst, NY: The Quality Leader Press.

Nightingale, F. (1859). *Notes on hospitals* (preface). London: Parker & Sons.

Pew Health Professions Commission. (1995). *Critical challenges: Revitalizing the health professions for the twenty-first century.* San Francisco: Pew Center for the Health Professions.

Prescott, P., Phillips, C.Y., Ryan, J., & Thompson, K.O. (1991, Spring). Changing how nurses spend their time. *Image: Journal of Nursing Scholarship, 23*(1), 23-28.

Prescott, P. (1993). Nursing: An important component of hospital survival under a reformed healthcare system. *Nursing Economic$, 11*(4), 192-199.

Princeton Research Survey Associates. (1996). *Nursing and the quality of patient care: 1996 survey.* Princeton, NJ: Author.

Rockey, L. (2000, January 19). Nurse-patient ratios. RNs demand adequate staffing to ensure quality of care. *The Chicago Tribune, NursingNews,* p. 1.

Rubach, L. (1995). Downsizing: How quality is affected as companies shrink. *Quality Progress, 28*(4), 8-14.

Serb, C. (1998, July 20). Is remaking the hospital making money? *Hospitals & Health Networks, 72*(14), 32-33.

Shamian, J. (2000). Re-energizing hospital care. *Reflections on Nursing Leadership, 26*(1), 24-26.

Shindul-Rothschild, J., Berry, D., & Long-Middleton, E. (1996). Where have all the nurses gone? Final results of the AJN patient care survey. *American Journal of Nursing, 96*(11), 24-30.

Shogren, E., Calkins, A., & Wilburn, S. (1996). Restructuring may be hazardous to your health. *American Journal of Nursing, 96*(11), 64-66.

Sigma Theta Tau International. (1999). New poll shows public concern about healthcare. *Reflections, 31*(4), 39.

Silvestri, G.T. (1997, November). Occupational employment projections to 2006. *Monthly labor review.* Washington, DC: Bureau of Labor Statistics.

Sloane, M. (1999, June 14). Survey says . . . more nurses needed. *Nursing Spectrum, 12*(12), 16.

Smith, R.N., & Panting, K. (1995, May). The changing and challenging ICU. *Nursing Dynamics, 4*(1), 10-15.

Sovie, M.D. (1995). Tailoring hospitals for managed care and integrated health systems. *Nursing Economic$, 13*(2), 72-83.

Stewart, M. (1999, September/October). Survey highlights nurses' concerns about health care. *The American Nurse, 31*(5), 3.

Tri-Council for Nursing. (1995). Statement on assistive personnel to the registered nurse. Author.

U.S. General Accounting Office. (1992). *Hospital costs: Adoption of new technologies drive costs growth.* Washington, DC: Author.

Ventura, M.J. (1999). Staffing issues. *RN, 62*(2), 26-31.

Woodhandler, S., Himmelstein, D., & Lewortin, J. (1993). Administrative costs in U.S. hospital. *New England Journal of Medicine, 329*(6), 400-403.

Wunderlich, G.S., Sloan, F.A., & Davis, C.K. (Eds.). (1996). *Nursing staff in hospitals and nursing homes.* Washington, DC: Institute of Medicine, National Academy Press.

Zimmermann, P.G., Nemeth, S., Bonalumi, N., Jones, S., Bachtel, I., Kaife, K., Huff, D., Williams, S., Treece, N., Anderson, D., & Roepe, L. (2000). Manager's forum: New/remodeled emergency departments. *Journal of Emergency Nursing, 26*(3), 254-258.

CHAPTER 39

Leadership in Transition

KARLENE M. KERFOOT

Health care is different than it was 10 years ago and promises to be more different in the years ahead. About every 5 to 10 years the health care industry has had to reinvent the way the work of health care is done. For example, the prospective payment system invented payment based on diagnosis-related groups (DRGs), which provided a predetermined rate of payment based on diagnoses irrespective of the costs of a particular patient. This was our first introduction to changing from cost-based pricing (in which the price is based on the cost) to price-based costing, in which the reimbursement is set regardless of the cost. The only option in this reimbursement scheme is to change the processes to take enough cost out of the system to match the price that the payers are willing to pay. Then came the managed care revolution, payment systems based on capitation, and now there are changes from the Balanced Budget Act of 1997 and implementation of the ambulatory payment system (APS) of 2000. All these reimbursement programs challenge us to cut costs to meet the price that the market is willing to pay. And new reimbursement systems continue to be developed.

Health care is also emerging from a small cottage industry made up of many small entities to large, consolidated organizations, the result of mergers and acquisitions, that place the leader in complicated roles across several diverse departments in large health care corporations. Physicians in solo practice are a rarity today, just as are stand-alone hospitals. The revolution that is in the making with the human genome project will quickly propel us further into the business of maintaining health rather than the repair shop mentality of trying to repair something that has broken.

We have nothing to look forward to in the future except enormous, rapid change. We are quickly moving from an industry built around disease and small, independent organizations into an industry focused on health and comprised of large corporate organizations. Each of these changes has made us totally rethink and reorganize the way we carry out the work of health care in this country and how we can lead the most effectively. Consequently the work of leaders in health care today must change rapidly to meet these challenges.

REVOLUTION IN HEALTH CARE

Many basic changes are happening in health care that will make us totally rethink the way we deliver health care in the next few years. It will be impossible for us to conceptualize these changes through the filters that we have learned in our professional socialization. We will have to abandon many old beliefs in order to make room for the new content that will drive our leadership models for the future. To absorb new technologies, we will have to be open to many new possibilities.

The Genetic Revolution

With the completion of the genome project and the mapping of the genetic structures upon which our lives depend, we will open the possibilities of many interventions that are now not even imaginable. At birth, one can conceivably be given a genetic map that will predict the future of our health. Health care will then be organized around preventing the inevitable by altering the genetic blueprint of our lives. Potentially many diseases we commonly know today will be eliminated. Cloning has been proven possible with the cloning of sheep and other animals. From this technology the cloning of body parts is potentially possible. An enormous number of possibilities for pharmaceuticals that can be developed quickly will be another outcome of the genetic revolution, as well as antiaging interventions.

Leaders will need to know the technical aspects of the genetic revolution in order to lead in this new world and also the implications of this revolution on the management of health care for our future. There will be many serious ethical debates about genetics and access to these new technologies will potentially create serious issues for our society. Health care leaders will be intimately involved in these ethical debates in the future.

Information Technology Revolution

With the incredible innovations in information technology will come tremendous social changes. In health care, the information revolution will put enormous amounts of information into the hands of the consumer that was formerly owned by the health professional. No longer will the health care profession be seen as the all-knowledgeable dispenser of information. Patients and the consumers of health will come to us with vast amounts of information about specific health care issues that will empower them to be much more knowledgeable consumers of health services. We will need to make the transition from the provider of information to the coordinator of information and the facilitator who helps guide the consumer through a morass of information.

Access to the World Wide Web will be in the hands of many as it becomes accessible through television sets and mobile telephones at relatively low cost. Becoming a virtual health care provider will happen as we interact with consumers through web sites, teleconferencing, e-mail, and other electronic media. Diagnostics will become sophisticated, as computer chips are developed to monitor continually a person's functioning. And innovations in computer technology with software will produce smart machines that can provide better diagnostics than humans can. We will be challenged to know about fuzzy logic and other systems that will propel the software of the future (Kosi, 1999).

Leaders in the future will be concerned not only about virtual relationships with the consumers of health care but also about those kinds of relationships with the people whom they lead. As organizations consolidate, and technology dictates that we can care for patients across a wide geographical divide, our people will also be dispersed in new and different ways. Leaders will need to know much about the technical side of information technology in order to make intelligent decisions for the future (Stis & Lacob, 1999). A leader's technical IQ will be important in the future. Leaders must also know the social implications of accomplishing work with patients electronically rather than in person, however, and must develop new models of effective, high-quality care in this new medium.

Consumerism. Consumers not only will be well informed about their health care but also will be demanding of a higher level of excellence and of their health care's being designed around their wants and needs. Consumers have become acutely aware of issues of patient safety and will demand the same level of attention to safety as other industries have implemented. Health care is complicated, but consumers will become absolutely intolerant of unnecessary patient safety issues. The use of complementary medicine will increase as consumers become better informed. Consumers will demand that the experience of health care be organized around their wants and needs and not those of the professionals.

Changes in Reimbursement

Reimbursement for health care is nothing short of chaotic and promises to remain that way in the future. Reimbursement for health care has been a strong battering ram for each political party to wield against the other in order to be elected. And now that more of our reimbursement comes from the governmental program of Medicare as our population ages, the arguments will only intensify. Leaders will need to be experts at financial management and change management to develop rapid cycle changes to adjust quickly to the ever changing reimbursement scene.

Accelerated Change

Information technology is propelling innovations in knowledge at an incredible speed. Coupled with the breakthroughs in genetics, we can look forward to rapid rates of change in the future (Gleick, 1999). Leaders will need to be masters at the science of change and develop many innovations to help people adjust to accelerated time frames of change. Building learning organizations that can cope with fast change will be an important role for the leader of the future, according to Senge (1990). It is impossible for the leader to continue to be the dispenser of information in the future. Staff members will need to adopt learning as their organizing framework and not depend on the leader for their knowledge. As important for learning is the task of forgetting. If organizations cannot forget the old paradigms that served them well in the past but that will not do so in the future, organizations cannot progress. Leaders must be masters at helping organizations and the people within them forget (Kerfoot, 1999).

LEADERSHIP IN HEALTH CARE

Obviously, from this brief discussion of a minute part of the drastic changes of the future, one can tell that leadership will need to change drastically to lead effectively in the future. As we face knowledgeable health care consumers, continual shortages of qualified health care professionals, and a rapidly changing health care system, the leader faces unique challenges.

Self-Management

Followers usually take on the characteristics of the leader. One of the easiest ways to effect change is for the leader to model the change. Leaders need to be visible learning machines who are always seeking out new information from which to operate better in their positions. If leaders can be the "CEO of their careers" and can help others seek experiences that will equip them for the latest innovation in health care, people will understand self-management. Managing oneself first will prepare one to achieve the desired outcomes.

Customer-izing

"One size fits all" doesn't apply in this new world of health care. Young staff members are concerned about their quality of life outside of work and other issues about which older workers have not been so vocal. Older workers want different things from the work site than those who are younger. Staff are diverse in their wants and needs. Successful leaders are those who can celebrate this diversity and develop programs to help the diverse groups achieve great satisfaction at work. We must build the work site around the wants and needs of the staff in order to meet the needs of affiliation and caring that the organization must adopt as its organizing framework in order to be successful. The successful leader of the future will be an expert at managing diversity and will be able to build work settings that are conducive to a variety of wants and needs. No longer do we see the workplace as a melting pot where everyone becomes homogenized into a certain mix. Instead the metaphor of a quilt that is made of many designs that together make a beautiful masterpiece is the goal.

The consumers of health care are telling us loudly that they expect their health care to be customer-ized, and not delivered in a cookie-cutter mode. Health care programs built around innovation will develop programs that can innovate around the customer. Health care consumers expect to not only be delivered of their problems but to also have a positive healing experience.

Accountability

As health care consumers become well informed about their care, they are demanding a higher level of accountability from us. Patient safety has become a factor in the public's concern about their health care. As we observe

other industries, we are learning to build in safeguards to make our environments safer. Leaders must build cultures where people can discuss their near misses and learn from them (Kerfoot, 1999). Leaders must build cultures in which the nurse not only is empowered to recognize potential problems but also has the authority in the organization to do what needs to be done to rescue the patient from potential harm.

Synergizing with Other Professionals and Patients

Nurses are traditionally seen as the coordinator of care. Effective nurses recognize this role as the key to providing good patient care. The nurse leaders of this new world of health care will be the leaders of other clinical disciplines. Unfortunately, nurses are often thrust in leadership positions of disciplines without a clear knowledge of the structures and process of these other disciplines. We must challenge ourselves to assume that the leaders of the future will lead patient care and not be exclusively devoted to the leadership of nursing. Connective leaders are those who can combine, connect, and build synergistic work teams (Lipman-Blumen, 1996).

In this new model of health care, synergistic teams that include the patient as an equal partner in health care decisions will be the norm. Nurses are well positioned to lead this model in the future. The leader of the future must have the talent to synergize professionals, patients, families, and communities in productive efficient teams.

Creating Sanctuaries of Caring and Sanctuaries of Healing

People will be demanding more from the workplace in the future. With many options available in health care, employees have become particular about how they spend their time at work. In health care, it is especially important to care for the caregiver at the work site. We know errors are caused by fatigue, stress, and interpersonally toxic work sites. The successful leaders in the future will create cultures of caring where nurses can come to work and feel safe, secure, and cared for in their work environment. Handy (1998) writes that our spirits are hungry for the kind of work environment in which our souls can grow and prosper. He notes that although most of the world values democracy and feels strongly that their voices need to be heard, the work site still remains a bastion of autocracy and hierarchical decision making. His advice to us is to pursue democratic process at work to build workplaces where people truly believe they can contribute and participate as a citizen of the corporation.

The consumers of health care will feel they have entered into a sanctuary of healing where they are supported both physically, socially, mentally, and spiritually by a team that can create the sanctuary they need for their healing processes. Health care is much more than the prevention or treatment of disease. It must also be an experience that satisfies. Crafting an environment that speaks "healing" to the patient and family nurtures perceptions that create the reality of health and healing. Companies like Starbucks and Disney sell an experience that satisfies (Flowers, 2000). Hospitals are not set up to be sanctuaries of healing. Consequently many patients don't experience their health care as healing. We know from information about the placebo effect that perception creates our reality. Consumers will demand the same "experience that satisfies" with health care as they do with Disneyland. Leaders of the future must create sanctuaries of healing where consumers can truly feel they have entered a healing reality.

LEADERSHIP TRANSITIONS FOR THE FUTURE

Leadership in this new world of health care will demand new skills. As the clinical practice of nursing transitions to genetics, wellness, and information technologies, lead-

ers will need to obtain advanced education in these areas. The new paradigms of complexity and chaos theory fit this future much better than the old linear models, but this means that future leaders need to be well schooled in these theories. Leaders will also need to be experts in creating the caring and healing cultures and in developing synergies between health care groups and patients and families.

There is much work to be done in health care. Hopefully nurses in the future will become involved in the creation of health policy and become politically active at the local, state, and national levels to advocate for the patient and the health of our nation.

REFERENCES

Flowers, J. (2000, January-February). What experience are you selling? *Health Care Forum, 43*(1), 12-17.

Gleick, J. (1999). *Faster.* New York: Pantheon.

Handy, C. (1998). *The hungry spirit.* New York: Broadway Books.

Kerfoot, K. (1999, July-August). Culture of courage. *Nursing Economic$, 17*(3), 238-239.

Kosi, B. (1999). *Fuzzy future.* New York: Harmony Books.

Lipman-Blumen, J. (1996). *The connective edge.* New York: Jossey-Bass.

Senge, P. (1990). *The fifth discipline.* New York: Doubleday.

Stis, G., & Lacob, M. (1999). *Who gives a gigabyte.* New York: Wiley.

CHAPTER 40

Nurses in Nonnursing Leadership Positions

BEVERLY L. MALONE

Nurses have a very special role in today's society. In addition to providing holistic care, nursing is the test case for women's issues in the 1990s. The interconnectedness of nursing and feminism places the nursing profession in the nonnursing leadership position for women's issues worldwide (Roberts & Group, 1995). As a profession, nursing is familiar with taking on nonnursing leadership positions; likewise, as individuals, nurses are growing accustomed to assuming nonnursing leadership positions in pursuing the development of their full potential.

With the complex interaction as women in a male-dominated society and as nurses in the traditional health care world—dominated by male hospital administrators and physicians (Moss, 1995)—nurses confront the issues of women who are pursuing careers of purpose. Not being a part of the dominant society places nurses in double jeopardy as a result of the compound factors of being both female and nurses. The consequences of society's myopic view of women and nursing can influence nurses and the nursing profession to choose powerless behavior reflective of an oppressed group rather than proactive behavior dedicated to change and growth.

Stereotypes of nurses flourish with images of the physician's handmaiden and a motherly, spontaneously altruistic, caregiver needing constant direction and supervision. Adding to the complexity are nurses who buy into these traditional stereotypes by their words and actions.

Interestingly, the real nursing leaders have never accepted these stereotypes but by their words and actions have negated them, thereby expanding the nurse's role into new territory. This chapter considers the acquisition of new territory or old space redesigned. While entitled, "Nurses in Nonnursing Leadership Positions," this chapter is about power.

To examine this expansionary strategy fully, the traditional roots of nursing are explored along with issues of leadership and power and nursing's ambivalent relationship with power. Finally, advantages and disadvantages of nurses in nonnursing leadership positions are presented.

THE TRADITIONAL NURSING LEADERSHIP POSITION

The nurse executive, vice president for nursing, or director of nursing is the chief nurse in a hospital. The individual in this position is ultimately responsible for all the nursing care—24 hours a day—that is provided in and more frequently out of the hospital. The educational preparation for these individuals usually includes a master's degree in nursing administration or business administration (Chitty, 1993). While supervising the largest group of health care personnel in the institution, nurse executives are frequently limited in their power base. These limitations may include exclusion from the board of trustees, where major policy decision making occurs, and less stature and clout than the chief of the medical staff.

While nurse executives are identified as leaders in health care settings, their origins are similar to all nurses, and all women, with the common bond of Victorian roots (Moss, 1995). From these Victorian roots grew branches of stereotypes that disqualified women from engaging in business with men outside the home. Some of these stereotypes were biologically based because women were perceived as not being intelligent enough to manage commerce or the professions (Altick, 1973). As Nightingale demonstrated in the reengineering of the military health care system of Britain, nurses can be brilliant, strategic administrators and leaders (Shames, 1993). However, the Victorian society transformed Nightingale from a gutsy, unrelenting visionary into a stereotypical ministering angel who reinforced the assumptions about women and their abilities.

These stereotypes are the underpinnings for the glass ceiling that serves as an unseen boundary to the career aspirations of nurses and women. Nurses in nonnursing leadership positions are frequently the first crack in the glass ceiling. Due to the invisibility of the glass ceiling and its lack of smell, taste, or other indications of its existence, nurses are usually surprised and confused when they bump or crash into the reality of the barrier.

The rumor of its existence has been shared throughout nursing folklore. However, the accomplished nurse leader who has surmounted obstacles ranging from irate and irrational physicians to the lack of adequate resources to provide optimum care is quite comfortable in tackling and overcoming barriers. Therein lies the surprise. The glass ceiling is an unusual barrier that has unique properties that attack the internal core self-esteem. The inability of nurses to break this barrier is typified by the following unstated areas:

- *Diagnosis:* Nurse leader dysfunction, with an origin based on being female, and early nurse-related social development
- *Symptoms:* Inability to run an organization or to make the hard decisions; lacking in depth, in critical thinking and fortitude in risk taking, and not fluent in the organizational culture's language
- *Treatment and prognosis:* Terminal unless the individual can reject the "nurse" descriptor and convert to the generic term of administrator/leader, which has a more acceptable, male-based origin.

All is not lost. This diagnosis is laced with sexism, which affirmative action guidelines began reproving and addressing in the 1960s and 1970s as a result of the Civil Rights and Women's Movements. These symptoms have not been documented in nurse leaders, and the mastery of leadership competencies is not gender-related. The prognosis is clearly not terminal and there exist other options than the rejection of one's nursing identity. In fact, the following action plan can allow one to crack the glass ceiling without capitulating one's nursing identity (adapted from Moss, 1995):

1. **Overcome hidden agendas.** Acknowledge the existence of an informal structure with unwritten expectations and stereotypes related to women, nurses, and others who are culturally different. Establish power networks of support both internal and external to the organization. Seek out mentoring relationships.

2. **Understand the existing power structure.** Learn the history of the corporate structure. Study the pathways and gatekeepers to organizational ascendancy. Develop your mentoring relationships.

3. **Learn the corporate language.** Moss (1995) suggests that corporate language stems from the military, sports, and sexual allusions. Developing a comfort level and familiarity with the language and its hidden meaning is a critical skill that does not necessarily require imitating men in the use of the language. While comprehending the language, a nurse leader can be selective but fluent in communicating the issues to colleagues.

4. **Memorize the play book.** For example, know the consequences of winning too frequently without sharing the perceived rewards with others. Underground societies have emerged to control the success of nurses and nursing departments who, in the eyes of the beholder, receive the lion's share of resources in the organization. One such organization rumored to exist is SPNGE, the *Society to Prevent Nursing from Getting Everything*. Develop a strategic plan to write new sections to the play book.

5. **Establish business and financial credibility.** Seek out validation of your business and financial skills from the head of the finance department. If these skills are absent, develop or polish them through continuing education or additional graduate study. In the interim, hire someone with the expertise required to affirm this critical area of knowledge.

6. **Utilize gender-specific communication styles.** This step involves acknowledging the basic differences in the communication of men and women. The premise is that men and women view the world differently: Men see the world as a hierarchical social structure while women view it as a network of connections. As a result, to men, dialogue is meant to achieve and maintain the upper hand; for women, it is a process meant to achieve closeness, confirmation, and support. Once these differences are acknowledged, one can choose the type of dialogue and the outcomes preferred. Heim and Galant (1993), on the other hand, suggest that women should limit rapport building with male colleagues to business topics because the discussion of personal experiences may leave a man feeling vulnerable. In other words, women should hide their differences. However, with today's global perspective and economic environment, diversity is being managed, not denied, through the acknowledgment and valuing of differences (Carnevale & Stone, 1994). Health care institutions and educational institutions have been the slowest learners in this new model of valuing diversity. In a recent study, six of six health care institutions were found to be lagging behind corporate industrial America in proactively managing diversity (Muller, 1994). Instead, these health care institutions were described as pluralistic organizations with compliance-ori-

ented strategies that address routine, modern human resource management practices. As the sociopolitical economic environment continues to demand management of diversity, health care institutions will choose to change or will not survive.

LEADERSHIP AND POWER: NURSING'S AMBIVALENT AFFAIR

While nursing is enamored with leadership, it is hesitant about its relationship with power. Nurses in nonnursing leadership positions must have a clear understanding of the intangible connectedness between leadership and power. Ambivalence is distracting and disempowering. Leadership and power are attached at their core, are inseparable, and are used most effectively with conscious, deliberate purpose. Leadership has been described as both a process and a property (Jago, 1982). The process of leadership is the use of power, the ability to move self and others toward a shared vision that becomes a shared reality. Depree (1989) describes leadership as an art form that empowers people to do what is required of them in the most effective and human way possible. Power is the action word for leadership.

As a property, leadership is a set of qualities attributed to those who are perceived as successfully achieving, with and through others, the outcome of a new shared reality. Nurses in nonnursing leadership positions need to have the following characteristics: vision, boundary management skills, risk taking, empowerment of followers, and mentoring (Bennis & Nanus, 1985; Grohar-Murray & DiCroce, 1992; Malone, 1984). A vision is a relative of a dream; it is not constrained by logic, time, or place. However, it is the sharable vision that is meaningful and achievable. In a study by Dunham and Fisher (1990), a nurse executive described the visioning process this way: "I always use the analogy of the artist who sketches a scene on a piece of canvas. It doesn't have to have all the colors. A tree doesn't have to have all the leaves" (p. 3).

Boundary management is of particular importance to nurses in nonnursing leadership positions. Nurses in these roles frequently exhibit cutting edge behavior. An edge is a boundary that separates entities and immediately alerts a leader to the need to design transactions across the boundary. Depree (1989) described living and dying edges. Nurses who have moved into nonnursing leadership positions are functioning at the living edge of the nursing profession. A nurse leader who was chief executive officer of an academic institution stated that a nurse in a nonnursing leadership position is an oxymoron. Once a nurse enters the position, it automatically becomes a nursing position, claimed new territory for the nursing profession.

Like all leaders, the nurse prior to or in a nonnursing leadership position must define the current reality, which includes the identification of existing boundaries. Once boundaries are located and noted, they are extended through risk taking. These nurse leaders are adept at temporarily overlapping boundaries with other entities while maintaining the integrity of their own boundaries.

The use and empowerment of followers is at the heart of nursing's reluctance to embrace the concept of power as an irretractable part of leadership. The idea of using and manipulating followers to achieve an outcome is not philosophically palatable to most nurses. Using followers implies a traditional hierarchical system of leadership that is based more on the male model than on a woman's way of knowing (Belenky, Clinchy, & Tarule, 1986). Yet in the process of leadership, the leader and followers are all used in service to the vision.

Perhaps what nurses uniquely bring to nonnursing leadership positions is the ability to achieve the outcomes of a new reality in a humanistic, caring manner. This requires not only the use of followers but also the empowerment of these followers. Depree (1989) used the term "roving leadership" to describe a participatory process that emphasizes situational leadership by empowered followers through the support and approval of the hierarchical leader. In support of this line of thought, Senge (1990) described leaders as designers, stewards, and teachers responsible for building organizations in which people continually expand their capabilities to understand complexity, clarify vision, and improve shared mental models. Nurses in leadership nonnursing positions come well prepared for this type of leadership behavior.

The final characteristic ascribed to a leader is mentoring. Mentoring is an intense career building, mutually beneficial relationship between two individuals of unequal power in an organization (Levinson, 1978). Nurses in nonnursing leadership positions require a mentor. The need a guide, coach, advocate, and sponsor in formal and informal settings who is committed to maximizing their success. At the same time, in order to continue the expansion of nurses in nonnursing leadership positions, the nurse leader must be mentoring other potential nurse leaders, preparing them for a successful encounter with the invisible glass ceiling of career opportunity.

ADVANTAGES AND DISADVANTAGES

The advantages of nurses in nonnursing leadership positions are multifaceted. There are rewards for both the individual nurse leader and for the nursing profession and humankind in general. These rewards include the affirmation of one's ability to lead, increased compensation potential, and increased political, policy, and decision-making power. These rewards result in an empowered and expanded image of the nurse.

Advantages: Affirmation, Compensation, and Power

Affirmation. For the individual nursing leader, the affirmation of one's ability to lead represents a step toward self-actualization, the ultimate building block in Maslow's (1954) hierarchy of needs. For nurses, who belong to a predominantly female profession, to be able to maximize their career potential within and beyond the traditional boundaries of nursing, thereby successfully breaking through the glass ceiling, is revolutionary. The individual nurse is affirmed. The profession, with all of its self-doubts about its professional status, is reaffirmed. Women, biologically different than men but capable of serving as leaders and partners in visionary organizational growth, are also affirmed.

Compensation. In concert with nursing's ambivalence to embrace power is the parallel reluctance to publicly value financial gain. Within every stratum of nursing (staff nurse, nurse manager, nurse director, school of nursing educator, and nurse executive), there is the issue of salary compression. Salary compression results in limited pay increases during a typical nursing career. Nurses tend to "top out" early in their careers, with more experienced nurses making little more than their less experienced counterparts. Chitty (1993) points out that salary progression in other professions is much greater than in nursing. For example, attorneys can expect a 226% salary progression during a typical career span, while nurses average a 69% progression. Moving nurses beyond the typical nursing career provides a greater opportunity for salary progression for all nurses as the "typical" nursing career is redefined with new and expanded boundaries.

The opportunity for greater financial compensation serves as an individual, professional, and public reward. The fact that 96% of the 2.2 million nurses in the United States are women translates into every step forward for nursing is a step forward for women throughout the nation and world.

Power: Policy Shaping and Decision Making. Nurses in nonnursing leadership positions are based in legislative bodies, major health care entities, academic settings, foundations, entrepreneurial small businesses, and industrial corporate institutions. For example, Eddie Bernice Johnson, Democratic State Representative from Texas, is the first nurse in Congress. Gloria R. Smith, past Director of the Michigan Department of Public Health and presently Program Director and Vice President—Program within the Kellogg Foundation, works from a national and international frame to empower communities by structuring partnerships in primary health care, healing, and learning between providers and consumers. Rhetaugh Dumas, past Deputy Director of the National Institute of Mental Health and Vice Provost of Health Affairs at the University of Michigan, has provided leadership in the expansion of nursing's image to include the successful management of complex health-related organizations that extend beyond nursing.

These nurse leaders affect the availability of resources and opportunities for other nurses and the general public. Nurses at the bedside benefit from deliberations occurring in the halls of Congress, hospital board rooms, and other decision-making forums that include nurses in nonnursing leadership positions. These nurses can advocate not only for other nurses but also most importantly for the individual consumer's quality of life.

Bringing a nursing perspective of healing and collaboration to a traditionally nonnursing leadership position has far-reaching consequences for the health of this nation. Whether the health of the nation is defined in physical, psychological, spiritual or economic terms, nurse leaders add value to organizations critical to its well-being.

Disadvantages: Tokenism, Competition, and Passing

Tokenism. The burden of tokenism is intense. As a token, the female nurse is brought in as an artificial, transitional intervention intended to give management a chance to correct an imbalance (Thomas, 1991). The nurse in the nonnursing leadership position may be identified as only one of few and thereby becomes representative of what women and nurses can do or becomes a stand-in for all women and nurses. While one may receive significant visibility in organizations in which success is dependent on becoming known, the more likely scenario is one of loneliness or exclusion. Kanter (1977, p. 207) describes it as "a stranger who intrudes upon an alien culture." Dumas (1985) describes the dilemmas of black female leaders in a way that is reminiscent of nurses in non-nursing leadership positions:

> There is a general resistance to having black women perform competently in formal, high status positions. . . . The black woman in leadership is expected to comfort the weary and oppressed, intercede on behalf of those who feel abused, champion the cause for equality and justice—often as a lone crusader. She is expected to compensate for the deficits of other members of her group, speaking up for those who are unable or unwilling to speak for themselves. . . . Expected to be mother confessor, she counsels and advises her superiors and peers as well as her subordinates, often on matters unrelated to the tasks at hand. [p. 326]

Bayes and Newton (1985) state that a woman given primary authority for an organization faces a basic incongruity between role requirements of the leadership position and the sex-linked role conception of a woman. This incongruity is magnified when a nurse occupies a nonnursing leadership position.

Competition. Nurses in nonnursing leadership positions are automatically in competition with other males, females, or nurses. The success of having cracked the glass ceiling is frequently envied rather than applauded and supported. Men assume that there is one less position available for them. Women have been socialized to compete with other women for favored positions with powerful men. It may appear difficult for women to join in supporting or protecting another woman who has achieved success (Bayes & Newton, 1985).

Competition is not necessarily negative. In corporate America, competition is the spice of organizational work life that leads to the prize. However, competition can be painful when the prize is gained only at the expense of other players. Nurses usually do not identify themselves as competitive. Therefore, they tend to be unaware of their own competitive urges and unprepared to compete in a healthy yet protective manner. Competition, especially from other female nurses, may be perceived as a malicious assault rather than a natural process of organizational life.

Passing. "Passing" is usually discussed in relationship to passing over the color line. In the days of slavery, children born to racially mixed parents, depending on the lightness of their skin color, had the opportunity to slip from the bonds of slavery into the mainstream of white America. This process was described as passing. For nurses in nonnursing leadership positions, the same opportunity is presented. By simply dropping the credential of Registered Nurse and all references to a nursing back-

ground, women and men are afforded the opportunity to wipe the presence of nursing from their career portfolio. This denial of one's educational and professional preparation eliminates another voice from being heard and identified as part of the nursing tradition. It nullifies the advantages that were discussed earlier and reinforces stereotypes of low status and mobility that surround the nursing profession. It is an individual decision with systemwide repercussions.

SUMMARY

Nurses in nonnursing leadership positions are of great value to the individual nurse, the profession, and society. These leaders clearly operate at the edge of the profession, balancing on the precipice of change and power. They have the opportunity to expand the dimensions of the profession, to be the holistic voice in redesigning the health care system, the welfare system, or other policy-shaping processes.

We in the nursing profession are aware of the potential isolation and loneliness for those who function at the edge of any activity. We must nurture our nurses in nonnursing leadership positions. Nursing and its organizations must find ways to continue to include our colleagues without demanding the sacrifice of their nonnursing positions; without requesting an exception from the role requirements of the position; and with an understanding that those who perform at the edge of the profession are just as essential to the wholeness of the profession as those who function at its core.

In nursing's role as an exemplar for women's issues worldwide, nurses must step forward to embrace this nonnursing leadership position. It is for the good of humankind that nursing must choose to lead.

REFERENCES

Altick, R. (1973). *The weaker sex in Victorian people and ideas.* New York: Norton.

Bayes, M., & Newton, P. (1985). Women in authority: A sociopsychological analysis. In A. Colman & M. Geller (Eds.), *Group relations reader 2.* Washington, DC: AK Rice Institute.

Belenky, M.F., Clinchy, B.M., & Tarule, J.M. (1986). *Women ways of knowing.* New York: Basic Books.

Bennis, W., & Nanus, B. (1985). *Leaders: The strategies for taking charge.* New York: Harper & Row.

Carnevale, A., & Stone, S. (1994, October). Diversity beyond the golden rule. *Training and Development.*

Chitty, K.K. (1993). *Professional nursing: Concepts and challenges.* Philadelphia: Saunders.

Depree, M. (1989). *Leadership is an art.* New York: Doubleday Currency.

Dumas, R. (1985). Dilemmas of black females in leadership. In A. Colman & M. Geller (Eds.), *Group relations reader 2.* Washington, DC: AK Rice Institute.

Dunham, J., & Fisher, E. (1990). Nurse executive profile of excellent nursing leadership. *Nursing Administration Quarterly, 15,* 1-8.

Grohar-Murray, M.E., & DiCroce, H.R. (1992). *Leadership and management in nursing.* Norwalk, CT: Appleton and Lange.

Heim, P., & Galant, S.K. (1993). *Hardball for women: Winning at the game of business.* New York: NAL/Dutton.

Jago, A. (1982). Leadership: Perspective training and research. *Management Science, 28,* 315-336.

Kanter, R. (1977). *Men and women of the corporation.* New York: Basic Books.

Levinson, D.J. (1978). *Seasons of a man's life.* New York: Knopf.

Malone, B. (1984). Strategies and approaches to policymaking: A nursing perspective. *Occupational Health Nursing, 32*(1), 24-27.

Maslow, A. (1954). *Motivation and personality.* New York: Harper & Row.

Moss, M.T. (1995). Developing glass breaking skills. *Nursing Administration Quarterly, 19*(2), 41-47: Aspen Publishers.

Muller, H. (Winter, 1994). Managing diversity in health services organizations. *Hospital & Health Services Administration,* 415-433.

Roberts, J., & Group, T.M. (1995). *Feminism and nursing. An historical perspective on power, status and political activism in the nursing profession.* CT: Praeger Publishers.

Senge, P. (1990). *The fifth discipline.* New York: Doubleday.

Shames, K.H. (1993). *The Nightingale conspiracy.* NJ: Enlightenment Press.

Thomas, Jr., R. (1991). *Beyond race and gender.* New York: American Management Association.

Community-Based Academic Health Centers

PATRICIA MAGUIRE MESERVEY

No longer is the focus primarily on the content and competencies that nursing faculty members believe students need to master. Rather, this conversation is now expanded, and thus fundamentally changed, by its focus on the development of new relationships requisite to community-focused practice which is characterized by quality and competency. —Forker and Yurchuck (1996)

Historians will describe the 1990s as the period of re-creating the health care system, overhauling a system established under the 1965 and 1967 big government acts of Medicare and Medicaid. These programs, while addressing critical health care needs, lacked the cost controls necessary for market forces to limit spending. And, when coupled with technological advances and consumer demands, they pushed health care costs to unprecedented levels. Health maintenance organizations found firm footing for new markets by promising low-cost, comprehensive services targeted to healthy individual consumers. As healthy individuals moved from traditional fee for service insurance models to capitated plans, hospitals turned to the unlimited funds of federal, state, and city governments to pay the bill for the high-risk consumer. These upwardly spiraling costs, combined with federal deficits and the end-stages of a recession, demanded a revamping of our entire health care financing and delivery system.

As the process of change begins to slow at the start of the new millennium, we have passed through vertical integrations, hospital closings, mega-mergers, and serious questions about the quality of our current health care. Although prevention, population-based health care approaches, and access were touted during the 1990s, we find little change in our health indicators. A few examples are our infant mortality rate, which is among the highest of developed countries, a life expectancy that ranks seventh, and the majority of premature deaths in the country being linked to behavior (e.g., substance abuse, smok-

ing, AIDS, cardiovascular disease). All this occurs despite the fact that the United States spends more money per person on health care than any other country in the world. Our health care system remains reactive, addressing illnesses and conditions once they appear, rather than seeking the causes of illness and conditions and providing the care and education necessary to prevent or minimize their effect. We do not have a health care system in the United States; we have a medical intervention system that is not providing the comprehensive health care our communities need.

As we continue the transformation of health care in our country, we are seeking a broader definition of health than the absence of illness. The concept of health includes the availability of resources for a family, the environment in which they live, the knowledge they possess to prevent disease, and the belief system guiding their choices. We are also likely to see a health care system that is more integrated, more intensively managed, more evidence based, more ambulatory or community based, and one that both uses and is dependent on the advances we are experiencing in information systems and technology (O'Neil, 1998). All these factors contribute to the health status of our society; all are aspects of health doctors, nurses, and social workers must know.

How then do we educate a workforce to attend to this broad definition of health? How do we teach the diagnosis and treatment of physical, mental, and social illness when the consumers are the population and not patients in a hospital bed? How do we validate our approaches to care, ensuring quality in both cost and care? How do we work together across disciplines to maximize the effectiveness of our care for our patients?

Health professional education and health services research must respond to the changing environment of health care by educating providers and researchers in the settings in which they will deliver care (Heller, Oros, & Durney-Crowley, 2000). No longer can medical, nursing, and social work education remain exclusively in the hospital institution. Students of all health professionals must learn their practice in the arena in which care will be rendered. Research must address the integration and application of knowledge in the broader community. Community-based academic health centers capture the functions of education, research, and service in close proximity to where people live, work, play, and pray, providing a new environment for discovery, learning, and care.

COMMUNITY-BASED ACADEMIC HEALTH CENTERS

> Preparation for the entry level professional nurse now requires a greater orientation to community-based primary health care, and an emphasis on health promotion, maintenance and cost-effective coordinated care that responds to the needs of increasing culturally diverse groups and underserved populations in all settings. [American Association of Colleges of Nursing, 1994]

Noting these changes emerging in the health care disciplines, the W.K. Kellogg Foundation developed the Community Partnership with Health Professions Education Initiative. The intent of this initiative was to reduce the gap between the culture of the community and the culture of academe and hospitals through partnerships (Richards, 1995). These partnerships would yield an organizational structure that would be academic, community based, and have a primary care focus. This community-based academic health center may take many forms (e.g., a nursing center, school-based health center, homeless shelter, or community health center). It shares common characteristics with the traditional academic health center through its role in education, research, and service. Yet it is the emphasis on the community and the implementation of education, research, and service in this setting that differentiates the community-based academic health center from its traditional counterpart.

Shifting education and research to the community requires significant change in our academic and health care

systems. First is a change in the orientation of health care from a system developed for providers and organizations to one centered on people, that is, communities. Communities must be engaged as full partners in health care and health profession education, providing greater assurances that the outcomes will address community needs.

A second change is developing the academic nature of the health center in the community environment. Historically many community health centers drew away from teaching programs because they resented the sense of being regarded as "teaching material" rather than as human beings (Zuvekas & Rosenbaum, 1995). More recently, health centers have recognized that for new practitioners to choose a community-based practice they must be exposed to and socialized into the practice arena. Further, students must view their community experiences as challenging and fulfilling, requiring community-based education to receive the same time and quality emphasis in curricula that institutionally based care receives. Universities and community-based health care centers must develop experience in partnership and focus on the essential knowledge and skills needed for the practice environment.

Community-based academic health centers should focus their practice in the areas of prevention and early intervention through a multidisciplinary model. It is important to bring health professionals together with the community to provide care. Much has been written about the advantages of teaming and coordinated care, yet most organizations promote a "turn" care system instead. Turn care is care delivered through patient panels that are shared by multiple providers, with some consultation across the disciplines. Multidisciplinary care blends the knowledge and skills that medicine, nursing, social work, and other health professions have to offer to improve health outcomes through a team approach, which reflects a true collaboration and coordination of care.

Community-based research is a shift from the traditional notion of research. As health service research has transformed our delivery system, community responsive research will bring the talents of the scientist to the pragmatic needs of the community. Boyer (1991) describes it as the scholarship of application. Taking knowledge believed to be true, applying it to practice in the community, and determining its effectiveness makes the scholarship of use to society.

Finally, there are large groups of people who are not receiving the health care services they need. Within the overall frame of the community-based academic health center is a focus on communities that are underserved and whose needs place them in high-risk health categories. This increases the services available in the community and socializes students to work in settings in which the clinical needs are high through a service learning approach. The assumption is that students will gain an appreciation for the strengths and challenges of both the communities and the providers who have chosen to serve them, thus increasing the likelihood of their choosing careers in underserved areas (Zuvekas & Rosenbaum, 1995).

CCHERS—A W.K. KELLOGG COMMUNITY PARTNERSHIPS PROGRAM

Boston's Center for Community Health, Education, Research, and Service (CCHERS, pronounced cheers) is a community-based academic health center, one of the 10 programs partially funded through the W.K. Kellogg Community Partnerships Initiative and the Graduate Medical and Nursing Initiative. The membership of CCHERS includes two universities, 12 health centers and their communities, a private hospital and the city's public health department. The primary purposes of this partnership are to create academic health centers in the community for primary care and to redirect health professional education into the primary care sector. These goals must be fulfilled with the full participation and involvement of the residents of these communities.

CCHERS is a nonprofit organization governed by a board of directors. The membership of the board includes representation from all constituents: universities, health centers, communities, hospitals, and the public health department. The board sets the policy direction, allocates resources, and oversees the implementation of the various programs of the organization. Reporting to the board is an executive director, who is responsible for the daily work of the programs. Each organization (health center, university, and health department) has a coordinator on site to facilitate the work of the program offerings and to ensure that the goals are met.

CCHERS is a community-based academic health system, with 12 participating health centers. Each health center has advanced its mission to include an active role in education and research to complement the strong service base that was their original mission. The communities served by the health center have active roles in the education and research of CCHERS. Many community-based organizations outside the health center join in educating students and participating in research endeavors.

Education

The lead educational activity of CCHERS has been participating in the curricula transformations and implementation for the undergraduate nursing program and the medical school. Inherent in the philosophy of the CCHERS partnership is the belief that the health services of the community are owned by the community and that the power of the community to direct its health and welfare is the right and responsibility of the community. Curriculum is owned by the university faculty with the faculty maintaining the responsibility for providing a sound educational experience for students. These two worlds converge because the curriculum must be designed to prepare graduates to meet the needs of the community's health.

The partnership enables faculty and community to share information, expectations, and limitations across traditional boundaries in order to create a responsive educational experience for students that benefits the community in both the short and long term. Residents of the neighborhoods are direct partners in the education of the students, in the development of service projects to meet community needs, and in the identification of research problems that the community wants and that need attention.

To accomplish the goal of community benefits in depth, clinical assignments are organized so that students return to the same community and neighborhood health center over the course of their educational program. In this manner a genuine partnership can be developed between the students and the families and clients they serve. Further, it is expected that the students will develop partnerships with each other and with community staff that is reflective of a genuine collaborative model (Meservey & Zungolo, 1995).

Extending beyond the nursing and medical programs, the community representatives of the CCHERS partnership sought opportunities for the children of the neighborhoods to have greater access to the university programs. It is their intent to "grow their own" and have the students in the health professions programs be the children of the community. In response to this need the CCHERS partnership has joined with the Boston School Department and Boston and Dorchester high schools to establish a Health Careers Academy. The academy is a full high school curriculum enriched with career exploration, mentoring, youth development, family supports, and academic enrichment. Students in the academy work with the medical and nursing students in the communities to learn about the opportunities in higher education and health professionals careers. It is expected that the academy will serve as a pipeline for inner-city children to pursue health careers.

Research

To achieve all the dimensions of an academic health center traditionally found in hospitals, the partnership must address other aspects of the shared relationship in addition to the learning experiences. The research-rich environment of traditional settings must be captured to enable the communities to attract top-notch clinicians for their centers and to communicate a value in the advancement of knowledge. Essential to these perceptions is the recognition of the void in knowledge about the efficacy of many current health practices, the effectiveness of interventions, the cost-benefit ratio of preventive therapies and diagnostic screenings, and the whole range of investigations necessary to explore the effectiveness of the health service delivery mechanisms. The role of the community residents in the approval and acceptance of research activities is pivotal to the success of the project as well as to the integrity of any research undertaking.

CHALLENGES OF A COMMUNITY-BASED ACADEMIC HEALTH CENTER

The community-based academic health center creates linkages that produce new organizations or at the least new, stronger relationships. There is a blurring of traditional boundaries that is a source of confusion, fear, and risk. There are differences in primary orientation between the health centers and universities. Universities have a primary mission to educate students while community health centers, nursing centers, and school-based health centers have as their primary mission to provide health services. The transition to the new organizational model demands a shifting of focus from the organization of origin to the partnership organization that has as its primary concern the blending of community and educational needs. Issues that will surface can be captured in the concept of a "boundaryless organization." The four principal boundaries to be considered are authority, task, political, and identity (Hirschhorn & Gilmore, 1992).

Developing strong communication, evolving trust, and creating positive organizational self-esteem are essential to the success of the new organization (Kawamoto, 1994). The traditional lines of authority are changed. The particular person or organization responsible for aspects of the work varies depending on the piece of work and how the work has changed with the new linkages of the

organization. This, as with the next arena of the task boundaries, creates tensions in the organization.

The task boundary is that of the work to be done. This may be the most directly threatening aspect of the new organization because an individual's or organization's past responsibilities are shifted in the new environment. The normal expectation that university faculty will do the teaching is changed. Community providers, community members, and a variety of other people participate in the new educational model. Similarly, delivery of care changes. The faculty and students are new additions to the community setting, and there are shifts of responsibility, authority, and control.

The new organization blurs our past definitions and creates a sense of confusion for the members of the original organizations. A new identity is needed. Emphasis on the common goals of the group and efforts to create a new model of both education and service are examples of strategies to foster the identity of "us." Multiple fields of expertise are needed. Neither of the original organizations alone could achieve the same level of success in the new model as could the combined talents of both health centers and universities. Excellence in each part of the organization is essential for the blended system to succeed, and the recognition of the need for collective excellence becomes the team's motivation.

The merging of organizations is difficult work and will certainly give rise to the question, What is in it for us? The common vision or shared goals are an essential element of the political boundary. Guiding the groups to an understanding of how mutual gains will be achieved and how, absent the new consortium, such gains could not be realized, is the basis for success in this area (Meservey & Zungolo, 1995).

PATHWAYS TO SUCCESS

Vision, leadership, and power are the key elements for success in the new health care organization. With these elements, the new model of education will find a new locus of operation that will interconnect the needs of communities with the learning needs, knowledge, and skills of students. Learning can occur as service is provided, yielding a gain-gain outcome for the organization.

Vision is the ability to move toward a collective goal. It requires an understanding that the principal orientation of each participating organization and individual will be shifting to a new arena. We do not know at this time what the future holds for health care. With change occurring at a rapid pace, the system is in chaos. In this environment, creating and holding a vision is challenging. The cornerstone of the community-based academic health center is understanding that however the system evolves there will be communities and the need to educate new health professionals and that these two needs can be mutually supportive.

Leadership plays a pivotal role in the success of these new organizations. Leadership must evolve from each part of the new organization including service, education, and community. Having a cadre of leaders who can understand the needs and demands of the multiple aspects of the organization and provide the bridge for the organization is important. Leaders can create a climate of openness in the organization to transcend the cultures of community and academe.

Finally, power and control over resources is essential. The current educational system is supported by a long tradition of funding pathways. This system must change to support community-based education, multiprofessional education, and primary care. To become a permanent part of the educational system, to be an essential care provider, the mainstream support must be redirected to provide the funds necessary for all aspects of education.

Outcomes sought with the new community-based academic health centers are an assurance of responsiveness and quality of services for the community. There must be a process of community assessment and mechanisms for community evaluation of programs. Because education is a cornerstone of such programs, ensuring quality education is also essential. The new community-based academic health centers facilitate the delineation of

new roles for health professionals, establish mechanisms for policy changes in health care systems, and determine outcome measures for successful programming.

REFERENCES

American Association of Colleges of Nursing. (1994). *Position statement: Nursing education's agenda for the 21st century.* Washington, DC: Author.

Boyer, E.L. (1991). *Scholarship reconsidered: Priorities of the professorate.* Princeton, NJ: The Carnegie Foundation.

Forker, J.E., & Yurchuck, E.R. (1996). Perspectives on assessment: Assessing outcomes of community-based nursing education. *Nurse Educator, 21*(2), 15-16.

Heller, B.R., Oros, M.T., & Durney-Crowley, J. (2000). The future of nursing education: 10 trends to watch. *Nursing and Health Care Perspectives, 21*(1), 9-13.

Hirschhorn, L., & Gilmore, T. (1992). The new boundaries of the boundaryless company. *Harvard Business Review,* May-June, 106-115.

Kawamoto, K. (1994). Nursing leadership: To thrive in a world of change. *Nursing Administration Quarterly, 18*(3), 1-6.

Meservey, P.M., & Zungolo, E. (1995). Out of the tower and onto the streets: One college of nursing's partnership with communities. In P.S. Matteson (Ed.), *Nursing in the neighborhoods: The Northeastern University model.* Philadelphia: Springer.

O'Neil, E. (1998). The changing health care environment. In E. O'Neil & J. Coffman (Eds.), *Strategies for the future of nursing.* San Francisco: Jossey-Bass.

Richards, R.W. (1995). From problems to solutions: A bridge between cultures. In R.W. Richards (Ed.), *Building partnerships: Educating health professionals for the communities they serve.* San Francisco: Jossey-Bass.

Zuvekas, A., & Rosenbaum, S. (1995). *Teaching community health centers: A guide.* Washington, DC: National Association of Community Health Centers.

Nursing Centers

New Opportunities and Continuing Challenges

SALLY PECK LUNDEEN

The health care system continues to be in a dynamic state of change. There are many examples of health care reform initiatives that tinker at the edges of system change. Most of these do not constitute a real paradigm shift. Nursing centers, however, have the potential to offer an alternative system of primary health care delivery. How do nursing centers fit into the emerging system of health care delivery? What is their relationship to the current paradigms of health care? What opportunities and challenges can be identified as nursing centers continue to develop and evolve as part of the changing health care landscape?

CURRENT NURSING CENTER DEFINITIONS

Built on the practice models of previous decades, nursing centers have emerged as a model of health care delivery that increases direct access to professional nurses (Glass, 1989). A definition of nursing centers and their characteristics has evolved over the past 20 years. The American Nursing Association (ANA) Task Force on Nurse-Managed Centers developed the first definition:

> Nursing centers—sometimes referred to as nursing organizations, nurse-managed centers, nursing clinics and community nursing centers—are organizations that give the client direct access to professional nursing services. Using nursing models of health, professional nurses in these centers diagnose and treat human responses to actual and potential health problems, and promote health and optimal functioning among target populations and communities. The services provided in these centers are holistic and client-centered, and are reimbursable at a reasonable fee level. Accountability and responsibility for client care and professional practice remain with the professional nurse. Overall accountability and responsibility remain with the nurse executive. Nursing centers are not limited to any particular or-

ganizational configuration. Nursing centers may be free-standing or may be affiliated with universities or other service institutions, such as home health agencies or hospitals. The primary characteristic of the organization is responsiveness to the health needs of the population. [Adylotte et al., 1987]

This definition of nursing centers, a number of national surveys, and other descriptions of nursing centers found in the literature identify common elements that define nursing centers as practice settings that:

- Provide consumers with direct access to nursing services (no referrals necessary)
- Provide nurse clinicians with a high level of professional autonomy when practicing in these centers
- Place professional nurses in administrative control
- Develop mechanisms for nurses to receive direct payment for nursing services
- Use nursing models of health as the core element of the conceptual service delivery framework

Although nursing centers are most definitely not limited to those developed in academic settings, most of the studies of nursing centers and the descriptions published in the literature have focused on those centers developed by faculty in professional schools of nursing across the country. Academic nursing centers (those supported by schools of nursing) have been developed to provide settings where the missions of research, teaching, and service can be integrated (Barger & Bridges, 1990; Lundeen, Friedbacher, Thomas, & Jackson, 1997; Rosenkoetter, Zakutney, Reynolds, & Faller, 1993). Nursing centers supported through the U.S. Public Health Service, Department of Health and Human Services (PHS, DHHS), Division of Nursing are developed to address the needs of communities through education and practice partnerships (Clear, Starbecker, & Kelly, 1999). More than 250 academic nursing centers are currently operated nationwide (American Association of Colleges of Nursing [AACN], 1998). These academic nursing centers also include two additional elements in their operational definitions: (1) provide opportunities for the education of nursing students and (2) promote the conduct of nursing research (Zachariah & Lundeen, 1997).

National surveys of nursing centers indicate that, where they are available, they have filled enormous gaps in care to the most vulnerable populations (Barger & Rosenfeld, 1993). These centers provide innovative health care delivery models that provide increased access for vulnerable populations to primary health care and the problems presented by individuals who chose to use these centers includes a wide range of issues related to health as well as illness (Kreuser, 1998). A recent multisite study of community nursing centers (CNCs) found that over 85% of the interventions provided in these settings are related to health teaching, counseling, case management, and coordination of care (Schoneman, 1999). Community nursing centers based on the WHO definitions of primary health care are located in convenient and accessible locations where people live, work, learn, and play (Farley, 1997; Lancaster, 1999; Lundeen, 1993, WHO, 1978). Initial planning in these centers begins with a dialogue between providers and potential clients. Lancaster (1999) identify the two basic questions to be addressed in the initial planning process: What do you need in the way of health care? and What kind of services would you use? This approach shifts the balance of power to include community residents and engenders community ownership and an increased impact on vulnerable persons is a direct result. In short, nursing centers are different kinds of health care organizations.

WHY DO WE NEED A NEW KIND OF HEALTH CARE ORGANIZATION?

A midpoint review of the outcomes of the *Healthy People 2000* objectives indicates that progress was slow in a number of areas (U.S. DHHS, 1995). Although 13% of HP 2000 targeted outcomes had been met or exceeded and 43% showed progress toward desired outcomes, 25% had either moved away from the target, showed mixed results, or remained unchanged, and another 14% could not be assessed as a result of inadequate data. Failure to achieve these benchmarks is certainly related to the larger societal issues such as poverty and race; however, it also may be a reflection of failures in the ways in which we organize and deliver care. In fact, a strong case can be made that the entire paradigm for the delivery of health care does not match the values of many populations (Lundeen, 1999).

This is the time for change. Seeking solutions that take into account the complexities of health care and health status are essential. Gaus and Fraser (1996) state that "there will never be a better time to learn what does and does not work in social policy and health care financing and organization." Curtin (1998) has observed that social conditions including poverty, class, poor nutrition, and "killing stress" have more to do with health status than biology and that we must learn how to manage the health of all if we are to find the money necessary to care for the chronically ill. Managing the health of all is a concept that does not resonate with much of this county's health care policy makers, who are focused almost exclusively on the management of illness. Even when a shift in paradigm to more prevention oriented care is espoused, health care providers frequently do not focus on maintaining health as much as curing illness. To complicate the issue further, many vulnerable clients present to the health care system with complex medical needs or at a more advanced stage of illness. The level of urgency and scope of their needs often replaces preventive health care as a priority. Also, preventive interventions require that individuals make lifestyle changes to lower risk for disease. This approach takes time and presents a challenge to health care professionals who want immediate, quantifiable results and to vulnerable clients who are, by necessity, time oriented in the present. There is a desperate need to find a balance between prevention and treatment for vulnerable populations if we are to affect health status outcomes long term. This author argues that community nursing centers have an opportunity to provide the missing link in a redefined health care delivery system that addresses the full continuum of health needs for all populations from primary prevention of illness to rehabilitation and even palliative care.

THE NEED FOR A SHARED CONCEPTUAL MODEL FOR NURSING CENTER PRACTICE

There is a great need to develop a shared conceptual model of nursing center practice models. This is perhaps our greatest challenge and our greatest opportunity related to nursing centers extant. The literature on nursing centers has suffered from inexact definitions and language and lack of clarity in the conceptualization of nursing enter practice models. To date, nursing leaders have not defined explicitly what the relationship of these nursing centers is, or should be, to the rest of the health care delivery system. Nursing centers across the country have adopted many different names including nurse-managed centers, nursing centers, nursing clinics, community nursing centers, and community nursing organizations. There appears to be no consensus about whether nurse practice models such as parish nursing or school-based clinics meet the criteria as nursing centers or if they even choose to identify themselves as nursing centers. It has even been questioned by some whether practice settings operated autonomously by nurses but not affiliated directly with schools of nursing or not participating directly in nursing education or research "qualify" as nursing centers. Likewise, the definition of the populations served by nursing centers need to be expanded. Many CNC participants come from predominantly underserved, low-income, urban communities; however, many of the health issues and concerns presented in these centers are just as applicable to rural populations and persons of all socioeconomic groups. It is time to revisit our definitions of nursing centers and differentiate more clearly the conceptual models on which their practice is built.

Nursing centers, by definition, are autonomous practice models that have moved beyond *dependent* models of practice, which require a physician's referral for nurses to provide care incidental to medical treatment. However, there have been limited attempts to describe systematically these innovative nursing models. Some see nursing centers as *independent* practice models that can operate side by side with traditional medical model providers, thereby giving consumers a real *nursing choice* in a growing smorgasbord of health provider and practice setting options. Others believe that nursing centers should be *interdependent* models, which attempt to bridge the current gaps in the health care delivery system and link multiple practice options and paradigms into a more coordinated and comprehensive system of care. Opinions on these definitions vary widely. It is not the purpose of this chapter to propose definitively what nursing centers should be. It is important, however, that nursing leaders from across the nation and around the world engage in this debate, and it is critical that some consensus be developed within the nursing profession about the core elements of nursing center models. For until conceptual clarity of nursing center model(s) emerges from the nursing professions, the potential for these centers to be discounted by nonnurses is maximized and the ability of nurses to successfully describe, evaluate, and "sell" nursing centers to policy makers at all levels is compromised.

Nursing centers are not all alike. In fact, the variability in nursing center models is currently great. Nursing centers are organized, staffed, and supported financially in different ways. They serve different populations and provide different services. They weight their investment to service, education of health professionals, and research differently. Different organizational structures and practice models have been developed that, at least implicitly, are grounded in different points of view about the role of the nurse. These differences are frequently deliberate and reflect the unique needs of the specific communities and populations served; however, it has not served nursing well in the larger political arena to operate as if all nursing center models are the same without clear descriptions of the practice models they represent. There is undoubtedly room for multiple nursing center models, but each should explicate the nature of nursing practice that sets it apart.

The work to define nursing center models from a theoretical perspective is far from finished. We must be able to articulate our differences as well as our similarities in order to move the nursing center political agenda forward. If we cannot define these differences within nursing, it will be difficult to differentiate nursing centers from other more traditional medical models of care. Without clear differentiation, it is nearly impossible to explain these models to the policy makers who make decisions about resource allocation. It is imperative that we lobby effectively for resources if we are to be a significant force in the improvement of health status for community residents.

Nursing centers have the potential to contribute significantly to the ultimate reconfiguration of the evolving American health care system in the next century (Weddle, 1996). The maturation of nursing centers as a practice model and their integration into the mainstream of health care policy and delivery systems in the United States and the world will occur only if nursing leaders seize the opportunities currently available. We must be aggressive in our quest for resources and partnerships in order to take advantage of the opportunities in the current health care arena.

One of the main areas of differences between nursing center models and medical models is the consistent focus on health promotion and coordination across the continuum of care. If nurses are successful in defining and describing models of practice that highlight the ability of nursing centers to contribute value in the areas of health promotion and coordination and continuity of care, nursing centers may well prove to be key in the development of a system of health care that begins to actually manage health rather than illness. In addition to articulating clear conceptual models of practice for nursing centers, we must seize the opportunity to design and develop collaborative partnerships, systematically document nursing practice in nursing centers, identify and measure nurse sensitive outcomes, expand our focus to include an international perspective, and disseminate our findings widely to other professionals, policy makers, and the public.

THE OPPORTUNITY TO DESIGN AND DEVELOP COLLABORATIVE MODELS OF CARE

There may be no single concept that is more often spoken and less frequently defined in health care today than collaboration. It also may be the most important concept to explicate and embrace if significant changes in the way health care is delivered are to be realized. The development and maintenance of truly collaborative practice models can be the most difficult and time-consuming aspect of nursing center work as well as the most important. Collaboration means much more than multidisciplinary case conferences or sharing clinical space and clients. True collaboration depends on the development of partnerships among relative equals. This means that nurses must be able to share power and influence with some partners who are less strong while asserting or leveraging influence with some partners who traditionally have held more power. Restructuring relationships among various health care professional groups, community residents and leaders, and other health and social service organizations in order to develop partnerships does not happen by accident and it does not happen quickly. Continuity of effort is critical. The development and maintenance of collaborative partnerships requires a high degree of interpersonal skills, knowledge of organizational theory and process, and the commitment to engage in this process over a long period of time. Although it is rarely reimbursed in the current health care delivery system, the individual and collective involvement of nurses in designing collaborative models of care will be a key factor in shifting the current delivery paradigm to one that embraces all health care providers and the community as participants in the quest for improved health and quality of life for all.

THE OPPORTUNITY TO DOCUMENT NURSING PRACTICE

Nursing center models must be clearly delineated from other practice models (Clark & Lang, 1992; Coenen, Marek, & Lundeen, 1996; McCormick et al., 1994). If this is not done, the subtleties of nursing practice so frequently

unheralded in terms of its impact on health status can be neither documented nor measured. Professional nurses always have advocated for community-based, accessible, affordable, quality care for all. Health promotion and disease prevention and population-based approaches to health are long-standing public health nursing principles. Yet, as the American health care system grapples with these issues anew, data on nursing practice and its impact on health care status of populations remains nearly invisible. Unless nursing scholars commit to the documentation of nursing practice, the likelihood that nursing centers will significantly affect the ways in which health care is delivered on a national or global level is dramatically reduced. The key here is the documentation of nursing practice in ways that actually capture its unique, as well as its shared, elements. This is rarely done. In spite of the fact that health care settings demand the capture of incredible amounts of data, nursing practice data remains unidentifiable in most of the industry. This is true for both institutional and community-based care. Because coding of both health problems and diagnoses and health providers' interventions and treatments and procedures is largely linked to the reimbursement process, the typical taxonomies used for coding practice are based on medical diagnostic (*International Classification of Diseases, Ninth Revision* [*ICD-9*]) and procedure (*Current Procedural Terminology* [CPT]) codes. The work of nursing is therefore typically coded as part of or incidental to the provision of medical care.

The unique and substantive interventions done by nurses in the areas of health promotion and screening, health education, counseling, care coordination, and individual and population surveillance are rarely captured in any delivery settings. With nursing as the largest health provider group in the world, this is a travesty that must be remedied. Nursing centers must commit to the development and implementation of nursing taxonomies, including the Omaha System, North American Nursing Diagnoses Association (NANDA), Nursing Interventions Classification (NIC), Nursing Outcomes Classification (NOC), and others, if we are to move toward a differentiated description of nursing practice that will have an impact on health policy decisions. To the extent possible, these documentation systems should be computerized and provide the ability to compare systematically nursing data sets across multiple and varied practice settings (Lundeen & Friedbacher, 1996). Data elements of interest must move beyond a focus on the individual client to include population-focused problems and interventions in order to document fully nursing practice.

There are new opportunities available to nurses. During the past year there have been several federal requests for proposal for funding that recognize the need for documentation of clinical data. Last year, the Agency for Healthcare Research and Quality (AHRQ, formerly Agency for Health Care Policy Research [AHCPR]) sought proposals related to the development of quality indicators of clinical practice with vulnerable populations. Even more recently, they called for proposals related to the development of practice-based research networks. Nurses who manage nursing centers are well positioned to take advantage of these new initiatives. Nursing centers are organizations that deal with the issues of quality for vulnerable populations. There is also a growing number of regional networks of nursing centers that could qualify as practice-based research networks. Nurses must capitalize on these opportunities for major federal funding to identify and document the nature of nursing practice in nursing centers.

THE OPPORTUNITY TO DEFINE AND MEASURE NURSE SENSITIVE OUTCOMES

In the final analysis, the viability of nursing centers as an integrated element in the mainstream health care delivery system will depend on the ability of those involved in these early developmental phases to demonstrate that they are effective and efficient models of care. Evaluation of the impact of nursing centers on the outcomes of individual clients and the communities they serve is the key to effecting significant and lasting change in the system. A broad health care perspective and creativity are essential to the success of this endeavor. Current outcome measures are frequently not sensitive to nursing interventions. These measures are largely based on an illness paradigm and seek to account for changes in clinical indicators or utilization for patient groups once diagnosed with some condition or disease. For nursing center programs and services that parallel or support the medical model, these indicators may be satisfactory; however, for nursing center practice activities focused on primary prevention, coordination of care, and the development of healthy communities, these outcome measures lack appropriate focus and the ability to discriminate outcomes based on unique nursing interventions. The evaluation of nursing center outcomes demands that more comprehensive measures be developed that are consistent with a health paradigm, population as well as individually focused interventions, and nursing practice models.

Again, opportunities for support of nurse investigators for these research activities have increased in recent years as federal initiatives have begun to focus on more comprehensive programs of research related to diverse population groups. It will continue to be a struggle to define outcome measures that are sensitive to the interventions of nurses in those health care organizations where the documentation of nursing practice is not separated from that of other health professional groups, but nursing centers are venues where *nurses* can define and document nursing practice and measures their impact. By seizing the opportunity to isolate and measure the impact of nursing practice on the health status of various high-risk populations, nursing centers could significantly increase the visibility of professional nursing as a major partner in both health care delivery and reform.

THE OPPORTUNITY TO EXPAND OUR INTERNATIONAL FOCUS

There is great interest in nursing centers internationally. In the past several years, this author has had requests for information on community nursing centers from representatives of Australia, Canada, Germany, Japan, South Africa, South Korea, Russia, Taiwan, and the United Kingdom. These conversations have led to articles published in international journals, presentations and workshops in foreign lands, faculty exchanges, student exchanges, postdoctoral fellowships, and joint international research projects. Other nurses involved in nursing centers have experienced similar interest. In 1999 the first International Conference on Community Nursing Centers was held in Milwaukee, Wisconsin. Cosponsored by the University of Wisconsin–Milwaukee Institute for Urban Health Partnerships, the U.S. PHS, DHHS, Division of Nursing, and the Independence Foundation, the conference expanded the boundaries of the discussion of nursing centers around the globe. There is a great opportunity to promote the establishment of nursing centers internationally and, by doing so, to affect health policy internationally. Make no mistake about it, we must be working toward policy changes that will support the integration of nursing centers into the mainstream of health care delivery worldwide. In fact, it is likely that the strong emphasis on primary health care in most of the rest of the world may make it possible for nursing center models with an effective primary prevention focus to gain stronger political support internationally than in the United States during the next decade. It is imperative that we broaden our vision and make linkages around the globe.

THE OPPORTUNITY TO DISSEMINATE OUR EXPERIENCE AND FINDINGS WIDELY

Finally, it is incumbent on us to create opportunities to disseminate our experiences and research findings widely. Dissemination of information about nursing centers must include the traditional methods of professional journal publications and professional presentations; however, these methods are not adequate. Nurses must also become more adept at sharing our stories with the general public and policy makers. We must make real the experience of nurses and the people and communities that we serve. Nurses serve families in ways that are unique and make a difference to real people. We must tell those stories as well.

Reprinted in this chapter are two vignettes developed by a long-time colleague and friend, Barbara Friedbacher, RN, MS, and other nursing staff and faculty at the University of Wisconsin–Milwaukee (UWM) School of Nursing (see box, pp. 310-311). These were first published in the *Wisconsin Journal of Medicine* and then reprinted in a special issue of *Nursing Matters,* a statewide nursing publication, that was circulated to state legislators and health care leaders in Wisconsin (Lundeen et al., 1997). The first vignette describes in minute detail a series of experiences that are common to many families that live in the communities served by community nursing centers; the second describes a process that is common to those families that are served by the four UWM nursing centers. This piece was developed to highlight our collective experiences in the real world of health care. It has been used successfully on a number of occasions to plead our case for change in the health care system. It is included here as an example that illustrates another way to disseminate the nursing center story.

Nursing center stories are important stories. They are the stories of nurses who have practiced in the community for decades, nurses who have highlighted the serious limitations of our current health care delivery system and then developed new models of care delivery, nurses who have identified problems with health care access in all segments of society and then moved in to provide services, nurses who have acknowledged the need for health professional educators to link more effectively with practice and research and then built integrated academic nursing center models to link these important missions, nurses who have discovered the need for a different kind of clinical documentation and have pioneered models to test it, and nurses who have heard the call for a more pop-

ulation-based focus in health care delivery and have responded to that call.

Nurses must recognize the need to interact with health policy makers and expend the extra time and energy to raise their levels of consciousness. Many of the challenges facing health care today may be new to many in the health care industry, but they are not new to nurses. It is important to acknowledge and extol what public health and community health nurses have done in this country for over a century. Those of us who are engaged in the development of nursing centers stand on the shoulders of giants. We should take every opportunity to share their stories as well.

CONTINUING CHALLENGES FOR COMMUNITY NURSING CENTERS

In order to assess the potential of community nursing centers to offer a real alternative to the current health care delivery paradigm, several challenging questions still must be answered: How do nursing centers provide a model of high-quality primary health care delivery that is accessible, acceptable, and affordable to urban and rural communities? Can nursing centers lay claim to a unique set of characteristics that are value added for health and health care delivery in America? Do these unique features contribute to improved health care delivery and health outcomes for targeted individuals and communities? The answer to these questions and others will come only if we meet the continuing challenges and seize the opportunities currently available to us. The opportunities are great, but nursing centers continue to face significant challenges. Maintaining a clear vision of a new health care delivery model while seeking the policy changes necessary to support it requires persistence and a conceptual clarity that is not easy to maintain. Developing and maintaining solid community partnerships requires time, patience, long-term commitment, and the maturity to understand the need to begin at the beginning in order to establish trust with communities who have been given little reason to trust health care providers in the past. Establishing interdisciplinary partnerships requires working through many long-ingrained patterns of social interaction in both the workplace and educational institutions and developing new ways for health and human service professionals to work together. The challenges created by the current health care payment systems are dramatic. Simply staying in business while attaining long-term fiscal stability in the current competitive marketplace has been difficult for many nursing centers. Integrating outcomes from the evaluation and research critical to the demonstration

CASE STUDIES

Case Study I: A Difficult Day in the Life of a Young Family

Ameshia, a 20-year-old mother of an 18-month-old daughter and 3-year-old son, presents at the Children's Hospital emergency room at 6:15 PM on a cold Wisconsin evening, stating, "My daughter started crying at 1 AM and has not stopped since." When asked why she brought the child to the emergency room instead of to the child's pediatrician, she described the following frustrating day. As an Aid to Families with Dependent Children (AFDC) recipient with Medicaid coverage, Ameshia and her children are assigned to an HMO. She had called the pediatrician's office at 9 AM and was told that although the first open appointment was in 2 days, the doctor would call her later in the day. Ameshia reported that she had to use a pay phone and asked when she could call the doctor back. The receptionist responded that early afternoon was best but that there was no guarantee when the doctor would be available. Cold and worried, Ameshia carried her daughter and led her young son the 3 blocks from the pay phone to her sister's apartment, where she was living temporarily. By this time both children were shivering and crying loudly. Her daughter continued to cry throughout the morning.

At 1 PM, with no one available to stay with the children, Ameshia bundled them up and again walked to the phone. A voice message at the doctor's office indicated that the office would reopen at 1:30 PM. After returning home the second time, Ameshia gave the children something to eat and was relieved that her daughter fell asleep for an hour. Ameshia reported that when she awakened at 2:15 PM, she was crying harder than ever and seemed very warm, although there was no thermometer available to check her temperature. Ameshia bundled the children up again and returned to the phone. The rushed receptionist at the doctor's office told her that he was swamped with sick patients and could not come to the phone. She suggested that Ameshia call back later. Exhausted, worried, frustrated, and cold, Ameshia decided to make the trip across town with her daughter to Children's Hospital. She returned to the apartment with her crying children to wait for her sister to come home, hoping she could borrow bus fare and ask her sister to take care of her son while she went to the hospital. It was the end of the month and Ameshia was out of money. To make matters worse, she had missed a WIC (Women, Infants, Children) appointment earlier in the week because it was 5° outside, too cold to take two buses to get to the public health department clinic. She had rescheduled the appointment for today, only to miss it again because of her daughter's illness. At 4:30 PM her sister arrived and gave her bus fare but stated she had to go somewhere and could not care for Ameshia's son.

Ameshia bundled up her tired and irritable children once again, walked to the bus stop, and began the 55-minute trip to Children's Hospital, where she was greeted by a waiting room full of parents and sick children. At the registration desk a receptionist could be overheard commenting to a coworker about her frustration with parents who wait all day with sick children and then show up in the evening at the short-staffed emergency room. Two hours later Ameshia's daughter was examined by a pediatric resident, who diagnosed the child with otitis media. Ameshia was given prescriptions for the child and instructions about follow-up care. After having the prescriptions filled at the hospital pharmacy, she began the long bus trip home. Because Ameshia had no money to purchase food at the hospital, she fed the children a supper of the few snacks she had quickly placed in her bag before hurrying out of her sister's apartment.

On the trip home Ameshia felt tired and wondered if it was possible that she was pregnant. She had continued a 4-year relationship with the father of her two children but remained the primary caretaker of the children. She worried about another child and whether she and the children would continue to receive health insurance coverage under the Pay for Performance welfare reform program which she had just been assigned to. Perhaps another child would jeopardize her welfare stipend. She knew she should make a doctor's appointment for herself, but that would have to wait until she found someone to answer her questions about her benefits. Both of the children were overdue for well child checkups with the pediatrician. Having moved a year ago to Milwaukee from Racine, the thought of finding a doctor for herself who would take her as a Medicaid client, scheduling appointments around her Pay for Performance work hours, and traveling by bus with two small children seemed overwhelming, especially after the day she had just spent. Although she knew prenatal care was important, it was hard to imagine fitting it in soon. All in all, it had been a bad day, an expensive day for the HMO and hospital, and a highly unsatisfactory day for the young mother, her children, and all involved providers.

Case Study 2: Another Kind of Health Care System Experience: The Community Nursing Center

Two months later Ameshia was directed to Silver Spring Neighborhood Center (SSNC) for her involvement in programs to meet the requirements of Pay for Performance, a welfare reform program. Although referred to the center specifically for welfare reform activities, Ameshia soon learned that neighborhood residents were welcome to participate in a wide array of family support programs and services. Ameshia was required by the state to spend 30+ hours per week at the center taking general equivalency diploma (GED)

CASE STUDIES Continued

classes and working in order to qualify for financial benefits for herself and her children. As a mother who is devoted to her children, she voluntarily participates in on-site parenting classes offered by the Family Resource Center (FRC), which is funded by the Children's Trust Fund of Wisconsin and operated jointly by SSNC and UWM Silver Spring Community Nursing Center (SS CNC). These parenting classes, which support welfare families in achieving self-sufficiency, provide Ameshia with 4 to 5 hours per week credit toward the Pay for Performance requirement while she increases her parenting knowledge and skills. The FRC also provides free, on-site child care for her two preschool children during all parenting classes and GED classes.

During her orientation to Pay for Performance activities, Ameshia received information about all SSNC on-site services, including the health care and social service programs offered by the interdisciplinary team of the SS CNC. She took advantage of a minihealth fair and cholesterol screening provided by the nurse clinicians, nursing students, and a medical student. One of the parenting classes she attended was facilitated by a family nurse practitioner (FNP) student who discussed prevention and early recognition of common childhood illnesses and described the things parents can do to promote their children's health. During class break, Ameshia talked with the FNP student about other services available in the SS CNC Clinic and requested an appointment for herself. Early the next week, during lunch break from her on-site work experience job, she kept her appointment and, among other services, received a pregnancy test. The positive test confirmed Ameshia's suspicions, and she willingly agreed to enrollment in the SS CNC Prenatal Care Coordination Pro-

gram. Because she had no health care provider in Milwaukee, she was offered the opportunity to receive her obstetrical care from the center's medical consultant who is on site at SS CNC one day a week. During her first visit with the physician, Ameshia, the physician, and the FNP student set health promotion goals for the pregnancy and agreed to work closely together to promote health for mother and baby. The FNP student and Ameshia scheduled a home visit for their next prenatal care coordination session and established a plan for Ameshia's on-site prenatal and childbirth education sessions. Subsequent visits with Ameshia enabled the FNP student to review the health care needs of her children and encourage her to follow through with well child exams with the children's pediatrician. With Ameshia's consent, she telephoned the pediatrician and established a plan for collaborating to meet the children's health care needs. The FNP also agreed to provide the children with their overdue immunizations.

During one visit at SS CNC, Ameshia was reintroduced by the FNP to the center social worker who had first met her when she facilitated a stress management workshop for the GED class. The two women struck up a brief conversation, giving the social worker an opportunity to further build a relationship with Ameshia. After other brief contacts with the social worker at the center, Ameshia made an appointment to discuss her concerns about welfare reform and her family's financial survival. Undoubtedly the challenges for Ameshia and her young family will be ongoing and their needs will change over time. At the same time, Ameshia will have access to the support of the SS CNC and SSNC interdisciplinary team with interventions that are both health promotion focused and geared toward increasing the family's self sufficiency.

---

of effectiveness into organizations with severely limited resources asks a great deal of both providers and communities. Telling our stories to each other, other professionals, policy makers, and the public requires an additional commitment of time and energy that may, at times, seem excessive. It is clear, however, that the development of nursing centers requires commitment, patience, maturity, wisdom, perseverance, and political savvy. The positive outcomes, however, for both communities and providers are significant. As nurses, we should celebrate our proud history, claim credit for the work we are doing in our dynamic present, and proclaim in a multitude of ways that nursing centers have met and will continue to meet the call for innovation in a challenging future.

REFERENCES

Adylotte, M., Bramstetter, E., Fehring, R., Lindgren, K., Lundeen, S., McDaniels, S., & Riesch, S. (1987). *The nursing center: Concept and design.* Kansas City, MO: American Nurses Association.

American Association of Colleges of Nursing. (1998). *Annual survey of baccalaureate schools of nursing.* Washington, DC: Author.

Barger, S.E., & Bridges, W. (1990). An assessment of academic nursing centers. *Nurse Educator, 15*(2), 31-36.

Barger, S.I., & Rosenfeld, P. (1993). Models in community health care: Findings from a national study of community nursing centers. *Nursing & Health Care, 14,* 426-431.

Clark, J., & Lang, N. (1992). Nursing's next advance: An international classification for nursing practice. *International Nursing Review, 39,* 109-111, 128-129.

Clear, J.B., Starbecker, M.M., & Kelly, D.W. (1999). Nursing centers and health promotion: A federal vantage point. *Family and Community Health, 21*(4), 1-14.

Coenen, A., Marek, K.D., & Lundeen, S.P. (1996). Using nursing diagnoses to explain utilization in a community nursing center. *Research in Nursing & Health, 19,* 441-445.

Curtin, L. (1998). The ethics of managing lives. Presentation at Quad Council of Public Health Nursing at American Public Health Association. In J. Schulte (Ed.), *Newsletter of the Association of Community Health Nurse Educators, 16,* 4, 3.

Farley, S. (1997). Developing professional-community partnerships. In J. McCloskey & H.K. Grace (Eds.), *Current issues in nursing* (5th ed., pp. 382-387). St. Louis: Mosby.

Gaus, C.R., & Fraser, I. (1996). Commentary: Shifting paradigms and the role of research. *Health Affairs, 15*(2), 235-242.

Glass, L.K. (1989). The historic origins of nursing centers. In National League for Nursing, *Nursing centers: Meeting the demand for quality health care* (pp. 21-31). New York: Author.

Kreuser, N.J. (1998). Access to primary health care: The nature of health problems and utilization for a vulnerable community nursing center population. (Doctoral dissertation, University of Wisconsin–Milwaukee, 1998). *Dissertation Abstracts International.*

Lancaster, J. (1999). "From the Editor." *Family and Community Health, 21*(4), vi.

Lundeen, S.P. (1993). Comprehensive, collaborative, coordinated, community-based care: A community nursing center model. *Family and Community Health, 16*(2), 57-65.

Lundeen, S.P. (1999). An alternative paradigm for promoting health in communities: The Lundeen community nursing center model. *Family and Community Health, 21*(4), 15-28.

Lundeen, S.P., & Friedbacher, B.E. (1996). Academic nursing centers and community-based nursing information systems. In E. Cohen (Ed.), *Nurse case management in the 21st century.* St. Louis: Mosby.

Lundeen, S.P., Friedbacher, B., Thomas, M., & Jackson T. (1997, June). Testing the viability of collaborative interdisciplinary practice in community-focused primary health care: A case study in change. *Wisconsin Medical Journal,* 30-36. Reprinted with permission in *Nursing Matters, 1997, 8*(11), 8-12.

McCormick, K.A., Lang, N., Zielstorff, R., Milholland, K., Saba, V., & Jacox, A. (1994). Toward standard classification schemes for nursing language: Recommendations of the American Nurses Association Steering Committee on Databases to Support Clinical Practice. *Journal of the American Medical Informatics Association, 1,* 421-427.

Rosenkoetter, M.M., Zakutney, M.A., Reynolds, B.J., & Faller, H.S. (1993). *A survey of academic nursing centers.* Wilmington, NC: The University of North Carolina at Wilmington School of Nursing.

Schoneman, D.J. (1999). Surveillance as a nursing intervention: Use in community nursing centers. Unpublished doctoral dissertation, University of Wisconsin–Milwaukee.

U.S. Department of Health and Human Services, Public Health Service, Agency for Health Care Policy Research. (1995). *Using clinical practice guidelines to evaluate quality of care. Volume 2: Methods* (AHCPR Pub. 95-0046). Rockville, MD: Author.

Weddle, C. (1996). A history of community nursing centers' influence on health policy since the 1970s. (Doctoral dissertation, University of Wisconsin–Milwaukee, 1996). *Dissertation Abstracts International, DAI-B, 57/12.*

World Health Organization. (1978). *Primary health care (WHO Alma Ata).* Geneva: Author. (Reaffirmed at Riga Conference, Geneva, 1988.)

Zachariah, R., & Lundeen, S.P. (1997). Research and practice agendas in an academic nursing center. *Image: The Journal of Nursing Scholarship, 29*(3), 255-260.

CHAPTER 43

Better Together

Developing Education-Community Linkages to Enhance Professional Practice for the 21st Century

ANNE S. BELCHER

Energized communities have the capacity to meet the health needs of people well into the 21st century. Nurses have a long history of supporting initiatives that empower individuals and communities aspiring to the goal of "health for all" (World Health Organization, 1978). Health care reforms have not embraced equal access to care for all, yet have provided opportunities for nurses to be proactive in communities and to collaborate with other professionals in addressing the health and social service issues of people living in these communities.

The challenge for faculty in institutions of higher education is to prepare professionals who are comfortable with the changing landscape of practice and equipped to address the challenges of the future. Advanced practice nurses must cooperate with communities and be skilled in collaboration at the community level for planning, implementing, and evaluating programs that make a difference. Partners in cooperative initiatives agree to work together to meet individual goals, but those using collaborative strategies "establish common goals and agree to use their personal and institutional power to achieve them" (Melaville & Blank, 1991, p. 15). Emphasis on the latter builds enduring relationships in communities and sustains programs over time.

Colleges and universities have been encouraged to renew their commitment to service and assume leadership roles in addressing the growing human needs evidenced in communities. Ernest Boyer (1994) urged universities to "respond to the challenges that confront our children, our schools, and our cities, just as the land grant colleges responded to the needs of agriculture and industry a century ago" (p. 48). The new pedagogy that addresses Boyer's challenge has been termed *service learning*.

Service learning has been defined as an instructional methodology built on a foundation of experiential learning and enhanced by critical reflective thinking. The definition of service learning used by the Corporation for National and Community Service (1994) states,

> [Service learning is] a method under which students or participants learn and develop through active participation in thoughtfully organized service that is conducted in and meets the needs of a community and is coordinated with an elementary school, secondary school, institution of higher education, or community service program, and with the community; helps foster civic responsibility; is integrated into and enhances the academic curriculum of the student's program or the educational components of the community service program in which the participants are enrolled; and includes structured time for the students and participants to reflect on the service experience.

Through community service learners have the opportunities to connect theory with application and practice in an environment that enhances civic and social responsibilities while developing critical thinking and group problem-solving competencies (Norbeck & Koerner, 1998). Service learning provides the opportunity to develop education-community linkages by taking curricular content and placing these concepts in the context of real-life situations.

Nurses have embraced a broader definition of health that goes well beyond the narrow framework of disease management. Nursing practice focuses on the enhancement of living systems and facilitates choices in individuals, families, and communities that lead to positive health outcomes. Nurses working in communities have a history of organizing successful programs that improve health and quality of life. Nurses and other professionals working in communities must understand that community empowerment is a process that enables but does not impose. Specific solutions to problems must be decided by citizens (Farley, 1997). Professionals with experiences in service learning have an appreciation of the reciprocity required for success. The exchange of giving and receiving between the participants minimizes the traditionally paternalistic approach to service and community work (Gibboney, 1997). This viewpoint chapter describes the design of an interdisciplinary university program to prepare students to work in urban schools and suggests that future professional nurses prepare themselves to enter into collaborative relationships with professionals and communities in order to evaluate the outcomes of service delivery at the community level.

Elementary, middle, and secondary schools provide a focal point in communities for the collaborative efforts of professionals to make a difference in the lives of its citizens. The roles, responsibilities, and challenges of working in city schools have changed tremendously in the past two decades. Educational health and human service needs of children and their families in urban settings have become more complex, causing many states to pass legislation fostering the coordination of health, social services, and education. In her book *Full Service Schools,* Joy Dryfoos (1994) describes a national movement to create integrated education, health, social service, and mental health programs to meet the needs of children and their families on school grounds or in easily accessible locations. She says, "The school building has emerged as *the place,* the one piece of real estate in declining communities that is publicly owned, centrally located, and consistently used, at least by children" (p. 139).

In response to the growing number of school-based and school-linked integrated service programs, university partnerships between schools of education, health, and social work are forming to prepare professionals with the necessary skills, knowledge, and dispositions to work collaboratively in urban neighborhoods (Knapp et al., 1994).

Indiana University Purdue University Indianapolis (IUPUI) is a doctorate-granting urban university created by a partnership between Indiana and Purdue universities to enhance the access to higher education for the citizens of Indiana's largest community. The university is located at the southern edge of the Indianapolis' United Northwest Area (UNWA), a neighborhood that is impoverished in some areas and more affluent in others. Deteriorating

and abandoned houses are rapidly replaced by new homes. The university student enrollments draws heavily from the broader Indianapolis region (69.3%) and is committed to serving the needs of the community. The university's mission, in part, is to serve as a model for collaboration and interdisciplinary activity in the state's capital city.

Several years ago, IUPUI embarked on a "strategic directions" long-range planning process that challenged faculty, staff, and administrators to envision the future. One of the projects that received funding as a result of the planning process was a collaboration among the schools of nursing, education, and social work and five Indianapolis public schools. The proposal called for development of an interdisciplinary program aimed at meeting the needs of the surrounding community.

During the initial planning of the interdisciplinary program, principals of the schools and community leaders were asked to engage in a series of deliberations to determine the parameters of the partnership. Discussions focused on beliefs, values, and logistical issues. Subsequent meetings were held with school teaching staff members, parents, leaders of community centers and organizations, and other service agencies. What came out of those meetings were plans for an interdisciplinary professional learning community that included nursing, education, and social work students. The learning community would incorporate experienced mentors involved in collaborative work, along with planned practicum experiences that included a reflective component. The structure was developed within the three schools of the university for the offering of an interdisciplinary elective, collaborative practice in the 21st century.

SCHOOL-LINKED SERVICES

Administrators, teachers, and parents requested that efforts be made to broaden the health services offered at the five schools. The larger school system does not provide nurses for these schools, and public health nurses from the local health department spend less than 2 hours per week at each school. The school of nursing developed a service learning experience for community health nursing students based on the Centers for Disease Control and Prevention's Comprehensive School Health Model (CDC, 1995). The student nurses addressed the need for basic health services in the schools, provided blood pressure screenings for the staff, as well as health counseling for students and staff. In addition the students developed, implemented, and evaluated educational programs requested by the schools.

Student nurses were in the schools 6 to 9 hours each week providing basic health services and collaborating with education and social work students to meet the needs of the children. Each week the nurses submitted a reflective journal based on their experiences, and seminar time offered the opportunity for faculty to facilitate students' thinking in new ways about the community, health, education, delivery of care, the root causes of complex health problems, and their roles as professional students in the settings.

Student nurses at the five schools completed 594 health service visits during the academic year. Health problems managed by the students included elevated temperature, ice application to injury, wound care, evaluation of sore throat, stomachache, headache, and exclusion for communicable diseases. In addition the students were case finders by completing lice, scoliosis, and vision screenings in their settings. Creative teaching strategies were used to promote positive health behaviors in children. Education offerings developed in collaboration with teachers were the Five-A-Day nutrition program, Bug Busters program for personal hygiene, and Growing Up, a primer on the expected changes during puberty. Students provided individual counseling to students, worked with teachers and social workers to identify behavioral problems, observed disruptive children in the classroom, and helped with anger control management. Community partnerships were developed with the university's school of optometry and the local health department's dental section to provide vision and dental screenings to children in the schools.

Outcomes reported by teachers and staff at the five schools included the following: "the students were so helpful and caring to everyone in the building"; "staff were more comfortable when the health professionals deal with health problems"; "student nurses have the expertise to treat the injuries and accidents"; "attendance improved and students remained in school"; and "our students see positive role models in the student nurses and believe that a college education might be possible to attain." Students in turn reported a high degree of autonomy, a greater understanding of community work, and satisfaction with their experiences in the urban schools.

Once each month students from the three disciplines met to discuss the on-site experiences and to share the professional perspectives of nursing, education, and social work students providing services in the schools. Prin-

ciples of interprofessional practice were developed in these sessions, including a focus on preventing problems; cultural competence; supportive development of youth, families and communities; and provision of high-quality services that met professional standards and addressed the needs expressed by the community. To enhance interprofessional practice, the expectation was that the future professionals would work in what is now popularly called an ecological, holistic way (i.e., viewing the K-12 student in the context of the family and larger community) (Melaville & Blank, 1991).

INTERDISCIPLINARY COURSE

The interdisciplinary elective meets weekly at the middle school in the UNWA area. University faculty, along with the "community faculty" (teachers, administrators, or individuals who have a long history of working the UNWA area) represent a multidisciplinary team of instructors who facilitate the learning, working together to deconstruct individualistic, autonomous ideas of practice and to construct a model of interprofessional collaborative practice. When students have completed the course, they have examined key themes and objectives that include

Communication and Collaboration
- Demonstrating effective communication at two levels: the interprofessional practice level and the student-family level. The students help each other to understand the language or professional jargon of each profession.

Cultural Competency
- Recognizing, analyzing, and critiquing his or her own personal and professional beliefs, cultural beliefs and biases, and evaluating the impact of these beliefs on interprofessional practice. The increasing diversity within schools is not limited to race and ethnicity. Students in urban schools come from different socioeconomic backgrounds and have differing abilities and disabilities; therefore, interprofessional practitioners must understand the meaning of culture and the effects it has on how people and groups live.

Public Policy and Policy Awareness
- Recognizing and evaluating the values, interests and concerns operating within schools and communities as important components for developing advocacy strategies and public policies.
- Analyzing the impact of policy on access, costs, quality of life concerns, and decision making in the respective practice settings.

Development and Coordination of Family, School, and Community Resources
- Identifying and assessing the range of resources available and needed within communities and collaborating to develop school and family partnerships to access resources and services.

Reflective Practice
- Developing critical thinking and inquiry skills to refine interprofessional practice by engaging in solo reflection, group deliberations, and cooperative inquiry.
- Locating and reviewing relevant literature and research findings for incorporation into one's own practice.

Leadership
- Envisioning, valuing, and influencing; calling colleagues' attention to the basic purpose of their work while thinking longer term; helping the site cope with conflicting requirements of multiple constituencies; negotiating power relationships with the community for the good of all parties.
- Leaders involved in university or school interdisciplinary professional preparation are crucial for organizational innovation and change because they act as compelling agents and sources of encouragement to think and act in different ways from the existing cultures of the individual professions.

SUMMARY

Developing education-community linkages provides a win-win situation for the professionals and communities involved. Nurses working in the communities of the 21st century must be equipped to respond to the fundamental root causes of complex health issues and social concerns facing individuals and families living in communities. Partnerships with urban schools have provided the landscape for addressing some of these social problems. These include:

- Perceived inadequacies in American education, not only in K-12th grade but also in higher education
- Increasing concern about youth's preparation to meet the responsibility of living in a democratic society and providing service to communities
- Addressing the lack of public funding for needed social and environmental services to enhance the health of the public (Gray et al., 1999)

In urban communities where professionals approach their work as nurses, teachers, social workers, therapists, or administrators, they are confronted by complex challenges related to providing appropriate services to indi-

viduals, families, and communities. These challenges include but are not limited to education, nutrition, health care, shelter, economic security, and child care. Increasingly, universities located in urban areas are working collaboratively with a number of agencies and especially schools and school-linked services to have a more powerful impact on urban communities, supporting family integrity and community cohesion. A commitment to ongoing research in the form of careful descriptions of organizational arrangements; the interface between the university teaching faculty, community faculty, school principals, experienced nurses and social workers and the coordination of their efforts; and the sharing of professional work, resources, and ideas is emerging (Murtadha-Watts, Belcher, Iverson, & Medina, 1999).

Questions to ponder include: How do we help people to work well together? How can we be sure to honor and benefit from the diversity of ideas and perspectives of others in the schools and larger communities? What processes will we use to resolve conflict and maintain trust? These questions begin to frame the assessment of a school's culture and the readiness for school and university collaboration.

Thus far students have evaluated the classes and service learning experiences in the schools as highly successful. One middle school principal pointed out that "Future professionals planning to work in urban settings must be committed to working with inner city populations. The mere fact that they are in the school building getting the direct experience helps. Too often they don't realize what really goes on in a family, a school building, or a community. The sooner they get to know this the better they will be for future job placements anywhere."

Educators who participate in the service learning pedagogical approach are providing service for the public good. Within nursing and the health professions this good is "public rather than simply for the learners themselves to the extent that the service is meeting real needs identified by the community and not just providing opportunities in a community based setting for students to practice clinical skills" (Gibboney, 1997, p. 23). As professionals in any discipline, we must encourage colleagues and students to serve in such a way that they are aware of the reciprocity of the relationship. Service recipients are also service providers. Gibboney (1997) writes, "The more we, as a society, are committed to serving each other, the less we will need to worry about broader issues of social justice, for a society that models true charity—not in the sense of giving hand outs but in the sense of voluntary action for the public good will be a just society."

REFERENCES

Boyer, E.L. (1994). Creating the new American college. *Chronicle of Higher Education, 41,* 48.

Centers for Disease Control and Prevention. (1995). *School health programs: An investment in our future: At a glance.* Atlanta: Author.

Corporation for National and Community Service. (1994). *Grant application guidelines for Learn and Serve America: Higher education.* Washington, DC: Author.

Dryfoos, J. (1994). *Full service schools: A revolution in health and social services for children, youth and families.* San Francisco: Jossey-Bass.

Farley, S. (1997). Developing professional-community partnerships. In J. McCloskey & H. Grace (Eds.), *Current issues in nursing* (5th ed., pp. 382-387). St. Louis: Mosby.

Gibboney, R. (1997). *Service learning: Lessons for and from nursing.* Paper presented at the Indiana University Conference on Nursing and Philanthropy. Indianapolis, IN.

Gray, M.J., Ondaatje, E.H., Fricker, R., Geschwind, S., Goldman, C.A., Kaganoff, T., Robyn, A., Sundt, M., Vogelgesang, L., & Klein, S.P. (1999). *Combining service and learning in higher education: Evaluation of the Learn and Serve America, higher education program.* Santa Monica, CA: Rand Education.

Knapp, M.S., Barnard, K., Brandon, R.N., Gehrke, N.J., Smith, A.J., & Teather, E.C. (1994). University-based preparation for collaborative interprofessional practice. In L. Adler & S. Gardern, *The politics of linking schools and social services* (pp. 137-151). Washington, DC: Falmer Press.

Melaville, A.I., & Blank, M.J. (1991). *What it takes: Structuring interagency partnerships to connect children and families with comprehensive service.* Washington, DC: Education and Human Services Consortium.

Murtadha-Watts, K., Belcher, A.E., Iverson, E., & Medina, M. (1999). City schools/city university: A partnership to enhance professional preparation. *National Association of Secondary School Principals Bulletin, 83*(611), 64-70.

Norbeck, J.S., & Koerner, J. (1998). *Caring and community: Concepts and models for service-learning in nursing.* Washington, DC: American Association for Higher Education.

World Health Organization. (1978). Declaration of Alma Ata. Report of the International Conference on Primary Health Care. Geneva: The World Health Organization and the United Nations Children's Fund.

Shared Governance Models in Nursing

What Is Shared, Who Governs, and Who Benefits?

MERIDEAN L. MAAS, JANET K. PRINGLE SPECHT

Governance, or self-regulation, has long been recognized as a privilege given to professions that earn the public trust by demonstrating accountability for their specialized practices (Crocker, Kirkpatrick, & Lentenbrink, 1992). To ensure that professionals do not misuse autonomy for their own interests, rather than those of their clients, society requires professionals to demonstrate accountability for their actions (Maas & Jacox, 1977). Nursing has developed many self-regulating mechanisms (e.g., codes of ethics, standards, credentialing and accreditation criteria, and guidelines for peer review) that demonstrate the ability to govern its members in the public interest (McCloskey et al., 1994); however, the privilege of governance has been slow in coming. Professional nursing governance in practice settings, where physicians and administrators who benefit from the subordinate employee status of nurses have dominated, has been especially constrained.

Although there are examples of the implementation of professional nurse practice models over several decades and there are current international examples (Horvath, 1990; Jacoby & Terpste, 1990; Johnson, 1987; Maas & Jacox, 1977; McDonagh, Rhodes, Sharkey, & Goodroe, 1989; O'May & Buchan, 1999; Rose & DiPasquale, 1990), recognition of the need for nurse governance became most focused in hospitals in the United States during the nursing shortage of the 1980s. The value of nursing to the delivery of health care in hospitals also became more visible as a result of relentless technological and medical advances and their associated costs. After a period of widespread use of registered nurses (RNs) to provide a variety of services to downsize other departments and workers, hospitals began to reconsider the best use of nursing knowledge and skills. The folly of using nurses to perform functions for which they are highly overqualified became clearer as the undersupply of nurses compared with de-

mand reached critical proportions. While the demand for nurses grew, increasing numbers of nurses demonstrated dissatisfaction with their jobs and careers by moving to part-time work, leaving nursing for other careers, or moving to other practice settings after a brief period of employment in one hospital (Prescott, 1987). A decreasing number of persons entered the nursing field owing to low pay, limited career advancement opportunities, and a greater number of other career options for women (American Nurses' Association [ANA], 1992). Finally, demands for more accountability for the outcomes of care accompanied the pressures to control costs. The result was an increasing number of nurse and hospital administrators who recognized that the staff nurse, at the point of contact with the patient, is in the critical position to ensure the delivery of quality care (Spitzer-Lehmann, 1989).

These and other factors encouraged nurse executives in hospitals to move to models of nursing practice that increased nurse autonomy for clinical decision making and participation in decision making throughout the organization. Shared governance models were a popular strategy in the 1980s and early 1990s to increase nurse job satisfaction and retention and to achieve cost-effective quality outcomes (Stichler, 1992).

Predictably, however, due to the efforts of nurse educators, the nursing profession, and health care and public policy makers, the supply of nurses increased in the mid-1990s. As concerns about nurse job satisfaction and retention waned with an oversupply of nurses, so did efforts to implement nurse shared governance in practice settings. Further, attention in hospitals shifted to cost reductions to maintain a competitive edge in managed care environments, resulting in downsizing of programs and staff. Shortened hospital stays, increased ambulatory care, and same-day surgeries reallocated health care that was previously provided in hospitals to community settings and families. Downsizing in hospitals was especially brutal in nursing departments. The consequences were another ebb in the number of admissions to nursing programs and many nurses who were laid off finding other employment, some in new community nursing opportunities and some in other fields. Again, as predicted, the new millennium dawned with another nurse shortage on the horizon. It is yet to be observed whether or not this shortage will result in another surge of interest in the implementation of nurse shared governance in hospitals.

Many nurse executives and nurses in hospitals have worked to maintain or continue to implement nurse shared governance. Nurse shared governance models also are beginning to appear in community-based settings, such as nursing homes and home health care (Ferguson-Paré, 1996; Melchior et al., 1997; Morrall, 1997). Nurses in these settings recognize that the aim of nurse shared governance models to empower nurses within the organization's decision-making system, particularly with regard to increasing nurses' authority and control over nursing practice, not only is important for nurses' job satisfaction but also for outcomes effectiveness. There are a number of issues, however, that need to be addressed as changes are made in organizations to implement shared governance. These issues include the lack of clearly defined criteria for shared governance, mixed motives for the implementation of shared governance, disagreement about how shared governance can and should be implemented, and concerns about the effects of shared governance on different roles within nursing and organization systems. The time is opportune to consider and resolve these issues in advance of increased interest in shared governance models that may accompany the current nursing shortage.

WHAT IS SHARED GOVERNANCE?

Clarification of the concept of shared governance and the structures and processes that must be in place for implementation in employing organizations is needed if the nursing profession is to honor its contract with society as described in the ANA's *Social Policy Statement* (ANA, 1980). The concept of shared governance comes from the recognition of the need to accommodate two systems of authority when professionals are employed in organizations. In organization, authority is ordinarily vested in positions arranged in a hierarchy, with positions higher in the hierarchy assigned a greater scope of authority than lower positions. Although professionals employed by organizations occupy positions with corresponding organizational authority, they also have au-

thority as a function of membership in their profession (Minzberg, 1979). For a profession, this authority is based on specialized knowledge. Society gives professionals autonomy to get important work done effectively by experts who also are competent judges of the needed expertise. When professionals are employed by organizations, there is always the danger that the societal needs that are entrusted to the profession will become subordinated to the organization's needs. This is the critical reason why governance shared by the organization and its employed professionals has evolved. Nurse shared governance is synonymous with professional nursing practice in organizations that employ nurses (Maas & Specht, 1990). In nursing, shared governance means that nurse employees and the organization are partners in meeting the goals of the organization and the mandates of the nursing profession (Porter-O'Grady, 1991a, 1991b). However, descriptions of the requisite structures and processes for claimed shared governance models are often incomplete or unclear. Professional nurse shared governance does not exist unless the authority and accountability of professional nurses is codified in the organization and decision-making structures and processes are in place that enable nurses to define and regulate nursing practice and share decisions with administrators regarding the management of resources.

As illustrated in Figure 44-1, specialized knowledge and commitment to a service ideal are the foundation for professional nurse autonomy and accountability (Maas & Specht, 1990). *Professional nurse autonomy* means that professional nurses have the authority to define and decide what services they will provide and what constitutes safe and effective practice. *Professional nurse accountability* means responsibility and answerability to authority for the services rendered. The profession must take action to ensure that the practice of its members is safe and effective. Thus, organizational structures of decision making, coordination, and control set forth in a constitution and bylaws, are needed (1) to enable nurse peer definition of the scope of nursing practice, standards of practice, nursing delivery systems, qualifications for the selection of staff, and knowledge and resources required and (2) to enable peer evaluation of the practice, promotion, and retention of individual nurses, evaluation of the department (collective) practice, peer consultation, dissemination of knowledge, and development of knowledge through research. Contrary to some definitions that describe shared governance as a structure for staff nurse autonomy (Pinkerton, 1988), the structure must enable professional autonomy and accountability of all profes-

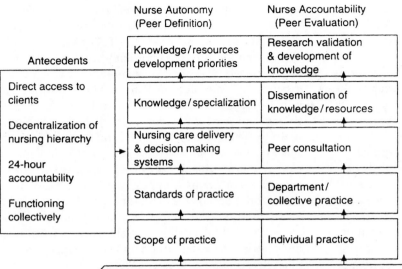

Antecedents

Nurse Autonomy (Peer Definition)

Nurse Accountability (Peer Evaluation)

Direct access to clients

Decentralization of nursing hierarchy

24-hour accountability

Functioning collectively

Knowledge/resources development priorities

Research validation & development of knowledge

Knowledge/specialization

Dissemination of knowledge/resources

Nursing care delivery & decision making systems

Peer consultation

Standards of practice

Department/collective practice

Scope of practice

Individual practice

Specialized Body of Knowledge & Commitment to Service Ideal

FIGURE 44-1 Iowa Veterans Home model of professional nursing practice. (From Maas, M.L. [1989]. Professional practice for the extended care environment: Learning from one model and its implication. *Journal of Professional Nursing, 5*[22], 66-76. © W.B. Saunders Company.)

sional nurses, as individuals and as a collective, if governance is to be shared by the organization and employed professional nurses (Maas, Jacox, & Specht, 1975). All RNs, regardless of their position in the organization (e.g., staff nurse, clinical specialist, nurse researcher, nurse educator, nurse manager, nurse administrator) must have professional autonomy and accountability as individuals and as a collective of peers (Maas & Jacox, 1977).

More than 1,000 hospitals in the United States implemented shared governance in the 1980s and early 1990s (Porter-O'Grady, 1994). As shared governance models continue to be applied in settings, it is important to note that there is much variation in the models implemented under this label. A number of different terms, such as participation in decision making, participative management, self-governance, empowerment, and professional practice are used at times to be synonymous with shared governance and at other times to indicate different organizational models with varying degrees of nurse participation in decision making. There appears to be consensus that shared governance means some amount or type of shared decision making by staff and nursing management. There is less clarity and agreement regarding what specific decisions are made or shared by nurses and managers, what staff are included in the shared governance, and whether nurses as individuals or as a collective have authority and accountability for certain decisions. Thus, models of practice implemented under the label of shared governance range from those with minimal, ad hoc, or informal participation by some or all nursing staff in a limited

number of decisions with little or no expectation for nursing staff accountability to models in which the profession and the organization truly share authority and accountability for the profession's mandates and the organization's mission.

Because all nursing staff do not have the specialized knowledge and socialization to the service ideal that professional nurses do, it should be obvious that democracy in the workplace is not nurse shared governance and vice versa. Nursing staff who assist RNs in the delivery of care are clearly not qualified to govern the profession, although they can and should participate in decision making in the organization.

There is increasing discussion of whole-systems shared governance (Evan, Aubry, Hawkins, Curley, & Porter-O'Grady, 1995; Porter-O'Grady, 1994; Wilson & Porter-O'Grady, 1999). Whole-systems governance are more similar to democracy in the workplace than to professional nurse governance. The basis for sharing in these models is doing the work rather than being a member of the profession. While whole-systems governance schemes increase participation in decision making for all workers, they do not address control of professional practice by the profession. Whole-systems shared governance reinforces the need for professional nurse shared governance, albeit complements governance by the profession, but does not supplant it. Both are important for the effectiveness of the organization; however, it is professional governance that enables the application of expert knowledge to best achieve quality outcomes.

The confusion between the concept of participation in decision making and professional governance has contributed to the view advanced by Porter-O'Grady (1994) and Wilson and Porter-O'Grady (1999) that whole-systems governance is a progression beyond nurse shared governance. This, however, is not the case. The goals of whole-systems shared governance and professional nurse shared governance are distinctly different. Integration, equity, and communication among disciplines within the organization are fundamental objectives of whole-systems governance, while nurse shared governance is a partnership between professional nurses and the organization to meet the mandates of the profession for autonomy and accountability of nurses for client welfare and the goals of the organization. These two approaches to governance come from different theoretical bases. From an organizational behavior perspective, whole-systems shared governance does not address the societal aegis and function of a profession as does nurse shared governance, which is derived from the sociology of professions literature. The two systems are not mutually exclusive and both can contribute positively to client outcomes and to effective organizations.

It is less obvious and quite controversial to assert that not all RNs are qualified to assume autonomy and accountability. All RNs share the profession's mandates; however, there is great variation in their knowledge, education, and experience. Implementation of shared governance requires that RNs who are expected to assume professional autonomy and accountability are prepared to do so. This means that the first shared decisions of the organization and nursing leadership must be the definition of criteria for admitting RNs to professional decision-making privileges and agreement on the programming and resources needed to assist RNs who desire to meet the criteria.

The controversy over what decisions professional nurses and organization management would make mostly focuses on a debate about whether nurses who are not managers can decide matters of resource distribution. This is simply a concern about loss of control on the part of managers and reflects a lack of commitment to professional nurse governance. The importance of this issue is underscored by the results of a survey of 1,100 RNs from 10 hospitals that was conducted from June 1993 to April 1994 (Hess, 1995). The study revealed that out of six aspects of governance, including control over professional practice, the nurses rated as most important the influence over organization resources that support practice. Another illustration of the importance of the issue is the recent downsizing of hospitals and elimination of nurse positions with limited participation and essentially no control over the decisions by nurses. In many instances nurses knew that the cuts were placing patients and nurses in jeopardy. It is only after serious effects occurred for some patients and collective action by some nurses that the recklessness of these decisions are now recognized and beginning to be reversed (ANA, 1999; California law requires staffing ratios, 1999; Minnesota nurses talk staffing, 1999).

Professional shared governance requires that all nurses in the organization develop a consensus about goals and priorities and the expectations that available resources will be allocated accordingly. All nurses are kept aware of the available resources, share the planning of their allocation, and share the responsibility to develop alternatives where there is shortfall. Specific areas of authority and accountability for difference roles (e.g., managers, educators, and clinicians) are defined, and control of decisions is placed with those who carry them out (Jenkins, 1991). Disagreements about decisions are resolved through negotiation. Although the development of the consensus, structures, and expectations for shared governance is not easy, resistance to doing it because of concern about who will make the decisions is most often a lack of commitment to professional nursing practice and an unwillingness to relinquish control.

Professional nurses participation in decision making, empowerment of nurse professionals, participative management, and work redesign each are coincident and necessary for professional nurse shared governance, but none is synonymous with it. The goals of work redesign are often to enhance the authority of nurses and rectify organizational problems that contribute to suboptimal use and turnover of professional nurses (Strasen, 1989). Thus, the goal of work redesign efforts may be directed toward implementation of shared governance models. The goals of many work redesign efforts, however, also are to increase the participation of nurses in decision making without providing the structures whereby they have professional authority and accountability for all decisions affecting nursing practice. Some work redesign efforts actually obscure nursing's identity as a professional discipline with obligations of accountability to clients for services rendered. The current emphasis on interdisciplinary efforts and team building, while laudable, often is interpreted as shared authority and accountability without recognizing the necessity of retaining mechanisms for demonstrating the accountability of disciplines other than medicine. A study of the implementation of nurse shared governance in one hospital described the concurrent implementation of patient-focused care, which resulted in the removal of the term "nursing" from all nurse shared governance documents (Ramler, 1995). Although patient-focused care is approaching the graveyard of other previously ill conceived models marketed by consultants who play to the desperations and priorities of administrators, it illustrates the lack of clear understanding of professional shared governance and its importance for quality outcomes that tends to prevail.

Many nurse executives have become vice presidents for patient care services (or some similar title), promoting the change in language from "nursing" to "patient care services" and in many instances eliminating departments of nursing (Specht, 1995). While most nurses applaud the need for a nurse executive to administer all patient services, few seem to analyze the implications critically. They do not appear to note the implications if the nursing department is not a visible and accountable entity. Nor do many appear to discern the need for nursing and each discipline to be autonomous and accountable for the practice of the discipline for interdisciplinary care to be a reality (McCloskey & Maas, 1998). It is in the circumstances of interpretation of interdisciplinary as negating the identities, unique perspectives, and obligations of individual disciplines that it is most critical to have professional nurse shared governance operational, but it is also when it is least likely to be implemented.

It is nurses who must be astute about the distinction among these concepts, so that they are not misled into believing that they are sharing governance with management as professionals, when in fact they are not equal partners in meeting the mandates of the profession or the goals of the organization. If the structures enabling professional autonomy and accountability outlined in Figure 44-1 are not implemented, nurse shared governance is not operational. Figure 44-2 provides one example of decision-making, coordination, and control structures defined in a constitution and bylaws that enable nurse shared governance in an organization (Maas & Specht, 1990).

We wondered earlier whether there will be a resurgence of interest in nurse shared governance as the current nursing shortage continues. Previously we noted that clarity about shared governance for nurses is essential if it is to be more than one more bandwagon jumped on without being anchored to a clear theoretical base and commitment to enabling professional nursing practice (Maas, Specht, & Ramler, 1997). Some continue to argue that nursing's knowledge base is insufficient to support control of practice as professionals and that the majority of nurses do not want professional authority and accountability. Others still complain that shared governance is little more than a philosophy, fad, or nursing self-aggrandizement and that there is no evidence that benefits accrue when nurses have

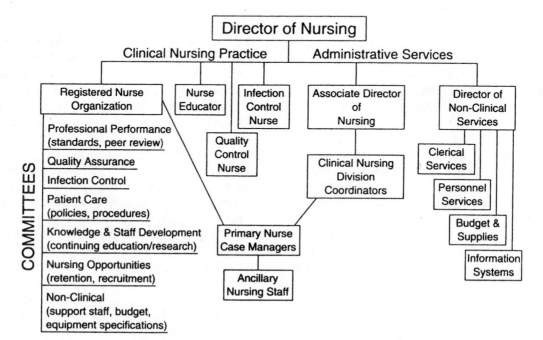

FIGURE 44-2 Iowa Veterans Home department of nursing. (From Maas, M.L. [1989]. Professional practice for the extended care environment: Learning from one model and its implication. *Journal of Professional Nursing, 5*[22], 66-76. © W.B. Saunders Company.)

more professional autonomy. A few assert that shared governance sounds like a religion when the converted argue its merits. Admittedly, the description of change to shared governance as "transformation" may sound a bit like "being born again," connoting a spiritual experience rather than a functional model of social organization derived from sound theory and validated empirically (Porter-O'Grady, 1992; Wilson & Porter-O'Grady, 1999). It is opportune that literature reporting the effects of nurse shared governance is mounting, which we review in a later section of this chapter.

The claim by some (Schwartz, 1990) that nurses are unwilling to exercise self-discipline and act in the public's behalf is unfounded. As a profession, nursing had demonstrated over and over that it is worthy of the public's trust and that it is able to govern its members in accord with that trust (Peplau, 1985). Nurse administrators who observe that staff nurses appear to be unwilling to assume professional authority and accountability are too often noting the behaviors of nurses who have been used and abused to benefit others. These nurses typically have experienced capricious changes, a lack of power and control over a heavy and often dangerously overwhelming workload, and a lack of socialization in the knowledge and skills needed for organizational and interdisciplinary politics. There is evidence that professional nurses welcome shared governance if it is implemented with their participation, with ample opportunity to gain the needed knowledge and skills for consensus decision making, and with the appropriate organizational structures for professional authority and control of practice in place (Maas, 1989). Further, there is evidence that nursing's knowledge base is sufficient to support control of practice and that nurses participate more actively in the development and dissemination of knowledge in a professional model of practice (Brooks, Olsen, Rieger-Kligy, & Mooney, 1995; Gulland & Payne, 1997; Maas, 1989; McDonagh et al., 1989; Skuback, Earls, & Botos, 1994; Wilson & Porter-O'Grady, 1999). The increased focus on outcomes effectiveness is an opportunity for nursing to demonstrate its accountability for client outcomes. It is regrettable that the structures and processes for the assessment of outcomes effectiveness are often not linked to the structures and processes for professional nurse shared governance.

MOTIVES FOR SHARED GOVERNANCE: IS IT AN OPIATE?

While it is assumed that the motives for implementing all shared governance models are to enhance the delivery of quality care, these motives are mixed in regard to the commitment to enabling the work of the professional nurse. Because shared governance remains an attractive aspect of the work environment for nurses, many hospitals boast shared governance as a desirable feature of their organizations. Yet there are often minimal structures of shared governance actually in place (Specht, 1995). In some cases, the motive seems to be to increase nurses' perceptions of empowerment for practice without actually divesting power from the organization hierarchy to nurses as professionals (Hess, 1995; Porter-O'Grady, 1991a, 1991b). Clearly, organization and nurse managers have been reluctant to relinquish power and control over decisions that influence nursing and the organization. Because of nurse dissatisfaction with the practice environment, collective bargaining and collective action have become more of a threat to nurse and hospital administrators (Kerfoot, 1992). The recent success of California nurses in obtaining legislation to specify minimum safe RN staff to patient ratios in hospitals is an example (California law requires staffing ratios, 1999). Administrators' decisions to implement shared governance may be based on a selection of the better of two less than desirable choices; shared governance or a less desirable form of collective nurse influence. When collective bargaining or some other collective threat is perceived, wise nurse administrators seek models that integrate the "threat" with structures of shared governance (Crocker et al., 1992).

Too often, nurses have had their hopes raised that they are gaining authority and control over the circumstances of their work and their ability to effect patient care priorities, only to have those hopes dashed by the whims of those who hold the real power in the organization. Implementation of shared governance may simply be a strategy to gain what management wants without actual gains in decision-making authority for nurses. Nurses may not initially recognize that what is portrayed as shared governance does not provide them with authority to control their practice or to enable nursing and the organization to meet the professional mandate and the organization's goals as partners with management. They soon recognize the lack of power and become frustrated and disillusioned. This is when nurses are apt to leave employment or withdraw to the safety of the traditional hierarchy, where they seek minimal accountability and investment of time, energy, and risk in their jobs. These circumstances underscore the importance of what shared governance entails in terms of nurses' authority and accountability for decision making as well as how shared governance is best implemented in organizations. Wilson and Porter-O'Grady (1999) write eloquently about the enlightened leadership that is needed to transform an organization for shared governance.

IMPLEMENTATION OF SHARED GOVERNANCE: IS THERE A BEST WAY?

It has been noted that shared governance models are not the same in all settings and that this variation is appropriate because of cultural and system operational differences (Porter-O'Grady, 1987; Wilson, 1989). There is debate, however, about whether implementation is best orchestrated from the top down or from the bottom up and whether shared governance can be operationalized as separate unit-based as opposed to organization-wide models. Certainly, there is agreement that the nursing and hospital administrations must be supportive of the changes in any case (Jenkins, 1988; Maas, 1989; Porter-O'Grady, 1991a, 1991b; Wilson & Porter-O'Grady, 1999). There is less agreement about how to involve the whole staff in the change process and about which is better: unit-by-unit implementation or simultaneous, phased-in implementation of shared governance throughout an entire nursing department (Carmanica & Rosenbecker, 1991; Fagan, 1991; Porter-O'Grady, 1991a, 1991b). Although unique issues must be addressed with each approach, either is appropriate, depending on the situation and assuming that principles of participative change and socialization are not violated.

Leadership from nursing administration and from clinical nurses who have a vision regarding nurse shared governance is essential. These persons must begin to define the objectives and expectations of nurses and create the organizational circumstances whereby all nurses participate to conceptualize and implement shared governance. Planned change, rather than directed change, is necessary (Hersey & Blanchard, 1986). Paradoxically, bureaucratic methods are used at the outset to reinforce expectations about professional practice, participation, and change. Participation, however, of all nurses to gain an understanding of shared governance and new organizational goals, develop new meanings about the nurse's role and work, and acquire new skills and behaviors needed to enact shared governance soon shifts the predominant decision-making methods to collaboration, negotiation, and consensus. Whether implementation of shared governance is top down throughout the whole organization or bottom up, unit by unit, nursing administrators and managers become consultants, teachers, coaches, and facilitators.

In either approach, nurses must learn the skills of confrontation, negotiation, collaboration, and consensus decision making (Maas, 1989). They also must understand the requirements of professional practice and what it means to be accountable as professionals (Wilson, 1989). Through consensus decision making combined with the expectation of accountability, nurses must develop shared beliefs and values about standards of practice and the structures and processes that will best ensure their enactment (Maas, 1989). Consensus decision making promotes collegiality and the responsible use of collective action by all nurses, regardless of position.

If the unit-based approach to the implementation of shared governance is chosen, one advantage is that more nurses involved in the change will likely be committed to it from the outset. Implementation is more focused and involves fewer nurses. Following success on one or more units, other units are apt to become interested, choose to implement shared governance, and profit from the experience of the pioneering units. Nursing administration and the nurses on the pioneering units will need to be cognizant of the effects of shared governance in one or a few units on the rest of the department and organization. Different patterns and models of communication and decision making will necessarily exist between the nurses on the units with shared governance and nurses on other units, nurse administrators and managers, persons in other departments, and members of other disciplines. Finally, the scope of shared governance implemented on single units will be constrained at the outset because collective authority and accountability cannot include all nurses in the organization. With unit-based shared governance, the collective, central power and influence of nursing is diluted. Nursing administration will need to retain the prerogative for any decisions that affect the nursing department or organization as a whole until all units implement shared governance and the partnership for decision between all nursing professionals and the organization is defined. For this reason, unit-based implementation may be more appealing to some nurse administrators who wish to dilute the collective power of nurses. Because of the limited scope of unit-based shared governance, progress to a full partnership of nurses and the organization may be slow and may never evolve. Shared governance is not fully implemented until there are structures for all professional nurses to make collective, department-wide decisions and negotiate these decisions with administration (Foster, 1992).

With the organization-wide approach, the issues focus on how to involve large numbers of nurses in the change process so that they learn the skills of consensus decision making, participate in decision making, developed shared meanings, and actualize the behaviors of professional autonomy and accountability. If shared governance is implemented throughout an entire system, individual nurses should be deprived of the choice not to participate and not to be accountable professionals. This can present difficult problems because nurses will have different amounts of understanding and commitment to professional practice. Further, the change process will necessarily occur within an environment that is usually not friendly to the investment of nurses' time in pursuits other than the patient care demands of the day. Nurse staffing is most often not planned to allow nurses much time to think and plan as a group. Nurse administrators therefore must expect all nurses, regardless of position, to plan and implement the changes needed for nurses to share governance with the organization and provide the circumstances whereby nurses are able to meet these expectations. In this regard, nurse administrators must depend on middle- and first-line managers to support the change to shared governance and to alter their roles to become facilitators, teachers, and consultants for staff nurses and each other. If middle managers are not committed to shared governance and resist the needed changes, many problems will ensue. The effects of shared governance on middle- and first-line managers, as well as on nursing and organization line and staff roles, staff nurse roles, and the roles of members of other disciplines, must be anticipated with plans carefully made to prepare position occupants for the needed changes and skills (Wilson, 1989).

ROLE AND SYSTEM EFFECTS OF SHARED GOVERNANCE

There are increasing reports of data about the effects of nurse shared governance models on the attitudes and roles of staff nurses, managers, and administrators, and on the structures and processes or organizational systems (Wilson, 1989). Discussions focus on the effects of shared governance on the attitudes and roles of the nurse manager and staff nurses with a consistent finding that nurse job satisfaction improves as nurse authority and control over practice is realized (Brodbeck, 1992; Brooks et al., 1995; DeBaca, Jones, & Tornabeni, 1993; Edwards et al., 1994; George, Burke, & Rogers, 1997; Hastings & Waltz, 1995; Kovner, Hendrickson, Knickman, & Finkler, 1993; Laschinger & Havens, 1996; Ludemann & Brown, 1989; Maas & Jacox, 1977; Porter-O'Grady, 1991a, 1991b; Relf, 1995; Song, Daly, Rudy, Douglas, & Dyer, 1997; Thrasher

et al., 1992; Westrope, Vaughn, Bott, & Taunton, 1995). An exception is a finding by Prince (1997) that job satisfaction of staff nurses decreased following implementation of unit-based nurse shared governance. Prince notes that the decrease in job satisfaction was likely due to increased time and workload commitments, increased stress, decreased budget, and reorganization and leadership transition. This finding is consistent with the emphasis on the importance of strong, committed, and skilled leadership to shepherd the change to shared governance and to create the organizational circumstances within which the change can best occur (Hastings & Walz, 1995; Havens, 1994; Maas & Jacox, 1977; Wilson & Porter-O'Grady, 1999).

A recent review of literature located 48 studies that either described or evaluated implementation of shared governance (O'May & Buchan, 1999). The studies reviewed confirm Haven's finding (1994) that confusion that exists regarding definition of nurse shared governance, makes it difficult to know for certain what is being evaluated. O'May and Buchan (1999) selected and reviewed the studies from organization management and business perspectives, including those that described or evaluated participative management, professional practice, and self-managed work team models. Shared governance models also included whole-system governance models that involved all staff in shared governance. Thus, the failure to delineate clearly models of nurse professional shared governance using criteria based on the sociology of professions and organizations leaves little remaining research that has evaluated the effects on staff, patient, and organization outcomes. What appears to be most consistently evaluated is the effects of participation in decisions on nurse and other staff attitudes.

There is agreement that management styles must change along with organizational structures to enable professional nurse shared governance (Maas & Jacox, 1977; Wilson & Porter-O'Grady, 1999). As stated earlier, the role of management becomes one of consulting, teaching, collaborating, and creating an environment with the structures and resources needed for the practice of nursing and shared decision making between nurses and the organization (Stichler, 1992). This new role is foreign to many managers. Nurse managers must become leaders who change who they are, what they do, and how they do it. To achieve nurse shared governance that is responsive to clients and organizations that are increasingly complex and fluid, nurse leaders must be an advocate of staff and model learning and changing (Wilson & Porter-O'Grady, 1999).

Although nurse managers will retain responsibility for specified functions, in a professional model they share accountability with all nurses and should act in accord with the consensus among nurse professionals about goals and priorities. Because rules about sharing decisions between management and professional nurses are ambiguous, managers experience stress and anxiety, especially in the early stages of implementing shared governance (Wilson, 1989). Managers also experience role stress because of the added time and costs required to enable consensus decision making among nurses. If not supported by organization and nursing administration, middle- and first-line managers—even though they are committed to shared governance—may not choose to expend the effort or take the risks needed to enable nurses to develop the needed consensus. Nurses need to be able to meet together for consensus decision making, and it is the manager/leader who must lead to facilitate their doing so. Administrators who understand the important gains from unleashing the expertise of professional nurses must lead to prepare managers for the new role and support them throughout the lengthy change process of relinquishing control of the decisions for which all professional nurses are accountable. In other words, nurse leaders must redesign their roles to serve the collective of nurse professionals, enabling professional autonomy and accountability for quality outcomes.

For staff nurses, the critical role changes with shared governance are increased accountability and risk. Problems are no longer blamed on others because all nurses share decisions and are accountable for the outcomes. As noted, new understandings and skills are needed. Perhaps most stressful to nurses is the accountability for knowledge to support the decision-making authority of professionals. Role conflict and ambiguity, however, also are stresses. An important example of role conflict with management is when resources are not considered appropriate for quality care (Porter-O'Grady, 1991a, 1991b). Rather than being avoided or ignored as sources of dissatisfaction, shared governance provides the organizational mechanisms for conflict resolution and role clarification through collaboration and consensus decision making.

Staff nurses should be salaried rather than paid an hourly wage, with salaries commensurate with the added accountability and investment required of a participant in shared governance (Johnson, 1987). Further, salaried staff nurses should have more flexible hours and greater control over their time, with accountability shared among nurses for patient care coverage but held as individuals for the care of specific clients throughout an episode of care. Staff nurses often fear being salaried because they believe administration may take advantage of them and make further inordinate demands on their time without adequate compensation. Administrators often resist paying staff nurses set salaries because they fear they will lose control and be unable to hold nurses accountable for an equitable exchange of investment for productivity. There also is resistance to individual nurses being accountable for specific clients throughout an episode of care. Adherence to the principle of accountability for specific clients is abandoned when an alternative appears to have greater short run benefits for the organization. Yet accountability is the bedrock of professional practice. Shared governance, with staff nurses salaried, provides the means for the most benefits to accrue to all parties—nurses, the organization, and patients—if nurses are afforded the rights and privileges ordinarily enjoyed by salaried professionals and are held accountable for cost-effective practice, as individuals and as a collective.

SUMMARY

Because almost all practicing nurses are employed, nurse shared governance in employing organizations is imperative if the profession is to fulfill its social contract (ANA, 1980). Nurse shared governance also is needed for organizations to perform best in the turbulent, managed care environment. The prediction that future provider contracts will be based on demonstrated quality outcomes should cause greater provider organization interest in nurse shared governance. This combined with the current RN shortage may produce more efforts to implement professional nursing models of practice in organizations. Implementation of shared governance models that enable professional nursing practice is jeopardized, however, when there is lack of clarity about what shared governance is and when shared governance is confused with other organizational innovations that are similar but not the same. Likewise, it is important that the motives of those who lead the implementation of nurse shared governance be consistent with professional authority and control over nursing practice so that the profession can meet its commitments to clients in all practice settings. As Hess (1995) noted, nurses and administrators need to agree on the meaning of shared governance and resolve their different views as to what aspects of authority and accountability are most important for nurses. Shared governance requires that nurses are accountable to define and control nursing practice. Nurses must also be accountable to understand what shared governance is, expect that the necessary structures and processes are present if implementation of shared governance is claimed, be discerning about the motives for implementation, and take the risks and develop the knowledge to support the privilege of professional practice. If the aim of all nurses in an organization is to implement structures and processes that enable the profession to define and control practice, unit-based versus organization-wide implementation does not matter. The critical imperative is that mechanisms for collective nurse decision making are developed for the organization as a whole at some point. Nurses committed to professional nursing practice also must be resolved to complete role adaptations and cope with corresponding stresses that accompany change to shared governance, recognizing the benefits of supportive collegial relationships and consensus decisions among nurses in all roles.

Finally, nurses also must be accountable for the outcomes of their interventions with clients. There is research linking shared governance to improved job satisfaction and social integration of nurses, but less that links shared governance to improved patient outcomes and least cost to organizations. Although there are increased efforts to study shared governance, more systematic evaluation and publication of the results are needed. As with all organizational innovations, strategies and tools must continue to be developed and tested so that nurse administrators and clinicians can conveniently and systematically evaluate the outcomes of shared governance (McCloskey et al., 1994). Foremost among the needed strategies is a standardized definition of the operations that must be observed for nurse shared governance to be implemented (Hess, 1995) and nursing clinical information systems containing uniform nursing languages that yield large databases for the evaluation of the effectiveness of nursing organization and clinical interventions. The use of effectiveness data to inform practice and policy decisions will empower nursing, prevent the adoption of every "new idea" presented as a panacea, and potentially interrupt the destructive cycles of nurse abundance and shortage that often accompany or prompt decisions for change that are made without evidence of the impact on nursing effectiveness.

REFERENCES

American Nurses Association. (1980). *Nursing: A social policy statement.* Kansas City, MO: Author.

American Nurses Association. (1999). *Principles for nurse staffing.* Kansas City, MO: Author.

American Nurses Association. (1992). Standards of nursing practice. Code for nurses with interpretive statement. The nursing shortage in the 1990's: Realities and remedies. In *Best sellers.* Kansas City, MO: Author.

Brodbeck, K. (1992). Professional practice actualized through an integrated shared governance and quality assurance model. *Journal of Nursing Care Quality, 6*(2), 20-31.

Brooks, S.B., Olsen, P., Rieger-Kligy, S., & Mooney, L. (1995). Peer review: An approach to performance evaluation in a professional practice model. *Critical Care Nursing Quarterly, 18*(3), 36-47.

California law requires staffing ratios. (1999). *The American Nurse, 31*(6), 11.

Carmanica, L., & Rosenbecker, S. (1991). A pilot unit approach to shared governance. *Nursing Management, 22*(1), 46-48.

Crocker, D.G., Kirkpatrick, R.M., & Lentenbrink, L. (1992). Shared governance and collective bargaining: Integration, not confrontation. In T. Porter-O'Grady (Ed.), *Implementing shared governance: Creating a professional organization.* St. Louis: Mosby.

De Baca, V., Jones, K., & Tornabeni, J. (1993). A cost-benefit analysis of shared governance. *Journal of Nursing Administration, 23*(7-8), 50-57.

Edwards, G.B., Farrough, M., Gardner, M., Harrison, D., Sherman, M., & Simpson, S. (1994). Unit-based shared governance CAN work! *Nursing Management, 25*(4), 74-77.

Evan, L., Aubry, K., Hawkins, M., Curley, T.A., & Porter-O'Grady, T. (1995). Whole systems shared governance: A model for the integrated health systems. *Journal of Nursing Administration, 25*(5), 18-27.

Fagan, M.J. (1991). Can unit-based shared governance thrive on its own? *Nursing Management, 22*(7), 104L-104P.

Ferguson-Paré, M.L. (1996). Registered nurses' perception of their autonomy and the factors that influence their autonomy in rehabilitation and long-term care settings. *Canadian Journal of Nursing Administration, 9*(2), 95-108.

Foster, B.E. (1992). Shared governance: Design and implementation. In T. Porter-O'Grady (Ed.), *Implementing shared governance: Creating a professional organization.* St. Louis: Mosby.

George, V.M., Burke, L.J., & Rodgers, B.L. (1997). Research-based planning for change: Assessing nurses' attitudes toward governance and professional practice autonomy after hospital acquisition. *Journal of Nursing Administration, 27*(5), 53-61.

Gulland, A., & Payne, D. (1997). Daisy chain power. *Nursing Times, 93*(34), 14-15.

Hastings, C., & Waltz, C. (1995). Assessing the outcomes of professional practice redesign: Impact on staff nurse perceptions. *Journal of Nursing Administration, 25*(3), 34-42.

Havens, D.S. (1994). Is governance being shared? *Journal of Nursing Administration, 24*(6), 59-64.

Hersey, P., & Blanchard, K. (1986). *Management of organization behavior: Utilizing human resources.* Englewood Cliffs, NJ: Prentice-Hall.

Hess, R.G. (1995). Shared governance: Nursing's 20th-century Tower of Babel. *Journal of Nursing Administration, 25*(5), 14-17.

Horvath, K.J. (1990). Professional nursing practice model. In G.G. Mayer, M.J. Madden, & E. Lawrenz (Eds.), *Patient care delivery models.* Rockville, MD: Aspen.

Jacoby, J., & Terpste, M. (1990). Collaborative governance: Model for professional autonomy. *Nursing Management, 21*(2), 42-44.

Jenkins, J.E. (1988). A nursing governance and practice model: What are the costs? *Nursing Economic$, 6*(6), 302-311.

Jenkins, J.E. (1991). Professional governance: The missing link. *Nursing Management, 22*(8), 26-30.

Johnson, L.M. (1987). Self-governance: Treatment for an unhealthy nursing culture. *Health Progress, 5,* 41-43.

Kerfoot, K. (1992, March). *Unit-based shared governance: The federation model.* Paper presented at Shared Governance: Sailing Towards Success, San Diego, California.

Kovner, C.T., Hendrickson, G., Knickman, J.R., & Finkler, S.A. (1993). Changing the delivery of nursing care: Implementation issues and qualitative findings. *Journal of Nursing Administration, 23*(11), 24-34.

Laschinger, H.K.S., & Havens, D. (1996). Staff nurse work empowerment and perceived control over nursing practice: Condition for work effectiveness. *Journal of Nursing Administration, 26*(9), 27-35.

Ludemann, R.S., & Brown, C. (1989). Staff perceptions of shared governance. *Nursing Administration Quarterly, 13*(4), 49-56.

Maas, M. (1989). Professional practice for the extended care environment: Learning from one model and its implementation. *Journal of Professional Nursing, 5*(5), 55-76.

Maas, M., & Jacox, A. (1977). *Guidelines for nurse autonomy/patient welfare.* New York: Appleton-Century-Crofts.

Maas, M., Jacox, A., & Specht, J. (1975). Nurse autonomy: Not rhetoric but for real. *American Journal of Nursing, 20,* 2201-2208.

Maas, M., & Specht, J.P. (1990). Nursing professionalization and self-governance: A model for long term care. In G.G. Mayer, M.J. Madden, & E. Lawrenz (Eds.), *Patient care delivery models* (pp. 151-163). Rockville, MD: Aspen.

Maas, M.L., Specht, J., & Ramler, C. (1997). Shared governance models in nursing: What is shared, who governs and who benefits? In J.C. McCloskey & H.K. Grace (Eds.), *Current issues in nursing* (5th ed., pp. 388-396). St. Louis: Mosby.

McCloskey, J.C. (1990). Two requirements for job contentment: Autonomy and social integration. *Image: The Journal of Nursing Scholarship, 22*(3), 140-143.

McCloskey, J.C., & Maas, M.L. (1998). Interdisciplinary teams. *Nursing Outlook, 46,* 157-163.

McCloskey, J.C., Maas, M., Gardner Huber, D., Kasparek, A., Specht, J., Ramler, C., Watson, C., Blegen, M., Delaney, C., Ellerbe, S., Etscheidt, C., Gongaware, C., Johnson, M., Kelly, K., Mehmert, P., & Clougherty, J. (1994). Nursing management innovations: A need for systematic evaluation. *Nursing Economic$, 12*(1), 35-45.

McDonagh, K.J., Rhodes, B., Sharkey, K., & Goodroe, J.H. (1989). Shared governance at St. Joseph's hospital of Atlanta: A mature professional practice model. *Nursing Administration Quarterly, 13*(4), 17-28.

Melchior, M.E.W., Van Den Berg, A.A., Halfens, R., Huyer Abu-Saad, H., Philipsen, H., & Gassman, P. (1997). Burnout and the work environment of nurses in psychiatric long-stay care settings. *Social Psychiatry and Psychiatric Epidemiology, 32*(3), 158-164.

Minnesota nurses talk staffing. (1999). *The American Nurse, 31*(6), 11.

Minzberg, H. (1979). *The structure of organizations.* Englewood Cliffs, NJ: Prentice-Hall.

Morrall, P.A. (1997). Professionalism and community psychiatric nursing: A case study of four mental health teams. *Journal of Advanced Nursing, 25,* 1133-1137.

O'May, F., & Buchan, J. (1999). Shared governance: A literature review. *International Journal of Nursing Studies, 36,* 281-300.

Peplau, H. (1985, February). Is nursing self-regulatory power being eroded? *American Journal of Nursing, 85*(2), 141-143.

Pinkerton, S.E. (1988). An overview of shared governance. In S.E. Pinkerton & P. Schroeder (Eds.), *Commitment to excellence: Developing a professional nursing staff.* Rockville, MD: Aspen.

Porter-O'Grady, T. (1987). Shared governance and new organizational models. *Nursing Economic$, 5*(6), 281-286.

Porter-O'Grady, T. (1991a). Shared governance for nursing. Part I: Creating the new organization. *Association of Operating Room Nurses Journal, 53*(2), 694-703.

Porter-O'Grady, T. (1991b). Shared governance for nursing. Part II: Putting the organization into action. *Association of Operating Room Nurses Journal, 53*(3), 694-703.

Porter-O'Grady, T. (1992). Shared governance: Looking toward the future. In T. Porter-O'Grady (Ed.), *Implementing shared governance: Creating a professional organization.* St. Louis: Mosby.

Porter-O'Grady, T. (1994). Whole systems shared governance: Creating the seamless organization. *Nursing Economic$, 12*(4), 187-195.

Prescott, P. (1987). Another round of nurse shortage. *Image: The Journal of Nursing Scholarship, 19*(4), 204-209.

Prince, S.B. (1997). Shared governance: Sharing power and opportunity. *Journal of Nursing Administration, 27*(3), 28-35.

Ramler, C.L. (1995). *Evaluation of the implementation of a professional nurse shared governance model.* Unpublished doctoral dissertation, University of Iowa, College of Nursing, Iowa City.

Relf, M. (1995). Increasing job satisfaction and motivation while reducing nursing turnover through the implementation of shared governance. *Critical Care Nursing, 18*(3), 7-13.

Rose, M., & DiPasquale, B. (1990). The Johns Hopkins professional practice model. In G.G. Mayer, M.J. Madden, & E. Lawrenz (Eds.), *Patient care delivery models* (pp. 85-96). Rockville, MD: Aspen.

Schwartz, R.H. (1990). Nurse decision-making influence: A discrepancy between the nursing and hospital literatures. *Journal of Nursing Administration, 20*(6), 35-39.

Skubak, K.J., Earls, N.H., & Botos, M.J. (1994). Shared governance: Getting it started. *Nursing Management, 25*(5), 80I-J, 80N, 80P.

Song, R., Daly, B.J., Rudy, E.B., Douglas, S., & Dyer, M.A. (1997). Nurses' job satisfaction, absenteeism, and turnover after implementing a special care unit practice model. *Research in Nursing and Health, 20,* 443-452.

Specht, J. (1995). *Shared governance: Development and features.* Unpublished doctoral dissertation, University of Iowa, College of Nursing, Iowa City.

Spitzer-Lehmann, R. (1989). Middle management consolidation. *Nursing Management, 20*(4), 59-62.

Stichler, J.F. (1992). A conceptual basis for shared governance. In T. Porter-O'Grady (Ed.), *Implementing shared governance: Creating a professional organization* (pp. 1-24). St. Louis: Mosby.

Strasen, L. (1989). Redesigning patient care to empower nurses and increase productivity. *Nursing Economic$, 7*(1), 32-35.

Thrasher, T., Bossman, V.M., Carroll, S., Cook, B., Cherry, K., Kopras, S.M., Daniels, L., & Schaffer, P. (1992). Empowering the clinical nurse through quality assurance in a shared governance setting. *Journal of Nursing Care Quality, 6*(2), 15-19.

Westrope, R.A., Vaughn, L., Bott, M., & Taunton, R.L. (1995). Shared governance: From vision to reality. *Journal of Nursing Administration, 25*(12), 45-54.

Wilson, C.K. (1989). Develop outcomes. *Journal of Nursing Administration, 26,* 14-19.

Wilson, C.K., & Porter-O'Grady, T. (1999). *Leading the revolution in health care* (2nd ed.). Gaithersburg, MD: Aspen.

Section Seven

Health Care Systems

System Reform

Opportunity or Threat?

JOANNE McCLOSKEY DOCHTERMAN, HELEN KENNEDY GRACE

The health care systems in the United States and many other countries are undergoing rapid change. Cost containment efforts and the move toward managed care have raised questions about everything, from the setting where care is delivered, to the provider of care, to the payer, and even to the status of the patient. The situation is creating a good deal of disturbing turmoil. Jobs are being threatened, and the security of the past is gone. During times of great change, however, there also is opportunity as people look for new solutions. What will nursing's attitude and behavior be during these next years of system change?

In the debate chapter for this section, Grace clearly outlines the old medical care system that we are slowly moving away from and the new comprehensive community-based health care system that we are evolving into. Grace demonstrates the wisdom of this evolution by presenting the arguments for both systems: first, she gives the reasons for keeping our current medical care system of illness treatment, then the reasons for refocusing toward health promotion and disease prevention. Arguments for keeping what we have include the following:

1. We know how to treat illness, and we do this well.
2. The education of our practitioners requires the challenges of complex medical problems.
3. Hospitals are efficiently designed to use the expertise of highly trained professionals.
4. The economic welfare of communities rests upon the viability of hospitals.
5. There are few proven alternatives.

Arguments for refocusing our efforts toward health promotion and disease prevention include the following:

1. More than half of all diseases are a product of unhealthy lifestyles.
2. Educating the young will result in healthier adults.

3. Community-based monitoring programs can detect problems at an early stage where intervention is most likely to have an effect.
4. The closing of some hospitals and the change in financing of health care would save money.

Grace puts forth the need for a more integrated health care system whereby there is less fragmentation of services. She finishes her chapter with an example of three communities in Michigan that are beginning the process of restructuring their health care. The importance of educating communities about health care is central to their revisioning of new systems and identification of barriers that constrain them. Grace believes that "quality affordable health care for all is an attainable goal" if community members are brought into partnerships with providers. This is a hard hitting and interesting chapter that is a must read for everyone.

Next, Walker, Barton, and Scott describe the need for business coalitions in this changing era. According to the authors, health care industries face three significant challenges: the impending shortages of knowledge workers, a need to provide culturally sensitive care, and the impact of technology. In addition, American higher education is undergoing dramatic change. The chapter will help readers understand how these changes and the resulting development of coalitions affect nurses. The chapter is a crash course on organizational structures and coalition building. Managed care coalitions offer opportunities for providers who can blend business knowledge with clinical practice. The authors challenge nurses to become active players in shaping the new health care organizations. Three interesting case studies complete the chapter and illustrate the new wave of coalitions. Distance education technology is at the center of some of these coalitions, and the reader will want to refer to the book's section on education.

The next chapter by Salmon makes the case that all nurses must take more responsibility for shaping the political forces that direct health care in the United States. Salmon wants her chapter to challenge each reader to examine his or her own participation in heath policymaking. It does. She begins by describing how the current health care system is a product of politics. The movement to a health care system that is market driven makes the politics less clear but perhaps more important. Although nursing has achieved a good deal of political sophistication in the past decade, Salmon says this is not enough. She calls for nursing to expand beyond our own boundaries and to make alliances with physicians and organized medicine and with consumers and communities. "The alliance of organized nursing with organized consumer groups is the political equivalent to the individual nurse serving as the patient's advocate." Salmon ends her chapter by reviewing the specific steps of public policymaking and places where nurses could take a more active role. Nurses need to help develop health agendas, not just influence legislation. Although the chapter relates to the political process in the United States, the message and ideas are relevant to nursing and the nursing profession worldwide.

The corporatization of health care is the subject of the next chapter by Beyers. Mergers and acquisitions use business approaches to achieve service goals. While each is unique and unpredictable, influenced by a number of factors, they all produce anxiety and require good communication and change skills. Beyers discusses the impact of mergers and acquisitions on employees, leadership, sponsors and owners, the community, the organization, the economy, and on nursing. There is little research to guide leaders through this process. Beyers believes that the movement from a public service to a business model can be to the advantage of nurses if we are prepared to be involved. During the merger process she urges nurses to continue to serve as the conscience of health care. This chapter gives a good overview of what to anticipate during a time of merger or acquisition.

Another change situation that provides opportunities for nurses is the proliferation of managed care. In the next chapter, Given describes the opportunities for nurse prac-

titioners. Nurses in advance practice, she says, must enhance their role involvement during this time of change. Given wants nurse practitioners to be proactive, to position themselves to be a major resource to managed care organizations. She says that to function in a managed care environment they need organizational, professional, and interpersonal skills. Given does a good job at describing opportunities and challenges in numerous roles of the nurse practitioner: direct primary care provider; prevention, health promotion, and demand management; disease management; patient advocacy and member services; care coordination; and outcomes management. Now is the time for nurse practitioners to expand their roles to meet the cost and quality goals of managed care. This is a helpful, thought-provoking chapter that should be required reading for all nurse practitioner students.

One mechanism for care provision in today's health care managed care system is the contract, a legal document that specifies services to be delivered and the payment for these services. In the last chapter in this section, Lamb and Zazworsky take the position that nurses must become skilled in negotiating and carrying out contracts for nursing services. With contracts, providers assume financial risk when they agree to provide services for a specific price. The authors do a good job of explaining contracts and the factors that contribute to success or failure. They argue that being able to price our services identifies the value of nursing. The authors urge nurses to take an active part in negotiating for contracts and to develop expertise in the business side of nursing. This is a chapter that all nurses should read.

Although the need for health care reform is obvious, the shape of the reform is not yet clear. Business practices and decision making are much more dominant. There is a definite movement from hospital-based and illness treatment care to community-based and health promotion care. Building coalitions among providers and with consumers is a part of this shift in emphasis. The changes are threatening to many, and politics plays a big part in the success or failure of new efforts. While the future shape of the health care system is unknown, it is clear that nurses must take an active role in being part of the solution.

From a Medical Care System for a Few to a Comprehensive Health Care System for All

HELEN KENNEDY GRACE

This is the story of a village on top of a mountain. The children of the village loved to play near the ledge at the top of the mountain, but they sometimes fell off the ledge to the bottom and suffered broken legs and other injuries. Eventually a hospital was built at the bottom of the mountain to treat the injured children. The doctors set up their offices and emergency care centers, and the parents would struggle to the bottom of the mountain to visit their injured children. One day at a meeting called for another purpose, the villagers began to reflect on the problem of the injured children. One young mother asked, "Why haven't we put a fence around the top of the mountain ledge so the children won't fall off?" After considerable discussion of how this might impair the panoramic view for the villagers, they agreed that an attractive fence could be built and that they could prevent the injuries. They did so, and eventually the hospital at the bottom of the mountain was closed and a comprehensive health care clinic opened in the village because the villagers, having solved the problems of children's injuries, then thought of numerous other ways that they might work together to keep their community healthy. They mounted a campaign to clean up the environment, paying special attention to toxic waste from the nearby chemical factory and testing of the water to be sure that it was pure. Every expectant mother had access to quality prenatal care that recognized the culture and values of the community, and there was a comprehensive immunization program so that all infants and children were protected from childhood illnesses. Every villager had access to a program of periodic monitoring of their health status, and whenever an illness was detected, the villagers were referred to the appropriate practitioner with expertise needed to address the problem. A small, efficient short-term-care hospital was part of the clinic, and a well-developed system of referral to the regional tertiary care center was in place. Use of information technology provided links between available knowledge and information to all within the network, and a system of transportation was in place to ensure that people in need of advanced medical treatment could access these services. The elderly were cared for in their homes through a comprehensive eldercare program. When they were unable to remain in their homes for some reason, they entered a nursing home that was located in the center of the village. The nursing home had a wide range of volunteer programs that brought the community—its young people and others—into partnerships to provide humane, caring services for the elders and served as a vital community communication link in transmitting the wisdom of the elders to future generations.

Is this utopia possible? Is it desirable? If so, how do we move from our current system of "hospitals at the bottom of mountains" (i.e., fixing problems only after they have developed) to one with a primary emphasis on keeping people healthy (i.e., preventing people from "falling off the mountain")? This chapter poses two sides of this argument. Should the emphasis be on maintaining and enhancing our current medical care system, or should the focus be shifted to health promotion and disease prevention? The closing argument suggests that we have both the capacity and the resources to merge our current medical care system into a comprehensive health care system and proposes steps that will move us down this road.

SUSTAIN AND IMPROVE OUR CURRENT MEDICAL CARE SYSTEM

The United States has the best medical care system in the world. We have the best-educated doctors and nurses and the most sophisticated hospitals in the world. Don't tinker with what isn't broken. We don't know how to prevent illness, but we do know to treat it. We just need to find a way to finance the existing system. Those who have the means should have the right to "the best."

Our current medical care system is a reflection of values in American society. No one should be denied access to the "best" care if they have the ability to pay or if insurance coverage is provided by their employers. These values are reflected in the way our society invests its resources. Over the years we have made substantial societal investments in scientific and medical research that has resulted in the most advanced knowledge related to the etiology and treatment of diseases. When organs are severely diseased and irreparable, we have the capacity for transplantation of hearts, livers, lungs, kidneys, or a combination of body parts. The ability to overcome the body's tendency to reject transplants has been addressed by a wide array of immunosuppressive agents. A great variety of drug treatments is available for the most complex of diseases. If a body part is "broken," our medical care system has a high level of capability for "fixing" it, either surgically or medically. We can keep people with a plethora of problems alive for prolonged periods of time. For example, cancer sufferers now have a much longer life span and a better quality of that life as a result of advances in the treatment agents given as well as those used to compensate for the numerous side effects of the treatment. Superpowerful antibiotics have given us the capability to overcome ever-increasing numbers of infectious diseases.

The training of medical doctors and nurses in the United States is the most sophisticated and arduous in the world. Extreme competition to get into medical schools in particular ensures that we are capturing the brightest minds in the country. These individuals need to be challenged continuously, both in their medical training and as they move into practice settings. The major challenges lay in finding ways to deal with the most complicated medical care problems. The medical school curricula, based on ever more complex decision-making trees, challenges the ability of the students to diagnose problems and devise treatment plans. Given the extensive investment of resources in medical education by the public, which supports most medical education through their tax dollars, and the extensive investment of time, energy, and money to support 4 years of postbaccalaureate study followed by residency programs, it would be a misuse of these dollars if specialty training were not the end product. This extensive an education to treat the commonplace colds, flus, broken arms, and aches and pains that plague most patients would be a misuse of these valued resources. The commonplace problems of people offer an insufficient challenge to the brilliantly honed minds of medical practitioners that is the end product of their rigorous education.

While in nursing there has never been the clamor to gain entrance to the field as there has been in medicine, many of the same arguments might hold. The "excitement" of an intensive care unit with its many sophisticated pieces of equipment, the challenge of interpreting the laboratory reports and correlating them to the clinical status of the patient, and the hovering over monitors to detect changes in the physiological status of the patient are all intellectually challenging. Investment in highly specialized advanced practitioner training dictates that this training be used in the intensive care environment of a hospital setting.

Hospitals are the centerpiece of our medical care system. They are the specially designed workplaces that use the expertise of our highly trained health professionals most efficiently. Further, they constitute a significant economic development resource in any community. With 6% of people employed in health-related fields, and the majority of these employed by hospitals, the economic welfare of communities frequently rests on the viability of hospitals and health-related institutions. Society has made a tremendous investment in the building of highly sophisticated hospitals with advanced technology equipment. It would be a tremendous waste of resources to see these facilities disintegrate or disappear; it is a wise investment to see that they are used to benefit all.

Perhaps one of the strongest arguments for maintaining and improving our current medical care system is that there are few proven alternatives. While some argue that it would be a better use of resources to invest in prevention, our highly trained health professionals and our highly developed technology are not designed to deal with health promotion and disease prevention. Most aspects of health promotion and disease prevention are contingent on the capacity of individuals to change their health-related behaviors, and it is in this area that highly educated medical practitioners are the most helpless. In addition, unless individuals are motivated to change their behavior, there is little that can be done. Our hospital facilities and our highly trained health professionals can be better utilized for the diagnosis and treatment of disease than in a misuse of this capacity in the area of health promotion and disease prevention.

REFOCUS OUR EFFORTS TOWARD HEALTH PROMOTION AND DISEASE PREVENTION

Despite our sophisticated technology and highly trained health care professionals, the efforts to diagnose and treat disease are far more costly than if the focus was on prevention of disease. Approximately 52% of all diseases are a product of unhealthy lifestyles and behavioral choices that result in ill health. Resources would be better used to focus on prevention of disease than on the costly approaches to treatment.

We should divert the large amounts of money going to research for the treatment of diseases and for development of technology to health promotion and disease prevention. For example, huge amounts of research and treatment dollars are spent on leukemia. The effects of the treatment approaches are limited at best, yet the cost of treating one leukemia patient can reach astronomical figures. Resources could be used much more effectively to reduce the toxic waste in our environment, control the use of chemicals that lead to bone marrow damage, and prevent disease rather than invest in treatments of unproved worth. We should spend some of the money that is currently being spent on medical care and research to clean up the environment.

Instead of our current focus on treatment, the emphasis should be shifted to education. We should focus on instilling within young people healthy lifestyles that will contribute to long and productive lives, and we should ensure that all citizens receive appropriate preventive health care. Every school curriculum in the country should contain content on the effects of the abuse of alcohol and drugs (including tobacco) and the impact of lack of exercise and poor nutrition on the health of the individual. A program designed to promote physical fitness in young people should be built into all educational programs. Fitness levels of school children should be tested periodically, and test scores should be reported much as academic achievement is now reported. Fitness trails, recreational facilities, and support groups that encourage healthy lifestyles should be part of each community.

Systematic programs of health monitoring should be set up in each community, with the expectation that different population groups would have periodic health screening to detect problems at the earliest possible stages and at the level at which intervention is most likely to have a profound effect. Prenatal care for expectant mothers, monitoring of both physical and psychological growth and development in children, adolescent health monitoring, periodic health examinations for adults, health and fitness assessment for seniors, and monitoring programs for chronic illnesses of the elderly would be components of this comprehensive preventive system.

The numbers of highly specialized health care providers should be decreased and the numbers of primary care practitioners increased. Additionally, practitioners from the education and behavioral science fields should be integrated into the health professions teams. Educational programs for health professionals should be refocused on early diagnosis and prevention and away from the heavy emphasis on physical sciences to a more balanced study of the behavioral sciences with a heavy emphasis on methods of teaching for adult learners.

The payment incentives within the system should provide rewards for keeping people well rather than paying for treatment of illnesses. This could best be achieved through funding on a capitated basis for communities. Because most public funds flow into communities through county governments, counties might well be the base for a capitated system. In instances in which a county is comprised of a large metropolitan area, the capitated system might be drawn along smaller geographic boundaries. The particular funding base for a community would need to be calculated based on the demographics of the particular area and would take into consideration the age spread of the population, the level of income and the racial and ethnic composition of the community, and the association of these demographics with known health risks. If the health care dollars flowing into the community were based on the numbers of people living in that community, the incentives would be to maintain the health of the people rather than to pay for treatment of costly illnesses. A capitated system that pays for building health promotion into the fabric of the community and one in which the health care "providers" are salaried rather than paid on a fee-for-service basis would be one way in which the incentive systems could be changed.

The majority of hospital beds in this country should be closed. Community hospitals in both urban and rural settings could become the hub for organizing the comprehensive system of health promotion and disease prevention activities across the community. A capitated system would dramatically decrease the numbers of people involved in the processing of paperwork related to financing the system (now estimated to be about 25% of health care dollars). These community hospitals would have facilities for short-term stays for "normal" conditions such as delivery of babies, handling of accidents and fractures, and simple surgery. The numbers of people displaced from paper-processing jobs could be absorbed into new, more productive roles within the community such as health promoters. A few highly specialized hospitals would remain to treat the limited number of acute care problems that develop despite all efforts at maintaining health in the community.

DEVELOP INTEGRATED COMPREHENSIVE HEALTH CARE SYSTEMS

This debate is posed most frequently as an either/or argument—that one must make a choice between a quality medical care system versus a system focused on the maintenance of health. The argument is generally made on the basis of available resources and is grounded on a premise that lack of resources constrains the system. The arguments develop based on what would appear to be a faulty premise, that is, that lack of resources are the problem. If one views the problem as one of lack of resources, the response is that of exerting efforts to get more resources out of the existing system. However, if one looks at the situation as one in which the problem is *use* of *existing* resources, the focus changes to looking at ways to achieve greater efficiency.

The United States spends more on medical care than any other country in the world. Yet our health indices do not reflect that this investment is paying off with the improved health of the people. Rarely is the question addressed from the perspective of how the resources flow and the use of these resources in the most cost-effective ways. Money for health and human services flows into communities through a wide array of funding tracks, each carrying with it its own rules and regulations, and a plethora of individuals is employed as gatekeepers to ensure "compliance." This results in inefficient use of the resources that are available in that funding "packages" are difficult to put together to meet the needs of individuals and families and that a disproportionate amount of the resources is used to pay for the paper processing to maintain all the separate funding streams. In a typical community there would of course be federally funded programs such as Medicare and Medicaid, but within these general programs there would be a variety of funding streams for a variety of programs. For example, prenatal care would have several components, often provided by multiple agencies. The Women, Infants, and Children programs are administered typically through health departments. A mother receiving prenatal care from a community health center may need to go to the public health department to receive funds from the Women, Infants, and Children program. If an expectant mother has other human service problems, such as being abused or abusing substances, she would then typically be referred to another agency that offers these programs. Most frequently the funding for these programs would be through a department of social services or mental health department. The department of child and family services might also be a possibility. All of these agencies, however, carry with them their own unique rules and regulations and a set of functionaries to maintain the multiple "systems." This results in fragmentation of services, difficulty for patients in obtaining the help that they need (frequently a case

manager is added to help the patient navigate through the morass), inefficient use of the human resources (the providers) within the system, and a plethora of paperwork that would be unnecessary if the system was put together as a system. In addition to publicly funded programs, multitudes of insurers provide several insurance plans to individuals and workers within the community. A typical community hospital may deal with up to 50 insurers, all with different reporting requirements and different forms to fill out. Hospitals have added to their financial and administrative staffs to process claims and to respond to the challenges. It is estimated that at least 25% of the resources within the system currently goes to administration. In private discussions with chief executive officers in community-based health service organizations such as visiting nurse associations it is estimated that up to one third of their resources are spent on administrative overhead to manage the multiple funding streams on which their survival depends. Noting how limited resources are used for health care in other countries and the misuse of our comparatively abundant resources within the United States, I find it hard to accept the premise that the problem is one of lack of resources.

Some might argue that use of human resources in the medical care system is integral to the economic well-being of communities and that therefore one should not tinker with the system. In a number of both rural and urban communities the health care sector is one of the major employers in the community. Closing a rural hospital is viewed as a major threat to the economy of the community, and these concern takes precedence over concerns for the impact of hospital closure on the health of the community. The health care industry is a major economic force within this country, and maintenance of the nonsystem may be crucial to our economic well-being. Seldom is this issue addressed in a straightforward manner, however. If we wish to have resources directed toward health as an industry and maintenance of the economy, it would be far better to address this issue directly rather than couching the arguments in terms of concern for the well-being of individuals who use the health care system. My personal argument would be that there are more productive ways of using the human resources that are now engaged in "paper processing," and that if we wish to develop integrated, comprehensive health care systems, some of the human resources need to be diverted to more productive lines of work that would have a more direct payoff in terms of improved health of people.

In recent years the W.K. Kellogg Foundation has provided funding to three communities in Michigan to begin the process of reconceptualizing and restructuring their health care to achieve a comprehensive integrated system. In one of these communities the total amount of funding coming into a county with 135,982 residents was $402,401,000, which translates to $3,000 per individual. A basic assumption underlying the Comprehensive Community Health Models (CCHMs) of Michigan's program is that these resources, if they were put together in a different way, would be adequate to fund a comprehensive integrated health care system that would be accessible to all. During the transition there may be a limited period of increased costs, but over time the benefits to be achieved from linking comprehensive health care to the current medical and human services, pooling the resources within the community to fund an integrated health care system, and placing the emphasis on maintaining the health of the community will result in a much more cost-effective system.

In the process of working with these three communities many lessons are being learned, the first and foremost of which is the importance of educating communities about health and medical care so that they can begin to exercise their decision-making power in a rational manner. A primary factor that inhibits significant change within the health related fields is the degree to which the system has been a mystery to the general public. By engaging in an extensive community "visioning" process the communities have begun to shift their views of health care away from the medical system as it is commonly defined toward a comprehensive health care system. For example, one of the results of this reconceptualization is that each of the three communities has placed a high value on the health of children and has concluded that an essential component of a comprehensive system is school nurses. In each community they have found ways of funding school nurses who are responsible for health monitoring and other health-related functions in the school. After defining a set of guiding values and identifying essential characteristics of a comprehensive health system, a process of electronic town meetings has been useful in building group consensus, identifying areas that are conflicting, and focusing discussions to resolve differences. As a wide range of community participants has become engaged in the visioning process, the tertiary medical care system is no longer the central focus, sometimes to the consternation of hospital administrators and physician specialists who view themselves as the center of the universe.

Each of these communities has engaged in a process of surveying the health of their residents, identifying pre-ventable health problems within their community, prioritizing areas of concern, and addressing ways in which problem areas might be addressed. As communities begin to understand that a comprehensive, integrated health care system includes comprehensive health promotion programs for target groups throughout the community (i.e., pregnant women, children, adolescents, working adults, women, impoverished groups, and elders), weaving health promotion into the fabric of the community becomes a major facet of the system. Health monitoring of key groups such as pregnant women, children, and adults and elderly then becomes another key component. As the focus shifts to health promotion and maintenance, the locus of services moves out of traditional health settings into community-based institutions such as schools, churches, Y centers, senior citizen centers, and worksites. The importance of primary health care providers also rises to the surface as communities build their vision of a comprehensive health care system.

As all sectors begin to come together around a common vision for health care in their community, a natural realignment of working relationships begins to occur. For example, the local public health department, which in most communities has become quite isolated from other sectors, becomes the source of data on the health of the community and has a key role to play in monitoring progress. As the health of all members of the community becomes the business of the community as a whole, no longer does the health department become relegated to being the providers of "last resort." Social service agencies and health providers find new ways of working together. Engaging members of the community in the dialogue and dealing with "real life" situations that people face in getting health care for themselves and their family members adds a new dimension to the discussion.

As these discussions progress, new voices emerge. In the community discussions in Michigan a wide array of "alternative health care providers" has emerged, adding yet another dimension to the discussions. For example, a young woman described her problem with migraine headaches. She could tell when a migraine was coming on, and if she went for massage therapy, the migraine could be averted. Her health insurance would not pay for massage therapy, however. If she went to her doctor, she couldn't get an appointment until the headache had developed, and she would need to take time off from work and take medication. Yet this much more costly (both physical and financial) course of action was reimbursable. This situation precipitated an interesting debate in the visioning process as to what should be reimbursable in an "ideal" health system. A prominent oncologist agreed that "only scientifically validated treatments" should be reimbursable. This was countered by a question of how many of his treatments were scientifically proven to be beneficial.

As the community becomes engaged in a new type of dialogue and the health of the community becomes "community business," the barriers that constrain the system inevitably become much more evident. Community governing boards have been constituted in the three communities involved in the CCHMs process. These boards become engaged in such ways that they may begin to have an impact on changing public policy, particularly that relevant to the funding for health and human services. An underlying premise of the CCHMs effort is that if communities could pool the dollars that are currently coming into communities through the funding stream and if this funding could be redirected to fund health promotion and preventive services as well as treatment for diseases, then there would be sufficient resources to ensure an adequate level of health care for all. Using state-of-the-art information technology and an understanding of how a comprehensive, integrated system works, the fragmented pieces that are currently out there could function in a much different way. In the end, then, each part of the system would be a "winner." Appropriate use of the expert skills of specialists, scaled-down hospitals, an organized system for monitoring health, a comprehensive health promotion program integrated into community-based organizations such as schools, churches, senior citizen centers, and a system in which community members and health workers work as a team to improve the health of the community would benefit all members of the community.

All can be winners. To achieve this goal, however, requires putting aside the traditional boundaries that have served to divide the "turf." Community members must be brought into the partnerships, and all parties must give up some additional areas of control. For example, physicians alone can no longer be the gatekeepers for the system. The health system of the future must be one in which the worth of all individuals—be they providers or patients—is valued and the human resources that collectively might work together are used to their full potential. Quality, affordable health care for all is an attainable goal.

Business Coalitions in an Electronic Age

Surviving in Local and Global Markets

PATRICIA HINTON WALKER, AMY J. BARTON, JILL SCOTT

The U.S. health care industry continues to experience rapid and significant change. Governmental intervention and consolidation throughout the health care system include mergers, alliances, and acquisitions between provider groups (such as hospitals, health maintenance organizations [HMOs], and preferred provider organizations [PPOs]), insurance carriers, suppliers, distributors, and other related industries. The big have become bigger, and the increase in alliances is growing at all levels of the value chain (Speckman & Isabella, 2000). Even the value chain is being defined in new ways as health care industries face three significant challenges: (1) impending global shortages of knowledge workers such as nurses and pharmacists, (2) the need to provide culturally sensitive services to future clients from a variety of cultures and communities, and (3) the impact of technology that will change the way all industries do business in the 21st century.

Managed care is still alive and well in the United States. Although many other countries around the globe have been managing care in an attempt to achieve the best health outcomes for individuals and communities, balancing cost and quality is still a significant challenge globally. Unfortunately the term *managed care* in the United States conjures up negative responses from provider groups and many consumers. The challenge of managing care for the best population-based outcomes is here to stay, however, so nurses need to develop and improve business knowledge and literacy in order to survive.

Managed care is still a term used to describe various coalitions, alliances, partnerships, and mergers whose goals are to increase market presence, manage provider practices, and improve patient flow. These organizations are still described as HMOs, such as Kaiser Permanente; as integrated delivery systems (IDS), which attempt to link hospitals, home health agencies, and group primary care practices; or as some form of PPO. Regardless of the particular model or approach, there are at least four common goals of any type of managed care organization:

1. To control costs, usually by controlling utilization of services
2. To use sound business approaches to ensure efficiency, which results in significant reductions in the health care labor force and work redesign
3. To ensure quality through the measurement of outcomes (clinical indicators, customer satisfaction, and cost)
4. To do all of the above by trying to form coalitions, alliances, or partnerships that will manage care across the wellness-illness continuum for a specified dollar amount (usually negotiated up front in a managed care contract)

Unfortunately, as competition has raged in markets experiencing high managed care penetration, the bottom line is driving many decisions that negatively affect the workplace environment, recruitment and retention of nursing staff, and the satisfaction of consumers.

To compound the effect of these changes in the health care industry, American higher education is also undergoing a transformation from largely government-run (state) institutions to market-driven systems that must appeal to new lifelong learners and to corporate and government purchasers of education and training. In the United States a total of $619 billion dollars (of which $60 billion is targeted to workplace training) is spent on education. Amazingly, this is 9.8% of our gross domestic product, which is second only to health care spending (14%) as a percentage of our gross national product (Meister, 1998).

These continuing changes in health care delivery and the emerging changes in the educational arena have significant implications for the nursing profession in practice, education, research, and administration. This chapter is designed to help nurses better understand how these changes in the "business" of health care delivery and the new market-driven education system affect nurses individually and collectively. Lastly, it is our hope that this chapter will provide incentives to look at this time of change as a time of great opportunity for nurses and the nursing profession. Changes in health care delivery continue to provide nurses with the opportunity to affect aspects of care that we have valued throughout history: coordinating care across the continuum, attention to prevention of disease and health promotion, attention to the role of the family and community, and empowering the voices of the patients (now clients/consumers/customers) in their own care. Because this is a market that is increasingly "bottom line" oriented, we must be creative and resourceful and prepared to understand the language and to master new competencies in finance, outcomes, and technology. Likewise with the changes in the education environment, we have the opportunity to bring reality to longstanding values of lifelong learning, relevance of research to practice, and competence in the workplace. Again this will require that nurses (individually and collectively) respond with creativity, some risk taking, and attention to the market forces that are driving education and corporate training in the context of an impending global nursing shortage.

CONTEXT FOR COALITIONS

When health care costs rose significantly in the 1980s, one of the ways that businesses and employers tried to control costs was through the development of coalitions (Rooney, 1992). Usually these coalitions were an attempt to contain costs on a community-wide basis and to control cost shifting from employer to employer. Although this approach met with marginal success, the use and development of many forms of coalitions to address many of the health care problems of today have continued. Now we continue to observe many forms of alliances and mergers including provider groups, hospitals, and buyer-supplier relationships. In this new century, new forms of alliances are developing to achieve the outsourcing of nonessential services, which brings unlikely businesses to the health care table; corporate-education contracts to ensure a competent current and future workforce; and technology access (Speckman & Isabella, 2000).

What is a coalition? How does it differ from alliances, partnerships, mergers, and networks? What do we need to

know about coalitions? And finally, how will this affect nursing and interdisciplinary practice, administration, and research?

The literature contains many references to coalitions but uses different terms to label them. A thesaurus lists alliance, network, partnership, affiliation, and consortium in connection with the use of the word *coalition*. Merriam-Webster (1994) specifically defines a coalition as "a temporary alliance of distinct parties, persons, or states for joint action." Partnership refers to a legal relationship usually involving close cooperation between parties with specified and joint rights and responsibilities; an alliance is an association that furthers common interests of members; and a consortium means an agreement, combination, or group formed to undertake an enterprise beyond the resources of any one member. For the purposes of this chapter these terms will be used somewhat interchangeably, depending on the particular reference.

Is a coalition an organization? Can we study coalitions and learn how to work within them and manage them in the same way we study traditional organizational structures? Can we better understand how to work in this newest evolution of organizational change in response to rapid changes in the delivery of health care and in education? The answers are yes, and it is even more important in this new millennium that nurses understand what is happening in organizations, particularly in the context of the rapid reshaping of health care and education with the growing number of alliances, coalitions, and mergers. Tichy (1983) indicates that we must understand organizational models to understand how organizations change. He describes a model as a set of assumptions or beliefs that guide managerial action, assist in diagnosing organizational problems, and focus the people that work in the organization. Three models—classic or mechanistic, human resource organic, and political—were described by Tichy (1983) and will sound familiar to most people who have lived and worked in organizations. First is the classic or mechanistic model, which focuses on structure, span of control, and specialized task functions. This model is like a typical bureaucratic organization with detailed job descriptions and a rigid chain of command, where decisions are made along vertical lines with minimum flexibility. The human resources organic model is more concerned about the human side, where there are more democratic decisions made, with lots of interaction vertically and laterally in the organization. Supervisors are usually motivators and facilitators who communicate through expectations rather than strict orders and tasks. There are clearly strengths and weaknesses within each of these two approaches. Third is the political model, which can be viewed as an arena in which multiple coalitions vie for control of the organization through ongoing processes of bargaining and negotiation. This model is best studied from the perspective of understanding internal (usually full-time employees) and external coalitions (partners, alliance members, networked groups) that make up the larger organization (Mintzberg, 1977). We need to better understand and learn how to influence these types of organizations in which change strategies are based on making political adjustments, understanding where the greatest power and influence is held, and mastering the skills of negotiation, bargaining, and coalition building (Tichy, 1983). The political model is developing rapidly in the health care field and increasingly in educational institutions in response to competition for consumers' dollars and market share because it is the most flexible, adaptive, and responsive model. Two weaknesses must be noted in this evolving model, however; sometimes the technical production, with attention to detail, and cultural problems are difficult to resolve between different organizations in a coalition. (Tichy, 1983, p. 49). Consequently attention to the structure, processes, and outcomes of quality care (production) and the merging of different organizational cultures or values may create problems in these new health care delivery structures.

PURPOSES AND REASONS FOR COALITION DEVELOPMENT

Why is the political model or the development of coalitions, alliances, and partnerships dominating the health care and education organizational structures at this time? Why do we even need to understand this new phenomenon? Again, we would look to the business literature for the answers because if we understand the nature of the organizational change that we are all participating in (either by choice, chance, or requirement), nursing can position itself as a profession and ourselves as professionals. The evolution of alliances, coalitions, mergers, and partnerships is an increasingly global phenomenon. Many companies in a variety of industries are choosing alliances, coalitions, and partnerships as vehicles for change in a tight market economy, and this phenomenon is occurring on a worldwide basis. Competition and rapid positioning are the name of the game, particularly with the rapid changes in technology. Internet access and the way this technology is changing business and education create significant challenges for the nursing profession. It is critical that nursing administrators in both health care and

educational settings increase nurse exposure and expertise in the use of computer technology. In a timely book, *Competing for the Future,* Hamel and Prahalad write that "competition for the future is competition to create and dominate emerging opportunities—to stake out new competitive space" (1994, p. 22). Further, the authors say, organizations not only must compete within the boundaries of existing industries (such as hospitals, home health, and insurance industries) but also must shape the structure of industries so they will be able to compete and dominate the market in the future. This means that "competition will take place within and between coalitions of companies, and not only between individual businesses" (Hamel & Prahalad, 1994, p. 23).

Why is it so important to understand these business trends anyway? It is clear that those nurses, other clinical professionals, and educators who are willing to abandon old ways and to assist the organization in its efforts to remain competitive will be valued and will also survive in a changing workforce. New competencies are needed. Meister (1998), in her book *Corporate Universities,* identifies competencies that Fortune 500 companies are now expecting of employees. These include leadership development, collaboration and communication skills, technological literacy, business literacy, learning to learn skills competency, and self-management of one's own career. Since competition is so high at this time in health care, education, and many other industries, no one organizational structure has evolved to be the solution. As nurses, if we understand that many companies are trying to "shape the structures" for managed care, and I believe we will see the term "managed education" in the future through development of different kinds of alliances and coalitions, then we can position ourselves within these evolving structures to have more influence on quality of care and consumer satisfaction, two of nursing's strengths. Consequently, regardless of the type of structure, it is important for nursing and nurses to decide to be active players shaping the organization and to contribute meaningfully to new ways of doing things.

One key to assisting our health care and education organizations in developing successful coalitions and alliances is to understand the reasons for coalition development and the process of building coalitions. Coalitions develop for several reasons, but most obvious is the reason that no one organization has all the required resources, skills, knowledge, and expertise to produce the product. In health care the product is to provide cost-effective quality care across the continuum. A second reason that coalitions are formed is for political advantage.

In some cases a coalition is a good way to co-opt potential future competitors or, through partnering, to prevent resources from getting in the hands of a competitor. A political coalition also may provide access to new markets. A third reason for coalition development is to share risks and costs. "Alliances allow participation in highly volatile industries, where knowledge spreads rapidly, at substantially lower investment and risk than would be the case for a single organization" (Kaluzny, Zuckerman, & Ricketts, 1995, p. 3).

Because many business coalitions are formed not only for political reasons but also to acquire resources, skills, and knowledge, they may seem to be linkages without logic. Coalition building follows no distinctive pattern. According to Bell and Shea (1998) partnerships are rapidly becoming the primary structure of contemporary business, as organizations partner with vendors, unions, customers, and even competitors to take advantage of market opportunities, leverage intellectual capital, and create more innovative enterprises.

The literature has evolved from a focus on describing coalitions, alliances, and partnerships to exploration of how to make them last. More alliances fail than succeed today, and this is evident to those who watch their employers change names, ownership, and partnerships frequently. Bell and Shea (1998) liken these evolving partnerships to the level of difficulty of a dance: the highest (most difficult) level of partnership is the tango (with very different partners who must move carefully and totally together); the waltz (tamed and simplified interaction); the square dance (with strict rules and protocols but little emotional intensity or closeness—actions called by outside forces); the twist (moving separately, but somewhat connected); and finally the line dance (partners are completely independent but moving in the same direction without entanglement). Bell and Shea focus on selection of the right partner, the building of trust, evolution of the relationship, and learning from mistakes to improve the dance over time. It would behoove many of us in health care and education to examine the nature of the partnership and the type of "dance" in order to prevent unrealistic expectations in the development and growth of the alliances and partnerships we experience in our work settings.

TYPES AND FORMATION OF COALITIONS IN HEALTH CARE

According to Kaluzny et al. (1995) there are two general types of alliances or coalitions, lateral and integrative.

Similar types of organizations come together to achieve economies of scale by pooling resources, sharing information and human resources, group purchasing, and increasing collective power. When this occurs, it is called a lateral alliance or coalition. Examples of this include hospitals merging or networking together based on type of service, geographic distribution, or religious preferences. Rural hospital networks or consortiums and community hospital partnerships are two specific examples. On the other hand, the integrative type is more related to market, strategic positioning, and competitive advantage. Kanter (1989) uses the term *stakeholder alliance* to describe linkages among buyers, suppliers, and customers. This type of alliance usually calls its members stakeholders. In these coalitions, both vertical and horizontal integration are evident and include clinical, administrative, financial, educational, and delivery components of the organization.

Case Studies Describing Three Alliances or Coalitions Relevant to the 21st Century

We have chosen three case studies that present examples of a new wave of alliances, coalitions, or partnerships. These three examples highlight important issues for nursing: the nursing shortage and recruitment of minorities into the profession, a global partnership addressing education and career development influenced by the use of the Internet and institutional purchasers of education, and a community-driven alliance designed to provide care to underserved populations and at the same time serve as an education and research site for the University of Colorado Health Sciences Center (UCHSC) School of Nursing. These business relationship examples will also demonstrate the types of dances described by Bell and Shea in their book *Dance Lessons* (1998).

CASE STUDY 1: A MODEL FOR ADDRESSING THE RURAL NURSING SHORTAGE

The UCHSC School of Nursing has a long-standing commitment to educating nurses in rural Colorado. Over 100 advanced practice nurses have been educated during more than 30 years of distance education. Recent curricular changes based on a set of principles that include nursing diversity, nursing cultural competence, relationship-centered, caring nursing practice competencies, and responsible social justice nursing practice competencies articulate our vision to serve ethnically rich and underserved rural Colorado.

The current dilemma is more daunting than how to educate those with a nursing license to reach the advanced practice level. The challenge today is how to provide new nurses to a rural workforce that is already struggling to maintain numbers, a workforce that cannot compete with the Denver market to find new nurses who are entering the workforce.

Research and experience show that health care professionals who were raised, live, or practice in rural areas—"homegrown" health care professionals—are more likely to stay and work in rural areas than those who originate in or go to school in urban areas. The challenge is how to connect with and educate those who are committed to remaining in rural communities.

To address the current challenge the school of nursing has proposed an innovative model for baccalaureate education with key partners. The partnership involves the school of nursing, two grant staff from the Area Health Education Center (AHEC) who are in midcycle with Robert Wood Johnson working on projects related to workforce issues, two regional AHECs located in the southeast and south central regions of Colorado, key clinical partners within the regions, affiliated regional community colleges, and community leadership.

The goal of this project is to develop new homegrown RNs with baccalaureate degrees and more culturally competent practicing nurses who use distance learning technologies while remaining in their communities for education, except for brief intervals. To date we have found no comparable effort anywhere in the United States that is focused on the rural nursing shortage, emphasizing new homegrown and minority (Hispanic) recruitment. We believe the project has the potential to become a national model.

This Colorado Rural Nursing Partnership (CRNP) proposes to design, pilot, and implement a community-based, technology-enhanced, culturally rooted bachelor of science (BS) in nursing within 22 rural southeastern and south central counties of Colorado.

A wide recruitment net will create a new kind of "pipeline": career changers with bachelors degrees who wish to become nurses, local associate degree (AD) community college students and graduates, local 4-year college students and graduates, and other allied health providers with substantial science backgrounds and health care experience. Local practicing RNs will be recruited to serve as mentors to the candidates.

An innovative five-part nursing education strategy will be implemented: (1) interactive video courses, (2) asynchronous Internet-based courses, (3) regional clinical scholars, (4) clinical intensives, and (5) community cluster support or focus groups and mentors. Access to higher education will be increased by redesigning the admissions process and delivering the curriculum to homegrown students where they live or work. Existing interactive video sites will be used for intersite communications and courses. Currently available computers will be loaned to all BS nursing students and selected clinical sites. The school of nursing will design and deliver additional Internet-based courses. Interactive video and the Internet will provide the vehicle for didactic course work. Clinical courses will be carried out locally with community-based clinical scholars functioning as on-site training managers. Brief clinical-intensive experiences will be arranged with Denver-based clinical partners to ensure depth

and breadth of clinical training. New cultural competency and mentoring components will be developed locally, within the community clusters, to meet the needs of each community with emphasis on the local Hispanic culture. For example, in the San Luis Valley, traditional Hispanic healing methods are combined with Western medicine; curanderas and herbalists provide many health care services. These approaches to healing will be shared with academic faculty, students, and practicing nurses.

This five-part nursing baccalaureate education partnership draws on the successful records of the partners, seeks to improve current practices, and increases responsiveness to community needs. Thus it is a true partnership that builds on the past to create an innovative new future for rural nursing education.

This partnership or coalition could be considered a waltz as described by Bell and Shea (1998). In this case the partnership is built on a smooth, longstanding, trust relationship, working together to achieve common goals. Trust has already been developed through many years of meeting the needs of rural practitioners and communities by the UCHSC School of Nursing (SON). The challenge for the future is to learn new ways to dance together, practice together, prepare for the performances (of recruiting and educating rural nurses), and learn from mistakes to continually improve the dance. The impending global nursing shortage will require new and different kinds of alliances and coalitions with unlikely partners if the profession is going to be successful in creating a diverse, distributed workforce for urban and rural communities.

CASE STUDY 2: A GLOBAL PARTNERSHIP FOR EDUCATION

The UCHSC-SON is developing a new innovative model for education by creating new types of coalitions or alliances. In this case the purpose is to provide education across traditional boundaries of countries and corporations. Instead of the consumer being the individual, whose personal goals dictate learning needs and career trajectories, this new model attempts to address both institutional (global university partners and corporate partners) needs and individual needs of nurses seeking further education in corporate America and abroad. In addition, another important member of this partnership, e-Vitro, Inc., and the Global Nursing Academy, is a relatively new business whose purpose is rapid development and distribution of courses in the corporate and global environments. As the education industry also experiences rapid change amid competition for market share and a shrinking population of knowledge workers such as nurses, new alliances such as the one described here will emerge. This unusual partnership includes an Internet development business, managed care companies who employ large numbers of nurses and are interested in continuing education, global nursing educational institutions seeking to develop advanced practice nursing roles and expand doctoral education, SON faculty, and individual students locally and globally.

With the growing demand for education from both corporate America and our colleagues in nursing from other countries, the UCHSC-SON is accepting its responsibility to provide leadership, particularly for RN-BSN education and doctoral education in the global expansion of the nurse practitioner movement. Many of the countries in the Pacific Rim have identified the need for innovative doctoral education programs. Countries and regions like Thailand, Hong Kong, Japan, and Korea historically have sent their young faculty to the United States or other countries for doctoral education. The economic crises in many of these countries, however, has made it difficult for these colleagues to leave home and take up residence in the United States for long periods of time. Through the development of Internet courses and plans for intensive study options, the UCHSC-SON has signed collaborative agreements with a number of institutions in countries and regions on the Pacific Rim, specifically Thailand, Hong Kong, and Japan. The arrangements vary and allow for a number of different options: a degree from the University of Colorado; a degree through collaborative educational programming from the students own country; development of a cohort of international students across country and region boundaries, with shared opportunities for intensive learning experiences in closer proximity to home for study; licensing courses to global educational institutions that have been developed on the Internet for individuals; and facilitating continuing education for faculty who need to update research, education, or practice competencies to develop new roles or refine current roles in these countries.

For the educational challenges in corporate America the faculty at the UCHSC-SON provide the intellectual capital, and e-Vitro and the Global Nursing Academy provide the development and distribution of Internet courseware. Copyright is maintained jointly by the University of Colorado Board of Regents and the faculty member. The win-win for all partners is that the course may be licensed with return on investment to the faculty member (similar to a royalty), a fee for the UCHSC-SON, and revenue for e-Vitro. Several options are possible: selected learners in the corporate setting could become tuition-paying students of the University of Colorado; courses could be licensed only with fees; or SON faculty could be additionally involved with train-the-trainer projects for other institutions interested in offering the Internet courses. Faculty might also be involved if another smaller college or university wanted to offer courseware and enter chat rooms as experts on the knowledge and competencies facilitated by the courseware.

This new model for coalitions or alliances and innovative partnerships is also intended for global distribution and will facilitate the goals of distribution of nurse practitioner education and doctoral education globally. According to Bell and Shea (1998) this model would best be described at this time as the twist. Each member of the coalition or alliance is independent and enters the dance on the basis of its own interest and its own "form of dance." All partners have many options, and as long as the options benefit the partnership, these entities will work together in loose-knit ways. Leadership and faculty in the UCHSC-SON believe that these types of partnerships will shape local and global education in this electronic age of the 21st century.

CASE STUDY 3: BUILDING COALITIONS TO PROVIDE ACCESS AND CARE THROUGH A NURSE-MANAGED CENTER

The Littleton Health and Wellness Clinic is a nurse-managed clinic in a southern suburb of Denver, Colorado. The clinic provides primary health care services to a largely indigent population. The clinic is staffed by a total of 2.3 full-time equivalents that include two family nurse practitioners (FNPs), a pediatric nurse practitioner (PNP), a certified nurse midwife (NMW), and a licensed practical nurse (LPN) with front office and back office responsibilities. The organizational structure is based on the human resources organic model. A democratic decision-making process is facilitated by monthly staff meetings. In addition, clinic staff are involved in community activities, serving as board members, consultants, and fund raisers.

Since it is a community nursing center, coalition building has been imperative for the clinic's survival. One reason coalitions are formed is to share risks and costs. The clinic was initially established via a grant from the U.S. Health Resources and Services Administration, the Division of Nursing. The 5 years of decremental funding helped the clinic establish a presence in the community and an administrative structure on which to build the business. This base has served as a catalyst to spur fund-raising efforts with private and public entities.

Coalitions for political advantage in this case are not necessarily directed at eliminating competition. There are not many providers standing in line to give care to the indigent. Rather, coalitions for political advantage are those that facilitate visibility within the community. One such coalition is with the mayor's office. This relationship has provided an entrée to other government and community-based resources. A second coalition of importance is that with the local health department, a significant referral base for the clinic.

The final reason for coalition development concerns capitalizing on the resources, skills, and knowledge of partners. The school of nursing has embarked upon such a relationship with Ergo Partners, Inc., a software development firm. Ergo's product, CareManager, was purchased for use in the clinic in an attempt to develop a prototype system for advanced nursing practice in ambulatory care. Clinic staff had collected standardized nursing data manually using the Omaha system for over a year. The CareManager product offered a point-of-care system incorporating both standardized nursing and medical language. The product did not incorporate the Omaha language. The vendor, however, was interested in partnering with us as a demonstration site.

This partnership may be most representative of the square dance described by Bell and Shea (1998). Because of the "calls" of outside forces—particularly economic forces and limitations imposed by access to providers in managed care networks—this coalition is made up of many different styles and types of partners who are dancing together. Protocols, procedures, and imposed structures are required to manage the different dimensions of this arrangement. The agreements in some cases have been made based on trust built over the past 5 years that the Littleton Clinic has been in existence. Other partnerships, however, are being based on economic and practice requirements influenced by managed care in the Denver area.

IMPLICATIONS FOR NURSES AND NURSING PROFESSION

Rosenstein (1994, p. 53) reports that "newer industry initiatives have begun to focus on the value for the health care dollar where large health care coalitions have begun to selectively contract with those providers who deliver more effective care." Is nursing ready for this challenge? Nurses have a unique opportunity to position themselves for places of influence in the development of new coalitions, alliances, and partnerships. New opportunities are emerging in both education and practice, but nurses must accept the challenge of exploring new frontiers, learning new competencies, and responding in entrepreneurial ways. We cannot afford to play the victim role; the future belongs to those who take charge of their own development. We must accept individual responsibility for mastering and teaching at least six of the competencies identified by Meister (1998) that global corporations will require in the future: (1) learning to learn new skills competence, (2) leadership development, (3) business literacy, (4) collaboration and team building, (5) technology literacy, and (6) management of one's own career. These ideas are not new but are more and more critical to our survival as individual nurses and as a profession in the 21st century. There are many roles in managed care, but nurses must be willing to work in and with this new market-driven business environment. Nurses are in many ways the best qualified to manage chronic illness with all of the psychoemotion and sociocultural challenges we are prepared to address. Disease management specialists and case managers are two roles that will continue to be important in the future. There are other opportunities emerging in the more mature managed-care markets, such as (1) coordination of care across the continuum, (2) education of providers and consumers regarding prevention and health promotion, (3) facilitating collaborative and interdisciplinary practice, (4) technology and informatics managers, and (5) clinical outcomes researchers in both clinical and educational settings.

Other new roles that are emerging are related to data and research needed to measure cost and quality out-

comes of care. Some disease management teams in mature managed care organizations have an expert in data and information analysis on the team as an equal player with the clinician. New roles for nurse informaticists are clear, particularly those interested in tracking and analyzing relevant data specifically related to the processes and outcomes of care. There are new roles for nurse researchers, particularly those interested in practice-based research and cost and quality outcomes research. More comparative studies demonstrating the cost-effectiveness of nurse-managed models of care such as birthing centers and nursing centers with sound methodological approaches are needed. Stone and Walker (1995) used decision analysis to demonstrate the cost-effectiveness of freestanding birthing centers versus traditional hospital care.

Primary care practice will also continue to be a challenge to maintain positive health outcomes. In some settings, advanced practice nurses are already managing primary care practices with physicians in a collaborative way. Many of our global nursing colleagues are preparing to implement some type of nursing role similar to that of the nurse practitioner in the United States in order to improve primary care outcomes. As a profession, we must find ways to assist our colleagues in their attempt to expand nursing roles, although they will not always look like the roles in the United States. We must also find creative, innovative, and cost-effective ways to facilitate learning across global boundaries. Technology is the answer but will require new ways of teaching, learning, and practicing.

Some managed care organizations are hiring nurses who have advanced knowledge and skills in information technology and business (master of business administration [MBA] or master of science in health administration) to manage some of the provider networks or coalitions associated with the managed care organization. There is a unique niche in the future for blending business, management of technology, clinical practice, and outcomes research. This is evidenced by the increasing numbers of physicians obtaining MBAs or law degrees in order to continue to control clinical decision making instead of just defaulting to the business expert in the organization.

"Many of tomorrow's most intriguing opportunities—interactive television, on-board navigational systems for cars and trucks, cell therapy, remote at-home medical diagnostics, satellite personal communication devices, a national video register of homes for sale, an alternative to the internal combustion engine—will require the integration of skills and capabilities residing in a wide variety of companies" (Hamel & Prahalad, 1994, p. 276). Business coalitions will be dominant in many global markets, including health care and education. The nursing profession must also step up to the challenge of educating its young and its aging workforce in business, law, technology, and leadership development to prepare for changes in the market.

Higher education faculty, administrators, and programs must become more flexible, adaptable, technologically focused, and competent. The challenge of educating for lifelong learning, of updating competencies of our current workforce, and preparing a workforce for the future is significant. New coalitions, alliances, and partnerships will be required. Learners and those organizations that employ lifelong learners are ready to become partners, just as consumers of health care and managed care companies have become our partners. How will we respond? Which dance will we want to perform? How will we prepare for the dance? Will we join the more complex dances that require significant knowledge and competence in the areas of building and maintaining alliances, coalitions, and partnerships, or will we just sit on the side lines while other professions assume many of the responsibilities that traditionally have belonged to nurses? We can just join the line dance, or we can create new dances for local and global challenges of partnership.

REFERENCES

Bell, C.R., & Shea, H. (1998). *Dance lessons.* San Francisco: Berret-Koehler Publishers.

Hamel, G., & Prahalad, C.K. (1994). *Competing for the future: Breakthrough strategies for seizing control of your industry and creating the markets of tomorrow* (p. 23). Boston: Harvard Business Press.

Kaluzny, A.D., Zuckerman, H.S., & Ricketts, T.C. III (with Walton, G.B.) (Eds.). (1995). Strategic alliances: A worldwide phenomenon comes to health care. *Partners for the dance: Forming strategic alliances in health care* (pp. 1-15 and 199-218). Ann Arbor, MI: Health Administration Press.

Kanter, R.M. (1989, August). Becoming PALs: Pooling, allying, and linking across companies. *Academy of Management Executives, 3,* 183-193.

Meister, J.C. (1998). *Corporate universities.* New York: McGraw-Hill.

Merriam-Webster Collegiate Dictionary (10th ed., p. 219). (1994). Springfield, MA: Merriam Webster.

Mintzberg, H. (1977). Policy as a field of management theory. *Academy of Management Review, 2,* 88-103.

Rooney, E. (1992). Business coalitions on health care: An evolution from cost containment to quality improvement. *American Association of Occupational Health Nurses, 40,* 342-351.

Rosenstein, A.H. (1994). Cost-effective health care: Tools for improvement. *Health Care Management Review, 19,* 53-61.

Speckman, R.E., & Isabella, L.A. (with MacAvoy, T.C.). (2000). *Alliance competence.* New York: John Wiley & Sons.

Stone, P.W., & Walker, P. (1995). Cost effective analysis: Birth center vs. hospital care. *Nursing Economic$, 13,* 299-308.

Tichy, N.M. (1983). *Managing strategic change: Technical, political and cultural dynamics.* New York: John Wiley & Sons.

CHAPTER 47

Nursing in a Political Era

MARLA E. SALMON

This chapter explores a fairly simple point of view: nurses have a professional responsibility for influencing health policy. This perspective reflects three premises that are fundamental to understanding nursing and health services in the United States. First, politics and public policy play major roles in shaping the current and emerging state of health care in the United States. Second, any shift toward a more health-oriented system will be driven largely by political and market forces. Third, professional nurses, whose primary orientation is toward promoting and protecting health, have a major stake in shifting the system toward one in which health is a primary goal.

The logic that flows from these premises leads to an important conclusion for nursing: if nurses are going to play a major role in health care in the United States, they will have to assume responsibility for shaping and directing the political forces that are driving this system. In other words, professional nursing practice cannot exist in a politicized health care system without nurses' engaging in the practice of politics and policy.

This chapter explores the notion of nurses practicing in the policy domain. The overall objective of this discussion is to challenge readers to examine their own engagement in this practice and, ultimately, their impact on the health of people.

THE HEALTH CARE SYSTEM AS A PRODUCT OF POLITICS

Historically the United States did not evolve as an organized mechanism for responding to the health care needs of the people. Rather, it reflects the tradition of individualism and entrepreneurialism that characterizes the overall development of this country. As a result, our health care system is anything but systematic. Whether this disorder is explained through the Norman Rockwell–like image of the fatherly physician guiding health care on a person-by-person basis or through a cacophony of forces

including professional dominance, shifting political agendas, and individual and corporate greed, it is clear that the delivery of health care in this country does not reflect a well-thought-out approach to meeting peoples' health care needs.

The rather chaotic nature of health care in the United States, however, is the very reason why politics and public policy are so important to its future. Throughout the last century, government has been asked repeatedly to fix the system in a number of ways, including providing health care for the elderly and poor, ensuring access to care for children, setting limits on how industry behaves, financing research to move health care forward, and constructing health care facilities, among others. Most recently safety and quality of health care have become key issues on the political agenda (Wakefield, 1998).

The involvement of government in health care, which actually began in 1798 with compulsory hospital insurance for merchant seamen (Mullan, 1989), initially focused on the development of public health interventions. Efforts to develop a social insurance–based system of health care in the early part of this century did not succeed (Starr, 1982). As a result, a pattern of fragmentation of financing and health care delivery was set into motion that has continued through the present. The role of government inevitably has been sporadic, ranging from active intervention to invisibility. This is not to say that there have not been forces driving what we see today. On the contrary, our health care "nonsystem" is the direct result of such factors as professional self-interest, corporate interest, and political action, none of which have been mutually exclusive. Political action has been the vehicle for both professional and corporate self-interest. In addition, it has been the single most important voice for the consumer, the mechanism by which the people can have a voice.

To understand how these forces have worked, one need only consider what has transpired with national health care reform since 1993. National health care reform was a major plank in the Clinton presidential campaign. With nearly 40 million Americans lacking health care insurance, millions of others uninsured, and growing concern about the runaway costs of health care, national health care reform was seen as critical for the United States. Americans seemed to want the federal government to "fix" the problems of health care. As a result the Clinton administration launched its Task Force on Health Care Reform and developed a proposal for comprehensive national health care reform that was formalized in the President's proposed Health Security Act.

The national debate on health care reform during that period was also heavily influenced by professional and corporate interest. Organized nursing, for example, was a vocal advocate for national reform and had made its interests known with the development of Nursing's Agenda for Health Care Reform in 1991 (American Nurses Association, 1991). Other professional groups were less supportive of overall health care reform. Many corporations with a financial stake in health care (e.g., insurers and pharmaceutical manufacturers) heavily influenced the final outcomes of the national health care reform effort.

One major lesson learned from the defeat of national health care reform was that health care unquestionably had become politicized. Through the political process the health care system of this country became a highly market-driven system in which the role of government became less, rather than more, involved in assuring its effectiveness.

MOVEMENT TO A HEALTH-ORIENTED SYSTEM

The overall goals of national health care reform in the early 1990s were aimed at increasing access, reducing cost, and ensuring quality of services. Since that time a market-driven health care system emerged that was not well equipped to address these goals in equal measure (Keepnews & Marullo, 1996). Initially the goal of reducing cost combined with the related interest in enhancing corporate gain and profit was the most prominent consideration in how health care was restructured. Many of health care's "marketers" believed that unleashing unregulated market forces not only would drive down the cost of health care but also would improve the overall quality of services because of the importance of quality in consumer choice. Others believed the overall reduction in the cost of health care would allow public resources to be stretched further to enhance access to services. A common theme across health care, however, was that a cost-and-profit-driven health care system would result in major systems change

and require provider organizations to encourage health promotion and disease prevention activities.

The critical question now, of course, is whether the wildfire corporatization of health care has actually enhanced the health of people. Unlike the national health care reform proposal of the Clinton Administration, the system that evolved over the last decade does not yet have clear mechanisms in place relating to quality of care and access. The traditional relationship between patient and provider, which was shaped by professional and legal checks and balances, has been overshadowed by a less well understood relationship between payers and health care organizations in which the legal latitude of the patient has changed. In the past, health professionals have been major determinants of the quality and nature of health care. Licensure, state practice acts, education, and professionalization have been seen as mechanisms for ensuring quality and expressing the public's endorsement of health professionals' roles.

With the movement away from provider-patient control of health care delivery, there is now widespread uncertainty on the part of patients and providers about who actually controls health care. As a result the concerns of citizens and providers alike have been expressed politically. An early indicator of this type of political activity was the passage of state legislation dictating the minimum length of hospital stays for new mothers and babies. Other political efforts seem to be aimed at putting into place some legislative checks and balances at state levels relating to accountability for quality and access. And the ongoing debate about the liability of individual and corporate providers of health care continues. The creation of President Clinton's Advisory Commission on Consumer Protection and Quality in the Health Care Industry in 1997 was a key indicator that all was not well with the health care system of the 1990s (Trossman, 1998; Wakefield, 1997).

The most recent signs that the health care system is floundering are particularly troubling. Most would agree that the goals of enhanced access and improved quality have not been achieved: we have more uninsured people than ever before, and there is serious public concern about health care quality. The recent news that costs are again on the rise (*Atlanta Journal-Constitution*, 2000) is perhaps the most troubling of all. Uncontrolled rising costs promise to create more chaos in the health care system as we once again try to find ways to contain cost. This has major implications for further public policy and political action. Whether one is an employer, provider, corporation, or individual patient, all will look to government in some form to address these serious issues. It is no accident that health care again was a major issue in the 2000 presidential campaign.

With health care back on the policy agenda, nurses and other health professionals will be crucial in shaping a system that ultimately serves the interests of those in need of care. We learned during the 1990s that a health care system in which market forces are the prominent drivers does not put the interests of patients or society in the forefront of concern. We also should have learned that public policy—*and its absence*—plays a key role in shaping our system of health care. Who will guide the policy agenda for health care in the future? Will it reflect advocacy for societal good? Will the concerns of quality, access, and cost be balanced in whatever equation emerges? Or will we see an even greater reliance on market forces to shape the system, hoping that further deregulation and movement away from the control of patients and health professionals creates new solutions to these challenges.

The profession of nursing has much to lose in the future. Clearly bread-and-butter issues of employment conditions and security have characterized the last decade of health care. But more importantly, nursing's professional role as advocate and effective caregiver is at stake. The extent to which nurses will be able to fulfill these roles rests with current policy and the policy that will emerge in the near future.

If this discussion creates some discomfort in the nurse reader, it should. Although nursing as a profession made major gains in the 20th century in its ability to function as a profession (Keeling & Ramos, 1995), its impact on the delivery of services may be in serious jeopardy. To be sure, there will always be nurses. The more important question is whether they will be able to play the roles for which they are prepared. The relationship between nurse, patients, and families is no longer simple. The major players in the health care system—care organization, payer, politics, and public policy—are increasingly determining whether a nurse even comes into contact with the patient and his or her family. If nursing has as its fundamental purpose the enhancement and preservation of the health of people, it can no longer do so only through the interactions of those people it "sees." Nursing must move its practice to a broader social level and involve itself with the forces that are, in fact, shaping that system.

NURSING AS A POLITICAL PROFESSION

The notion that politics and health are intrinsically linked is not new. In fact, Nightingale herself clearly made the connection between the political decisions of Parliament in England and the conditions in which soldiers found themselves in the Crimea. American nursing has also known of this link and has involved itself in shaping the political forces that affect health. Health policy in the early part of the century was influenced by the voices of such remarkable nurses as Sanger, Wald, and Dock, who understood clearly that the plight of those whom they hoped to serve was influenced heavily by the presence or absence of sound public policy (Hall-Long, 1995). They were consummate political activists who were clear that their advocacy was on behalf of the people whom they served. Their common goal was to enhance the health of these people through constructive public policy.

The realization of the importance of political activism in nursing has not been restricted to the notables of the early 1900s. The last century of nursing's history saw a dramatic increase in the number of professional organizations and the rise in organized political activism in nursing. Nursing has recognized the importance of political activism to its own survival and to the health of the people it serves. Nursing's prominence in the national health care reform debates at the end of the 20th century was a strong indicator of nursing's political successes (Clinton, 1993; "Health Care Reform," 1993; Sprayberry, 1993).

Given nursing's political sophistication, one might question why it is now necessary to call for political action on the part of nurses. The imperative rests in the recognition that this emerging health care system is unlike any we have seen before, and it is seriously flawed. The roles of nurses and other health professionals—and even patients—in the system are increasingly less clear, and the impact of this system on the health of people has not been favorable. In short, the stakes are high for both the health of people and the future of nursing.

So what should nursing do? First, it is essential that nursing accept political responsibility for the current and future health care system. This is not to say that nurses alone are responsible for what has or will transpire. Rather, if nursing is to play a crucial role in the health of people in the future, it must assume responsibility for the system on a larger societal level. It is not enough to be responsible for only those people we touch in the everyday delivery of care. Because the marketplace and politics are key venues for making an impact, nursing must weigh in politically. Because so much of the political action in health care will occur at state and national levels, these should be the primary foci for major nursing political activity.

Secondly, nursing must examine critically what it has done in the area of political action and where it wishes to go. The tradition of nursing political action has been one in which nursing has focused largely on unifying its own political forces within the profession and on issues relating to the profession itself or to specific proposed legislative agendas. It is important to analyze these dimensions of political activity carefully.

There are a number of examples of nursing's unification to strengthen its political clout. Perhaps the most prominent is the formation of the Tri-Council for Nursing in 1981, composed initially of the American Nurses Association, the National League for Nursing, the American Association of Colleges of Nursing, and, later, the American Organization of Nurse Executives. This alliance and others have been instrumental in galvanizing the various interests across organized nursing into consolidated political action. As individual professional organizations face challenges relating to their own identities and viability, presenting a unified front becomes problematic. If nursing is to be effective now and in the future, its organizations will need to supersede organizational self-interest and continue to forge key, strategic political alliances across nursing groups.

Although nursing has become more sophisticated about alliances across nursing and consolidating its own political power, the political challenges facing the profession call for expanding effectively beyond nursing's boundaries. Although nursing has at times developed alliances with other groups in both state and national political arenas, this has not been the hallmark of its ongoing political activism. This must change. As the impact of the marketplace increasingly overshadows the roles that health professionals and patients play in the determination of care, two types of natural alliances seem to be emerging.

The first natural alliance is probably the least comfortable for organized nursing and its potential counterpart, organized medicine. Although the longstanding chasms in the political landscape between the two groups are clear, there is a rapidly expanding common ground that needs to be cultivated by both. Nursing, medicine, and other health professional groups are experiencing major threats to both their professional autonomy and the quality of care for which they traditionally have been responsible. If the emerging health care system is to achieve a reasonable set of checks and balances in which cost is part of a larger equation that includes quality and access, it will be because of social and political activism. It makes great sense that nursing and medicine should lead in these efforts, given their longstanding shared social mandate of caring for the health of people.

The second natural alliance is with consumers and communities. As our health care system emerges, major changes are taking place in the ways in which care is delivered and its impact on communities. For example, the community hospital or clinic may be an important institution to the community in which it is located. Unfortunately these resources have been imperiled or have ceased to exist in the face of new ways of delivering service. So also is the case with the individual physician or other provider. Systems of service also mean systems of providers. The fabric of communities increasingly will be affected by the changes in the overall system.

For the individual consumer the emerging health care system also indicates major change. As individual concerns become more public, individual activism also will become better organized. The history of health policy nationally is one in which consumers have organized and weighed in on the debates. One only need examine the debates around the restructuring of Medicare and the grave and growing concerns about the financing of health care for older Americans to see this type of consumer activism.

As the concerns and involvement of consumers become better organized, nursing has an opportunity to amplify and focus its own political power. Nursing has claimed that one of its key roles is that of patient advocate. The alliance of organized nursing with organized consumer groups is the political equivalent of the individual nurse's serving as the patient's advocate.

Let us look again at what nursing should be concerned with politically. The themes of the Clinton health care reform agenda are still compelling and valid: high-quality, affordable health care for all people. Nursing's political agenda should continue to focus on these key goals, and it should do so in partnership with others who share those commitments.

NURSING'S ACTIVISM IN HEALTH POLICY: GOING BEYOND A NARROW VIEW OF POLITICAL ACTIVISM

Any discussion of the impact of nursing on a societal level must go beyond the rather restrictive view of political activism. Nurses need to see themselves as politically responsible, well beyond the basic function of voting. Nursing must also see itself as politically responsible beyond influencing the legislative process through lobbying and grassroots efforts. These are certainly essential and a part of all that has been discussed here. Nursing, however, must view itself as engaged in all of the processes that result in public policy relating to health. This is a far broader agenda and requires consideration of ground that probably is not familiar to nurses.

Perhaps the easiest way to describe where nurses should weigh in is to describe the dimensions of public policy that affect health care today. The first is the identi-fication of problems that need policy solutions. Surely there is no better time than now to begin to identify what is not working well in the emerging system of health care. It is important to note here that initially identifying prob-lems in a politically relevant way is frequently best done through use of the media and anecdotal evidence. This is not to say that one should not attempt to document problems carefully. Rather it is to suggest that the politi-cal system is highly media sensitive and tends to be more responsive to those issues that receive the attention of the media. Now is the time for nurses to tell their stories and the stories of those they serve. One cannot expect policy-makers to become concerned about problems that are not brought to their attention. This is an area in which nurses should become better equipped. For better or worse, Americans look to media such as talk-radio, exposé re-porting, and afternoon talk shows to inform their opin-ions. Nurses need to become fluent in the ways in which people get and give information.

Once problems are identified, the transition to devel-oping viable policy agendas can be difficult. Effective agenda setting for health policy depends on having people in public office and public service who understand the problems related to health care delivery and who are knowledgeable about and committed to health issues. Nurses need to participate actively in the development of health agendas, not just in influencing legislation. Because these agendas generally precede the development of legis-lation and involve policymakers, nurses should become involved in key advisory roles that are directly related to this process at all levels. For example, the recent highly in-fluential President's Advisory Commission on Consumer Protection and Quality in the Health Care Industry had nurses who served as members. This group has had an im-pact on agenda setting for national health policy in Con-gress and elsewhere. Membership in such groups is an im-portant vehicle for nursing's voice. As well, serving in Congress or state legislatures in elected or staff positions is a key role that nurses should be playing. The message here, of course, is that nurses should consider public service as an important avenue for having a professional impact.

Once a policy agenda is developed, it may then move to the stage of developing program proposals and sup-portive legislation. In the area of health this means that nurses should be playing active roles in developing the ac-tual strategies for addressing the problems and imple-menting an agenda. Again, active, ongoing roles in Con-gress and state legislatures are important for nursing involvement. As proposals and actual legislation move

forward, it is also important that nurses be prepared to serve as experts in informing the process by providing testimony and input to legislators. (If this were all that nurses did, however, it simply would not be enough.)

It is important to note here that not all policy is en-acted through legislation. Most presidents and governors come into office with their own policy platforms and seek to accomplish these through both the executive and leg-islative branches of government. Their choices of political appointees for key positions can have a major impact on the nature of governmental action. Nurses should seek political appointment and understand the type of politi-cal activism required for one to become positioned for these types of appointments.

For policy that is enacted through legislation, the stage following enactment is one in which nursing should also play a key role. The actual implementation of legislation moves the law into the "machinery" of government and relies on the bureaucracy to do what is intended legisla-tively. There is usually latitude in the interpretation and implementation of legislation; most laws are not micro-scopic in their language. The old adage that "the devil is in the details" is very true when it comes to actually making laws work. Implementation of health legislation can ben-efit greatly from the advice and involvement of nurses. Most nurses probably do not consider moving into careers in government. The important knowledge and skills that nurses can bring to moving legislation into actual imple-mentation should not be overlooked, however. Nurses in-terested in policy should consider both the executive and legislative branches of government as career options.

Finally, laws that have been enacted generally have some requirements or expectations for assessment of im-pact. Frequently, assessments of this type are undertaken as studies or projects by contractors outside the govern-ment itself. This is an area in which nurses can also play roles. Schools of nursing, for example, might begin to look at evaluation research contracts as an area in which their nurse researchers might be involved. Nurse re-searchers themselves should consider conducting health services research that can shed light on the impact of pol-icy on the delivery and effectiveness of health services. Nurses should actively seek opportunities to become in-volved in all dimensions of the assessment of government program effectiveness.

SUMMARY

The ability of nurses to have a positive impact on health is no longer primarily determined by the capabilities of the individual nurse and the health status of individual patients and families. Nursing, as with all that is health care today, is being shaped by the societal forces found in the marketplace and the public policy arena. If nursing is to be all that it claims—the patient's advocate and a profession with a commitment to achieving, protecting, and preserving health—it must strive to direct those forces that are shaping the system of health care delivery in this country. In other words, the practice of nursing at all levels should include the practice of public policy.

REFERENCES

American Nurses Association. (1991). *Nursing's agenda for health care reform.* Kansas City, MO: Author.

The Atlanta Journal-Constitution. (2000, February 29). Health care costs (p. C1).

Clinton, H.R. (1993). Nurses in the front lines. *Nursing & Health Care, 14*(6), 286-288.

Hall-Long, B.A. (1995). Nursing's past, present, and future political experiences. *Nursing & Health Care: Perspectives on Community, 16*(1), 24-28.

Health care reform: A politically high-risk venture, Washington focus. (1993, May). *Nursing & Health Care, 14*(5), 236-237.

Keeling, A.W., & Ramos, M.C. (1995). The role of nursing history in preparing nursing for the future: Nursing policy forum. *Nursing & Health Care: Perspectives on Community, 16*(1), 30-34.

Keepnews, D., & Marullo, G. (1996). Policy imperatives for nursing in an era of health care restructuring. *Nursing Administration Quarterly, 20*(3), 19-31.

Mullan, F. (1989). *Plagues and politics* (p. 14). New York: Basic Books.

Sprayberry, L.D. (1993). Nursing's dual role in health care policy. *Nursing & Health Care, 14*(5), 250-254.

Starr, P. (1982). *The social transformation of American medicine* (p. 241). New York: Basic Books.

Trossman, S. (1998). Quality managed care: A nursing perspective. *American Journal of Nursing, 98*(6), 56-58.

Wakefield, M. (1998). Engaging in the policy dialogue. *Journal of Professional Nursing, 14*(2), 68.

Wakefield, M. (1997). MNA member appointed to national commission on health care quality. *Maryland Nurse, 16*(1), 1.

The Corporatization of Health Care

Mergers and Acquisitions

MARJORIE BEYERS

Few business approaches illustrate the effects of corporatization on health care as well as mergers and acquisitions do. The context of this chapter is corporatization of health care as characterized by application or adaptation of generic business approaches to health care. These business approaches are apparent in the way health care is financed, organized, managed, and delivered and in the use of terms such as *the health care industry* or the *enterprise*. An underlying theme in the discussion of impact of mergers and acquisitions is that corporatization of health care has disrupted long held beliefs that the business of health care should be kept separate from patient care (Beyers, 1999). Mergers and acquisitions challenge this philosophy by using business approaches to achieve service goals.

A cautionary word about mergers and acquisitions is useful. Each merger or acquisition is unique (Pritchett, 1997). Because the impact of mergers or acquisitions is unpredictable, a succinct or specific analysis is not possible. Therefore insights into mergers and acquisitions are presented with the intent that they be applied as appropriate to specific situations. Many factors can influence the response to and eventual impact of a merger or an acquisition. For example, the impact of a hostile merger is very different from the impact achieved when the involved groups mutually agree on the merger or acquisition from the early stages onward. The perspective of individuals or groups also influences the impact, as does the meaning the merger or acquisition has for the individual or group. The reasons for change, the degree of support and acceptance by stakeholders, and the leadership are other factors influencing the impact.

Mergers and acquisitions, once rare and anxiety producing in health care, are now more common but no less anxiety producing. The very mention of mergers and acquisitions produces anxiety because they signal signifi-

cant change that has uncertain outcomes. They have been compared to marriages; some work and some do not. Every situation of merger or acquisition has to be analyzed for its own characteristics including the organizational cultures, the relationships of the organizations to the community, the financial status of the organizations, and the community's perception of service and accessibility. Different individuals or groups may respond differently to the merger or acquisition. What some view as a positive move may be perceived by others as negative. Few individuals or groups are untouched by a merger or an acquisition.

THE MAIN IMPACT: WAS THE MERGER OR ACQUISITION SUCCESSFUL?

The chief reason for mergers and acquisitions is to further the strategic achievement of business goals. Formerly the primary purpose of mergers and acquisitions was to achieve economies of scale and scope through consolidation. Resources and services were consolidated to improve cost effectiveness through increasing the critical mass of users, reducing redundancy, standardizing work processes, and targeting outcomes (Baker et al., 1999; Zelman, 1998). The improvement through economies of scale and scope has not consistently met the expectations. Over time, some mergers have not proved beneficial, resulting in revisiting and renewing the terms of the merger. In some situations the merger is turned around. Some mergers or acquisitions are irrevocable.

Despite concerns about the outcomes of past mergers or acquisitions, they continue to be a strategy for the times. A merger or acquisition may now mean survival for a health care entity. In today's "new economy," growth and expansion are critical to success in business. Mergers and acquisitions provide a way to become more competitive in the market place through increased capacity to respond to customers (Kingman & Prehein, 1999). Mergers and acquisitions can be used to acquire capital to stabilize or grow the organization (Carey, 2000). Recognizing that it is difficult to accomplish anything by yourself in these times, many health care organizations are reviewing their strategic plans and objectives and evaluating their resources and level of technological strength to identify strategies for faster development and implementation (Davidson, 1996; Weaver & Sorrells-Jones, 1999).

IMPACT ON EMPLOYEES

Mergers and acquisitions bring about periods of intense change and challenges for people. Leadership is needed to help employees navigate the change. Information is key, as is having a champion for the change. It can be expected that each of the involved organizations has an established pattern of change. Bringing different change patterns together in the process of early integration helps one understand how the changes will be made over time. How change is made influences the readiness and willingness of employees to participate (Weaver & Sorrells-Jones, 1999). Because employees are stressed in relation to their jobs and future, communication is essential to overcome the hurdles of gaining commitment to change and participation to identify the best change strategies (Kanter, 1997). Each situation needs to be assessed to determine the readiness levels of employees and the best strategies for change information and communication.

The impact of mergers and acquisitions on everyone is more likely to be positive if the purposes are achieved. Acquisitions particularly are highly visible in the community, and the perception of failure can be devastating (Carey, 2000). Early involvement of employees and community members fosters acceptance of the merger or acquisition, which may eventually influence the outcomes. It is easier to involve community members when the decision to merge or acquire is made through extensive debate and deliberation with key stakeholders in the community and the involved organizations. Involvement is difficult in highly competitive situations in which decision making is not as open.

Although mergers and acquisitions achieve similar purposes, they are somewhat different. Both are complex, but acquisitions tend to be more straightforward than mergers. Mergers usually involve integration of two or more similar businesses into one organization to secure its future or to support growth. In comparison to the processes of acquisitions, the processes of merging are

long term and often diffuse. The impact of the merger is colored by the reasons for the merger, conditions of the merger, and negotiated terms such as the percentage of ownership and protections for the community and employees. Acquisitions are usually undertaken to expand a business. The acquired business becomes a component of the parent, and the extent of integration varies. In some cases the acquired business may continue in its present state with no major changes other than reporting relationships. In other cases the financial and management structures may change, but the expertise and work processes of the acquired entity remain much the same, largely because the work is different from that of the new owner.

A key question in acquisitions is, Should we acquire something that now exists elsewhere, or should we make our own? Current assets and services and organizational capacity are assessed to answer the "make or buy" question (Carey, 2000). Acquiring existing assets, products, or services allows an organization to expand its products and services to customers. Another reason for acquisitions is to establish new distribution channels or expand customer bases useful to build comprehensive services, as in the patient care continuum.

IMPACT OF MERGERS AND ACQUISITIONS ON LEADERSHIP

Leadership is critical to the success of mergers or acquisitions. Both strain leadership to its limits. One of the complicating factors is that leaders are stretched to deal with the merger or acquisition and often do not have sufficient time to work effectively with employees. Because there is a paucity of research findings to guide decisions in mergers and acquisitions, most leaders must forge their way through the complex processes of planning, implementing, and sustaining a merger or an acquisition. At the same time they must keep the organization functioning, which is difficult enough in the turbulent health care system.

Resources for these leaders include consultation, anecdotal information from peers and colleagues, case studies of other mergers or acquisitions, and business analysis. The capability to work diligently to achieve an effective merger or acquisition challenges leadership. Positive attitudes toward change and the ability to support others in the change processes are required to lead employees and community members in the changes associated with mergers or acquisitions. Many leaders must overcome their personal responses to the change to effectively help others accept and adapt to the new changes (Davidson,

1996). This leadership is taxing, particularly when the leader usually has the most tenuous job future.

Mergers and acquisitions present a leadership challenge. While leaders are negotiating the terms of mergers and acquisitions over time, they must also be providing clear communication to those affected (Parsons, Murdaugh, & O'Rourke, 1998). Ambiguity is not well tolerated in times of merger and acquisition. Providing appropriate information in a timely way can be complex, particularly if the negotiations are limited to a few people behind closed doors because of competition or other issues. The phases of negotiation can be communicated. Usually mergers and acquisitions are negotiated in phases, beginning with the business portfolio, followed by integration of people and processes of the organization. Most employees and many community members have difficulty waiting for the business side to be completed because their future is at stake in the people and processes phases. Generally the organizational integration begins with computer services, financial systems, and evaluation and data systems.

A strategy to gain participation and support of employees is to begin the work of integration in the planning phases. Two considerations in support of early integration are retaining key employees and maintaining consistency in community services during the change. Incentives are needed to retain talent during times of change. Another compelling reason for retaining employees is that employees throughout the organization have the priceless "organizational memory." Employee memory recently has been rediscovered as a valuable commodity in organizations. This employee memory is closely aligned with employee loyalty, a valuable asset in any organization (Cross & Baird, 2000). Key employees can ask the right questions about the logic of the change and about the work processes, which can save time and resources as the merger or acquisition unfolds.

Early management structures for integration include provision for evaluation of level of performance, dealing with inevitable loss of identity, adapting and changing cultures to become a new organization, and assessing the strengths and talents throughout the involved organizations. In many instances, consultants are retained to assist with the change processes (Weaver & Sorrells-Jones, 1999). Other reasons to support early integration management strategies are to help employees deal with the inevitable loss of identity, to help them adjust to management styles of consultants and merger or acquisition teams, and to learn new roles or functions. Nurturing trust in leadership and helping people separate culture from work processes are important early integration objectives.

Some mergers or acquisitions are highly emotional, but all are made on the basis of analyzing the business options available. For example, partnerships and strategic alliances may be used to achieve some of the same business goals as mergers and acquisitions, such as enhancing services, pooling resources, sharing risk, combining strengths, or expanding customer bases while achieving their respective identities (Pollard, 2000). The existing services, willingness to partner or align, and agreement on common goals and mutual benefit all influence whether partnerships or strategic alliances are viable options. These options involve complex change in organizations in different ways and in varying degrees, but mergers and acquisitions have potential for more permanent and penetrating change in the involved organizations.

INTEGRATION: AN ACHIEVABLE GOAL?

The success of mergers or acquisitions is often evaluated on the degree of integration achieved. Some mergers or acquisitions are successful; some are not. When two or more organizations merge or when an organization is acquired, a process of integration is used to create a new organization. The goal is to improve productivity, cost-effectiveness, quality, and consistency in the production of services or to expand services to offer a continuum of care that is accessible and user friendly for patients and their families.

Review of the business literature indicates that mergers are more successful with "widget"-producing type businesses than with those that are knowledge intensive (Carey, 2000). The knowledge-intensive businesses are more volatile with shifting opportunities. They grow and change rapidly with little attention to quality. Health care, although not as volatile as some high-technology companies, is essentially a knowledge business. The integration of financial aspects of the organization, for example, is generally more successful than integration of clinical services. This difference may be attributed to the fact that nurses, doctors, and others are knowledge workers. Other anecdotal information on mergers and acquisitions indicates that success or failure is often related to the responses from the key stakeholders affected by the change.

In some of the early mergers or acquisitions within health care there was an expectation that clinical integration would follow naturally once the financial and organizational leadership issues were resolved. This expectation did not prove to be the case in practice. Clinical integration continues to be difficult. The various cultures and financial aspects of clinical services are often barriers to integration. A key issue is lack of clarity on the meaning of clinical integration (Formella & Balner, 1999). In some cases, clinical integration refers to the integration to form a continuum of care services including acute, long-term, home, and hospice care (Schaffner et al., 1999). In other cases, clinical integration refers to standardization of clinical processes and analysis to reduce variance and to improve quality. In yet other cases, clinical integration involves formation of multidisciplinary care teams (Parsons et al., 1998; Williams, 1998). The variation in cultures and operational processes within health care entities continues to confound the issue of clinical integration.

IMPACT OF MERGERS AND ACQUISITIONS ON SPONSORS AND OWNERS

The ultimate decision to merge, to acquire, or to be acquired rests with the sponsors or owners of the organization. Boards may drive action toward mergers and acquisitions, or they may be one of the first key stakeholder groups engaged in the discussions. In either case the board members are key stakeholders and leaders in determining the vision and strategies for the organization that guide decision making (Pritchett, 1997). Work on continuity to sustain the changes is an important factor, as is dealing with the complex issues of implementation. Board members usually have a significant personal stake in keeping an organization going. They may serve to connect people prepared to represent the interests of stakeholders, shareholders, and management in mergers. A challenge to sponsors and boards in mergers and acquisitions is creating a new identity for the organization being formed through the merger or acquisition. Creating a new identity implies that existing identities may be lost. Efforts to retain connection with the existing organizations may prevail through incorporating something from each of the organizations in the name or logo. In other instances the dominant organization's name may be used. It is not uncommon to "transcend" the merged organizations' identity by creating an entirely new identity for the new organization.

In all of these scenarios it is easier to be the acquiring than the acquired. Many health care organizations have deep historic roots that are meaningful not only within the organization but also in the community (Kanter, 1997). The situation leading to the decision to merge colors the impact. Sponsors often take the attitude that they honor the accomplishments of past leaders by ensuring the future of the organization's mission through the merger or acquisition. Gaining consensus at the sponsor or owner level may be contentious, and to some degree the decision to change causes disruption, pain, and loss, even when it is clear that the change is the right thing to do. Sponsors or owners, knowing that once the change is begun, it cannot be undone, often push for conservative approaches to meet the current resource needs. The future is unpredictable, and decades of commitment and work can be lost in communities when the service identity is changed or services are disrupted. The sponsors or owners may prevent a merger or acquisition or may complicate the merger or acquisition processes before, during, or after they unfold. The attitude of these leaders influences responses of others and thus the impact of the change.

IMPACT OF MERGERS AND ACQUISITIONS ON COMMUNITY

Health care is local. People in a community usually have strong feelings about their health care and consider health care organizations a community asset. Health care organizations not only provide essential community services but also are a driver of financial strength in a community. Health care organizations, particularly hospitals, are a source of jobs, thus directly influencing the community's economy and support of public services such as schools, churches, and community services. On the other hand, the community is the market place and source of consumers. The unique interdependence between communities and their health care organizations is grounded in the interchange between the health care organization and the community. Health care is an essential community service, providing help and support. Many hospitals have reached out to the community to learn about key health issues and population needs for health care and have established projects to improve community health (Price, 1998). As a result of mergers, these initiatives may continue or may be interrupted or discontinued.

Because health care is integral to the community life, mergers or acquisitions evoke community response and reactions. Again the situation of the change influences the response. Community leaders may block a merger or acquisition or may fully support the change, depending on their perspective. A key issue is whether community needs will continue to be met at the same or better level. If the community needs take second place to the merger goals, the merger or acquisition may be perceived, appropriately, as a loss of essential community services. The community accountability is a strong countervailing force in deliberations about mergers and acquisitions.

IMPACT OF MERGERS AND ACQUISITIONS ON THE HEALTH CARE ORGANIZATION

The impact of mergers and acquisitions on the organization depends on the perceived and real benefits. Benefits of mergers include survival, increased market share, improved service delivery, and improved quality through improved logistics and coordination. The key to positive attitudes and cooperation in mergers and acquisitions is mutual trust and mutually agreed on processes and objectives. Involvement of all parties in analysis of business objectives and transition planning encourages understanding and fosters commitment (Formella & Balner, 1999). It is easier but no less complex to be the acquirer rather than the acquired: the holder of 51% or higher of the merged organizations. The work of mergers encompasses agreeing on common goals and working together to resolve problems and remove obstacles. Transferring customer loyalty to the new organization and sustaining relationships are ongoing processes throughout all phases of the merger (Cross & Baird, 2000). Achieving mutual trust, commitment, consensus, and involvement challenges leadership (Coile, 2000). The work of mergers and acquisitions challenges leadership at every level of the organization.

Because research findings to guide decisions in mergers and acquisitions are sparse, most leaders must forge their way through the complex processes of planning, implementing, and sustaining a merger or an acquisition (Baker et al., 2000; Williams, 1998). Resources for these leaders include consultation, anecdotal information from peers and colleagues, case studies of other mergers or acquisitions, and business analysis.

ECONOMIC IMPACT

The economic impact of mergers and acquisitions is complicated. Job security is a major issue for individuals whose jobs are affected by mergers and acquisitions. Job identity is as strong an issue for many when they perceive that their role or function will be significantly altered in the merger or acquisition. Typically, administrative and management positions are most vulnerable in mergers or acquisitions, but employees in all types of positions usually share feelings of vulnerability about their jobs, relationships, and future employment. The economy of the community may also be affected when a merger or acqui-

sition leads to downsizing or significant loss of jobs in the area. In many communities the hospital or health care system is a financial driver, and any changes in the hospital or health system are likely to affect other aspects of the community economy.

IMPACT ON NURSING

Nursing has been affected significantly by mergers and acquisitions. The established model of nursing practice in any organization represents commitment and a sense of ownership that is difficult to give up. When two or more nursing departments are merged, the professional practice models are often integrated. As with the identity, this integration may involve blending by taking the best of each and forming a new whole, by establishing the nursing model of the dominant organization as the "corporate" model, or by creating a new model. Also often affected are aspects of the organization that support nursing practice including clinical support systems of education and quality improvement and policies and practices for ongoing education. Work processes, forms, and general procedures may also change as part of "standardization" in mergers, requiring adaptation of the nursing staff. Nursing leadership is challenged to provide direction, to keep the focus on professional nursing practice, and to ensure that the standards of clinical nursing practice are upheld as the tools, procedures, and supports are assessed and adapted to the new organization. Another leadership challenge is to analyze the change and to identify or recognize opportunities to strengthen or enhance clinical patient care.

Given the essential nature of nursing in health care delivery, it is inconceivable that nursing has not realized its strong potential to be a countervailing force in change. Nursing's significant, unrealized potential to affect the health care infrastructure and financing is a factor in how mergers and acquisitions progress through implementation. Corporatization of health care provides an entrée for nursing to strengthen and expand the clinical care role of nurses (Beyers, 1999). Recent challenges to traditional roles and functions such as who can prescribe medications, changes in reimbursement, and societal trends toward consumer participation create a new environment for nursing practice. New technology has heralded new roles and functions for health professionals, as have initiatives such as total quality management and integrated work processes (Williams, 1998).

Nurses are in a good position to design patient care services, to evaluate the quality of patient care services, and to debate the issues of health care rights. Nurses are also well positioned to debate the issues of not only how to finance health care but also of how the resources should be deployed in the evolving health care system. The movement from a public service to a business model can be used to advantage by nurses ready and willing to lead nursing toward a new future. To move toward this future, nursing will be pressed to ensure a strong financial and business base for nursing services. As with any service, the success of the financial and business base depends on the quality of the service. Designing quality patient care services continues to be a key, essential role for nurse administrators. The business and finance aspect can be viewed as tools to accomplish the goals of the patient service design.

Nurses are also aware of the "human condition" in the communities they serve. In many cases, people in these communities require health services that do not have a cost or price. These services, which may be categorized as public or community service, are just as important as the reimbursed services. Consequently, nurses should carefully consider whether it is prudent to fully buy-in to the business approaches that achieve health care corporatization. Some community health care services such as the outreach programs do not fit the corporate business model. Yet these services are important to the health care mission. Nurses have long served as the conscience of health care. Nurses are with patients 24 hours a day, in every setting where health care is delivered. Patients trust nurses. Nurses are perceived to be patient advocates because they put the patient first. Nurses understand what patients experience in their health care complexity. Nurses know that some of the most salient aspects of health care do not have a price, cannot be packaged or branded, and would not be considered useful for leverage or other business purposes. Nurses relate to and speak for the human condition, which transcends corporatization.

REFERENCES

Baker, C.M., Ogden, S.J., Prapaipanich, W., Keith, C.K., Beattie, L.C., & Nickleson, L.E. (1999). Hospital consolidation: Applying stakeholder analysis to merger life-cycle. *Journal of Nursing Administration, 29*(3), 11-19.

Baker, C.M., Messmer, P.L., Gyurko, C.C., Domagala, S.E., Conly, F.M., Eads, T.S., Harshman, K.S., & Layne, M.K. (2000). Hospital ownership, performance, and outcomes: Assessing the state-of-the-science. *Journal of Nursing Administration, 30*(5), 227-240.

Beyers, M. (1999). In R.W. Gilkey (Ed.), *The 21st century health care leader* (pp. 278-289). San Francisco: Jossey-Bass.

Carey, D., moderator. (2000). Lessons from master acquirers: A CEO roundtable on making mergers succeed. *Harvard Business Review, 78*(3), 146-166.

Coile, R.C., Jr. (2000). *New century healthcare* (pp. 225-249). Chicago: Health Administration Press.

Cross, R., & Baird, L. (2000). Technology is not enough: Improving performance by building organizational memory. *The Sloan Management Review, 41*(3), 69-78.

Davidson, D.R. (1996). The role of the nurse executive. In B. Brown (Ed.) and R. Anderson (Guest Ed.), Corporatization of health care. *Nursing Administration Quarterly, 20*(1), 49-53.

Formella, N.M., & Balner, J. (1999). Role transitions for patient care vice presidents: From a single entity to a system focus. *Journal of Nursing Administration, 29*(4), 11-17.

Kanter, E.R. (1997). Restoring the heart in the organization of the future. In F. Hesselbein, M. Goldsmith, & R. Beckhard (Eds.), *The organization of the future* (pp. 139-150). San Francisco: Jossey-Bass.

Kingman, M., & Prehein, G. (1999). Longitudinal evaluation of professional nursing practice redesign. *Journal of Nursing Administration, 29*(5), 10-20.

Parsons, M.L., Murdaugh, C.L., & O'Rourke, R.A. (1998). *Interdisciplinary case studies in health care redesign*. Gaithersburg, MD: Aspen.

Pollard, C.W. (2000, Spring). Immersion as an organizing principle. *Leader to Leader, 16*, 17-21.

Price, H.B. (1998). Gaining equal access in economic power. In F. Hesselbein, M. Goldsmith, R. Beckhard, & R.F. Schubert (Eds.), *The community of the future* (pp. 213-222). San Francisco: Jossey-Bass.

Pritchett, P. (with Robinson, D., & Clarkson, R.). (1997). *After the merger: The authoritative guide for integration success* (revised ed.). New York: McGraw-Hill.

Schaffner, J.W., Alleman, S., Ludwig-Beymer, P., Muzynski, J., King, D.J., & Pacura, L.J. (1999). Developing a patient care model for an integrated delivery system. *Journal of Nursing Administration, 29*(9), 43-56.

Weaver, D., & Sorrells-Jones, J. (1999). Knowledge workers and knowledge-intense organizations, Part 2. *Journal of Nursing Administration, 29*(9), 19-25.

Williams, M.B. (1998). *Changing roles and relationships in nursing and health care*. St. Louis: Warren H. Green.

Zelman, W.A. (1998). *The changing health care marketplace: Private ventures, public interests*. San Francisco: Jossey-Bass.

Nurse Practitioners

Issues Within a Managed Care Environment

BARBARA A. GIVEN

Managed care as an approach to health care delivery has proliferated in the past two decades and has had complex repercussions for nurses within managed care. The transition from the fee-for-service approach to managed care has changed the way health care is organized, delivered, and financed for all health care providers. Many health care professionals see managed care as a threat to their professional autonomy and to their ability to deliver quality care, whereas others see these changes as an opportunity for health care professionals to alter the way they practice, with increased emphasis on quality of care. Despite the day-to-day controversies, most consumers with managed care coverage give managed care a high satisfaction rating (Blendon et al., 1998).

In general, managed care involves capitated arrangements with networks of health care professionals, hospital and health care systems, and supportive care facilities. The intended focus is to deliver to groups of individuals quality care that is readily accessible and cost-effective. This involves more than simple cost control. In the decades ahead managed care will continue to evolve and be affected not only by managed care organizations (MCOs) and employer groups but also by consumers, government, and health care professionals. Now that length of hospital stay as a cost-containment approach has been achieved, new initiatives to cost containment will be designed as health care costs continue to rise.

Today the consumer is more knowledgeable about health care than in the past, and specific coverage and benefits have become important commodities. There is a certain amount of distrust of health plans by the consumer because the cost-containment initiatives lead to a perceived lack of choice and restriction in benefits. In response to consumer pressure to these perceptions, government, at both the state and federal levels, is responding to consumer fears of managed care efforts to contain costs

and manage utilization (Robinson, 1999). Consumer protection and consumer rights legislation has burgeoned for federally funded programs, for example, Veteran's Administration, the military, and Medicare and Medicaid. These efforts are likely to bring change to the non-government-supported managed care systems as well. Nurses in advanced practice need to seek opportunities for enhanced role involvement in managed care during this time of change (Barber & Burke, 1999; Barger, 1997).

As a result of the evolution in the managed care industry and of the frustration and chaos in managed care, consumers, health care professionals, and health plans are beginning to realize that there must be collaboration among all participants involved in the delivery of health care if there is to be an effective system. Successful collaboration and partnerships between health care professionals and consumers are needed to ensure that the key components of quality, choice, and access are not compromised and remain priorities despite continued efforts to contain costs. Recognition of this need provides numerous opportunities and challenges for the advanced practice nurse in the delivery of health care in a managed care environment (Cohen & Juszczak, 1997, 1998).

HEALTH MAINTENANCE ORGANIZATIONS

For the purpose of this discussion, we will describe health maintenance organizations (HMOs) as the paradigm in which the recommendations for nursing practice occur, since HMOs are the most common type of managed care plan. The HMO benefit package includes prevention as well as inpatient and outpatient care after the onset of symptoms or illness. HMOs contract with providers (e.g., community agencies, tertiary hospitals, and health care providers) to provide care to their enrolled subscribers.

Managed care programs use control mechanisms such as coordination of care by primary care providers (PCPs), provisions for prevention and screening, utilization review, drug formularies, and quality assurance programs. These services enable HMOs to contain costs and to pass savings on to plan members. The providers are at financial risk for the care provided and therefore have an incentive to provide cost-effective, high-quality care. HMO enrollees select a PCP who manages total care by seeing them for their primary care and authorizing specialist visits, hospitalization, and other supportive care services. Models of HMO plans include the staff model, group model, and open panel (independent practice association) (Kongstvedt, 1995; Satinsky, 1996). Managed care programs are becoming more open to allowing consumers to have choice and receive point of service coverage.

NURSES IN MANAGED CARE: OPPORTUNITIES AND CHALLENGES

Although nurses have often reacted negatively to the controversies and chaos of managed care, the reader is encouraged to think about how some of the basic tenets of managed care can be positive for nursing roles. The emphasis that managed care places on health promotion, disease prevention, integrated systems, quality, and a comprehensive continuum of care is consistent with the goals and values of nursing practice. These aspects of managed care will require a proactive approach, innovation, and empowerment on the part of the advanced practice nurse (APN). Nurses in this managed care environment will need to be proficient in organizational, professional, and interpersonal skills. It will be necessary to function comfortably when roles are ambiguous and negotiable and to work autonomously when needed and to interact with multiple professionals both within and outside the organization. The managed care environment gives nurses in advanced practice a significant opportunity to participate in the health care system using their critical thinking and decision-making capabilities (Harrison, 1999).

APNs are as yet an untapped resource for managed care systems to achieve the stated goal of cost-effective, quality care. Nurses must strategically position themselves to be a major resource at the forefront of managed care. Opportunities for APNs in a managed care environment include, but are not limited to, providing (1) direct primary care, (2) prevention, health promotion, and demand management, (3) disease management, (4) patient advocacy for member services, (5) care coordination, (6) edu-

cation, (7) quality improvement, and (8) outcomes management. Each of these opportunities will be discussed.

Direct Primary Care

Nurses who deliver direct care will become more visible in the provider panels in managed care, and their value as primary care providers will be recognized. The lack of provider billing numbers, lack of prescriptive authority, and limited reimbursement all contribute to nurses' current invisibility. Nurses need to market the benefits they provide to consumers and to other health care professionals and plan administrators. Nurses already use their clinical judgment, critical thinking skills, and expertise to safely and effectively manage patients across the continuum of care spanning practice boundaries with a minimum of supervision (Barter, Graves, Phoon, & Corder, 1995; Harrison, 1999). The contribution of nurse practitioners to clinical patient outcomes is well documented (Lorig et al., 1999; Moody, Smith, & Glenn, 1999; Mundinger et al., 2000; Rice & Stead, 1999). Primary health care, coordination and management of chronic illnesses, lifestyle management, and life-stressors management are easily delivered by nurse practitioners. In the direct care role they provide health promotion and disease prevention, information, and education; successful performance of health histories, physical examinations, and diagnosis and treatment of common primary care problems are well documented. Patient education and counseling and guidance regarding lifestyle behaviors and self-care skills are common role components (Aubert et al., 1998; Brown & Grimes, 1993; Moody et al., 1999; Mundinger et al., 2000; Stuart-Shor et al., 1999).

There is evidence from studies over the last two decades that nurse practitioners provide primary care comparable to that of physicians (Brown & Grimes, 1995). The most recent article by Mundinger et al. (2000) supports findings through a randomized clinical trial for primary care, follow-up, and ongoing care. These authors conclude that where nurses had the same authority, responsibility, productivity, and administrative requirements as physicians had, the patient outcomes were comparable. These patients did not differ in self-reported health status, physiological measures, satisfaction measures (except for one measure), and in health services utilization. The high level of consumer satisfaction adds to the marketability of this role within the managed care system (Sox, 2000).

Integral to the direct care role, and acknowledged as an important resource in managed care, APNs must demonstrate their capacity to implement cost-effective primary care (Schaffner & Bahomey, 1999; Stone, 1998). Comprehensive quality patient care is important, but this must be balanced with the cost containment that is a part of the practice environment in which care is delivered; cost-effective care is critical. APNs in a managed care environment need clinical and financial skills and the knowledge and insight to combine them (Buerhaus, 1994). The nurse must be concerned at all times with the correlation between the *process of appropriate care* that she or he is delivering and clinical *patient outcomes.* Cost consideration is placed right at the heart of clinical decision making for APNs (Blanchett & Flarey, 1995; Doerge & Hagenow, 1995; Malloch & Porter-O'Grady, 1999; Mohr & Mahon, 1996).

This cost containment goal, along with the clinical outcome goal, may be hard to reconcile and consider, but the relationship between delivery of care and financing is complex and intertwined. APN-MD collaboration needs to be expanded to achieve both the cost and quality outcome. Nurses should seek to document how this collaboration contributes to improved patient outcomes, improved patient satisfaction, enhanced plan image, and health team effectiveness, all of which lead to cost containment. If nurses in advanced practice want a *visible* leading role in direct care within a managed care environment, they must reconcile this juxtaposition and focus on and balance the cost-effective and quality components of care.

Prevention, Health Promotion, and Demand Management

Nurses have an important role to play in developing partnerships with patients so that patients are able to assume greater self-care responsibility in prevention, health promotion, and demand management within managed care (Harrison, 1999; Moody et al., 1999). To date, however, many HMOs have not put emphasis on these areas of health services, focusing instead on restricting access to services (Pronk, Goodman, O'Connor, & Martinson, 1999). As costs continue to escalate and preauthorization practices fall from favor, HMOs will foster and encourage members to assume more responsibility for self-care, disease prevention, and health promotion (Healthwise Communities, 1999). The public has come to expect more prevention services and more support. Although patients will continue to be sick, they also will expect greater efforts in prevention and curative and long-term care. Nurses can come forward, assume a leadership role, and offer their skills in the management of these three "product lines." Educating consumers and other health

care professionals about the expertise of nurse practitioners in prevention, early detection, and health promotion is important. Nurses partner effectively with patients to help them assume greater responsibility for self-care (Harrison, 1999; Moody et al., 1999) as it relates to screening practices and healthy lifestyle choices such as smoking cessation, physical activity, and proper nutrition (Aubert et al., 1998; Becker et al., 1998; Lorig et al., 1999; Mandelblatt et al., 1999).

The concept of demand management, which includes self-care health promotion, health education, and prevention, has become an important approach in managed care systems (Lorig et al., 1999; Vickery & Lynch, 1995). Demand management is a series of in-person and telephone contacts intended to help reduce the need to access more expensive medical interventions by focusing on education in self-care, including appropriate use of health care resources. This approach includes prevention and wellness services to reduce general health risks and promote healthy lifestyle behaviors. Self-management of health as well as the management of minor episodic illness promotes personal responsibility for health and the appropriate use of health services. Risky behaviors (drug abuse, smoking, unprotected sex, violence), lack of preventive health practices (e.g., poor nutrition, lack of exercise), or choosing not to access care even when it is available are all part of patient responsibility. This systematic approach helps reduce calls and inappropriate care, since self-care strategies are used as the first line of care rather than more expensive services (Musich, Burton, & Edington, 1999).

Informed consumers who understand the underlying basis for quality of care can make confident informed decisions that are within guidelines or standards of care and advocate for themselves (Lorig et al., 1999). When patients are treated as partners in health care decisions, they assume more responsibility for their health outcomes. Thus patients will become more accountable for the health consequences of their own behavior in the face of available, accessible, affordable, and appropriate health services and information.

Nurses can assume the leadership for a broad array of activities associated with demand management, prevention, and health promotion that include educational seminars, public service programs, special mailings, and lifestyle-modification programs. Information services, self-care handbooks, nurse telephone advice lines, and patient workshops help build the member-provider partnerships needed to implement demand management. Providing health care information to members to enable them to manage their own health, to identify their health goals, to promote healthy lifestyle behaviors, and to assist them to resolve problems and advocate for their needs is essential to achieving the goals of demand management. Demand management recognizes that knowledge and information alone do not affect demand management but that cognitive skills, social support, self-efficiency, and cultural norms also affect self-care. Nurses can work as partners with patients to help them gain access to self-care interventions with competence and confidence in self-care skills and to perceive less need for formal care as they exercise their own choices. These interventions alter utilization behavior and choices by changing patient knowledge and perception.

Demand management, if delivered properly, can assure that the wisest choices for care are made for both the patient and the system. Providers must actively enable patients to be participants in their own care, including decision making. Patient empowerment will help to maximize members' roles within the managed care system. The practice of the future must successfully manage the health of members who present themselves to the system, but it must also be concerned about those members who have not yet presented themselves.

Demand management needs to be expanded if we are to be successful in achieving cost containment and quality of care goals in managed care (Medical Alliances, 1998). Nurse practitioners are well positioned to assume the first line in demand management, to assist with the coordination and appropriate and timely referral of patients, and to encourage self-care. Carving out this area as a domain for nursing practice is important, as in the next decade the task of managed care will be to help optimize health over a lifetime, that is, to sustain maximum physical, mental, and emotional capacity of their members.

Disease Management

Disease management within managed care occurs for complex chronic diseases and health problems. It is based on risk appraisal and is used to clinically manage the disease and its complications for patients in a manner that assumes optimal outcomes and most effective use of system resources. Diabetes, asthma, congestive heart failure, arthritis, chronic obstructive lung disease, and cardiovascular disease are major areas for concern for preventing complications and costly care and have been the prime focus of disease management programs. Management of these chronic problems examines the clinical interfaces necessary for risk adjustment, diagnostic appropriateness, disease treatment, and prevention of complications

and recidivism. The goal of disease management is to help the patient reduce the disease complications and manage the demand for illness-related services by educating the patient about risk behaviors, complications, and self-management of symptoms and behaviors (Wagner, Austin, & Von Korff, 1996; Ward & Rieve, 1997).

Disease management consists of assessment, enhanced education, information support, medical management, and evaluation following designed treatment algorithms and focused visits to ensure adherence to the therapeutic plans. Evidenced-based guidelines are used by professionals, patients, and families for decision support in prevention, early detection of complications, treatment, and follow-up services using appropriate levels of care (Woolf, 1999). Nurses can assess patients' responses to treatment and implement the educational, psychosocial, and physiological interventions that lead to physiological and psychosocial stability for patients with chronic conditions as evidenced by a number of randomized clinical studies that document the value of the clinical management by nurse practitioners (Aubert et al., 1998; Lorig et al., 1999; Stuart-Shor et al., 1999). A registry of patients in these programs is recommended to ensure adequate follow-up and to evaluate practice patterns and guideline compliance (Wagner et al., 1996).

Although the focus in managed care is on disease and demand management, another important role of the nurse that needs to be exploited and that could be combined with the disease management role in managed care is symptom management. For many *episodic* problems there is a need to assist patients and their families to properly manage symptoms. Plans need to consider the expertise that nurses bring to the management of the symptoms such as fatigue, depression, pain and discomfort, sleep disturbance, diarrhea, fever, difficulty breathing, stress, and decisional conflict that often affect chronic disease (Kelly, 1999). These symptoms are frequently reasons for patients to increase their use of health care resources such as urgent care visits, hospital readmission, or extended care. These are often acute, self-limiting problems that need to be systematically managed, perhaps as a special variation of disease management. Nurses are successful in assisting patients with symptom management using education and counseling and non-prescriptive and prescriptive therapy and should assume a major role in the management of common symptoms.

Patient Advocacy and Member Services

There are numerous accounts indicating that members of managed care plans often do not understand the breadth of benefits and entitlement available in their plans; thus they do not optimize the appropriate use of benefits and services. This lack of understanding may lead to a perception of restrictions and dissatisfaction when care expectations are not met. Enrollees who are new participants in managed care plans are often confused by the rules and regulations of their health plans; they look not only to plan member relations departments but also to providers to clarify the requirements and benefits for access, referral, and reimbursement. Nurses who understand both primary care and managed care can do much to interpret for plan members the various programs, benefits, and services that will be available to them. Many members may take advantage of more expensive programs or expect more services because they simply do not know and understand the benefits that can accrue from the less expensive and more effective approaches.

Nurses in advanced practice could carve out an important role for themselves in this area of advocacy and member services to help the members use the plan in an appropriate way. Nurses can be central in helping patients understand demand management programs, for example, in those with asthma so that they can learn to read peak flow meters rather than going to the emergency department and in persons with diabetes to record and act on blood sugar levels. Or nurses could help educate patients about home care and alternative community services such as the availability of physical fitness programs, Weight-Watchers, or senior services.

Nurses with teaching and coaching experience are well suited to be in member services areas to help consumers understand and tailor the use of available benefits for their own needs. Capitated systems could benefit from having nurses act as patient advocates by alerting members to available services and facilitating their appropriate use of them. Reaching out to members who have not used the system will be an important role if the overall health and well-being of the plan membership is to be maintained.

Care Coordinator

Within a managed care context, primary care delivery has even broader implications than in a nonmanaged care environment. PCPs, often called "gatekeepers," not only provide direct care but also coordinate appropriate referrals and ensure that enrollees for whom they are responsible have access to a variety of wellness, prevention, and health promotion services and to disease-specific or chronic care services. Supportive care such as home care and long-term care require that the PCP understand eligibility criteria. As care shifts away from the acute care

setting, the ability of the PCPs to manage enrollees' total health care requires familiarity with many health-related services, settings, and intervention techniques and an awareness of the benefit of services for each level of required care. In the future this gatekeeping role will broaden and will include more care coordination and case management than gatekeeping (Bodenheimer, 1999; Coile, 1995; Fagin & Binder, 1997; Fagin & Schwartz, 1993; Weiss, 1998).

The care coordinator as outlined here is distinct from the disease and demand manager, although related. The key is to match the resources to the level of care and to tailor services to need, not merely to move patients through the system according to a general guideline. The intent of the care coordinator is to provide comprehensive, continuous, nonfragmented care to individuals with complex medical problems needing *multiple* services. Care coordinators perform at least the following tasks: assessment, planning, facilitation, intervention, monitoring, negotiation, advocacy, and evaluation. Care coordinators use sound judgment to move patients across the health care continuum, bridging the gap as patients move across levels of care. The focus of case management should be on reducing high cost and managing complex problems that serve the goals of both cost-effectiveness and quality care. Ineffective tailoring at the appropriate level of care by case mangers can actually add to the cost of care (Buerhaus, 1994; Coile, 1995).

By virtue of their advanced knowledge, clinical judgment, and experience in acute, home, and long-term care, APNs are well suited to facilitate both internal and external linkages for care coordination. We need to ensure that nurses with the most knowledge and skills assume these roles so that the care activity goes well beyond the phone triage and referral so prevalent today. For many of the complex chronic diseases, or the frail elderly, the key reason for needing the expert practitioner is to tailor the follow-up and services at the appropriate level of care. Untailored services may lead to inappropriate and costly care along with inappropriate understanding and utilization, which does not lead to desired outcomes.

Nurses should assume a major role in risk management programs that identify those chronically ill patients at high risk for complications and hospitalization and then provide programs of education and treatment to alter unhealthy habits, encourage good health behavior, and prevent high-cost utilization patterns (Coile, 1995). This level of care coordination may not be at the same level of intensity as that for the chronically ill and frail elderly but can do much to contain costs by its efforts to reduce the level of risk and prevent complications. There is a place for this within the overall care coordination role, although this role might be integrated into the disease or demand management activities of a plan. There is little literature that makes this role a component of long-term care management, yet it appears to be a part of that care continuum. Further exploration of the value of such a role within managed care plans is needed.

The care coordinator in a managed care system is as concerned with the individual patient as with the system of care. In the management of patients across the seamless continuum of care, there must be considerations for quality, standardization of the process of care, and determination of the appropriate level of care across the multiple settings. System-focused care facilitates efficient, quality care services to improve patient outcomes. It also enhances appropriate selection and mobilization of services by the high-risk population while controlling the high cost of specialized care. The role of case manager to meet these goals can be effectively filled by an experienced nurse who can conduct the appropriate in-depth assessment to determine the needed level of care using clinical judgment.

Education

There are important opportunities for patient education within each of the roles already discussed, especially the direct care role. It is important, however, to expand that activity within the managed care environment. Moody et al. (1999) note that, "APNs appear far more likely than physicians to provide teaching and counseling services. They were more likely to provide nutrition counseling, more likely to provide exercise counseling, almost three times as likely to provide smoking cessation counseling, slightly more likely to provide weight reduction counseling, and fifty times as likely to provide family planning counseling" (p. 100). There remains a need for special, distinct educators to be responsible for patient and family education in the overall plan and to assume responsibility for groups as well as individual education. Some education programs are likely to exist within a plan; other programs will need to be evaluated for feasibility and value. Educational programs will need to be created or changed depending on the standards and practice guidelines selected by the plan for their members. APN skills can add much to the value of the plan by developing the curriculum materials, implementing the program, and evaluating the overall educational component of the disease, demand, and risk-reduction management programs. Keeping programs current with state-of-the-art

guidelines is a critical feature of this role so that the plans can remain competitive.

The APN as an educator in managed care coordinates education activities for patients and families but also has an important role in professional staff education to help them implement the standards and guidelines and thus meet the quality improvement goals of the plan. The nurse educator can ensure staff development and education so that practice performance goals of the plan can be achieved.

Quality Improvement

There is increased emphasis on quality and performance review for system, patient, and provider outcomes within the health care system. Nurses in advanced practice, because of their understanding of quality care, can assume a major role in both documenting and contributing to continued performance improvement. Nurses in advanced practice scored as well as or higher than physicians on quality of care measures that included patient satisfaction, patient education and confidence, and clinical outcomes (Brown & Grimes, 1993; Mundinger et al., 2000). The big challenge in managed care is to identify which clinical activities or processes of care result in quality outcomes so that the unnecessary use of costly diagnostic tests, treatment plans, and procedures can be reduced or eliminated. Nurses currently assume major roles within managed care to collect, document, and analyze data on the outcomes for quality improvement departments. Expanded efforts in this realm can assist with the interpretation of performance indicators—such as the Health Plan Employer Data and Information Set (HEDIS) by the National Council on Quality Assurance (1999a, 1999b, 1999c) and the accrediting body for HMOs (Rustia & Bartek, 1997)—for both the plan and the professional provider.

To achieve the highest quality care requires more precision and less variation from the highest standards; practitioners, individually and in the aggregate, must learn to improve the care they provide through continued analysis of patient outcomes. As they receive feedback about their performance, clinicians will analyze their practices and compare them with those of their colleagues and with national benchmarks. Clinical decision support systems through quality programs will aid greatly in implementing best practices by promoting the provider with key information at the time care decisions are made. Given the concern for quality, reduction in errors, and improved performance indicators, creativity must be brought to the quality improvement efforts of the managed care systems. Given the history of nurses' involvement in quality improvement, they are in a unique position to develop new initiatives to deliver the best quality health care possible.

Outcomes Management

Outcomes management is a variant of care coordination and disease management, but the focus for this discussion is directed to utilization of outcomes assessment information to enhance the clinical, quality, and financial outcomes for patients *and* the system through full integration and coordination of services (Houston & Luquire, 1997). Outcomes management is based on a belief that achieving positive health status outcomes will improve the quality and cost of care. Targeting outcomes results in implementing the appropriate care guidelines and process of care to minimize complications, side effects, and unmanaged symptoms that prevent timely discharge or that add to readmission and admission rates or utilization of urgent care services (Saks, 1998). In the managed care system, clinical paths and evidenced-based practice guidelines with specified outcomes form the basis of what is used to determine the outcomes plan approach within a managed care plan.

Outcome management across the continuum of care ensures use of the appropriate level and location of care to achieve the desired patient outcome and the best use of the financial resources of the plan (Houston & Luquire, 1997). This role facilitates the management of outcomes for a specified population, which may be a particular DRG, HEDIS guideline, service line, or chronic disease. This focus does not ignore the specific patient but rather is oriented to group or population outcomes. Outcome managers apply the desired outcome paths and guidelines and outcome measures and have the authority to suggest the changes and refinements needed in the system in response to the analysis for this population. The outcomes manager monitors the outcomes of all cases in a designated population and implements systems to assist providers to implement the essential process components of care. The outcomes manager ensures the coordination of the levels of care and contracted services needed to link the needs of the targeted group with the outcomes that are desired.

This role serves as a liaison among patients, families, clinicians, administrators, vendors, and payers with the goal of improving the designated outcome. These professionals must be strategically located within the organization so that they have the authority to implement system changes needed to accomplish the desired clinical and fi-

nancial outcomes for the given targeted patient population (Moss, Steiner, Mathnke, & Cohen, 1998). The APN is well situated to serve in this role.

SUMMARY

There are numerous other roles the nurse can seek within the managed care environment; this discussion has provided a few examples of focused roles for the APN beyond that of direct care. With the complex and changing health care system, it is critical that nurses take a proactive approach to expand their role and opportunity in the managed care system. Nurses can have a direct impact on an organization's fiscal bottom line by generating revenue through such roles as practitioner or case manager and also indirectly through other roles such as outcomes or demand manager. These roles are not new, but nurses generally have not taken a leadership role within the system to show the "value added" to meet the goals of managed care. APN effectiveness can translate into both cost-effectiveness for the system and patient outcome, both goals of managed care.

Nurse practitioners must take advantage of opportunities in managed care and align themselves with managed care organizations to be valuable, visible resources. Nurses in advanced practice need to articulate the myriad contributions that the APN can make to managed care systems, plan executives, physicians, other providers, state and federal officials, the media, and consumers (Mason, Cohen, O'Donnell, Baxter, & Chase, 1997).

Nurses working within the managed care organization can do much to ensure access across the full continuum both in types and level of care by assuming more active, visible involvement. Nurses need to document their value for patient outcomes and cost reduction by improved patient satisfaction and enhancement of the plan's image. Nurses need to be visible and diligent in integrating these roles into the changing managed care system. There are many opportunities for nurses in the future of managed care.

REFERENCES

Aubert, R., Herman, W., Water, J., Moore, W., Sutton, D., Peterson, B., Bailey, C., & Koplan, J. (1998). Nurse case management to improve glycemic control in diabetic patients in a health maintenance organization. *Annals of Internal Medicine, 129*(8), 605-612.

Barber, P., & Burke, M. (1999). Advanced practice nursing in managed care. In M. Mezey & D. McGiven (Eds.), *Nurses, nurse practitioners* (pp. 203-218). New York: Springer Publishing.

Barger, S. (1997). Building healthier communities in a managed care environment: Opportunities for advanced practices nurses. *Advanced Practice Nursing Quarterly, 2*(4), 9-14.

Barter, M., Graves, J., Phoon, J., & Corder, K. (1995). The changing health care delivery structure: Opportunities for nursing practice and administration. *Nursing Administration Quarterly, 19*(3), 74-80.

Becker, D., Raquerno, R., Yook, R., Kral, B., Blumenthal, R., Moy, T., Bezirdjian, P., & Becker, L. (1998). Nurse-mediated cholesterol management compared with enhanced primary care in siblings of individuals with premature coronary disease. *Archives of Internal Medicine, 158,* 1533-1539.

Blanchett, S.S., & Flarey, D.L. (1995). *Reengineering nursing and health care: The handbook for organizational transformation.* Gaithersburg, MD: Aspen.

Blendon, R.J., Brodie, M., Benson, J.M., Altman, D.E., Levitt, L., Hoff, T., & Hugick, L. (1998). Understanding the managed care backlash. *Health Affairs, 17*(4), 80-94.

Bodenheimer, T. (1999). Primary care physicians should be coordinators, not gatekeepers. *JAMA, 281*(21), 2045-2049.

Brown, S.A., & Grimes, D.E. (1993). *Nurse practitioners and certified nurse midwives: A meta-analysis of studies on nurses in primary care roles.* Washington, DC: American Nurses Association.

Brown, S.A., & Grimes, D.E. (1995). A meta-analysis of nurse practitioners and nurse midwives in primary care. *Nursing Research, 44,* 332-339.

Buerhaus, P. (1994). Economics of managed competition and consequences to nurses. Part II. *Nursing Economic$, 12*(2), 75-80.

Cohen, S., & Juszczak, L. (1997). Promoting the nurse practitioner role in managed care. *Journal of Pediatric Health Care, 11*(1), 3-11.

Cohen, S., & Juszczak, L. (1998). Focus groups reveal perils and promises of managed care for nurse practitioners. *The Nurse Practitioner, 23*(6), 48-77.

Coile, R. (1995). Integration, capitation and managed care: Transformation of nursing for 21st century health care. *Advanced Practice Nursing Quarterly, 1*(2), 77-84.

Doerge, J., & Hagenow, N. (1995). Management restructuring: Toward a leaner organization. *Nursing Management, 26*(12), 32-37.

Fagin, C., & Binder, L. (1997). Dangerous liaisons: Nursing, consumers, and the managed care marketplace. In J.C. McCloskey & H.K. Grace (Eds.), *Current issues in nursing* (5th ed., pp. 444-451). St. Louis: Mosby.

Fagin, C., & Schwartz, M.R. (1993). Can APNs be independent gatekeepers? *Hospitals and Health Networks, 67*(11), 8.

Harrison, J. (1999). Influence of managed care on professional nursing practice. *Image: Journal of Nursing Scholarship, 31*(2), 161-166.

Healthwise Communities. (1999). Smarter Medicaid consumers saving Idaho millions by being wise about their health. Retrieved January 15, 2000, from the World Wide Web: http://www.healthwise.org/22onth.htm.

Houston, S., & Luquire, R. (1997). Advanced practice nurse as outcomes manager. *Advanced Practice Nursing Quarterly, 3*(2), 1-9.

Kelly, J. (1999). Rheumatology NPs outscore MDs in pain management study. *Clinician News, 3*(9), 18. Retrieved January 29, 2000, from the World Wide Web: http://www.medscape.com/CPG/ClinNews/1999/v03.n09/cn0309/cn0309.08.html.

Kongstvedt, P. (1995). *Essentials of managed care.* Gaithersburg, MD: Aspen.

Lorig, K., Sobel, D., Stewart, A., Brown, B., Bandura, A., Ritter, P., Gonzalez, V., Laurent, D., & Holman, H. (1999). Evidence suggesting that a chronic disease self-management program can improve health status while reducing hospitalization. *Medical Care, 37*(1), 5-14.

Mandelblatt, J., Traxler, M., Lakin, P., Thomas, L., Chauhan, P., Matseoane, S., & Kanetsky, P. (1993). A nurse practitioner intervention to increase breast and cervical cancer screening for poor, elderly black women. *Journal of General Internal Medicine, 8,* 173-178.

Malloch, D., & Porter-O'Grady, T. (1999). Partnership economics: Nursing's challenge in a quantum age. *Nursing Economic$, 17*(6), 299-307.

Mason, D., Cohen, S., O'Donnell, J., Baxter, K., & Chase, A. (1997). Managed care organizations' arrangements with nurse practitioners. *Nursing Economic$, 15*(6), 306-314.

Medical Alliances. (1998). Demand management generates bottomline results. Retrieved February 27, 1998, from the World Wide Web: http://www.medsource.com/providers/pro6.html.

Mohr, W.K., & Mahon, M.M. (1996). Dirty hands: The underside of marketplace health care. *Advances in Nursing Science, 19*(1), 17-20.

Moody, N., Smith, P., & Glenn, L. (1999). Client characteristics and practice patterns of nurse practitioners and physicians. *The Nurse Practitioner, 24*(3), 94-103.

Moss, J., Steiner, K., Mathnke, K., & Cohen, R. (1998). A model to manage capitated risk. *Nursing Economic$, 16*(2), 65-68.

Mundinger, M.O., Kane, R.L., Lenz, E.R., Totten, A.M., Tsai, W., Cleary, P.D., Friedewald, W.T., Siu, A.L., & Shelanski, M.L. (2000). Primary care outcomes in patients treated by nurse practitioners or physicians. *JAMA, 283*(1), 59-68.

Musich, S.A., Burton, W.N., & Edington, D.W. (1999). Costs and benefits of prevention and disease management. *Disease Management Health Outcomes, 5*(3), 153-166.

National Council on Quality Assurance. (1999a). The Medicare health outcomes survey (formerly Health of seniors survey): Questions and answers. Washington, DC: Author. Retrieved November 28, 1999, from the World Wide Web: http://www.ncqa.org/pages/policy/hedis/health%20of%20seiors/hosq&a.htm.

National Council for Quality Assurance. (1999b). *HEDIS/Report Cards.* Retrieved September 1999 from the World Wide Web: http://www.ncqa.org/pages/policy/hedis/newhedis.htm.

National Council on Quality Assurance. (1999c). HEDIS 2000 list of measures. Washington, DC: Author. Retrieved November 28, 1999, from the World Wide Web: http://www.ncqa.org/pages/policy/hedis/h00meas.htm.

Pronk, N., Goodman, M., O'Connor, P., & Martinson, B. (1999). Relationship between modifiable health risks and short-term health care charges. *JAMA, 282*(23), 2235-2239. Retrieved February 8, 2000, from the World Wide Web: http://jama.ama-assn.org/issues/v282n23/abs/joc90579.html.

Rice, V.H., & Stead, L.F. (1999). Nursing interventions for smoking cessation. *Cochrane Review Abstracts, 3.* Retrieved January 29, 2000, from the World Wide Web: http://www.medscape.com/cochrane/abstracts/ab001188.html.

Robinson, J. (1999). Blended payment methods in physician organizations under managed care. *JAMA, 282*(13), 1258-1263.

Rustia, J., & Bartik, J. (1997). Managed care credentialing of advanced practice nurses. *The Nurse Practitioner, 22*(9), 90-103.

Saks, N. (1998). Developing an integrated model for outcomes management. *Advanced Practice Nursing Quarterly, 4*(1), 27-32.

Satinsky, M. (1996). Advanced practice nurse in a managed care environment. In J. Hickey, R. Ouimette, & S. Venegoni (Eds.), *Advanced practice nursing: Changing roles and clinical applications* (pp. 126-145). Philadelphia: Lippincott-Raven.

Schaffner, R., & Bohomey, J. (1998). Demonstrating APN value in a capitated market. *Nursing Economic$, 16*(2), 60-74.

Sox, H. (2000). Independent primary care practice by nurse practitioners. *JAMA, 283*(1). Retrieved January 5, 2000, from the World Wide Web: http://jama.ama-assn.org/issues/v283n1/full/jed90087.html.

Stone, P. (1998). Methods for conducting and reporting cost-effectiveness analysis in nursing. *Image: Journal of Nursing Scholarship, 30*(3), 229-234.

Stuart-Shor, E.M., Skinner, S., McCleary, N., Clark, S., Waldman, H., & Kemper, A. (1999, November). A nurse-directed, community-based, integrated multiple cardiac risk reduction program: Physiological and behavioral outcomes. Presented at the American Heart Association 72nd Scientific Sessions, Atlanta, Georgia.

Vickery, D., & Lynch, W. (1995). Demand management: Enabling patients to use medical care appropriately. *Journal of Emergency Medicine, 273*(1), 551-557.

Wagner, E., Austin, B., & Von Korff, M. (1996). Organizing care for patients with chronic illness. *The Milbank Quarterly, 74*(4), 511-544.

Ward, M.D., & Rieve, J.A. (1997). The role of case management in disease management. In W.E. Todd & D. Nash (Eds.), *Disease management: A systems approach to improving patient outcomes.* Chicago: American Hospital Publishing.

Weiss, M. (1998). Case management as a tool for clinical integration. *Advance Practice Nurse, 4*(1), 9-15.

Woolf, S. (1999). The need for perspective in evidence-based medicine. *JAMA, 282*(24), 2358-2365. Retrieved February 2, 2000, from the World Wide Web: http://jama.ama-assn.org/issues/v282n24/full/jpp90034.html.

Contracting for Nursing Services

GERRI S. LAMB, DONNA ZAZWORSKY

The thought of contracting for nursing care is unsettling for many nurses. Contracts are associated with a business model of health care. They raise images of compromising the nurse-patient relationship for a financial transaction. It is not uncommon to hear, "I became a nurse to serve patients. Money has no place in nursing care." In this view, contracts, which represent the exchange of payment for service, should not be a part of nursing practice, nor of concern to nurses. We disagree.

Viewpoint. The ability to contract directly for nursing services and to receive payment for services delivered is essential for the survival of professional nursing practice. Contracting is directly tied to recognition for nurses' contributions to health care outcomes, to control over practice, and to decision making over allocation of scarce health care resources. The ability to contract directly for nursing care is the difference between nurses' remaining invisible in health care or shaping the future of our health care delivery system.

WHAT IS A CONTRACT?

Most simply, a contract is a legal document between two or more parties that specifies services to be delivered and the payment for those services. The context for the services is usually defined in great detail, including where the services will be provided, how often they will be provided, the penalties for nondelivery of services or missing agreed-upon time frames, insurance coverage for liability for adverse outcomes, and processes for dispute resolution and termination.

In health care today, contracts are the major vehicle for health care organizations to provide care to a target population and be paid for it. Hospitals, home care agencies, skilled nursing facilities, and physician groups alike contract with a variety of entities like government agencies, employers, insurance companies, and health maintenance organizations (HMOs) to provide one or more compo-

nents of the full continuum of health care services. Without contracts, it is possible to provide health care services, but it is unlikely that the service will be reimbursed.

Individuals and organizations that enter into health care contracts agree to deliver services or to pay for them. Depending on the type of reimbursement, both provider and payer of services may take on varying degrees of financial risk. For example, fee-for-service payment is not associated with substantial risk for a hospital or health care organization as long as the agreed-upon payment allows a certain margin of profit. The hospital or health care organization just needs to make sure that it maintains sufficient volume of services to cover costs and make a profit.

In contrast, contracts that use capitated payment are common in managed care arrangements and may be associated with significant financial risk for providers of care. Under capitated payment, providers are reimbursed in advance for the delivery of a defined set of services for a certain population. For example, a primary care physician is assigned 1,000 patients from a certain HMO. The HMO agrees to pay the physician $10 per member per month (PMPM). Thus the physician receives $10,000 each month to provide primary care services to this group of patients *whether or not the patients use any primary care services.*

It is possible to make or lose substantial sums of money in capitated contracts depending on the extent to which services covered in the contract are used. No matter how much service the population uses, whether more or less than estimated, the contracted provider remains financially responsible for delivering services under the terms of the agreement of the contract. Providers who enter into capitated contracts, also called risk contracts, do so with the premise that they will be able to manage service use and costs and thus have dollars remaining from the prospective capitated payment at the end of the month.

Today, health care professionals and organizations can enter into a variety of different types of contracts, each associated with different amounts of financial risk. For profit and nonprofit organizations alike, the goal is to deliver quality services and to make enough money to continue and expand services and pay stockholders investing in the organization.

Contracting is considered both art and science. Although many of the financial components of a contract, like costs and expected use of services, can be estimated with some degree of accuracy, there are numerous factors that contribute to the success or failure of health care contracts. The mix of contracts held by an organization, the health needs of patients covered by the contract, and service use patterns all affect profitability. Not surprisingly, as health care professionals participate more in contract negotiations and share more of the financial risk, their interest in mastering the skills of contracting has grown tremendously. The health care literature contains numerous articles with advice on how to negotiate and manage contracts, especially capitated or risk contracts (Gallagher, 1997; Knight, 1997; Potter, 1999).

NURSES AND CONTRACTS

In many practice settings, nurses have owned businesses and entered into contracts for decades. In the early 1900s, Lillian Wald, the visionary leader of the Visiting Nurse Service of New York, contracted with several benefit societies on the lower east side of New York City to provide home nursing care to the members (Denker, 1993). In 1909, Wald initiated an experiment with Metropolitan Life Insurance Company that ultimately led to the first national system of insurance coverage for home-based care. She managed not only to convince insurers about the benefits of home nursing care but also to negotiate a successful capitated contract almost a century ago.

Following on the heels of the success of leaders like Lillian Wald, numerous nurses have chosen to become entrepreneurs. Today, nurses own and manage small businesses as well as large health care companies. In competitive arenas like home care and case management, they provide skilled nursing services for health care organizations and insurers. Their businesses rely on contracts and direct payment for nursing services for income and survival.

Today, however, there continues to be a number of settings that do not bill directly for nursing care. In hospitals and nursing homes, for example, nursing care is typically included in the price of room and board. In many primary care settings, nurse practitioner services are billed under the physician's payment code.

What difference does it make whether nursing services are paid for directly or indirectly? As long as nurses can provide good nursing care and get paid, why make an issue of nursing' being included in contracts or receiving direct payment?

When you go into a grocery or department store and pay for an item of food or clothing, do you think about the skill sets or time of different individuals whose work went into the production of that item? Do you distinguish any specific group for their contributions to the quality of the item or demand that their seal of approval come with the purchase?

In settings that do not bill directly for nursing care the purchasers may be aware that nursing is included in the negotiated price but usually have limited knowledge of the expertise they are buying. Contract discussions usually revolve around the cost of hospital care, not skilled nursing care, even though skilled nursing care is the largest component of hospital expenses. When patients receive their hospital bill or notification of insurance payment, more often than not they do not associate the bill with the quality of the nursing care they received. In effect, nursing is invisible to payers and the public.

In our society the willingness to pay for services is directly tied to the value placed on the service. Consumers do not pay for services they do not value. Conversely, we need to ask, do consumers value services they are not aware they are paying for? If payers and the public do not link the hospital or primary care bill to the outstanding nursing care they received, what is the likelihood that they will demand that nurses receive payment commensurate with their expertise? How likely are they to become involved in issues that affect the quality of nursing care? Invisibility has been and continues to be costly to the profession of nursing.

For nursing, the ability to contract (and thus, be paid) directly for nursing services:

- Reflects the value placed on nursing care by consumers and payers
- Recognizes that nurses offer a distinct service
- Provides control over nursing care decisions and resulting dollars
- Permits public evaluation of nursing's contribution to care
- Generates dollars to serve vulnerable and underserved groups
- Improves the contracting process

Our willingness to pay for a service or product is associated with the value we place on it. Individuals and insurers pay for health insurance and services because they want and value health care or their customers demand it. Although there is ongoing debate about the extent to which health care follows typical market principles, the way that health care dollars are allocated still reflects the value placed on varying services. Services that are exchanged for payment at the contract table are those that the payer wants and is willing to pay for.

Inclusion of nursing care in contracts indicates that nursing is recognized as a distinct and valuable service. Specific identification of nursing as a covered service indicates that the payer wants the service, is willing to pay for it, and holds the organization accountable for the quality of that care. Most other health care professionals, like physicians or therapists, are named in contracts and thus have the opportunity to negotiate the terms under which their services are delivered. Invisibility at the contract table means not only having nursing services sold for unacceptable rates but also a missed opportunity to educate and reeducate contractors and payers about nursing.

When payment is hidden, included in the room fee or attributed to another professional, nurses lose a critical opportunity to demonstrate their contribution to health care. In primary care settings that bill services delivered by a nurse practitioner incident to physician services and under the physician's name, data about the services included on the billing statement are connected to the physician not the nurse practitioner. Mason and colleagues (1999) note, "Reimbursement under the physician PIN [provider identification number] may generate more profit for the practice but it eliminates recognition of the nurse practitioner as the service provider and clouds accountability" (p. 207).

The ability to contract and thus generate direct revenue has major implications for participation in decision making and control over allocation of health care resources. Nursing directors in hospitals and nursing homes oversee areas associated with the largest component of hospital budgets. In fact, without nurses, hospitals and nursing homes would not exist. Yet across the country, nursing directors are being moved further and further from the seat of power and decision making. We must ask, Would this be happening if nursing directors controlled all access to nursing resources and were the primary negotiators for nursing care during contracts? How might this affect nursing's ability to take control over nursing delivery models?

Clearly, most nurses are not in nursing for money or to make a profit. Nurses have a distinguished record of serving vulnerable and underserved populations. The reality, however, experienced by many nurses who have been involved in caring for these groups is that it is extremely difficult to maintain funding for even the most essential programs.

Contracting is a vehicle to generate dollars that can be used to pay for services for which there is no reimbursement. Community nursing centers have done an extraordinary job maintaining services for uninsured and vulnerable populations by increasing income from contracts (see box below). There is a common saying in health care

---

TODAY'S COMMUNITY NURSING CENTERS: CONTRACTING WITH PETER TO PAY FOR PAUL

Community nursing centers emerged more than three decades ago to serve individuals and populations without access to traditional health care services. Today there are estimated to be over 300 community nursing centers (CNCs) across the United States in both inner-city and rural settings providing care to individuals of all ages and ethnic groups (Watson, 1996).

Most of the CNCs started in academic health centers and received funding through federal grants. Grants from the Department of Health and Human Services Division of Nursing have been instrumental in enabling nursing faculty to set up innovative community care models.

Although grant funding is an excellent vehicle to jump-start much needed community-based health initiatives, eventually grants end and programs are faced with finding the money to continue operations. CNCs are particularly challenged in this regard, since they typically serve populations for whom there is limited or no reimbursement for services. Much of the current literature on CNCs addresses their economic viability and survival.

Today, many of the mature CNCs, that is, those that have been around for a long time, report an important new step toward long-term financial survival. They have diversified their funding streams to balance expenses associated with reimbursable and nonreimbursable care. Income from Medicare, Medicaid, and state contracts augments grant support, and together they permit successful CNCs to continue to carry out their mission of service for vulnerable populations.

Without a funding menu that includes contracts, CNCs could not continue to provide health care services to the thousands of uninsured and vulnerable individuals and families they see each year. For CNCs the ability to compete for and win contracts is essential to reaching out and responding to unmet community needs.

that goes, "No margin, no mission." Nurses in community health centers and other settings have demonstrated that successful contracting prevents this unacceptable cycle.

Finally, nursing involvement in contracts is an important way to improve health care contracts. Individuals who negotiate health care contracts for most large health care institutions and insurance companies are not usually clinicians or practitioners. Although they may be expert at the financing of health care, they often do not understand the operational dynamics of service delivery or the interdependence of health care services. Contracts that appear to be reasonable financially often result in frustration and financial losses because they do not work clinically or overlook essential services or incentives that make the whole package work better. For example, any nurse who works in a hospital knows how critical the services that follow hospitalization are to preventing subsequent admissions and emergency department visits. Yet some contracts create incentives to minimize or delay the use of postacute services. Having skilled nurses at the contract table avoids perverse scenarios that diminish quality of care and ultimately increase expenses.

GETTING TO THE CONTRACTS TABLE

Participation in contracts requires expertise and data. Contract negotiations incorporate the art of bargaining and compromise and the science of finance and economics.

Nurses who engage in contracting come prepared. They are able to:

- Define the services for which they are to be reimbursed
- Specify the costs of the services, for example, cost per visit
- Provide data about the quality of their service
- Assume the responsibility and risk associated with the terms of the contract
- Walk away from the contract when it is unacceptable

In some settings, nurses can readily generate the necessary information to engage in contracts. Financial and information systems are sufficiently developed to capture major outcomes and expenses associated with the delivery of nursing care. In other settings, considerable effort and capital must be infused into developing the infrastructure needed to support this effort.

There is no getting away from the fact that credible data are a requirement for successful contracting. Settings that are unwilling or unable to allocate resources to documenting nursing outcomes and costs in a systematic and ongoing way must be considered suspect in their commitment to deliver nursing services. Without data and contracts, nursing programs may continue to exist at the whim of the current administrators and remain extremely vulnerable.

To successfully negotiate with all the knowledge, experience, and data necessary for contracts, nurses must work to put to rest the "nurses should not deal with money" issue and any associated issues related to feelings about competition. Expertise and experience on the business side of health care is a necessary means to a desired end of better health care for the persons nurses serve. The refusal to deal with money or competition is also a refusal to participate at the level that critical decisions about allocation of health care resources are made.

In addition, nurses need to actively work to remove other barriers to participating in contracts and receiving equitable reimbursement for their services. Legislative advances like the Balanced Budget Act of 1997, which mandated Medicare reimbursement for advanced practice nurses, are essential to level the playing field for nurses. Hopefully, future legislation will rectify issues related to equal pay for equal work for nurses.

CONCLUSION

Every nurse must come to terms with the role that money plays in health care today. Whether the nurse works as employee or independent practitioner, someone or some organization is paying, either directly or indirectly, for the services nurses provide. The distance between the payment for services and the paycheck may be short or long, but nurses fool themselves if they ignore the fact that money and financial incentives drive much of our behavior and decisions in health care. Just watch what happens when Congress changes the methods for reimbursing Medicare or Medicaid if you have any lingering doubt.

For a growing number of nurses this strong message about the importance of reimbursement and contracting is a case of preaching to the converted. All too many, however, still have a long way to go. The need to bring nurses into the 21st century of health care represents a critical opportunity for nursing educators and administrators to work together to shape the future of nursing and health care. It would be a national tragedy if professional nursing goes the way of the dinosaur because it refused to learn and master the lesson of integrating business and mission.

REFERENCES

Denker, E.P. (1993). *Healing at home: Visiting Nurse Service of New York*. New York: Visiting Nurse Service.

Gallagher, R.M. (1997). What APRNs need to know about contracting with managed care organizations. *Nursing Trends & Issues, 2*(6), 1-8.

Knight, W. (1997). *Managed care contracting: A guide for health care professionals*. Gaithersburg, MD: Aspen.

Mason, D., Alexander, J.M., Huffaker, J., Reilly, P.A., Sigmund, E.C., & Cohen, S.S. (1999). Nurse practitioners' experiences with managed care organizations in New York and Connecticut. *Nursing Outlook, 47*(5), 201-208.

Potter, L. (1999). The managed care contract: Survival or closure? *Nursing Administration Quarterly, 23*(4), 58-62.

Watson, L.J. (1996). A national profile of nursing centers. *Nurse Practitioner, 21*(3), 72-80.

Section Eight

Health Care Costs

A Concern for Costs

JOANNE McCLOSKEY DOCHTERMAN, HELEN KENNEDY GRACE

It's an interesting fact that, even though cost containment is the driving force in health care, we always have a difficult time identifying people who can write good chapters about health care costs related to nursing. Not many nurses have developed programs of research or careers around nursing economics. Until recently, this was not a subject that was taught in many schools of nursing or a source of concern for many nurses. Things have changed. The concern for costs is determining a number of decisions that affect nurses and our patients. This section introduces some of the issues around the costs of nursing and health care.

In their debate chapter, Seefeldt, Garg, and Grace overview the two major approaches to the control of health care costs: regulation and competition. This is a very informative chapter and contains a clear overview of a number of cost-control initiatives. Total U.S. health expenditures grew from $41.9 billion in 1965 to $425 billion in 1985. The authors review the various regulatory (government intervention) initiatives of the past 30 years: certificate of need, economic stabilization program, professional standards review organization, prospective rate setting, and prospective payment systems. In the past two decades competitive approaches, such as competitive contracting, managed care and health maintenance organizations, preferred provider organizations, cost sharing, medical savings accounts, and managed competition, have been used to supplement or supplant regulatory approaches. Each of the regulatory and competitive approaches is described with some information about its advantages and disadvantages. Despite all of the approaches, the major problems remain: escalating costs, increasing numbers of individuals without any insurance, and uneven access and quality of care. The Medicare population is using resources at a much higher rate than their contributions; the Medicaid program is now funding more elderly care than care of children. The solutions to the problems, according to the authors, do not lie with

government or insurers or providers or employers, but with the consumers of health services. Yet, they point out, the consumer is not part of the debate. Seefeldt, Garg, and Grace want to end the outdated model of health care in which "professionals are the all-knowing" and empower the people. They believe that until the consumer becomes an active partner in the system, the problems are insoluble. The chapter provides an excellent overview of past measures to control costs and raises many important issues that should be carefully digested and debated.

In the first viewpoint chapter Maddox examines the evolution of managed care, the financial factors that have created the current health care system, and the impact of the changes on nursing. The chapter contains numerous financial facts. For example, in the past the categories of services generating the most growth in expenditures were hospitals and physician cost, but since 1998, the fastest rising spending category is prescription drugs. Maddox demonstrates that the federal government is increasing its role in the financing of U.S. health services. She covers the evolution of the third-party pay system and clearly explains the functions of Medicare and Medicaid and prospective payment systems. She overviews the different models of managed care and discusses in some detail the preferred provider organization (PPO) and the health maintenance organization (HMO). She spends the last half of her chapter discussing the impact of managed care and current reimbursement methods on hospitals, ambulatory and outpatient services, long-term care, nurse staffing, and selected nursing roles such as the advance practice nurse and the nurse manager. Three utilization management strategies are discussed: prospective, concurrent, and retrospective. The Balanced Budget Act of 1997 brought several changes, including the recognition of nurse practitioners, clinical specialists, and physician assistants as authorized Medicare providers, eligible for direct reimbursement. But with this new role comes increased responsibility for the provider. This is an informative chapter about the history and current issues related to reimbursement trends in the United States and the impact on health care and nursing.

The cost of home care for a person with a disability is the topic of the next chapter by Aronow. This is an increasingly important topic in nursing because the number of persons in society with a disability is growing. The increase is due to the aging of society and the better survival rate of those with a disability. As Aronow states, the reorganization of care away from large institutions and toward home care and homelike residences requires a clear analysis of services and costs to the disabled community. Aronow structures her chapter by four types of care in the home: short-term recovery, long-term care, technology-supported care, and end of life care. For each type of care she presents a patient example and discusses the components of cost. She concludes her chapter with a discussion of the responsibilities of professionals. Whereas the home has become a viable alternative for care of persons with disabilities, the cost of home care is not well understood. She believes that the nurse has some responsibility to help explain costs associated with alternative choices and that the nurse should be prepared to become a part of the family negotiations that involve the patient and the informal caregivers. The chapter provides an excellent overview of the financial and care burden issues related to caring for a variety of diverse patients in the home.

As the previous chapter illustrates, it is more important than ever that nurses understand the business aspects of health care. A different example of this is illustrated in the next chapter by Klemczak and Dontje, who discuss the need for sound business practices in the development and conduction of nursing centers. A nursing center is an organization, controlled by nurses, whose primary mission is to provide nursing services. Although nursing centers have existed for many years, usually attached to schools of nursing, most of them were supported by grants and did not have to be concerned about income generation. As these grants are being reduced or eliminated, the centers are left with commitments and few funds to deliver services. With the 1997 Balanced Budget Act that changed the Medicare law to designate advance practice nurses (APNs) as reimbursable Part B providers, nursing centers that employ APNs can seek new types of funding. Klemczak and Dontje urge existing nursing centers to expand the services they offer to include a complete set of primary health care services, including health screening, testing, prescribing, treatment, referral, case management, and patient teaching. They discuss reimbursement of these services

under capitation contracts. The last part of their chapter is a case study of the development of a nurse-managed center at the College of Nursing at Michigan State University. The college has a contract with the Office of Veterans Affairs in Battle Creek to provide primary care services to veterans living in the surrounding community. The authors discuss this experience and conclude with related issues and challenges.

Reimbursement for nurses and other nonphysician providers is the subject of the chapter by Lee. The proliferation in consumer use of alternative therapies, such as autogenic training, biofeedback, massage, acupuncture, Ayurvedic techniques, and reflexology, to name a few, has resulted in the recognition that there needs to be a way to document the use of such therapies and bill for reimbursement as they become more accepted. Consumer demand for alternative therapies has been so dramatic that they are increasingly being included in mainstream practice and medical journals. In 1996, the Health Insurance Portability and Accountability Act called for the setting of a national standard to communicate with all providers (not just physicians) electronically in a standardized way. This act combined with the widespread and growing dissatisfaction with the *Current Procedural Terminology (CPT)*, currently the only coding system approved for Medicare reimbursement by the Health Care Financing Administration (HCFA), opened the door for the development of the *Complete Complementary Alternative Medicine Billing and Coding Reference*. The *Reference*, published for the first time in 1999, includes Alternative Billing Codes (ABC Codes) developed by a group known as Alternative Link in Las Cruces, New Mexico. In this *Reference*, alternative is defined as any provider other than an allopathic physician and the treatments provided by these providers. Thus, nursing is included (although most nurses do not think of themselves as alternative providers). The ABC Codes do include interventions from the Nursing Interventions Classification (NIC), the Home Health Care Classification (HHCC), and the Omaha System. Although the system has not yet been adopted by HCFA for reimbursement, the ABC Codes have been included in the *American National Standards Implementation Guideline* and the National Library of Medicine Unified Medical Language. The system not only includes language for thousands of alternative therapies, it provides the legal scope of practice for multiple practitioner groups. It will be interesting to see future developments in this area. Will HCFA approve the use of this *Reference* for reimbursement to alternative providers? If not, how will the growing use of alternative therapies be documented?

The last chapter in the section by Schmidt overviews the financial skills needed by patient care managers. As the role of the nurse manager has grown and become more challenging, the need for financial skills is essential. Schmidt discusses the prerequisite computer skills including spreadsheet applications. She overviews the budget measures of volume, revenue, and labor and nonlabor expenses. She shows how to operationalize the budget with a staffing plan. Several types of productivity measures are defined and four types of analyses are reviewed that can be used to help evaluate cost and productivity performance. These are staffing-to-demand analysis, productivity benchmarking, use of labor dollars analysis, and workforce composition. Schmidt's chapter provides an excellent overview of the financial skills a nurse manager must have to be an effective leader and manager in the ever evolving complex health care environment.

Nursing's ability to identify and deal with economic issues has come a long way in the past decade. More and more, all nurses and nursing students are gaining knowledge about costs of health care, but nursing is still not a major player in health care cost-containment efforts. We need to make the concern for costs a nursing concern and voice this concern and appropriate actions whenever the opportunities arise.

CHAPTER 51

Controlling Health Care Costs

Regulation vs. Competition

F. MICHAEL SEEFELDT, MOHAN GARG, HELEN KENNEDY GRACE

The issue of controlling health care costs hits at the heart of a major social dilemma that grows out of the American character and the values surrounding the practice of medicine: the rights of the individual versus responsibility for the larger social group. The tensions between balancing individual rights against the common social good become compounded in the area of medical care because the physician and, more recently, the provider organization become the arbiter between the individual and society. Although there was a time when the physician could make decisions largely on the basis of what was deemed best for the patient, today's concerns over the rising costs of medical care services and the large numbers of people without access to these services have made it increasingly difficult to practice in this simplistic manner. With the costs of medical care rising far more rapidly than those of other parts of the economy, the concern for controlling these costs has become an increasing preoccupation in recent years.

Before the 1960s, most medical care costs were covered by insurance that was provided as part of the benefits package paid by employers for their workers. This system worked effectively for those who were employed and provided reimbursement to physicians and hospitals in a satisfactory manner. Over the years, however, an aging population, increased numbers of people who are not part of the workforce, and increasing costs of insurance to employers have resulted in a situation open for governmental intervention. The enactment of Medicare and Medicaid legislation in 1965 signaled the beginning of a new chapter for medical care in this country. The intent behind Medicaid and Medicare was to provide health care to the two most vulnerable groups: the elderly and the indigent who were not covered by employer-provided health care insurance and were unable to pay out of

pocket. In effect, the federal government became the insurer for these uninsured populations. Soon after the enactment of these programs, it was realized that health care expenditures were rising much faster than the economy, and initiatives were undertaken to address the issue. The agreed payment system based on "reasonable" costs for hospitals and "reasonable prevailing charges for physicians" provided little incentive for patients or providers to control health care costs. Over the past 30 years a variety of legislative approaches have been taken to try to control escalating costs. A systematic display of major initiatives is presented in Figure 51-1. These approaches can be classified either as competitive, describing a condition of the workings of the free market in which the unfettered private sector forces of supply and demand determine the most efficient allocation of resources, or regulatory, which assumes that market forces function imperfectly and that government intervention is required to control costs. This chapter reviews the approaches taken and encourages the reader to consider the pros and cons of regulation vs. competition in controlling medical care costs.

REGULATORY APPROACHES

The reimbursement system of Medicare and, to some extent, Medicaid, which was based on "reasonable charges," created intense inflationary pressure on health care costs. Earlier, much of the health care for the elderly had been offered as charity and was not reimbursable. In addition, there had been no incentives to add new expensive procedures before Medicare. That changed dramatically. Substantial reimbursement was available for increasing hospital revenue for providing additional procedures requiring new staff and equipment. By creating a surplus of income over revenues, this money went back into fur-

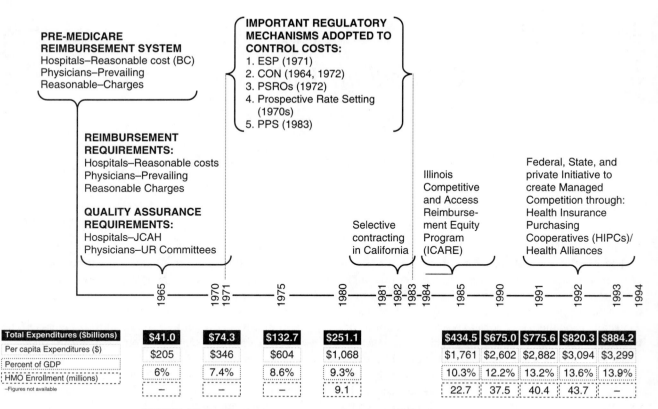

FIGURE 51-1 An overview of cost-control initiatives in U.S. health care.

ther expansion of facilities and staff, ultimately resulting in increased cost.

This increased cost, which was not retrievable from public sources, was then passed on to private patients and their insurers, creating inflationary pressures on the entire system. Total health expenditures grew from $41.9 billion in 1965 to $425 billion in 1985. This increase occurred despite governmental efforts to control costs. From 1971 to 1983 the major efforts to control costs were through regulatory efforts. None appreciably slowed the growth in total health care costs (Fig. 51-2).

Certificate of Need

One type of intervention used the strategy of controlling the structure of medical care (i.e., the settings and instruments available and used for the provision of care) by limiting the development of hospital capacity. Built on a certificate of need (CON) law initiated in New York State in 1964, Congress in 1972 passed amendments to the Social Security Act to give planning agencies more authority. In 1974, Congress passed the National Health Planning and Resources Development Act, which required

every state to pass a CON law allowing it to review plans by any institutional provider for capital expenditures over $150,000 or a change in the number of beds and services. The impact of CON programs was minimal. A number of studies indicate that the review boards passed nearly everything that was brought to them (Begley, Schoeman, & Traxler, 1982; Lewin Associates, Inc., 1975; Salkever & Bice, 1976; Sloan & Steinwald, 1980). However, one side effect of the CON program was that hospitals gained sophistication about market conditions, long-range planning, and resource use-expertise easily adapted to a competitive market.

Economic Stabilization Program

This program, introduced during the Nixon administration, was developed in two phases. Phase 1 (August 15, 1971, to November 13, 1971) involved a 90-day freeze on all wages and prices, and phase II (November 14, 1971, to April 30, 1974) limited institutional health care providers to a 6% annual limit in price increases in aggregate revenue, subject to cost justification. These controls applied to both hospital and physician fees. The Economic Stabilization Program appears to have moderated both the increase in average cost per hospital day (Salkever, 1979) and also the growth of physician fees; but there is some evidence that while fees were frozen, physicians classified visits into more expensive categories, thereby holding the line on price while allowing revenues to increase (Holahan & Scanlon, 1978).

Professional Standards Review

The quality, quantity, and cost of hospital care provided under Medicare was to be monitored primarily through mandatory establishment of utilization review committees in participating hospitals Through review processes conducted under the supervision of physicians, their function was to control medical services such as admissions, diagnostic investigations, and therapeutic interventions provided by physicians to their hospitalized patients. A 1970 Senate Finance Committee Report judged the utilization reviews to be of a token nature and ineffective as a curb to unnecessary use of institutional care and services. The criticism of the utilization review led the American Medical Association to propose a Medicare peer review system to be controlled by the medical societies. Legislative action led to the establishment of professional standards review organizations with responsibility to review hospital care under their jurisdiction, with particular emphasis on the appro-

priateness of admission and the length of stay for hospitalization. Evaluations of the program are mixed, with one study concluding that the savings to Medicare and Medicaid exceeded the cost of the program by 10% to 15% (Smits, 1981), whereas another study concluded that it cost Medicare and Medicaid an estimated $1.80 for every $1 the program spent (Alpem, 1980).

Prospective Rate Setting

By 1980, most states had some form of hospital rate-setting program, but the programs varied considerably. Most were voluntary, with hospitals choosing whether to participate or comply. Only eight states had programs that involved mandatory review and compliance with rates set by a rate-setting authority. Mandatory rate-setting programs initiated by several states resulted in slowing the rate of growth of expenditures per patient day.

Prospective Payment Systems

In 1983, Congress established the Medicare Prospective Payment System (PPS), which replaced retrospective cost-based reimbursement for hospital care. The primary objective was that of controlling escalating hospital costs. Under the PPS, inpatient hospital services for Medicare eligibles were bundled into 468 diagnosis-related groups, each with a fixed reimbursement schedule. Adjustments

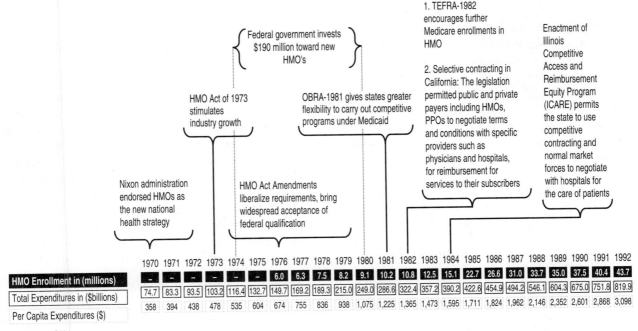

FIGURE 51-2 An overview of legislative initiatives and the emergence of managed care and accompanying escalation of cost.

were made for important factors such as case severity; rural, urban, and regional labor cost differentials; teaching costs; and disproportionate shares of uncompensated care. During the first 3 years of the PPS, inflation in hospital expense was reduced by about 5% to 7% from the pre-PPS double-digit levels.

Despite these major regulatory programs, health care costs continued to escalate at a higher rate than the general economy. Expenditures for health care in 1985 totaled $420.1 billion compared with $74.4 billion in 1970. The share of health care expenditures as a percentage of the gross national product increased from 7.3% in 1970 to 10.5% in 1985, with hospital expenditures accounting for 40% of all health care spending.

COMPETITIVE APPROACHES

As health care costs have continued to escalate in the past two decades, attempts to contain costs by restructuring the health care market to make cost-effective competition possible have supplemented, and in some cases supplanted, the regulatory programs described previously. For economists, competition in a perfectly competitive or "free" market implies rivalry between sellers of comparable goods for customers. Customers will then choose the goods that cost less, knowing that they are not sacrificing quality, and thus the operation of the market encourages suppliers to keep prices down. The model of free market competition fully applies only when all product attributes other than prices are standardized. Obviously, many of the products in health care are not standardized.

A modified form of competition can occur between suppliers of noncomparable products in a particular market, but there is no guarantee that this kind of competition will result in lowered prices. This modified form of (nonprice) competition did occur among health care providers during the regulated era that followed the enactment of Medicare in 1965. During this period, hospitals competed for doctors and patients primarily on the basis of availability of sophisticated diagnostic and therapeutic technology. Patient comforts such as food quality, friendliness of staff, and cleanliness also played a major role in attracting patients to a particular facility. Despite nonstandardized "products" (in this case medical services), prices may have played a role in the competition if patients paid their own bills. However, during this period most patients had insurance, so price did not play any role in their choices. Thus, relevant competitive variables included service offerings and amenities but not price. Furthermore, as third-party payers, health insurance companies did not

promote price competition because they were not able to exclude providers on the basis of price. Hospitals and physicians were reimbursed on a "reasonable costs" and "reasonable charges" basis, respectively, but there was no competitive mechanism preventing "reasonable costs" from rising over time. Several factors such as collusion within the medical profession promoted increasing costs.

Competitive Contracting

In 1982 the State of California enacted legislation providing a mandate for "selective contracting." This approach was designed to reshape the health-care market by enabling third-party payers to legally exclude providers from their list of participants without significant risk of antitrust prosecution. Under this legislation, both private and public payers, including health maintenance organizations (HMOs) and preferred provider organizations (PPOs), could negotiate terms and conditions with specific providers such as physicians or physician groups and hospitals, who they would reimburse for services to their subscribers. Two hundred fifty hospitals negotiated agreements with the state to provide services to Medi-Cal eligibles (Medicaid) and accepted reductions in their normal payments ranging from 5% to 20%. As a consequence of the selective contracting, California saved an estimated $470 million in fiscal year 1983-1984 (Iglehart, 1984). Following the trend set by California, other states began to follow various forms of competitive contracting.

Managed Care and HMOs

The main feature of managed care that distinguishes it from retrospective and fee-for-service payments is that payment under managed care is prospective and capitated. Under such a system the financial risk no longer resides with the patient or the third-party payer as distinct from the provider; instead the managed care entity becomes a financial risk bearer, as well as a patient care provider. This means that the organizational focus of care shifts from individual illness care to concern for the health of a defined population: the membership of the plan or HMO. The incentives shift from performing unreviewed, high-intensity patient care to a case management function in which primary care providers coordinate all care and limit access to costly specialization and hospitalization.

Preferred Provider Organizations

Changes in state insurance laws have permitted payers to contract selectively with providers such as hospitals and physicians' groups, including those not run by HMOs. Under such schemes most payers have started identifying a subset of hospitals and physicians to be "preferred providers" on the basis of a predetermined rate of reimbursement. Patients are steered to those hospitals and physicians through financial incentives such as lower co-payments and deductibles. The providers sign agreements with payers to deliver services to their enrollees and are designated as preferred providers, and the organizations are designated as preferred provider organizations. To select these preferred providers, payers generally demand price discounts or strict utilization review procedures from the providers.

Cost Sharing

Cost sharing through increased coinsurance and larger deductibles is a relatively simple plan for providing disincentives for overuse of the system by insured individuals by requiring them to pay more out of pocket. This approach addresses the concern that third-party payment shields the patient from the costs of his or her care.

Medical Savings Accounts

If cost sharing means that individual consumers have to pay more out of their own pockets, it becomes a matter of concern how deep those pockets are. Cost sharing as a form of cost containment will not work if consumers cannot pay their bills. The concept of medical savings accounts (MSAs) was developed as a type of cost-sharing program that encourages people to save to pay for their own health care costs, thus ensuring that the money to pay health bills will be there when they need it. This is how the MSA would work. Currently, on average, nearly $4,500 per year per worker is paid by employers for health insurance. Of this amount the employer would put $3,000 annually into each employee's MSA, which the employee would use to pay the first $3,000 of his or her medical costs. For the remaining $1,500 the employer would purchase an insurance policy that would take care of medical expenses above $3,000. It is recommended that (1) an MSA would be the personal property of the employee, so that it would be portable if the individual changed jobs, (2) an MSA would be allowed to grow tax free, and (3) the employee would draw from it to pay for medical expenses. Under this arrangement, MSAs will provide consumers with built-in incentives to control health care expenditures because they will benefit directly if they spend less.

Problems of Competitive Systems

In a competitive environment, it is the firm or organization that maximizes profits that succeeds at the highest level. Health insurance companies wishing to maximize their profits can do so either by operating at a higher level of efficiency and effectiveness than their competitors or by practicing risk aversion to the highest level possible. Finding ways to avoid insuring the few very sick people can be very rewarding. Insurers practicing risk aversion as their main profit-making approach exclude individuals on the basis of preexisting conditions or by having coverage canceled midtreatment when unexpected illnesses become too large a financial liability to the firm. HMOs are accused of taking only young, healthy members of the workforce, whereas some firms have had their coverage canceled if one worker or his or her dependent is too great a financial risk.

The costs of health insurance have escalated commensurate with increases in the cost of care. An increasing percentage of the population has no health insurance coverage. Of those earning less than $10,000 per year, 32% are uninsured (Wicks, Curtis, & Haugh, 1994). Many businesses that once provided health insurance can no longer do so. Increasing numbers of individuals are employed on a part-time basis, and thus employers avoid paying costly health insurance benefits. A considerable proportion of the increased costs are a result of the inefficiencies in the system and the high administrative costs for managing the plans. It is estimated that one third of all fees paid for health insurance are used for costs other than for the direct provision of coverage. Finally, one of the most commonly voiced concerns of the public is the lack of choice of plan or of provider. The rise of managed care systems, with restrictions on self-referral to specialists by employing a given panel of generalists as gatekeepers, increasingly diminishes individual choice, a value ingrained in the American ethos.

MANAGED COMPETITION

In the late 1980s the dynamics and difficulties described earlier became increasingly problematic, and health care costs continued to escalate despite the innovations in health care financing. A proposal was made by Enthoven on behalf of an ad hoc group called the Jackson Hole Group, espousing a concept called "managed competition." Under managed competition, costs would be controlled by reshaping the health care market through establishing health alliances (sometimes called health insurance purchasing cooperatives), which would represent large groups of consumers. These purchasing cooperatives would have the clout to negotiate lower costs with providers. Furthermore these health alliances would offer not just one health care plan but a variety of plans, providing consumers with adequate information to choose between plans based both on cost and on standardized benefit levels. This would foster price competition and more inclusivity, what Enthoven (1993) calls "value-for-money" competition at the level of individuals making choices about plans. Value-for-money competition emphasizes that what cost-conscious health consumers seek isn't simply the least expensive health care services or health care package available, but the ones that give them the most for their money. The ability of the consumer to make informed choices is crucial. If consumers do not have adequate information, available in a form that makes comparing alternatives easy, then competitive market processes cannot work effectively in containing costs and promoting high-quality health care.

Limitations of Managed Competition

One of the major limitations of managed competition grows out of the fact that it requires competing health plans to work. Where this is a population insufficient to support several health plans functioning independently without collusion, this model cannot apply. Although information technology could be used to overcome some of the problems of serving isolated communities, transportation technologies are also important when it comes to getting people to tertiary care in a timely fashion or for paying specialists to be flown to remote areas when needed. In all of these plans there would be a mandated minimum benefit package. Those who choose the low-cost benefit package will be those who cannot afford a higher level of coverage or those who believe that they do not need more. This leaves room for a new type of "adverse selection," even within managed competition. A further concern is found in the fact that managed competition relies on managed care to achieve much of its savings. Data on the effectiveness of doing so is far from definitive or complete. Although it is clear that HMOs operate at lower costs than traditional fee-for-service plans, it is not yet clear how much of the savings they achieve are due to higher levels of efficiency and how much is due to selection bias (enrolling healthier members) in the markets where they exist. Low-income individuals will still be at a relative disadvantage.

Other Models

President Clinton made health care reform a major element in his election campaign. In the summer of 1993 he revealed his plan for national health care reform, which he titled the Health Security Act. This act was based on the model of health insurance purchasing cooperative-driven managed competition, employing regional health alliances (to be established by the states) and large-firm (more than 5,000 employees) corporate alliances as market managers. Among the key features of this proposal were universal coverage for all Americans, portability of coverage from employer to employer, and payment by means of a mechanism called "employer mandate," by which all employers would be required to provide health insurance for their employees, with subsidies to small businesses to help absorb the costs. As proposed, the Health Security Act was extremely complex, attempting to embrace virtually every aspect of the health care delivery system in the United States. Its complexity and the problems in communicating it to the public, together with the successful lobbying efforts of the insurance industry and others who felt their interests threatened by the bill, led to the failure of the Act or any of the comprehensive reform proposals that came out of congressional committees to gather enough votes to pass in either house of Congress.

HEALTH CARE REFORM ON HOLD

With the federal effort for reform at a standstill, local states and communities moved into the vanguard of innovation. A number of states (e.g., Minnesota, Washington, California, Florida, Tennessee) and local communities (Rochester and Cleveland) are taking a variety of approaches to address the problems.

The major problems that remain are escalating health care costs despite efforts at control through management or competition, increasing numbers of individuals without any health insurance (15% of the population, with most of that group the working poor), and uneven access and quality of care dependent on ability to pay. With capitated health care plans and greater financial monitoring of health care in general, the uninsured find fewer health care providers open to them. In addition, constant market segmentation by risk-averse health insurers, whether operating in a managed care environment or not, means the number of uninsured and underinsured is increasing. This places an increasing burden on the few health care providers willing to provide expensive emergency care to the uninsured or underinsured; these costs, one way or another, get passed on to the rest of the community.

Corporatization

The deregulation of the health industry initiated during the early 1980s and the collapse of the Clinton plan provided a fertile ground for corporatization of the American health care system. At present, the system is more fragmented and profit oriented than ever before. The role of employer-based insurance has declined, government expenditures have increased and so also has the number of uninsured. The U.S. health care system is still the most expensive and inadequate system in the developed world and even among the seven richest countries of the world (Canada, France, Germany, Italy, Japan, United Kingdom, and the United States). An examination of the per capita health expenditures and percent of government-assured health insurance in 1997 (Table 51-1) among the seven richest countries puts the United States in an indefensible position (Anderson & Poullier, 1999). Despite spending almost $4,000 per capita in 1997, the United States provided government-assured health insurance to only 33.3% of its population. The population assured government health insurance primarily includes Medicare and Medicaid eligibles and government employees including military personnel. But nearly 16.1% of the population had no health insurance in 1997, and quite a few have limited coverage. Moreover, the uninsured population is increasing at the rate of about 100,000 per month. The rest of the population is either self-insured or insured through employers.

On the expenditure side, the national health expenditures grew at a very slow rate during the period from 1992 to 1997, the lowest in the last 35 years. However, *government* expenditures for health care increased to $507 billion in 1997 (46% of the total) from $283 billion (or 40% of the total) in 1990. Compared with this, payments made by *private* resources for health care declined to 54% of the total or $585 billion in 1997 from 60% of the total or $416 billion in 1990 (Levitt et al., 1997). In 1997, nearly 75% of all the persons covered under private health in-

surance were enrolled in managed care plans dominated by for-profit corporate entities. These organizations treat health care as a commodity and try to maximize profits by avoiding insuring high-risk patients and controlling utilization of health services by capitating physicians.

Insurance Coverage

One of the most important observations of the health coverage in the United States during the period from 1990 to 1997 is the slow but steady erosion of health insurance coverage. This has happened despite the fact that the government has tried to fill the gap by introducing new programs such as Medicare + Choice, the Health Insurance Portability and Accountability Act, expansions of state Medicaid programs, and the $24 billion Children's Health Insurance Program in 1997. All these attempts have failed to arrest the increasing number of uninsured in the country. The percentage of Americans without insurance increased from 14.2% in 1995 to 15.3% in 1996 and to 16.1% in 1997. In 1997, 43.4 million were uninsured, and their rank is increasing at the rate of about 100,000 per month (Kuttner, 1999).

Some of the reasons for such trends are:

- Increasing premiums for health insurance for those who could afford it
- A move in the national work force toward temporary and part-time jobs
- Reduction in health care coverage, specifically for prescription drugs
- Managed care organizations' attempts to reduce covered usual health service by creating financial disincentives for physicians and hospitals (This leads to denial of care and shifting cost to patients.)
- A trend toward moving patients from traditional HMOs to point of service and PPOs, but with increasing deductibles and coinsurance, thereby shifting cost to the patient
- Decline of Medicaid coverage due to welfare reform and increasing cost of "Medigap" coverage for the elderly

Employer Health Insurance

In 1997 nearly 167.5 million Americans were covered under private health insurance, and of these, 151.7 million were covered by their employers. Since 1993, employers adopted several methods to reduce health care expenditures incurred on behalf of their employees. The employers achieved a reduction in their contributions for health care by (1) replacing family coverage by employee coverage, (2) shifting cost to the employees through limiting

TABLE 51-1 Per Capita Expenditures and Governmental Coverage

Country	Per Capita Expenditure ($)	Percent Population with Government-Assured Health Insurance
Canada	2,095	100.0
France	2,051	99.5
Germany	2,339	92.2
Italy	1,589	100.0
Japan	1,741	100.0
United Kingdom	1,347	100.0
United States	3,925	33.3

their choice of providers and increasing coinsurance and deductibles, and (3) forcing the managed care organizations to adopt rigorous cost-containment measures to control utilization of health services. All Fortune 500 companies provide health insurance, but only 49% of companies with less than 200 employees provide health insurance. Smaller companies provide less comprehensive health services, and 30% of companies with less than six employees provide no health insurance.

GOVERNMENTAL COVERAGE FOR SPECIAL POPULATIONS

With 38.6 million Medicare eligibles the problems of governmental coverage are of a different nature compared with the 167.3 million covered under private health insurance. The federal government spent $214.6 billion to provide health services to Medicare eligibles in 1997 compared with $21.5 billion in 1977, almost a 10-fold increase. The Medicare population is using health resources at a much higher rate then their contributions to the system. For example, a retired couple in 1998 contributed about $16,790 (excluding employers contributions) to the pool compared with their expected utilization of about $109,000. At present, about 89% of the revenues for Medicare comes from the population under 65 years of age and 11% from Medicare eligibles. The federal government is therefore dipping into the revenues currently contributed by the working population. If nothing is done, the federal government is expected to run out of Medicare funds by the time the first baby boomer is eligible to receive benefits in 2010.

As a stop gap arrangement, the federal government enacted the Balanced Budget Act of 1997 that would reduce Medicare expenditures by $116.6 billion during 1998-2002. But all the savings will be achieved by reducing payments to the providers—hospitals and physicians—sparing the beneficiaries of additional financial responsibilities. Although BBA-1997 has resolved the problem until 2002, the debate continues to find long-term solutions to make Medicare fiscally sound. One proposal under serious consideration of the National Bipartisan Commission on the Future of Medicare is to replace defined benefits with a "premium support system" that will enrich the pool.

With almost 42 million eligibles in 1997, Medicaid is the largest health services provider. A total of $159.9 billion was spent to provide health services to the recipients—$95.4 billion by the federal government and $64.5 billion by the states. States set their own stan-

TABLE 51-2 Distribution of Medicaid Expenditures

Category	Population (%)	Expenditures (%)
Elderly	9.9	27.3
Blind and disabled	16.2	36.4
Adults	22.3	10.9
Children	51.5	15.6
Disproportionate hospital share	Not applicable	9.7

dards regarding benefits under federal guidelines and receive matching funds from the federal government varying from a minimum of 50% to 83% depending on the per capita income of the state. Eligible children comprise more than half of the Medicaid population, but only 15.6% of the total expenditure (Table 51-2). One of the primary aims of the program was to provide health insurance to children of needy families, but, over time, other groups were added and support for children has declined. For the present, elderly, the blind, and the disabled consume about two thirds of the resources. The major Medicaid expenditures are for nursing homes services provided to eligible elderly. Nearly 42.5 billion or 27% of the total was spent on the institutional care of the elderly, far exceeding the expenditure on providing health services to children. In addition to a shift in population characteristics, Medicaid was besieged by a high rate of inflation. During 1989-1993, Medicaid expenditures increased by an average of 21.2%; this rate of increase declined to an average of 6.1% during 1993-1997. To control expenditures under Medicaid, states started moving Medicaid eligibles to managed care. For the present, 48% of Medicaid eligibles are enrolled in managed care plans. Its outcome, however, is still being evaluated.

SUMMARY

The history of health care reform can be divided into three major periods (1) from 1965 to the early 1980s, (2) from the early 1980s to 1994, which includes President Clinton's promise to provide universal health care to its collapse, and (3) from the collapse of the Clinton plan to the end of the 20th century. The first period was strictly governed by the two regulatory principles: payments to hospitals on their reasonable costs and to physicians on reasonable—usual—customary charges. Under this arrangement, hospitals were able to expand their services, incorporate state-of-the-art medical technology, add graduate medical education programs, provide health care to the uninsured, and shift costs to other third-party insurers. Physicians enjoyed almost total autonomy to make decisions on behalf of their patients without consideration of the cost-effectiveness of their decision. In fact, the patient was in the driver's seat, and physicians and hospitals tried to cater to the patient by providing the latest health services with little attention to costs and outcome. This regulatory process no doubt was primarily responsible for most of the advances that American medicine made during two decades after the enactment of Medicare and Medicaid in 1965. But this brought with it an inflationary trend that defied each regulation intended to bring it under control. The prospective payment system was introduced for inpatient service for Medicare eligibles as an attempt to control costs, and introduction of waivers under OBRA-1981 permitted states to buy health care for their Medicaid eligibles though the competitive bidding process. California was the first state to obtain the waiver and used it and in doing so extended it to the other third-party payers as well. It took almost a decade for the health care industry to understand the newly created opportunities to corporatize American health care. Enrollment in for-profit HMOs increased from 42% in 1987 to 62% in 1997. In addition, during the 1990s, many of the hospitals, HMOs, home health care agencies, hospices, and nursing homes became for-profit entities publicly traded on the stock exchanges. Initially, these new entities were able to make good profits by aggressive cost cutting and through controlling utilization, rationing care, and reducing physician autonomy. However, a persistent demand to lower health insurance by employers forced these organizations to dip into profits, thereby reducing profitability resulting in declining stock prices. Two of the major health care plans—Columbia/HCA and the Oxford Health Plan—sustained large losses. Oxford lost $291 million in 1997. The publicly traded health care companies are predicted to have large losses for the next few years. Despite problems with for-profit health companies, a relentless move toward profit continues. Besieged by mounting losses, the for-profit entities are in search of profitable combinations primarily by mergers and acquisitions. If successful, a few companies would control large markets, diminishing competition and starting a new cycle of squeezing health through draconian measures. All said, there are two primary issues that presently draw the attention of the public and the private sector. The private sector wants to hold on to the low inflation rate it enjoyed over the last few years. The government's main interest, echoed through the two current presidential candidates, lies in finding a solution to re-

duce the number of 43.4 million uninsured Americans and to add prescription drug coverage to Medicare. In the opinion of many experts, a permanent solution lies only in universal coverage. However, the national leadership is afraid to revisit this issue in view of what happened to the Clinton Plan. The reformers had to wait 30 years from the enactment of Medicare and Medicaid in 1965 to the introduction of a universal plan by President Clinton, and probably they will have to wait another 30 years for emergence of a leader who would be able to muster the consensus to carry it through the legislative process. What happens until then is anyone's guess.

Are there any answers to these dilemmas? The answers do not lie within the federal government, for-profit corporate health care organizations, insurers, physicians (who in the debate are synonymous with providers), or employers, yet these are the only people sitting around the decision-making tables. It is noteworthy that the biggest stakeholder of all, the consumer of health care services, is rarely mentioned as part of the debate. The problems are defined consistently as those having to do with the financing of health care, without any examination of health care per se. As long as there is such excess capacity within the system—too many specialists, too many hospital beds, overuse of highly trained specialists for work that could more effectively be managed by other practitioners (i.e., nurse practitioners)—and as long as the consumer is left out of the equation, the problems cannot be solved. As a society we are in conflict over health care as an industry serving as a major place of employment for large numbers of people versus health care as a needed service for all people. As long as industry is running the debate, the problems will not be solved. If the public becomes an informed part of the solution, however, rather than being perceived as part of the problem, a whole new dynamic may be brought to bear on the system. As we look to the 21st century as a time of massive shifts from an industrial to an information and increasingly diverse society, in which increasing numbers of people will not be employed or employable in the way to which we have become accustomed, the "third sector" of nongovernmental organizations and community volunteers becomes a potent political force for change. Solving the problems of infant mortality, adolescent pregnancy, and young people who die as a result of violence in their communities will not be achieved through our current health care system no matter how much we invest. The costs of emergency department care for the teenager shot in a gang fight will continue to escalate until we engage communities in a new way to become part of the solution. In a country as wealthy as the United States, to take a posture that we cannot afford to provide access to health care for all is reprehensible. As long as we use an outdated model of health care in which the "professionals" are the all-knowing and controlling seers, we will be unable to solve our problems. If people can be empowered with knowledge, and communities empowered as caring networks of people who will not tolerate the drug dealers and the gangs that would rob them of their children, then we can begin to solve our problems. Our problems are not those of financing the outdated system that currently exists, but to reconstruct a health care system that truly emphasizes the maintenance of health for all people. It is only when we have a health system for all that our problems can be solved.

REFERENCES

Alpem, D. (1980). Reagan, new directions. *Newsweek,* 1-33.

Anderson, G.F., & Poullier, J.-P. (1999). Health spending, access and outcome: Trends in industrialized countries. *Health Affairs,* *18*(3), 178-192.

Begley, C.E., Schoeman, C., & Traxler, H. (1982). Factors that may explain interstate differences in certificate of need decisions. *Health Care Financing Review, 3,* 87.

Enthoven, A.C. (1993, Fall). Why managed care has failed to contain costs. *Health Affairs,* 27-43.

Holahan, J., & Scanlon, W. (1978). *Price controls, physician fees and physician incomes.* Washington, DC: The Urban Institute.

Iglehart, J.K. (1984). Cutting costs of healthcare for the poor in California. *New England Journal of Medicine, 311*(11), 745-748.

Kuttner, R. (1999). The American healthcare system—Health insurance coverage. *New England Journal of Medicine, 340*(2), 163-168.

Levitt, K., Cowan, C., Braden, B., Stiller, J., Sensenig, A., & Lazenby, H. (1998). National health expenditures in 1997: More slow growth. *Health Affairs, 17*(6), 99-110.

Lewin Associates, Inc. (1975). *Evaluation of the efficiency and effectiveness of Section 1122 Review Process. National Technical Informational Service.* Washington, DC: U.S. Department of Commerce.

Salkever, D., & Bice, T. (1976). The impact of certificate of need on hospital investment. *Milbank Memorial Fund Quarterly, 54,* 185.

Salkever, D.S. (1979). *Hospital-sector inflation.* Lexington, MA: Lexington Books.

Sloan, F.A., & Steinwald, B. (1980). *Insurance, regulation and hospital costs.* Lexington, MA: Lexington Books, DC Heath and Company.

Smits, H.L. (1981). The PSRO in perspective. *New England Journal of Medicine, 305*(3), 253-359.

Wicks, E.K., Curtis, R.E., & Haugh, K. (1994). *Designing health purchasing alliances/cooperatives: Federal policy issues and options.* Washington, DC: Institute for Health Policy Solutions.

Managed Care, Prospective Payment, and Reimbursement Trends

Impact and Implications for Nursing

PEGGY JO MADDOX

Rapidly increasing costs of health care services, coupled with the lack of universal access, are prompting health care policymakers to consider serious structural reform of the U.S. health system. The federal government's highest priority is to reduce the budget deficit without creating new taxes. State and local governments are responding to similar public pressures amid budget constraints. Since the 1980s, almost all government programs have refused to cover the increasing costs of health care. In the private sector, employers are increasingly concerned about the cost of purchasing health insurance and are demanding that insurers be more aggressive in their efforts to reduce the rate of premium increases. They are using managed care products at a growing rate and are passing some percentage of health insurance costs on to employees.

These trends mean that managers in the health care industry will face continued pressures from all parties to offer quality services at the lowest possible costs. It also means that the financial consequences of actions will become increasingly important in management and clinical decision processes, and managers and clinicians alike must adopt more sophisticated optimization, management, and planning skills.

In the last decade, economic pressures have created the momentum for change, much of it related to restructuring. Factors cited as primary motivation for restructuring have included rising costs, prospective payment (PPS), consumer expectations, the quality movement and regulatory avoidance (Christiansen & Bender, 1994; Kreuger Wilson & Porter-O'Grady, 1999; Sovie, 1995). Health care service organizations have responded by eliminating excess capacity—improving economies of scale by integrating services or merging or consolidating—and by attempting to become more efficient (Buerhaus & Needleman, 2000). The focus of this chapter is twofold: to examine the evolution of managed care and the demographic, economic, and financial factors that have served as the motivation for changing the U.S. health system and to examine selected impacts that managed care and economic pressures have exerted on nursing in recent years.

ECONOMIC TRENDS AND THE U.S. HEALTH SYSTEM

The U.S. health care system is a diverse collection of subindustries, which are involved directly or indirectly in the provision of health care services. The major players in the industry are health professionals who provide health care services, pharmaceutical and equipment suppliers, insurers (public/government and private), managed care plans (health maintenance organizations [HMOs] and preferred provider organizations [PPOs]), and other entities such as educational institutions, consulting and research firms, professional associations, and trade unions. Today, the health care industry is large and pervasive, with characteristics and operational differences that vary widely between geographical and rural or urban areas. It is the second largest industry in the United States following the real estate industry.

In 1996 the United States spent $1,035 billion on health care, 13.6% of the nation's gross national product (GNP). The United States spends more on health care than any nation in the world, averaging $3,659 per person. The infrastructure of the U.S. health system and current eco-

TABLE 52-1 Health Care Expenditures 1950-1996: Total, Per Capita, and Percent GNP

Calendar Year	Total Health Expenditures (in Billions)	Per Capita Expenditures (Private)	Per Capita Expenditures (Public)	Percent Gross National Product
1950	$ 12.7	$ 60	$ 22	4.4%
1960	26.9	106	35	5.1
1970	74.7	212	129	7.1
1980	249	606	446	8.9
1990	675	1597	1094	12.2
1996	1035.1	2005	1754	13.6

From Health Care Financing Administration, Office of the Actuary, National Health Statistics Group. (1996). *Health Care Financing Review, 19*(1).

nomic conditions has evolved rapidly since the 1950s. Growth in health expenditures has also increased during this time. The largest increases in health-related expenditures occurred between 1960 and 1990, attributable primarily to the advent of Medicare and Medicaid programs.

In 1950 U.S. health expenditures averaged $82 per person (per capita) and accounted for 4.4% of the GNP. By 1996, per capita expenditures increased to $3,759 and health services accounted for 13.6% of GNP. Table 52-1 depicts the growth of expenditures in the U.S. health system since 1950.

Analysis of health care expenditures by service category points to high-cost service areas that have recently attracted the interest of the public and our elected representatives. These services have been the focus of increasing and more rigorous regulatory oversight and more restrictive financial arrangements. To appreciate the nature of economic growth, further category-specific economic data are provided. Table 52-2 identifies selected categories of health-related expenditures and their actual and projected levels from 1970 through 2007.

Data through 1990 illustrate that the categories of services generating the most concerns about rising costs have been hospital and physician related. Expenditures follow the proliferation of hospital and physicians during this period.

Since approximately 1998, prescription-related expenditures have replaced these categories as the most rapidly increasing spending category. Public discussion reflects emerging concerns about the pharmaceutical industry and policy change options for managing publicly funded pharmaceutical costs.

DEMOGRAPHICS AFFECTING HEALTH CARE COSTS

Demographic changes are underway in the United States, including the aging of the population and AIDS and chemical dependency epidemics. These changes have implications for providers' health services and have an impact on the overall costs of health care. Because most of the aged and other special populations receive services though publicly funded programs, the impact of growing health needs among these populations has considerable impact on financing arrangements and providers associated with Medicaid and Medicare programs.

TABLE 52-2 National Health Expenditures by Selected Service Category 1970-2007

Spending Category	1970	1980	1990	1993	1997*	1999†	2001†	2007†
National expenditures (billions)	$73.2	$247.3	$699.4	$898.5	$1,092.4	$1,228.5	$1,403.6	$2,043.1
Hospitals	28.0	102.7	256.4	323.0	371.1	401.3	447.5	624.9
Physicians	13.6	45.2	146.3	185.9	217.6	241.5	275.9	391.8
Home health	0.2	2.4	13.1	23.0	32.3	33.8	38.3	60.2
Nursing home	4.2	17.6	50.9	66.4	82.8	90.1	99.2	141.5
Prescriptions	5.5	12.0	37.7	50.6	78.9	100.6	124.4	223.0
Administration	2.7	11.9	40.5	53.7	50.0	65.1	79.6	97.2
Research	2.0	5.5	12.2	14.5	18.0	19.7	21.6	30.1

*Revised health expenditures.
†Projected.
From Health Care Financing Administration, Office of the Actuary, National Health Statistics Group.

TABLE 52-3 Percent Increase in Population Estimates by Age Cohort: 1995-2030

Age and Period	Lowest Estimate (%)	Middle Estimate (%)	Highest Estimate (%)
65+			
1995-2010	10.8	17.5	24.2
1995-2030	75.6	106.8	136.4
75+			
1995-2010	14.5	24.1	35
1995-2030	71.8	116.2	164
85+			
1995-2010	37.9	56	79.1
1995-2030	59.1	132.7	235.1

From U.S. Bureau of the Census. National Aging Information Center, 1999.

The aging population is, however, expected to have more of an impact on health services than any other demographic factor. In 1950, more than half of the U.S. population was less than 30 years of age; in 1994, half of the population was 34 years of age or older. In 1990, 65-year-olds comprised 12.5% of the population; by 2030 they are estimated to comprise up to 21% of the population. That is, one in eight Americans were 65+ in 1990; one in five are projected to be 65+ in 2030. In addition, the number of persons 85+ is expected to double between 1990 and 2030. Table 52-3 indicates projections for growth in aged cohorts projected through 2030.

Although many elderly are independent and active, they are likely to experience multiple chronic conditions that may become disabling. The elderly are admitted to hospitals three times more often than the general population, and their average length of stay is more than 3 days longer than the average. The elderly visit physicians more often and constitute a larger percentage of nursing home residents. Table 52-4 illustrates the economic impact of funding health services for those older than age 65.

Life expectancy and health status have been increasing in the United States. The elderly continue to con-sume a disproportionate share of financial resources, however.

Health care providers are also concerned about the growth in the elderly population because public funding sources have not been increasing their reimbursement rates sufficiently to cover inflation, and thus, providers earn a smaller return on elderly patients each year.

The aging of the population also spurs concerns about funding their health expenditures because of changes in the ratio of employed to retired persons; this as participants in the work force pay the most income taxes and all social security payroll taxes. The funding base for Medicare decreases as the population ages and as retirement rates increase.

Macrodemographic indicators termed *dependency ratios* inform policymakers about the need for economic and physical support of the elderly. The elderly support ratio is the number of persons 65 years and older, divided by the number of persons age 20 to 64 (primary age of the workforce), multiplied by 100. It is an indicator of requirements necessary for economic and physical support. As Table 52-5 indicates, the elderly support ratio is projected to increase sharply over time. As a result, some policymakers believe that Medicare and system reforms are needed to ensure adequate financing and delivery of health care services to an aging population.

Policy-related reform options under consideration include increased age limits for Medicare eligibility, means testing for Medicare eligibility, increased availability and coverage for long-term care insurance, increased incentives for prevention, and less expensive and more efficient delivery arrangements and care settings (i.e., managed care arrangements). Meanwhile, the debate continues as to how to best handle the future funding of the growing Medicare program.

FUNDING U.S. HEALTH SERVICES

Since the 1960s, U.S. health care services have been funded by both private and public (federal, state, and local government) sources. Although total spending by all

TABLE 52-4 U.S. Health Spending for the Elderly, 1995*

% Total Health Spending on Elderly 1995	Ratio of Health Spending for Persons >65 and <64	Estimated % GDP Spent on Health for the Elderly	% GDP Spent on Health	Health Spending per Capita 1997
38	3.8	5	13.6	$12,090

*Data from O.E.C.D. Health Data 1999.
From Anderson, G.F., & Hussey, P.S. (2000). Population aging: A comparison among industrialized countries. *Health Affairs, 19*(3), 195.

TABLE 52-5 Elderly Support Ratio by Age: 1990-2050

Year	65-74 Years	75+ Years
1990	12.4	8.9
2050	16.5	21.7

From Bureau of the Census. Hobbs, F.B., & Damon, B.L. (1996, April). Current Population Reports Special Studies, 65+ in the United States.

sources has increased, the percentage of total expenditures attributable to private sources has decreased in relation to public sources from 1950 to 1990. Among public sources, the percentage paid by the federal government is increasing the most rapidly. In fact, the percentage of expenditures covered by state and local sources has remained about the same during the 40-year period. Increased participation by the federal government in funding health services is attributable to Medicare and Medicaid programs. The rate of public expenditure increases slowed and was stabilized compared with prior decades. This stabilization is largely attributable to the impact of prospective payment system (PPS) and managed care policies.

An analysis of trends in funding sources identifies the increasing role of the federal government in financing U.S. health services. In 1980, private funding sources accounted for 57.6% of health-related expenditures; the federal government funded 29.1%; state and local government funded 13%. By 1997, public sources of expenditures increased. Private sources accounted for 53.7% of health care expenditures, federal government for 33.6%, and state and local government for 12.8%. Table 52-6 summarizes the funding sources for health-related services from 1970 projected through 2007.

TABLE 52-6 National Health Expenditures by Source of Funds, Selected Years 1980-2007

Source of Funds	1970	1980	1990*	1993*	1997*	1999†	2001†	2007†
National expenditures (billions)	$73.2	$247.3	$699.4	$898.5	$1,092.4	$1,228.5	$1,403.6	$2,176.6
Private funds total	45.5	142.5	416.2	513.2	585.3	669.2	774.9	1,102.2
% Distribution		57.6	59.5	57.1	53.6	54.5	55.2	53.9
Private insurance	16.3	69.8	239.6	306.8	348.0	403.7	474.2	677.5
		28.2%	34.3%	34.1%	31.9%	32.9%	33.8%	33.2%
Out-of-pocket	24.9	60.3	145.0	167.1	187.6	208.8	236.5	334.1
		24.4%	20.7%	18.6%	17.2%	17.0%	16.8%	16.4%
Public funds total	27.7	104.8	283.2	385.3	507.1	559.3	628.7	940.9
% Distribution		42.4	40.5	42.9	46.4	45.5	44.8	46.1
Federal total	17.8	72.0	195.2	275.4	367.0	399.8	447.7	664.5
% Distribution		29.1	27.9	30.6	33.6	32.5	31.9	32.5
Medicare	7.7	37.5	111.5	148.7	214.6	230.1	257.4	376.1
		15.2%	15.9%	16.6%	19.6%	18.7%	18.3%	18.4%
Medicaid	2.9	14.5	42.7	76.8	95.4	108.0	122.7	198.6
		5.9%	6.1%	8.6%	8.7%	8.8%	8.7%	9.7%
Other	7.3	19.9	41.0	49.8	57.1	61.6	67.6	89.9
		8.1%	5.9%	5.5%	5.2%	5.0%	4.8%	4.4%
State/local total	9.9	32.8	88.0	110.0	140.0	159.5	181.0	276.4
		13.3%	12.6%	12.2%	12.8%	13.0%	12.9%	13.5%
Medicaid	2.5	11.6	32.7	44.9	64.5	74.0	84.0	137.1
		4.7%	4.7%	5.0%	5.9%	6.0%	6.0%	6.7%
Other	7.4	21.2	55.3	65.1	75.6	85.5	97.0	139.3
		8.6%	7.9%	7.2%	6.9%	7.0%	6.9%	6.8%

*Revised national expenditures.
†Projected.
From Health Care Financing Administration, Office of the Actuary, National Health Statistics Group, and U.S. Department of Commerce, Bureau of Economic Analysis.

FINANCING TRENDS IN THE U.S. HEALTH SYSTEM

National health expenditures are projected to total $2.2 trillion in 2008, growing at an average annual rate of 6.5% from 1997. This will represent an increase in health care's share of the GNP to 16.2%. Three patterns of economic growth for the health sector were projected by the National Health Statistics Group, Office of the Actuary, Health Care Financing Administration (HCFA) (Smith, Heffler, & Freeland, 1999): (1) a rising share of GNP devoted to health care, but at a lower rate than was experienced from 1960 to 1992; (2) cyclical growth in private spending for health care, with accelerated growth expected from 1998 to 2001 and decelerated growth expected from 2002 to 2008; and (3) diverging patterns of growth in private and public spending from 1998 to 2002. These projections are based on implementation of the Balanced Budget Act (BBA) of 1997 and projected restraints on the growth in Medicare spending. If BBA rollbacks take place, public spending for Medicare is expected to increase significantly, and public spending will outpace private source spending.

In terms of funding sources, the United States has developed and maintained a dependence on private source funding for health services. Although public funding has been and continues to increase, it is useful to examine some of the factors that have accounted for the development and growth of all third-party payers; this, as the payer system sets the economic climate and determines the threats and opportunities health care organizations and providers must respond to.

Evolution of the Third-Party Payer System

Most nurses are familiar with the dramatic changes in health care that have occurred as a result of scientific and technical advances since the 1950s. Over this period, hospitals became the dominant locus for the diagnosis and treatment of disease. It is the 1930s, however, a period in which the United States experienced both increasing costs for health care and the Great Depression, that explains the motivation for our insurance dependence. During the depression, physicians and hospitals (through the American Hospital Association) encouraged the development of insurance plans, primarily Blue Cross and Blue Shield. As a result, private health insurance developed and grew rapidly through the period after World War II. In 1966, Medicare and Medicaid programs were established as government-sponsored "insurance" programs for the elderly and the poor. The impact of these programs and the changing focus of their management have served as the

primary locus for discussion and action concerning health care cost containment and health reform efforts in recent years.

Medicare and Medicaid. Medicare is a federal insurance program designed to cover health care services for persons 65 years and older. In 1990, almost 35 million persons were enrolled in Medicare. Future concerns about the solvency of the Medicare Trust Fund come from both projections about the growth of the aged in the U.S. population and the continued growth of health care costs (the rate of annual cost increases continues to outpace the rate of inflation). Some predictions call for bankruptcy of the Medicare system by 2015 unless substantial changes are made.

Medicare has two parts, each with its own federal trust fund designed to ensure that adequate funds are available. The health insurance portion (Part A) pays for inpatient hospital care, posthospital skilled nursing care, home health services, and hospice care. Supplemental medical insurance (Part B) covers physician services, hospital outpatient services, and selected other services. Medicare is primarily funded through payroll taxes and by Part B charges to enrollees.

Federal and state governments jointly fund Medicaid. The federal government establishes the minimum requirements for Medicaid eligibility and defines essential services that must be provided. States design the scope of their own programs, using federal requirements as a minimum. States receive roughly one dollar from the federal government for each dollar of coverage. Some policymakers believe that this has created incentives for states to expand Medicaid coverage because they bear only about half of the costs. In 1990, about 25 million persons received some type of Medicaid benefit, with most benefits directed toward the aged, blind, and disabled.

Prospective Payment Systems. The most significant change in Medicare has been associated with adoption of the prospective payment system. As part of the Tax Equity and Fiscal Responsibility Act (TEFRA) of 1982, Congress established the rationale for hospital payment based on cost per case. In 1983 amendments to the Social Security Act further defined the case payment system. These amendments created a revolutionary payment of reimbursement to hospitals for treating Medicare patients based on diagnosis-related groups (DRGs). The PPS applied to hospitals in fiscal years beginning on or after October 1, 1993. Under this system, hospitals are paid a preestablished amount per case treated with payment rates varying by type of case. Initially DRGs classified patients into 23 major diagnostic categories, with 490 subcategories.

Specialty hospitals, such as children's long-term care, rehabilitation, and psychiatric hospitals were exempt from PPS. States with approved alternative payment systems (New Jersey and Maryland) were also exempt.

Medicare's DRG payment system applies only to a portion of the cost of treating patients (inpatient operating costs). Payments for direct medical expenses, capital, and hospital outpatient expenses were not included in the DRG prospective payment system. Capital and related costs were paid for on a "reasonable cost" basis until October of 1991, when prospective payment for capital and related costs went into effect. PPS capital payment regulations use a standard federal rate for these costs based on the estimated fiscal year 1992 national average Medicare cost per discharge. Incremental payments are made under PPS for indirect medical education costs and for outlier cases (cases involving atypical costs).

Federal rates are updated annually. Actual rates for DRGs are calculated on the base year with an annual update factor. Specific urban and rural payment rates are established for each of the nine geographical regions, in addition to national, urban, and rural payment rates. The federal DRG payment rate is usually published in June and finalized in September. Congressional intervention related to deficit reduction has in recent years delayed the annual determination until November or December.

As of June 1, 1999, skilled nursing facilities (SNFs) providing subacute care for Medicaid patients were subject to yet a different PPS. Medicare's skilled nursing facility PPS follows the intent of the Balanced Budget Act of 1997, which mandates that SNF PPS work on a per diem payment system modified by case adjustments. The PPS per diem reimbursement covers all routine, therapy, and capital-related costs except certain approved education activities. Separate adjustments exist for urban and rural areas and geographical differences in labor costs (Knapp, 1999).

The SNF PPS uses resource utilization groups (RUGs), which measure resident characteristics and staff care time for various categories of patients. RUGs have seven categories of patient severity. Caregivers derive classifications from assessments recorded in the Minimum Data Set (MDS) assessment instrument, required at specified intervals for days 5, 14, 30, 60, and 90 during a Part A stay. A 3-year phase-in of facility-specific, cost-based, and national per diem PPS rates applies to all facilities that were paid on or before October 1, 1995 (Knapp, 1999). The federal per diem rate is derived from 1995 cost reports and is adjusted for area wage differences and case mix, with no exception or exemption amounts. The federal per diem includes drugs and therapies covered under Part B, as well as necessary laboratory tests, x-ray examinations, and ambulance services provided during the skilled nursing care stay.

Managed Care

Managed care is an approach to managing the quality and cost of health care. In the current environment, there is no single definition of managed health care. Among the varieties of managed care arrangements there are two common characteristics: an authorization system and provider restrictions. From least to most restrictive the different models of managed care include:

- Indemnity insurance with precertification, mandatory second opinion, and large case management
- Service plan with precertification, mandatory second opinion, and large case management
- Preferred provider organization (PPO)
- Point-of-service (POS) plan
- "Open access" HMO
- Traditional HMO
  - Open panel
    - Individual practice association (IPA)
    - Direct contract
  - Network model
  - Closed-panel HMO
    - Group model
    - Staff model

The two most prevalent types of managed care arrangements are HMOs and PPOs. The PPO evolved during the early 1980s. Typically, they are considered a hybrid of HMOs and traditional health care insurance. They use many of the cost-saving strategies developed by HMOs, such as utilization review and reduced reimbursement by volume service contracting. However, PPOs do not require beneficiaries to use providers with which the PPO has discounted fee contracts. Unlike HMOs, PPOs do not require beneficiaries to use preselected gatekeeper physicians who serve as the initial contact and authorize all services. PPOs are less likely than HMOs to provide preventive services, and they do not assume any responsibility for quality assurance because the enrollees are not limited to using only PPO providers.

The HMO is organized on the premise that the current fee-for-service system creates perverse incentives that reward providers for treating patients' illnesses while offering few or no incentives for providing prevention and rehabilitation services. Full-risk HMOs combine the financing and the delivery of comprehensive health care services into a single system and theoretically have an incentive to focus on the prevention of illness over treatment. In recent years, HMO incentives have come under attack amid allegations of withholding treatment to manage costs or increase operating margins.

There are many different types of HMO structures with varying arrangements for ownership and financial incentives (risk). HMOs use a variety of methods to control costs, including limiting patients to particular providers, gatekeeper physicians who must authorize specialized services, utilization review to ensure that services rendered are appropriate, discounted rate schedules from providers, and payment methods that transfer some risk to providers. In general, services are not covered if beneficiaries bypass their primary care (gatekeeper) physician or provider or use non-HMO providers. The cost of providing services and the quality of service provided also vary among HMOs nationwide. Managed care plans reflect the current movement to control health care spending by combining providers and insurers into a related entity.

Managed Care Trends. Managed care arrangements have proliferated, and enrollment in them has grown rapidly since the 1980s. Hybrids of HMOs and PPOs such as exclusive provider organizations and point-of-service (POS) plans have enjoyed considerable growth in public and private sectors. It is estimated that about one third of the insured population is currently enrolled in some form of a managed care plan. Among large firms, enrollment in managed care plans grew from 5% in 1984 to 50% by 1993 (Gabel, Ginsburg, & Hunt, 1997).

Between 1993 and 1997, HMOs and PPOs dominated employer plan offerings and enrollment in both small and large organizations. The percent enrollment by type of managed care offering and size of employer is presented in Table 52-7.

In an effort to achieve the potential cost savings of HMOs and PPOs, conventional insurance companies have started to apply HMO and PPO strategies to their own plans. Such plans, called managed fee-for-service plans, are using preadmission certification, utilization review, and second surgical opinions to control inappropriate utilization. Although the differences between HMOs, PPOs, and conventional plans were once distinct, considerable overlap now exists in the strategies and incentives they use. Thus the term *managed care* now describes a continuum of managed care organizations or arrangements, which vary significantly in their approaches to providing combined insurance and health care service programs.

SERVICE DELIVERY TRENDS IMPACTED BY MANAGED CARE

Before the 1980s, most health care organizations were freestanding and not formally linked with other organizations. Those that were linked tended to be part of horizontally integrated organizations that controlled a single type of health care facility, such as nursing homes. During the 1990s, many health care providers have diversified and become vertically integrated. The benefits of providing hospital care, ambulatory care, long-term care, and

TABLE 52-7 Utilization of Managed Care Arrangements by Organizational Size 1993-1997*

Employer Size	HMO Only (%)	POS Only (%)	PPO Only (%)	Indemnity Only (%)	Managed Care and Indemnity (%)	Other Combinations (%)
<50 employees						
1993	15	3	23	49	7	3
1997	34	6	34	17	3	6
50-499 employees						
1993	13	3	23	34	16	11
1997	29	6	29	11	10	15
>500 employees						
1993	6	3	13	29	37	12
1997	8	12	19	12	22	27
All employers						
1993	10	3	18	34	25	10
1997	19	9	25	12	15	20

*Data from National Employer Health Insurance Survey and 1997 Robert Wood Johnson Foundation Employer Health Insurance Survey.
From Marquis, S.M., & Long, S.H. (1999). Trends in managed care and managed competition, 1993-1997. *Health Affairs, 18*(6), 83.

business and support services through a multi-institutional arrangement are the motivation for vertical integration. Some of the obvious benefits include keeping patients in the corporate network of services, acquiring access to managerial and functional specialists (i.e., marketing specialists), effective use of information systems, greater access to capital, and an enhanced ability to recruit and retain management and professional staff. Although delivery settings are discussed as separate entities, common corporate integration is recognized as key to organizational stability in establishing more powerful collectives, strengthening patient referrals, and increasing profitability.

Hospitals

Hospitals provide diagnostic and therapeutic services to persons who require more than several hours of care, although most hospitals also provide ambulatory services as well. Hospitals differ in function, length of patient stay, size, and ownership. These factors affect the type and quantity of fixed assets, programs, and management requirements and often determine the type and level of reimbursement available.

Recent environmental and operational changes have created significant challenges affecting the management of hospitals. From 1980 to 1990, hospitals experienced a decrease in admissions and reduced average lengths of stay. At the same time, hospitals were pressured to reduce annual growth in patient charges, as well as assume risk in their contracts with third-party payers. The impact on U.S. hospitals is that operating margins have been declining. Urban and rural hospitals find it particularly difficult to achieve retained earnings after paying for operating expenses. Current projections on U.S. hospital operating margins are illustrated in Table 52-8.

In addition to financing expensive new technology, staff payroll and benefit expenses are usually the largest recurring operating expense hospitals incur. Of these

TABLE 52-8   Total Margin, Length of Stay (LOS), and Discharge Cost Changes: U.S. Hospitals, 1997-1999

Year	Margin	LOS Change	Discharge Cost Change (%)
1997	6.0	−3.4	0.5
1998	3.9-4.3	−2.7	1.5
1999	2.7	−4.5	Not available

Data from Green, T. (2000, March). Presentation to MedPAC Commission.

nursing service personnel (registered nurses [RNs] and others) usually comprise the largest cost object. Thus interest has evolved in recent years in reducing nursing service costs as one method of improving the short-term economic performance of hospitals.

Ambulatory and Outpatient Services

Ambulatory and outpatient care services encompass services including medical practices, hospital outpatient departments, and emergency departments. In the 1980s substantial growth in new ambulatory care settings, such as home health care, ambulatory surgical centers, urgent care centers, diagnostic imaging centers, rehabilitation and sports medicine centers, and clinical laboratories was observed. In general, these new settings offer patients increased convenience compared with hospital-based services, and in many situations the new centers provide services at lower costs than hospitals do.

Although many factors account for the expansion of ambulatory services, technology and cost containment are the leading contributors. Patients who once required hospitalizations because of the complexity, intensity, invasiveness, or risk associated with certain procedures can now be treated in outpatient settings. In addition, third-party payers have encouraged providers to expand their outpatient services through mandatory authorization for inpatient services and by payment mechanisms that provide incentives to perform services on an outpatient basis. Finally, fewer regulatory requirements are associated with building and managing outpatient services compared with establishing new programs and services in long-term care or hospital facilities.

Long-Term Care

Long-term care entails health care and personal services provided to individuals who lack some degree of functional capacity. Long-term care usually covers an extended period, and it includes both inpatient and outpatient services, many of which focus on mental health, rehabilitation, and nursing home care. Long-term care is concerned with levels of independent functioning with activities of daily living and mobility. Individuals become candidates for long-term care when they become too mentally or physically incapacitated to perform the tasks necessary to live independently and when their family members are unable to provide the services needed. Long-term care is typically a hybrid of health and social services. Three levels of nursing home care exist: skilled nursing facilities, intermediate care, and residential care facilities. Medicaid dominates the list of payers for nursing home care, followed by private pay and then Medicare. As the percentage of elderly in the U.S. population grows, demand for long-term care is expected to grow. The elderly are disproportionately high users of health services and major users of long-term care.

UTILIZATION MANAGEMENT STRATEGIES

Because health care costs are thought to vary as a function of price and volume, utilization management has become a particularly important goal that is directly or indirectly related to the expansion of managed care. The management of utilization in this regard is divided into three types of efforts: prospective, concurrent, and retrospective.

Prospective utilization management involves such efforts as health risk appraisals, demand management, referral services, and institutional services. Demand management involves managing the demand for medical services before use. The most common approaches involve providing home care manuals, increasing access to preventive services, and nurse advice lines. Prospective institutional service management involves authorization or approval before accessing services in inpatient or outpatient settings (e.g., preadmission authorization). Clinical criteria for authorizations are commercially available, or plans may develop their own. Nurses are often the vehicle for implementing institutional service management programs.

Efforts related to concurrent review are typically applied to inpatient care and large case management. Interventions include inpatient care and continued stay review, large case management, and disease management. Large case management refers to the management of catastrophic or chronic cases that exceed routine costs and in which active intervention by nurses can make a significant difference. Cases such as AIDS, transplants, diabetes, and psychiatric disorders often benefit from nurses who are able to coordinate the many aspects of care in order to improve the quality of care and reduce costs. Disease management is a special form of large case management. It typically involves selected clinical conditions and works proactively with the patient to control the course of the disease. Disease management differs from preventive care activities in that the diagnosis is clear, and cost savings occur by improving individual outcomes.

Retrospective management typically involves managing utilization after services have been provided. Two categories of activity are common: case review and pattern analysis. In case review, individual cases are examined for appropriateness of care, billing errors, or other problems. Pattern analysis involves the review of large amounts of utilization data to determine whether patterns exist. Medical practice profiling is one such example.

Although none of these falls into the exclusive domain of managed care, all are potentially useful methods of reducing unnecessary variation in practice. As a result, managed care arrangements typically provide the environment that is most receptive to the oversight and accountability embedded in these efforts.

LEGISLATIVE INTERVENTIONS FOR HEALTH CARE COST CONTAINMENT: THE BALANCED BUDGET ACT OF 1997

Although most efforts at cost containment in recent years have been focused on changing delivery systems and financial incentives, some have been legislated. The most recent and far-reaching legislative intervention to focus on health care cost containment is the Balanced Budget Act of 1997. Implementation of the BBA began in 1998 amid initial estimates by the Congressional Budget Office (CBO) that Medicare spending could be cut by approximately $112 billion from 1998 through 2003. Some 300 provisions in the legislation were expected to provide a complex array of new preventive benefits and payment system reforms designed to promote Medicare service access and efficiency, many of which are achieved through payment reductions.

Significant reductions are targeted for the home health industry. Reimbursement for home health services has been severely curtailed by the BBA, as the HCFA adopts a PPS to replace the interim payment system (IPS). This provision is expected to produce an estimated savings of $40 billion in Medicare payments alone. Additional savings are expected to come from skilled nursing facilities' (SNFs) prospective payment. As SNFs have received higher acuity patients from hospitals and have offered higher levels of care, they are now caught between new Medicare payment rules and a new SNF PPS with rates based on average industry costs for different types of care. In addition to these features, the BBA closed loopholes that allowed nursing homes to clear 30% profit margins on respiratory, physical, and occupational therapy.

As a result of full BBA implementation, an increase in negative Medicare operating margins was projected by hospitals, with rural hospitals expected to be hurt the most. According to the American Hospital Association, negative operating margins for Medicare outpatient services was projected to range from −4.4% to −7.8% annually. Outpatient PPS rules were expected to reduce outpatient service margins under Medicare to between –20.3% and –28.8%.

BBA Impact: Nonphysician Practitioners

Among the diverse provisions of the BBA, many are associated with nonphysician practitioners. The BBA extends to nonphysician providers, including advanced practice nurses (APNs), new opportunities and responsibilities. A number of BBA provisions and implementation features are of particular significance to APNs. First, NPs, clinical nurse specialists (CNS), and physician assistants (PAs) were recognized as authorized Medicare providers, eligible for direct reimbursement. A HCFA ruling associated with this provision subsequently defined only APNs and CNSs with a master's degree in nursing to be qualified to receive payments from Medicare Part B services. The revision allows for a grace period before the minimum education rule is enforced in 2003 (Buppert, 1999).

The BBA standardized NP reimbursement at 85% of the physician's Medicare fee schedule, regardless of where services are provided. This represents up to a 20% increase in reimbursement for providing services such as those rendered as a first surgical assistant. APN enrollment in the Medicare program carries with it increased personal responsibility. Medicare has the most aggressive fraud and abuse guidelines of any insurance plan. It is essential that APNs become familiar with billing for services (*International Classification of Diseases [ICD]-9* and *Current Procedural Terminology [CPT]* codes) and using evaluation and management codes (E and M codes). These codes are the only method that the payer can use to substantiate that the level of service provided was equal to the severity and complexity of the presenting problem (Towers, 1999).

In addition, the BBA cedes supervision and legislative scope of practice back to the individual states. This provision effectively removes the requirement for a physician to see a Medicare patient first or be in the office when services are billed under the APN's provider number. However, APNs must be familiar with state supervision requirements (Table 52-9).

The BBA also permits APNs to develop independent contractor arrangements with medical practices and provider entities (called 1099 arrangements). This provides considerable employment flexibility but shifts the income-tax responsibility from the practice or organization to the independent contractor (Mazzocco, 2000). Here, APNs must be familiar with tax and employment contract responsibilities.

Although these BBA provisions have done more to influence the course of advanced practice nursing than any other single piece of legislation in the 1990s, the ramifications are many and far reaching. In other aspects related to APN use and reimbursement, the BBA is limited. The BBA has no effect on private insurance carriers; it only permits APNs to enroll as Medicare providers. Each private insurance plan has its own policies and authorized list of providers. When plans do not recognize APNs to be eligible for direct reimbursement, some practice situations may fall back on "incident to" billing techniques. "Incident to" is an old billing method that permits practices to bill for APN services under the supervising physicians billing number at 100% of the physician's fee schedule as long as the physician is present in the office at the time services are rendered.

Concerning regulation and interpretation, HCFA has little enforcement capability over its carriers. Individual medical directors have the ability to exercise a wide degree of flexibility in interpreting the regulations (including down coding of services provided by APNs).

Although much of the impact associated with the 1997 BBA is related to reducing Medicare costs though reductions in payment rates to hospitals, ambulatory clinics, and so forth, other features have introduced unprecedented opportunities for nonphysician providers such as

TABLE 52-9   Number of States Reimbursing Advance Practice Nurses

	Medicaid Reimbursement	Private Insurance Mandates	Medicare Reimbursement
Nurse practitioners	48	29	Yes
Certified nurse midwives	49	37	Yes
Physician assistants	49	3	Yes
Certified registered nurse anesthetists	36	22	Yes
Clinical nurse specialists	36	0	Yes

From Cooper, R.A., Henderson, T., & Dietrich, C. (1998). Roles of nonphysician clinicians as autonomous providers of patient care. *Journal of the American Medical Association, 280*(9), 799. Copyrighted 1998, American Medical Association.

APNs. Current reactions to implementation have been uniformly negative concerning the adverse impact on organizations. As a result, legislation is pending that alters implementation considerably.

IMPACT OF MANAGED CARE AND CURRENT COST CONTAINMENT EFFORTS

One of the main reasons for the growing popularity of managed care among health insurance purchasers (including employers and public sector programs) has been its emphasis on cost containment in an era of rising health care spending. Savings have been derived largely from decreased use of inpatient hospital services. Research on this topic has indicated that compared with fee-for-service plans, HMO enrollees have lower hospital admission rates and lengths of stay and less use of expensive tests and procedures (Weinick & Cohen, 2000). Many PPOs and POS plans use the same types of utilization controls as HMOs (i.e., requiring precertification for an approved length-of-stay and plan review for medical necessity) while increasing consumer choice.

Growth in managed care plan enrollment and increased managed care plan options have experienced changes in the types of persons enrolling in managed care plans over time. On average, managed care populations have become less healthy, and managed care's advantage with respect to hospital use and expenses has been attenuated. Recent evidence from HMOs financial performance and premium increases suggest support for this notion.

In addition, local markets have been affected by managed care expansion. Competitive pressure to reduce expenses by decreasing hospital use and so on has been extended to fee-for-service plans. Weinick and Cohen examined existing national survey data for managed care enrollment and hospital use in 1987 and 1996. In 1987 statistically significant hospital use differences were found between managed care and nonmanaged care enrollees, with managed care rates being lower. The differences were no longer statistically significant by 1996 because changes were attributable to decreased hospital use among nonmanaged care enrollees.

The study also observed shifts in the characteristics of managed care–enrolled populations. Publicly insured populations were more likely to be enrolled in a managed care organization. The proportion of managed care enrollees who were in fair or poor health did not change over time. However, nonmanaged care enrollees were less likely to be in fair or poor health in 1996. These shifts may help explain decreased hospital use among those covered by nonmanaged care plans. Practice pattern changes adopted by providers and plans were also identified as a possible influencing factor (Weinick & Cohen, 2000).

Regardless of whether the changes observed are attributable to shifts in the composition of managed care populations or changes in plans' or providers' behavior, findings suggest that the competitive advantage of managed care organizations with respect to inpatient hospital use was eroded by 1996. Thus the ability to generate further cost savings in hospital care through increasing managed care enrollment may be limited as we approach convergence in utilization between managed care and nonmanaged care plans.

With or without full BBA implementation the U.S. health system continues to undergo considerable change. Whether these changes will be attributable to legislative initiatives designed to reduce costs or to managed care remains to be seen. There is, however, considerable consensus about cost-reduction strategies and interventions designed to respond to the competitive managed care environment. In general, two approaches are advocated: the shift of services away from hospital-based delivery systems to ambulatory, home health, and long-term care systems and sector-specific interventions related to improving cost-containment and the quality of health-related services (Buerhaus & Staiger, 1996; Shortell, 1993; Sovie, 1994; Weinick & Cohen, 2000).

Selective contracting and legislation mandating PPS have led to many changes in hospital care: fewer inpatient admissions, lower average lengths of hospital stay, more serious patient acuity (Dranove, Shanley, & White, 1993; Guterman, Eegers, Riley, Greene, & Terrell, 1988). In addition, because nurse wages are the largest single item in the hospitals operating budget, incentives exist for hospitals to adjust nurse staffing as a cost-reduction strategy.

Managed Care and Nurse Staffing

The effect of HMOs and PPOs on the staffing of nursing personnel and hospitals is a source of growing concern. Recent newspaper articles report that hospitals reduced their use of RNs by replacing them with unlicensed assistant personnel in response to cost-cutting pressures caused by the growth of HMOs (Kunen, 1996; Rosenthal, 1996; Shuit, 1996). Patient advocates, nursing unions, and other observers have argued that staffing changes are reducing the quality of care provided by hospitals. In response to these claims of reduced nurse staffing and reduced quality of care, some state legislatures are attempting to regulate hospital employment of nursing personnel. Legislation has been introduced in several states, including Massachusetts, Nevada, California, and Florida, to establish minimum staffing levels for the nurses and other staff.

Unions and hospitals have engaged in heated debate about whether nurse-staffing levels have in fact been reduced and whether such reductions adversely affect the quality of care. Union contract disputes have drawn additional public attention to nurse staffing changes and nurse's assertion that the quality of care in hospitals is adversely affected (Hall, 1998; Hercher, 1997). Little research has been published to date on staffing and staffing ratios. And the research that has been done to date presents contradictory findings. Some researchers have reported finding a reduction of full-time equivalent employment of hospital nurses per patient day (Aiken & Fagin, 1997); others report increased hours worked in hospitals (Anderson & Kohn, 1996; Spetz, 1998, 1999). Buerhaus and Staiger (1996) conducted a cross-state comparison of RN employment and HMO penetration, identifying slower rates of RN employment growth in states with higher HMO penetration. Spetz (1999) examined the effects of managed care and the PPS on hospital employment of RNs, licensed practical nurses (LPNs), and unlicensed assistive personnel (UAP) in California from 1994 to 1997. She reported that HMOs used fewer LPNs and UAPs and that HMOs did not reduce RN demand. Additional findings included managed care having a smaller affect on RN staffing in medical-surgical units than in daily hospital service units as a whole, and PPS was not found to have a statistically significant effect on nurse staffing changes. The author noted that organizational changes created in response to PPS might have an impact on care delivery systems and affect the quality of care. This study reinforced the link between characteristics of HMO organizations and the quality of care (Spetz, 1999).

In considering skill mix staffing levels, the effect on nursing personnel use and impact on quality of care is often questioned. The Institute of Medicine examined the adequacy of nursing personnel staffing and found little research that systematically examined the relationship between skill mix and quality of care (Wunderlich, Sloan, & Davis, 1996). Contradictory findings were reported in two other studies examining the association between nurse staffing and patient outcomes (Aiken & Fagin, 1997; Mitchell & Shortell, 1997). Aiken and Fagin reported a possible effect between certain organizational characteristics and their impact on quality of care that may be more important than staffing levels alone (Aiken & Fagin, 1997). Buerhaus and Needleman (2000) conducted a review of federally funded nursing workforce studies and research efforts that investigated the relationship between hospital nurse staffing and patient outcomes sensitive to nursing. He identified that there remains an insufficient body of empirical evidence that links changes in hospital nurse staffing to adverse effects on the quality of patient care, particularly for purposes of mandating minimum staffing levels.

Managed Care and Nursing Roles

The direct and indirect impact of managed care and PPSs on nursing roles is considerable. Although an extensive discussion about impact on advance practice roles (clinical and administrative) and changing RN roles in acute care and other settings is beyond the scope of this chapter, an overview of impact trends is provided. A summary of impact related to use and roles of clinicians and managers follows.

Nonphysician clinicians (NPCs) are becoming increasingly prominent as health care providers. A study conducted by Cooper, Henderson, and Dietrich (1998) and Cooper, Loud, and Dietrich (1998) examined NPCs including nurse practitioners (NPs), physician assistants (PAs), and certified nurse midwives (CNMs). The aggregate number of NPCs graduating annually in 10 NPC disciplines doubled between 1992 and 1997 and was expected to increase by 20% through 2001. The greatest growth in the 1990s was projected among those nonphysician providers who provided primary care services, such as PAs and APNs (nurse practitioners, certified nurse midwives, certified registered nurse anesthetists, and clinical nurse specialists).

Until 1977 the reimbursement of APNs (NPs, CNMs, clinical nurse specialists [CNSs]), and PAs by Medicare and Medicaid was governed by the "incident to" provision. This allowed nonphysician clinicians who were employed by physicians to be reimbursed by means of payment to the employer. In 1977 the Rural Health Clinic Act permitted Medicare and Medicaid to directly reimburse PAs and NPs working in free-standing, physician-directed rural clinics located in health professions shortage areas. This was subsequently expanded to cover care provided in other locations, and on-site physician supervision was waived unless it was a requirement of the state. The BBA of 1997 further expands direct Medicare reimbursement for PAs, NPs, and CNSs to include all nonhospital sites and removes the requirement for physician involvement. Although nonphysician clinicians are authorized to provide a range of physician services, often in an independent manner, and can be reimbursed for that care, marked variation has been identified in their scope of practice, independence, and reimbursement (Schaffner, Ludwig-Beymer, & Wiggins, 1995).

The number of practicing nonphysician clinicians also varies substantially from state to state, and the number is expected to grow in anticipation of managed care demand. Provider organizations, such as clinics, physician group practices, and HMOs have reported increased use of nonphysician clinicians in their practices or offering independent practice agreements (Cooper, Henderson, & Dietrich, 1998).

Regardless, the use of advance practice nurses to support population-based health management interventions such as critical pathways (also called clinical pathways) are one method of planning, assessing, and evaluating the cost-effectiveness of patient care. Critical pathways are predetermined courses of progress that patients should be making while undergoing diagnosis and treatment for specific health-related problems, and patient progress is monitored against established critical pathways indicators. Analysis of clinician's interventions and patient progress is conducted to identify cost-effectiveness and optimize clinical outcomes.

Among the most significant changes associated with managed care have been changes in the use of registered nurses in a wide variety of organizations and health sectors to manage and improve clinical outcomes. Numerous reports of nursing contributions in the management of patient outcomes is found in the literature for nursing roles that are associated with both registered nurses and advance practice nurses (Madden & Reid Ponte, 1994; Maddox, 1999).

Impact of Managed Care and Nurse Manager Practice

A lengthy discussion of the impact of managed care on nurse manager practice is beyond the scope of this chapter. However, the challenges managed care and PPOs payment systems pose to managers in acute and postacute care sectors are tremendous. Since the 1980s, nursing and other health system managers have been implored to learn how to prepare their facilities and staff for prospective payment and, more importantly, how to provide the leadership to carry out a strategic plan for survival. Longfest (1998) and others have identified a variety of competencies required for senior managers in the rapidly changing health system. These competencies include conceptual, technical, managerial, clinical, interpersonal, collaborative, political, commercial, and governance skills that are different from those espoused before the 1970s.

Initially, the focus of efforts was motivated by a need to reduce operating expenses. More recently, efforts have focused on improving customer service and satisfaction, along with overall quality of care (while operating efficiently). New leadership sensitivities and skills associated with managing competing stakeholder relations, allocating scarce resources, and changing organizational culture have been called for (Maddox, 1999; Sovie, 1994; Stahl, 1998). The era of managed care has had considerable impact on nursing and has demanded considerable change in the management and leadership that nurses provide to organizations and the direct provision of services in all sectors of the U.S. health system.

As outpatient care consumes an increasing portion of the health care dollar and efforts to control outpatient spending are enhanced, the traditional operations role of the ambulatory manager is changing. In the past, ambulatory care managers have typically met the needs of physician owners by ensuring adequate billing, collections, staffing, scheduling, and patient relations, whereas physicians have tended to make the long-term business decisions. Changes in reimbursement systems, including managed care contracts, however, now require a higher level of management expertise. In the future, increasing competition, as well as the increasing complexity of the health care environment, will force managers of ambulatory care facilities to become more sophisticated in making business decisions, including financial management decisions.

SUMMARY

The "graying of America" is resulting from increased longevity, coupled with the aging of post–World War II baby boomers. The trend is of major concern to policymakers, because the elderly use a disproportionately high share of health care services, most of which is funded through public sources.

Managing the financial viability of the health care organization involves a collection of processes for subsystems to obtain funds for the organization and to make optimal use of those funds once obtained. Most hospitals receive a substantial amount of the revenue from regulated payers such as Medicare and state Medicaid programs.

Managed care continues to evolve, as does the U.S. health care system. Economic and regulatory forces as described in this chapter will also influence practice patterns among managed care and nonmanaged care providers. Nevertheless the desire to provide access to high-quality, affordable health care will continue to motivate the use of cost-containment and cost-reduction strategies that have been the cornerstone of managed care.

Nurses have played a pivotal role in implementing care management strategies in particular, and nurse managers are a critical resource in health care organizations in balancing competing demands on limited resources. Whether it be the use of APNs as nonphysician providers, the intervention of nurses in case management, or the intervention of nurse managers in resource allocation decisions, nurses must possess the knowledge, skills, and abilities to participate in a health system that demands greater accountability and the delivery of high-quality, efficient health services.

REFERENCES

Aiken, L., & Fagin, C. (1997). Evaluating the consequences of hospital restructuring. *Medical Care, 35*(suppl 10), OS1-OS4.

Anderson, G.F., & Hussey, P.S. (2000). Population aging: A comparison among industrialized countries. *Health Affairs, 19*(3), 191-203.

Anderson, G.F., & Kohn, L. (1996). Employment trends in hospitals 1981-1993. *Inquiry, 33*(1), 79-84.

Buerhaus, P., & Needleman, J. (2000). Policy implications of research on nurse staffing and quality of patient care. *Policy, Politics, and Nursing Practice, 1*(1), 5-15.

Buerhaus, P., & Staiger, D.O. (1996). Managed care and the nurse workforce. *Journal of the American Medical Association, 276*(18), 1487-1497.

Buppert, C. (1999). HCFA revises criteria NP Medicare billing. *Clinician News, 3*(8), 29-30.

Cooper, R.A., Henderson, T., & Dietrich, C. (1998). Roles of nonphysician clinicians as autonomous providers of patient care. *Journal of the American Medical Association, 280*(9), 795-801.

Cooper, R.A., Loud, P., & Dietrich, C.L. (1998). Current and projected workforce of nonphysician clinicians. *Journal of the American Medical Association, 280*(9), 788-794.

Cristiansen, P., & Bender, L.H. (1994). Models of nursing care in a changing environment: Current challenges and future directions. *Orthopaedic Nursing, 13*(7), 64-70.

Dranove, D., Shanley, M., & White, W.D. (1993, April). Price and concentration in hospital markets: The switch from patient-driven to payer-driven competition. *Journal of Law and Economics, 36*, 179-204.

Gabel, J.R., Ginsburg, P.B., & Hunt, K.A. (1997, September-October). Small employers and their health benefits, 1988-1996: An awkward adolescence. *Health Affairs*, pp. 103-110.

Guterman, S.P., Eegers, P.W., Riley, G., Greene, T.F., & Terrell, S.A. (1988). The first 3 years of Medicare prospective payment: An overview. *Health Care Financing Review, 9*(3), 67-77.

Hall, C. (1998, February 5). Evidence doesn't back Kaiser nurse's claims. *San Francisco Chronicle*, p. A1.

Hercher, E. (1997, August 21). Nurse talks focus on staff levels. *San Francisco Chronicle*, p. A17.

Knapp, M.T. (1999). Nurses' basic guide to understanding the Medicare PPS. *Nursing Management, 30*(5), 14-15.

Kreuger Wilson, C., & Porter-O'Grady, T. (1999). *Leading the revolution.* Gaithersburg, MD: Aspen.

Kunen, J. (1996). The new hands off nursing. *Time, 148*(16), 56-57.

Longfest, B. (1998, March/April). Managerial competence at senior levels of integrated delivery systems. *Journal of Health Care Management*, p. 119.

Madden, M.J., & Reid Ponte, P. (1994). Advance practice roles in the managed care environment. *Journal of Nursing Administration, 24*(1), 56-62.

Maddox, P.J. (1999). Management skills. In J. Lancaster (Ed.), *Nursing issues in leading and managing change* (pp. 415-431). St. Louis: Mosby.

Marquis, S.M., & Long, S.H. (1999). Trends in managed care and managed competition, 1993-1997. *Health Affairs, 18*(6), 75-88.

Mazzocco, W.J. (2000). The Balanced Budget Act of 1997: Reimbursement in the advanced practice nurse. Medscape, Inc. Available: www.Medscape.com.

Mitchell, P.H., & Shortell, S.M. (1997). Adverse outcomes and variations in organization of care delivery. *Medical Call, 35*(11), NS19-NS32.

Rosenthal, E. (1996, August 19). Once in big demand, nurses are now targets for hospital cutbacks. *New York Times*, p. A16.

Schaffner, J.W., Ludwig-Beymer, P., & Wiggins, J. (1995). Utilization of advanced practice nurses in health of the care systems and multispecialty group practice. *Journal of Nursing Administration, 25*(12), 37-43.

Shortell, S.M. (1993). Creating organized delivery systems: The barriers and facilitators. *Hospital & Health Services Administration, 38*(4), 447-456.

Shuit, D.P. (1996, July 1). Hospitals feel pain of health systems restructuring. *Los Angeles Times*, pp. A1, A17.

Smith, S., Heffler, S., & Freeland, M. (1999). The next decade of health spending: A new outlook. *Health Affairs, 18*(4), 86-95.

Sovie, M.D. (1995). Tailoring hospitals for managed care and integrated systems. *Nursing Economic$, 13*(2), 72-83.

Spetz, J. (1998). Hospital use of nursing personnel: Has there really been a decline? *Journal of Nursing Administration, 28*(3), 20-27.

Spetz, J. (1999). The effects of managed care and prospective payment on the demand for hospital nurses: Evidence from California, Part I. *Health Services Research, 34*(5), 993-1007.

Stahl, D.A. (1998). PPS challenges and postacute care. *Nursing Management, 29*(8), 10-14.

Towers, J. (1999). Medicare reimbursement for NP's. *Journal of the American Academy of Nurse Practitioners, 11*(7), 289-292.

Weinick, R.M., & Cohen, J.W. (2000). Leveling the playing field: Managed care enrollment and hospital use, 1987-1996. *Health Affairs, 19*(3), 179-184.

Wunderlich, G.S., Sloan, F.A., & Davis, C. (Eds.). (1996). *Nursing staff in hospitals and nursing homes: Is it adequate?* Washington, DC: National Academy Press, Institute of Medicine.

Cost of Home Care for Persons with Disability

HARRIET UDIN ARONOW

Persons with disability are as diverse as the ways in which individuals can be impaired and temporarily or permanently unable to perform activities of daily living (ADL). Disability can be lifelong, acquired in youth or middle age, or appear as frailty in old age or terminal illness. Indisputably, the number of persons living with disability in our society is growing, and this demands a clear analysis of the cost to provide health services and long-term care to this population.

The greatest contributor to the burden of disability on individuals and society is the ever-increasing number of persons who are surviving into very old age. Persons older than age 85 comprise the fastest growing age group in this country. As well, because of advancements in technology (e.g., trauma care, surgical and drug interventions) a growing number of persons disabled by illness or injury are surviving into older years. The life expectancy of persons with developmental disability is also extending, and those who survive into their forties and older are experiencing early onset of frailty and other sensory and cognitive impairments associated with old age.

The cost of home care for this population is an issue not only because of growing numbers making demands on family caregivers and the formal health and long-term care systems but also because of the reorganization of the delivery system in the past two to three decades. The social movement away from large institutions has vastly increased the demand for home care and homelike residences for persons with many severe disabilities, including those with chronic, disabling mental illness. A shift in payment for acute and postacute care has motivated the rapid increase of all kinds of health services previously provided in institutional medical settings to be offered in the home.

When one asks how much does home care for the disabled cost, one must qualify the response by asking cost to whom and examining the components of the cost. Decisions about where a person with disability should live and who should take care of him or her should always take these factors into account. Although home health care was embraced by patients, caregivers, health professionals, and policymakers in the 1980s, and the home health industry has grown significantly since that time, evidence of an impact on health, prevention of nursing home placement, and cost savings has been variable (Cummings & Weaver, 1991; Hughes et al., 1997).

WHO BEARS THE COST?

The dollar cost of disability is measured first and foremost as a cost to society. One might think that private insurance and government programs—Medicare, Medicaid, Social Security Disability, Supplemental Security Income—bear the largest proportion of formal home health and long-term care for the disabled. The larger cost to society can be measured in the lost productivity and out-of-pocket expenses of family and other informal caregivers, however, who may forgo full employment to provide care in the home.

Early in the 1990s there was concern in policy circles that the growth of payment mechanisms for home care would diminish the contribution made by unpaid family members and community services (Hanley, Wiener, & Harris, 1991; Tennstedt, Crawford, & McKinlay, 1993). A more recent study confirmed that the economic value of informal caregiving services (at $196 billion in 1997) far outweighed the dollar cost of either formal home health care ($32 billion) or nursing home care ($83 billion) (Arno, Levine, & Memmott, 1999).

Health care economists have argued that the value of informal caregiver services and the time and resources spent by patients and informal caregivers should always be included in the research and policy decisions concerning alternative settings for health and long-term care services for persons with disabilities (Brouwer, Koopmanschap, & Rutten, 1998; Smith & Wright, 1994). When knee-to-knee with patients and families making decisions about care, it is also the responsibility of the health care provider—nurse, care manager, physician—to consider emotional and financial costs to patients and caregivers (Holicky, 1996).

WHAT ARE THE TYPES OF CARE AND COMPONENTS OF COST?

Short-term Recovery in the Home

When my mother is discharged from the hospital after her planned total knee replacement, she will likely need some continued outpatient rehabilitation. She will not be able to fully take care of herself. But she lives nearby, and she would rather recover at home than in a nursing home. Her Medicare HMO will arrange to have a nurse and a physical therapist visit her on a regular basis to provide follow-up care and therapy.

I plan to take off work for a week to be available to help with daily personal care. We will arrange for meals-on-wheels and for a retired neighbor to come in to clean the house, prepare other food, help me with my mother's personal care and transferring from the bed to her chair (none of us are getting any younger), and to keep her company when I go back to work. After 2 or 3 weeks of this arrangement, we anticipate that my mother will be getting around her house fairly well. But I will probably still be concerned about her consistency and therefore her safety.

I will go back to work. My daughter will check in with her and visit after school. Our neighbor will accompany my mother by senior/disabled transportation to the HMO outpatient rehabilitation center for continued physical therapy. After a few weeks my mother will resume driving, and we will be able to return to living our lives pretty much the way we did before her surgery, although somewhat more wary and watchful over her well-being.

For an acute episode like this the disability is temporary and the cost for care in the home is largely made up of the postacute nursing and therapy services that are needed. With the exception of the week of personal time off taken by the daughter, the remainder of the personal care, food, transportation, and watchful monitoring is relatively low cost.

The trend toward substituting home care for inpatient acute and skilled nursing care has been examined for its cost-effectiveness. The results have been equivocal, leading researchers to recommend more careful evaluation research and a focus on cost outcomes, as well as health outcomes (Sheppard et al., 1998; Soderstrom, Tousignant, & Kaufman, 1999).

Long-term Care in the Home

A colleague of mine has a 21-year-old daughter with Down syndrome. He and his wife live among her tight-knit family. His mother-in-law recently died, and the family is worried about his father-in-law's growing frailty. He is estranged from his own father, who recently wrote him a letter asking his forgiveness for being physically abusive 40 years earlier and would he consider beginning to see him now that he is old and frail. My colleague is faced with providing lifelong care for his daughter and for planning for the growing care needs for his aging parents.

The second typical scenario of home care for persons with disability focuses on the long-term care needs of persons with onset of permanent disability or lifelong disability. This population may or may not have higher risk of acute medical problems. If serious acute medical events do occur, they are treated with the same options of hospital vs. home vs. skilled nursing setting, although an episode of acute care may have a more protracted recovery than for a person with no prior disability.

In a study of families caring for an adult member with mental retardation, researchers estimated that out-of-pocket expenses for care was slightly less than 10% of annual income (Fujiura, Roccoforte, & Braddock, 1994). Although wealthier families spent more, there was a fixed lower limit that resulted in poorer families spending a significantly larger proportion of their income to support their disabled family member. The costs of caring for the individual with permanent disability in the home setting have profound implications for cost to caregiver and society.

By force of demographics the cost of long-term care provided in home settings is largely a phenomenon associated with aging. Even for those persons who acquired a disability in youth or from birth, aging brings challenges in the cost of long-term care associated with early onset of frailty and the aging of the caregiving social support network.

The cost of care for disabled elderly, including both formal services and informal caregiving, was estimated to be slightly less than $10,000 per year in 1995 (Harrow, Tennstedt, & McKinlay, 1995). The greater the disability, the higher the cost and the more likely the older person was to live with his or her caregiver and to become institutionalized. In almost all cases, the combined annual cost to provide care in the home was less than the average cost of 1 year in a nursing home.

New models of community-based residential care have begun to appear, in part related to the independent living movement led by younger persons with disabilities. Persons of all ages, however, will likely benefit from the right to choose among different options for residential long-term care. There are increasing options being tried in residential care facilities for the elderly and for persons with developmental disability. For example, cluster care facilities offer the opportunity for people to live independently in apartments arranged in clusters with central services and care providers (Feldman, Latimer, & Davidson, 1996; Kane, 1995). In long-term care outside institutions the necessity and cost of environmental modifications and equipment become an added consideration affecting choices. Because environmental modification and equipment costs are nonrecurrent, if they directly substitute for the cost of human labor, they can be cost beneficial over the long run (Manton, Corder, & Stallard, 1993).

Technology-supported Care in the Home

At the rehabilitation hospital where I currently work there is a program to wean patients from ventilator-supported breathing. These patients have typically failed weaning in the intensive care unit of an acute hospital and face an uncertain future in institutional care. If they can be weaned in our program and the family trained in respiratory care, they are more likely to return to the home setting.

A third type of care for persons with disability is that provided to children and adults who are in some way dependent on technology for life support. This is most commonly breathing support. There have been a few studies of the cost of home vs. institutional care for technology-dependent children and adults. A study in Germany in 1997 reported nearly double the cost to care for ventilator-dependent spinal cord injury patients at home than in the hospital (Botel, Glaser, Niedeggen, & Meindl, 1997). On the other hand, results of a cost analysis of rehabilitation of ventilator-assisted individuals in New York (Bach, Intintola, Alba, & Holland, 1992) suggested that by enabling patients to use noninvasive methods of ventilatory support, one could reduce nursing cost substantially in the home setting and bring the daily cost to about one third the cost of institutional care.

The impact on the caregiver, and, in the case of families with a technology-dependent child, on the family

must be considered in the measure of cost and benefit of the home setting for care of these individuals. On the one hand, an advantage of the home setting for technology-dependent persons is seen to be the increased control individuals can have over their lives in the home setting (Bingley, 1993). On the other, a study of technology-dependent children suggested that there is significant variation in the degree of impact on financial burden, the family social system, and personal strain, depending on the type of technology dependence of the child (Fleming et al., 1994).

End of Life Care in the Home

Shortly before her 76th birthday, my neighbor's mother discovered she had lung cancer. The tumor had metastasized, and she was given a poor short-term prognosis. Having been socially and politically active in an area of Los Angeles with a large gay community affected by AIDS, she booked a room with a local hospice provider. Although not technically in her own home, the house was owned by a family who had converted their garage into a single room private hospice service with a lovely wall of glass looking out into a quiet green garden. In this home-like setting she lived out her remaining weeks among her friends and relatives nearby in the community, while hospice workers visited as needed, and the host family provided basic personal care services.

Home hospice care has been embraced as an option for persons at the end of life who are no longer able to care for themselves. Palliative care can be provided in the home and has been shown to reduce the number of hospital days and high cost interventions (Maltoni et al., 1997; Maltoni, Nanni, Naldoni, Serra, & Amadori, 1998). In a meta-analysis of the impact of home care on the use of hospital days, it was noted that home care for terminally ill patients consistently lowered hospital use, whereas other studies of home care for nonterminal patients showed variable effects (Hughes et al., 1997).

Responsibilities of Professionals

Persons with disabilities and their families have greatly expanded choices available for where and how to arrange for health and long-term care needs. The home has become a viable alternative for a wide range of disabilities and care scenarios. But the issues of the cost of care in the home are not, as yet, well explored or understood. Until such time as all the economic implications are defined, the health care professionals working with the person with disability and his or her family bear some responsibility to help explain costs associated with each alternative choice. In addition, the health care professional should be prepared to become a part of the intimate negotiations that go on among the person being provided care and his or her network of informal and formal caregivers. This ombudsman-like role will require that professionals educate themselves about the costs and trade-offs among the choices, so they can in turn educate the consumer and assist in the open communication among caregivers, care recipients, and others in the social support network.

REFERENCES

Arno, P.S., Levine, C., & Memmott, M.M. (1999). The economic value of informal caregiving. *Health Affairs, 18*(2), 182-188.

Bach, J.R., Intintola, P., Alba, A.S., & Holland, I.E. (1992). The ventilator-assisted individual. Cost analysis of institutionalization vs rehabilitation and in-home management. *Chest, 101*(1), 26-30.

Bingley, J.D. (1993). Southport experience with domiciliary ventilation. *Paraplegia, 31*(3), 154-156.

Botel, U., Glaser, E., Niedeggen, A., & Meindl, R. (1997). The cost of ventilator-dependent spinal cord injuries—patients in the hospital and at home. *Spinal Cord, 35*(1), 40-42.

Brouwer, W.B., Koopmanschap, M.A., & Rutten, F.F. (1998). Patient and informal caregiver time in cost-effectiveness analysis. A response to the recommendation of the Washington Panel. *International Journal of Technology Assessment in Health Care, 14*(3), 505-513.

Cummings, J.E., & Weaver, F.M. (1991). Cost-effectiveness of home care. *Clinics in Geriatric Medicine, 7*(4), 865-874.

Feldman, P.H., Latimer, E., & Davidson, H. (1996). Medicaid-funded home care for the frail elderly and disabled: Evaluating the cost savings and outcomes of a service delivery reform. *Health Services Research, 31*(4), 489-508.

Fleming, J., Challela, M., Eland, J., Hornick, R., Johnson, P., Martinson, I., Nativio, D., Nokes, K., Riddle, I., & Steele, N. (1994). Impact on the family of children who are technology dependent and cared for in the home. *Pediatric Nursing, 20*(4), 379-388.

Fujiura, G.T., Roccoforte, J.A., & Braddock, D. (1994). Costs of family care for adults with mental retardation and related developmental disabilities. *American Journal of Mental Retardation, 99*(3), 250-261.

Hanley, R.J., Wiener, J.M., & Harris, K.M. (1991). Will paid home care erode informal support? *Journal of Health Politics, Policy, and Law, 16*(3), 507-521.

Harrow, B.S., Tennstedt, S.L., & McKinlay, J.B. (1995). How costly is it to care for disabled elders in a community setting? *Gerontologist, 35*(6), 803-813.

Holicky, R. (1996). Caring for the caregivers: The hidden victims of illness and disability. *Rehabilitation Nursing, 21*(5), 247-252.

Hughes, S.L., Ulasevich, A., Weaver, F.M., Henderson, W., Manheim, L., Kubal, J.D., & Bonarigo, F. (1997). Impact of home care on hospital days: A meta analysis. *Health Services Research, 32*(4), 415-432.

Kane, R.A. (1995). Expanding the home care concept: Blurring distinctions among home care, institutional care, and other long-term-care services. *Milbank Quarterly, 73*(2), 161-186.

Maltoni, M., Nanni, O., Naldoni, M., Serra, P., & Amadori, D. (1998). Evaluation of cost of home therapy for patients with terminal diseases. *Current Opinions in Oncology, 10*(4), 302-309.

Maltoni, M., Travaglini, C., Santi, M., Nanni, O., Scarpi, E., Benvenuti, S., Altertazzi, L., Amaducci, L., Derni, S., Fabbri, L., Masi, A., Montanari, L., Pasini, G., Polselli, G., Tonelli, U., Turci, P., & Amadori, D. (1997). Evaluation of the cost of home care for terminally ill cancer patients. *Support Care Cancer, 5*(5), 396-401.

Manton, K.G., Corder, L., & Stallard, E. (1993). Changes in the use of personal assistance and special equipment from 1982 to 1989: Results from the 1982 and 1989 NLTCS. *Gerontologist, 33*(2), 168-176.

Sheppard, S., Harwood, D., Jenkinson, C., Gray, A., Vessey, M., & Morgan, P. (1998). Randomized controlled trial comparing hospital at home care with inpatient hospital care. I: Three month follow up of health outcomes. *British Medical Journal, 316*(7147), 1786-1791.

Smith, K., & Wright, K. (1994). Informal care and economic appraisal: A discussion of possible methodological approaches. *Health Economics, 3*(3), 137-148.

Soderstrom, L., Tousignant, P., & Kaufman, T. (1999). The health and cost effects of substituting home care for inpatient acute care: A review of the evidence. *Canadian Medical Association Journal, 160*(8), 1151-1155.

Tennstedt, S.L., Crawford, S.L., & McKinlay, J.B. (1993). Is family care on the decline? A longitudinal investigation of the substitution of formal long-term care services for informal care. *Milbank Quarterly, 71*(4), 601-624.

Paradigm Shift

Taking Care of Patients and Taking Care of Business

JEANETTE C. KLEMCZAK, KATHERINE DONTJE

The recent passage of direct Medicare reimbursement for NPs reflected public policymakers' continuing support for NPs as primary care providers.
— Harper and Johnson (1998, p. 158)

There is no such thing as "free" health care. Although advanced practice nurses (APNs) are well intentioned, writing off services to patients may not benefit the practitioner or the patient. Nurses have traditionally believed that we need not concern ourselves with payment for our services. Our goal was to "care" for the patient, but in the present day health care system, to care for the patient we need to also understand the business of health care.

Our nursing culture often views dealing with the financial issues of health care as unprofessional and getting in the way of taking care of the patient. However, we need only pick up a newspaper or view the evening news to learn how the health care world is dealing with these "unprofessional" issues of finance. Hospitals are looking at ways to cut costs, and nursing is often one of the areas that is hit the hardest, partially because we do not have data to define the "care" of nursing. Organizations are merging, closing their doors, or declaring bankruptcy. HMOs are canceling contracts for their Medicaid patients, leaving thousands of individuals with no access to care. Medicare will pay thousands of dollars for a hospitalization but not reimburse for nursing services in the home or clinic that might have prevented that hospitalization or long-term care.

The cataclysmic state of our health care system demands that nurses understand the business, financial, and reimbursement aspects of the patient care they are delivering. Nursing leaders inform us that nursing practice is changing drastically as a result of radically shifting reimbursement methods in health care (Mundinger, 1997). As employees of health care systems, nurses have not always understood health care finance or their role within the organization. In the midst of hospital downsizing and layoffs of thousands of nurses, the United States Department of Labor awarded a grant to develop a program and curriculum to prepare hospital nurses to transition into community-based practices (U.S. Department of Labor, 1995). One of the most disturbing findings of this grant was that when asked why they were losing their jobs, the staff nurses from two major health care systems were unable to articulate what had happened. They believed that as long as they provided "good nursing care" that they would always have a job. Obviously, that is not enough in today's health care world. In 1991 the National League for Nursing surveyed nearly 250 community nursing centers. When they were asked about payment for services, some centers reported that they did not want to charge clients even if it meant the centers would not financially survive (Lockhart, 1995).

Nursing values access to holistic quality care for all individuals. These values cannot be translated to practice without first understanding the "business" of patient care. This chapter will focus on issues central to the practice of nursing centers using a model of practice led by APNs. Emphasis will be placed on the establishment of sound financial and reimbursement strategies in the development and implementation of nursing centers.

CURRENT CLIMATE

The ability for APNs to enroll as independent providers and receive reimbursement for their services is increasing in both the public and private insurance sectors. This represents revenue opportunities that allow for independent nurse-managed health care centers, resulting in the potential for increased access to care. Reimbursement also allows tracking data that document the contribution and outcome of nursing care.

In the late 1980s the Omnibus Budget Reconciliation Act required states to enroll and directly reimburse pediatric and family nurse practitioners and certified nurse midwives in their Medicaid programs. Additional groups of APNs could also be reimbursed at the states' option (e.g., adult APNs, geriatric APNs). In 1997 the federal Balanced Budget Act effected a statutory change in the Medicare law designating APNs as fully qualified (and reimbursable) Medicare Part B providers. Commercial insurers have taken the lead of Medicaid and Medicare and in some states provided leadership (Blue Cross of Michigan, for example) in enrolling and directly reimbursing APNs for primary care.

When nursing services are included in the general health care charges, it is not possible to measure the cost/benefit ratio of nursing services. In the past most APN services were simply billed under the physician provider number whether the physician was directly involved or the nurse was functioning independently. This is one of the most powerful arguments for APNs to obtain individual provider numbers in as many public and private insurance programs as possible. Nurses and their data are invisible unless they are billing under their own provider members.

Changes in reimbursement in health care are highly charged issues. The current climate of controlling, if not reducing, health care costs and the "pocketbook" (competitive) concerns among other health care providers are major factors in determining how much change can be achieved. Data and cost information must be used to document the effectiveness of the nurse-managed model and inform reimbursement issues. To act, policymakers must have the data to document the impact on patient care costs, patient satisfaction with the model of practice, and patient outcomes. The data clearly document that APNs provide excellent quality, increase access, and maintain or improve outcomes in nurse-managed primary care centers (Brown & Grimes, 1995). The challenge is to make certain the information is available to the appropriate decision makers and the stakeholders. Nursing must be po-

litically wise and well positioned to work with the politics involved with change. Change is incremental, and nursing must provide data and documentation at each incremental step, using information to maintain momentum toward the ultimate policy goal of reimbursement for nursing services.

DEFINITIONS AND PURPOSE OF NURSING CENTERS

Nursing centers serve many purposes and include many different models of care. If we are to expand public understanding of the contributions of nursing centers and build the legislative support to have an impact on policy, we must seek professional consensus about the definition and purpose of nursing centers. In 1990 the National League for Nursing Council on Nursing Centers adopted a broad working definition of nursing centers. "A nursing center is defined as an organization whose primary mission is to provide nursing services, may provide other services, and is owned, operated or controlled by nurses" (National League for Nursing, 1994).

Historically, nursing centers derived their primary purposes from meeting the health care needs of the community. Nursing centers have often been developed to increase access to care to populations otherwise not served. Thus, they contribute a safety net for the uninsured and vulnerable populations (Brown, 1995; Matherlee & Skydell, 1998). APNs in the primary care setting provide services similar to those of primary care physicians, including care of chronic diseases and routine acute conditions. In addition, APNs bring the unique characteristics of nursing to their patients with a focus on health promotion, disease prevention, patient education, and a holistic view of the patient.

In the past many of these nursing centers have rather narrowly defined the focus of services to include limited services such as immunizations, breast and cervical screening, school health, or health promotion activities. The authors advocate for a model of care that provides a full range of primary care services. The full scope of primary care is within the ability of the APN and is well defined in the Institute of Medicine definition: "Primary care is the provision *of integrated, accessible health care services by clinicians* who are *accountable* for addressing a large *majority of personal health care needs,* developing a *sustained partnership* with *patients,* and practicing in the *context of family and community*" (Donaldson, Yordy, Lohr, & Vanselow, 1996). APNs are prepared to practice the entire scope of primary care providing comprehensive services to clients in consultation and collaboration with other disciplines. The model of care has been supported by numerous studies, including an early study by the U.S. Office of Technology Assessment (U.S. Office of Technology Assessment [OTA], 1986) and more recently the Columbia study (Mundinger et al., 2000).

If access to care and continuity are values for nursing and nursing centers, the goal must be to provide a wide range of continuous care. It is proposed that nursing centers strive to provide a complete set of health care services to the client, including health screening, assessment, testing, prescribing, treatment, referral, care management, joint decision making, patient teaching, and education. These components are a part of the primary health care needs of individuals and families. This is the comprehensive model that is recommended for nursing centers.

REIMBURSEMENT OF NURSING CENTERS

Dedication to a comprehensive continuous patient care model requires defining the model and using new reimbursement strategies. Strategies need to include a business plan that ensures long-term viability. Reimbursement for services provided in nursing centers has taken many forms. One of the main sources of funding was grants from federal, state, and local government agencies. These funds allowed nursing centers to provide a specific service such as breast and cervical cancer screening or immunizations. However, these funds are often reduced or eliminated as governments move on to new areas of health interest. Nursing centers have been left with ongoing commitments to patients without the financial resources to provide these services.

Nursing centers need to develop business plans that include a variety of payment sources to cover the cost of operation (Potash, 1997). This is a change in the culture of nursing requiring nurses to consider the financial cost of their services. For most centers, the strategy should be focused on public and private third-party reimbursement, including managed care and capitated contracts. Centers may include a mix of community partnerships and other sources to deliver comprehensive and continuous service.

Some centers become providers in traditional government and private insurance programs. Provider reimbursement under these plans has been labeled fee-for-service, with each patient visit reimbursed at a specific amount. This type of reimbursement is tied to the number of patients seen and procedures done. For nurses who tend to do more education and preventive services this is not the ideal model of reimbursement.

Capitation within managed care is another model of reimbursement that ties the services provided to the overall care of the individual. Capitation can be defined as a "fixed dollar amount that covers the costs of healthcare services based on the membership of healthcare services plan; usually refers to a negotiated per capita rate paid periodically to providers; often expressed in units of care per member per month" (Nash, 1997). Nursing centers can negotiate a contract with managed care organizations to provide a comprehensive set of services to patients based on a capitation rate. This is often expressed as a "per member/per month" rate. The managed care organization pays the nursing center a specific amount of money per client enrolled per month. For example, a capitation contract may pay a nursing center $30 per member per month for 12 months. The center agrees to care for 1,000 patients over a year. The center would receive $30,000 of revenue each month. The provider organization, in this case the nursing center, receives payment each month for the patient whether the patient uses any services or not. This allows nursing to provide services in a variety of nontraditional ways such as phone management, case management, and home visits. Many of the ideas of managed care such as health promotion and disease prevention fit the model of nursing care better than the fee-for-service model. Capitation allows the APN to offer services that will best meet patient needs and result in more positive outcomes.

For nurse-managed centers, the danger with capitation is twofold. One concern is that patients may use more visits and services than the total amount received from the managed care organization for the year. The more this situation occurs, the greater the danger that a center will lose money on its contract. An additional danger lies in nursing's tendency to provide services without recognition of actual costs and resources.

With a capitated model the APN must continue to be aware of cost of services and outcomes achieved. The nursing center model can serve to reduce the number of visits and use of services required by patients by implementing its unique model of care. Developing relationships with the patient and partnering with the patient in decision making can reduce care demands and improve compliance and outcomes. These are the essential ingredients in a cost-effective model of practice.

CASE STUDY

Knowledge of financial information and data helps nurses understand how they contribute to both the cost and the revenue of health care. This is true for nurses involved in a nursing center as administrators or nurse practitioners, or employed in ambulatory care. Financial savvy can help nurses build a case for their practice, negotiate a more favorable contract for their employment, and provide more efficient, evidence-based care for their patients. These issues may be better understood in the context of a case study.

This case study involves the development of a nurse-managed health center as part of a wholly owned business of a College of Nursing Faculty Practice at Michigan State University.

The faculty in the college of nursing had long been committed to faculty practice. Over the years faculty had been involved in a variety of models of practice, including working with local health departments and providing services in senior public housing. Practices yielded little or no reimbursement. The faculty involved in clinical practice determined that the model of practice most desirable would be one owned and operated by the college. This model would allow control over the model of care, practice decisions, service delivery, and student placements. Faculty, providers, and students would be able to deliver health care within the context of this nursing practice in a model consistent with the core concepts of the undergraduate and graduate programs. It would provide opportunities for both graduate APN students and undergraduate community nursing students to work together and learn from each other. It also offered the opportunity to develop research initiatives that could test the model of nursing primary care. A project is underway at Michigan State University College of Nursing, in collaboration with the United States Department of Veterans Affairs (DVA), to develop a research initiative based on the nurse-managed model of care.

The ability to develop the nursing center stemmed from the convergence of a number of internal and external opportunities and resources at a time when the college was ready to move forward with developing this model of faculty practice. We like to think of this as having had the heavenly stars in the right alignment.

• Practice faculty embraced the concept of developing a practice site under the ownership of the college.
• The goals of the nursing center include the key missions of the college: teaching, practice, research, and service.
• A community hospital system was seeking opportunities for partnership with the college of nursing. The

hospital system had an obligation to fund services for indigent members of the community. They were willing to refer and reimburse patients based on the center's fee schedule.
• The college received a grant from the W.K. Kellogg Foundation as part of a four-university consortium. A portion of the funding was available to develop sites for nurse practitioner–provided primary care services to low-income populations. Some of these funds provided startup funds for the center.
• The DVA approached the college to contract for providing primary care services for veterans in the community. The DVA is committed to APN-provided primary care at the national policy level.
• The university offered resources to ensure that legal, risk management, financial, and business plan issues were addressed before any contractual commitment.
• The University Provost's Office agreed to establish a line of credit for the college, with interest, and a repayment schedule. This allowed the college to ensure meeting payroll and other operations costs should cash flow issues occur during the startup period.
• The Ingham County community developed funding to provide primary preventive health care for uninsured adults. The local health department reached its full capacity to serve uninsured residents and approached the college to serve a group of these adults in a second capitated contract called the Ingham Health Plan. This is a second innovative reimbursement contract for the center.

The initial insurer contract for this nursing center was with the United States Department of Veterans Affairs, Battle Creek, Michigan. It is a capitated 3-year agreement to provide primary care services to veterans living in the community within a tricounty area. The contract covers a minimum of 1,000 patients in the first year operation. The capitated contract with the DVA provides an excellent opportunity for a nursing center because of the extensive referral system available for consultation and referral to specialists as needed. DVA physician specialists are required, under the contract, to accept referrals from the APN provider. This allows the APN to provide the primary care services knowing the patients have access to specialty health care.

The DVA patient demographics are primarily men older than 55 years of age with multiple chronic illnesses. The business plan was based on the projected number of visits and time required with each client. Provider productivity standards are an essential component of the business plan. The faculty were aware of the necessity of a fiscally sound contract to ensure ongoing care to the clients.

A business plan was developed for the new center at the same time that the DVA capitated contract was being prepared. The business plan included capital costs, personnel, supplies, laboratory, radiology, and contracts for physician collaboration agreements. The model of care for the center needed to be developed to identify the appropriate personnel required. For example, staffing mix, ratio of provider to client, and support staff direct personnel costs. Creative linkages and partnerships can be useful. For example, the center has linked with the community health nursing students for home visits to provide patient education and medication setups and monitoring. The patient care benefits derived from these home-based services are leading us to develop a nurse case manager role for the veteran population. This position will be proposed in year 2 of the DVA capitated contract.

The clinical faculty providers have gained new skills, experience, and knowledge during the process of developing the nurse-managed center. Support received from the university and community, as well as the DVA, has been essential for the viability of the center. Most importantly, high-quality health care is being provided, the center is fiscally sound, and the model of practice supports the teaching and research missions of the college. The innovative reimbursement strategy of the DVA capitation helps ensure the viability of the center.

ISSUES AND CHALLENGES

This is an exciting time for nurses in the health care arena with many opportunities and challenges. As the number of nursing centers increase, the "lessons learned" can make an impact on health care delivery in the future. To maximize opportunities, key issues must be addressed and key challenges must be met including:

Changing the culture of nursing: The profession must be a leader in addressing the issues of health care delivery. The practice of nursing must demonstrate a sound business model without jeopardizing the "caring" component of nursing to position the profession to make this contribution.

Educating nursing students to provide care and be informed, contributing members of the health care industry: Nurses need to understand and be able to articulate their role and function in relation to the organizational goals, financial realities, and societal needs. This requires full understanding of reimbursement issues, health care delivery issues, organizational goals, and mission. This knowledge must be incorporated into nursing curricula but also made broadly available to practicing nurses through continuing professional education.

Documenting nursing practice to develop a comprehensive database: Nursing must continue to build the data necessary to document the contributions of nursing to patient outcomes. The data must include cost and benefit. In acute care settings, this may require repositioning nursing costs and outcomes to be independently accounted for and monitored. This also requires unique provider enrollment as an APN in insurance and other payer programs. These data will not only identify the strengths of nursing but also provide the information needed to improve nursing care in the future.

Informing policy: Nursing has traditionally remained in the background of health care policy issues. Although the largest health care profession, nursing has not reached its potential as a cohesive and powerful force for change. The key issues of cost, quality, and access are central to the delivery of nursing care and ones the profession can and must take leadership in addressing.

Broadening our partnerships: To achieve the goals related to documentation, culture change, education, and policy change will require broad collaboration across nursing practice, nursing education, policymakers, politicians, health care delivery systems, health care purchasers, consumers, and others. Nursing must partner with other health professions, identify strong stakeholders in industry and government, and get to the decision-making table with creative solutions for the difficult issues of our health system.

The challenges facing nursing are old, but the options now available to nursing are new. New reimbursement streams are emerging for APN services. Nursing centers are an important ingredient in positioning nursing to be a leader in the business of health care delivery. The challenges can be met and must be met if nursing is to move forward to achieve its goals.

Although there is, indeed, no free health care, nursing is free to identify and access reimbursement opportunities, which will create the ability to serve more community members in need.

REFERENCES

Brown, N. (1995). Health reform and the role of nursing centers. In B. Murphy (Ed.), *Nursing centers: The time is now* (pp. 19-32). New York: National League for Nursing Press.

Brown, S.A., & Grimes, D.E. (1995, November/December). A meta-analysis of nurse practitioners and nurse midwives in primary care. *Nursing Research*, pp. 336-337.

Donaldson, M.S., Yordy, K.D., Lohr, K.N., & Vanselow, N.A. (Eds.). (1996). *Primary care: America's health in a new era.* Washington, DC: National Academy Press.

Lockhart, C.A. (1995). Community nursing centers: An analysis of status and needs. In B. Murphy (Ed.), *Nursing centers: The time is now* (pp. 1-19). New York: National League for Nursing Press.

Matherlee, K., & Skydell, B. (1998). *Providing community based primary care: Nursing centers, CHC's and other initiatives.* National Health Policy Forum Site Visit Report: March 30-31, 1998, Philadelphia. Washington, DC: The George Washington University.

Mundinger, M.O. (1997). A philosophy of scholarly faculty practice. In L.N. Marion (Ed.), *Faculty practice: Applying the models* (pp. 63-64). Washington, DC: National Organization of Nurse Practitioner Faculties.

Mundinger, M.O., Kane, R.L., Lenz, E.R., Totten, A.M., Tsai, W., Cleary, P.D. (2000). Primary care outcomes in patients treated by nurse practitioners or physicians. *Journal of the American Medical Association, 483*(1), 59-68.

Nash, D.B. (Ed.). (1997). *The managed care manual: Updated first edition.* Boston: Total Learning Concepts.

National League for Nursing. (1994). *Council for nursing center membership directory.* New York: Author.

Potash, M. (1997). A guide to faculty practice. In L.N. Marion (Ed.), *Faculty practice: Applying the models* (pp. 107-121). Washington, DC: National Organization of Nurse Practitioner Faculties.

United States Department of Labor, Employment and Training Administration. (1995). *Health workers retraining program.* Grant # N-5526-5-00-87-60.

United States Office of Technology Assessment. (1986). *Health technology case study 37: Nurse practitioners, physician assistants, and certified nurse-midwives: A policy analysis* (OTA Study). Washington, DC: Congress of the United States.

Reimbursement for Alternative Providers

JUDY LEE

An examination of the fairly recent history of consumers' demands for complementary alternative medicine (CAM) calls for the inclusion of developing data on professional nursing's positive contributions to patient outcomes and costs. In the history of nursing, there was never a mechanism that allowed for development of this information. Historically, nursing charges have been lumped into untrackable "day charges" or vague time-based "visit" charges, without documentation of what was actually being done for the patient.

DOCUMENTING NURSING'S CONTRIBUTIONS

Nursing interventions, recorded in actuarial data as part of a "package of services," do not allow for validation of the actual value of nursing's contribution to patient outcomes. Having this hard data made available for the first time in the history of nursing makes a major, positive impact on the nursing profession as a whole by (1) giving the profession the measurable credibility it has long deserved, (2) developing actuarial data that will allow insurance companies to underwrite independent nursing services as plan benefits, (3) increasing the potential for development of independent, entrepreneurial, nursing practices, (4) leveling the playing field for reimbursement for those services, (5) increasing consumers' access to independent nursing services, and (6) expanding services to medically underserved areas of the nation.

OVERVIEW OF THE HISTORY OF CAM

It is a fact that healing approaches that incorporate emotional and spiritual elements have been around for years, in one form or another. But the mainstream has treated them like poor stepchildren and relegated them to the fringes of alternative medicine (Pert, 1997). Nurses are actually on the forefront of incorporating CAM techniques into traditional allopathic models. Early on, many nurses received education and inaugurated Therapeutic Touch into their practices. The American Holistic Nurses Association (AHNA) was already founded by 1980. *Nursing Interventions Classification (NIC)* (McCloskey & Bulechek, 1996), which is reflective of advanced practice nursing, for many years has included "alternative therapies" such as autogenic training, biofeedback, calming techniques, hypnosis, meditation, simple guided imagery, and simple relaxation therapy. In the most recent edition the *NIC* included forgiveness facilitation, spiritual growth facilitation, religious addiction prevention, and others as alternative therapies (McCloskey & Bulechek, 2000).

Naturopathy, osteopathy, and chiropractic practitioners, who once had a large following, were effectively squelched in the United States by serious, concerted efforts of the AMA (Coulter, 1995). Strong consumers' demand for these and other CAM services, however, became even more widespread during the 1970s and 1980s. CAM became a virtual health care buzzword by the early 1990s, so much so that consumers choosing nonallopathic options could not be ignored. Over these three decades, increasing numbers of consumers realized that wellness-oriented systems were more beneficial and cost-effective than illness-oriented models. Consumers began to vote with their pocketbooks, seeking out these services without the blessing or support of traditional third-party reimbursement models. They paid for most of the services primarily out of their own pockets. In 1990 alone, 44% of Americans used CAM providers, and the resulting 425 million visits translated into more than $12 billion dollars spent (Eisenberg et al., 1993).

There was a resurgence of the classic models of chiropractic and acupuncture benefiting many Americans, and both were being creatively expanded. An innovative combination of chiropractic and acupuncture techniques was pioneered in the West by Dr. George Goodheart, founder and developer of Applied Kinesiology. Significant contributions were seen with the development of Network Spinal Analysis (NSA) (Association for Network Chiropractic website). Dr. Devi Nambudripad's NAET (Nambudripad Allergy Elimination Technique) also drew significant international attention to both professions with effective, nonimmunization allergy desensitization in large populations (Nambudripad, 1999a). Amazing improvement of allergy-related autism also warranted further study (Nambudripad, 1999b). Another example is demonstrated by statistics collected nationally for many years by the Midwives Alliance of North America (MANA). These data documented the dramatically reduced cesarean section rates—3.4% aver-

age—for planned out of hospital births with midwife attendants (Davis & Johnson, 1999). This significant reduction occurred while cesarean section rates were spiraling upward of 28% throughout the nation. The modalities of chiropractic, naturopathy, midwifery, homeopathy, and Western and Oriental herbs were regularly being bantered about in social discourse and discussed in great depth in the popular press. The dramatically changing view of the consumer concerning "health and healing" in all areas of life is well reflected in Dr. Donald Epstein's Social Myths chart (Table 55-1) in *Healing Myths Healing Magic* (2000).

TABLE 55-1   Social Myths

The Tree of Knowledge	The Tree of Life
The Supreme Agency The conscious mind through the gaining of knowledge. The intellect can be used to solve every problem or challenge that might ever occur.	Life itself, through a fuller, richer experience of life. Life contains all the miracles and wisdom of the universe, and all solutions to every challenge that might ever occur.
How Success Is Achieved By manipulation of the environment and others. Insulation of the individual from unwanted events, circumstances, and situations is vital.	By being sensitive to the timing and rhythms of nature, as well as the rhythms, pulsations, and vibrations of our body. Every step in life then becomes obvious and requires little work other than to be awake and aware.
Relationships Valued for what they can offer us in achieving personal advancement or success.	Valued for expanding our participation in the world; for nurturing, and being nurtured by, the people and opportunities that come into our life.
Physical Symptoms Viewed as annoyances or interruptions in life, to be eliminated, controlled, or avoided.	Viewed as gifts that have an important message to give us, and that guide us toward healing and a deeper experience of life.
Health The state in which the individual is not deterred from living a normal life. Achieving our personal goals without physical limitations or discomfort.	The state of optimal physical, emotional, mental, social, and spiritual well-being. Health is associated with gaining a deeper connection with the vibrations, pulsations, and rhythms of life through our bodymind.
Solutions Chosen Exclusive, competitive, and logical. More is better. The more complicated, the higher the educational degree, the more difficult to master, or the more sacrifice, money, or risk is involved, the greater the dividend or benefit. A greater result requires greater intellect or force.	Inclusive, noncompetitive, and illogical. Those that magically appear or become self-evident at the time of need. Internal biological and spiritual forces guide the process, which may not always be logical. Solutions often include unexpected gifts that life presents us.
Avoidance Avoid the unexpected, chaotic, emotional, or spiritual unless prior planning allows it to be controlled.	Avoid ideas, practices, and situations that do not seem to work in our life, including attitudes and actions that separate us from other people, or our bodymind and its feelings, rhythms, and sensations. Avoid whatever detracts from our experience of wonder and awe for the power of life.

From Epstein, D.M. (2000). *Healing myths, healing magic: Breaking the spell of old illusions, reclaiming our power to heal.* San Rafael, CA: Amber-Allen Publishing.

CONSUMER DEMANDS

Consumer demands have been so dramatic, even mainstream medical journals such as the *Journal of the American Medical Association (JAMA)* dedicated an entire issue to alternative medicine (December of 1998). *Advance for Nurse Practitioners* regularly carries articles such as "Alternative Health Trends" (Cozic, 2000). Even massage therapy services have become mainstream, creating a strong demand for books such as *The Medical Massage Office Manual* (Callahan & Luther, 1999), which provides effective instruction on properly filing insurance claim forms. In the second edition of the popular textbook *Massage during Pregnancy* (Waters, 1999), certified nurse-midwife Bette L. Waters added a full three-page addendum instructing massage therapists on how to become preferred providers on managed care networks. The face of health care delivery in the United States has rapidly changed and is continuing to do so.

PHYSICIANS' RESPONSES

"In recent years, holistic providers have faced hostile medical boards and organized opposition from segments of the biomedical community," stated internationally renowned attorney Michael H. Cohen (1998) in *Complementary and Alternative Medicine: Legal Boundaries and Regulatory Perspectives*. Pioneering physicians like Ted Rozema, MD, and many others, integrating CAM techniques into their own allopathic practices, have often been subjected to personal and professional attack by peers, perhaps even more cruelly than other providers. For example, despite formal physician protocols, rules of conduct and positive outcome studies, ethylene diamine tetraacetic acid (EDTA) chelation therapy providers came under peer attack. "Like all pioneering ventures in virtually any field, turf battles have to be fought, sometimes for years before acceptance comes" (Lonsdale, 1997). This delicate phrasing was used by the American College for Advancement in Medicine when referring to some of the ongoing attacks.

The conservative estimates of out-of-pocket expenses of *$34.4 billion* in 1997 for CAM was comparable to total out-of-pocket monies spent for *all physician services in the United States* (Eisenberg et al., 1998). Following the money, if not the many years of consumers' demands, medical doctors all over the country are gradually beginning to implement some of these alternative modalities into their own practices. By the late 1990s, chelation therapy, acupuncture, homeopathy, Ayurvedic techniques, and referrals to massage therapists, reflexologists, and herbalists became somewhat more common. The lack of a standardized language describing this myriad of CAM services was a major problem. Providers, even within the same profession, often were not using the same words to describe the same procedures. The problem was compounded significantly by cross-profession conversations and documentation efforts.

NEED FOR STANDARDIZATION

Further nightmares were created daily as insurance companies and providers incorporated CAM and tried to communicate in the existing vague and nonstandardized vocabularies. They were faced with an urgent need to track efficacy and costs because insurers cannot take the financial risk of fully underwriting a plan benefit until actuarial data are accumulated. Early attempts to address this problem further complicated the intent. Local (in-house) billing code sets and dummy billing systems proliferated across the country as managed care organizations rushed to provide these alternative services. Because one system could not talk with the other, claims processing was all but impossible, and no nationally valid data could be developed. Imagine trying to use an ATM card if each bank in the world spoke in its own native "dialect" and was unable to interpret the electronic data "language" of another bank to do business. Also imperative was the need for any new electronic messaging format adopted for CAM to be easily incorporated into the existing health care model. Even a minor change to any existing field on the Health Care Financing Authority (HCFA) 1500 (the Medicare-Medicaid, industry-standard insurance billing claims form) would make them electronically unreadable and would likely cost the industry and all stakeholders hundreds of billions of dollars. Yet standardization would save all stakeholders money in the long run according to a *Wall Street Journal* article in January of 2000 (Gentry, 2000).

GOVERNMENT'S RESPONSE

The Health Insurance Portability and Accountability Act of 1996 (HIPAA)* was the response by the U.S. Congress to contain costs and address many varied health-related issues. The act implicitly called for setting a national stan-

---

*104th Congress of the United States. (1996). Health Insurance Portability and Accountability Act, Public Law 104-191. Washington, DC: *Congressional Record, 142,* 1-180.

dard to effectively communicate with *all providers* electronically in a common "language." In an attempt to eliminate the proliferation of local code sets, it required the Secretary of Health and Human services to "name" a national electronic standard no later than August 2000. Work on implementation of the many mandates in HIPAA proceeded very slowly with regular and ongoing delays. The urgency to continue was highlighted by many surveys in 1998 and 1999, that reported 70% to 86% of the nation's largest health maintenance organizations (HMOs) were covering or stated their intention to incorporate and pay for some type of alternative modalities by 2000 (Goodwin, 1999).

THE AMERICAN MEDICAL ASSOCIATION

Throughout this period, the American Medical Association (AMA) apparently had good financial reasons to basically ignore CAM models of practice. They had issued only four chiropractic and two acupuncture billing codes, and this did not occur until the mid-1990s. By then much work had been done by several nursing organizations to classify and create a taxonomy for nursing procedures and to gain national licensing. National licensing efforts remained in the embryonic stage into the new millennium. This put nursing in the same boat as all other "alternative" providers, who had differing scopes of practice and licensing requirements in every state. Despite traditional allopathic provider status and ongoing efforts to secure them, nurses had not been blessed with any *Current Procedural Terminology (CPT)* billing codes, which are developed and owned by the AMA.

AMA's membership roles dropped significantly over the last two decades of the century, and the membership that remained were frequently engaged in ongoing challenges of both leadership and policies. When questioned in 1999 by its own members about "using brute force and domination," Board Chair D. Ted Lewers said "we recognize the fact that we have acted like an 800-pound gorilla" (Boothe, 1999). Even the AMA's role in controlling the CPT Standard for Electronic Transaction and Codes Sets was being challenged publicly by its own members and the Association of American Physicians and Surgeons (AAPS). During the 1998 public comment period to the HIPPA Act and the HCFA proposed response (Proposed Rule HCFA-0149-P), the president of the AAPS made several significant points:

> Even most members of the AMA—who constitute a small fraction of physicians—have no meaningful rights to partic-

ipate in the decision making of the leadership. . . . The Proposed Rule allows the AMA to revise the CPT coding system at its discretion without any procedural safeguards. . . . The AMA has a financial incentive to perpetuate ambiguities and complications . . . , so that physicians will be required to purchase from the AMA and its licensees publications . . . [contributing] $100 million per year in CPT-related revenue. . . . Indeed physicians are not even allowed to attend the meetings at which revisions are considered, and the AMA decision makers are neither elected by nor accountable to the vast majority of physicians affected. [AAPS, 1998]

Although physicians all over the country were attacking the perceived arrogance and lack of inclusiveness of the AMA, alternative providers were voicing concerns that a conflict of interest existed by having the AMA develop billing codes for nonallopathic models. The AMA did not request from the Department of Health and Human Services (HHS) the right to do so by the formal 1998 deadline.

THE MISSING LINK IS FINALLY FOUND

As fate would have it, inside a small, nondescript building in Las Cruces, New Mexico, a curious mixture of insurance specialists, lawyers, health care administrators, midwives, massage therapists, accountants, acupuncturists, marketing executives, physicians, and computer geeks had been laboring doggedly to put the finishing touches on this exact "missing link" for CAM reimbursement (Hudson, 1998). Melinna Giannini, a licensed and credentialed third-party health administrator, and Marion Stone, a self-described "grandmother/entrepreneur," had first begun assembling the strange mix of experts in 1996, well before the HIPAA Act was published. With input from their "experts" and state and national provider associations and credentialing bodies, by late 1998, Alternative Link, LLC, was able to birth the ABC Codes for billing. These 4,000 totally new billing codes met the intent and criteria of the HIPAA Act to contain costs while accurately reflecting the actual patient encounter with all providers. In the 1996 edition of the *Nursing Interventions Classification,* editors McCloskey and Bulechek stated, "Indeed, reimbursement to nurses is a key issue in the reduction of health care costs." In 1998, as Director of Research for Alternative Link, LLC, I was able to incorporate most of the NIC interventions into the system. In addition, Home Health Care Classification (HHCC), the OMAHA System, and Sexual Assault Nursing Examinations (SANE) were also integrated into the billing system by the year 2000.

BECOMING A NATIONAL STANDARD

Alternative Link cleared numerous hurdles and met the HHS's 1998 deadline for submitting this billing code set for consideration as a national standard. This was the only code set submitted that included alternative medicine providers and procedures and met all the criteria outlined by HHS. As mentioned previously, the Secretary of Health and Human Services had already been required by the HIPAA Act to "name" an electronic billing coding set that would cover the activities of all providers by August of 2000. A U.S. Patent was awarded in 1998 for the Alternative Billing Concepts (ABC Codes) Coding System, "A Coding System for the Billing and Reimbursement of Alternative Medicine Services." Patent pending filings had also been obtained in 90 other countries. While awaiting HHS adoption as a national standard, in 1999 the American National Standards Institute (ANSI-X12N) voted the ABC Codes system into their Implementation Guide. An official optional code set can be used immediately by any payer. Unique coding information on nursing and alternative interventions was included in the Unified Medical Language System of the National Library of Medicine, where the AMA's CPT codes for allopathic medicine also reside.

The Complete Complementary Alternative Medicine Billing and Coding Reference (Hall, 1999) was prepared for use, with related patented information, to expand the existing capabilities of current allopathic coding systems. This was accomplished by uniquely addressing (the complex and changing clinical and legal) varying state-specific requirements governing providers and payers in the area of CAM and nursing. The ABC Codes are paired with terminology and definitions that accurately describe what is said, done, ordered, prescribed, or distributed by 13 practitioner types (see box, right). The system is a living document and was purposely designed for easy expandability to include more treatments and more licensed providers. More than 11 million code combinations are possible within the structure to support emerging services, and more than 1,200 modifiers can be added to support future licensed providers *without any costly additions to the health care industry or any stakeholders*. The system was built on the belief that the codes will greatly improve entrance of CAM into mainstream health care. The codes provide the infrastructure needed for payers of all types to measure the effectiveness and costs of CAM services side by side with conventional medicine, thus facilitating responsible patient access to integrated health care.

THIRTEEN PROVIDER TYPES IN THE 2000 EDITION OF ABC CODES WITH BILLING CODE MODIFIERS*

AN	= Advanced nurse practitioner
CN	= Clinical nurse specialist
DC	= Doctor of chiropractic
DO	= Doctor of osteopathy
MD	= Holistic medical doctor
MT	= Licensed massage therapist
ND	= Naturopathic doctor/physician
NM	= Certified nurse midwife
OM	= Doctor of Oriental medicine/acupuncturist
PA	= Physicians assistant
PN	= Licensed practical nurse or LVN
RM	= Registered midwife or CPM
RN	= Registered nurse

*Other licensed providers can easily be added to the system by request of State Provider Associations.

© Alternative Link, LLC, 1999, Las Cruces, New Mexico.

BENEFITS FOR NURSING PRACTICES

Until the advent of the ABC Codes system, no standardized coded data for CAM existed that allowed cost and outcome data to emerge. With this system, the insurance industry can incorporate CAM and nursing into plan benefits and broaden availability to the public. Equally important, underwriters can now compare CAM and allopathic coded treatment patterns to assess the costs and benefits associated with the addition of these services.

Beta site testing of the Alternative Link system to make it user-friendly was accomplished in 1998 and 1999. It began to be gradually introduced on a state-by-state basis into other payer systems, starting in early 2000. When looking closely at how the system works, one can see the inherent elegant solution for both the providers and the payers. Figure 55-1 shows the life of an electronic claim. As any billing clerk knows, "kick backs or pending of claims" (not paying for a service while asking the provider for more information) occurs at many junctures in this process. Requests for more information such as Narrative Reports and S.O.A.P. notes takes place regularly with all current allopathic coding systems. Because of design oversights that have not been corrected, to date no in-depth allopathic information is able to be transmitted electronically. Payment or cash flow to providers is stopped at each point more information is requested. Be-

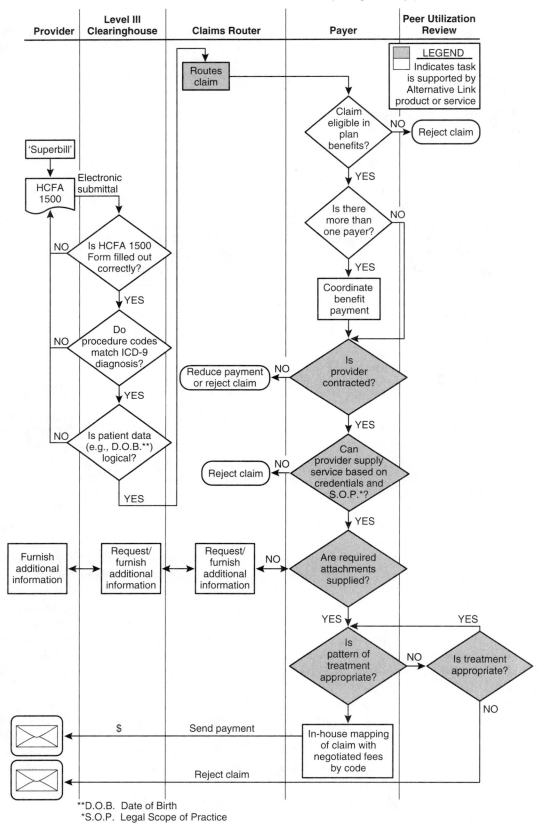

THE LIFE OF A CLAIM: ELECTRONIC COMMERCE (averages 14 days)

| Provider | Level III Clearinghouse | Claims Router | Payer | Peer Utilization Review |

LEGEND
Indicates task is supported by Alternative Link product or service

Routes claim

Claim eligible in plan benefits? — NO → Reject claim

'Superbill'

HCFA 1500 — Electronic submittal

Is HCFA 1500 Form filled out correctly? — NO

YES

Do procedure codes match ICD-9 diagnosis? — NO

YES

Is patient data (e.g., D.O.B.**) logical? — NO

YES

Is there more than one payer? — NO

YES

Coordinate benefit payment

Is provider contracted? — NO → Reduce payment or reject claim

YES

Can provider supply service based on credentials and S.O.P.*? — NO → Reject claim

YES

Furnish additional information ↔ Request/furnish additional information ↔ Request/furnish additional information ← NO — Are required attachments supplied?

YES

Is pattern of treatment appropriate? — NO → Is treatment appropriate? — YES

NO

Send payment ← $ — In-house mapping of claim with negotiated fees by code

Reject claim

**D.O.B. Date of Birth
*S.O.P. Legal Scope of Practice

FIGURE 55-1 The life of a claim: electronic commerce (averages 14 days). (© Alternative Link, LLC, 1999, Las Cruces, New Mexico.)

TABLE 55-2 An Expanded Definition

1. Supports submission of electronic claims with attachments the payer needs to "pass" on claims.
2. Builds precise communication between the provider and payer, thus saving time and money for both.

ABC Code	Description	Expanded Definition
CCAAA	Block technique, general, chiropractic services, practice specialties	The application of wedge blocks to specific anatomical sites before, after, or as manipulation.
CCAAB	Educational kinesiology, 15 minutes, general, chiropractic, practice specialties	Fifteen-minute period of applying specific exercises, ranges of motions, and/or strengthening procedures to rehabilitate a compromised joint.

© Alternative Link, LLC, 1999, Las Cruces, New Mexico.

cause of the ease of playing these "pending games" in their favor, payers have long collected enormous sums of interest by holding monies owed to providers. Writing and reading nonstandardized reports is also costly to all parties both in staff time and money. Furthermore, it is in direct conflict with the HIPAA Act mandate to reduce paperwork.

The designers of the ABC Codes were aware of the many problems in the existing arcane allopathic models used for health care billing. They purposely circumvented old design flaws with the inclusion of solutions. In electronic format an "expanded definition" was attached to each billing code and explains, in a formalized set manner, to both providers and payers, exactly what transpired or is being billed for (Table 55-2). This is of great value to the provider because it (1) eliminates claim "pending" by a payer (who will not pay for a service that has already been rendered until receiving more information from the provider), (2) reduces the possibility of inadvertently "unbundling" global fee types of services (some services must be billed as a package only) or "upcoding" (charging for a similar but not identical procedure that pays a higher price), (3) reduces the possibility of HCFA-levied fines of up to $10,000 per claim (endnote) for "not reflecting the actual patient encounter" appropriately, and (4) speeds up reimbursement, thereby improving provider cash flow and profit margins of the practice. This method of transferring accurate billing data will allow for electronic direct deposit of insurance monies into the provider's account, further speeding up the influx of monies to practices.

Not only does the ABC Code system describe the actual patient encounter accurately, more importantly, it explains to all payers that the service being billed is, or is not, within the legal scope of practice of that provider. A Training Standard was also electronically attached to each code, indicating legal scope of practice details (see box, p.

418). This information is state-by-state specific for all provider types covered by the system. The amount of ongoing research that is required to keep up with this rapidly changing area of health care delivery in all 51 regions of the United States is impossible to describe here. Expansion to include other providers is an integral part of the system design. In 2000, along with CAM providers, the system also included legal state-specific scope of practice information for practical nurses, registered nurses, nurse midwives, advanced nurse practitioners, and clinical nurse specialists.

HOW IT ALL WORKS

Alternative Link's code books, databases, and support tools are designed for providers, payers, claims adjusters, medical managers, provider network developers, third-party payers, and software producers throughout the health care industry. The products support both paper and electronic claims. The system was created to save health care entities time, money, and the risk of potential legal liability. A "technical" summary indicates that providers and payers, connected by the Alternative Link system, gain the following benefits (Giannini & Koshewa, 2000):

- Providers file accurate descriptions of the patient encounter on standard claim forms.
- Payers use the same information as the provider filing the claim, thus enhancing communication.
- Claims adjusters have references for each claim filed to ensure compliance with state laws.
- Payers develop cost and outcome data (without needing to purchase new software system).
- Payers underwrite insured benefits for CAM based on the cost and outcome data.
- Providers and payers save time and money by not having to create or interpret written reports.

TRAINING STANDARDS*

ABC Code CEAAB†: Certified Nurse Midwife Training Standard

If practicing in a regulated state, territory, or possession of the United States, licensure, certification, or registration as required by law, or successful completion of nurse midwifery program or an education program accredited by the American College of Nurse Midwives or successfully completed certification process of the American College of Nurse Midwife Certification Council, Inc.

ABC Code CEAAB: Registered Midwife Training Standard

If practicing in a regulated state, territory, or possession of the United States, licensure, certification, or registration as required by law. If practicing in an unregulated jurisdiction, current active certification as certified professional midwife (CPM) by the North American Registry of Midwives (NARM) or certification by the American College of Nurse Midwife Certification Council, Inc. (ACC) or current licensure, registration, or certification as midwife in another state.

ABC Code CEAAB: Naturopathic Doctor Training Standard

If practicing in a regulated state, territory, or possession of the United States, licensure, certification, or registration as required by law and licensed as midwife in that state or hold current active midwifery certification by the American College of Naturopathic Obstetricians. If practicing in an unregulated jurisdiction, current active certification by and passing scores received on naturopathic physicians licensing exam (NPLEX) in naturopathic medicine; or current licensure, registration, or certification as a naturopathic physician in another state, territory, or possession of the United States; and license as a midwife in another state, territory, or possession of the United States; or hold current active midwifery certification by the American College of Naturopathic Obstetricians.

---

*Training standards for different practitioner types are contained in machine-readable format by code.
†Note the 5-digit, all alpha format of the ABC Codes. Training standards vary on a state-by-state basis for each provider type for legal use of the *same* code.
© Alternative Link, LLC, 1999, Las Cruces, New Mexico.

- Providers and payers reduce the risk of liability of claims falling outside the scope of practice laws.
- Provider networks negotiate fees with payers in any locale using existing business models.

NUTS AND BOLTS

In plain English, all of this is much more simple. For the first time in the history of U.S. health care, with the use of the ABC Codes, payers can compare apples and apples when it comes to patients' costs and outcomes. Information develops stemming from the identical source of warehoused allopathic data, the *International Classification of Diseases, Ninth Revision (ICD-9),* diagnosis code. If thousands of patients have an identical diagnosis and one group is treated using typical allopathic methods and the other is treated using nursing and alternative medicine, costs and outcomes develop and can be compared. Reliable information quickly tells payers which providers contain costs while helping patients stay well longer or get well more quickly. Managed care organizations, in particular, are looking for ways to enhance their bottom line. The historical emphasis of CAM has been on preventive activities that are designed to keep people well and to avoid costly crisis intervention–type health care, as much as possible. The savings on visits to emergency departments and in-patient services alone could be astronomical. Documenting the monies that are saved by using chelation therapy to avoid bypass surgery, in and of itself, should also prove to be very interesting. Anecdotal evidence has shown most CAM procedures to be significantly less costly in general than much of allopathic medicine. An analysis of data from malpractice insurers from 1990 through 1996 stated, "We found that claims against these (CAM) practitioners occurred less frequently and typically involved injury that was less severe than claims against physicians during the same period" (Studdert et al., 1998). There is now a way to demonstrate which providers and which modalities contain costs while providing excellent outcomes. Simple, but not easy, until the Alternative Link was established.

Access and inclusiveness to the system have been guaranteed, by Alternative Link policy. Provider associations can easily request additional codes or inclusion of additional provider types simply by submitting a form to Alternative Link (www.alternativelink.com). Typically there is no charge for this service and expansions can be implemented in a timely manner. A nonprofit organization called the Institute for Comprehensive and Alternative Nomenclature (ICAN) is expected to be operational in 2000. ICAN's mission is to assist state and national associations with legislative languaging, political action strategies, member education, and to level the playing field for third-party reimbursement for providers.

CHALLENGES

Consumers are now much more well-educated and well-armed than ever before. Patients *will* be showing up in your office with a proliferation of articles and "studies" pulled from popular press and off the World Wide Web. Be prepared to discuss the pros and cons of all options in depth. Now is an appropriate time to educate yourself, and perhaps decide which of these alternative modalities might be appropriate to incorporate into your own practice. Nurses, particularly nurse practitioners who are trained in alternative therapies, are in a unique position to enhance patients' well-being and help them take realistic charge of their own health and future.

Using this system, nurses will quickly be designing incredibly creative studies that will play a major role in a healthier and happier population. Nonpharmaceutical pain relief or outcomes associated with including massage as part of routine prenatal care are only two interesting areas worthy of exploration.

REFERENCES

American Holistic Nurses Association website. Available: http://ahna.org.

Association of American Physicians and Surgeons, Inc. (1998). Proposed rule HCFA-0149-P. Baltimore: *Comments on standards for electronic transactions and code sets* (070198)-64 of 184.

Association for Network Chiropractic website. Available: http://www.associationfornetworkcare.com.

Boothe, B. (1999, September 6). AMA leaders promise more collaboration with specialties. *AMNews.*

Callahan, M.M., & Luther, D.W. (1999). *The medical massage office manual* (2nd ed.). Steamboat Springs, CO: Callahan/Luther Partnership.

Cohen, M.H. (1998). *Complementary and alternative medicine: Legal boundaries and regulatory perspectives.* Baltimore: Johns Hopkins University Press.

Coulter, H. (1995). *Use divided legacy* (vol. 4). Washington, DC: The Center for Empirical Medicine.

Cozic, A. (2000). Complementary health care, alternative therapies, tools for the new millennium. King of Prussia, PA: *Advance for Nurse Practitioners, 8*(1), 64-66.

Davis, B., & Johnson, K. (1999). Hospital procedures for 9,966 intended home and birth center births—MANA 1999. *Midwives' Alliance of North America Newsletter, XVII,* 6-14.

Eisenberg, D.M., Davis, R.B., Ettner, S.L., Appel, S., Wilkey, S., Rompay, M.V., & Kessler, R.C. (1998). Trends in alternative medicine: Use in the United States, 1990-1997. *Journal of the American Medical Association, 280,* 1569-1575.

Eisenberg, D.M., Kessler, R.C., Foster, C., Norlock, F.E., Calkins, D., & Delbanco, T. (1993). Unconventional medicine in the United States. Prevalence, costs, and pattern of use. *New England Journal of Medicine, 328,* 246-252.

Epstein, D.M. (2000). *Healing myths, healing magic: Breaking the spell of old illusions, reclaiming our power to heal.* San Rafael, CA: Amber-Allen Publishing.

Gentry, C. (2000, January 3). Health-care firms face costly change. *Wall Street Journal,* pp. 3A-4A.

Giannini, M., & Koshewa, C. (Eds.). (2000). *The complete complementary alternative medicine billing and coding reference* (2nd ed.). Newton, MA: Integrative Medicine.

Goodwin, J. (1999). A health insurance revolution. *New Age Journal, 6*(1), 66-69.

Hall, D. (Ed.). (1999). *The complete complementary alternative medicine billing and coding reference.* Newton, MA: Integrative Medicine.

Lonsdale, D. (1997). Special issue protocols for chelation therapy. *Journal of Advancement in Medicine, 10*(1), 3.

McCloskey, J.C., & Bulechek, G.M. (Eds.). (1996). *Nursing interventions classification (NIC)* (2nd ed.). St. Louis: Mosby–Year Book, Inc.

McCloskey, J.C., & Bulechek, G.M. (Eds.). (2000). *Nursing interventions classification (NIC)* (3rd ed.). St. Louis: Mosby.

Nambudripad, D.S. (1999a). *Say goodbye to illness.* Buena Park, CA: Delta Publishing Co.

Nambudripad, D.S. (1999b). *Say goodbye to allergy-related autism.* Buena Park, CA: Delta Publishing Co.

Pert, C.B. (1997). *Molecules of emotion.* New York: Scribner.

Studdert, D.M., Eisenberg, D.M., Miller, F.H., Curto, D.A., Kaptchuk, T.J., & Brennan, T.A. (1998). Medical malpractice implications of alternative medicine. *Journal of the American Medical Association, 280,* 1610-1615.

Waters, B.W. (1999). *Massage during pregnancy* (2nd ed.). Mesilla, NM: Bluwaters Press.

Financial Management for Patient Care Managers

DONNA YOUNG SCHMIDT

The health care environment is changing rapidly to address the government and consumer demand for access to cost-effective, quality health care. Within provider organizations, managers face significant challenges to effectively manage the delivery of cost-effective patient care. The manager's responsibilities are daunting: managing clinical teams, maintaining staff satisfaction, meeting physician needs, and achieving the organization's business goals. At the center of care delivery, the manager has been identified as the lynchpin in the delivery of quality and cost-effective patient care (Eubanks, 1992), the "nerve center" of the patient unit (Mintzberg, 1994), and the most visible and influential culture bearer on the unit (Horvath, 1994).

Today, a patient care manager has a broad span of responsibility based on number of units, number of employees, and size of operating budget. The boundaries of accountability have expanded, and the manager is often responsible for unit-based clinical teams that include nursing staff, other health care professionals, and support personnel. Organizational structures based on a continuum of care process need managers who can effectively operate primary care settings, outpatient facilities, inpatient units, and nonnursing services, such as ancillary or support departments. The increasing complexity of the health care delivery system and the management role requires that the manager function at a higher level of financial and operational performance. Eubanks (1992) states that the manager "is responsible for creating the significant change in the way patient care is delivered and in the cost to the institution of delivering that care" (p. 22). Oroviogoicoechea (1996) identified six financial management skills needed by the successful manager. These financial skills include proficiency with cost containment, productivity measurement, budget forecasting, cost benefit analysis, unit budget control measures, financial resource procurement, and financial resource monitoring.

What knowledge and skills are required for the patient care manager to be successful? The critical job skills of the manager role have been well documented in the literature (Boston & Forman, 1994; Chase, 1994; Everson-Bates, 1992; Kirk, 1987). The importance of financial management and decision making is often understated, however. The manager has primary authority to set goals and plan for the effective and efficient use of human, financial, and material resources (Mark, 1994). The manager also has responsibility for market assessment, strategic planning, and program development. The competent and successful manager has strong financial management skills and uses financial data to evaluate unit performance, develop new clinical programs, and achieve the organization's business goals.

Some studies have found that financial and operational management skills were low on the list of important management skills identified by chief nurse executives (CNE) and managers (Patz, Biordi, & Holm 1991). However, there is significant literature that identifies these skills as essential to the manager role. Boston and Forman (1994) found strong consensus among CNEs that good managers need both strong fiscal skills and clinical competence.

CSC Healthcare conducted a survey of chief nurse executives to identify key management skills for patient care managers and to describe the actual performance of managers (CSC Healthcare Survey, 1998). Less than 60% of the CNEs reported that managers are successful in implementing organizational change and managing to operational standards. Approximately one third of the executives reported that their managers were unsuccessful with skills, including managing financial standards, using data to improve clinical performance, and using information technology to improve performance. The manager's use of these skills directly ties to the organization's capability to demonstrate exceptional outcomes in operational and financial performance. It is a critical challenge to strengthen managers' skills in financial management and financial management decision making.

LEADERSHIP DEVELOPMENT

Most managers have had little formal education and have acquired their skills with on-the-job training (Boston & Forman, 1994; Everson-Bates, 1992; Haas & Hackbarth, 1997). It has been demonstrated that leadership development is effective in improving knowledge and ability in managerial role functions. Krejci and Malin (1997) found that the perception of understanding and ability increased after leadership development programs and was sustained for 3 months. Henninger (1994) demonstrated that patient care managers achieved a higher degree of independence in meeting performance standards after participating in a leadership development program. These findings have demonstrated the necessity and benefits of formal leadership development in graduate school and on the job.

Financial and operational management skills are addressed in most management development programs and graduate education programs. However, managers and CNEs continue to identify a need for increasing the manager's financial management skills. Few managers in the Boston and Forman study (1994) indicated that they ever received education or training in this area. Patient care managers have had considerable continuing education, but the content is related mostly to personnel development or unit management skills (Edwards & Roemer, 1996). Most managers have had little formal education that sufficiently improves their capability and confidence in managing financial and operational standards.

The increasing complexity and importance of the management role makes it imperative that organizations provide opportunities for coaching managers to develop the critical skills that will make them successful. The effectiveness of leadership development is enhanced and sustained when the manager has a relationship with a mentor or coach. This partnership provides an opportunity to problem solve financial and operational challenges and evaluate how critical situations were managed with a more experienced manager who has "been there, done that."

COMPUTER SKILLS

In this age of information technology, web technology, and electronic commerce, there are nurses that still have not developed confidence in their computer skills. Most financial and operational analyses are performed with spreadsheets. The use of basic spreadsheet applications can enhance the manager's ability to evaluate data and proposed business solutions. There are basic formulas within the spreadsheet that perform simple arithmetic. More complex calculations (e.g., standard deviation, mean, and average) can also be performed. Although managers do not need to be expert computer analysts, it is important to have an understanding of what a spreadsheet is and how to set up simple analyses (e.g., staffing to demand). With this tool the manager has the capability to perform analyses that are required to evaluate unit performance.

A flexible staffing tool can be developed with a spreadsheet. The staffing tool is a guide for the manager and staff to adjust staffing as patient volume changes. The tool can be used to project the budget impact of different staffing scenarios. The staffing grid can be easily revised when the productivity standard changes. This staffing tool enables the manager to project the budget impact of personnel resource decisions.

BUDGET FORECASTING AND CONTROL

Managers are responsible for developing, monitoring, and achieving a unit budget. The budget is a financial tool to project workload, identify labor and nonlabor resources required for the delivery of patient care, and monitor unit financial performance. When addressing financial performance, a lot of attention is paid to budgets and budget performance. However, it is important to remember that although financial performance is essential, the budget is only one dimension of unit performance. It does not provide information needed to evaluate quality of patient care, including patient outcomes and service targets.

The budgeting process varies greatly among organizations. Hospital budgets may be developed for functional departments (e.g., an inpatient unit or pharmacy) or product lines (e.g., heart center and cancer center). Every budget is developed, however, using measures that define volume, revenue, and the expenses that are required to provide the service (e.g., patient care or ancillary services).

Projecting Volume and Revenue

Projecting workload volume (e.g., patient days, number of tests or number of procedures, and workload requirements) is the foundation for developing the unit budget. Future volume projections can be estimated by reviewing internal volume trends and understanding changes in the local market. These projections must be modified on the basis of anticipated events that would change the assumptions (e.g., new programs or projected decrease in length of stay [LOS]). Volume is translated into budgeted revenue by multiplying volume and the expected charge per unit of service (UOS) (e.g., patient day or laboratory test).

It is important to understand that gross revenue is not the actual reimbursement for providing a service. First, payers do not reimburse the provider for total charges. Most payers, including governmental programs such as Medicare and Medicaid, reimburse by established rates for a diagnostic category (diagnosis-related group [DRG]) or procedure. Second, projecting gross revenue is a budget exercise, and it is only an indicator of projected work volume and potential financial reimbursement. Therefore, the manager needs to know the actual reimbursement for providing the service by payer type. Successful financial performance is achieved when the cost per UOS is managed to expected actual revenue collection.

Labor Expenses

Labor expense is the single largest cost in a hospital or patient unit budget and accounts for approximately 60% of the budget. Personnel requirements and associated expenses must be projected accurately to achieve the organization's financial goals and to ensure that sufficient resources are available to deliver the service.

The labor budget for a patient unit is complex and is based on the total number of hours and cost per labor hour. The total number of labor hours consists of direct worked hours, worked hours that are not direct care, and paid hours not worked. The direct worked labor hours needed to provide patient care are calculated by multiplying the projected volume, or UOS, by the established productivity standard. For example, when the budgeted productivity standard is 5.6 hours per patient day (HPPD) and the projected patient volume is 12,500 days, the hours required to provide direct patient care is 70,000 labor hours.

Units of service × Productivity standard = Direct worked hours

The labor expense also includes worked hours that are not direct care (orientation, education, and management time) and paid hours not worked, including vacation, holiday, and sick leave. Other wage expenses include overtime, differentials, and on-call pay. Each wage expense is itemized and monitored regularly to assess actual labor expenses compared with budget.

Nonlabor Expense

Nonlabor expenses account for approximately 40% of the total budget. These expenses include supplies and minor equipment used for patient care and unit management. Education and travel costs to support professional development are included.

Establishing priorities for using the unit's financial resources is a challenging and difficult responsibility. Nonlabor expenses are often perceived as "discretionary" and are curtailed or eliminated when the budget is not being maintained because of unexpected increases in labor costs. Education and professional development are as essential to the quality of patient care delivery as the direct care staffing, and therefore, managing all resources judiciously is critical to exceptional unit performance.

DEVELOPING THE BUDGET INTO AN OPERATIONAL PLAN

An operational plan is developed that translates the unit budget into a position control "roster" and a unit staffing plan. Using an inpatient unit as the example, the position control "roster" defines the number of positions and the hours worked by each individual. The composition of full-time and part-time employees is optimized to provide sufficient staff to meet the unit staffing needs while creating market-competitive positions. The manager determines the total number of positions and the full-time–part-time mix needed to effectively meet patient care needs and provide adequate coverage for each shift.

The next step in developing the unit operational plan is to create a staffing plan (Table 56-1). The staffing plan defines the number of staff that are required to meet patient care needs at various census levels by shift, while maintaining the budgeted productivity and labor expense. The staffing plan enables the manager to confirm whether the position control roster and the staff composition of full-time and part-time staff provide the maximal coverage and flexibility. The staffing plan is used to project the required personnel resources based on the census.

A unit schedule template is created from the staffing plan. The schedule template is a management tool to minimize management time spent creating routine unit schedules. The template can then be modified by staff who self-schedule or by the manager to accommodate those requests that are not routine. Automated management systems are available that will generate the schedule

TABLE 56-1 Patient Unit Flexible Staffing Pattern (Labor Hour Standard 5.6 HPPD)

Volume	15	16	17	18	19	20	21	22	23	24	25	26	27	28	29	30	31	32	33	34	35	36	37
7-3 Shift																							
CN	1	1	1	1	1	1	1	1	1	1	1	1	1	1	1	1	1	1	1	1	1	1	1
RN	3	3	3	3	4	4	4	4	4	4	5	5	5	5	5	6	6	6	6	6	7	7	7
LPN	0	0	0	0	0	0	0	0	0	0	0	0	0	0	0	0	0	0	0	0	0	0	0
NA	1	1	1	1	1	1	1	1	2	2	2	2	2	2	2	2	2	2	2	2	2	2	2
Scheduled hours	40	40	40	40	48	48	48	48	56	56	64	64	64	64	64	72	72	72	72	72	80	80	80
Required hours	33.6	35.8	38.1	40.3	42.6	44.8	47.0	49.3	51.5	53.8	56.0	58.2	60.5	62.7	65.0	67.2	69.4	71.7	73.9	76.2	78.4	80.6	82.9
3-11 Shift																							
CN	1	1	1	1	1	1	1	1	1	1	1	1	1	1	1	1	1	1	1	1	1	1	1
RN	2	2	2	2	2	2	2	2	2	3	3	3	3	3	4	4	4	4	4	4	4	5	5
LPN	0	0	1	1	1	1	1	1	1	1	1	1	1	1	1	1	1	1	1	1	1	1	1
NA	1	1	1	1	1	2	2	2	2	2	2	2	2	2	2	2	2	2	2	2	2	2	2
Scheduled hours	32	32	40	40	40	48	48	48	48	56	56	56	56	56	64	64	64	64	64	64	64	72	72
Required hours	31.9	34.0	36.2	38.3	40.4	42.6	44.7	46.8	48.9	51.1	53.2	55.3	57.5	59.6	61.7	63.8	66.0	68.1	70.2	72.4	74.5	76.6	78.7
11-7 Shift																							
RN	2	2	2	2	2	2	2	2	2	2	2	2	2	2	2	2	2	2	2	2	2	3	3
LPN	0	0	0	0	0	0	0	0	0	0	1	1	1	1	1	1	1	1	1	1	1	1	1
NA	1	1	1	1	1	2	2	2	2	2	2	2	2	2	2	2	2	2	2	2	2	2	2
Scheduled hours	24	24	24	24	24	32	32	32	32	32	40	40	40	40	40	40	40	40	40	40	40	48	48
Required hours	18.5	19.7	20.9	22.2	23.4	24.6	25.9	27.1	28.3	29.6	30.8	32.0	33.3	34.5	35.7	37.0	38.2	39.4	40.7	41.9	43.1	44.4	45.6
Total scheduled hours	96	96	104	104	112	128	128	128	136	144	160	160	160	160	168	176	176	176	176	176	184	200	200
Total required hours	84.0	89.6	95.2	100.8	106.4	112.0	117.6	123.2	128.8	134.4	140.0	145.6	151.2	156.8	162.4	168.0	173.6	179.2	184.8	190.4	196.0	201.6	207.2
Variance	(12.0)	(6.4)	(8.8)	(3.2)	(5.6)	(16.0)	(10.4)	(4.8)	(7.2)	(9.6)	(20.0)	(14.4)	(8.8)	(3.2)	(5.6)	(8.0)	(2.4)	(3.2)	(8.8)	(14.4)	(12.0)	(1.6)	(7.2)

HPPD = hours per patient day.

templates and eliminate the manager's time developing the core schedule.

Manager orientation programs frequently focus on budget development, and most financial textbooks describe the fine points of developing a budget. Proficiency in understanding financial reports is greatly valued in organizations. However, the most challenging management task is to understand what is driving cost and productivity performance. The manager must know what data are needed to evaluate unit performance, leading to potential solutions and exceptional financial and operational performance. The competent manager understands how to actively manage to reduce costs and improve results (Dreisbach, 1994).

Assessing Financial and Operational Performance

The patient care managers' success will be measured by their ability to identify and balance cost and quality issues effectively while managing staffing under a varying patient census and demanding patient acuity (Dreisbach, 1994). The key to effective monitoring is access to information necessary to make the right management decisions regarding financial and personnel resource use. Management systems are needed that will provide access to accurate and timely data. Tracking key performance indicators allows the manager to proactively respond when financial or operational indicators are not meeting established standards.

Unit Cost Indicators

The primary indicator for operating expense is cost per unit of service. Unit of service is the measure of workload demand (e.g., number of tests, procedures, patient days, or discharges). Patient discharge is the standard indicator for operating performance in the hospital setting. Cost per discharge measures the total resources used during the episode of care and the cost impact of length of stay. Most hospital performance measures are based on adjusted patient discharges (e.g., cost per adjusted discharge) to recognize the volume of outpatient activity. The outpatient adjustment factor is calculated by dividing the sum of total inpatient and outpatient revenue by total inpatient revenue.

PRODUCTIVITY MEASUREMENT

Productivity measures are routinely monitored to evaluate use of personnel resources and total paid labor expenses. HPPD or hours per patient discharge is the standard productivity indicator. Productivity measures that can be monitored to assess operational performance are listed in Table 56-2.

Four key management analyses can be made to assess cost and productivity performance. These analyses are staffing-to-demand, productivity benchmarking, use of labor dollars, and workforce composition.

TABLE 56-2   Definitions of Productivity Measures

HPPD Measures	Definitions	Data Included	Data Not Included
Total direct RN hours	All RN hours providing direct patient care	All worked hours spent in direct patient care, including charge nurse roles	Orientation, education, meetings, management hours, and paid time off
Total worked RN hours	Total worked hours for all RNs, including "charge roles"	All worked hours including orientation, education, meetings	Management hours and paid time off
Direct patient care hours	Total labor hours providing direct care—for all caregivers, e.g., LPN, patient care assistant (unit-based)	All direct care hours for unit-based caregivers	Orientation, education, meetings, management hours, clerical, and paid time off
Total patient care worked hours	Total worked hours for all unit-based caregivers	All worked hours including orientation, education, meetings	Management hours, clerical hours, and paid time off
Total RN paid hours	All RN paid hours	All RN worked hours and paid time off, e.g., vacation and illness benefit	Management hours
Total patient care paid hours	All unit-based caregiver paid hours	All worked hours and paid time off, e.g., vacation and illness benefit	Clerical hours and management hours

HPPD = hours per patient day; LPN = licensed practical nurse; RN = registered nurse.

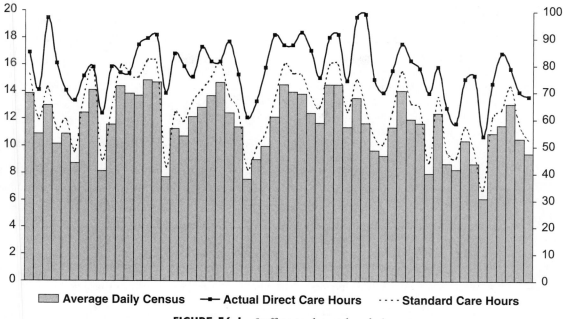

FIGURE 56-1 Staffing-to-demand analysis.

Staffing to Demand

Staffing to demand is an analysis that tracks staffing resources and census variation. Plotting patient census and actual staffing resources used by day demonstrates the effectiveness of flexing staffing resources to variation in patient volume. In units where census varies significantly by hour of the day (e.g., emergency or labor and delivery), the staffing to demand analysis will provide a more accurate assessment when performed by hour of day. Although the census and staffing data may not routinely be collected hourly, a 2- or 3-week concurrent sample can provide an initial assessment.

Figure 56-1 demonstrates a surgical unit that experiences wide fluctuations in daily census and decreasing workload on weekends. In this example, short-stay patients are "admitted" to the unit during the week, creating unexpected staffing demands during the shift. Elective surgical patients are usually discharged on weekends. The staffing curve demonstrates that staffing resources are adjusted to follow the census trend. However, it also demonstrates that the actual staffing hours do exceed the required hours, which are based on budgeted HPPD standards. This analysis demonstrates that there is some opportunity for enhanced operational performance if scheduled staffing hours were better matched to actual patient census. Therefore, the potential solutions for achieving improved performance include adjusting the core schedule to better match the census trends and de-

veloping a staffing complement that provides higher flexibility to meet the wide and unexpected fluctuations in patient volume.

Benchmarking

Most hospitals participate in a benchmarking system that provides managers with performance data from units that have similar characteristics. Internal trends within the same hospital or health system can be used to ensure that similar staffing resources are available to the same patient populations (e.g., med-surg). External benchmarking provides a general assessment of performance relative to other organizations. However, there is less precision with this comparison on the basis of variations among institutions (e.g., case mix, types of services).

There are many debates about the value of benchmarking. Most benchmarking systems are based on performance indicators (e.g., HPPD or cost per day). This information does not provide the manager with "how" unit performance is achieved. However, the performance metrics are one data point that a manager can use to evaluate unit performance.

The manager must understand the characteristics of units within the benchmarking database. Table 56-3 lists factors that will affect the productivity measures and should be considered when using benchmark data to evaluate unit performance.

TABLE 56-3 Benchmarking

Patient Care Area	Factors to Consider

All areas	Patient care roles
	• Which roles are included in direct hours, worked hours, and paid hours?
	   – Are management roles included?
	   – Are "charge nurse" or "lead nurse" roles included in direct care?
	   – Are clerical roles included in worked hours?
	• Are agency and traveler resources included?
	• What ancillary/service tasks are performed by unit staff, e.g., ECG, phlebotomy, and housekeeping?
	RN skill mix
	• Cost savings are achieved with a balance between RN mix and HPPD. For example, a "higher" RN skill mix and "lower" HPPD may achieve the same cost performance as "lower" RN skill mix and "higher" total HPPD

Intensive care units	• Does the organization have step-down units or transitional care units? The level of severity in the ICU may be higher when a step-down area is available, resulting in the need for higher patient care hours • Are monitor technician roles used and are they included in HPPD? • Are assistive personnel included in HPPD?
Medical-surgical units	• What are the patient demographics of each unit? Is the unit general med-surg or more specialized, e.g., orthopedics, pulmonary? • What is the admission/transfer/discharge (ATD) ratio or pattern? A unit with a high number of encounters per day will need more RN resources to meet the needs of admission assessments and discharge procedures • Where are telemetry patients located, e.g., specialized monitoring unit or within the med-surg units? • Where are observation patients? Units that provide care for observation patients require more RN resources to meet the demands of constant observation and rapid admit and discharge
Obstetrics/nursery	• What is the model of obstetrical care, e.g., traditional L&D, LDR, or LDRP units? • What is the policy for "rooming-in"? How many hours per day do most normal newborns spend in mother's room? • What is the LOS? The more aggressive or lower the LOS, the more resources may be needed to provide required care needs

ECG = electrocardiogram; HPPD = hours per patient day; ICU = intensive care unit; L&D = labor and delivery; LDR = labor, delivery, rooming-in; LDRP = labor, delivery, rooming-in, postpartum; LOS = length of stay; RN = registered nurse.

If the benchmarking data indicate that the unit's productivity performance is lower compared with similar units, the manager must carefully assess opportunities to provide patient care at a more cost-effective operational level without quality suffering. As most managers have experienced, however, it is difficult to reduce patient care hours without changing the way the staff work. Assessing current processes and evaluating technology enablers to minimize time not spent in direct care goes beyond the scope of this chapter. It is, however, the important next step when faced with the challenge of providing quality care with less staffing resources.

Labor Dollar Utilization

Labor dollar utilization demonstrates what is driving labor costs and the potential opportunities to control labor costs. The HPPD may be maintained within budget standards, but the budget will not be achieved if the labor hour cost exceeds expected standards. Direct care worked hours usually account for 70% of the labor hours. Hospital policy and benefits determine paid time off and differential costs.

Premium paid staffing—overtime, agency use, and other staffing incentives—increases the labor hour cost significantly, and aggressive management is required to minimize these costs. Labor hour and labor dollar analyses provide data needed to determine the drivers of labor expenses (Fig. 56-2). For example, when overtime expenses exceed the industry standard of 3% to 5% of total labor costs, the reasons for overtime must be identified. Potential solutions for decreasing overtime costs will vary depending on the reason for overtime.

Figure 56-3 demonstrates that overtime is used primarily to replace scheduled shift vacancies. There is no

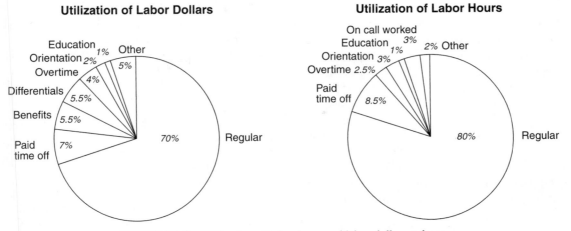

FIGURE 56-2 Utilization of labor hour and labor dollar analyses.

simple solution to accessing adequate staffing resources. A high percentage of overtime used to replace scheduled vacancies, however, leads the manager to assess productivity performance, review staffing and scheduling procedures, and evaluate the composition of staff positions, especially part-time and per diem employees.

End of shift documentation is the second contributing factor to overtime use. Addressing documentation processes and technology to streamline documentation will be more effective than increased supervision of personnel working overtime hours.

Workforce Composition

Staffing flexibility is achieved with the appropriate composition of full-time, part-time, and per diem or casual employees. A full-time–part-time mix that has a greater ratio of part-time employees will improve staffing flexibility and maximize the number of employees available to share weekend and vacation coverage. Units that experience significant variation in daily census (e.g., obstetrics and intensive care units) benefit from a higher ratio of part-time staff, such as 50% of the employees working part-time hours.

UTILIZING THE DATA

Chase (1994) suggests that a shift is needed from financial management to "financial management decision-making and problem solving." Collecting data and conducting the appropriate analyses will lead to hypotheses

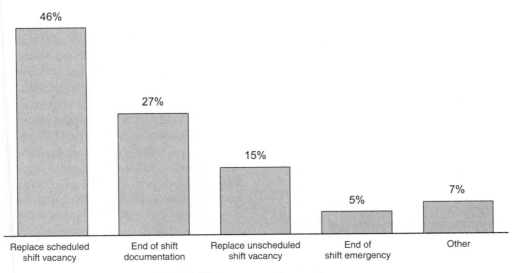

FIGURE 56-3 Reasons for overtime use.

but does not answer questions nor solve the problem. The manager requires competence in using the data and analytical results to generate potential hypotheses and solutions. It is not unusual to get "data-crazed," constantly seeking more data to provide assurance that the data are accurate or that the potential solution is the correct one. Data integrity is important, and management systems are required that collect and report accurate and timely data. Data are never perfect, however, and analyses provide direction, not solutions. On the basis of the data available, the manager must move forward, problem solving and generating possible solutions to address the critical issues that will have an impact on the unit's performance.

SUMMARY

The financial and operational responsibilities of the management role are challenging and difficult. Managers may not be confident in their roles because of lack of proficiency with the financial skills that are required. Often the manager is faced with the uncomfortable role and moral dilemma of balancing patient care quality with limited financial resources. The manager is the critical "lynchpin" between the delivery of quality and cost-effective patient care. Arming the manager with the requisite financial skills will not eliminate the difficult choices that must be made, but competent and highly successful managers will make those choices for the patients and the organization.

REFERENCES

Boston, C., & Forman, H. (1994). A time to listen. *Journal of Nursing Administration, 24*(2), 16-18.

Chase, L. (1994). Nurse manager competencies. *Journal of Nursing Administration, 24*(4S), 56-64.

CSC Healthcare Group. (1998). Computer Sciences Corporation Patient Care Executive Survey.

Dreisbach, A.M. (1994). A structured approach to expert financial management: A financial development plan for nurse managers. *Nursing Economic$, 12*(3), 131-139.

Edwards, P.A., & Roemer, L. (1996). Are nurse managers ready for the current challenges of healthcare? *Journal of Nursing Administration, 26*(9), 11-17.

Eubanks, P. (1992). The new nurse manager: A lynchpin in quality care and cost control efforts. *Hospitals, 66*(8), 22-29.

Everson-Bates, S. (1992). First-line nurse managers in the expanded role: An ethnographic analysis. *Journal of Nursing Administration, 22*(3), 32-37.

Haas, S.A., & Hackbarth, D.P. (1997). The role of the nurse manager in ambulatory care: Results of a national survey. *Nursing Economic$, 15*(4), 191-203.

Kirk, R. (1987). Management development: A needs analysis for nurse executives and managers. *Journal of Nursing Administration, 17*(4), 7-8.

Krejci, J.W., & Malin, S. (1997). Impact of leadership development on competencies. *Nursing Economic$, 15*(5), 235-241.

Mark, B. (1994). The emerging role of the nurse manager. *Journal of Nursing Administration, 24*(1), 48-55.

Mintzberg, H. (1994). Rounding out the manager's job. *Sloan Management Review, 36*(1), 11-26.

Oroviogoicoechea, C. (1996). The clinical nurse manager: A literature review. *Journal of Advanced Nursing, 24*, 1273-1280.

Patz, J.M., Biordi, D.L., & Holm, K. (1991). Middle nurse manager effectiveness. *Journal of Nursing Administration, 21*(1), 15-24.

Section Nine

Role Transitions

Colleagues and Conflict

JOANNE McCLOSKEY DOCHTERMAN, HELEN KENNEDY GRACE

As is demonstrated in other sections of the book, health care is undergoing many changes, some unwelcome and all challenging. In response to the changes, old roles are evolving and new roles are emerging. These roles involve both collaboration and conflict, two topics that are explored in some detail in the chapters in this section.

The debate chapter for the section is about collaboration between nurses and physicians. Nurse leaders have long desired more collaborative roles and relationships with physicians, but do these exist? Baggs begins her assessment of the situation by noting that the terminology of collaborative practice has different meanings in medicine and nursing. Most of the writing related to collaborative practice has been done by nurses. Loss of power by physicians and gaining of power by nurses is a threat to traditional medical practice. Although collaborative practice was advanced through the National Joint Practice Commission some 30 years ago, only some of the guidelines developed then have been implemented in practice settings today. Despite evidence that collaborative practice results in improved patient outcomes, an astoundingly low percentage of physicians and nurses report use of collaborative problem solving in clinical settings. Obstacles to collaborative practice include traditional communication patterns, decision-making prerogatives of physicians, and reluctance on the part of nurses to accept greater responsibility for decision making. Changes in educational programs to promote collaborative learning and changes within practice settings to facilitate collaborative problem solving are beginning to emerge but, as Baggs concludes, "collaboration is not the usual mode of practice." This chapter contains an excellent and comprehensive review of the literature on nurse-physician collaboration.

The changing roles of nurses reflect the changing roles of women in society. In the first viewpoint chapter, Chinn explains that because most nurses are women and be-cause nurses' role of caring for the sick has been assigned to women world wide, feminism and nursing are inextricably connected. Chinn structures her chapter around a statement by Florence Nightingale: "Passion, intellect, moral activity—these three have never been satisfied in women." Chinn discusses these three values historically and in modern times. She relates passion to feminism as a culture grounded in women's experience and a political stance to right injustices against women; intellect to feminism as a discipline seeking to give voice to women's experience; and moral activity to feminism as an ethic of valuing women and women's experience. Feminism, she says, is not an ideology but a perspective that values diversity. She concludes her chapter with a set of suggested readings and questions to explore further some of the ideas that she has raised. Chinn's chapter is highly recommended for all women and men in nursing who value the contributions of both sexes.

The unique perspective and contribution that nurses bring to the patient is labeled by Pike in the next chapter as "nurses voice." Pike urges nurses to choose colleagueship over silence. She says that nurses' voices have been silenced by both external and internal forces. Among the new external constraints is the restructuring in health care in the United States. These constraints, says Pike, have inflicted wounds on nurses' professional self-esteem. Rather than acting out the appealing victim role and remaining silent and blaming physicians, Pike urges nurses to speak out, to define themselves as colleagues. The taking up of the conflict requires, she says, an understanding of the uniqueness of nursing, a breadth of clinical experience, a language to communicate to others the nature of nursing, and an understanding of the constraints imposed on nurses. Using two case studies, she illustrates that nurses' silences have significant implications for patient care as well as for nurses' role and satisfaction. All nurses should read and act on this thought-provoking and important chapter.

Edwards addresses collaboration between nursing and medicine in the delivery of services to the community. Community-based care, says Edwards, requires a shift in power from the hospital and expert professionals to community members. A new collaborative approach to the education of medical and nursing students is necessary in order to embrace the new philosophy. Edwards says that collaboration is about three things: empowerment, relationships, and synergy. She discusses some of the societal, professional, and economic forces that work against collaboration between doctors and nurses. A few successes of effective collaboration are beginning to be documented. In the second part of her chapter, Edwards describes the 10-year successful collaborative education model at East Tennessee State University designed to provide health care to the Blue Ridge Mountain Community. A large community need and a series of grants from the W.K. Kellogg Foundation have enabled community leaders and health professionals in the colleges of medicine, nursing, and public and allied health to work together and establish a successful multidisciplinary education and practice model. While the setting and driving forces may not be the same as other parts of the country the accomplishments of this group are clearly visionary and admirable. In this day of rapid change in health care and recognized need to refocus our education and services to the community, everyone should read this chapter.

A specific case where collaboration is needed is between nurse practitioners (NPs) and physician assistants (PAs). In the next chapter, Williams, who is both a NP and a PA, makes the case that these two providers, more similar than different, should work together. She reviews the origins of each role and then compares the current status in several areas, including education and skills. In January 2000 a master's degree in nursing was required for national certification for NPs; in January 2003 the Health Care Financing Administration (HCFA) will require a master's degree for obtainment of a Medicare billing number. Williams says that despite an independent license, the majority of NPs practice with physician supervision. She despairs about the negative comments made by one group (usually the NPs) about the other. She says nurse practitioners and physician assistants are like twins, looking alike and sounding the same, yet have some differences. She urges the "long lost siblings" to embrace and work together to accomplish patient care goals.

The difficulties that are inherent in collaboration are demonstrated in the next chapter by Keenan, Kocan, Lundy, Averhart, and Aebersold. This group of nurse collaborators set out to improve nurse-physician relationships in their institution. The process they used to accomplish this was to design an intervention to assist nurses and physicians to collaborate with each other. The research study they designed and implemented to evaluate the intervention showed that the goal of collaboration between nurses and physicians was achieved. In the process, however, the study group itself became divided by conflict. The chapter reviews both the lessons learned from the intervention study and the lessons learned from the study group interaction. The authors advise that it "is prudent to expect conflict to occur within groups comprised of very different stake holders and to be prepared to handle conflict constructively when it arises." They overview the win-win process of "mutual gains," which they used to manage different interests and repair relationships. As collaborative efforts increase on numerous fronts, others will discover, as these authors did, the challenges of group work. This chapter can help others to be prepared to work through the challenges.

Conflict and its resolution is also the subject of the last chapter by Kritek. Kritek says that conflict is so endemic to nursing that it is often not recognized as conflict. Her chapter is a personal philosophical reflection on the nature of conflict in nursing and ways that nurses handle conflict. She raises questions such as Why is it so pervasive? Do we like our solutions? She suggests some good reading materials and briefly overviews the philosophical viewpoints of Toulmin and Anderson. Nurses, she says, are multilingual at conflict management. We keep multiple perspectives about conflict alive and we have good conflict management skills, but we often choose to act as codependents and smooth over or polarize conflicts instead of using the skills we have. Kritek wants nurses to think of themselves as people who can creatively and constructively assist in the resolution of conflicts. The first step she says is to recognize that we are at an "uneven table" and that what we are doing now is harmful. Kritek says that conflict in health care will increase, and she wants nurses to transform their current behavior to that which is "beyond mere manipulation." This is a thoughtful, challenging chapter, one that should be read several times by many of us.

Collaborative practice for nurses is closer to reality than in the past because of the changes in society and in health care delivery. But collaboration requires certain skills and a risk-taking attitude. And, in a sense, the opportunity for collaboration creates conflict. When we choose collaboration, we choose conflict. This realization and knowledge of strategies to deal with conflict may move us closer to a preferred future.

Collaboration Between Nurses and Physicians in the 21st Century

What Is It? Does It Exist? Why Does It Matter?

JUDITH GEDNEY BAGGS

Collaboration is an ethical responsibility of highest priority. —Myra E. Levine (1989)

COLLABORATION BETWEEN NURSES AND PHYSICIANS: WHAT IS IT?

To collaborate is to "work together, especially in a joint intellectual effort" (*American Heritage Dictionary*, 1992, p. 371). Indeed, working together is the essence of the meaning of collaboration as we use it in nursing to describe a type of working relationship we value with physicians. However, working together is not a specific enough definition. Working together could mean working in parallel, without communicating or planning together, or simply working in the same geographical area.

The concept of collaboration has been analyzed several times (Baggs & Schmitt, 1988; Corser, 1998; Henneman, 1995a, 1995b; Sullivan, 1998). In addition, a number of conceptual models of collaboration have been developed to guide understanding of the term collaboration. Thomas (1976) proposed that collaboration is a form of handling interpersonal interactions that combines cooperativeness (concern for the other's interests) with assertiveness (concern for one's own interests). His framework has been used to guide much of the nursing research and theorizing about the concept. It may be time to reassess the value of this framework to us as a profession (Baggs, 1998b; Corser, 1998).

More recently nurses have developed at least five other conceptual models that describe antecedent conditions and outcomes of collaboration. King, Lee, and Henneman (1993) proposed a theoretical model with the antecedents of conflict resolution, cooperation, assertiveness, collaboration, and integration. The outcomes identified were decreased patient morbidity and mortality, more nurse and patient satisfaction, and improved costs. Baggs and Schmitt's (1997) empirically based model was developed in a grounded theory study of ICU nurses and resident physicians. In their model the antecedent conditions of availability and receptiveness precede working together as a patient-focused team, which is followed by the outcomes of improved patient care, job satisfaction, and cost control. Corser's model (1998), based on a literature review, combined antecedent conditions of personal/interpersonal influences with organizational/professional influences to predict collaborative interactions. His identified outcomes were clinical goal achievement, fewer negative patient outcomes, coordinated planning, care provider job productivity and satisfaction, and more interdisciplinary problem solving and decision making. Keenan, Cooke, and Hillis (1998) modeled conflict between the professions, which they saw as key to understanding collaboration. Their model, which was supported in an empirical study, predicts that the likelihood of a nurse's collaboration with a physician is based on the nurse's expectation of whether the physician will collaborate and on the nurse's assessment of work group norms for collaboration. Sullivan's model (1998) is based in systems theory and describes the collaboration system and subsystems for partnership and practice. It includes patient, provider, and organizational outcomes. Any of these models could be used to structure research or a description of collaboration between nurses and physicians.

In the nursing literature the critical attributes of collaboration have been identified as sharing in planning, decision making, problem solving, goal setting, and responsibility; working together cooperatively; coordinating; and communicating openly (Baggs & Schmitt, 1988). Based on these critical attributes and the Thomas model, one definition of collaboration is "nurses and physicians cooperatively working together, sharing responsibility for solving problems and making decisions to formulate and carry out plans for patient care" (Baggs & Schmitt, 1988, p. 145).

Does collaboration mean the same thing to physicians as it does to nurses? The construct of collaboration is addressed more often by nurses than by physicians, as evidenced by an examination of the primary library indexes for the professions. The *Cumulative Index to Nursing and Allied Health Literature (CINAHL)* has had a subject heading for collaboration since 1989. In the 1998 on-line version of this index, that heading contained 490 citations. The *Index Medicus* does not use collaboration as a subject heading; rather one must look under interprofessional relations, patient care team, or cooperative behavior, all of which also are found in the *CINAHL*.

Most of the literature about collaboration between physicians and nurses has been written by nurses (e.g., Baggs & Schmitt, 1988; Corley, 1998; Corser, 1998; England, 1986; Fagin, 1992; Gardner & Cary, 1999; Henneman, 1995a, 1995b; Larson, 1999; Steel, 1986; Stichler, 1995; Styles, 1984; Weiss & Davis, 1985) or by nurses and physicians together (Batalden, Cronenwett, Brown, Moffatt, & Serrell, 1998; Evans & Carlson, 1992; Hansen, Biros, Delaney, & Schug, 1999; Harvey, Fujii, & Carlson, 2000). In a MEDLINE search of publications on the topic of nurse-physician relationships between 1990 and 1995, Larson (1999) found 61 citations, 64% of which had been published in nursing journals. A cross-disciplinary group has written of the importance of cooperation, but their definition, "working together to produce mutual benefit," is similar to collaboration (Clemmer, Spuhler, Berwick, & Nolan, 1998, p. 1004). Physicians occasionally have written about the construct (Michelson, 1988).

Other articles by physicians have discussed collaboration, although it was not the primary focus of their work. For example, Stein, Watts, and Howell (1990) updated Stein's classic article on the "doctor-nurse game" (1967), noting that the earlier relationship between the professions had changed. In the past, nurses could only have input by convincing physicians that the physicians had initiated any decision making themselves (Stein, 1967). Stein et al. (1990) believe that nurses are now more highly ed-

ucated with a defined area of expertise, functioning more as autonomous health professionals. These authors characterized the new relationship between physicians and nurses as one of "mutual interdependency" (p. 547). They cited movement toward collaboration and collegiality as less hierarchical and more open than in the past. They indicated the possible positive and negative aspects of this new relationship but generally approved of the direction it is taking.

Greenfield (1999) wrote about the "troubled partnership" of nurses and physicians, noting that, particularly for nurse practitioners and physicians, roles are becoming less distinct. He predicted an end to the stereotypes of the "omnipotent physician and subservient nurse" (p. 288) and recognition that it is essential if nurses and physicians are to collaborate in care delivery. Similarly Grumbach and Coffman (1998) stressed the importance of collaboration between physicians and a group they called "non-physician clinicians." All these physicians appear to be speaking of collaboration with a definition comparable to the term used in the nursing literature.

Despite this evidence of comparability of definition, there is also evidence of differences in implications and assessment of collaboration for the two professions. In the 1980s Styles (1984) noted that physicians often feel threatened when nurses discuss collaboration because they see the process as an invasion of their position of authority and power. Indeed, a secondary definition of collaboration is "to cooperate treasonably, as with an enemy occupation force" (*American Heritage Dictionary*, 1992, p. 371). Some physicians sense a collapsing hierarchy. In the past physicians seen to be collaborating with staff nurses may have been the primary source of this threat. More recently physician concerns have been stimulated by perceptions about competition for patients with nurse practitioners, whom some view as physician substitutes.

Stein et al. (1990), in their description of the negative aspects of collaboration, identified physicians' loss of the security in the old hierarchy and the potential for competition and disputes. Indeed, the movement toward interdisciplinary team care, a construct related to collaboration, was described as a move by nurses to make interprofessional relations more egalitarian and less hierarchical (Brown, 1982). Physicians who were comfortable with the older, castelike system (Wesson, 1966) in which nurses were subordinate are not likely to welcome collaboration in practice (Campbell-Heider & Pollock, 1987; Prescott & Bowen, 1985). Fagin (1992) noted that "physicians, more often than not, do not value or demonstrate collaboration in their work with nurses" (p. 295).

Nurses too may feel threatened by the increased responsibility and accountability involved in collaborative practice (Cape, 1986; Prescott, Dennis, & Jacox, 1987). For nurses to fulfill the assertive aspect of collaboration they need to assume accountability and increased authority in practice areas.

Katzman (1989) studied the different perceptions by nurses and physicians of areas of appropriate nursing authority. She asked nurses and physicians from a southwestern hospital to rate their agreement or disagreement as to whether specific nursing roles, functions, and behaviors reflect the current status of nursing authority. She then asked them to rate the same behaviors in an ideal situation. The area of greatest difference between ratings from nurses and physicians in the current situation concerned the statement that nurses are not serving primarily as physicians' assistants. The nurses agreed, and the physicians' responses were neutral to disagree. In the ideal ratings the greatest difference concerned whether nurses should have equal say in health policy making. The nurses agreed to strongly agreed; physicians disagreed. Some of the areas of greatest disagreement concerned nursing care, with physicians according nurses less authority in both current and ideal situations. In an ideal situation nurses strongly agreed that they should have authority to decide standards of nursing care, while physicians were neutral. In determination of nursing care for patients, nurses' rating was strongly agree, physicians' was neutral. Perhaps in other settings and with other groups of providers some of these differences would diminish, but these disagreements about nursing authority suggest difficulties in moving to more collaboration in practice.

Benner, Hooper-Kyriakidis, and Stannard (1999) noted the difficulties in communicating across disciplinary lines, particularly when there are status and power inequities, as there generally are between nurses and physicians. They found nurses who "continue to use indirect patterns of communication and deference to physicians in order to avoid conflict" (p. 412). However, they proposed that those patterns be "abandoned for forthright communications" (p. 412). They also found evidence that the old patterns are changing in favor of clear communication, good listening, and collaborative skills. Another team-building skill they recommended was debriefing after communication breakdowns, to avoid similar problems in the future.

There is research evidence for different interpretations or observations of collaboration. In a medical intensive care unit (ICU), staff nurses and medical residents were given the same definition of collaboration and asked to report how much collaboration was involved in making decisions about transferring about 300 patients out of the medical ICU. The correlation between their reports of the amount of collaboration in making decisions was only $r = .10$ ($P = .10$; Baggs, Ryan, Phelps, Richeson, & Johnson, 1992). In a similar but larger study involving three ICUs and over 1,400 patients the correlation was .09 ($P < .05$) both for nurses with resident physicians and for nurses with attending physicians (Baggs, unpublished data).

Somehow these clinicians are not seeing the same interactions or are assessing them differently. Work that was conducted on collaboration between social workers and physicians may shed some light on how nurses and physicians have different perceptions. Abramson and Mizrahi (1996) found that both professions valued communication in collaboration. Social workers more than physicians valued respect, understanding of the other's role, acknowledgment of capability, positive style, inclusion in decisions, degree of emotions, noninterference with autonomy, and positive personality traits. Physicians more than social workers valued capability and independent functioning by the collaborator. The authors' conclusion was that social workers valued interactional factors more than physicians, which is probably true for nurses as well.

In ethical decision making too there is evidence of a lack of collaboration. Hierarchical rather than collaborative decision making was the third ranked ethical issue in a study of almost 800 hospital nurses (Omery, Henneman, Billet, Luna-Raines, & Brown-Saltzman, 1995). Researchers in several studies have demonstrated nurse and physician differences about how aggressively patients should be treated (Eliasson, Howard, Torrington, Dillard, & Phillips, 1997; Farber et al., 1985; Frampton & Mayewski, 1987; Walter et al., 1998; Wolff, Smolen, & Ferrara, 1985). In three studies, nurses perceived ethical decision making as a problematic area in their interactions with physicians (Erlen & Frost, 1991; Gramelspacher, Howell, & Young, 1986; Holly, 1989). Nurses have been shown to perceive less communication about patient care decisions between the two professions than do physicians (Frampton & Mayewski, 1987; Webster, Mazer, Potvin, Fisher, & Byrick, 1991). Several authors have stressed the importance of a collaborative working relationship between nursing and medicine as essential to ethical, compassionate patient care (Aroskar, 1998; Corley, 1998).

In a study involving interviews of administrators in medicine and nursing about interdisciplinary team care, the goals for team care differed for each profession. Physicians expected nurses to act as physician extenders, while nurses expected to use their knowledge to direct patient care (Temkin-Greener, 1983). Although there was agreement about the definition of a team (people with differing expertise working together to provide patient care), there was conflict about leadership and authority in decision making and concern about territory.

There is evidence of common ground. During interviews of 10 medical residents and 10 ICU nurses, members of both professions defined collaboration similarly and valued it highly (Baggs & Schmitt, 1997). Both were clear that collaboration benefited patient care and made their work more satisfying. One physician said, "I think it takes less time to work as a team. You are smoother. If everybody is clear on what is going on . . . where we're going, and how to get there, then you get there faster and better" (Baggs, 1998a, p. 187). A nurse said, "Things the MD is going to miss along the way, the nurse is going to pick up on, and then the patient will be totally cared for" (p. 187).

The definitions of collaboration appear similar for nursing and medicine, but there appear to be differences in the implications of the term for each profession (Baggs & Schmitt, 1997). Not too surprisingly, the loss of power by physicians and the gain of power by nurses that are inherent in collaboration in practice lead the two professions to approach such a move differently. Nurses and physicians also may observe or interpret interactions differently in assessing how much collaboration has taken place.

COLLABORATION BETWEEN NURSES AND PHYSICIANS: DOES IT EXIST?

One of the first groups to promote the notion of collaboration between physicians and nurses in practice was the National Joint Practice Commission (NJPC), which was established in 1971 "to make recommendations concerning the roles of the physician and the nurse in providing high quality health care" (NJPC, 1981, p. 1). The commission, founded by the American Medical Association and the American Nurses Association, was composed of equal numbers of physicians and nurses. They proposed five guidelines for the development of what they termed joint or collaborative practice: establishment of a joint practice committee, primary nursing, encouragement of nurses' individual clinical decision making, integrated patient records, and joint patient care record reviews. Several model collaborative practice units were established implementing these five practices. Although data obtained were primarily subjective opinions of participants, increased quality of care, patient satisfaction, and

nursing job satisfaction were reported (Devereux, 1981a, 1981b, 1981c; NJPC, 1981). Unfortunately, the NJPC no longer exists.

Currently, about 30 years after these guidelines were developed, many of them, particularly integrated patient records, have been implemented in various institutions. Does their implementation mean that collaborative practice is a reality? Work by Prescott and Bowen (1985) suggests that we are not yet at that point. They used the Thomas model to classify the modes of handling disagreements reported by nurses and physicians in acute care settings. They found that only 14% of physicians and 7% of nurses reported using collaborative problem solving; the primary mode used by both providers was competition (Prescott & Bowen, 1985).

Further analyses of data from the same study suggest that the staff nurse role in clinical decision making about patient care is, at best, interdependent rather than truly collaborative, with physicians accepting nurses' input but handling final decision making themselves in most situations (Prescott et al., 1987). The nurses in the study were generally satisfied with this arrangement, provided they believed their input was listened to and valued by physicians. Many of the nurses did not want more responsibility for decision making. Physicians were willing to cede to nursing only decisions they considered unimportant. In fact, they did not view them as decisions at all.

This represents less the new collaborative mode promoted in nursing and more the older "doctor-nurse" game, with the change being that nurses now may make suggestions openly. A recent publication on physicians' failure to use ethics consultation may shed some light on their reluctance to collaborate (Davies & Hudson, 1999). The researchers found that most of their physician subjects believed that their role as attending physician meant that they should be the primary decision makers, that it was integral to their leadership of the health care team. They believed that shared decision making was an intrusion into their relationship with their patients and an abdication of responsibility. This attitude presents a barrier to collaborative care.

Prescott believes we have not gone far enough toward collaboration, despite many nurses' satisfaction with the status quo. She sees collaboration as important in the development of professional practice and financially in the management of hospital care (Prescott, 1989; Prescott et al., 1987; Prescott, Phillips, Ryan, & Thompson, 1991). Professional practice is enhanced by nurses who have independence in some decision making, such as in decisions about administering analgesics for headache or changing diets as tolerated. Enabling nurses to make some decisions frees them from wasted and expensive time spent looking or waiting for physicians. Such decision making supports the assertive aspect of collaboration.

Collaboration in practice is not yet a reality for most nurses. Obstacles to collaborative practice come from both the nursing and medical professions. Collaboration is missing in some of the areas where we would most expect to find it, such as in primary care teams of nurse practitioners and physicians, where the nurses are highly educated in their area of practice. Lamb and Napodano (1984) audiotaped interactions between team members on two teams. They found that only 23% of the interactions qualified as collaborative, although the providers rated themselves as collaborating 59% of the time. McLain (1988a) said, "The research literature is strikingly devoid of studies that have demonstrated the actual existence of collaborative practice as a predominant pattern between nurses and physicians" (p. 391). She found that both physicians and nurses promoted distorted communication and nonmeaningful interactions that blocked collaboration (McLain, 1988a, 1988b). The inability of the Cochrane Collaboration, a large database of systematic reviews of research, to find any randomized controlled trials of interventions to promote nurse physician collaboration suggests an urgent research need (Zwarenstein, Bryant, Bailie, & Sibthorpe, 1999).

COLLABORATION BETWEEN NURSES AND PHYSICIANS: WHY DOES IT MATTER?

Larson has said that "Failure of physicians and nurses to work together, to share decision making, and to communicate is not only undesirable but actually unethical because such behavior fails to focus on patient needs and can produce harm" (1999, p. 39). A number of authors have summarized reasons to support collaboration (Fagin, 1992; Larson, 1999; Miccolo & Spanier, 1993). Sorrells-Jones and Weaver (1999) discussed the synergistic performance of effective interdisciplinary teams, essential as part of the new "knowledge work" in health care, and the barriers to implementation. Collaboration has been identified, along with primary nursing, as one of the two concepts from nursing and health care over the past 20 years that has been promoted as having a positive effect on patient care and provider satisfaction (Alpert, Goldman, Kilroy, & Pike, 1992). Aiken, Sochalski, and Lake (1997) identified a high level of hospital nurse autonomy and a good relationship between nurses and physicians as key elements in patient outcomes.

It is not just nurse authors who have identified collaboration as crucial to health care delivery. Christensen and Larson (1993) see collaboration as a way of maximizing both the sharing of information unique to different professional participants and of creating the opportunity for each to learn more about the other's knowledge and talents, thereby improving future collaboration. McMahan, Hoffman, and McGee (1994) noted that collaboration has become part of most quality improvement programs.

Prescott et al. (1991) noted the importance of collaboration as a way of improving patient outcomes. There are a number of empirical studies that support such a belief. Studies of interdisciplinary teams in long-term care have demonstrated that team care leads to a slower rate of deterioration in patients with chronic diabetics (Feiger & Schmitt, 1979; Schmitt, Watson, Feiger, & Williams, 1981) and lower mortality in geriatric patients (Rubenstein et al., 1984). Outcomes of collaboration in acute care hospital general units include lower costs (Koerner & Armstrong, 1984) and increased patient satisfaction (Koerner, Cohen, & Armstrong, 1985). Investigators in ICUs have found collaboration to be associated with better than predicted mortality (Knaus, Draper, Wagner, & Zimmerman, 1986; Mitchell, Armstrong, Simpson, & Lentz, 1989), decreased risk of death or readmission to the ICU (Baggs et al., 1992; Baggs et al., 1999), more provider satisfaction, and improved nurse retention (Baggs et al., 1992; Baggs et al., 1997; Mitchell et al., 1989). On surgical services coordination of work responsibilities and better, more frequent interactions between surgeons and nurses was associated with better patient outcomes (Daley et al., 1997; Young et al., 1997). Lack of collaboration may be associated with poor outcomes. For example, poor communication between nurses and physicians in the ICU was associated with dangerous errors (Donchin et al., 1995).

Collaboration between nurses and physicians may also support improved bioethical decision making in health care. Nurses' closeness to and communications with patients (Luce, 1990) and their support for patient autonomy (Davis & Jameton, 1987; Ott & Nieswiadomy, 1991; Ouslander, Tymchuk, & Rahbar, 1989; Zorb & Stevens, 1990) make their inclusion in ethical decision making important. Nurses tend to use a style of decision making that identifies the importance of personal relationships, while physicians are more concerned with rights and rules (Haddad, 1991). The combination of perspectives may enrich ethical decision making. In addition, Pike (1991) proposed collaboration as a way to overcome the moral distress that arises when providers encounter institutional barriers to carrying out what they see as the morally appropriate action.

Critical care nurses have identified collaboration with physicians as their most important professional issue (Hartwell & Lavandero, 1991). For both ICU nurses and residents collaboration is significantly associated with satisfaction with the decision-making process (Baggs & Ryan, 1990; Baggs & Schmitt, 1997; Baggs et al., 1992; Baggs et al., 1997). The Joint Commission on Accreditation of Healthcare Organizations has supported development of more collaborative care, with an article proposing methods for clinicians to move their practice in that direction (Batalden et al., 1998).

Some authors have developed new care delivery models to promote collaboration (King, Lee, & Henneman, 1993). One example is a special care unit in Cleveland that was developed for treatment of the chronically critically ill (Daly, Phelps, & Rudy, 1991; Daly, Rudy, Thompson, & Happ, 1991). In this unit a nursing case management model using protocols for common patient problems, such as ventilator weaning, has decreased costs using a less hierarchical, more collaborative interdisciplinary approach to care. Care is organized around the patient, not around a physician team leader. Another example was a unit developed in Boston (Alpert et al., 1992), which unfortunately no longer exists. The unit was focused on provision of intensive nursing care, with participation by nurses and physicians committed to collaborative practice.

A common intensive care unit activity that can promote collaboration but that is no longer practiced in many hospital units is interdisciplinary rounds (Briones, Thompson, & Daly, 1996; Bryan-Brown & Dracup, 1998). This provides a time for members of different disciplines to present their perspective and goals about each patient and for the team to plan activities. On units without a physician consistently present and in settings outside of the hospital, it may take some creative thought to develop an equivalent activity, but it is likely to be worth the effort.

Another idea that has been proposed to improve physician-nurse collaboration is to begin with nursing and medical students to implement elements into the curriculum so that they learn together from the beginning (Kenneth, 1969; Mason & Parascandola, 1972; Shumaker & Goss, 1980; Yeaworth & Mims, 1973). Model programs have been described (Anvaripour, Jacobson, Schewiger, & Weissman, 1991; Barnum, 1990; Cloonan, Davis, & Burnett, 1999; Vanderberg & Springle, 1998). Such programs could assist the two professions to have a better idea of each other's roles, supporting cooperation and promoting respect for assertion of the individual

professional perspective in patient care situations. Understanding the other's role and "lived experience" has been identified as central to building collaborative relationships (Baker & Diekelmann, 1994). Learning together is one way for such understanding to develop.

There is support both conceptually and empirically for collaboration in practice between nurses and physicians, and there are some examples of it. Some writers believe that collaboration is already occurring in practice, particularly in ICUs (Ames & Perrin, 1980), but there is still work to be done in understanding and promoting collaboration in practice. On the whole, it continues to be true that collaboration is not the usual mode of practice.

REFERENCES

Abramson, J.S., & Mizrahi, T. (1996). When social workers and physicians collaborate: Positive and negative interdisciplinary experience. *Social Work, 41*, 270-281.

Aiken, L.H., Sochalski, J., & Lake, E.T. (1997). Studying outcomes of organizational change in health services. *Medical Care, 35*(11, suppl), NS6-NS18.

Alpert, H.B., Goldman, L.D., Kilroy, C.M., & Pike, A.W. (1992). 7 Gryzmish: Toward an understanding of collaboration. *Nursing Clinics of North America, 27*(1), 47-59.

American Heritage Dictionary. (1992). Boston: Houghton Mifflin.

Ames, A., & Perrin, J.M. (1980). Collaborative practice: The joining of two professions. *Journal of the Tennessee Medical Association, 73*, 557-560.

Anvaripour, P.L., Jacobson, L., Schweiger, J., & Weissman, G.K. (1991). Physician-nurse collegiality in the medical school curriculum. *Mount Sinai Journal of Medicine, 58*(1), 91-94.

Aroskar, M.A. (1998). Ethical working relationships in patient care: Challenges and possibilities. *Nursing Clinics of North America, 33*, 313-324.

Baggs, J.G. (1998a). Nurse-physician collaboration: The challenge of collaboration. In A.L. Suchman, R.J. Botelho, & P. Hinton-Walker (Eds.), *Partnerships in healthcare: Transforming relational process.* Rochester, NY: University of Rochester Press.

Baggs, J.G. (1998b). Response to "A conceptual model of collaborative nurse-physician interactions: The management of traditional influences and personal tendencies." *Scholarly Inquiry for Nursing Practice: An International Journal, 12*, 343-346.

Baggs, J.G., & Ryan, S.A. (1990). Intensive care unit nurse-physician collaboration and nurse satisfaction. *Nursing Economic$, 8*, 386-392.

Baggs, J.G., Ryan, S.A., Phelps, C.E., Richeson, J.F., & Johnson, J.E. (1992). The association between interdisciplinary collaboration and patient outcomes in medical intensive care. *Heart and Lung, 21*, 18-24.

Baggs, J.G., & Schmitt, M.H. (1988). Collaboration between nurses and physicians. *Image: The Journal of Nursing Scholarship, 20*, 145-149.

Baggs, J.G., & Schmitt, M.H. (1997). Nurses' and resident physicians' perceptions of the process of collaboration in an MICU. *Research in Nursing & Health, 20*, 71-80.

Baggs, J.G., Schmitt, M.H., Mushlin, A.I., Eldredge, D.H., Oakes, D., & Hutson, A.D. (1997). Nurse-physician collaboration and satisfaction with the decision-making process in three critical care units. *American Journal of Critical Care, 6*, 393-399.

Baggs, J.G., Schmitt, M.H., Mushlin, A.I., Mitchell, P.H., Eldredge, D.H., Oakes, D., & Hutson, A.D. (1999). The association between nurse-physician collaboration and patient outcomes in three intensive care units. *Critical Care Medicine, 27*, 1992-1998.

Baker, C., & Diekelmann, N. (1994). Connecting conversations of caring: Recalling the narrative to clinical practice. *Nursing Outlook, 42*, 65-70.

Barnum, B.J. (1990). At New York University, the Division of Nursing develops a model for nursing and medical school collaboration. *Nursing & Health Care, 11*(2), 89-90.

Batalden, P.B., Cronenwett, L.R., Brown, L.L., Moffatt, C., & Serrell, N.P. (1998). Collaboration in improving care for patients. *Journal on Quality Improvement, 24*, 609-618.

Benner, P., Hooper-Kyriakidis, P., & Stannard, D. (1999). *Clinical wisdom and interventions in critical care.* Philadelphia: Saunders.

Briones, J., Thompson, K.S., & Daly, B.J. (1996). Case management of patients with chronic critical illness. *Critical Care Nurse, 16*(6), 59-66.

Brown, T. (1982). An historical view of health care teams. In G.J. Agich (Ed.), *Responsibility in health care* (pp. 3-21). Dordrecht, Holland: D. Reidel Publishing Co.

Bryan-Brown, C.W., & Dracup, K. (1998). The patient is turned every 2 hours. *American Journal of Critical Care, 7*, 165-167.

Campbell-Heider, N., & Pollock, D. (1987). Barriers to physician-nurse collegiality. *Social Science and Medicine, 25*, 421-425.

Cape, L.S. (1986). Collaborative practice models and structures. In D.A. England (Ed.), *Collaboration in nursing* (pp. 13-26). Rockville, MD: Aspen.

Christensen, C., & Larson, J.R. (1993). Collaborative medical decision making. *Medical Decision Making, 13*, 339-345.

Clemmer, T.P., Spuhler, V.J., Berwick, D.M., & Nolan, T.W. (1998). Cooperation: The foundation of improvement. *Annals of Internal Medicine, 128*, 1004-1009.

Cloonan, P.A., Davis, F.D., & Burnett, C.B. (1999). Interdisciplinary education in clinical ethics: A work in progress. *Holistic Nursing Practice, 13*(2), 12-19.

Corley, M.C. (1998). Ethical dimensions of nurse-physician relations in critical care. *Nursing Clinics of North America, 33*, 325-337.

Corser, W.D. (1998). A conceptual model of collaborative nurse-physician interactions: The management of traditional influences and personal tendencies. *Scholarly Inquiry for Nursing Practice: An International Journal, 12*, 325-341.

Daley, J., Forbes, M.G., Young, G.J., Charns, M.P., Gibbs, J.O., Hur, K., Henderson, W., & Khuri, S.F. (1997). Validating risk-adjusted surgical outcomes: Site visit assessment of process and structure. *Journal of the American College of Surgeons, 185*, 341-351.

Daly, B.J., Phelps, C., & Rudy, E.B. (1991). A nurse-managed special care unit. *Journal of Nursing Administration, 21*(7/8), 31-38.

Daly, B.J., Rudy, E.B., Thompson, K.S., & Happ, M.B. (1991). Development of a special care unit for chronically critically ill patients. *Heart and Lung, 20*, 45-51.

Davies, L., & Hudson, L.D. (1999). Why don't physicians use ethics consultation? *The Journal of Clinical Ethics, 10*, 116-125.

Davis, A.J., & Jameton, A. (1987). Nursing and medical student attitudes toward nursing disclosure of information to patients: A pilot study. *Journal of Advanced Nursing, 12*, 691-698.

Devereux, P.M. (1981a). Essential elements of nurse-physician collaboration. *Journal of Nursing Administration, 11*(May), 19-23.

Devereux, P.M. (1981b). Does joint practice work? *Journal of Nursing Administration, 11*(June), 39-43.

Devereux, P.M. (1981c). Nurse/physician collaboration: Nursing practice considerations. *Journal of Nursing Administration, 11*(Sept.), 37-39.

Donchin, Y., Gopher, D., Olin, M., Badihi, Y., Biesky, M., Sprung, C.L., Pizov, R., & Cotev, S. (1995). A look into the nature and causes of human errors in the intensive care unit. *Critical Care Medicine, 23*, 294-300.

Eliasson, A.H., Howard, R.S., Torrington, K.G., Dillard, T.A., & Phillips, Y.Y. (1997). Do-not-resuscitate decisions in the medical ICU. *Chest, 111*, 1106-1111.

England, D.A. (1986). *Collaboration in nursing.* Rockville, MD: Aspen.

Erlen, J.A., & Frost, B. (1991). Nurses' perceptions of powerlessness in influencing ethical decisions. *Western Journal of Nursing Research, 13*, 397-407.

Evans, S.A., & Carlson, R. (1992). Nurse/physician collaboration: Solving the nursing shortage crisis. *American Journal of Critical Care, 1*(1), 25-32.

Fagin, C.M. (1992). Collaboration between nurses and physicians: No longer a choice. *Academic Medicine, 67*, 295-303.

Farber, N.J., Weiner, J.L., Boyer, E.G., Green, W.P., Diamond, M.P., & Copare, I.M. (1985). Cardiopulmonary resuscitation values and decisions. *Medical Care, 23*, 1391-1398.

Feiger, S.M., & Schmitt, M.H. (1979). Collegiality in interdisciplinary health teams. *Social Science and Medicine, 13A*, 217-229.

Frampton, M.W., & Mayewski, R.J. (1987). Physicians' and nurses' attitudes toward withholding treatment in a community hospital. *Journal of General Internal Medicine, 2*, 394-399.

Gardner, D.B., & Cary, A. (1999). Collaboration, conflict, and power: Lessons for case managers. *Family Community Health, 22*(3), 64-77.

Gramelspacher, G.P., Howell, J.D., & Young, M.J. (1986). Perceptions of ethical problems by nurses and doctors. *Archives of Internal Medicine, 146*, 577-578.

Greenfield, L.J. (1999). Doctors and nurses: A troubled partnership. *Annals of Surgery, 230*, 279-288.

Grumbach, K., & Coffman, J. (1998). Physicians and nonphysician clinicians: Complements or competitors? *Journal of the American Medical Association, 280*, 825-826.

Haddad, A.M. (1991). The nurse/physician relationship and ethical decision making. *Association of Operating Room Nurses Journal, 53*, 151-156.

Hartwell, J.L., & Lavandero, R. (1991). What's important to critical care nurses? *Focus on Critical Care, 18*, 364-371.

Hansen, H., Biros, M.H., Delaney, N.M., & Schug, V.L. (1999). *Academic Emergency Medicine, 6*, 271-279.

Harvey, M.A., Fujii, T., & Carlson, R.W. (2000). Building bedside collaborative practice. In A. Grenvik, S.M. Ayres, P.R. Holbrook, & W.C. Shoemaker (Eds.), *Textbook of critical care* (4th ed., pp. 2015-2023). Philadelphia: Saunders.

Henneman, E.A. (1995a). Collaboration: A concept analysis. *Journal of Advanced Nursing, 21,* 103-109.

Henneman, E.A. (1995b). Nurse-physician collaboration: A poststructuralist view. *Journal of Advanced Nursing, 22,* 359-363.

Holly, C. (1989). Critical care nurses' participation in ethical decision making. *Journal of the New York State Nurses Association, 20*(4), 9-12.

Katzman, E.M. (1989). Nurses' and physicians' perceptions of nursing authority. *Journal of Professional Nursing, 5,* 208-214.

Keenan, G.M., Cooke, R., & Hillis, S.L. (1998). Norms and nurse management of conflicts: Keys to understanding nurse-physician collaboration. *Research in Nursing & Health, 21,* 59-72.

Kenneth, H.Y. (1969). Medical and nursing students learn together. *Nursing Outlook, 17,* 46-49.

King, M.L., Lee, J.L., & Henneman, E. (1993). A collaborative practice model for critical care. *American Journal of Critical Care, 2,* 444-449.

Knaus, W.A., Draper, E.A., Wagner, D.P., & Zimmerman, J.E. (1986). An evaluation of outcome from intensive care in major medical centers. *Annals of Internal Medicine, 104,* 410-418.

Koerner, B., & Armstrong, D. (1984). Collaborative practice cuts cost of patient care: Study. *Hospitals, 58*(10), 52-54.

Koerner, B.L., Cohen, J.R., & Armstrong, D.M. (1985). Collaborative practice and patient satisfaction. *Evaluation and the Health Professions, 8,* 299-321.

Lamb, G.S., & Napodano, R.J. (1984). Physician-nurse practitioner interaction patterns in primary care practices. *American Journal of Public Health, 74,* 26-29.

Larson, E. (1999). The impact of physician-nurse interaction on patient care. *Holistic Nursing Practice, 13*(2), 38-46.

Levine, M.E. (1989). The ethics of nursing rhetoric. *Image: Journal of Nursing Scholarship, 21,* 4-6.

Luce, J.M. (1990). Ethical principles in critical care. *Journal of the American Medical Association, 263,* 696-700.

Mason, E., & Parascandola, J. (1972). Preparing tomorrow's health care team. *Nursing Outlook, 20,* 728-731.

McLain, B.R. (1988a). Collaborative practice: A critical theory perspective. *Research in Nursing & Health, 11,* 391-398.

McLain, B.R. (1988b). Collaborative practice: The nurse practitioner's role in its success or failure. *Nurse Practitioner, 13*(5), 31-38.

McMahan, E.M., Hoffman, K., & McGee, G.W. (1994). Physician-nurse relationships in clinical settings: A review and critique of the literature, 1966-1992. *Medical Care Review, 51,* 83-112.

Miccolo, M.A., & Spanier, A.H. (1993). Making collaborative practice work. *Critical Care Clinics, 9,* 443-453.

Michelson, E.L. (1988). The challenge of nurse-physician collaborative practices: Improved patient care provision and outcomes. *Heart and Lung, 17,* 390-391.

Mitchell, P.H., Armstrong, S., Simpson, T.F., & Lentz, M. (1989). AACN demonstration project. *Heart and Lung, 18,* 219-237.

National Joint Practice Commission. (1981). *Guidelines for establishing joint or collaborative practice in hospitals.* Chicago: Author.

Omery, A., Henneman, E., Billet, B., Luna-Raines, M., & Brown-Saltzman, K. (1995). Ethical issues in hospital-based nursing practice. *Journal of Cardiovascular Nursing, 9,* 43-53.

Ott, B.B., & Nieswiadomy, R.M. (1991). Support of patient autonomy in the do not resuscitate decision. *Heart and Lung, 20,* 66-72.

Ouslander, J.G., Tymchuk, A.J., & Rahbar, B. (1989). Health care decisions among elderly long-term care residents and their potential proxies. *Archives of Internal Medicine, 149,* 1367-1372.

Pike, A.W. (1991). Moral outrage and moral discourse in nurse-physician collaboration. *Journal of Professional Nursing, 7,* 351-363.

Prescott, P.A. (1989). Shortage of professional nursing practice: A reframing of the shortage problem. *Heart and Lung, 18,* 436-443.

Prescott, P.A., & Bowen, S.A. (1985). Physician-nurse relationships. *Annals of Internal Medicine, 103,* 127-133.

Prescott, P.A., Dennis, K.E., & Jacox, A.K. (1987). Clinical decision making of staff nurses. *Image: The Journal of Nursing Scholarship, 19,* 56-62.

Prescott, P.A., Phillips, C.Y., Ryan, J.W., & Thompson, K.O. (1991). Changing how nurses spend their time. *Image: The Journal of Nursing Scholarship, 23,* 23-28.

Rubenstein, L.Z., Josephson, K.R., Wieland, G.D., English, P.A., Sayre, J.A., & Kane, R.L. (1984). Effectiveness of a geriatric evaluation unit. *New England Journal of Medicine, 311,* 1664-1670.

Schmitt, M.H., Watson, N.M., Feiger, S.H., & Williams, T.F. (1981). Conceptualizing and measuring outcomes of interdisciplinary team care for a group of long-term, chronically ill, institutionalized patients. In J.E. Bachman (Ed.), *Interdisciplinary health care: Proceedings of the third annual conference on interdisciplinary team care* (pp. 169-181). Kalamazoo, MI: Center for Human Services Western Michigan University.

Shumaker, D., & Goss, V. (1980). Toward collaboration: One small step. *Nursing and Health Care, 1*(11), 183-185.

Sorrells-Jones, J., & Weaver, D. (1999). Knowledge workers and knowledge-intense organizations: Implications for preparing healthcare professionals. *Journal of Nursing Administration, 29*(10), 14-21.

Steel, J.E. (1986). *Issues in collaborative practice.* Orlando: Grune & Stratton, Inc.

Stein, L.I. (1967). The doctor-nurse game. *Archives of General Psychiatry, 16,* 638-642.

Stein, L.I., Watts, D.T., & Howell, T. (1990). The doctor-nurse game revisited. *New England Journal of Medicine, 322,* 546-549.

Stichler, J.F. (1995). Professional interdependence: The art of collaboration. *Advanced Practice Nursing Quarterly, 1,* 53-61.

Styles, M.M. (1984). Reflections on collaboration and unification. *Image: The Journal of Nursing Scholarship, 16,* 21-23.

Sullivan, T.J. (Ed.). (1998). *Collaboration: A health care imperative.* New York: McGraw-Hill.

Temkin-Greener, H. (1983). Interprofessional perspectives on teamwork in health care: A case study. *Milbank Memorial Fund Quarterly, 61,* 641-658.

Thomas, K. (1976). Conflict and conflict management. In M.D. Dunnette (Ed.), *Handbook of industrial and organizational psychology* (pp. 889-935). Chicago: Rand McNally College Publishing Company.

Vanderberg, A., & Springle, R. (1998). Nurse/physician collaboration—The "Buddy Program." *Nursing Management, 29*(7), 65.

Walter, S.D., Cook, D.J., Guyatt, G.H., Spanier, A., Jaeschke, R., Todd, T.R.J., & Streiner, D.L. (1998). Confidence in life-support decisions in the intensive care unit. *Critical Care Medicine, 26,* 44-49.

Webster, G.C., Mazer, C.D., Potvin, C.A., Fisher, A., & Byrick, R.J. (1991). Evaluation of a "do not resuscitate" policy in intensive care. *Canadian Journal of Anaesthesia, 38,* 553-563.

Weiss, S.J., & Davis, H.P. (1985). Validity and reliability of the collaborative practice scales. *Nursing Research, 34,* 299-305.

Wesson, A.F. (1966). Hospital ideology and communication between ward personnel. In R. Scott & E. Volkhart (Eds.), *Medical care* (pp. 458-475). New York: Wiley.

Wolff, M.L., Smolen, S., & Ferrara, L. (1985). Treatment decisions in a skilled-nursing facility. *Journal of the American Geriatrics Society, 33,* 440-445.

Yeaworth, R., & Mims, F. (1973). Interdisciplinary education as an influence system. *Nursing Outlook, 21,* 1973.

Young, G.J., Charns, M.P., Daley, J., Forbes, M.G., Henderson, W., & Khuri, S.F. (1997). Best practices for managing surgical services: The role of coordination. *Health Care Management Review, 22,* 72-81.

Zorb, S.L., & Stevens, J.B. (1990). Contemporary bioethical issues in critical care. *Critical Care Nursing Clinics of North America, 2,* 515-520.

Zwarenstein, M., Bryant, W., Bailie, R., & Sibthorpe, B. (1999). Interventions to promote collaboration between nurses and doctors. *The Cochrane Database of Systematic Reviews, 2.*

Feminism and Nursing

Reclaiming Nightingale's Vision

PEGGY L. CHINN

Passion, intellect, moral activity—these three have never been satisfied in woman. In this cold and oppressive conventional atmosphere, they cannot be satisfied. To say more on this subject would be to enter into the whole history of society, of the present state of civilization. — Florence Nightingale (1979, p. 29)

These words were written by Florence Nightingale in 1852, just after she pursued her nursing training at Kaiserswerth. They appear in an essay titled "Cassandra." For years in her young adulthood, Nightingale yearned to pursue a social calling to serve people, but as a Victorian woman her options were severely restricted. Her essay "Cassandra" is an outcry against the plight of Victorian women like herself and reflects her strong conviction that women had many lost talents and abilities that could be developed.

Nightingale's quote illustrates several aspects of feminism that are equally important today. Even though much has changed for women in many parts of the world since Nightingale's time, "passion, intellect, and moral activity" are three key aspects of women's experience that are still being addressed by feminists today. Her observation that these three "have never been satisfied in woman" is a fundamental premise of feminist activism. Today, some women in the world can exercise these capacities, but many more remain constrained by the same kinds of social forces that existed in Nightingale's day. Feminist activists seek to right the wrongs and injustices that persist against women, not only through equal opportunity, but also through seeking to understand women's experience in the world and to break down the barriers to valuing that experience. Finally, Nightingale's observation that "to say more on this subject would be to enter into the whole history of society, of the present state of civilization" summarizes precisely what feminist authors have set

about to accomplish in the past several decades. In other words, feminism is not the singular, polemical, or fanatical fad that is portrayed in the media. Rather, feminism encompasses many perspectives that have entered the whole history of society and the present state of civilization (Young, 1997).

Feminist thought and action is grounded in women's experience and take stances that assume that women's experience is real and valuable. Feminist thought and action is inherently political. It challenges the prevailing attitudes that tend to devalue and discount women. The actions and writings that come from feminist thinking are motivated by a desire to benefit women, with the underlying conviction that if it is not good for women, it is not good. Because what affects women affects the world, and what affects the world affects women, feminist concerns are as broad as the world, even the universe.

Nursing and feminism, regardless of definitions of either concept, are inescapably connected because of the presence of women. Not only are most nurses women, but nursing's social role—to care for the sick—is one that historically has been assigned to women worldwide. Therefore many of the actions and concerns that nurses assume in their day-to-day work are those that are associated with being female in gender. The *American Heritage Dictionary* gives the following as one of the definitions of "nurse": "One that serves as a nurturing or fostering influence or means" (American Heritage Talking Dictionary, 1994). Generally, those who nurture are women,

441

and when men provide formal nurturing roles in society, they usually enter social realms where women predominate. What are usually not associated with nurturing roles are precisely the three concerns that Nightingale addresses: passion, intellect, and moral activity. Caring for others and fostering their growth is generally viewed as ordinary—something that anyone can do—and certainly not requiring intellectual interest or ability. Furthermore, caring for others is generally prescribed to women by the dominant culture; therefore, exercising independent moral activity is not presumed to be required (Reverby, 1987). While the world has changed remarkably for women in the Western world since Nightingale's time, women remain tied to their socially accepted female roles, and the roles associated with women are devalued. Even more striking is the fact that worldwide, not much has changed for women since the time of Nightingale.

I will explore feminist perspectives on Nightingale's three concerns—passion, intellect, and moral activity—and will show how these perspectives can assist nurses to move toward changes that are consistent with what is good for nurses, for women, and for all people. These concerns are interrelated. They have distinct aspects, but when you turn to the suggested readings listed at the end of this chapter, you will find that they weave together to form a whole, a global concern.

PASSION

> When shall we see a life full of steady enthusiasm, walking straight to its aim, flying home, as that bird is now, against the wind—with . . . calmness and . . . confidence? [Nightingale, 1979, p. 36]

For Nightingale, the idea of passion included powerful emotion, even sexual desire—all of which were severely restricted for women in her time. Her primary interest, however, was what she termed "high sympathies," which in her view need to be fed and nurtured in order to serve society well. She said,

> If, together, man and woman approach any of the high questions of social, political, or religious life, they are said (and justly—under our present disqualifications) to be going "too far." That such things can be! [Nightingale, 1979, p. 28]

Activists and theorists of the feminist movement of the second half of the 20th century began to recognize the oppressive dynamic of being ridiculed with accusations of going too far (Morgan, 1968), when in fact they could see clearly that women had not gone far enough. And so women began, with an intensity and seriousness never

before seen in human history, to approach the high questions of social, political, and religious life.

In speaking of passion, Nightingale (1979) stated that "poetry and imagination begin life" (p. 30). Nightingale believed that women begin life with vivid and rich imaginations and that their dreams and imaginations hold a key to developing the intellect and moral activity that is required for meaningful social action. She speculated, however, that women learn early to subdue their imaginations because it is so dangerous. Young girls and women receive messages early that society does not want, and that she cannot want, to fulfill her imaginations and dreams.

Nightingale identified the daily circumstances of women's lives that restrict them from developing the seeds of social action that lie dormant in their imagination: lack of time, time consumed by service to the home, time constantly interrupted. Speaking of the constant demands made on women's time by anyone and everyone, Nightingale stated,

> Yet time is the most valuable of all things. If they had come every morning and afternoon and robbed us of half-a-crown we should have had redress from the police. But it is laid down, that our time is of no value. [p. 35]

Indeed, when the feminist movement of the second half of the 20th century began, women realized that they must gain control over their own time in order to begin to change social and political structures that held control over their lives. They began to meet together in small groups to form the art and imagination that is necessary for social activism. The method of feminism—consciousness-raising—was developed in small group processes. In sharing stories of their lives, women began to discover patterns in their lives and among their lives. They began to see individual circumstances of a woman's life in the context of the social and political patterns that sustain women's oppression. And thus was born the idea that the personal is political.

The insight that "the personal is political" represents recognition of the interrelatedness of all things. It is an insight that is expressed in many forms, calling for the joining together of what has been torn apart by centuries of patriarchal dominance. Passion, which is presumed to reside in the personal realm, is actually in all aspects of life. It is the necessary fire that gives energy to sustain action in the public world when all seems futile. It is through passion that the life of thought and the life of action can be brought together.

The enterprise of bringing together that which has been torn apart is a cultural and political enterprise. Culture teaches and reinforces the values that are thought by its members to be good and right. Politics is the ability to enact those values in a social arena. Take, for example, the cultural norm that sustains different moral codes for the personal life from those of the public life. Undertaking to bring together a single moral code for all of life is a project of huge proportions, requiring enormous energy, vivid imagination, and commitment to action.

In nursing, the splits are many: mind-body splits, practice-theory splits, real-ideal splits, public-private splits, work-home splits. Feminist ideas and historical models provide a framework from which to begin to understand the origins of these splits, to understand how they are sustained, and to begin to form action to bring them together into one (Chinn, 1989).

INTELLECT

> What wonder if, wearied out, sick at heart with hope deferred, the springs of will broken, not seeing clearly *where* her duty lies, she abandons intellect as a vocation and takes it only, as we use the moon, by glimpses through her tight-closed window-shutters? [Nightingale, 1979, p. 37]

Nightingale reasoned that the sphere in which women were required to remain—the private sphere of home and family—was much too narrow a field for development of the mind. Speaking of the systematic ways in which women's lives and interests were curtailed, she said: "This system dooms some minds to incurable infancy, others to silent misery" (p. 37).

Nightingale had a strong conviction that women have the mental abilities to achieve whatever they wish to achieve: compose music, solve scientific problems, create social projects of great importance. But the material limitations on women's lives robbed them not only of the time to devote to such activities but also of the development of the mental and physical skills required to achieve socially meaningful actions. Out of this conviction came her resolve and action to establish nursing as a profession, whereby women could develop the intellectual abilities to contribute meaningful service to society.

Over a century later, as feminist thought and action developed, nursing began to be seen in different contexts. Feminists began to recognize the hazards of sustained sex-segregation in occupations and ways in which this social and cultural pattern sustained women's oppression (Greenleaf, 1980). Feminists also challenged the unquestioning acceptance by women of their nurturing and caring roles in society, and often saw nurses as sustaining this unquestioning acceptance (Chinn & Wheeler, 1985).

However, out of a commitment to value women and women's experience, feminist insights also began to give new meaning to the nature of nurturing and caring and to recognize the essential value of the attitudes, skills, and knowledge that are required to be in relation with others in a caring and nurturing way (Gilligan, 1982; Larrabee, 1993; Noddings, 1984, 1999).

Nursing as a profession did accomplish what Nightingale envisioned: it provided an avenue for nurses to leave the relatively restricted environment of home and family and to enter a broader world of social service. It has provided, worldwide, an avenue for women's education. For many women, becoming a nurse has been the only way to obtain an education, to develop the intellect. But has this been enough? What has been the nature of this education and has it served women well?

Jo Ann Ashley, feminist nurse historian, studied the history of nursing education in hospitals. She concluded that not only were nurses not served well by apprenticeship education but also that all nurses continue to suffer the remnants of attitudes and beliefs that continue to influence the content and the processes of nursing education and of nursing (Ashley, 1976, 1980).

Consider, for example, the persistent language that sustains nursing's subservience to medicine. The phrase "physician's orders," which nurses are still legally responsible to follow, has not been changed or replaced since the earliest days of nursing as a profession. There have been alternatives suggested (e.g., physician prescription, medical treatments). The alternatives suggest the nature of physician work and relationship with the patient compared to the implications of the physician-nurse relationship in the phrase "physician orders." But nurses are still being educated, in many parts of the world, in ways that differ little from the earliest days of nursing to follow physician orders and, more importantly, not to question the terminology, practices, or orders themselves.

MORAL ACTIVITY

> Women dream of a great sphere of steady, not sketchy benevolence, of moral activity, for which they would fain [sic] be trained and fitted, instead of working in the dark, neither knowing nor registering whither their steps lead, whether farther from or nearer to the aim. [Nightingale, 1979, p. 38]

Nightingale has been criticized for her insistence on the moral character requirements that she imposed on the earliest nurses and the heritage of emphasis on character that the profession inherited from her early views. Many of these criticisms are well founded from the perspective of more recent contexts; moral and ethical necessities change over time. However, it is now possible to also consider sustained values in her views on moral activity. Her essential concern in the essay "Cassandra" was that women's perspectives are not valued. She believed that when women's values are not realized, society suffers. She decried the waste of human resources when women are denied the circumstances in which they can develop and know their own moral sense of what is good and what is right.

For Nightingale, two circumstances are required to develop moral activity: time for learning and reflection (bringing together passion and intellect) and sustained experience in applying or acting on what is reflected upon, or experience. She states,

> Women . . . long for experience, not patch-work experience, but experience followed up and systematized, to enable them to know what they are about and *where* they are "casting their bread" and whether it is "*bread*" or a stone. [Nightingale, 1979, p. 39]

She speculated how any profession or occupation could be developed at odd times, which is what women are generally required to do in developing anything. She wonders how an art can be developed if it is only viewed as an amusement, which is how women's arts are typically viewed. She likened the situation of women's sketchy opportunities for development of the intellect and moral activity to starvation and saw it as serious a situation as if we were physically starved of food for the body. She viewed women's unquestioning acceptance of prescribed social roles as a moral problem:

> With what labour women have toiled to break down all individual and independent life, in order to fit themselves for this social and domestic existence, thinking it right! And when they have killed themselves to do it, they have awakened (too late) to think it wrong. [Nightingale, 1979, p. 42]

Nightingale's criticism about women's unquestioning acceptance of their social and domestic existence in her day is a serious issue that deserves consideration today. Consider how her words would read if revised to apply to nursing today:

> With what labor nurses have toiled to break down all individual and independent life, in order to fit themselves for this social and professional existence, thinking it right! And when they have killed themselves to do it, they have awakened (too late) to think it wrong.

Today, nurses do have models and frameworks with which to begin to judge what is right and what is wrong in their nursing practice (Fry, 1992). However, much of what is practiced in nursing is not questioned, and if it is questioned, it feels much too dangerous to act on the insight. So now we turn to the question, What is a nurse to do?

FEMINIST PERSPECTIVES ON BEING, KNOWING, AND DOING

> Nothing can well be imagined more painful than the present position of woman, unless, on the one hand, she renounces all outward activity and keeps herself within the magic sphere, the bubble of her dreams; or, on the other, surrendering all aspiration, she gives herself to her real life, soul and body. For those to whom it is possible, the latter is best; for out of activity may come thought, out of mere aspiration can come nothing. [Nightingale, 1979, p. 50]

Today, the choice of action does not require women to also surrender all aspiration. A multitude of possibilities for action have emerged out of the dreams and imaginations of feminist activists and theorists of the past few decades. In fact, the disjunction between thought and action has been directly opposed by feminists, and healing that disjunction is a major enterprise of feminist activists and theorists. Feminist activists in the second half of this century struggled with the choice of whether to develop theory or whether to take social and political action. Not everyone did both, but the prevailing practice that emerged was to be sure that both theory (thoughtful reflection) and action always characterize feminist enterprises (Redstockings, 1975).

Table 58-1 summarizes definitions of feminism and the concerns—both in aspiration and in action—that feminism has developed in this century. The Suggested Readings at the end of this chapter provide classic and recent resources where you can find additional information on each of these concerns. The following sections describe the various definitions linked with Nightingale's ideas of passion, intellect, and moral activity and provide a sketch of ways in which women have actually claimed places in society to exercise these three.

Passion: Feminism as a Culture Grounded in Women's Experience

Feminist writers, scholars, and activists have indeed entered the whole history of society and the present state of civilization. They have developed extensive cultural resources from which to change women's experience and

TABLE 58-1   Definitions and Characteristics of Feminism

Definitions	Characteristics
A culture grounded in women's experience	• Reclaims women's heritage in history, religion, culture • Reclaims women's personal and social power • Reclaims women's wisdom • Celebrates women as healers, artists, creators, statespersons
A political stance to right injustices against women and the earth	• Acts on the premise that the personal is political • Connects gender socialization and women's roles with larger political issues, including restoring the earth's ecology • Critiques the institutionalization of patriarchal norms • Seeks an end to private and public violence • Seeks balance of power in economic and political terms
A discipline seeking to give voice to women's experience	• Critiques patriarchal norms, practices, and theories • Relates the diverse experiences of women to social, political, philosophic, and scientific interests • Explores the dynamics by which women are silenced and ways to end the silence and invisibility of women • Explores women's health and development • Revises criteria of worth for scholarship and for what counts as knowledge about women
An ethic of valuing women and women's experience	• Critiques "malestream" morality and ethics • Develops ethics of caring and relationship • Reunites as one the public/private ethic • Redefines meanings of responsibility, truth, right, justice, good, beauty

from which to change the patriarchal tendencies of the dominant culture. Consistent with other social movements, a major concern has been to reclaim women's heritage in history, religion, the arts, and the emergence of civilization. Feminists have been persistent in asking, "Where were the women, and what were they doing?" in every period of known human history. Out of this question has come new appreciation of women as healers, artists, statespersons, creators, and inventors.

From knowledge of women's heritage, women have reclaimed women's personal power to create, to shape the values of the culture, to bring women's wisdom to bear on the higher questions of society.

Passion: Feminism as a Political Stance to Right Injustices

No other perspective has remained so persistent and broad-based in its concern for righting injustices. While women's well-being is a central focus, feminist insights link the rights and well-being of women with children, all people (particularly other oppressed groups), and the earth. Women's historical and current situation in the family and society are linked with such far-reaching issues as economics, agricultural, industrial production,

war and other forms of social violence, ecological health, and prevailing patterns of political violence. Feminist writers have shown how women's roles in the family and society are sustained by the larger political patterns and, in turn, sustain the nature of local, national, and global political patterns.

Feminist examination of political issues and creation of new theories of politics have given rise to new meanings for such political concepts as equality, justice, rights, peace, and diversity. For example, rather than merely accepting the prevailing notion that "equality" means "equal to white middle-class males," feminists seek carefully to construct meanings, criteria, and standards for "equality" that examines what is "good" for all. Out of these insights and committed to bringing together the personal and the political, feminist activists have taken significant local, regional, national, and international stands.

Nurses and nursing have particularly benefited from feminist political activism that demanded equitable pay for women's work. For example, the landmark case of nurses in Denver who fought to be paid more than tree trimmers established the idea that work should be paid in accord with its educational and skill requirements, not in accord with the gender of the person who typically performs it.

Intellect: Feminism as a Discipline Seeking to Give Voice to Women's Experience

Feminism has developed as a discipline that seeks to give voice and understanding to women's experience. One focus is the plight of women in the patriarchy and the search to find ways for women to change their existence in the patriarchy, as well as ways to change the patriarchy or to create a different world order based on women's aspirations. Another aspect of feminism as a discipline is consideration of the biology-culture debate, addressing questions concerning the extent to which women's experience is shaped by biology and to what extent it is shaped by culture or experience.

Women's health and development is a large area of concern for feminist scholars. Feminists pose questions such as how women's health and development, particularly mental health and development, have been defined, distorted, created, or shaped by the patriarchy. Redefining what health is and what healthy development is for women is a major feminist enterprise. Redefinition does not occur in an ivory tower vacuum; rather, it happens in conjunction with experience, with practice, with action. An example of the redefinition of women's health and development is the work of the Boston Women's Health Book Collective, producers of many books for women about women's health.

Another important area of study for feminist scholars has been discovery of the ways in which women have been silenced, their work rendered invisible in society, and exploring ways to change women's experience so that they know what it is to be valued, to be heard, to be strong and courageous, to act in the world. Related to explorations of women's silence has been work that is directed toward revising the criteria by which something is judged to be worthy of scholarly attention or worthy to count as knowledge. Feminist scholars have insisted that what concerns women cannot any longer be excluded as worthy of scholarly attention.

Moral Activity: Feminism as an Ethic of Valuing Women and Women's Experience

Feminist ethics is both thought and action directed toward values that sustain life, well-being, peace, nurturing, and growth for all. It includes critique of "malestream" morality and ethics, particularly the prevailing patriarchal morality that differentiates standards of ethical behavior at home and in the workplace. Feminist ethics seeks to reunite as one the public and private ethic.

Explorations of the relationship between gender and moral development has led to a better understanding and valuing of women's experience, as well as valuing of the perspectives that tend to emerge when women's values are taken into account. Women tend to value relationships and perceive personal and social obligations in terms of relationships and the well-being of significant others. This perspective redefines what it means to be responsible, to act justly, or to know what is good or right.

Much of the tension that nurses experience in their work lives involves difficult ethical dilemmas for which there are no resolutions if only the traditional patriarchal perspectives of justice and worth are considered. This is largely because patriarchal ethics does not take into account that which most concerns nurses—the quality of relationships and the meaning of caring. As nurses embrace more fully perspectives of feminist ethics, it will be possible to embrace ethical sensibilities that more closely align with the fundamental values of nursing.

SUMMARY

Contrary to popular perception, feminism is not an ideology. Feminism embraces many ways of viewing the world that bring women, women's experiences and perspectives, into focus. It embraces perspectives that value seeing clearly the diversity that exists among all women, not an attempt to define "woman." As you think about what I have presented and as you explore some of the suggested readings, ask yourself the following questions:

• In what ways do I value women? Who am I in relation to women?

• Do my views and values benefit women and in turn all people?

• What do I know about women and nurses in history? Are my assumptions about women and nurses in history accurate and well conceived?

• What do I know about the experience of women who are not like myself in economic status, culture, ethnic background, or belief?

REFERENCES

American Heritage Talking Dictionary (Windows, Mac). (1994). Cambridge, MA: Softkey International.

Ashley, J. (1976). *Hospitals, paternalism, and the role of the nurse.* New York: Teachers College Press.

Ashley, J. (1980). Power in structured misogyny: Implications for the politics of care. *Advances in Nursing Science, 2*(3), 3-22.

Chinn, P.L. (1989). Nursing patterns of knowing and feminist thought. *Nursing Outlook, 10*(2), 71-75.

Chinn, P.L., & Wheeler, C.E. (1985). Feminism and nursing. *Nursing Outlook, 33*(2), 74-77.

Fry, S.T. (1992). The role of caring in a theory of nursing ethics. In H.B. Holmes & L.M. Purdy (Eds.), *Feminist perspectives in medical ethics.* Bloomington, IN: Indiana University Press.

Gilligan, C. (1982). *In a different voice: Psychological theory and women's development.* Boston: Harvard University Press.

Greenleaf, N.P. (1980). Sex-segregated occupations: Relevance for nursing. *Advances in Nursing Science, 2*(3), 23-37.

Larrabee, M.J. (1993). *An ethic of care: Feminist and interdisciplinary perspectives.* New York: Routledge.

Morgan, R. (1968). *Going too far: The personal chronicle of a feminist.* New York: Vintage Books.

Nightingale, F. (1979). *Cassandra.* New York: The Feminist Press.

Noddings, N. (1984). *Caring: A feminine approach to ethics and moral education.* Berkeley, CA: University of California Press.

Noddings, N. (1999). Care, justice, and equity. In M.S. Katz, N. Noddings, & K.A. Strike (Eds.), *Justice and caring: The search for common ground in education* (pp. 7-20). New York: Teachers College Press.

Redstockings. (1975). *Feminist revolution: An abridged edition with additional writings.* New York: Random House.

Reverby, S.M. (1987). *Ordered to care: The dilemma of American nursing, 1850-1945.* Cambridge: Cambridge University Press.

Young, S. (1997). *Changing the wor(l)d: Discourse, politics, and the feminist movement.* New York: Routledge.

SUGGESTED READINGS

Achterberg, J. (1990). *Woman as healer.* Boston: Shambala.

Alcoff, L., & Potter, E. (Eds.). (1993). *Feminist epistemologies.* New York: Routledge.

Bunch, C. (1987). *Passionate politics: Feminist theory in action.* New York: St. Martin's Press.

Cheatham, A., & Powell, M.C. (1986). *This way daybreak comes: Women's values and the future.* Philadelphia: New Society Publishers.

Chinn, P.L. (1995). *Peace and power: Building communities for the future.* New York: NLN Press.

Daly, M., & Caputi, J. (1987). *Webster's first new intergalactic wickedary of the English language.* Boston: Beacon Press.

Edwalds, L., & Stocker, M. (Eds.). (1995). *The woman-centered economy: Ideals, reality, and the space in between.* Chicago: Third Side Press.

Freeman, J. (Ed.). (1995). *Women: A feminist perspective* (5th ed.). Mountain View, CA: Mayfield Publishing.

Frye, M. (1983). *The politics of reality: Essays in feminist theory.* Freedom, CA: The Crossing Press.

Hine, D.C. (1989). *Black women in white: Racial conflict and cooperation in the nursing profession: 1890-1950.* Bloomington, IN: Indiana University Press.

Holmes, H.B., & Purdy, L.M. (Eds.). (1992). *Feminist perspectives in medical ethics.* Bloomington, IN: Indiana University Press.

Hooks, B. (1990). *Yearning: Race, gender, and cultural politics.* Boston: South End Press.

Humm, M. (1995). *A dictionary of feminist theory.* Columbus, OH: Ohio State University Press.

Johnstone, M.-J. (1994). *Nursing and the injustices of the law.* Philadelphia: Harcourt Brace & Co.

MacKinnon, C.A. (1989). *Toward a feminist theory of the state.* Cambridge, MA: Harvard University Press.

Rich, A. (1986). *Of woman born: Motherhood as experience and institution* (10th Anniversary ed.). New York: W.W. Norton.

Roberts, J.I., & Group, T.M. (1995). *Feminism and nursing: An historical perspective on power, status, and political activism in the nursing profession.* Westport, CT: Praeger.

Spender, D. (1982). *Women of ideas and what men have done to them.* Boston: Routledge & Kegan Paul.

Stanley, L. (Ed.). (1990). *Feminist praxis: Research, theory and epistemology in feminist sociology.* New York: Routledge.

Tong, R. (1998). *Feminist thought: A more comprehensive introduction* (2nd ed.). Boulder, CO: Westview Press.

Tuana, N. (1989). *Feminism and science.* Bloomington, IN: Indiana University Press.

Entering Collegial Relationships

The Demise of Nurse as Victim

ADELE W. PIKE

Scholars of women's development have observed a uniqueness in women's ways of thinking, of knowing, of relating to others, and of being (Belenky, Clinchy, Goldberger, & Tarule, 1986; Gilligan, 1982; Miller, 1976). They refer to this uniqueness as "women's voice." Their metaphor of voice is borrowed here and applied to nurses. "Nurses' voice" thus refers to the unique perspectives and contributions that nurses bring to patient care. Disturbingly, this voice is often silent, and that silence is seriously demoralizing to nurses. For patients the consequences are more grievous because the silence denies them the integration of the nursing perspective into the care they receive.

The factors involved in silencing—in censoring—nurses affect the way nurses define their professional self-concept, often leading them to perceive themselves as helpless victims. Most of the factors are rooted in cultural and social mores that, despite being outdated and no longer applicable in present-day health care, are deeply etched in memory. Despite the persistence of their legend, the power of these traditions to silence nurses should be rendered invalid.

For this to occur, nurses must appreciate that they are presented with opportunities for choice: the choice to remain silent or to become essential colleagues in the health care team. This chapter presents an analysis of the factors that suppress nurses' voice and of the significance of the choice nurses make with regard to making their voices heard. In discussing the implications of this choice, critical incidents (Benner, 1984) depicting patients and families facing ethical dilemmas are used in order to contrast

The critical incidents published in this chapter initially appeared in Pike, A.W. (1991). Moral outrage and moral discourse in nurse-physician collaboration. *Journal of Professional Nursing, 7*, 351-363. Used with permission.

two divergent outcomes that result from the different ways in which nurses choose to exercise their voice.

SILENCING OF VOICE

Numerous forces affect nurses' voice. Many of these forces are external, such as the historical role of nurse as handmaiden, the hierarchical structure of health care organizations, the perceived authority and directives of physicians, hospital policy, and the threat of disciplinary or legal action. Alarmingly, the current restructuring of health care in this country imposes additional and powerful constraints to nurses' voice. Changes in health care financing and reimbursement have led to reductions in staff and consequent work speed-ups, leaving nurses little time for reflection and discourse. Additionally, health care "reform" has led to the closing of nursing units, displacements of nurses, and layoffs (Pike & Alpert, 1994). The real threat of job loss, combined with the turmoil that accompanies downsizing of health care systems and institutions, can quickly and insidiously lure articulate professionals into the perceived safety of being but a cog in a bureaucratic wheel.

Equally ominous and plentiful are the internal forces that constrain nurses' voice. Characteristics such as role confusion, lack of professional confidence, timidity, fear, insecurity, or sense of inferiority lead nurses to *choose* silence as often as external forces impose silence on them (Pike, 1991; Yarling & McElmurry, 1986).

These internal and external constraints inflict wounds on nurses' professional self-esteem. These wounds deepen and expand the innate capacity for self-doubt that nurses, like all individuals, have. Having been wounded, nurses experience great difficulty believing in their own capacity, ability, and right to contribute to patient care as vital and essential professionals. Their ambitions and aspirations are stifled. Their vision grows myopic, and they fail to recognize both their opportunities and their obligation for self-advancement. Such an inclination establishes a pattern in which nurses perceive themselves as inferior and unable to change their lot (Steele, 1990).

This poor professional self-concept sabotages any possibility of collaboration between nurses and other care providers because it identifies nurses as embattled victims and customarily marks physicians as their antagonists. Such a relationship urges an adversarial stance in which the victims place the onus of responsibility for the problematic relationship on their perceived aggressors rather than accepting responsibility and accountability for who they are and what they want to be (Steele, 1990).

The stance of victim is seductive; there are many incentives for maintaining this role. Victims are perceived as innocent, and by assigning the locus of their control to external forces, they avoid responsibility and accountability. Victims are spared the stress of change because in the matrix of victimization it is the oppressor who must change for the victim's condition to improve (Cooper, 1991; Steele, 1990).

There can be no argument that in the past nurses were the victims of oppression and were made to suffer the subjugation of physicians and hospital administrators. They had little choice but to be exploited as conveniences, as loyal and obedient servants. Today, nurses must grapple not only with the memory of this exploitation but also with the real threat that the current crisis in health care economics will drive them back into a role of subservience. It will take tremendous courage and strength of professional character for nurses to maintain and further the success that advances in nursing practice, education, research, and administration have made toward unraveling the traditional socialization of health care providers and culture of health care organizations. Nurses are thus faced with a critical choice: to consider themselves helpless victims of past injustice and present-day economic threats or to define themselves as full-fledged and essential members of the health care team (Pike & Alpert, 1994).

The choice is not easy given the unconscious incentives to remain victims (Cooper, 1991). Defining oneself as an equal professional means being responsible and accountable, which are stressful, difficult, and frightening burdens. The definition obligates nurses to exercise their voice, to articulate their unique knowledge of patients and their responses to illness, and to participate with other health care professionals as colleagues rather than as subordinates. It means overcoming self-doubt and timidity and resisting the forces that threaten to corrupt

nurses' obligations to patients. Overcoming the internal and external constraints that inhibit the voice, aspirations, and talents of nurses requires relentless effort. Although the choice to exercise nurses' voice is risky, the choice to remain silent is an unacceptable alternative (Pike & Alpert, 1994).

BEING A COLLEAGUE

Part of the difficulty for nurses in defining themselves as colleagues of other health care professionals is that so little is known about how best to operationalize the role (Alpert, Goldman, Kilroy, & Pike, 1992; Petro, 1992; Prescott & Bowen, 1985; Stein, 1967; Stein, Watts, & Howell, 1990). Colleagueship involves entering into a collaborative relationship that is characterized by mutual trust and respect and an understanding of the perspective each partner contributes. Collaboration involves a bond, a union, and depth of caring about one another and about the relationship. The colleagueship this breeds obliges individuals to put aside their feelings of interprofessional competition and antagonism that are rooted in history so that the work and expertise of all participants may be integrated and patient care maximized (Alpert et al., 1992; Aradine & Pridham, 1973; Pike, 1991; Weiss & Davis, 1985).

Colleagues openly acknowledge that they share a common goal: the health and comfort of patients in their care. They recognize their interdependence and, accordingly, share responsibility and accountability for patient outcomes. Collegial relationships are safe. Each participant accepts the other as someone who is well-intentioned and trying to do his or her best. When conflict arises, it is addressed at its source and not escalated up a hierarchical chain of authority (Alpert et al., 1992; Mangiardi & Pellegrino, 1992; Pike et al., 1993).

Colleagueship has many characteristics of a caring relationship, as defined by the ethic of care. It dispenses with hierarchical habits of relating, replacing dominance and rank with mutual respect and shared decision making. As colleagues, persons attend to each other's growth and development, protect each other from belittlement, and enhance each other's professional dignity (Gadow, 1985; Mayeroff, 1971; Noddings, 1984; Watson, 1988).

Incorporating the concept of colleague into one's professional identity is a developmental process that requires critical self-reflection. To collaborate with others, a nurse must understand and value the unique perspective that nursing offers. Being a colleague requires a breadth of clinical experience that solidifies professional confidence. Nurses who define themselves as colleagues must develop a language that allows them to articulate their unique perspective to nonnurses so that they will be understood. This definition of professional self also requires the maturity to recognize the incentives to remain victimized and to reflect on how one might be seduced by these incentives. Additionally, one must understand the historical and cultural roots to the internal and external constraints imposed on nurses and appreciate that their influence can quickly subjugate nurses at a time when patients can ill afford a silencing of nurses' unique perspectives. Nurses who choose to define themselves as colleagues must overcome these constraints and learn to manage their backward pull.

Operationalizing the concept of professional self as equal colleague frees nurses from the internal constraints that contribute to the silencing of their voice. Once the influence of these internal forces is curtailed, nurses can question, challenge, and overcome external constraints. Colleagueship is difficult work fraught with anxiety, confusion, and frustration, but it is also a fruitful enterprise offering tremendous promise and benefits to both nurses and patients (Pike, 1991).

CONSEQUENCES OF CHOICE

The way in which nurses choose to construe their professional selves has significant implications for both patient care and nurses' role and satisfaction. The consequences of their choice are particularly dramatic in the care of patients and families in the throes of ethical uncertainty. Consider the following critical incident involving Mr. S. This incident describes a dilemma not unfamiliar to nurses, and it leaves powerful images of morally unacceptable care.

Mr. S. was a 72-year-old man admitted to the hospital from a nursing home as a result of his failure to thrive and a severe infection. On admission he was frail, cachectic, and minimally responsive. He had a temperature of 101.8° F, heart rate 160 beats per minute in atrial fibrillation, respiratory rate of 28 breaths per minute, and an unstable blood pressure. His blood tests suggested severe dehydration.

Mr. S.'s peripheral veins were small and fragile, and repeated attempts to start an intravenous line in his arms were unsuccessful. A line was finally established in his foot, and intravenous fluids and antibiotics were administered.

Long before his admission, Mr. S. had made it known that he did not want "heroic measures" taken to prolong his life in the event of a grave illness. It was documented and well known that "do not resuscitate" applied in his case.

We were unable to determine the source of his infection. Even gentle attempts to provide hydration exacerbated his congestive heart failure and atrial fibrillation. His kidneys failed,

and his lungs, damaged by years of smoking, were barely able to meet the increased demands of his illness. It seemed clear that Mr. S. was dying. His nurses worked to minimize any pain or distress he might suffer during his terminal illness.

On his fourth hospital day, Mr. S.'s intravenous line infiltrated and another peripheral line could not be placed. On the following day, the physicians involved in Mr. S.'s care felt obliged to establish a central intravenous line, since in the absence of peripheral access, Mr. S. was not receiving any fluid or antibiotics. At the time no one openly questioned this decision, despite the fact that his nurses considered such an invasive, aggressive intervention to be wrong in the context of Mr. S.'s illness and wishes.

During the central line insertion Mr. S. suffered a pneumothorax, and an emergency chest tube was inserted. At this point he exhibited notable signs of pain and discomfort, which had been absent during the earlier days of his admission.

Mr. S.'s family was called, and they were distressed that invasive interventions had been carried out. They requested that no further aggressive treatment be used in his care.

Mr. S. was given oxygen and morphine for comfort. He died less than 2 days later, but continued to show signs of respiratory distress throughout this period.

The nursing staff agonized over the pain and suffering he experienced. We began to place blame and among ourselves spoke of the callousness, aggressiveness, and insensitivity of physicians . . . of their ability "only to cure, not to care." We felt anger, frustration, pain, remorse, and guilt.

The story of Mr. S. is one of moral failure and moral outrage that resulted in large measure from the silencing of nurses' voice. Mr. S.'s nurses encountered a moral dilemma while they cared for him about whether to place a central line and continue hydration or forgo the line and allow him to die. Faced with this dilemma, the nurses reasoned that Mr. S. was at the end of his life and wanted to prevent his pain and suffering.

Mr. S.'s physicians, faced with the same dilemma, reached a different decision. Tragically, there was no discourse and the authority and directives of the physicians took precedence over the nurses' plan. The physicians' actions were seen as unquestionable, and this perception served as a constraint to the nurses who had legitimate concerns about Mr. S.'s suffering. The physicians' response—and the nurses' willingness to subjugate their own moral reasoning—effectively censored the nursing perspective.

It is true that the physicians acted in an authoritative manner and never solicited nursing advice, but they had accomplices in this censorship. The nurses caring for Mr. S. chose to be silent: "No one openly questioned this decision." The words used by the nurse reporting this incident suggest that she and her peers were disturbed, even horrified, by the physicians' decision. Yet no nurse spoke up.

The nurses responded to their silencing with moral outrage. An emotional response to the inability to carry out moral choices or decisions, moral outrage is characterized by demoralizing frustration, anger, disgust, and a sense of powerlessness (Pike, 1991). The nurses were furious about the moral failure of Mr. S.'s care, yet they only blamed the physicians, failing to recognize their own contribution to this tragedy. Had any one of Mr. S.'s nurses defined herself as a colleague, instead of as a helpless victim, a nurse's voice would have been heard; moral outrage would have been averted; and moral discourse would have ensued. In the end, Mr. S. most likely would have received more morally appropriate care.

In contrast, the following case illustrates the morally acceptable care that resulted from a nurse's choice to see herself as an integral and full-fledged colleague of physicians.

Mrs. H. had been a healthy, active 65-year-old woman until she suffered massive intracranial bleeding. She showed severe neurological impairment, with only occasional and minimal responses to noxious stimuli. The prognosis for neurological recovery was grim. Mrs. H. had prepared a handwritten statement 2 years earlier, at the time of her husband's death from cancer. It was a request that her life not be sustained in the event of an irreversible illness or injury. A photocopy of this statement hung on the bulletin board in her room.

Mrs. H.'s children, however, expressed their desire to pursue every treatment possible. They were adamant that they wanted their mother resuscitated in the event of a cardiac arrest. Mrs. H.'s physician felt obliged to comply with her children's wishes. I understood and respected his feeling of obligation, but found it morally conflicting. I suspect he did also.

Mrs. H. was deteriorating daily. Aggressive, invasive care continued. I had to leave the room more than once during invasive procedures due to the assaultive nature of the treatments. I saw them [as being] clearly in opposition to Mrs. H.'s wishes.

I spoke with her children and her physician each day. Although I could see and appreciate the agony they were experiencing in light of the massive ethical issues facing them, it was as if we were all speaking in different dialects of the same language. We needed a three-way conversation to help us understand the perspectives each of us brought to the situation.

I arranged a conference during which the patient's family, [the] physician, and I reviewed Mrs. H.'s condition and prognosis, and elaborated care plan options. Her family spoke of their grief and their feelings that they would be abandoning their mother if invasive treatments were discontinued. The physician and I explained that their mother would never be abandoned. We discussed how we could provide care for her in accordance with her wishes, and what the specifics of that care would be. In the end Mrs. H.'s family decided to change the aim of care and keep her comfortable until she died.

This is a difficult and poignant story. There was clearly a dilemma and clearly conflict. At an earlier point in her professional development, Mrs. H.'s nurse might have taken on the role of helpless victim and remained silent. The conflict would have simmered and bred moral outrage. Instead this nurse chose to see herself as a colleague who had the right, the duty, and the ability to facilitate discourse among all involved parties. In doing so she not only avoided her own moral distress but also transformed the meaning of the situation from conflict to miscommunication. Her actions prompted a discussion that allowed all perspectives to be integrated into Mrs. H.'s care. Her exercise of nurses' voice changed the nature of the care for this patient, making it more consistent with the patient's wishes and more comfortable for her family.

SUMMARY

These critical incidents strongly suggest that the choice a nurse makes about how she defines her professional self affects not only her morale but also the nature of care her patients receive. When a nurse identifies herself as the victim of deeply rooted social and economic constraints she increases the probability that her voice will be silenced. The stance of victim can lead to feelings of moral outrage and denies patients the benefits of the nursing perspective. When a nurse makes the choice to define herself as a colleague, however, participating in patient care as an integral member of the health care team, she seizes opportunities for professional fulfillment while affording patients the benefits of integrated care.

The responsibility and accountability for defining oneself as a colleague resides in individual nurses. Perhaps it does not seem fair that nurses, because they have inherited internal and external constraints to their professional identity, autonomy, and aspirations, now have to rescue themselves from subjugation. Perhaps it would seem fairer if those whose predecessors exploited nurses made concessions. Fairness aside, history shows that members of dominant groups do not generally offer restitution to those whom they have exploited (Steele, 1990). While growing numbers of physicians are to be commended for enlightened attitudes and behaviors, nurses will only grow increasingly frustrated waiting for past injustices to be repaid.

While the issue of fairness will always linger, it is, ironically, fortunate that compensation is not forthcoming.

For the possibility of compensation keeps the responsibility for collegiality with physicians and leads to the familiar slogan among nurses, "We're ready to be colleagues just as soon as the doctors change." Making colleagueship dependent on changes among physicians maintains nurses as victims; it asks nonnurses to exercise nurses' voice. The only one who can declare herself an essential colleague is the individual nurse, and to do so she must emancipate herself from both internal and external constraints.

Nurses' choice to define themselves as colleagues, as full-fledged vital members of the health care team, holds great moral significance for nursing and for patient care. In making this choice, nurses take the opportunity to overcome subjugation and to assume a stance of empowerment. By defining themselves as colleagues nurses initiate a move on their own behalf and on behalf of their patients to make their voices heard (Cooper, 1991). Such a professional self-concept is a prerequisite for, as well as a driving force in, the development of collaborative relationships with physicians, health care administrators, and, in this era of managed care, even third-party payers. Collaboration unifies the contributions of all involved in patient care, making that care more efficient, effective, and comprehensive (Aiken, 1990; Knaus, Draper, Wagner, & Zimmerman, 1986; Pike, 1991; Prescott & Bowen, 1985). By choosing to make their voice heard nurses afford patients not only the advantage of the nursing perspective but also the full benefit of integrated care. The promise this holds for advancing the care delivered to patients and families cannot be underestimated.

REFERENCES

Aiken, L.H. (1990). Charting the future of hospital nursing. *Image: The Journal of Nursing Scholarship, 22*(2), 72-78.

Alpert, H.B., Goldman, L.D., Kilroy, C.M., & Pike, A.W. (1992). 7 Gryzmish: Toward an understanding of collaboration. *Nursing Clinics of North America, 27*(1), 47-59.

Aradine, C.R., & Pridham, K.F. (1973). Model for collaboration. *Nursing Outlook, 21*(10), 655-657.

Belenky, M.F., Clinchy, B.M., Goldberger, N.R., & Tarule, J.M. (1986). *Women's ways of knowing.* Boston: Basic Books.

Benner, P. (1984). *From novice to expert.* Menlo Park, CA: Addison-Wesley.

Cooper, M.C. (1991). Response to moral outrage and moral discourse in nurse-physician collaboration. *Journal of Professional Nursing, 7*(6), 362-363.

Gadow, S.A. (1985). Nurse and patient: The caring relationship. In A.H. Bishop & J.R. Scudder (Eds.), *Caring, curing, coping: Nurse-physician-patient relationships* (pp. 31-43). Birmingham: University of Alabama Press.

Gilligan, C. (1982). *In a different voice.* Cambridge, MA: Harvard University Press.

Knaus, W.A., Draper, E.A., Wagner, D.P., & Zimmerman, J.E. (1986). An evaluation of outcome from intensive care in major medical centers. *Annals of Internal Medicine, 104*(3), 410-418.

Mangiardi, J.R., & Pellegrino, E.D. (1992). Collegiality: What is it? *Bulletin of the New York Academy of Medicine, 68*(2), 292-296.

Mayeroff, M. (1971). *On caring.* New York: Harper Collins.

Miller, J.B. (1976). *Toward a new psychology for women.* Boston: Beacon Press.

Noddings, N. (1984). *Caring: A feminine approach to ethics and moral education.* Los Angeles: University of California Press.

Petro, J.A. (1992). Collegiality in history. *Bulletin of the New York Academy of Medicine, 68*(2), 292-296.

Pike, A.W. (1991). Moral outrage and moral discourse in nurse-physician collaboration. *Journal of Professional Nursing, 7*(6), 351-363.

Pike, A.W., & Alpert, H.B. (1994). Pioneering the future: The 7 North model of nurse-physician collaboration. *Nursing Administration Quarterly, 18*(4), 11-18.

Pike, A.W., McHugh, M., Canney, K., Miller, N., Reilly, P., & Seibert, C.P. (1993). A new architecture for quality assurance: Nurse-physician collaboration. *Journal of Nursing Care Quality, 7*(3), 1-8.

Prescott, P.A., & Bowen, S.A. (1985). Physician-nurse relationships. *Annals of Internal Medicine, 103*(127), 127-133.

Steele, S. (1990). *The content of our character.* New York: St. Martins Press.

Stein, L.I. (1967). The doctor-nurse game. *Archives of General Psychiatry, 16*(6), 699-703.

Stein, L.I., Watts, D.T., & Howell, T. (1990). The doctor-nurse game revisited. *New England Journal of Medicine, 322*(8), 546-549.

Watson, J. (1988). *Nursing: Human science and human care.* New York: The National League for Nursing.

Weiss, S.J., & Davis, H.P. (1985). Validity and reliability of the collaborative practice scales. *Nursing Research, 34*(5), 299-305.

Yarling, R.R., & McElmurry, B.J. (1986). The moral foundation of nursing. *Advances in Nursing Science, 8*(2), 63-73.

Collaboration Between Medical and Nursing Education in Community-Based Settings

JOELLEN B. EDWARDS

Health care delivery systems in the United States have undergone unprecedented change in recent years. Assumptions long held by the public, legislators, insurers, and health professionals themselves about health care systems have been shaken. Providers and educators have been challenged to greater fiscal accountability, efficiency, and improved quality at less cost through the rise of managed care. The acute care setting, once the focal point for health professions education and practice, has given way to health care delivery that takes place in myriad settings, far beyond institutional walls. Integrated systems aim to contain costs, improve quality and satisfaction, and coordinate care across multiple types of delivery sites. Along with this shift in the place of health care services, a set of powerful systemic forces have brought about examination of the way in which health professionals are educated for practice in the emerging health care system.

The Pew Health Professions Commission provided a succinct statement of the competencies that would be needed by health professionals in the future, including the ability to care for the community's health and an ability to work in interdisciplinary teams (O'Neil, 1993). Professional organizations such as the American Association of Colleges of Nursing (1995), the National League for Nursing (1993), and the Council on Graduate Medical Education (1997) added their support to these concepts. Nursing, medicine, and a variety of allied health professions are beginning to rise to the challenge of preparing graduates who can work together as teams to meet the health needs of the community. Funding to support such efforts has been offered by leading philanthropic foundations such as the W.K. Kellogg Foundation and the Robert Wood Johnson Foundation and by numerous federal initiatives.

Our students become what we teach them. A community-based, interdisciplinary approach to the learning process in the education of medical and nursing profes-

sionals, leading to the competencies proposed by the Pew Commission, has been suggested as a foundation for meaningful and lasting change in the way health care is structured and operationalized in this country (Holmes & Osterweis, 1999). While strides have been made in some institutions, educators and practitioners in all academic health professions must take a hard look at values, beliefs, traditions, and structure of educational programs. The present patterns for training nurses and physicians maintain persistent barriers to the kinds of learning experiences our graduates need to prepare them for today's practice.

NURSING AND MEDICAL EDUCATION

Both nursing and medicine arose from the tradition of caring for the health and illness needs of people. However, as the disciplines became formally recognized, distinct difference in their educational patterns became institutionalized. After the Flexner Report in 1910, the medical profession organized schools at the graduate level in university settings, creating the only path to the legal right to practice medicine. Nursing, even after the Goldmark Report in 1934, remained, for many years, closely aligned with hospital training schools. The autonomy and societal acceptance of medicine as a profession was readily established, while recognition of nursing as a profession was stifled until far into the 20th century. Medical schools fostered the development of autonomy and the idea that the physician was the sole decision maker and responsible party in all patient care. Until the relatively recent past, nursing schools fostered the development of subservience, strict adherence to policies and procedures, and support of the singular authority of the physician (Kalisch & Kalisch, 1977).

The historical dominance of the medical profession in health care continues today. This trend influences the continuation of educational practices that isolate both professions, and deflects attempts at collaborative practice. Other educational factors, such as faculty support of the traditional patterns and relationships, perceived curricular conflicts between the two professions, unfounded beliefs that accreditation processes prohibit changes in educational patterns, and university structures that foster isolation contribute to the barriers between nursing and medical education (Baldwin, 1996; Bulger, 1995; Bulger & Bulger, 1992; Cook & Drusin, 1995; Erikson, McHarney-Brown, Seeger, & Kaufman, 1998; McEwen, 1994; Zungolo, 1994).

Nursing and medicine maintain different philosophical approaches to the education of students. Although some changes are on the horizon, medicine has been found to value content, rationality, data, and assimilation of scientific information in their educational strategy over attention to the social and relational aspects of health care (Bloom, 1988; Greenlick, 1992). Nursing, on the other hand, has been shown to value and teach a more holistic and relational approach to caring for well and ill persons (Lindeman, 1995). The values of the profession are transmitted through educational approaches. A study by Wolf (1989) identified the core values of nursing as "persons as individuals" and "wholeness in life." Medicine's core values were identified as "responsibility" and "human life." These core values are reflected in the differing strategies for education, and thus practice, between the two disciplines.

One similarity between nursing and medical education stands out. The focus for educational experiences for both groups, since the emergence of the institution, has been the hospital as the predominant training site. Hospital care has made significant contributions to the preservation of human life and offers ample opportunity for health professions students to learn to care for the extremely ill. Yet, today's students also need to practice the competencies needed to prevent illness, promote health, provide primary care, address environmental issues, and help individuals and families cope with the effects of their chronic illness in their own life setting. Health professions students need the opportunity to find their place outside hospital walls and to both participate in and lead efforts to positively influence the community's health. Community-based, interdisciplinary approaches to learning can make a significant difference in the expectations for practice created in educational programs.

COMMUNITY-BASED EDUCATION AND PRACTICE

Community-based education and practice tends to be perceived and defined differently by medicine and nurs-

ing in a way that is consistent with each profession's implicit and explicit values. Nursing tends to view "community based" as the incorporation of the whole of the community—homes, schools, shelters, stores, day care centers, primary care practices, and others—into the education of nursing students and as sites for professional practice (Oerman, 1994). Medicine, outside the community-oriented primary care movement (Nutting, Wood, & Conner, 1985), more often views "community based" as the incorporation of precepted ambulatory care experiences in physician offices into the medical school or residency curricula, and community-based practice as a physician enterprise outside the university setting.

If the voice of prominent health care foundations, professional organizations, and national leadership is heard, community-based practice and education will evolve to be about far more than the place of clinical learning or care delivery. Community-based care will require a shift in power from institutions and expert professionals to community members and the creation of accessible, affordable, and acceptable health services that will meet the needs of the population. People in communities, in partnership with professionals, will need to define the health needs to be met and maintain control of the strategies for meeting those needs. This pattern is in direct opposition to the current system of education and practice, in which health care organizations and expert professionals decide what the community needs and maintain control of services offered.

If students are to emerge from health professions education programs ready to participate fully in a delivery system that meets basic health needs of the population, significant changes in the approach to medical and nursing education to embrace and incorporate community-based philosophy will be necessary. True collaboration between the disciplines and their communities will be the key to success.

COLLABORATION

Differences in the perception of the meaning of collaboration can be seen between medical and nursing professionals, also congruent with intraprofessional values and core beliefs. Nurses and other health professionals tend to perceive that collaborative relationships mean that different professionals complement each others' equally valued skills in a setting or patient care situation; physicians tend to perceive collaboration as directing other professionals who extend the domain of medicine (Abramson & Mizrahi, 1996; Brown & Chamberlin, 1996; Hojat et al., 1997).

Collaboration in health care could be more positively approached if it were viewed as a relationship in which individuals become increasingly invested in each others' success, to the benefit of both the professionals and their clients. Collaborators are willing to share information, alter their activities for the betterment of all concerned, share resources to accomplish a common goal, and willingly enhance the capacity of another to achieve a common purpose.

Several themes emerge from this description of collaboration that apply to nursing and medicine in educational and practice settings. These themes are empowerment, relationship, and synergy. Empowerment is the ability of each involved party to find the strength within to do what needs to be done for self or others. Empowerment is about mutual support of involved parties to find and exercise that power within (Rappaport, 1984).

Communication expresses relationship, and no communication exists outside the context of the relationship of the communicators (Coeling & Wilcox, 1994). Collaboration is only possible in relationships that are mutually respectful, open, direct, and assertive. Collaboration creates synergy that makes possible the achievement of a common goal in a way that is greater than the sum of the contributions made by each party. The knowledge and expertise of each person involved in the collaborative effort is recognized and valued, and is freely given and accepted among collaborators.

COLLABORATION BETWEEN NURSING AND MEDICINE

The idea that the two most predominant health professions would not collaborate is almost incomprehensible. Yet, societal, professional, and economic forces militate against collaboration in education and practice. Power relationships between the two disciplines have historically remained inequitable, with the clear balance of traditional forms of power in the hands of physicians (Barr, 1997; Bradford, 1989; Bulger & Bulger, 1992; Doering, 1992; Kalisch & Kalisch, 1982). Issues such as sex role stereotyping, socialization processes in nursing and medical training, and social class differences between medical and nursing career aspirants, contribute to power differences. These differences pose significant barriers to collaboration (Fagin, 1992). Evidence exists that traditional forms of physician power are eroding. Physicians are acutely aware of threats to their autonomy and previously unquestioned professional privileges (Butler, 2000; Friedman, 1994).

Relationships between nurses and physicians are expressed through communication, and have been studied as they influence the possibilities for collaboration. Stein (1967) documented communication styles, naming the dominant physician-deferential nurse pattern of the "doctor-nurse game." A follow-up study by Stein, Watts, and Howell (1990) found that historical patterns of submissiveness by nurses had given way to a more direct, confrontational style. Communication patterns can be a barrier or a facilitator to effective collaboration.

Barriers to the synergy created through collaboration exist as well. Medicine and nursing are likely to differ in the areas of problem identification and mutual goal setting, important elements of collaboration. The differing value systems of nursing and medicine can contribute to disparity rather than cohesiveness in goal setting in patient care situations.

In spite of the barriers, collaboration among health professionals has been shown to positively affect the outcomes of several indicators in the health care system. A variety of studies involving a wide range of patient care settings from intensive care units to chronic care management have shown the value of interdisciplinary collaboration in decreasing costs, improving patient outcomes, improving satisfaction of professionals with their jobs, better continuity of care, and improved professional identity (Baggs, Ryan, Phelps, Richeson, & Johnson, 1992; Baggs & Schmidt, 1997; Baggs et al., 1997; Burl & Bonner, 1991; Hansen, Bull, & Gross, 1998; Larsen, 1995; Le, Winter, Boyd, Ackerson, & Hurley, 1998; Maguire, 1994; Middleton & Whitney, 1993; Pacheco et al., 1991; Pugh et al., 1999; Stichler, 1995).

The idea of collaborative approaches to health and health care systems is an ideal increasingly espoused by health professions educators and practitioners. Interdisciplinary collaboration between medicine and nursing is possible and is working in some institutions (Holmes & Osterweis, 1999). The beginning of the adoption of collaboration as the norm rather than the exception starts with the education of nursing and medical students, as well as students from other health disciplines (Fagin, 1992; Forbes & Fitzsimmons, 1993; McEwen, 1994).

COLLABORATION AMONG HEALTH PROFESSIONS AND THE COMMUNITY

The establishment of a collaborative relationship between members of health professions and communities has remained as elusive as among health professionals from various disciplines. Health professionals have been notorious for their domination of the planning and implementation of health care systems (Osborne & Gaebler, 1992). Health care services are organized on the turf of professionals, offered at times convenient to professionals rather than users, and often implemented without regard for the true needs of the population to be served. A narrow focus on illness and acute care is more common than attention to the health promotion and illness prevention strategies sought by community members. The ability to be reimbursed for the service is more often the driving force in determining what health care is available than true need.

Health professionals hold expert power in medicine or nursing and often positional power in comparison to those they serve. Implementation of a power rather than empowerment model has created an imbalance in the power relationships between health care providers and users of health care systems. Educational and economic gaps between providers and communities impose an additional barrier to collaboration. Community members may believe they have nothing to offer or are unable to influence highly educated experts in health fields.

Relationships between community members and health professionals, expressed through communication, can be problematic. Health professionals maintain their own language that sometimes excludes those who do not understand medical terminology. Professional jargon, or conversely, colloquial terminology, can lead to unshared or misinterpreted meanings among potential collaborators. Values, beliefs, and priorities can be highly divergent (Cortes, 1986). Difficulty in valuing and appreciating the contributions of both community members and professionals can arise. Collaboration with community, like collaboration among professionals, is a process of sharing power and appreciating diverse expertise. Palmer (1990) defines community as "a gift to be received, not a goal to be achieved" (p. 4). The power of collaboration with the community can only be realized by the willingness of those who hold traditional power to give it away (Richards, 1993).

COLLABORATION AMONG NURSING, MEDICINE, AND OTHER HEALTH PROFESSIONS IN COMMUNITY-BASED SETTINGS: CASE STUDY OF A 10-YEAR EFFORT

East Tennessee State University (ETSU), a comprehensive, regional university with a specific mission focus in the education of health professionals, is one institution that has attempted to improve collaboration in the education of its health professions students in community-based settings. The division of health sciences is an organizational unit of the university that, since 1989, has united the colleges of medicine, nursing, and public and allied health toward common goals and purposes, under a vice president for health affairs.

In 1990, the colleges of nursing and medicine at ETSU were approached by business and governmental leaders from rural Johnson County for assistance in rebuilding their shattered health care system. Unemployment had skyrocketed to 35%, the small rural hospital had closed, and only three physicians, one in part-time practice, remained in the county. These leaders believed that a viable health care system was foundational to attracting new industry and business to the rugged mountain community. The division of health sciences, with its focus rural primary care, was a natural ally.

The community's request brought medicine and nursing to the community to serve in two different settings. One was a traditional medical clinic, operated by the department of family medicine; the other was a primary care practice, open in the evening and on weekends, operated by nurse practitioner faculty from the college of nursing (Edwards, Kaplan, Barnett, & Logan, 1998). Significant investment in the form of facilities, equipment, moral support, advice, and direction for the endeavor was extended by the community. Nursing and medicine began tentative steps toward collaboration (Pullen, Edwards, Lenz, & Alley, 1994).

In 1991 the health sciences division competed for and received a 5-year, $6 million grant from the W.K. Kellogg Foundation, Community Partnerships for Health Professions Education. With its purpose to educate medical, nursing, and public health professionals together in communities over an extended period of time, the opportunity offered the three health sciences colleges the support they needed to make their leaders' goal of meaningful collaboration possible.

The first grant year was spent building the primary care practices in the county; learning to work together and with the community; analyzing the health needs of the population; refining the administrative structure; and creating the interdisciplinary, rural, community-based curriculum. Twenty-five percent of the bachelor of science in nursing and medical school content was offered in this format, for a maximum of 25% of the students. Bachelor's level students from public and allied health were vital participants, although their numbers were smaller.

All disciplines recruited faculty who would live as well as work in the rural communities, thus increasing the human connections that made this endeavor successful. Community boards, set up to guide and direct the project, were key to the recruitment process. In 1992 the first cohort of students entered the "rural primary care track"; in 1993 another cohort was added in the second partner community, Hawkins County. Students continue through the present to enter this track in both rural sites, and many, particularly medical students, come to the institution from across the country specifically for that purpose.

At times, the problems faced in interdisciplinary and community collaboration in the implementation of this unique and challenging effort seemed overwhelming. Every barrier to collaboration, particularly between nursing and medicine, was encountered. Faculty who did not know each other were thrown into an intense year of negotiation over what content was appropriate for the interdisciplinary classes. Language was a barrier in the beginning. Physicians were "trained"; nurses were "educated." People receiving care were "patients" to physicians and "clients" to nurses. Hands-on techniques for gathering data about the patient/client were "physical examinations" to physicians and "physical assessments" to nurses. Myths, stereotypes, and cherished ways of doing almost everything had to be surrendered on all sides. Some gave up the ghost easily; some died hard; and some reappear from the grave, even after 10 years, to haunt us occasionally! The intense level of emotion associated with these seemingly small details, as well as major turf and professional issues, had to be addressed.

Stereotypes held by the community about academe and academe about the community had to be given up as well. Myths about "ivory tower university types" came tumbling down as deans, faculty, and community members worked side by side physically and intellectually to prepare space, move equipment and supplies, and launch the students successfully into the community. Any idea that rural people were not interested in planning for the health of their community or were shy and backward about offering their input was quickly dispelled. Respect and true friendship grew rapidly among representatives from the university and community members.

The project achieved successful outcomes (see box, right). Even today, long after the funding period ended, medical, nursing, and public health students continue to enter and graduate from the rural cohorts; faculty live and work in the communities; and learners and community members continue to benefit from the collaboration (Behringer, Bishop, Edwards, & Franks, 1999).

The integration of the innovation into the culture of the division made the next logical step in the progression of increased collaboration, the expansion of the interdisciplinary, community-based effort to include graduate students, both desirable and possible. In 1996, again

funded by the W.K. Kellogg Foundation, a plan to bring together family medicine residents, graduate family nurse practitioner students, and graduate public health students was implemented (Edwards & Smith, 1998). Graduate students and residents attend seminars, join in interest groups to further their knowledge base and collaborative skills in a clinical area (school health, palliative care, migrant health and occupational health are a few examples) and, when schedules can be arranged, practice together in sites that model exemplary interdisciplinary care.

The success of the collaborative, community-based efforts of the division of health sciences has impacted the entire university. In 1998 an additional project, the Expanding Community Partnership Program, was funded, again by the W.K. Kellogg Foundation. This project brings the potential for every academic unit on campus to participate in community-based, interdisciplinary education. Two additional rural counties, Unicoi and Hancock, joined the partnership, and the governance structure was widened to incorporate all areas and colleges. In this effort, community members from all four partner counties engage with faculty and students to enrich student learning and implement projects, both short and long term, that will benefit all participants. Examples of partnership projects to date include the development of a leadership program for rural youth, economic development in a rural county still plagued by an unstable industrial base, and the production of an original historical drama about a town in Johnson County that was a unique and moving experience for community members and students alike.

SELECTED SUCCESSES OF RURAL, INTERDISCIPLINARY PROJECT

- Total curriculum of nursing, medicine, and public and allied health influenced and improved
- 10 years of consistent, high-quality primary care by nurse practitioners and family physicians in rural, underserved areas
- Improved health status in communities
- Student performance equal to traditional students on standardized professional examinations (USMLE, NCLEX)
- 96% of medical graduates chose primary care residency
- 58% of BSN graduates chose practice in rural, underserved, or community-based settings
- Influence of graduate medical education funding and nurse practitioner reimbursement in the state

The impact on the individual colleges, the division as a whole, the university, and the surrounding communities cannot be overstated. Efforts at collaboration, viewed as enhancing each others' success for the benefit of all, continue to mature. The numbers of spontaneous interdisciplinary projects within the university have grown, crossing lines that were not imagined in the past. Examples include a collaboration among nursing, public health, and business to educate graduate students in health administration; a graduate certificate in gerontology involving public health, communicative disorders, nursing, medicine, sociology, nutrition, and others; unique ventures between history and theater; and many others. The community is increasingly integrated into the university, and the university is increasingly open to the community. Community leaders in the health partnerships and the broader university partnerships have shaped student learning and outcomes in their own counties. Empowerment of students, faculty, and community members is evident. Students have taken an increasingly active role in shaping the experiences of their own and following cohorts.

Relationships, expressed through communication among participants, have changed over the years of working together intensely. Faculty have taught together, conducted research and practice projects, published, made presentations, argued publicly and privately, gone to lunch, learned about each others' lives outside the university, in short, become acquainted as human beings. Interpersonal conflict still occurs, and turf battles still occasionally arise. When a conflict occurs, however, it is most often about individual differences rather than a professional stereotype. The synergy of the collaboration has achieved outcomes that no unit would have been able to achieve alone.

The focus on interdisciplinary, community-based education continues to expand. Current efforts at refinement within the health sciences division includes the expansion of the interdisciplinary communication course to include all health professions students, development of a series of projects with partner communities in which at least 50% of health students will participate, and strengthening the health leadership focus in the curriculum. At the university level, the 1999 revision of the mission and purpose statement identified interdisciplinary, community-based education as a major area of emphasis for the institution (see box, left).

MAJOR EVENTS IN COLLABORATION OVER A DECADE

1990	• Community requests collaboration
	• Primary care clinics established, Johnson County
1991	• Community-University governance formal structure
	• "Community Partnerships for Health Professions Education" grant awarded for medical students, BSN students, and BS public and allied health students
1992	• Community input into interdisciplinary curriculum
	• First Johnson County cohort of nursing, medicine, and public health students enter
1993	• Primary care clinic established, Hawkins County
	• First Hawkins County cohort of nursing, medical, and public health students enter
1996	• Community students, faculty, refined interdisciplinary curriculum
	• "Graduate Health Professions Education" grant awarded for family medicine residents, graduate nursing, and public and allied health students
1998	• Unicoi and Hancock counties join partnership
	• "Expanding Community Partnerships" grant awarded for all disciplines on campus
2000	• Health professions, university, and community collaborations continue
	• University mission statement revised to focus on community-based, interdisciplinary collaboration

---

SUMMARY

Community-based, interdisciplinary education and practice for health professions students is the way of the future. It is a strategy that will enable the health needs of populations to be better met. Health care economics, professional altruism, and the voices of the people who need accessible, affordable, and acceptable health care will not allow isolationism to continue. Entering into a commitment to collaborate to improve health outcomes of populations requires patience, persistence, communication skill, willingness to trust past opponents, incredibly hard work, and, most of all, an unshakable inner belief that it is the right thing to do. When it works, the results are beyond highest hopes.

REFERENCES

Abramson, J.S., & Mizrahi, T. (1996). When social workers and physicians collaborate: Positive and negative interdisciplinary experiences. *Social Work, 41*(3), 270-281.

American Association of Colleges of Nursing. (1995). *Position statement: Interdisciplinary education and practice.* [On-Line]. Available: http://www.aacn.nche.edu/Publications/positions/interdis.htm.

Baggs, J.G., & Schmitt, M.H. (1997). Nurses' and resident physicians' perceptions of the process of collaboration in the MICU. *Research in Nursing and Health, 10*(1), 71-80.

Baggs, J.G., Ryan, S.A., Phelps, C.E., Richeson, J.F., & Johnson, J.E. (1992). The association between interdisciplinary collaboration and patient outcomes in a medical intensive care unit. *Heart and Lung, 21*(1), 18-24.

Baggs, J.G., Schmitt, M.H., Mushlin, A.I., Eldredge, D.H., Oakes, D., & Hutson, A.D. (1997). Nurse-physician collaboration and satisfaction with the decision-making process in three critical care units. *American Journal of Critical Care, 6*(5), 393-399.

Baldwin, D. (1996). Some historical notes on interdisciplinary and interprofessional education and practice in health care in the USA. *Journal of Interprofessional Care, 10*(2) 173-187.

Barr, O. (1997). Interdisciplinary teamwork: Consideration of the challenges. *British Journal of Nursing, 6*(17), 1005-1010.

Behringer, B., Bishop, W., Edwards, J., & Franks, R. (1999). A model for partnerships among communities, disciplines, and institutions. In D. Holmes & M. Osterweis (Eds.), *Catalysts in interdisciplinary education: Innovation by academic health centers* (pp. 43-58). Washington, DC: Association of Academic Health Centers.

Bloom, S. (1988). Structure and ideology in medical education: An analysis of resistance to change. *Journal of Health and Social Behavior, 29,* 294-306.

Bradford, R. (1989). Obstacles to collaborative practice. *Nursing Management, 20*(4), 72I, 72L-72M, 72P.

Brown, G.F., & Chamberlin, G.D. (1996). Attitudes toward quality, costs, and physician centrality in healthcare teams. *Journal of Interprofessional Care, 10*(1), 63-72.

Bulger, R.J. (1995). Generalism and the need for health professional education reform. *Academic Medicine, 70*(1 suppl), S31-S34.

Bulger, R.J., & Bulger, R.E. (1992). Obstacles to collegiality in the academic health center. *Bulletin of the New York Academy of Medicine, 68*(2), 303-307.

Burl, J.B., & Bonner, A.F. (1991). A geriatric nurse practitioner/physician team in a long term care setting. *HMO Practitioner, 5*(4), 110-115.

Butler, L. (2000). Nonphysicians gain clout. *American Medical News* [On-Line]. Available: http://www.ama-assn.org/sci-pubs/amnews/pick_00/gv110117.htm.

Coeling, H., & Wilcox, J. (1994). Steps to collaboration. *Nursing Administration Quarterly, 18*(4), 44-45.

Cook, S.S., & Drusin, R.E. (1995). Revisiting interdisciplinary education: One way to build an ark. *Nursing and Healthcare: Perspectives on Community, 16*(5), 260-264.

Cortes, E. (1986). Organizing the community. *The Texas Observer, 10*(16).

Council on Graduate Medical Education. (1997). *Preparing learners for practice in a managed care environment.* Washington, DC: U.S. Department of Health and Human Services.

Doering, L. (1992). Power and knowledge in nursing: A feminist post-structuralist view. *Advances in Nursing Science, 14*(4), 24-33.

Edwards, J., Kaplan, A., Barnett, J.T., & Logan, C.L. (1998). Nurse managed primary care in a rural community: Outcomes of five years of practice. *Nursing and Health Care Perspectives, 19*(1), 20-25.

Edwards, J., & Smith, P. (1998). Impact of interdisciplinary education in underserved areas: Health professions collaboration in rural Tennessee. *Journal of Professional Nursing, 14*(3), 144-149.

Erikson, B., McHarney-Brown, C., Seeger, K., & Kaufman, A. (1998). Overcoming barriers to interprofessional health sciences education. *Education for Health, 11*(2), 143-149.

Fagin, C. (1992). Collaboration between nurses and physicians: No longer a choice. *Nursing and Health Care, 13*(7), 354-363.

Flexner, A. (1910). *Medical education in the United States and Canada.* Boston: D.B. Updike, The Merrymount Press.

Forbes, E., & Fitzsimmons, V. (1993). Education: The key for holistic interdisciplinary collaboration. *Holistic Nursing Practice, 4*(7), 1-10.

Friedman, E. (1994, December 2). The power of physicians: Autonomy and balance in a changing system. *National Health Policy Forum, 659,* 1-9.

Goldmark, J. (1934). *Nursing and nursing education in the United States.* New York: Macmillan.

Greenlick, M. (1992). Educating physicians for population based clinical practice. *Journal of the American Medical Association, 267*(12), 1645-1648.

Hansen, H.E., Bull, M.J., & Gross, C.R. (1998). Interdisciplinary collaboration and discharge planning communication for elders. *Journal of Nursing Administration, 29*(9), 37-46.

Hojat, M., Fields, S.K., Rattner, S.L., Griffiths, M., Cohen, M.J., & Plumb, J.D. (1997). Attitudes toward physician-nurse alliance: Comparisons of medical and nursing students. *Academic Medicine, 72*(10, suppl 1), S1-S3.

Holmes, D., & Osterweis, M. (1999). What is past is prologue: Interdisciplinary at the turn of the century. In D. Holmes & M. Osterweis (Eds.), *Catalysts in interdisciplinary education: Innovation by academic health centers.* Washington, DC: American Association of Academic Health Centers.

Kalisch, B., & Kalisch, P. (1977). An analysis of the sources of physician-nurse conflict. *Journal of Nursing Administration, 7*(1), 50-57.

Kalisch, B., & Kalisch, P. (1982). *Politics of nursing.* Philadelphia: Lippincott.

Larsen, E.L. (1995). New rules for the game: Interdisciplinary education for health professionals. *Nursing Outlook, 43*(4), 180-185.

Le, C.T., Winter, T.D., Boyd, K.J., Ackerson, L., & Hurley, L.B. (1998). Experience with a managed care approach to HIV infection: Effectiveness of an interdisciplinary team. *American Journal of Managed Care, 4*(5), 647-657.

Lindeman, C. (1995). *Refocusing undergraduate nursing education.* Atlanta: Southern Council on Collegiate Education in Nursing with the Southern Regional Education Board.

Maguire, D. (1994). Multidisciplinary collaboration in neonatal intensive care. *Nursing Administration Quarterly, 18*(4), 18-22.

McEwen, M. (1994). Promoting interdisciplinary collaboration. *Nursing and Health Care, 15*(6), 304-307.

Middleton, E., & Whitney, F. (1993). Primary care in the emergency room: A collaborative model. *Nursing Connections, 6*(2), 29-40.

National League for Nursing. (1993). *A vision for nursing education.* New York: Author.

Nutting, P., Wood, M., & Conner, E. (1985). Community oriented primary care. *Journal of the American Medical Association, 253*(12), 1763-1766.

Oerman, M. (1994). Reforming nursing education for future practice. *Journal of Nursing Education, 33*(5), 215-219.

O'Neil, E. (1993). *Health professions education for the future: Schools in service to the nation.* San Francisco: Pew Health Professions Commission.

Osborne, D., & Gaebler, T. (1992). Community-owned government: Empowering rather than serving. In *Reinventing government: How the entrepreneurial spirit is transforming the public sector* (pp. 49-75). Reading, MA: Addison-Wesley.

Pacheco, M., Adelsheim, S., Davis, L., Mancha, V., Aime, L., Nelson, P., Derksen, D., & Kaufmann, A. (1991). Innovation, peer teaching, and multidisciplinary collaboration: Outreach from a school-based clinic. *Journal of School Health, 61*(8), 367-369.

Palmer, P. (1990). Scarcity, abundance, and the gift of community. *Community Renewal Press, 1*(3), 1-5.

Pugh, L.C., Tringali, R.A., Boehmer, J., Blaha, C., Kruger, N.R., Capauna, T.A., Bryan, Y., Robinson, J., Belmont, D., Young, M., &

Xie, S. (1999). Partners in care: A model of collaboration. *Holistic Nursing Practice, 13*(2), 61-65.

Pullen, C., Edwards, J., Lenz, C., & Alley, N. (1994). A comprehensive primary health care delivery model. *Journal of Professional Nursing, 10*(4), 201-208.

Rappaport, J. (1984). Studies in empowerment: Introductions to the rescue. *Prevention in Human Services, 3,* 1-7.

Richards, R. (1993). Observations on the redirection of an iceberg: Leading educational reform in medical schools. *Annals of Community-Oriented Education, 6,* 207-217.

Stein, L. (1967). The doctor-nurse game. *Archives of General Psychiatry, 16*(6), 699-703.

Stein, L., Watts, D., & Howell, T. (1990). The doctor-nurse game revisited. *New England Journal of Medicine, 322*(8), 546-549.

Stichler, J.F. (1995). Professional interdependence: The art of collaboration. *Advanced Nursing Practice Quarterly, 1*(1), 53-61.

Wolf, B. (1989). *Nursing identity: The nursing-medicine relationship.* Denver, CO: Denver Bookbinding Co., Inc.

Zungolo, E. (1994). Interdisciplinary education in primary care: The challenge. *Nursing and Health Care, 15*(6), 288-292.

Nurse Practitioners and Physician Assistants

Separated at Birth

RITA M. WILLIAMS

The history of the practice of modern medicine has all the makings of a classic novel. There are mystery, suspense, fear, and despair within the quest for a happy ending. The main characters seem never to change. The patient is the victim of a sinister disease. Nurses play the supporting role. And the hero, the physician, saves the day!

Like many classics, someone usually writes a screenplay. And like most, the movie is never like the book. The basic story is unchanged. It includes a victim, the villain, a supporting cast, and, of course, the hero. The current elements of health care provide the latest screenplay based on the classic practice of medicine. Patients are still victims, diseases are still the villain, and nurses still play a supporting role. But the leading role of the hero is changing. Two new players, nurse practitioners and physician assistants, are vying to share the leading role. Each one has auditioned well for this role. The final casting has not been decided, but it may result in two or three heroes in this plot.

ACT I: THE BIRTH OF A CONCEPT

The concept of a nurse practitioner or physician assistant was borrowed from the 17th and 18th century European military. Peter the Great introduced the idea, known as feldshers, to the Russian military. These individuals provided health care to the Russian troops and eventually to rural Russian communities of Alaska in the 1800s. Experienced feldshers could diagnose, prescribe, and begin emergency care (Ballweg, 1999).

In the 20th century, a similar provider was developed in China. The 1965 Cultural Revolution resulted in a health care provider known as the barefoot doctor. Chairman Mao directed the redistribution of the health care system, resulting in the training of 1.3 million barefoot doctors over the following decade (Ballweg, 1999). They were originally designed to function independently, although they were trained and supervised by local hospital medical staff.

In the United States, this concept began in the 1930s with military corpsmen. They were used in the federal prison system to extend the services of the prison physicians. During World War II, the Coast Guard trained purser mates as health care providers on merchant ships. In the late 1950s, Eugene Stead, MD, in collaboration with Thelma Ingles, who was training master's prepared nurse practitioners, developed a program at Duke University Hospital to extend nursing capabilities. Unfortunately, the National League for Nursing proposed that it was inappropriate and potentially dangerous for nurses to assume medical tasks (Bliss & Cohen, 1977) and believed it moved these nurses into the medical model and out of the nursing model (Ballweg, 1999). Therefore, accreditation of this graduate program was denied on three different occasions, and the collaboration was discontinued. This was likely the beginning of the unfortunate divide between the professions of nursing and medicine. After the dissolution of this concept, Stead went on to develop the first physician assistant program at Duke University, utilizing other clinically trained personnel, military corpsmen (Fowkes & Mentink, 1997). In 1961 the concept was introduced to the American Medical Association by Charles Hudson, MD. He proposed these individuals would work in a dependent relationship with the physician, performing procedures such as intubation, lumbar puncture, or suturing (Ballweg, 1999). Eventually, in 1965, Colorado baccalaureate nurses were trained to care for disadvantaged pediatric populations in a collaborative project by Loretta Ford, a registered nurse, and Henry Silver, a physician. This became the cornerstone for the Child Health Association PA program and the nurse practitioner movement (Ballweg, 1999). This same year, Duke University's physician assistant program accepted its first four students.

The Duke University program's philosophy was to provide education and skills similar to family physicians or internists to meet the needs of the growing health care crisis. The physician assistant was the first to penetrate the barrier around the practice of medicine and to share its knowledge base. Although nursing maintained its nursing model, a collaboration with medical knowledge finally developed.

ACT II: THE FORMATIVE YEARS

The educational process of nurse practitioners and physician assistants has many parallels. Two programs in California include nurse practitioners and physician assistants in the same curriculum. All nurse practitioners are registered nurses who have had advanced education to broaden their knowledge base and develop advanced clinical decision-making skills. Their educational focus is on health promotion and disease prevention; utilization of communication skills, counseling, and community resources; and patient education to manage disease. Since the early to mid-1960s the nursing profession has been discussing the level of education necessary for entry into practice. Over the years, nurse practitioner programs, all associated with a school of nursing, have provided several educational tracks. These are certificate, associate degree, bachelor's degree, and master's degree programs. For nurse practitioners, a master's degree in nursing soon will be the required level of education in all states. Effective January 1, 2000, national certification requires a master's degree in nursing. On January 1, 2003, the Health Care Financing Administration (HCFA) payment policy and application for a Medicare billing number will require a master's degree. Nurse practitioners without a master's in nursing will be grandfathered in some cases.

The physician assistant, as the nurse practitioner, has four different educational tracks. These include certificate programs, associate degree programs, bachelor's degree programs, and master's degree programs. Most are affiliated with medical schools. The physician assistant curriculum is the same in all four academic pathways with a concentration in primary care medicine, patient education, and utilization of community resources for underserved populations (Hammond, 1999). Current proposals for entry into practice at the master's degree level are being discussed by physician assistant organizations and their members.

Another common factor in the education of each of these providers is the crossover of the faculty. Physicians, nurse practitioners, and physician assistants provide lectures, clinical skills training, and preceptoring at all levels in both profession's programs, thus reinforcing the interrelationship of these three professions.

ACT III: ARE THEY TWINS?

Over the past several years of the author's career as a nurse practitioner and a physician assistant, there have been several comments made by her colleagues in each of the respective professions about the other profession. With more than two decades of experience as a registered nurse before becoming a nurse practitioner and physician assistant, it's saddening that most of the negative comments are made by nurse practitioners toward physician assistants. She is quick to set them straight that their comments are incorrect, explaining the two professions are similar in education and practice (Table 61-1).

Demographics

The physician assistants profession was originally a male-dominated profession composed of mostly medics from the military. This trend has changed, however, with nearly 50% of the profession men and 50% women (Grumbach et al., 2000). As described in the Fifteenth Annual Report on Physician Assistant Educational Programs in the United States, 1998-1999, the proportion of men to women students enrolled in a physician assistant program from 1983 to 1999 has remained fairly constant, with women a slight majority at 55.1% to 62.8% of the total. Alternatively, nurse practitioners are predominately women. This comes as no surprise with only 7% of registered nurses being men (Grumbach et al., 2000).

Practice Areas

In the NP/PA/CNM Report by the Office of Statewide Health Planning and Development and the Center for California Health Workforce Studies at the University of California, San Francisco, the majority of nurse practitioners and physician assistants practice primary care medicine and 39% are providing care to populations either in underserved areas of the country, county facilities, or community health centers. Nurse practitioners and physician assistants are also found practicing in other specialties such as orthopedics, pediatrics, ob/gyn, emergency medicine, and other subspecialties of internal medicine. Physician assistants are more commonly found assisting in surgery than are nurse practitioners (Grumbach et al., 2000).

TABLE 61-1 Provider Comparisons

	Nurse Practitioner	Physician Assistant
First training program	1965	1965
Education		
Certificate	Yes	Yes
Associate degree	Yes	Yes
Bachelor's degree	Yes	Yes
Master's degree	Yes	Yes
Program affiliation	Nursing school	Medical school or department of family medicine
Registered nurse	Required	Not required (many are both RN and PA)
Skills		
Patient history	Yes	Yes
Physical examination	Yes	Yes
Medical diagnosis	Yes	Yes
Treatment plan	Yes	Yes
Patient education	Yes	Yes
Community referrals	Yes	Yes
Perform procedures	Yes	Yes
Prescriptive privileges	Individual state guidelines	Individual state guidelines
Primary specialty	Family/general medicine	Family/general medicine
Physician supervision	Individual state guidelines	Yes—required in all states
Professional license	Yes—RN and NP	Yes—PA, most states
Professional certification	Not required	Required in all states to begin practice (recertification requirements per individual state guidelines)
CME recertification requirements	75 hours every 5 years	100 hours every 2 years

Certification and Licensing

Nurse practitioner programs vary in length and credentialing. Shorter programs result in an associate degree or certification only. Longer programs are usually bachelor's or master's degree programs. Any one or all three of the educational tracts may be available to a potential applicant within a state. Nurse practitioners must have a license to practice regardless of the state they live in. Licensure renewal requirements vary from state to state and are usually established by the state's Board of Registered Nursing (BRN). National certification is not required, although many nurse practitioners are certified. A nurse practitioner may be certified in any one of a variety of areas such as family practice, gerontology, pediatrics, community health, women's health, and many others. Certification is maintained with 75 hours of BRN-approved continuing educational credit hours every 5 years (Buppert, 1999b).

The licensure and certification process for a physician assistant also varies in each state. All states require a physician assistant to graduate from a program accredited by the Commission on Accreditation of Allied Health Education Programs. In addition, they must pass the arduous 6-hour Physician Assistant National Certifying Ex-

amination. Certification is renewed every 2 years by completing 100 hours of continuing medical education (CME) approved by the American Academy of Physician Assistants (AAPA, 1999). Recertification by written examination is necessary every 6 years, although some states do not require continued certification to practice. States not requiring continued certification do require documentation of completion of CME classes (Pedersen, 1999).

Managed Care

The impact of managed care on the practice of medicine and the delivery of care to patients has affected both the nurse practitioner and the physician assistant. Both professionals are recognized for their advanced skills and level of knowledge, with the ability to deliver safe and appropriate care to a variety of patients resulting in increased utilization because of these abilities and their proposed cost-effectiveness (Jones & Cawley, 1994). The focus away from a physician provider has resulted in competition for jobs among the three disciplines (Oransky & Varma, 1997; Cooper, Henderson, & Dietrich, 1998). Several studies have compared the skills and patient outcomes of these providers and found them to be similar. These studies may have been weakened by the interactive role of the physician, however, thus failing to provide a true evaluation of the independent skills of a nurse practitioner or a physician assistant. It must be realized that, according to state guidelines and the definition of a physician assistant, physician supervision is required for this professional to practice medicine (American College of Physicians, 1994). Many state guidelines allow a nurse practitioner to practice independently without physician supervision. Despite these guidelines, the majority of nurse practitioners do practice with physician supervision. In light of these state requirements and actual practice relationships, it is unclear whether an accurate comparison can be made among these three providers. Although there are many similarities among the groups, one must not forget the few but significant differences among them, their collaborative relationship, and the value that each provider's philosophical orientation can bring to a practice (Cooper, Henderson, & Dietrich, 1998). Whether a comparison of independent practice is necessary will depend on the goals for practice of each profession.

ACT IV: UNITED WE STAND

The adverse comments made by nurse practitioners pertaining to physician assistants, and physician assistants regarding nurse practitioners are counterproductive to both disciplines and give me reason for concern. Each day there are more similarities between the two professions. Their scope of practice is identical, as well as the populations they serve. The educational track is similar, with two programs in California providing training in both disciplines within the same curriculum. Even the demographics for each provider group are similar. State and federal legislation and insurance companies are recognizing the similarities between these two groups. Recent gains in prescriptive privileges have been made because of collaboration between the legislative arms of each discipline's professional organization. If the professional representatives can work together to advance both professions on a large scale, it seems reasonable to assume that individuals within each group should be able to support and assist each other within either a geographical area or an individual practice. Collaboration has already resulted in combined postgraduate educational forums. Within an individual practice, the physician assistant could assist in surgical procedures while the nurse practitioner could provide outpatient office procedures. The list of collaborative projects is limited only by one's imagination.

SUMMARY

Nurse practitioners and physician assistants are like identical twins. They look and sound the same, but there are subtle yet significant differences. And, like many twins have discovered, collaboration is much more productive. Both professions will continue to improve and be able to provide the best possible care to their patients whether there is collaboration or not. The difference will be in the speed with which these advances occur and the mood of the environment in which they occur. The experience the nursing profession has had with its antagonistic relationship with organized medicine should reinforce the need to banish any adversarial feelings between nurse practitioners and physician assistants. The goal of these two disciplines should be to strive for collaboration between the professions. Nurse practitioners and physician assistants are encouraged to recognize their common ground, embrace it and each other like the long-lost siblings they are, and reach together toward that common goal, the patient. They need to work together and with their physician colleagues to meet the patient's needs in the most effective manner possible. After all, isn't that why we all do what we do?

REFERENCES

AAPA Physician Assistant Census Report: 1999 [electronic database]. (1999). Alexandria, VA: American Academy of Physician Assistants [Producer and Distributor].

American College of Physicians. (1994). Physician assistants and nurse practitioners (position paper). *Annals of Internal Medicine, 121*(9), 714-716.

Ballweg, R. (1999). History of the profession. In R. Ballweg, S. Stolberg, & E. Sullivan (Eds.), *Physician assistant: A guide to clinical practice* (2nd ed., pp. 1-23). Philadelphia: Saunders.

Bliss, A., & Cohen, E.D. (1977). *The new health professionals: Nurse practitioners and physician assistants.* Germantown, MD: Aspen Systems Corp.

Buppert, C. (1999a). Legal scope of nurse practitioner practice. In C. Buppert (Ed.), *Nurse practitioner's business practice & legal guide* (pp. 39-103). Gaithersburg, MD: Aspen.

Buppert, C. (1999b). What is a nurse practitioner? In C. Buppert (Ed.), *Nurse practitioner's business practice & legal guide* (pp. 1-38). Gaithersburg, MD: Aspen.

Cooper, R., Henderson, T., & Dietrich, C. (1998). Roles of nonphysician clinicians as autonomous providers of patient care. *Journal of the American Medical Association, 280*(9), 795-802.

Fowkes, V., & Mentink, J. (1997). Nurses and physician assistants: Issues and challenges. In J. McCloskey & H. Grace (Eds.), *Current issues in nursing* (5th ed., pp. 545-551). St. Louis: Mosby.

Grumbach, K., Coffman, J., Mertz, E., Rosenoff, E., Gonzalez-Leiva, P., Desmarais, B., Mendoza, E., & Florida, M. (2000). *NP/PA/CNM Report.* San Francisco: University of California, San Francisco, Office of Statewide Health Planning and Development and the Center for California Health Workforce Studies.

Hammond, J. (1999). Education. In R. Ballweg, S. Stolberg, & E. Sullivan (Eds.), *Physician assistant: A guide to clinical practice* (2nd ed., pp. 24-36). Philadelphia: Saunders.

Jones, E., & Cawley, J. (1994). Physician assistants and health system reform: Clinical capabilities, practice activities, and potential roles. *Journal of the American Medical Association, 271*(16), 1266-1272.

Oransky, I., & Varma, J. (1997). Nonphysician clinicians and the future of medicine. *Journal of the American Medical Association, 277*(13), 1090-1091.

Pedersen, D. (1999). Credentialing: Accreditation, certification, and licensing. In R. Ballweg, S. Stolberg, & E. Sullivan (Eds.), *Physician assistant: A guide to clinical practice* (2nd ed., pp. 37-46). Philadelphia: Saunders.

Conflict and Collaboration

Relationships and Challenges

GAIL M. KEENAN, MARY JO KOCAN, FRANCENE LUNDY, VICTORIA AVERHART, MICHELLE AEBERSOLD

Recently a physician colleague's presidential address on the topic of nurse-physician relations appeared in the *Annals of Surgery* (Greenfield, 1999). In his remarks to the American Surgical Association, Greenfield conveyed a deep concern about the impact of a "troubled partnership" between nurses and physicians on patient care and his resolve to take action from his newly elected position. The opinions shared were based on his formal assessment of the situation and years of experience as a physician. Greenfield is to be applauded for this bold move. Heretofore the adverse impact of poor nurse-physician relations has generally gone unnoticed by physicians. Nurses, on the other hand, have long recognized the troubled partnership and have worked to improve it and written about it extensively (Aiken, 1990; Baggs, 1994; Coeling & Wilcox, 1994; Fagin, 1992; Feiger & Schmitt, 1979; Keenan, 1995; Keenan, Cooke, & Hillis, 1998; Lamb & Napadano, 1984; Pike [see Chapter 59, this text]; Prescott, Dennis, & Jacox, 1987; Weiss, 1985). Greenfield's message, however, reinforces why nurses and physicians must work together to change the relationship.

Strategies created solely by nurses or physicians just do not generate the interest and commitment of the other needed to bring about desired change in the relationship. Such efforts on the part of one professional group can be likened to the dynamic that occurs in a troubled marriage when one partner works feverishly to reconcile a relationship problem while the other is oblivious to it. There is little chance that the marriage will be improved if this dynamic operates regularly when mutual problems arise. Thus regardless of whether or not one agrees with all of Greenfield's remarks, he deserves credit for his attempts to raise physician awareness and motivation to collaborate with nurses to improve patient care. We, however, have learned through our experiences that successful collaboration requires much more than awareness and motivation.

Several years ago our group set out to improve nurse-physician relations and pilot tested an intervention that produced successful collaboration between nurse and physician clinicians. Misunderstandings, however, developed among stakeholders and created a major challenge. Subsequently, our group reflected on the experience and was energized by what we discovered. In the following chapter, we share our lessons learned and suggestions for engaging in successful collaborative partnerships.

BACKGROUND

The experiences reported are part of a larger effort that consisted of eight phases ranging from Preparatory to Dissemination (Table 62-1). Phase I began when an upper-level physician administrator approached the top-level nursing administrator of the university health system indicating a desire to improve nurse-physician communication at the patient care level. The nursing administrator then held a series of meetings with the physician and the nursing director responsible for that division to establish what "improved communication" should look like and how it might be achieved. When a clear idea and plan failed to materialize over a period of time, the nurses involved took additional steps to move forward. A subgroup was formed consisting of the nursing director of surgical units, the director of nursing research, two nurse managers, and two clinical specialists. Building on the previous discussions, the subgroup decided it would be fruitful to do a research study and began to lay the groundwork for this. During this time, a nurse scientist and new member of the university's school of nursing was approached by the director of nursing research and asked to participate in the project study. The nurse scientist agreed to contribute her expertise and by so doing extend her doctoral and postdoctoral work on collaboration. This began phase II.

TABLE 62-1   Project Phases

Project Phase	Description
Phase I: Preparatory	Initial activities of parties interested in improving nurse-physician communication that led to the study (phases II through VIII) on two surgical units
Phase II: Planning	Study designed to produce and evaluate effectiveness of formal collaboration between nurse and physician clinicians on each unit
Phase III: Baseline Assessment	Data collected to determine the baseline status of nurse-to-nurse, physician-to-physician, and nurse-to-physician communication and identify problems of mutual concern to colleagues who provided care on each unit
Phase IV: Intervention—Task groups convened	Small, expert-facilitated, nurse-physician task group convened for each unit and charged (time limited to four 2-hour sessions) to: • Reach agreement on a problem of mutual concern • Develop a solution to the problem • Develop implementation plan • Select an evaluation mechanism
Phase V: Evaluation of intervention process	Immediate postintervention assessment of task group member satisfaction with intervention process
Phase VI: Implementation of task group solution	Implementation of task group's solution, the 6-month period following the end of each task group's formal meetings
Phase VII: Evaluation of intervention effectiveness	6 months after intervention, baseline survey repeated, status of task group solution evaluated, data analyzed, and results interpreted
Phase VIII: Dissemination	Results reported, distributed, and applied

The nurse researcher met regularly with the nursing director, nurse managers, and clinical specialists of the two study units who had been members of the subgroup. This group of six members became the study team and together developed and coordinated the research activities of phases II through VII. Building on the nurse scientist's research, the group designed an intervention to assist nurses and physicians to collaborate with each other on an issue of common concern. The ultimate goal of the intervention was to orchestrate a situation that would demonstrate to clinicians that nurse-physician collaboration is both possible and desirable.

The study design consisted of a pretest, intervention, and posttest (Table 62-2). Phase III was the pretest period in which the perceived quality of communication within and between nurses and physicians who worked together on a given unit was assessed. The intervention, phase IV, involved the use of a task group consisting of an expert facilitator, two nurses, and two physicians. The specific charge of a task group was to select an issue from a peer-identified list and develop and implement a solution to the issue. The facilitator was responsible for assisting the group to develop a workable solution to a problem that both groups would feel had been achieved through compromise and collaboration.

TABLE 62-2   Design and Data Collection Points of Nurse-Physician Collaboration Study

	Baseline Survey	Appointment of Task Group	Intervention/Task Group Meetings (Four 2-Hour Sessions)	Evaluation Satisfaction with Intervention Process (Immediately After Intervention)	Evaluation Intervention Effectiveness (6 Months After Intervention)
Work Group A	X	X			X
		Task Group A	X	X	X
Work Group B	X	X			X
		Task Group B	X	X	X

Work Group A = All nurse and physician clinicians of unit A.
Work Group B = All nurse and physician clinicians of unit B.
Task Group A = Two nurses and two physicians from Work Group A.
Task Group B = Two nurses and two physicians from Work Group B.

TABLE 62-3   Nurse and Physician Type of Involvement by Employment Category

	Nursing Top Management	Nursing Upper Management	Nursing Line Management	Nursing Clinicians*	Nursing Scientist	Medicine Top Management	Medicine Upper Management	Medicine Line Management	Medicine Clinicians
Phase I	D	D	D	D	—	—	D	—	—
Phase II	I	D	D	D	D	—	I	I	—
Phase III	I	I	I	D	D	—	I	I	D
Phase IV	I	I	I	D	D	—	—	I	D
Phase V	I	I	I	D	I	—	—	I	D
Phase VI	I	I	I	D	D	—	—	I	D
Phase VII	I	D	D	D	D	—	I	I	I

Key: D = direct involvement; I = indirect involvement; — = no involvement.
*Includes staff nurses and clinical nurse specialists.

Nurses and physicians were carefully selected to participate in a task group and possessed the following qualifications: motivation to collaborate, excellent reputation as a clinician, known as an informal leader, and comfortable with expressing disagreement. Meetings were videotaped, limited to four 2-hour sessions, and held off-site. In phase V, member satisfaction with task group process was evaluated immediately following the final task group meeting. Phase VI was the 6-month period following the task group work, during which the group's solution was implemented on the unit. An evaluation, phase VII, of the effectiveness of the intervention was carried out at 6-month posttask group meetings and included assessments of work group compliance with the task group's plan and impact on work group communication. Data were analyzed in preparation for dissemination of findings in phase VIII.

During the eight phases of the overall project, the mix of participants on the full project team and the type and level of their involvement varied (Table 62-3). Top- and upper-level management were more directly involved in phase I and less so thereafter. Nurse and physician clinicians and line managers, those closest to the issue, were naturally more heavily involved in phases II through VII. The nurse scientist assumed primary responsibility for the activities of phases II through VII, believing this was the expectation of project leaders and commensurate with her expertise. She secured external funds to support the study and prepared and submitted the materials required for institutional review board (IRB) approval to protect study subjects. She prepared and coordinated distribution of study surveys, located space and scheduled task group meetings, hired the group facilitator, and videotaped all task group sessions. When the study was completed, the nurse researcher conducted preliminary analyses of the data and distributed the information in a series of reports to study team members and project ad-

ministrators. She then participated in a study team presentation of findings to physician and nurse administrators of the full project team.

Study team members supported the nurse researcher with numerous aspects of the research. In phase II they provided historical context information and assisted with locating subject names and addresses, acquainting subjects with the study, and distributing surveys. In preparation for phase III, group members helped to identify and recruit appropriate nurse and physician task group members. The managers and clinical specialists were also instrumental in adjusting staffing to accommodate nurse task group members' participation in meetings at the designated times. Their level of commitment to the study was demonstrated on the occasion when a study unit was in extreme crisis and in need of the help of a task group member during a prescheduled meeting. The nurse manager and clinical specialist of the unit, recognizing the importance of the nurse's presence at the meeting, worked diligently to ensure the nurse's attendance at the meeting. The study team also assisted with editing the letter and consent forms sent to the IRB and attended to internal communication to project members outside the core group.

LESSONS LEARNED FROM THE STUDY INTERVENTION
What Worked Well

The intervention was successful for both task groups. Each addressed the issue of streamlining day-to-day communication flow between nurses and physicians but tailored the solution to fit the unit environment and culture. One developed a structured face-to-face rounding solution, and the other developed a written method of communicating patient information between nurses and physicians on centrally located clipboards. Both solutions remain in place today. Task group participants reported high satisfaction with the process and outcomes of their meetings and indicated an eagerness to participate in the same type of group in the future. Also noted was an increase in the quality of communication among task group members in the clinical setting that facilitated discussion and resolution of patient-related issues.

There were a number of factors that contributed to these positive outcomes. The issues addressed by the task groups had a direct impact on their collective work and had been selected from previously compiled lists of colleagues' suggestions. All members of the task groups were motivated to participate in the group and pleased with the meeting arrangements. The four sessions were held off-site in a friendly atmosphere where food was served and distractions were limited. A facilitator and ground rules were in place to balance member input and maintain focus on the group charge, relieving members of the responsibility for coordinating and directing the meetings. Meetings were held only if all members were in attendance. The rule had been invoked to emphasize the importance of each member's contribution and eliminate the need to reorient an absent member at a subsequent meeting. The rule was easy to administer because there were only five participants to a task group, and each recognized the importance of the rule.

The nurse manager, clinical specialist, and physician specialty administrator of a unit directly supported task team activities. This support was particularly important in phase VI, Implementation of Task Group Solution. Although overtly simple, the solutions required educating numerous clinicians, encouraging their compliance with the procedures, and troubleshooting until the mechanism was firmly established. Members of a respective task group, the nurse manager, clinical specialist, and the physician, collectively assumed responsibility for these tasks. Their collective efforts were no doubt instrumental to solution compliance and in large part explain why the solutions remain in place today.

The study provided a golden opportunity for team members to focus on the numerous constraints to effective nurse-physician communication and collaboration within the hospital setting. Nurses and physicians generally do not understand the nature of each other's work. Moreover, the structure of care in the fast-paced environment of the hospital setting frequently results in nurses and physicians not knowing or communicating with each other. Communication and understanding, however, are the foundation to effective collaboration. Nurses and physicians therefore must be given the time and support to engage in dialogue that will lead to successful collaboration. The intervention tested in this study effectively addressed the gap.

What Needs Improvement

In the evaluation of the intervention, the study team reflected on what might be done better when repeating the intervention. It was noted that although task groups were provided a list from which to select a problem of focus, an inordinate amount of time was dedicated to isolating the problem area. The study team recommended that whenever possible, the task group's charge should be made as specific as possible to reduce the time needed by the group to refine a focus. This, however, need not preclude the use of the task group as a mechanism to isolate a problem that might later be addressed by another task group. Another area that might be improved is staff awareness of task group activities. In the evaluation it was found that most of the clinicians were unaware that their colleagues designed the new communication tool that had been instituted. Thus members were also unaware that successful nurse-physician collaboration had taken place. It is suggested that efforts be directed at promoting awareness through regular updates to clinicians and by soliciting their input to inform task group work. Moreover, showcasing the specific contributions of physicians and nurses to task group solutions could further enhance staff buy-in and provide visible proof that collaboration improves patient care.

LESSONS LEARNED FROM STUDY TEAM ACTIVITIES
What Worked Well

It is clear that the work completed in the Preparatory phase was critical and instrumental in laying the groundwork needed to develop and implement the study successfully. The need and desire to improve nurse-physician communication was first introduced by upper management and, at the time this study began, had appropriately filtered to the level closest to the problem, the primary work unit of nurses and physicians. The study team had been empowered to take action as they saw fit without the intense scrutiny of upper management. Members of the team had been included in the early project work and therefore recognized the support of upper management and were motivated to carry out the full project team's intentions. Thus as phase II began, it appeared to all involved parties that this was a golden opportunity for practice and research to partner on a common interest and capitalize on each other's perspectives and expertise.

What Needs Improvement

As was noted earlier, all study team members were deeply motivated to work together to improve nurse-physician collaboration from the onset. The nurse researcher, the newest member of the team, reported having felt clear about her role on the project from the start. She believed that she would meet her own interest and that of the project team by assisting them to implement a strategy that improved nurse-physician collaboration. Not fully understood at the time, however, was the powerful impact that various stakeholders' norms and perspectives would have on team processes and relations over time. Tension between the nurse researcher and other study team members began to surface during phase VII, the 6-month postintervention evaluation and data analyses period. It may be recalled that the nurse scientist had assumed responsibility for data analyses and had reported results in pooled form to maintain subject confidentiality. Study team members who represented the different units in the pilot were naturally interested in examining unit level data. The nurse researcher declined this request, feeling that the response sets were such that the release of unit-specific data would threaten to violate subject confidentiality. The other members of the study team disagreed and felt that unit-level information would not violate confidentiality on some of the response sets. Eventually, the researcher did release some unit-specific data that did not violate confidentiality. By this time, however, the researcher had completely exhausted the study resources and was frustrated by the circumstances.

Further misunderstandings occurred when the study team members presented findings to the full project team. Unbeknownst to the researcher at the time, members of the full project team were upset with the nurse researcher for not including the names of all team members on her slides and handouts. Several months later, top- and upper-level nursing administrators on the project team met with the researcher. In the meeting they firmly reiterated their prior requests for the study data and also asked that the researcher assist the team in preparing a related manuscript. In addition, the researcher was told that her behavior in the presentation had been offensive. The researcher explained that she could not release the data and that there were no resources available for further work. She felt the team had no right to make further demands on her time. Deeply hurt by the incident, she withdrew from the relationship.

After a sustained time the study team reopened communication, having recognized a common desire among members to pursue a more favorable outcome. Both sides had felt the adverse impact of the separation. During the year-and-a-half period, dissemination of findings was halted, work to build knowledge in the area ceased, and the team received no positive reinforcement for their accomplishments. Ironically the experience provided the nurse researcher an opportunity to identify firsthand conditions under which forcefully asserting one's own position may be counter to one's goals. In her dissertation on nurse-physician conflicts, Keenan (1995) had examined the circumstances under which nurses favored being proactive in asserting their ideas. She found that two types of norms were associated with nurses' preferences for using the proactive conflict management styles in physician-nurse scenarios: (1) achievement oriented and affiliative and (2) power oriented and oppositional. On the basis of these findings, Keenan recommended training and supporting nurses to use forceful and confrontational behaviors to promote their ideas with physicians. This suggestion, however, was specifically directed at replacing the ineffective traditional pattern of nurse deference toward the physician with one that was more effective. As the study team learned, the use of forceful and confrontational behaviors is not always appropriate and may create major adverse consequences if it is viewed to be out of line with the receiver's normative expectations.

Another revelation for the team was that all stakeholders did not and could not have been expected to understand fully the other's interests at the onset. The team processes were dynamic and most facets of the study gradually unfolded over time. Consequently, the data interests of the study team only became clearer across time. In retrospect, no one could have easily predicted the conflict that developed around the data and subject confidentiality. So, too, the researcher could not have been expected to correctly estimate the magnitude of the interest of the top-level nursing administrator who intervened directly into team conflict during phase VII. It was also not clear from the onset that the researcher's willingness to assume responsibilities for a majority of the study details would result in members' inability to appreciate fully the scope of this effort.

The group learned a number of lessons through reflection on the team's processes. First, reflection was a valuable exercise and helped members uncover what went wrong and why. The experience raised awareness of the need for project members to be clear in their communication with each other, define terms, explain intent, and outline roles, responsibilities, and authority. Equally important is for individual members to take responsibility for seeking clarification of others' words and intentions when these are unclear. Persons with different perspectives do not always know when others perceive them to be unclear. The most important lesson learned, however, was that it is prudent to expect conflict to occur within groups comprised of diverse stakeholders and to be prepared to handle conflict constructively when it arises. Serious conflict was not anticipated by the team and consequently was poorly managed, resulting in the breakdown that occurred. It was agreed that, although the exact nature of the conflict could not have been foreseen, the development of conflict within the group was predictable. It thus is recommended that individuals who intend to work together agree at the onset on a conflict management process that they will use to manage disagreements as they arise. The study team subsequently adopted such a process to assist members to handle differences and misunderstandings constructively.

SUMMARY

The study team's experiences have thoroughly acquainted members with the complexities and challenges of communication and multilevel, multistakeholder collaboration. Numerous stakeholder perspectives were represented on the full project team including managerial, clinical, academic, professional, and multiple combinations of the aforementioned. Collaboration in theory is desirable because the process is directed at combining individual perspectives and expertise into a whole that is much greater than the sum of the parts. Thus, differences are the foundation of effective collaboration. As the team discovered, however, weaving the multiple differences into a cohesive whole is the major challenge. A lesson learned from the study intervention was that controlling the process of collaboration is associated with positive outcomes. Building on this lesson, the team decided to adopt a formal collaborative process to more effectively manage group member differences and conflicts. Several members of the team had used a process called mutual gains to manage differing group interests (Moore, 2000). The team engaged in this process to decide how to proceed and have adopted it as the formal process to be used to address conflicts that arise within the study team in the future.

Mutual gains is based on the win-win strategy outlined by Fischer and Ury (1991) of the Harvard Negotiation Project. The objective of the strategy is to resolve problems together. Interests of parties are the central focus rather than positions. A position is something decided on, whereas interests are the desires and concerns

behind positions that motivate people. Fischer and Ury maintain that looking at interests makes it possible to find solutions that meet mutual needs.

The mutual gains process adopted by the study team includes three successive rounds of discussion with corresponding decision points. The first level involves the identification and ranking of topics. For example, the team members participated in this exercise to determine how they might move forward together on the project. A number of topics were generated by members and then ranked to determine the topic of greatest interest to members. The topic ranked the highest by the study team was dissemination of findings. This topic was moved to the second round of discussions that entailed explicating each party's interests in the topic. Fisher and Ury pointed out the importance of being aware, however, that individuals are not always conscious of their interests and oftentimes need encouragement and support to disclose their interests. Sensitivity coupled with consistently asking why and why not questions facilitates this process. In the study team exercise the following interests were identified:

- Package and market the intervention process used in the study
- Write and publish additional articles about the study
- Repeat the intervention on the same units focusing on different problems
- Repeat the study focusing on different problems and collect additional types of data
- Share the intervention and process with colleagues in the institution
- Make the work of the project and outcomes more visible
- Celebrate our success

Once interests have been explicated, the group moves to a third round of discussions. The round involves the identification of options to meet interests and a consensus decision on the options to pursue. Participants are directed to concentrate on inventing solutions that meet one's own interest and the interests of the others. Members of the study team developed a series of plausible options to meet parties' expressed interests. The following were some of these options:

- Generate a list of potential target publications
- Schedule a four-hour block of time to develop a publication strategy
- Schedule a time for a dinner party to celebrate our success

- Develop a standard "road show" to roll out the intervention and process hospitalwide and at the school
- Nurse scientist to produce rough draft of data analysis article and circulate among team members for review, input, and coauthorship
- Schedule a second meeting to identify a new study and topic
- Study team to collaborate on producing first data analysis publication

The final step in the mutual gains process is to connect options to interests and then collectively decide on what option or combination is feasible and one all members can embrace. The consensus decision arrived at by the study team was, "*Schedule a 4-hour block of time to develop a publication and presentation strategy and celebrate our success.*" Members also agreed to prepare and distribute material prior to the meeting to improve the efficiency of the session.

As we have outlined, our group originally convened with the purpose of improving nurse-physician communication and collaboration at the patient care level. We successfully achieved this goal, but in the process learned the challenges of communication and collaboration with members of our own team. Unfortunately we failed to manage the conflict that subsequently occurred before it resulted in damage to our relationship. Fortunately we persisted in trying to heal the relationship and to move forward through the use of the mutual gains process. We recommend this process, outlined above, to others as a way of improving group effectiveness.

REFERENCES

Aiken, L.H. (1990). Charting hospital nursing. *Image: Journal of Nursing Scholarship, 22*(2), 72-78.

Baggs, J.G. (1994). Development of an instrument to measure collaboration and satisfaction about care decisions. *Journal of Advanced Nursing, 20,* 176-182.

Coeling, H.V., & Wilcox, J.R. (1994). Steps to collaboration. *Nursing Administration Quarterly, 18,* 44-55.

Fagin, C.M. (1992). Collaboration between nurses and physicians no longer a choice. *Nursing and Health Care, 13*(7), 354-363.

Feiger, S.M., & Schmitt, M.H. (1979). Collegiality in interdisciplinary health teams: Its measurement and its effects. *Science and Medicine, 13*(A), 217-229.

Fischer, R., & Ury, W. (1991). *Getting to yes* (3rd ed.). New York: Penguin Books.

Greenfield, L. (1999). Doctor and nurses: A troubled partnership. *Annals of Surgery, 230*(3), 279-288.

Keenan, G. (1995). Nurse management of conflicts with physicians in emergency rooms. *Dissertation Abstracts International* (9B), 3817. (University Microfilms No. 9506547.)

Keenan, G., Cooke, R., & Hillis, S. (1998). Norms and nurse management of conflict: Keys to understanding nurse-physician collaboration. *Research in Nursing and Health, 21,* 59-72.

Lamb, G.S., & Napadano, R.J. (1984). Physician-nurse practitioner interaction patterns in primary care practices. *American Journal of Public Health, 74,* 26-29.

Moore, P. (2000). Resolutions Incorporated, 34 Holyoke Street, Suite 200, Boston, MA 02116.

Prescott, P.A., Dennis, K.E., & Jacox, A.K. (1987). Clinical decision making of staff nurses. *Image: Journal of Nursing Scholarship, 19,* 56-62.

Weiss, S.J. (1985). The influence of discourse on collaboration among nurses, physicians, and consumers. *Research in Nursing and Health, 8,* 49-59.

Some Reflections on Conflict Resolution in Nursing

The Implications of Negotiating at an Uneven Table

PHYLLIS BECK KRITEK

If one were to inquire among practicing nurses about their familiarity with conflict, the responses, ranging from anguish to hilarity, would document something so pervasive that nurses frequently fail even to call the presence by its name: conflict. They may tell you about their most recent experience with conflict, the difficulties they have experienced, and the outcomes they have achieved, charged alternately with chagrin or triumph. They would not, however, customarily open the dialogue by asking, "Have I told you about my latest conflict?" The presence of conflict in the work life of the practicing nurse is so endemic and integral it is simply not labeled as conflict. More often, it is simply perceived as a given, perhaps even a central fiber, in the tapestry of professional nursing activity.

Asked to document the locus of conflict, the list would be long and comprehensive: patients, families, other nurses, administrators, physicians, other health care providers, third-party payers, persons controlling access to services, alternative care institutions, professional organizations, the maintenance man in charge of light bulb replacement, the ambulance driver, the list can seem endless. If you ask nurses how they resolve these conflicts, their responses show equally rich variance, ranging from a serious reply about negotiation to descriptions of aggressive action or covert manipulation to a wink about who really knows "what's going on in this place!"

It is therefore not surprising that when you invite a group of nurses to learn more about conflict resolution, their eyes often glaze over and they drift to the next option on their menu. After managing conflict each day, as best one can, and feeling stressed or overwhelmed by the magnitude of the task, one does not welcome platitudinous advice that lacks awareness of the complexity of the problems nurses confront or, alternately, that provides a set of useful provisions that may disrupt the current carefully crafted and sustained practices of a given nurse. It is not a place where we go seeking advice, counsel, and the opportunity for transformative change.

These, too, are commonplaces that most nurses recognize when I describe them in workshops on conflict resolution: Nurses know what I mean and they readily see themselves in this picture. The commonplaces themselves warrant some reflection. More concretely, Why is so much of a nurse's day focused on conflict? Why are nurses expected to or expecting themselves to resolve conflicts in their work environments? Whose conflict is it? and Why are nurses so reluctant to subject their models of conflict management to scrutiny? Do nurses manage conflict or resolve it? More subtly, are the models of conflict management that nurses use those that deal with the temporary flare-up and fail in the long run to address more substantive issues? If this is true, even part of the time, what are the substantive issues nurses fail to address? Why do they fail to address them? Can or will any of this change? If so, how?

These are the questions that led me along a personal path that involved training in conflict resolution during a National Kellogg Leadership Fellowship, giving me an opportunity to study with some of the key national leaders in conflict resolution in the United States. This fellowship has resulted both in a book on conflict resolution that explores the nature of uneven tables (Kritek, 1994) and in the redirection of much of my energy toward the field of conflict resolution. It seemed to me then, as now, that the noble ideals and commitments of practicing nurses get twisted and sullied in the world of conflict management as they live it. I was in search of some tools that might help, and it was my hope to share those tools with other nurses. The journey has been instructive.

Part of the journey has involved interdisciplinary study, training, dialogue, writing, and collaboration, resulting in a second book with my collaborators (Marcus, Dorn, Kritek, Miller, & Wyatt, 1995). The experiences that resulted in that book have shaped me in myriad ways, taught me lessons that Walt Disney's Pocahontas would say "I never knew I never knew." I have also had the opportunity to teach my collaborators things they did not know. Together, we have struggled and celebrated our way through the morass of health care conflicts and wondered that we are able to do so much good in the midst of so much conflict. We have been able to bring diverse groups of health care providers together to resolve conflicts, to study conflict resolution, and to become negotiators of health care conflicts. It has been gratifying work and has unveiled for me the windows on conflict that others have—windows that in some ways are not unlike those nurses look through yet in other ways differ dramatically.

Part of the journey has, however, been more solitary and involved the reflective effort to think through the nature of conflict for the practicing nurse. I have listened to and studied the stories of nurses and have heard conflict descriptions from a variety of situations and perspectives. Some things seem consistent. A large number of practicing nurses see the management of conflict as a central dimension of their job. When it shows up, they feel obligated to do something about it; nurses do not ignore conflict. In addition, competent practicing nurses, if they create conflict, tend to have lengthy explanations for why they did so; they do not create conflict lightly and their reasons tend to tap into important values and passions. Most interesting to me, however, is that these same nurses accept that all sorts of other folks appropriately create conflicts for them to resolve. It is simply accommodated, like moon cycles and deciduous trees. It can leave the uncomprehending listener with the sense that the competent professional nurse is a conflict magnet. Concurrently, one senses that this conflict magnet is also fairly conflict-aversive, creating conflicts only as a last resort while identifying and busily smoothing over everyone else's conflicts as quickly and expeditiously as possible.

There are some tempting platitudes that emerge: It is because nurses are women, or socialized to be conflict-aversive, or essentially conservative, or primarily healers, or inherently nurturant. These seem to me to beg the question. Such platitudes are also further confounded by the recent emergence of nursing manager elites, nurses who perceive their role in nursing as leaders but who more often appear to struggle to achieve some identification with the control-management-success idiom of our culture, sometimes with a frenzy. Much as our histories of science, theory, education, and research have emerged from imitations of other groups we perceive as "correct" or "successful," we now have a generation of nursing manager elites who mimic the prevailing discourse of the organizational and business idiom. Many of the members of this elite group appear to be neither nurturant nor healing nor conflict-aversive. Indeed, they are increasingly identified by some practicing nurse groups as the locus of new, sometimes more pernicious, conflicts.

A disclaimer may prove helpful here. These are observationally based generalization, the musings of a thoughtful student of the culture of nursing in the United States. They are meant neither to condemn nor condone. I view neither as useful investments of my energy. Rather, they raise questions and activate my curiosity. Exactly what is nursing's relationship with conflict? Why is it so pervasive in our nursing culture? What do we intend to do about it? Do we like our solution?

The first and perhaps most difficult observation that compels me through this exploration is the honest recognition that the values, beliefs, hopes, and dreams of nurses and their convictions about what ensures health, wholeness, and healing for humans is not the prevailing world view guiding health care decision making in the United States, nor has it been for the life span of even the oldest among us. We have spent a good deal of time and energy as a health care subculture contesting this fact, trying to assure ourselves that someday our world view will prevail or sneaking it in the back door, but the reality is that the world Nightingale envisioned is not the overriding perspective guiding health care decision making. An equally compelling honest recognition is the fact that as a collective of health care providers, while we are the group with the largest numbers, we are at least second and often third and fourth to other groups in health care when it comes to status, power to control outcomes, income, influence, and the freedom to exercise moral agency. Because these are measures of import in the larger social system, clearly knowing our position in the health care hierarchy (and it is a hierarchy, no matter how nervously we wish otherwise) is a critical insight.

These seem truisms to me, yet I am continually amazed at the number of nurses who become uncomfortable confronting them. They of course lead to the next worrisome observation: Given our scope of impact on health care and the critical role we play in people's lives, we would be wise to admit honestly that we are disadvantaged in negotiating health care conflicts, and that disadvantage is one that just about everyone but nurses consents to and intends to sustain. This, in short, makes us aptly described as a group that is systematically discriminated against. There are implications for this in the land of conflict and its resolution.

Although much has been developed over the last 30 years on the behaviors that emerge from systematic discrimination, I think few writings capture the candor of Allport's (1958) early work on the theme. He noted that groups that are systematically discriminated against can become either intropunitive or extropunitive. It has seemed to me that nurse "smoother overs" are behaving in a fairly intropunitive fashion and nurse "elite controllers" are acting in an extropunitive fashion. This is an oversimplified distinction, but it helps one to begin to understand some of the most overt dimensions of nurse-managed conflict. The former use an array of manipulative tools to contain conflict and keep themselves in a state of relative, albeit compromised, safety from what they perceive as external threats. The latter become party to and members in the external threats to the best of their ability. In both cases, pleasing powerful others may be the most compelling motive. Likewise, the simple effort to diminish the discomfort associated with conflict is more compelling than some honest recognition of the nature of the conflict and some honest effort to responsibly identify, address, experience, explore, and resolve the conflict. Consequently it is sustained. Accommodation is not resolution, and it is not transformative.

It is not my interest, in confronting these givens in the world of nursing, to engage in the country's current inclination to blame some evil other or to excuse inappropriate personal behaviors with elaborate explanations of abuse by others. I further do not wish to be party to the trivialization of the real pain and struggle involved in systematic oppression. There is some tenuous path of balance in this exploration that is difficult to achieve, but it is my goal. I am convinced that the game victims and victimizers play is a dangerous and pathological one, and I am not interested in playing. I am interested in alternatives.

This returns me to my interest in conflict resolution, one of the few tools I have been able to locate that provides me with a potential pathway to an alternative. The first and most obvious option confronting nurses is to learn what experts in the field are doing these days. The literature is ample; workshops abound. For the curious

reader who wants to begin the process, I can comfortably recommend those I find most useful and acceptable to nurses. Fisher and Ury's classic *Getting to Yes: Negotiating Agreement without Giving In* (1981) is always a good starting point. Moore's (1986) comprehensive and morally sensitive discussion of the mediation process is the one I find most congruent with nursing's values. Ury's *Getting Past No: Negotiating with Difficult People* (1991) seems to have a particular appeal for the kinds of conflicts nurses confront. These are useful tools and can activate a learning process. They will guide you to more demanding texts if your curiosity peaks.

Merely absorbing the guidance from expert others, however, seems to me only a partial solution. Indeed, it can easily become one more case of imitating the "correct" or "successful" others without an honest scrutiny of fit with nursing's unique realities. None of the books I have studied in conflict resolution honestly confronts the issue of systematic discrimination and the intent to sustain it, which is the focus of my book. The struggle to find these alternative perspectives and articulating them is for me the more compelling and fascinating task in any honest exploration of conflict in health care.

Because I am by inclination and gifts a nurse philosopher, these alternatives are for me first embedded in philosophical discourse. Because the descriptor nurse is central to my approach to philosophy, these alternatives are necessarily focused on action, on the practical and the pragmatic meaning of my philosophical discourse, here and now, with real nurses doing real nursing today. Those two perspectives make me reluctant to be prescriptive for others without a basket of disclaimers, so the alternatives are for me personal ones I can elect to share with others in an honest fashion but without the presumptive hook that they must then change or elect to do things my way.

SOME REFLECTIONS OF THE PHILOSOPHER

When I slogged through my doctoral education in the late 1970s, Kuhn's (1970) insights had not yet infected the programmatic discourse, and I was left feeling assaulted by a picture of reality that was deeply incongruent with portions of the reality I knew. The received view was still alive and well in nursing, and those of us slow to embrace that view were a troublesome lot, resistive to the thrills of certitude and finality. As I prepared to develop a doctoral program, however, Kuhn came to my aid, along with Rorty (1979), Gale (1979), Laudan (1977), Reason and Rowan (1981), and a host of others. Postmodernism was edging its way into the nursing dialogue.

It is still edging, from what I can tell. Toulmin (1990) more recently has completed an analysis of the origins and potential future of modernity. He posits that the first phase of modernity was actually the Renaissance with its distinctively humanistic focus, and the second, the more familiar referent, the Cartesian era we call the Enlightenment. He posits that postmodernism can also be referred to as the third phase or modernism, where the promise of both the Renaissance and the Cartesian era will serve as a springboard to something new in the next millennium. The next generation of doctoral students in nursing will chew on this menu.

His analysis is noteworthy, however, because he delineates four distinct shifts that occurred during the transition from the Renaissance to the Enlightenment eras: from the oral to the written, from the particular to the general, from the local to the universal, and from the timely to the timeless. He then posits some bringing together of these perspectives in the future. In describing this future, one of his contentions is that "scientific inquiry will increasingly shift from abstract laws of universal application to particular decipherments of the complex structures and detailed processes embodied in concrete aspects of nature" (Toulmin, 1990, p. 204). I hope he's right. Certainly all the evidence says that's where we're headed, and that can only be good news for nurses since the unique worldview they bring to our culture is not the prevailing one. The prevailing view is, of course, deeply Cartesian in character, even when it tries not to be. We are creatures of habit and we are having a good deal of difficulty letting go. Nurses intuitively seem to know that the Cartesian world view has served us well, and is also limited in its applicability to all that can be known.

Anderson (1995), who has compiled a wonderful collection of readings on postmodernism, attempts to draft an efficient map of the evolutionary path from premodernity through modernity and into postmodernity. With the arrival of postmodernity, he posits that there are now "at least four distinguishable worldviews," each with a distinct culture and an epistemology (p. 110). He describes them as follows: (1) the postmodern-ironist, which sees truth as socially constructed; (2) the scientific-rational, in which truth is "found" through methodical, disciplined inquiry; (3) the social-traditional, in which truth is found in the heritage of American and Western civilizations; and (4) the neoromantic, in which truth is found either through attaining harmony with nature or spiritual exploration of the inner self. Each of these views has its own set of truths and its own ideas about what

truth is—where and how you look for it, how you test it, and how you prove it.

By now you may be wondering if I got lost in the philosophy section of the library; what has this to do with nursing and conflict? All of these world views are active in nursing in the United States today and shape our dialogue both among ourselves and with others who are equally diverse. Most of us, however, were neither educated nor trained to live in a pluralistic world without certainty, fraught with ambiguity, and awash in social constructs where we are unable to locate the social constructors and take them to task for their products. Indeed we are the constructors and the products, and this worries us some. Anderson (1995) posits that the postmodernists "are the wave of the future, the people you want to study to see where the world is going" (p. 115). He notes that "some people seem to be completely organized around one way of understanding truth, are deeply threatened by the others, and repress their own tendencies to wander into the forbidden worlds of postmodernism or neo-romanticism" (p. 115). He concludes that the optimal location, knowing we are all slowly becoming postmodernists, is multilingualism, being "able to think rationally and understand science, able to appreciate and draw on a social heritage, and able to drink from the well of ecological and spiritual feeling that is being tapped by new-romanticism" (p. 116).

As I noted, all these perspectives abide in nursing. Indeed, the competent balanced nurse distinguishes himself or herself by being multilingual in exactly this way. In this sense we are a bit of a national resource because we have somehow been working at keeping all four of these perspectives concurrently alive in the body politic, with compelling reasons for all four. We seem un-self-conscious of the richness, unable to get enough distance from ourselves to think of ourselves as valuable. In addition, we often collapse before the pressure by one or another external authority to treat the four world views as if they were some sort of competition in which one must prevail. This propensity for edging backward is characteristic of humans dealing with monumental change. Indeed, Toulmin (1990) posits that the 1980s in this country were "a time for nostalgia rather than imagination" (p. 205), a longing look backward in search of an illusion of certainty that is no longer available. This requires a bit of compassion for us all.

This is the context for conflict in health care today. It is an attempt to provide an alternative forest, where the trees of managed care or the leaves of a physician or pharmacist do not distract us unduly from the actual process we are collectively experiencing and the reasons for its discontents. In particular, most of the humans cutting their path through this change were taught to believe that being right was imperative and that there was only one right answer. This equips us poorly for postmodernity. When the issues at stake are or seem to be life-and-death issues, the stakes go up. We would be wise to assume conflict will endure and even worsen on occasion as we struggle culturally through this morass to the future we are collectively birthing, sometimes against our will.

Pulling these threads together, it seems to me nurses would be wise to become a bit more conscious and self-aware about the global, national, local, and institutional contexts in which the conflicts they confront occur. We find an ease in the extremely local and personal aspects that make us lose contact with the bigger picture, which might serve us well. In addition, we might be startled to find that we are skillful at analyzing conflicts in part because we are a fairly multilingual lot, schooled through education and experience in all four world views and living out some nervous tension of them as best we can. We might further take the daring leap of thinking of ourselves not so much as persons who alternately smooth over or polarize conflicts to people uniquely equipped in some dimensions to creatively and constructively assist in the resolution of these conflicts. That could be good news for everyone.

SOME REFLECTIONS OF THE PRAGMATIST

Which raises the obvious question: If we have these gifts and insights, why aren't we using them more constructively? The postmodernists would have us survey the current language systems that inform our understanding of human behavior gone awry. Today in the United States, this idea is most often reflected in a body of literature that springs from the self-help movement. Any casual trip though a local bookstore will document this fact. While the established health care community flounders with regard to the vagaries of human behavior, hoping to reduce all manner of human vulnerabilities to simple physical phenomena, the public has crafted and implemented an enormous structure designed to address the real problems of real humans today. Where we have failed, self-help groups have done strikingly successful things. Using this paradigm for understanding our reluctance to solve our own struggles with conflict management might prove useful. Its most powerful voice is the 12-step types of program groups.

In November 1989 the *American Journal of Nursing* published an article by Hall and Wray entitled "Codependency: Nurses Who Give Too Much." The article did not cause a national moment of self-honesty, although it might have been good news if it had. I admire Hall and Wray for raising the issue so candidly. The codependency literature itself often identifies nurses as a specific group trained and reinforced to be codependent. It is unquestionably part of my education, and I find it unwise to ignore this fact. I also believe I have never worked in an organization among nurses where the insights of Schaef and Fassel (1988) describing the addictive organization didn't fit.

I bring up this topic with some trepidation. There are dimensions to this literature and to the proponents who espouse it that are deeply uncomfortable for me: too facile, too dogmatic, too simplistic, too prescriptive. As a good postmodernist willing to look at emerging neoromantic world views, however, I have elected to tackle this powerful voice-shaping public life. Whitfield (1991), one of my preferred authors on the topic, posits that multiple definitions of codependence are desirable but provides this description, among others, that has served me well: "We become codependent when we turn our responsibility for our life and happiness over to our ego (our false self) and to other people" (p. 3). I like this description because it highlights my sense of nursing's role in health care conflicts: All sorts of other people have the power and make the decisions; we just carry them out and smooth over the fracas created as necessary.

On September 22, 1989, a group of experts in the field generated the following consensus description or definition: "Co-dependency is a pattern of painful dependency on compulsive behaviors and on approval from others in an attempt to find safety, self-worth and identity. Recovery is possible" (Wegscheider-Cruse & Cruse, 1990, p. 8). While the latter statement in the definition is purportedly good news, it is surely of little worth and value if the presence of the problem is denied or ignored. In nursing we have fretted about our oppressed status without much willingness to look at the primary mechanisms we use to deal with this status. Those who study the phenomenon are not so reticent; most identify nurses as one of the groups that manifest and perpetuate codependency. This is worrisome news.

The community of practitioners and proponents of this world view is, like us all, evolving. For nurses struggling with the insights of this particular world view, Kasl (1992) provides a stabilizing antidote that may prove useful. In her critique of the pervasive mystique surrounding twelve-step programs and their related ideas about addiction and codependency, she examines both social and personal contexts with particular emphasis on internalized oppression. She encourages alternate pathways. What is useful is her clear-headed recognition of and willingness to tackle the problems that current solutions have engendered without escaping the original stimulus: the codependency and the addictions.

Once more pulling these threads together, it seems that for me as an individual (and for the vast majority of my colleagues), the socialization I have historically and even currently experienced as a nurse encourages me to engage in codependent behaviors. I can rebel against the program—and have—but it changes neither the system nor me. Rebellion is not resolution. Indeed, I have slowly leaned it is merely a different face to entrapment. The critical key is questioning the system, beginning to understand better how it operates and what it asks of me. Cooptation wears many costumes and requires reasoned scrutiny. In engaging in such scrutiny, what I find is a system nostalgically looking backward more than forward, often hoping that the nurses will smooth over the inevitable conflicts that emerge from that incongruity. The repeated effort to find new ways to deal with this system was for me a significant impetus in writing a book about alternate ways of being at an uneven table. The first step in meaningful conflict resolution, however, is the willingness to see the uneven table, to know you are at one, and to make clear decisions about what you are now doing that is harmful and what you might do in the future that is more constructive.

In the book I call these "ways of being," and list 10 exemplars that I believe, interactively, can change how we negotiate as nurses. They presuppose that we will have climbed over the habits of the codependent heart, one way or another, and faced the way we "do" conflict now, usually with complex skill arrays of manipulations and maneuverings that serve to harm ourselves and others and keep the conflict and the source of conflict afloat. We have some choices to make here.

SOME OBSERVATIONS OF A PERSONAL NATURE

What I have written here is, in a good postmodernist fashion, a personal appraisal of the situation as it looks to me from where I am sitting. I have no corner on this market, nor do I purport to have one. What I have learned has stood me in good stead and may prove useful to some others. That would please me. What is clear to me is that the frequency and depth of conflict we will experience in

health care settings and among nurses are likely to increase, not decrease, and we are ill prepared for that eventuality. It is equally clear to me that if nurses elected to tap into their considerable conflict management skills, transformed them with honesty and moral courage so that they move beyond mere manipulations, we could be a formidable force in enhancing the health care environments we inhabit and create. I have no wisdom on whether we will elect to do that, or to what degree. I love the imagination of it, however, and when I list my personal collection of rainbow-level hopes and dreams, I always include it with a smile.

REFERENCES

Allport, G.W. (1958). *The nature of prejudice.* Garden City, NY: Doubleday.

Anderson, W.T. (1995). Four different ways to be absolutely right. In W.T. Anderson (Ed.), *The truth about the truth, de-confusing and re-constructing the postmodern world* (pp. 115, 116). New York: G.P. Putnam's Sons.

Fisher, R., & Ury, W. (1981). *Getting to yes: Negotiating agreement without giving in* (2nd ed.). New York: Penguin Books.

Gale, G. (1979). *Theory of science.* New York: McGraw-Hill Book Co.

Hall, S.F., & Wray, L.M. (1989). Codependency: Nurses who give too much. *American Journal of Nursing, 89*(11), 1456-1460.

Kasl, C.D. (1992). *Many roads, one journey: Moving beyond the 12 steps.* New York: HarperCollins.

Kritek, P.B. (1994). *Negotiating at an uneven table: Developing moral courage in resolving our conflicts.* San Francisco: Jossey-Bass.

Kuhn, T.S. (1970). *The structure of scientific revolutions* (2nd ed.). Chicago: The University of Chicago Press.

Laudan, L. (1977). *Progress and its problems, towards a theory of scientific growth.* Los Angeles: University of California Press.

Marcus, L.J., Dorn, B.C., Kritek, P.B., Miller, V.G., & Wyatt, J.B. (1995). *Renegotiating health care: Resolving conflict to build collaboration.* San Francisco: Jossey-Bass.

Moore, C.W. (1986). *The mediation process: Practical strategies for resolving conflict.* San Francisco: Jossey-Bass.

Reason, P., & Rowan, J. (Eds.). (1981). *Human inquiry, a sourcebook of new paradigm research.* New York: John Wiley & Sons.

Rorty, R. (1979). *Philosophy and the mirror of nature.* Princeton, NJ: Princeton University Press.

Schaef, A.W., & Fassel, D. (1988). *The addictive organization.* San Francisco: Harper & Row.

Toulmin, S. (1990). *Cosmopolis.* Chicago: The University of Chicago Press.

Ury, W. (1991). *Getting past no: Negotiating with difficult people.* New York: Bantam Books.

Whitfield, C.L. (1991). *Co-dependence, healing the human condition.* Deerfield Beach, FL: Health Communications.

Wegscheider-Cruse, S., & Cruse, J. (1990). *Understanding co-dependency.* Deerfield Beach, FL: Health Communications.

Section Ten

Cultural Diversity

Diversity in Nursing

A Formidable Challenge

JOANNE McCLOSKEY DOCHTERMAN, HELEN KENNEDY GRACE

Throughout history nursing has been a pathway for social mobility, especially for women. With relatively few career options outside of the home, acceptable career choices for women were in the fields of teaching, nursing, and secretarial work. White women, first from rural backgrounds, found nursing an acceptable and safe field in which they might advance economically. Ironically, this has not been the case for women from minority groups. Women from underrepresented groups have been relegated primarily to roles of servitude within the health care system either as nursing aides or as practical nurses. Entrance into the system in these roles has severely limited the ability to advance within the mainstream of nursing.

Since the 1960s considerable advances have been made in their increasing participation in all levels of society by previously underrepresented groups. But in nursing the situation has remained static, with little advancement on the part of nurses of color. For a profession that prides itself on being an advocate for the rights of patients of all creeds, colors, or national origins, the lack of diversification of the nursing work force has received only minimal attention. As we move into the 21st century, the diversity of the population of the United States is increasing significantly. Ethnic minorities currently comprise 28% of the general population. This percentage is projected to increase to 37% by the year 2025. While the percentage of minorities within the general population continues to increase, nursing continues to lag substantially behind with only about 10% minority representation within the profession. This problem is compounded in that the largest number of minorities entering the profession enter through associate degree programs. Advancement to higher education, particularly to the doctoral level, is difficult to achieve. And without a substantial number of

nurses prepared at the doctoral level, leadership within the profession is limited.

Why does this situation remain unchanged? All of the usual reasons can be offered, and they are presented in this section: the image of nursing; difficulty in recruiting students into the profession; difficulty in retaining them through the educational programs; and once into practice, encouraging their career development. While these are all valid observations, why isn't there more of a concern for the future of the profession if this situation is not reversed dramatically? How can nursing continue to be an advocate for patients, when the majority of nurses are white, middle-class, while the populations they serve are increasingly becoming people of color?

In the opening debate chapter, Warda addresses the question of racism and genderism in nursing. Is the lack of representation of minority groups in nursing a result of lack of motivation on the part of potential students to enter the field or a reflection of biases within the profession that create barriers to entrance and progression? Warda provides an overview of the statistics that show the nursing profession falling far behind in diversity to match that of the general population and addresses the implications of these data related to the appropriateness of care for patients. She then outlines some of the factors that serve as barriers for entrance to the field and the ways in which these might be addressed. One of the major problems is that most students from underrepresented groups enter the field at the lowest end of the career hierarchy, as practical nurses or through associate degree programs. Educational progression then becomes more difficult, and the percentages of nurses from underrepresented groups becomes even sparser in leadership roles within the profession. With few faculty members and nurses in visible leadership positions, the role models for potential students wanting to advance in the profession are extremely few. Without a concerted effort on the part of the nursing profession as a whole the prospects for change are limited.

Castiglia addresses the issues of racial diversity in academic programs and the importance of cultural competence in the preparation of nurses. She argues that the delivery of culturally competent care requires that the nurse understand the culture of the patient. If there are no nurses representative of the culture of the patient, this understanding is severely limited. "How this situation (lack of minorities in nursing) has evolved, where the profession is today in recruiting and retaining minority students and faculty, and the remediation strategies employed may well determine the relevance of the nursing profession for the complex emerging health care system of the 21st century." Issues related to the recruitment, retention, and progression of minority students, particularly Hispanics, are addressed and suggestions made as to the support systems necessary to address these inequities.

On a more positive note, Bullough addresses the issue of men in nursing and notes the increased percentage of males enrolled in nursing educational programs. Tracing the historical roots of genderism in nursing, Bullough notes that women will remain the dominant force in nursing for the foreseeable future and men will have to be aware of the anxieties and fears that women have about men. One of these fears relates to advancement of men more rapidly into leadership positions, particularly into administration. As men increase within the profession and their relative power increases, it is important that the strengths of men and of women join to work together. In the future, Bullough posits "men will undoubtedly help change nursing but they will be joining with women to do so."

Dennis addresses issues related to African Americans in nursing. Inclusion of the "world view" of the African American patient and tailoring nursing actions appropriately are essential in giving good care. Particular cultural beliefs and values of African Americans are described. Health disparities between African Americans and whites are presented. Dennis notes that 70% to 90% of recognized illnesses in blacks are managed outside the formal health system. Because of the history of exploitation and experimentation, there is an understandable suspicion of health care providers. If health care for African Americans is to improve, and if the patterns of disease and mortality are to be ameliorated, increased numbers of African American nurses providing culturally competent care are an important part of the solution.

Asians and Pacific Islanders now constitute one of the fastest growing minority groups within this country. Noting that this categorization masks wide differences between groups, Inouye details the differences in incidence of disease of particular groups. Asian distrust of Western medical care stems from their long history of herbalist or shamanistic healing. Provision of care to Asians and Pacific Islanders needs to be sensitive to the other cultural values, such as the importance of the family and the reverence for elders. Only 4.4% of the nursing profession are of Asian or Pacific Island origin, and the majority of that group practice in acute care settings. A model of community-based care is recommended as a way of increasing the health of the Asian and Pacific Islander population. For such a care model to be effective, increased numbers of Asian and Pacific Islander nurses would be essential in providing culturally relevant care.

Torres and Castillo address the challenge of adequately addressing the demographic changes occurring within this country, particularly the "browning" of America. Although the Hispanic/Latino population in the United States is expected to increase to about 13% of the population by 2010 and to 23% by 2050, only 1.6% of nurses in the United States are of Hispanic origin. Because of the economic plight of this population, the few Hispanic nurses in the profession enter largely through the associate degree programs. The numbers that advance to graduate education and to doctoral preparation in particular are few. This creates a problem of lack of role models and mentors that might be effective in encouraging more to enter the profession. A comprehensive program of recruitment, support systems, and mentoring are recommended as a way to begin to redress the complex problems of increasing the numbers of Hispanics/Latinos in the nursing profession.

In the final article in this section, Keltner, Smith, and Slim address the issue of bridging of cultures with Native American communities and nursing. They caution us to build a framework for developing bridges rather than a blueprint and note that "we are eager to embrace technology so long as it does not short circuit the soul. The missionary mindset is brought by people of science streaming onto the reservations and urban settings with solutions to problems they have identified." The authors then describe the assaults upon Native Americans through time: relocation from areas that had been home to remote and desolate areas of the country; taking children away to place them in boarding schools that served to separate them from their families and communities; and the taking away of freedom and self-determination.

The natural characteristics of Native Americans include their strength and resilience as a people, strong family bonds, and religious rootedness. In providing care it is important to reinforce these values rather than undermine them. Treatment needs to be treatment of the whole person. In providing health care it is important to link health care to the culture. An increase in the numbers of Native American nurses would do much to bridge cultures and produce culturally relevant care. The authors note that "white professionals tend to talk too much and listen too little." Bridging cultures will require true partnerships rather than the more traditional paternalistic approach of health care professionals, including nurses.

This section is a combination of "good news" and "bad news." The bad news is that so little progress has been made in altering the overall diversity in the field of nursing. This is even more problematic given the perception of many nurses of color that within the profession there is a backlash against nurse leaders of color as they become effective leaders. The good news is that strong leadership is emerging and new voices are being heard as evidenced by the stimulating articles in this section.

Why Isn't Nursing More Diversified?

MARIA R. WARDA

Diversity has always been a major strength of American society. Although the United States remains "a nation of immigrants," socioeconomic stratification and discrimination have limited the benefits that a diversified population can bring to society. In the United States there is incongruity between the increasing number of racial and ethnic groups and their power to influence and access health care. Recent immigrants, members of ethnic minority groups, and the poor are adversely affected because they lack the income to purchase health services, the knowledge of which services to purchase, and the knowledge of how to use the services (Funkerhouser & Moser, 1990). Ensuring the cultural competence of all health care workers and increasing the diversity among health care professionals are key strategies that could address some of these inequalities.

Diversity includes consideration of race and ethnicity, socioeconomic class, gender, age, religious and spiritual beliefs, sexual orientation, and physical disability (American Association of Colleges of Nursing [AACN], 1998). From its beginnings the United States has struggled with the ways that values and value conflicts relate to diversity. Early ideology in the evolving United States focused on cultural homogeneity. Immigrants were asked to forsake their cultural and ethnic identities and become assimilated into the mainstream (Bessent, 1997). The current shift in U.S. demographics has proved more effective in promoting a multicultural society than the institutional summons for cultural homogeneity. The realities of the demographics of the future mandate greater attention to embracing and celebrating diversity in our communities.

As this nation debates issues of equal access, opportunity, and representation, the chosen course of action takes on a more serious urgency in the 21st century. The growth in the number of ethnic minority groups is reshaping the composition of future student pools and the labor force in the United States. In this new millennium, ethnic minorities are expected to comprise an estimated 28.2% of the U.S. population and to increase to 37% in the year 2025 (U.S. Census Bureau, 1999). The increasing numbers of ethnic minorities will continue to create social and political changes throughout society, particularly in health care, where demands on the financing and delivery systems will increase to equalize the health status between minorities and the majority population.

The data from the National Sample Surveys of Registered Nurses (NSSRNs) showed that in 1996 there were about 246,000 RNs from minority backgrounds compared with 120,000 in 1980. The almost 10% of RNs that come from ethnic minority backgrounds are made up of African Americans (4.2%), Asians and Pacific Islanders (3.4%), Hispanics (1.6%), and American Indian and Alaskan Natives (0.5%) (U.S. Department of Health and Human Services, 1996). Thus the proportion of RNs from racial and ethnic minority groups in the total RN population still falls far short of the proportion of minorities in the total U.S. population. The rhetoric of nursing's problem of recruitment and retention of minorities into the profession has failed to result in action to adequately address the issues.

To address the question Why isn't nursing more diversified? this chapter explores the presence of racism in nursing and nursing's pervasive disinclination to take assertive action to assure diversity in the profession. The point being debated is whether nursing will become internally driven to action in diversifying the profession or whether it will remain a passive witness to the demographic changes taking place in our social and academic systems.

DIVERSITY IN NURSING

The NSSRNs that have been carried out for the period of 1980 to 1996 indicate that the economic and social environment of the nursing profession has undergone many changes. The significant changes affecting nursing are increased participation of women in the nation's workforce, increasing numbers of minorities among the country's population, periods of recession and inflation, technological innovations in health care, increasing concerns about health care costs, and restructuring of the health care delivery system (U.S. Department of Health and Human Services, 1996).

Other significant findings related to ethnic diversity of the nursing workforce indicated that RNs from minority backgrounds were more likely to be employed in nursing than nonminority RNs were and that minority nurses were also more likely to be employed full time. With the exception of RNs from an Asian or Pacific Islander background, the distribution of RNs in each of the racial and ethnic categories according to their initial nursing preparation is similar in that they were likely to have graduated from either a diploma or associate degree program. When both the initial and post-RN education are taken into account, however, African Americans and Asians and Pacific Islanders were more likely than Hispanics and nonminorities to have at least baccalaureate preparation. Among African Americans, 12% had a master's or doctoral degree compared with about 10% of the nonminority nurses and approximately 7% of the Hispanic and Asian nurses. The data support the benefits to the U.S. population of promoting the advanced preparation of minority nurses. The potential outcome of more minorities entering nursing is an increase in the number of actively employed nurses and in the number of nurses that hold advanced degrees.

As informative as the data from the NSSRNs are in describing the characteristics of the nursing profession in the United States, they do not offer insights into why nursing is not more diversified. A critical examination of public policy in the United States can be especially helpful in understanding ethnic inequalities in nursing.

SOCIAL POLICY

Generally, "policy" refers to a course of action or inaction selected from among alternatives in the context of given conditions to guide present and future decisions and implementation of those decisions. Public policy consists of a course of action chosen by government (Kalisch & Kalisch, 1982). All public policy issues involve ethical and value dimensions that often are not considered explicitly in debate that focuses on how needs and interests of individuals and society will be reconciled. American society is characterized by a delicate interplay between equity and inequity. Inequity is less acknowledged but is, in fact,

more frequently practiced (Felton, 1987). Evidence of a national policy based on supremacist ideologies and practices can be identified from the time of establishment of the Thirteen Colonies. From its beginnings, the United States enlisted its educational institutions as tools for shaping and preserving cultural homogeneity or the Anglo-Saxon conception of righteousness (Bessent, 1997).

The support of legalized discrimination remained until the mid 20th century, with laws that kept people of color from equal access and participation in education and employment. The 1964 Civil Rights Act led to legislative, executive, and judicial influences that placed pressure on corporations and universities to increase the participation rates of underrepresented minority groups. Affirmative action had its origins in the same period. In 1961 President Kennedy issued Executive Order No. 10,925, which directed federal contractors to take affirmative action measures designed to achieve nondiscrimination (Helms, Anderson, & Theis, 1998). The policy of affirmative action was promulgated largely to encourage aggressive means to overcome the negative effects of past discrimination in employment and college admission practices. Precise measures of implementation were not spelled out, and there have been numerous applications including adoption of goals (quotas), specialized training, revising the use of selection criteria, or other approaches to remedying past discrimination of targeted groups. Affirmative action is a controversial measure that continues to be challenged to this day.

Richardson and Skinner (1996) noted that the civil rights movement created a coalition between those who sought a fair process or equal educational opportunity and those concerned about fair outcomes or distributive justice. In the 1980s, social action shifted from assuring fair process to achieving fair outcomes. The prospect of achieving fair outcomes with "color-free" strategies has led to higher college admission standards, and the assessment movement (application of test scores for selection and admission purposes).

The main debate regarding affirmative action efforts is that they may unduly burden other groups or have the potential for "reverse discrimination." Opponents of affirmative action assert that preferential treatment and other remedies result in the selection of unqualified individuals. Taylor (1997) discussed how arguments that are cast in terms of individual merit (microjustice) versus general societal good (macrojustice) take on a tone of "authenticity" when they come from African American conservatives. These attacks on quality and diversity share the underlying premise that rewards should be proportional to the individual's merit or qualifications (Goll-fredson, 1988; Sackett & Wilk, 1994; Steele, 1990).

The quality initiatives of the current individual interest (microjustice) cycle have had an adverse impact on the participation and achievement of ethnic minority students in majority institutions. It has been determined that black-white differences in ratings of job performance tend to be small, whereas differences in black-white performance on standardized tests are large (Dawes, 1993). Thus, if job selection or college admission is based solely on standardized tests results, then testing is a means of securing preferential selection of whites. The empirical research on affirmative action provides little guidance on its effects on the measurement of qualification in the selection process (Taylor, 1994).

With affirmative action hanging by a thread, one might assume that educators, as gatekeepers of opportunity and privilege, would look for solid evidence about the benefits of diversity. However, academic researchers devoted far more attention to examining the problems that minority students experience on campus than to the benefits of diversity. Fortunately over the past few years academic researchers have now conducted several studies that provide credible and convincing evidence that affirmative action is beneficial to students, higher education institutions, and society. Bowen and Bok (1998) examined grades, test scores, choice of major, graduation rates, careers, and attitudes of 45,000 students at 28 of the most selective schools in the U.S. The study begins by documenting the problem clearly: blacks who enter elite institutions do so with lower test scores and grades than those of whites, and black students receive lower grades and graduate at a lower rate. But after graduation, the study found, these students achieve notable success. They earn advanced degrees at rates identical to those of white classmates. Black students are even slightly more likely than whites from the same institutions to obtain professional degrees in law, business, and medicine. Black and white participants reported fairly substantial social interaction at college, which they said helped them relate to members of different racial groups later in life.

One commonly voiced objection to affirmative action is the assertion that since minorities admitted through race-sensitive policies do not keep up with their white colleagues, they end up failed and stigmatized (Themstrom & Themstrom, 1997). But Bowen and Bok (1998) found that the black dropout rate for the elite institutions practicing affirmative action was 25%, much lower than the national black dropout average of 60%. The more selective the college, the lower the black dropout rate. The study findings support the notion that diversity is a valu-able aspect of education for all races. Still, researchers should make further contributions to the affirmative action debate before the country makes the critical choice about broadening the applicant pool or denying entry to its elite universities to members of minority groups.

At its core the discussion of diversity in the formulation of social policy calls upon us to revisit questions about sensitivity, knowledge, and skills needed for constructive relations among people who are different, and the principles that underlie a just and democratic society. The gift that diversity gives is the insistent invitation to ask hard questions about what we mean by access and opportunities for education, how we teach, which people should be included as students and teachers, and what we are accomplishing in our schools and universities. The next section offers a focused discussion of the role of ethnic diversity in nursing education.

NURSING EDUCATION

The critical underrepresentation of minorities in the nursing profession raises concerns about minority enrollment in nursing education. Thus discussions of minorities in nursing must address recruitment and retention of students in higher education. More than 20 years have passed since the enactment of the 1964 Civil Rights Act, and higher education has made real progress in opening up our nation's campuses to minority students. But progress since then has slowed, and national commitment to equality and access seems to have faltered. Black and Hispanic enrollment in nursing schools has remained stagnant since 1993 (U.S. Department of Health & Human Services, 1996). This is not to say that institutions have failed to address the problem; indeed, nursing schools across the nation have put into place a variety of programs and policies to promote the recruitment and retention of minority students, faculty, and staff. The gap between the participation rates of white students and minority students is growing, however, particularly in graduate education, and attrition is a major problem. What, then, has gone wrong? Why isn't nursing more diversified?

There are several possible answers to the questions. The barriers to diversity enhancement in nursing education fall under three categories: negative perceptions of nursing as a career, use of traditional approaches to recruitment, and the school's culture and climate (retention).

Negative Perceptions of Nursing

The literature has identified several factors related to the shrinking pool of nursing students: (1) the negative view of nursing as a career choice, (2) the increase in nontraditional students (those that are older, studying part-time, working, and supporting families), and (3) the changing role of women in society that has allowed intellectually capable women to pursue professions such as business, medicine, and computer science (Bednash, 1997; Farrell, 1988; Norbeck, 1995).

The problem of declining enrollment in schools of nursing has been linked to the pervasive image of nursing as a powerless profession with low salaries and poor working conditions. Two studies have reported on high school students' perceptions of nursing as a career. Stevens and Walker (1993) surveyed high school seniors to determine why nursing is not selected more frequently as a career. The findings indicated that the decision to choose or not to choose nursing was significantly influenced by past experiences with nursing and illness, and characteristics preferred in a future career. Students who chose nursing as a career found it important to be helpful to others in their job, to work as a team member, to use scientific information, and to follow the orders of others. Those not choosing nursing indicated dislike of dying people and the salary as the main reasons for choosing another career. Interestingly, the important job characteristics identified by non-choosers were being in demand, being able to see the results of their work, being respected and admired for their work, and doing important work. A high percentage of the respondents did not know that nurses worked with computers or high-technology equipment, that they directed programs, or held management positions. A large percentage of those who chose nursing knew a nurse personally (68.6%) or had someone close to them who died (71%) or had had a serious illness (78.2%).

A survey of 300 high school junior students explored the relationship between the experience of having a nursing role model and the decision to consider nursing as a career (Grossman, Arnold, Sullivan, Cameron, & Munro, 1989). The results indicated that this sample of high school students seemed to have a lack of knowledge about expanded roles and opportunities for advancement in the nursing profession, and there was a significant relationship between the experience of having a nursing role model and students' decision to consider nursing as a career. In addition, less than 20% were considering nursing as a career.

The concept that minority parents hold negative views of nursing has received limited attention in the nursing literature. Orque, Bloch, and Monrroy (1983) found that nursing was viewed negatively by black parents. Many parents considered nursing to be a menial job with low prestige and were not supportive of nursing as a career choice for their children. It can also be hypothesized that many new immigrant parents may bring views of nursing as servile role, with low pay and minimal or no educational requirements. The nursing profession needs to further investigate minority parents' perceptions of nursing as a career choice for their children. In addition, precollege recruitment efforts of minority students may need to incorporate family involvement and support strategies.

The changing economic, social, and demographic conditions in the United States are reshaping the composition of student pools. A number of individuals are returning to college for new careers with greater potential for economic security (Bednash, 1997). Some nursing schools have already restructured their programs to meet the emerging trends in nursing student pools. One example is the master's entry programs for college graduates with nonnursing degrees. These "accelerated" programs were controversial when first established. Felton (1987) saw the master's entry model as a threat to the educational mobility of disadvantaged and minority students because of the high qualifications associated with such programs. However, the University of California School of Nursing reports that their master's entry program in nursing averages over 20% minority enrollment. Recent efforts at assessing the merits of generic master's programs for nonnurses by a cohort of nursing schools in Northern California will further illustrate the impact of these programs on the number of minorities in advanced practice nursing roles (S. Ziehm, personal communication, February 18, 2000).

The diversity of career opportunities available to women is negatively affecting enrollment in nursing schools. How can we view this as a negative outcome? It brings an end to years of oppression and inequality for women. The feminists' profession of nursing needs to support the progress of women while directing efforts to improving the image of nursing. The design of nursing programs that are creative, flexible, and that reflect the needs of untraditional and emerging majority students will bring more diverse individuals into the nursing profession. The infrastructure necessary for the recruitment and retention of the changing pool of candidates is addressed next.

Barriers to Recruitment

Two major issues related to minority recruitment have been identified: (1) the significant imbalance in the distribution of minority enrollment between associate and

---

BARRIERS TO COLLEGE EDUCATION FOR MINORITIES

Negative perceptions of nursing
Inadequate secondary school preparation and counseling
Cultural/environmental barriers
Fewer successful role models
Cost of higher education
Limited access to higher education information
Lack of familiarity with the admission process
Restrictive admission process
Perceived and actual racial biases

---

baccalaureate programs and (2) the relatively slow growth in the recruitment of minority students coupled with continuing problems with their retention (Naylor, 1997; Weekes, 1997). A study by the National Association of Hispanic Nurses (NAHN, 1998) revealed that those participants that entered nursing at the ADN (associate degree in nursing) level indicated the affordability of the associate degree, lack of sufficient financial aid for baccalaureate education, and the pressure to begin earning money as important considerations in their decision to enter an ADN program. The lack of counseling to pursue college education in general and nursing in particular, and the tracking of many Hispanics into vocational or non-college-bound programs were also cited as barriers to entry into baccalaureate education (NAHN, 1998). Since the baccalaureate degree is the most direct route to graduate education in nursing, it can be concluded that minority registered nurses prepared at the diploma or associate degree level will have added barriers to achieving advanced degrees.

Barriers faced by minority applicants to health care professional schools have been widely investigated across disciplines (Dowell, 1996; Naylor, 1997; NAHN, 1998; Snyder & Bunkers, 1994; Weekes, 1997). Refer to the box above for a comprehensive list of barriers to college education for minorities. Thus the questions to be considered, knowing as much as we do, are Why is there so little sustained progress in increasing the number of minorities in nursing education? Why isn't nursing more diversified?

Recruitment Approaches

Increasing the ethnic diversity in the nursing workforce has been identified by government, professional nursing, and community groups as a means of enabling access to culturally appropriate health care (Broadnax, 1993). Cur-

rent nursing literature offers little help in identifying effective approaches to recruitment and retention of minority students, and few studies have focused on assessing the effectiveness of such programs (Dowell, 1996). Many schools are still using traditional recruitment efforts such as open houses, personal contacts with faculty and alumni, and distribution of brochures at career fairs and conferences. However, a variety of innovative strategies is being adopted by some schools, including using minority alumni and current students as recruiters, forming partnerships with high schools and 2-year colleges, offering summer programs on campus, obtaining financial aid in the form of work-study or work-grant programs in collaboration with potential employers, and implementing accelerated pathways to the master of science in nursing for second-degree students (Dowell, 1996; Green, 1989; Naylor, 1997). The main characteristic inherent in these approaches is the attention to the unique sociodemographic and cultural dimensions of many minority applicants. First, the use of minority alumni and current students will provide needed role models and access to program information. An added benefit to the use of student recruiters is that many potential applicants would like to know "what it is like to be a student at your institution," and this is particularly important to minority applicants.

Second, health professions schools typically have competed against each other and with other professional schools in recruiting minority students. The fundamental problem is that the overall pool of minority students from which everyone is trying to recruit is too small (Ready, 1997). Instead of focusing primarily on how to out-compete other schools in recruiting students from the too-small applicant pool, it would be better if health professions schools collaborated with each other and with educational institutions at earlier stages of the "pipeline." This collaboration would substantially increase the number of minority students who are both interested in and academically prepared to pursue a career in one of the health professions. The lack of attention to the issue of early academic outreach to elementary school children is a fundamental flaw found in the nursing profession's approach to recruitment. Educational theorists suggest that elementary school children should be targeted for career education because by the time they reach adolescence, they have formulated decisions and attitudes toward career choices (Naylor, 1997). A framework that links universities and K-12 (kindergarten through 12th grade) schools as partners in facilitating career education, academic experiences, and mentoring has great potential for closing the minority-white enrollment gap in higher education (Hayward, Brandes, Kirst, & Mazzeo, 1997).

Third, an examination of the literature regarding outreach programs found a high degree of agreement across programs on the key barriers to higher education for large numbers of historically underrepresented groups (Hayward et al., 1997; Ready, 1997). A list of the barriers to educational mobility for minority students is found in the box on page 487. The final "ingredient" missing from the list is the opportunity to get to know health professionals personally in order to better understand what it is like to be a nurse, doctor, or a dentist, and what it takes to get there. Summer intern programs can provide direct contact with nursing care environments, thus improving the knowledge of college-bound high school students about the nursing profession. The opportunity to interact personally with practicing nurses, faculty, and nursing students has the potential to influence more favorable opinions about nursing. It will demonstrate to the participants and other minority and underrepresented students that come in contact with them that nurses do important work, are respected by other health professionals and patients, use scientific information, and receive competitive salaries.

Fourth, it is not uncommon to graduate from nursing school (even in diploma and associate degree programs) with debt ranging from $10,000 to $15,000. Students from ethnic or racial minorities will generally have greater need for financial assistance than those in the majority (Green, 1989). It will then prove more attractive to all applicants to provide them with work-grant programs and fewer loans. Last, the availability of master's entry programs for nonnurses has the potential to reach a wider population of minority undergraduates than the existing 10% segment of the RN population.

Adequate financial and manpower resources are required to ensure the implementation and evaluation of these innovative recruitment approaches. Stipends should be provided for students who participate in summer programs to replace lost summer earnings and to encourage students to enroll (Naylor, 1997). Hiring nursing students as part-time recruitment assistants, and assigning them to work with college admission officers or recruitment coordinators can provide needed role models for individuals making career choices. Nursing leadership is required to influence state and public policies supportive of funding outreach and recruitment approaches aimed at enhancing the diversity of the nursing workforce.

Several authors have discussed the critical importance of obtaining total organizational support for improving the minority recruitment situation. Green (1989) identified successful recruitment strategies as those that garner commitment from leadership and staff, allocate sufficient resources, provide incentives, are explicit and outcome oriented, and that set manageable, realistic goals. While enhancing minority enrollment must be everyone's agenda, leadership and oversight must reside with one senior individual with the accountability and resources to obtain targeted outcomes. The move to centralize overall administrative responsibility for recruitment and retention initiatives in one individual is widely practiced in general college campuses but is rarely present in the organizational structure of schools of nursing.

Organizational vision of recruitment needs to be explicit and to incorporate the diverse perspectives of the groups being addressed into institutional policies, procedures, and curricula and be based on commitment to eradicate all forms of discrimination (Thomas & Ely, 1996). In Bessent's survey (1997) of recruitment and retention status in the nation's major research universities, the responders failed to identify marketing and nursing recruitment strategies that addressed cultural dimensions directly. The integration of cultural, organizational, and marketing theories and principles in planning recruitment and retention activities is rarely considered in the nursing profession.

Contemporary nursing publications advocating for diversity in the profession continue to focus on strategies to assist the ethnically diverse student to "adapt" to the educational system (Davidhizar, Dowd, & Giger, 1998). Minimal attention is given to considering educational system changes or adjustments required to develop culturally based recruitment and retention strategies. Effective recruitment efforts need to respond to changes in American society and the nursing profession by enhancing access for an increasingly broader range of students and by developing academic structures, policies, and practices that can accommodate differences in cultural values.

Barriers to Retention

Successful recruitment is ultimately a failure if the applicants do not gain admission, are not provided with enriching academic and personal experiences, and fall short of graduation. To address the high rate of attrition among minorities enrolled in schools of nursing, several authors have grouped significant factors under three categories: personal, environmental/cultural, and academic/system (Jeffreys, 1998; Snyder & Bunkers, 1994; Weekes, 1997). The box on page 489 lists the major factors related to retention as reported in the literature.

MAJOR FACTORS RELATED TO RETENTION AMONG MINORITY STUDENTS IN SCHOOLS OF NURSING

Personal
Self-efficiency
Determination
Study skills
Grade point average
Language proficiency
Precollege education

Academic
Lack of faculty support
Unavailability of mentors
Lack of program flexibility
Inadequate academic services
Lack of financial aid
Devalued cultural perspectives
Lack of peer support
Pressures to conform

Cultural/Environmental
Family support
Family responsibilities
Hours of employment

Personal Factors

Jeffreys (1998) examined the influence of self-efficacy and select academic and environmental variables on academic achievement and retention among underrepresented and ethnic minority students in an associate degree program. For the participants in this study, the environmental variables (e.g., finances, work, and family responsibilities) were perceived as influencing academic achievement and retention more so than academic variables (e.g., academic advising). The at-risk students in the sample were those "supremely" efficacious individuals who overestimated their academic supports and underestimated their need for preparation. The researcher recommended that nurse educators should actively engage in early identification of the at-risk student to allow for interventions aimed at maximizing strengths, recognizing weaknesses, and preparing for future educational challenges. Weekes (1997) and Yoder (1996) have warned against making the stereotype judgment that all minority students will have the same problems and needs. For example, the faculty may hold the view that minority students will do poorly in mathematics, science, and writing. Steele (1995) suggested that stereotypical world views, when communi-

cated to the student (either overtly or covertly), can influence performance anxiety in the student. The most promising approach is not to assume that differences are disadvantages that need to remedied, while focusing on assessing all students' performance and offering timely interventions to at-risk individuals.

Other personal factors that should be further investigated are perseverance and self-determination. The National Association of Hispanic Nurses study (1998) described the participants who succeeded in obtaining nursing education as having inner strength, power, and determination. A qualitative study of minority nursing students in a master's program identified an important facilitator for success as the fulfillment of personal ambition, determination, and self-confidence (Snyder & Bunkers, 1994). These attributes of resilience are necessary for the minority student to gain access and successfully "cope" in majority white institutions. Barbee (1993) stated that minority nursing students and nurses are acutely and chronically aware of racism in the profession and in health care generally. They spend much time and energy combating institutional discrimination and racism, whereas a segment of European-American nurses spend as much time and energy denying that racism exists. Until nursing schools are transformed into educational systems that welcome and celebrate diversity, minority students may need to rely on characteristics of personal strengths almost exclusively.

Environmental/Cultural Factors

Increasingly, the family environment has been addressed as an important factor influencing academic achievement and retention. Environmental barriers may include family members who discourage aspirations for college education, family responsibilities such as child care, and the need to negotiate day-to-day transactions for relatives with limited English proficiency. Paradoxically, family environment has also been described as a facilitator to educational mobility. Minority students have described the importance of having the encouragement and support of parents, siblings, husbands, and friends (NAHN, 1998; Snyder & Bunkers, 1994). The stress of having to balance full- or part-time employment, school, and home responsibilities has also been identified as a major barrier to success in nursing school (Snyder & Bunkers, 1994).

Academic System Factors

Campus climate/environment embraces the culture, habits, decisions, practices, and policies of the educational institution. It is the sum total of the daily environment and central to the "comfort factor" that students, faculty, staff, and administrators experience on campus (Green, 1989). Traditionally nursing has been a middle-class, female, nonminority profession. To be accepted in nursing education programs, minority students are expected to adjust to an institution designed by traditional majority faculty (Yoder, 1996). European-American values of individualism, self-confidence, and straightforwardness are powerful influences in the development of nursing school curricula and grading criteria. Ethnically diverse students are likely to espouse values related to mutual interdependence and a group versus individual focus; congruent attributes that support these values are the preference for smooth interpersonal relations, cooperation, tolerance, and accommodation of others (Pacquiao, 1995). In the generic approach to education the minority students feel that they are required to conform to European-American behaviors but that they are given no assistance in assimilating. The negative consequences that the students experience in adverse academic environments are listed in the box on page 489.

Retention Approaches

A study that evaluated a supplementary university-wide program to promote black students' retention in a health sciences campus supported the benefit of devoting time and energy resources to combining several retention approaches in a coordinated effort (Hesser, Pond, Lewis, & Abbott, 1996). The cornerstone activity evaluated in the study consisted of a special advisory effort through which help with academic, personal, social, financial, career, and other concerns (e.g., racial prejudice) was available. Other supplementary activities included (1) an 8-week summer nonmatriculated program for high-risk students whose admission was contingent upon their full participation in the program, (2) a special new student orientation, (3) reading skills–study skills workshops, and (4) quarterly advising meetings.

Participants in a study of the facilitators and barriers for minority students in master's nursing programs suggested the provision of a strong faculty mentorship program, an expanded orientation program for new minority students, the availability of tutors and editors, and respect for diversity as essential strategies for enhancing retention of minority students (Snyder & Bunkers, 1994).

Norbeck (1995) identified the implementation of ethnic support groups within a school of nursing and sensitivity training for faculty as retention strategies. She described the establishment of the Faculty Mentor Program

as an approach to ensure that a broad base of faculty assume responsibility for the needs of students from diverse backgrounds.

The lack of a critical mass of minority students, a lack of academic support services, a lack of mentor programs, and the lack of a culture of diversity demonstrate the "real" attitude of colleges and universities to their minority students (Justiz, Wilson, & Bjork, 1994). These factors contribute to the interpretation by students of a hostile environment and result in feelings of isolation, which in turn interfere with academic and personal achievement. A curriculum that pointedly ignores the contributions and the lifestyle of a significant part of its population contributes to the belief that anything we know about diverse groups is knowledge about a subculture or deviant, nonnorm behavior.

A critical aspect of changing institutional climate and culture is increasing the number of minority faculty and administrators. The presence of minority faculty and administrators enhances the minority students' bonds with the institution and demonstrates to all students that minorities can serve in leadership roles, thus providing a basis for future acceptance and expectation. Therefore an examination of campus culture must also include an evaluation of its hiring and recruitment policies.

Few nursing studies have addressed the issue of retention of disadvantaged or minority students, and there has been little effort to document the outcomes of retention approaches. The profession of nursing has historically demonstrated a preference for homogeneity in its faculty and student population and in approaches to curricula (Barbee, 1993). This inertia in regard to taking aggressive steps toward diversifying the profession will ensure its homogeneity and traditions (e.g., individual orientation, avoidance of conflict). The goal to enhance diversity in nursing needs to be viewed by all nurses as one of the most important professional issues for the 21st century. The challenge is to ask not, Why isn't nursing more diversified? but, How can we bring diversity into nursing?

SUMMARY

The current shift in demographics in the United States is increasing awareness of the ethnic disparity in the nursing profession. It is estimated that almost 10% of the 2,558,874 registered nurses in this country come from ethnic minority backgrounds. The percentage of minority RNs is not representative of the ethnic minority composition of the general population. In addition, most ethnic minority nurses have graduated from diploma or associate degree programs.

The United States has historically preferred cultural homogeneity, and educational institutions have played a critical role in promoting the supremacy of European-American values. In the 1960s the Civil Rights Act and the policy of affirmative action were intended to overcome the effects of past discrimination practices in employment and in college admissions. Since its inception, affirmative action has been a controversial policy. The debate centers on the premise that rewards should be proportional to the individual's merit and qualifications and that affirmative action efforts may negatively affect other groups (reverse discrimination). Recent studies have supported the notion that diversity is an invaluable aspect of education for all races.

The barriers to diversity in nursing education are grouped under three categories: negative perceptions of nursing as a career, use of traditional recruitment approaches, and the presence of aversive academic environments. Evidence exists that many high school students lack knowledge of contemporary roles of nurses, and advanced practice roles in particular. The nursing profession's involvement in early academic outreach efforts from elementary to high school holds promise to increase enrollment in nursing programs.

Explicit and well-tested recruitment strategies that incorporate socioeconomic and cultural dimensions are scarce in nursing. Effective recruitment efforts need to be clearly identified, incorporate the diverse perspectives of the target groups, and represent academic structures and policies that value diversity.

The personal attributes of self-efficacy, perseverance, and self-determination have been identified as important facilitators for minority students' success in nursing programs. The irony is that these attributes are necessary because minorities must learn to "cope" in majority institutions. The perceived or actual environment of discrimination is a contributor to poor quality of academic life and to high attrition levels.

The complex personal, academic, and environmental/cultural factors related to the lack of diversity in nursing deserve the immediate collaboration of educators, researchers, practitioners, and students of all races and ethnic groups. More students and faculty members need to verbalize, research, and document their experiences with diversity as an invaluable aspect of nursing education. We may discover that there is a great deal more hope than we expect for genuine progress in diversifying nursing.

REFERENCES

American Association of Colleges of Nursing. (1998). Diversity and equality of opportunity. *Journal of Professional Nursing, 14*(3), 189-190.

Barbee, E.L. (1993). Racism in nursing. *Medical Anthropology Quarterly, 7*(4), 346-362.

Bednash, G.P. (1997). The changing pool of students. In J.C. McCloskey & H.K. Grace (Eds.), *Current issues in nursing* (5th ed.). St. Louis: Mosby.

Bessent, H. (1997). Closing the gap: Generating opportunities for minority nurses in American health care. In H. Bessent (Ed.), *Strategies for recruitment, retention, and graduation of minority nurses in colleges of nursing.* Washington, DC: American Nurses Publishing.

Bowen, W., & Bok, D. (1998). *The shape of the river: Long term consequences of considering race in college and university admissions.* Princeton, NJ: Princeton University Press.

Broadnax, W. (1993). Moving the health care agenda forward through partnerships and coalitions. In *Caring for the emerging majority: Empowering nurses through partnerships and coalitions.* Washington, DC: Division of Nursing, Bureau of Health Professions, Health Resources & Services Administration, and Office of Minority Health, Office of the Assistant Secretary.

Davidhizar, R., Dowd, S.B., & Ginger, J.N. (1998). Educating the culturally diverse health care student. *Nurse Educator, 23*(2), 38-42.

Dawes, R.M. (1993). Aptitude tests can't be neutral to experience because aptitude itself isn't neutral to experience. *Academe, 79*(3), 31-34.

Dowell, M.A. (1996). Issues in recruitment and retention of minority nursing students. *Journal of Nursing Education, 35*(7), 293-297.

Farrell, J. (1988). The changing pool of candidates for nursing. *Journal of Professional Nursing, 4*(3), 145, 230.

Felton, G. (1987). Obstacles to nursing's preferred future. *Nursing Outlook, 35*(3), 126-128.

Funkerhouser, S.W., & Moser, D.K. (1990). Is health care racist? *Advances in Nursing Science, 5*(5), 279-282.

Gollfredson, L. (1988). Reconsidering fairness: A matter of social and ethical priorities. *Journal of Vocational Behavior, 33*(2), 293-319.

Green, B. (1989). *Minorities on campus: A handbook for enhancing diversity.* Washington, DC: American Council on Education.

Grossman, D., Arnold, L., Sullivan, J., Cameron, M.E., & Munro, B. (1989). High school students' perceptions of nursing as a career: A pilot study. *Journal of Nursing Education, 28*(1), 18-21.

Hayward, G.C., Brandes, B.G., Kirst, M.W., & Mazzeo, C. (1997). *New directions for outreach.* San Francisco: University of California, Outreach Task Force.

Helms, L.B., Anderson, M.A., & Theis, S. (1998). A legal primer on affirmative action in nursing education. *Journal of Professional Nursing, 14*(4), 234-241.

Hesser, A., Pond, E., Lewis, L., & Abbott, B. (1996). Evaluation of a supplemental retention program for African American baccalaureate nursing students. *Journal of Nursing Education, 35*(7), 304-309.

Jeffreys, M.R. (1998). Predicting nontraditional student retention and academic achievement. *Nurse Educator, 23*(1), 42-47.

Justiz, M.J., Wilson, R., & Bjork, L.G. (1994). *Minorities in higher education.* Washington, DC: American Council on Education, Oryx Press.

Kalisch, B.J., & Kalisch, P.A. (1982). *Politics of nursing.* Philadelphia: Lippincott.

National Association of Hispanic Nurses. (1998). *Bridges and barriers: Educational mobility of Hispanic nurses.* Washington, DC: Author.

Naylor, M.D. (1997). Recruitment of students into nursing. In J.C. McCloskey & H.K. Grace (Eds.), *Current issues in nursing* (5th ed.). St. Louis: Mosby.

Norbeck, J. (1995). Who is our consumer: Shaping nursing education to meet emerging needs. *Journal of Professional Nursing, 11*(6), 325-331.

Orque, M., Bloch, B., & Monrroy, L. (1983). *Ethnic nursing care: A multicultural approach.* St. Louis: Mosby.

Pacquiao, D. (1995). Multicultural issues in nursing practice and education. *Issues, 16*(2), 4-12.

Ready, T. (1997). Educational partnerships for diversity in the health professions. In *Proceedings of the Nurse Leadership 97 Invitational Congress* (pp. 37-55). Denver: U.S. Department of Health & Human Services Bureau of Health Professions Division of Nursing.

Richardson, R.C., & Skinner, E.F. (1996). *Achieving quality and diversity: Universities in a multicultural society.* Washington, DC: American Council on Education, Oryx Press.

Sackett, P.R., & Wilk, S.L. (1994). Within-group norming and other forms of score adjustment in preemployment testing. *American Psychologists, 49*(7), 929-954.

Snyder, D.J., & Bunkers, S.J. (1994). Facilitators and barriers for minority students in master's nursing programs. *Journal of Professional Nursing, 10*(3), 140-146.

Steele, C.M. (1995, August 26). Black students live down expectations. *The New York Times,* p. A12.

Steele, S. (1990). *The content of our character: A new vision of race in America.* New York: St. Martin's Press.

Stevens, K.A., & Walker, E.A. (1993). Choosing a career: Why not nursing for high school seniors? *Journal of Nursing Education, 32*(1) 13-17.

Taylor, D.A. (1997). The qualifications dilemma. In H. Bessent (Ed.), *Strategies for recruitment, retention, and graduation of minority nurses in colleges of nursing.* Washington, DC: American Nurses Publishing.

Taylor, M.C. (1994). Impact of affirmative action on beneficiary groups: Evaluation from the 1990 General Society Survey. *Basic and Applied Social Psychology, 15*(2), 143-178.

Themstrom, S., & Themstrom, A. (1997). *America in black and white.* Boston: Simon & Schuster.

Thomas, D.A., & Ely, R.J. (1996). Making differences matter: A new paradigm for managing diversity. *Harvard Business Review,* pp. 79-90.

U.S. Department of Health & Human Services. (1996). *The Registered Nurse Population* (Findings from the National Sample Survey of Registered Nurses). Washington, DC: Bureau of Health Professions Division of Nursing.

U.S. Census Bureau. (1999). Tables: Resident population of the United States: Estimates by sex, race, and Hispanic origin, with median age; resident population of the United States: Middle Series Projections 2015-2030, by sex, race, and Hispanic origin, with median age. [On line]. Available: www.census.gov.

Weekes, D. (1997). Identifying the barriers facing prospective minority nurses in today's climate. In *Caring for the Emerging Majority: Nurse Leadership 97 Invitational Congress* (pp. 67-75). Denver: U.S. Department of Health & Human Services Bureau of Health Professions Division of Nursing.

Yoder, M.K. (1996). Instructional responses to ethnically diverse nursing students. *Journal of Nursing Education, 35*(7), 315-321.

Minority Representation in Nursing Education Programs

Increasing Cultural Competence

PATRICIA T. CASTIGLIA

It is estimated that ethnic minorities constitute 25% of the U.S. population in 2000 and that this number will increase to 51.1% by the year 2080 (Andrews, 1992). There are approximately 19.8 million Americans (8%) who were born in foreign countries, and 32 million are estimated to speak languages other than English ("The numbers game," 1993). Nursing education programs are challenged by these demographics as they strive to prepare graduates for a comprehensive health care system. Graduates must master core competencies for practice, including effective interpersonal relationships. It is well recognized that language and cultural barriers can create misunderstandings that may result in ineffective health care practice and treatment. Despite this recognition, the impact of culture has not always been incorporated into practice by nursing education programs as reflected in recruitment and retention strategies. Since 1990, affirmative action programs, many of which began in the 1960s, have been a subject of considerable continuous and escalating debate. Civil rights protests, including marches on Washington, did much to formulate more proactive policies to assist members of minority groups into schools and positions formerly closed to them. For 2 years, Lamar Alexander, Education Secretary in the Bush administration, studied the legality of minority scholarships and developed a draft document of guidelines that would have barred them (Jaschik, 1993).

The current debate emphasizes the idea of reverse discrimination, that is, that qualified whites are being denied access to academic programs and jobs because they do not have minority status. The Bakke decision in 1978 (*Regents of the University of California vs. Bakke*) endorsed the use of race as one factor in admissions decisions. In the case of Podberesky, a Hispanic student, the U.S. Court of Appeals for the Fourth District ruled that the University of Maryland at College Park had failed to meet the legal tests for offering a minority scholarship. This suit challenged a scholarship for black students at the university, and that decision is the only one at the appellate level that deals with a minority challenge. The ruling stated that past discrimination was not sufficient cause for a race-based remedy and that such discrimination must exert some present effect (Jaschik, 1993). The Adarand decision in June 1995 held that race could only be used for preferential treatment if it can withstand "strict scrutiny" by the federal courts (Michaelson, 1995). As it is interpreted, this decision affects higher education because all colleges and universities are, to some extent, governed by state and federal civil rights laws in order to receive federal and state money. Therefore, "strict scrutiny" would have a far-reaching effect. Both California and Michigan are currently engaged in legislative processes to ban or severely modify affirmative action in those states. In 1996 the Adarand decision was used when the federal Fifth Circuit Court ruled on a suit brought by law students at the University of Texas at Austin regarding preferential treatment given to minority applicants. The ruling on the case, *Hopwood vs. U.T. Austin Law School,* stipulates that universities in the Fifth Circuit jurisdiction cannot use race or ethnicity as factors in determining admission to the university, to special programs, or for scholarships or financial aid (Kauffman, 1996). Admissions can be made for example, on the basis of economic disadvantage, bilingual ability, or regional or geographical needs. This legislation means that educational institutions must find new or additional ways to continue to improve diversity in our student bodies. After 3 years, however, The University of Texas at Austin has almost the same percentage of minority students that it had when it ended affirmative action programs in 1996. This is purported to be attributable to stronger recruiting efforts and new financial aid programs (Carnevale, 1999). The Hopwood case may have far-reaching effects in other states and on the federal level. The National Science Foundation (NSF) and other funding agencies have modified or are modifying their guidelines to encourage recruitment and selection strategies.

In relation to health care in the United States, it is obvious that minority populations are greatly underserved. Since the 1960s the federal government has increased efforts to provide accessible, cost-effective care to underserved populations; the Department of Health and Human Resources plays a major role in that effort. Among the programs that have been developed are the National Health Service Corps, the Health Careers Opportunity Program, Centers of Excellence in Minority Health, and Student Assistance Programs (U.S. Department of Health and Human Services [DHHS], 1991). The underlying assumption of these programs is that the recruitment and support of minority students in the health professions will assist in meeting the health care needs of underserved minority communities. It must be noted, however, that the Minorities in Higher Education, 1995-96 Fourteenth Annual Status Report found that high school completion rates increased for African Americans but declined for Hispanics; women completed high school at higher rates than men, with a 6% difference for Hispanics, a 6.3% gap for African Americans, and a 3.9% gap for Caucasians; the total college enrollment declined slightly; all four major ethnic groups showed enrollment growth in colleges, with Hispanics increasing 6.9% and Asian Americans increasing 7.5%; and the number of faculty of color increased 43.7% from 1983 to 1993. White faculty members increased 6.4% during the same period (Carter & Wilson, 1996). Curtailing affirmative actions might seriously impact on the ability to prepare minority students who have a vested interest in serving underserved minority communities.

CULTURAL COMPETENCE

Over the last 40 years various contracts have evolved that have sought to recognize, define, and develop section plans for the multicultural, multi-ethnic population of the United States. Nurse educators, as well as nurses in direct client service, have struggled with these contracts as they evolved from cognition to practice. Terms such as multiculturism, cultural sensitivity, cultural awareness,

and transculturism (Leininger, 1994) have evolved to the more popular and broader conceptualization in 2000 of cultural competence. Leininger has been among the most prolific authors urging culturally congruent care as one of the highest priorities in nursing. The impact of this growing realization is evident in Medicare contracts that mandate the ability to offer linguistically and culturally appropriate care in awards to managed care institutions (Salimbene, 1999).

The construct of cultural competence has developed because awareness, sensitivity, and cultural knowledge are not sufficient. Culture is a system of learned patterns of behavior shared by members of a group. It does not refer exclusively to ethnicity and could include a variety of cultures (MacDonald, 1998). Culture molds personal needs and expectations as well as group needs and expectations (Salimbene, 1999).

Wells (1996) developed the Multicultural Competency Education Model. This model incorporates three major areas: self exploration, knowledge, and skills. It also identifies the components of attitudes, behaviors, and perceptions as assimilated in the learning process. The Culturally Competent Model of Care was proposed by Campinha-Bacote (1994). This model includes cultural awareness, cultural knowledge, cultural skill, and cultural encounters as essential components.

Salimbene (1999) states that equal care does not mean the same care in a multicultural society. It is necessary to commit to increasing the cultural and linguistic awareness of members of the profession. Certain skills and abilities were identified as essential for cultural competence. These 10 competencies emphasize awareness, sensitivity, and tolerance as well as understanding, knowledge, and skills that are culturally relevant. The final criterion is "confidence in one's ability to offer care to patients of other cultures" (Salimbene, 1999, p. 31).

Cultural competence is not only relevant for patient care and for nursing education that defines that care, but also for the profession of nursing. Minority representation in the profession of nursing has been a concern for many years. How this situation has evolved, where the profession is today in recruiting and retaining minority students and faculty, and the remediation strategies employed may well determine the relevance of the nursing profession for the complex emerging health care system of the future.

MINORITY REPRESENTATION IN NURSING

Job opportunities are expected to rise faster than the norm in the next decade. Nursing can no longer sustain itself without incorporating, to a greater extent, diverse minority groups into the profession. Interwoven with the issues related to minorities in nursing are a number of issues that reflect societal views toward women, toward subcultures in our society, and toward demographic changes that have occurred over time. Although the number of men in nursing has increased, the profession remains predominantly female (approximately 96%). Therefore gender socialization has played and continues to play a major role in both the continuation and the development of nursing. Stereotypes related to both gender and ethnicity cannot be separated artificially when examining the past, present, and future considerations of minorities in nursing.

Basic influences when selecting a career relate to one's beliefs about oneself. Where do I belong or fit? What is an acceptable career from the viewpoint of my family and my social group? Where can I find personal fulfillment? Financial reward? Advancement? Security? Ability to be mobile, yet permanence in a career?

All statistics related to minority status are self-reported. Students indicate their ethnic status as they perceive it. For federal government reports the usual categories are black non-Hispanic, white non-Hispanic, American Indian or Alaskan Native, Asian or Pacific Islander, Hispanic, and race or ethnicity unknown (Borden, 1995). In 1996 there were 2,558,874 licensed reported registered nurses (RNs) in the United States. In 1992 less than 10% (approximately 207,000) were identified as being of a minority background: blacks (90,600), Asian or Pacific Islanders (76,000), Hispanics (30,400), and American Indian or Alaskan Natives (10,000) (Moses, 1993); the 1996 figures are expected to be similar. When these data are compared with data collected by the Division of Nursing in 1988 (U.S. Department of Health and Human Services [DHHS], 1990), it appears that the growth in the number of minority RNs has probably kept pace with the growth of the total number of nurses, but the proportions of minority nurses have not increased. The 10% minority population in nursing is less than the 25% representation of minorities found throughout the United States. The only equal representation appears with those of Asian or Pacific Island backgrounds (Moses, 1993).

It should be noted that there is a difference in the type of education for nursing for minority groups. There are 1,508 basic RN programs in the United States: 109 diploma programs, 876 associate degree programs, and 523 baccalaureate programs. A decline in admissions to nursing programs began in 1992-1993, with the result that 10,700 fewer students were admitted to nursing pro-

grams in 1995-1996 (National League for Nursing [NLN], 1997). Completion of associate degree programs is the prevalent mode for 46% of Hispanic nurses and 42% of African American nurses. Although baccalaureate programs have higher proportions of minority students than do associate degree programs, because associate degree programs tend to produce more graduates than do baccalaureate programs, the actual numbers of associate-degree graduates in the nursing population is greater (Moses, 1993). An analysis of educational levels for minority nurses also indicates that about 10% of black nurses have master's or doctoral degrees compared with 8% of white nurses and 6% of Hispanic and Asian nurses (Justiz, 1995). It is important to note that Hispanics remain underrepresented at the collegiate level. Only 2.9% of Hispanics are awarded baccalaureate degrees, and only 1.8% receive doctoral degrees (Justiz, 1995). From 1989 to 1994 the number of Hispanic and African American students graduating from basic RN programs has decreased, whereas Asian graduates have increased (NLN, Part III, 1997).

These figures must be related to what is occurring in nursing education. Obvious questions to be investigated include the following: Are members of minority groups attracted to nursing? Do they successfully complete programs of study? Do they remain in the profession? Why should we be concerned about the representation, or rather lack of representation, of significant numbers of minorities in nursing? What directions should we pursue?

CURRENT STATUS OF MINORITIES IN NURSING EDUCATION PROGRAMS

Nursing is not unique among the professions, which traditionally have attracted predominantly white students. This has persisted despite efforts at equal opportunities for the culturally diverse segments of American society. It is indeed incongruous when one considers Hodgkinson's 1985 study of demographic trends and their impact on our educational system. That study concludes that by the current year, 2000, one in every three citizens will be nonwhite. Harris (1990) predicts that by the 21st century one third to one half of all students will be students of color. The nursing population is not a predominantly young group. In 1984, 20% of all graduates were younger than 30 years of age, and in 1988 this had decreased to 15.6%. The average age of a new nursing graduate is 29 years (NLN, Part III, 1997). The average age for all RNs is 43.1 years, with Hispanic nurses being somewhat younger (39.7 years) than those of other groups (Moses, 1993).

During the 1980s declining enrollments in nursing education programs encouraged schools to actively pursue minority candidates. The Nurse Training Act of 1964 and subsequent revisions provided special funding to increase the number of disadvantaged and minority students in schools of nursing. In 1965 the Sealantic fund (Rockefeller brother's fund) began sponsoring a program in nursing education for disadvantaged students. This project emphasized recruitment, counseling, summer enrichment programs, and financial assistance. The American Nurses Association Minority Fellowship program and the Kellogg Fellows program are other examples of attempts not only to improve the numbers of minority nurses but also to assist minority nurses to advance in the profession.

In 1963, the National Student Nurses' Association developed the Breakthrough to Nursing project, which focused on recruiting minorities into the nursing profession. Federal funding for this project was obtained in 1971 and again in 1974. The Breakthrough project emphasized the establishment of one-to-one relationships with prospective candidates and also included a planned tutoring-advocacy-counseling component (Carnegie, 1988). Despite this 37-year effort in nursing, the racial-ethnic composition in nursing education programs remained the same as that reported for all higher education students in 1988, with the number of blacks being marginally higher for nursing (11.4%) than for all students (10%). In 1990 Carter reported increases in American Indian, Hispanic, and African American students in 2-year institutions, whereas there were more Asians enrolled in 4-year institutions.

The tracking of nursing students by the NLN clearly illustrates that the minority composition of nursing students varies across geographical areas of the country. A variety of sources verifies this geographical distribution. For example, approximately 73% of African American RNs are employed in the Northeast and South, with about 47% of African American nurses working in the South. Seventy percent of all employed RNs are found in the western or southern regions of the country (36% in the West and 33.5% in the South). Asian nurses are usually employed in the West (38%) and Northeast (32%) (Moses, 1993). As in earlier reports, the Midwest has the fewest minorities in all categories.

The NLN Research Annual Survey for 1995 found that minority enrollment in licensed vocational nurse (LVN) programs increased and represented 29.9% of the total enrollment. Hispanic and American Indian enrollments continued to increase, 6.3% and 1.8%, respectively. Asian enrollment was unchanged at 3.1% (NLN, 1997).

Men continue to represent only a small minority in nursing, and because the recruitment efforts in nursing focus on ethnic minorities, it is expected that this representation will continue. Although the national average for male enrollment is reported as 3.3% by Moses (1990), enrollment in geographical areas varies. In west Texas, for example, men constitute anywhere from 15% to 18% of the student nursing enrollment. It may be that the increased enrollment of men in this region is a reflection of their viewing nursing as a route upward in the social and economic structure, the acceptance in these communities of men in a predominantly female profession, or the great need for nurses in this area.

Statistics related to minority enrollment in nursing programs become of even greater concern when considered in relation to the enrollment in specific types of nursing programs. At the baccalaureate level, for example, Hispanics constitute 2.9% of the total enrollment, but at the master's and doctoral levels their enrollments are only 1.7% each. Although African Americans generally represent the largest minority in nursing, it is worth noting that of all African American nursing students, 8.8% are enrolled in generic baccalaureate programs, 7.4% in RN baccalaureate programs, 5.2% in master's programs, and 4.3% in doctoral programs. Only 1 of 14 postdoctoral students was African American (American Association of Colleges of Nursing [AACN], 1990). Figures reported by the National League for Nursing in 1997 verify a consistency in the distribution of minorities enrolled.

Factors Influencing the Need to Change Minority Ratios

A persistent decline in the number of young people eligible for college admission has been documented nationwide. Concurrently there has been an increase in the number of older students (those over 25 years of age) who are interested in pursuing college careers, including nursing.

Applications to nursing programs recovered from the 1980s' slump as a result of the compounded impact of the nursing shortage, a lack of access to health care for many Americans, an aging population, a shift in emphasis to primary community health care, cost containment efforts by hospitals (including the use of diagnostic-related groups [DRGs]), and a movement to break down barriers between the health professions through expanded reimbursement by Medicaid, Medicare, and third-party insurers for specifically prepared nurses. These factors have forced the health care system to upgrade salaries and benefits for nurses. When adequate financial reimbursement occurs in a profession, members of that profession develop an increased sense of self-esteem and colleagues in other professions develop an increased respect. Despite increased salaries and the efforts by hospitals to recover from failed downsizing attempts, enrollments of entry-level nursing students fell by 5.5% in the fall of 1998, and master's degree enrollments fell slightly by 2.1% compared with the previous year (AACN, 1999). As health care moved to a managed care system, there occurred a downsizing of beds and nursing staff in hospitals. Unfortunately, adequate remuneration has not extended to areas of need beyond hospital settings. Public health nursing salaries, school nursing salaries, and salaries in extended care facilities still lag. This is a serous manifestation of the blatant lack of provision for quality health care to the poor, to rural and urban underserved and underinsured citizens, and to minority populations, and particularly a diminished commitment to health promotion and disease prevention activities. The Division of Nursing of the U.S. Department of Health and Human Services projects that the rising demand for RNs will outstrip the supply by 2010.

The question of quality in nursing practice continues to be a factor that must be considered carefully. In the past, nursing schools were tempted to make exceptions to admissions requirements in order to maintain programs through sustained enrollments. Now the pendulum may swing toward admitting only the most highly qualified applicants in relation to quantitative measures such as American College Test (ACT) scores, Scholastic Aptitude Test (SAT) scores, or grade point average (GPA). Because of the increased applicant pool, admissions committees may be tempted to fill classes with only the best students as measured by traditional criteria. If efforts are not made on elementary, middle, and high school levels to better prepare minority students, we may find that the equal opportunity access has been thwarted. Most admissions evaluations cannot accommodate all minimally prepared applicants, so admissions committees seek to select the students with the most potential for success (Boyle, 1986). If this is carried to the extreme, minority students may suffer because they will not be afforded the opportunity to attempt to succeed. To make matters worse, several schools have closed nursing programs either completely, for example, Niagara University, or for undergraduate nursing education, as did the University of Rochester. Both of these nursing programs are in the Northeast, and both are in western New York State. The Northeast has reported an oversupply of RNs. Other programs have cut back on enrollment, for example, the University of Cincinnati.

Traditionally, minority students have been classified as high-risk students because they often experience higher attrition rates than white students. The most frequently used criteria on which admission to nursing is based include high school grade point average (GPA), high school rank, interviews, health data, college GPA, ACT assessment scores, SAT scores, and autobiographical essays. There have been a number of conflicting studies regarding the usefulness of these criteria for the prediction of success in a nursing program. Dell and Halpin (1984) recommend the use of high school GPA, SAT scores, and National League of Nursing (NLN) scores as effective for use with all ethnic groups.

The Boyle (1986) study found that the ACT score was the strongest and most effective predictor of state board examination achievement and of final GPA. Entering GPA was the only variable that was found to account for program completion, but it did not accurately predict program dropouts. The higher the entering GPA, however, the greater the likelihood of program completion. The predictive power for blacks was less than that for other minorities, but an earlier investigator (Schwirian, 1977) maintained that less than 50% of attrition is really related to academic difficulty and that attrition may rather be due to greater social and economic disadvantages. A study by Schmidt, Pearlman, and Hunter (1980) sought to evaluate the validity and fairness of employment and educational tests for Hispanics. The results of this study indicate that there is strong evidence that the tests are neither differentially valid for, nor unfair to, Hispanics. The validity and slope differences were found to be the result of chance, as reported in an earlier study by Bartlett, Bobko, Mosier, and Hannon (1978) of African Americans and whites.

In recent years, women have been attracted to professions other than the traditional occupations of nursing and teaching. The attractiveness of the nursing profession has been enhanced during the past 30 years, however, by the development of new and expanded roles in nursing. These new roles are characterized by increased autonomy and by increased appreciation and recognition from the public and from professional colleagues. Efforts have recently been increased by Sigma Theta Tau International and the National Student Nurses' Association to raise the consciousness of the general public and particularly junior high school students to nursing as a profession (Fitzgerald, 2000).

High school students today have a broad range of career choices. The AACN (1990) report dealing with enrollment management found that a large percentage of students cited nursing as a career objective and that parents exerted the most influence on student career choice. When students were asked why they had an interest in nursing, they cited the following desires: (1) to help others, (2) to work directly with people, and (3) to work with life-and-death situations. The reasons they lacked interest in nursing were related to the requirements to (1) work in high-pressure situations, (2) work in stressful situations, and (3) work different shifts. Parental goals for their children were reported as follows: (1) to be financially secure, (2) to do rewarding work, and (3) to have time to spend with family. These items were rated number 11, 2, and 10, respectively, by parents in relation to the nursing profession (AACN, 1990).

The Hispanic Student in Nursing

The term *Hispanic* includes those of Spanish, Mexican American, Puerto Rican, and Cuban descent. The greatest numbers of Hispanics in the United States are Mexican American (Chicanos). Rojas (1994) cites data from the *Laredo Morning Times* of December 5, 1992, that estimates that 33% of the U.S. population growth from 1992 through 2000 will be a growth in the Hispanic population. From 1989 to 1994 the number of Hispanic RN graduates decreased from 3.1% in 1989 to 3% in 1994 (NLN, Part III, 1997). This growth is predicted to accelerate to 57% from 2030 to 2050. Hispanic students rely heavily on financial aid for college expenses because almost 25% of Hispanic students come from families with an annual income of less than $10,000. An additional 20% of Hispanic students come from families earning between $10,000 and $20,000 annually (Dutko, 1994). Despite this great need, the average financial aid award to Hispanic students ($3,466) is less than that for other groups, including Asians ($4,383), African Americans ($3,788), and non-Hispanic whites ($3,524) (Dutko, 1994). Over half of all Hispanic students attend 2-year programs, and almost half of all Hispanic students attend school part-time.

A study by Vasquez (1982) found that sex-role restrictions and low socioeconomic status rather than culture or language partially accounted for the relatively low number of Chicanas (Mexican American women) in postsecondary education. Chicanas are no different from other people in wanting education as a means to socioeconomic mobility and independence. Unfortunately, these women, who are often the first in their families to attend college, experience dissonance in relation to their expected role in Mexican American society as wife, mother, and subservient person to the man; all these factors exert an influ-

ence to diminish professional career expectations. Unfortunately, Mexican American students are often steered into taking noncollege preparatory courses in high school. This may be promulgated by the family as a means of keeping women in less demanding work, which in turn is perceived as having a less negative impact on the woman's traditional role. Such advice from family members may be reinforced by educators who often stereotype Mexican American students as unable to prepare for more challenging careers. Most of these students need financial assistance, as their parents are generally unable to contribute as much to their education as white parents can (Vasquez, 1982). Therefore they generally rely heavily on scholarships and work-study programs and, to a lesser extent, on loans. Because of the difference in cultures and the difficulty in acculturation, many of these minority students feel more comfortable in smaller colleges or community colleges. Support systems such as associations and organizations that can recognize, promote, and reinforce cultural values are important for student adjustment regardless of the size of the educational setting.

Financial difficulty and discomfort in the setting, while problematic, are not the primary factors for leaving educational programs. A study by Cope and Hannah (1975) found that the motivation to finish college was influenced in great measure by the family's emotional support of the student. This may be a comforting fact to relay to parents who fear "losing" their child when she or he pursues higher education. Because parents do influence their child's choice of a career, some reassurance from an individual's ethnic group—such as continued inclusion in family and community activities—has been found to be a necessary positive component of adjustment and success in college. This finding may reassure Mexican American parents of their continued important role. In fact several researchers, including Ramirez and Castaneda (1974), have found that participating in two or more cultures may provide for a more flexible adjustment.

It would appear to be self-evident that Hispanic students, like other students, would tend to persist in their education when their parents have higher educations and when parental occupations result in higher incomes. Low family income, for many students, results in their dropping out of school. Because Mexican American families generally have lower incomes and either larger or extended families to absorb those incomes, their children are at risk for attrition. Efforts must persist, therefore, to obtain scholarships and grants to attempt to alleviate some of this financial pressure. In 1991 the DHHS instituted a new scholarship program called Scholarships for

Disadvantaged Students. These scholarships recognize that the concept of being disadvantaged is not necessarily tied to ethnicity alone, but rather is tied to socioeconomic factors including deficits in a particular school district's ability to offer enriched programs for students.

The African American Student in Nursing

Almost 15% of the graduates of licensed practical nurse (LPN) or LVN programs and only 6.8% of the graduates of RN programs are African American (NLN, Part III, 1997). African American graduates fell from 9.2% in 1989 to 6.8% in 1994 (Rosella, Regan-Kubinski, & Albrecht, 1994). Only 7.1% of all RNs are African American. This is significant because African Americans, in terms of general health, tend to be sicker than the general population. Whereas European Americans have a life expectancy of 76 years, the average life expectancy of African Americans is 69.2 years (National Center for Health Statistics, 1992). African Americans die 6.6 times more often from homicide than European Americans do, and hypertension occurs in 2% of the African American population and in only 0.1% of European Americans (Rosella et al., 1994). These statistics are important examples because the low numbers of African American nurses present a barrier to treatment because of the lack of integration of the cultural beliefs, values, and practices of African Americans. Thus, despite the fact that numerous studies have shown that African Americans' compliance to treatment is affected by cultural values (Berg & Berg, 1989), there are few African American nurses to positively affect the integration of cultural values.

Nursing education has historically provided one of the few avenues for African American women to acquire a respected profession. For many years, however, that education was primarily obtained in African American hospitals and colleges. New graduates worked only with African Americans. As the nursing profession evolved, an elitist system developed in which most white schools had racial quotas. An early effort to recruit African American nursing students was stimulated during World War II by the Cadet Nurse Corps program. Today the emphasis is on attracting African American and other minority students, not to fill quotas but to develop a cohort of professional nurses who better represent the general population.

Between 1976 and 1982 the National Advisory Committee on Black Higher Education and Black Colleges and Universities studied the admission and retention problems of African American students at seven predominantly white universities. Although this committee no longer exists, the problem it faced—the retention of African American baccalaureate nursing students—persists (Allen, Nunley, & Scott-Warner, 1988).

African American students, like other minority students, often receive a poor secondary education. Their self-esteem has been low and the university setting has generally been perceived as hostile to them. Not only high school counselors have failed in encouraging African American students to pursue higher education but also university counselors who have not been able to effectively thwart the feelings of loneliness and alienation that African American students frequently experience. Inadequate financial aid has been found to be a barrier to both the admission and the retention of African American nursing students (Allen et al., 1988).

Graduate Nursing Education and the Minority Student

Minority enrollment in graduate nursing programs has consistently been a small segment of the total enrollment. Total graduate enrollment of all minority groups fell slightly from 1994 to 1995, and African Americans continue to have the highest representation (6.3%); Asians are next at 3.7%, Hispanics at 2.7%, and American Indians at 0.5%. Graduations of minorities also decreased in this time period by 0.8% (NLN, Part III, 1997). Graduate education in nursing continues to grow, as indicated by an 8.1% increase in master's degree graduates from 1989 to 1990 (NLN, 1991). In addition, the number of doctoral programs rose to 50 in 1990 (NLN, 1991). In 1995, 30 new master's programs were established. Master's programs now total 306 (NLN, Part III, 1997). The expansion of advanced educational preparation in nursing is related to increased specialization in the practice arena, necessitating increased preparation in terms of the complexity and competency needed to administer quality nursing care and to pursue relevant research.

Funding for students to attend graduate programs is always subject to the legislators' awareness of the importance of and need for such funding. Federal monies distributed as a result of the Nursing Education Act are primarily allocated for nurses pursuing advanced preparation as nurse practitioners, nurse-midwives, nurse anesthetists, and advanced clinical specialists.

As in undergraduate education, geographical distribution differences exist, with the largest number of graduate minority students found in the South and the smallest number in the West (NLN, 1991). Almost two thirds of all master's graduates prepare for advanced clinical practice, 9% prepare for administration, and 12% prepare for teaching. Of those nurses prepared at the graduate level,

13.2% are members of minority groups; 6.3% are African American, 2.7% are Hispanic, 3.7% are Asian, and 0.5% are American Indian. The number of those who actually complete graduate programs is somewhat lower (NLN, Part III, 1997).

Between 1989 and 1990, the number of nursing doctoral degrees awarded in the United States dropped from 324 to 295. The NLN (1991) speculated that this may be a result of increased numbers of part-time students, decreased funding for dissertation research, and a lack of doctorally prepared faculty to work with students. Since 1991-1992 there has been an increase in doctoral degrees conferred, with 425 new graduates in 1994-1995 (NLN, Part III, 1997). The number of doctoral programs in nursing has increased to 64. Four new programs were added from 1994 to 1995 (NLN, Part III, 1997). Minority enrollment in doctoral programs has been reported as 1.1% or lower for American Indians or Alaskan Natives, 1.7% for Hispanics, and 4.3% for African Americans. All minority groups are represented by lower percentages at the graduate level as opposed to those at the baccalaureate level. This is in contrast to the white students, who increase in percentage at the graduate level: Whites account for 81.9% of all baccalaureate students, 86.1% of all master's students, and 83% of all doctoral students. It should be noted that at the doctoral level 2.6% (more than Hispanics and Asian or Pacific Islanders) are nonresident alien students, and 5.3% are of unknown heritage (AACN, 1992).

What do these data mean? It is obvious that the numbers of minority students seeking higher education in nursing are not representative of the general population, especially in the case of Hispanics. Therefore these nurses are not able to move within the profession to positions of leadership and power. Why does this happen? Once again a variety of factors interact. The following interpretation is a premise for those of Hispanic origin. Because of the low economic status of most Mexican American families, when the student completes the basic nursing program, she or he is expected to go to work immediately, often the day after graduation, to contribute to the family's finances. In more than one instance, the graduate is expected to put the next child through college. In addition, at this stage in their lives, marriage and child rearing become a focus. The Mexican American family culture frowns on leaving children at day-care centers or in the care of nonfamily caregivers. In addition, the basic cultural value of the dominant male figure often overrides a career drive. In other words, the nurse resumes life in a culture that generally does not encourage advanced preparation. Survival of the family unit is the primary motivator. This is not to judge that value but rather to acknowledge that it exists and that it may be a factor that discourages minority nurses from pursuing graduate education.

STRATEGIES TO IMPROVE THE ETHNIC MIX IN NURSING

It is predicted that the population of the United States will increase to 300 million shortly after 2010 and may increase to 394 million by 2050 (a 50% increase from 1995). The Hispanic population, which grew 37% from 1995 to 2000, is predicted to grow 44% from 2000 to 2020 and 62% from 2020 to 2050. The non-Hispanic white population during these same years is predicted to fall steadily from 74% of the population in 1995 to 64% in 2020, to 53% in 2050. By 2050 the African American population is predicted to nearly double its 1995 size to 61 million (U.S. Bureau of Census, 1996, pp. 1 and 15). Other races (Asians, Pacific Islanders, and American Indians) are predicted to triple in number by 2040 (a growth of 16 million) (U.S. Bureau of the Census, 1986, p. 1). One successful program designed to help the retention of minority students is PLUS (Partnership in Learning for Utmost Success) implemented at the Saint Xavier College School of Nursing in Chicago, Illinois. It includes a comprehensive assessment plan, the PLUS program of studies (six 1–credit hour academic courses in nursing), faculty development, and partnerships for learning (mentoring) (Lockie & Burke, 1999).

Mexican Americans comprise the second largest minority in the United States and can be found not only in the Southwest but also in urban areas throughout the United States. Therefore increased representation of these minority groups must be a priority. As these populations grow, there will be an increased need for nurses who can relate to, understand, and be accepted by the community. Two important roles will be (1) assisting people who have been deprived of access to health care to participate in the existing health care system and (2) molding the future health care system to be responsive to their needs.

In order to accomplish these goals, federal, state, and local financial support must be available. Inequities in public education must be addressed. Local public school boards must direct resources toward the goal of quality educational opportunities for all children. Poor school tax districts must receive assistance from the state.

Factors inhibiting minority members from attaining a career in nursing include feelings of powerlessness; inadequate academic preparation, especially in the sciences; financial costs and the actual and projected decrease in financial aid; inadequate career counseling; and more and better recruitment strategies by other disciplines. At the postsecondary level, institutions must provide counseling and tutorial services as well as financial aid. Retention of minority students may be negatively affected by "stereotype vulnerability." In this situation, minority students disengage themselves from the anxiety of performance; that is, they accept the view that they lack the ability to succeed (Davidhizar, Dowd, & Giger, 1998).

A major problem in nursing education is the few members of minority nursing faculty. Less than 9% of nursing faculty were minority members in 1992: 5.9% were African American, 0.9% Hispanic, 1.6% Asian, and 0.3% Native American or Native Alaskan (NLN, 1993). The composition of nursing faculties must reflect an ethnic mix, not only for token representation or to reflect a specific community but also to become a living model of diversity in collaboration, a model that stresses competence, academic ability, caring, and true equality. Potential minority faculty members must be identified as early as possible in their academic careers and supported in their efforts to obtain graduate degrees. In one possible system, they could pay back the institution's financial support through a committed service period.

These young faculty members, like all junior faculty, must be nurtured through a mentoring program. They have the potential to serve as role models for minority students and, in time, can serve as mentors themselves. It is unfortunate that research by minority faculty members is often not only unappreciated but also denigrated. For example, colleagues in nursing may look despairingly upon research concerning American Indian rites related to health or African American nutritional practices. If culturally based research is not valued, minority faculty members may not be tenured. This prevents career advancement and limits contributions to that particular program (Campbell & Sigsby, 1994).

There is currently a greater proportion of African American faculty members in nursing compared with their representation in all other colleges. There is a smaller percentage, however, of all other minority groups in nursing faculty compared with that in all other colleges. Regional population differences exist, with more African Americans in the South and more Asians and Hispanics in the West. Associate-degree programs appear to have more faculty diversity (NLN, 1991). This may be related to the minimal academic credential of a bachelor's degree that is required to teach in an associate-degree program. Additionally, fewer than 8% of the chief administrators of nursing programs are designated as members of a minority group (NLN, 1991). These figures are similar for all nursing administrative positions.

In recent years there have been philosophical discussions about whether there should be organizations for minorities in nursing, such as the Hispanic Nurses' Association or the National Black Nurses' Association. It would appear that these organizations provide support and networking for minority nurses who may not be able to take advantage of opportunities in the major nursing organizations because of their small numbers. Therefore until the minority nurses themselves feel that a need no longer exists, local chapters of these organizations should be encouraged. Professional nursing success, which is necessary to advance in the profession, can be interpreted as psychological success whereby an internalized goal includes ego involvement. Psychological success increases self-esteem and strengthens a commitment (Hall, 1976). A supportive social network is a means of minimizing the threat to one's sense of self-worth and fostering career enhancement.

Nursing education has a direct responsibility to educate practitioners for the future. The demographics of the United States have changed. Spanish has become a second language in many parts of the country, and we must educate our own to meet these changes.

SUMMARY

Health care reform issues mandate minority representation in all health professions. The new health care system must reflect the community, and as care moves into the community, health care provider-community partnerships are formed. It has also been reported that ethnic minority health care providers are more likely than non-ethnic minority health care providers to practice in culturally diverse settings after graduation (U.S. Department of Health and Human Services, 1992).

There is considerable literature on recruiting and maintaining minority representation in nursing. Some educational institutions recruit very heavily from minority institutions. They offer excellent financial assistance to students and woo faculty members with high salaries. The fact that many of these programs experience difficulty in retaining minority students and faculty members should send a message to everyone. The issue of minority representation in nursing is complex. Unless efforts are made to integrate the values, beliefs, and cultures of minority populations into the curricula and into support programs, there will be no success. Minority students must be encouraged to share their diversity. They must select what is important to them from their own culture and adapt to the educational environment.

Multiple strategies are required, and financial assistance, while very important, is not solely sufficient. Unless strategic planning for minority recruitment and retention is implemented, all efforts will be doomed. For example, hiring minority faculty members, without mentoring and assistance in the assumption of leadership roles, will not be successful as a long-term strategy. For both students and faculty, support services, formal and informal, can assist in resolving cultural dissonance. Such strategies must be incorporated throughout the curriculum. Content areas such as interpersonal skills, communication skills, leadership ability, and professionalism must be blended.

It is amazing that we are still grappling with racial and ethnic issues as we head into the 21st century. If we do our job well, however, these issues will become extinct.

REFERENCES

Allen, M.E., Nunley, J.C., & Scott-Warner, M. (1988). Recruitment and retention of black students in baccalaureate nursing programs. *Journal of Nursing Education, 27*(3), 107-116.

American Association of Colleges of Nursing. (1990). *Enrollment management for programs in nursing education* (Pub. No. 19-2419). Washington, DC: Author.

American Association of Colleges of Nursing. (1992). *1991-1992 Enrollment and graduations in baccalaureate and graduate programs in nursing* (Pub. No. 91-92-1). Washington, DC: Author.

American Association of Colleges of Nursing. (1999). *1998-1999 Enrollment and graduations in baccalaureate and graduate programs in nursing.* Washington, DC: Author.

Andrews, M.M. (1992). Cultural perspectives on nursing in the 21st century. *Journal of Professional Nursing, 8*(1), 7-15.

Bartlett, C.J., Bobko, P., Mosier, S.B., & Hannon, R. (1978). Testing for fairness with a moderated multiple regression strategy: An alternate to differential analysis. *Personnel Psychology, 31,* 233-241.

Berg, J., & Berg, B.L. (1989). Compliance, diet and cultural factors among Black Americans with end-stage renal disease. *Journal of National Black Nurses' Association, 3*(2), 16-28.

Borden, V.M.H. (1995, June). Analysis of postsecondary degrees conferred to minorities. *Black Issues in Higher Education,* pp. 38-73.

Boyle, K.K. (1986). Predicting the success of minority students in a baccalaureate nursing program. *Journal of Nursing Education, 25*(5), 186-192.

Campbell, D.W., & Sigsby, L.M. (1994). Increasing minorities in higher education in nursing: Faculty consultation as a strategy. *Journal of Professional Nursing, 10*(1), 7-12.

Campinha-Bacote, J. (1994). Cultural competence in psychiatric mental health nursing. *Nursing Clinics of North America, 29,* 107.

Carnegie, M.E. (1988). Breakthrough to nursing: Twenty-five years of involvement. *Imprint, 35*(2), 55-56, 59.

Carnevale, D. (1999, September 3). Enrollment of minority freshmen nears pre-Hopwood levels at University of Texas at Austin. *The Chronicle of Higher Education,* p. A71.

Carter, D.J. (1990). Racial and ethnic trends in college participation: 1976-1988. *Research Briefs (American Council on Education), 1*(3).

Carter, D.J., & Wilson, R. (1996). *Minorities in higher education, 1995-96.* Fourteenth Annual Status Report (pp. 1-93). Washington, DC: American Council on Education.

Cope, R.G., & Hannah, W. (1975). *Revolving college doors: The causes and consequences of dropping out, stopping out, and transferring.* New York: Wiley-Interscience.

Davidhizar, R., Dowd, S.B., & Giger, J.N. (1998). Educating the culturally diverse healthcare student. *Nurse Educator, 23*(2), 38-42.

Dell, M., & Halpin, G. (1984). Predictors of success in nursing school and on state board examinations in a predominantly black baccalaureate nursing program. *Journal of Nursing Education, 23*(4), 147-150.

Dutko, K. (1994). Enrollment rise: Will aid follow? *Hispanic, 16*(7), 14.

Fitzgerald, T. (2000, January 10). Nurse appeal: Profession tries new tactics to woo next generation of nurses. *Health Week,* p. 15.

Hall, D.T. (1976). *Careers in organizations.* Pacific Palisades, CA: Goodyear.

Harris, R.L. (1990). Recruiting Afro-Americans into the graduate school pipeline. *Perspectives, 28*(1), 6, 11-12.

Hodgkinson, H.L. (1985). *All one system: Demographics of education, kindergarten through graduate school.* Washington, DC: Institute for Educational Leadership.

Jaschik, S. (1993, February 10). Supporters say threat to minority scholarship outlasts the Bush years. *The Chronicle of Higher Education,* p. A25.

Justiz, M.J. (1995). Hispanics in higher education. *Hispanic, 8*(5), 96.

Kauffman, A.H. (1996, August). The Hopwood Case—What it says, what it doesn't say, the future of the case and the rest of the story. *Intercultural Development Research Association (IDRA) Newsletter,* pp. 7-8.

Leininger, M. (1994). Transcultural nursing education: A worldwide imperative. *Nursing and Health Care, 15*(5), 254-257.

Lockie, N.M., & Burke, L.J. (1999). Partnership in learning for utmost success (PLUS): Evaluation of a retention program for at-risk nursing students. *Journal of Nursing Education, 38*(4), 188-192.

MacDonald, R. (1998). What is cultural competency? *British Journal of Occupational Therapy, 61*(7), 325-328.

Michaelson, M. (1995, July 28). Building a comprehensive defense of affirmative action programs. *The Chronicle of Higher Education,* p. A56.

Moses, E.B. (1990, June). *The registered nurse population. Findings from the National Sample Survey of Registered Nurses, 1988.* Rockville, MD: U.S. DHHS, PHS, HRSA, Bureau of Health Professions.

Moses, E.B. (1993). *Nurse leadership: Caring for the emerging majority: Empowering nurses through partnerships and coalitions* (pp. 15-26). Bethesda, MD: U.S. Department of Commerce.

National Center for Health Statistics. (1992, January 7). *Monthly Vital Statistics Report, 40*(8; suppl 2). Hyattsville, MD: U.S. Public Health Service.

National League for Nursing. (1991). *Nursing data source: Vol. 3. Leaders in the making: Graduate education in nursing* (Pub. No. 19-2422). New York: Author.

National League for Nursing, Division of Research. (1993). *Nursing data review* (Pub. No. 19-2529). New York: National League for Nursing Press.

National League for Nursing. (1997). *National League for Nursing Final Report. Commission in a workforce for a restructured health care system* (Parts I, II, III, IV). New York: National League for Nursing Press.

The numbers game. (1993, Fall). *Time, 142*(21), 14-15.

Ramirez III, M., & Castaneda, O. (1974). *Cultural democracy, bicognitive development and education.* New York: Academic Press.

Rojas, D. (1994). Leadership in a multicultural society: A case in role development. *Nursing and Health Care, 15*(5), 258-261.

Rosella, J.D., Regan-Kubinski, M.J., & Albrecht, S.D. (1994). The need for multicultural diversity. *Nursing and Health Care, 15*(5), 242-246.

Salimbene, S. (1999). Cultural competence: A priority for performance improvement action. *Journal of Nursing Care Quality, 13*(3), 23-25.

Schmidt, F.L., Pearlman, K., & Hunter, J.E. (1980). The validity of fairness of employment and education tests for Hispanic Americans: A review and analysis. *Personnel Psychology, 33*(4), 704-724.

Schwirian, P. (1977). *Prediction of successful nursing performance: Part 2. Admission practices, evaluation strategies and performance prediction among schools of nursing* (HEW Pub. No. HRA 77-27). Washington, DC: U.S. Government Printing Office.

U.S. Bureau of the Census. (1986). Spencer, G. Projections of the Hispanic population: 1983 to 2080. *Current Population Reports,* series P-25, No. 995. Washington, DC: U.S. Government Printing Office.

U.S. Bureau of the Census. (1996). Day, J.C. Population projections of the United States by age, sex, race, and Hispanic origin: 1995 to 2050. *Current Population Reports* (pp. 25-1130). Washington, DC: U.S. Government Printing Office.

U.S. Department of Health and Human Services. (1990). *The registered nurse population: Findings from the national sample survey of registered nurses, March 1988.* Washington, DC: Author.

U.S. Department of Health and Human Services. (1991). *Nursing: Health personnel in the United States, 1991: Eighth report to Congress.* Prepublication Report. Washington, DC: Author.

U.S. Department of Health and Human Services. (1992). *Health status of minorities and low-income groups.* Washington, DC: Author.

Vasquez, M.J.T. (1982). Confronting barriers to the participation of Mexican-American women in higher education. *Hispanic Journal of Behavioral Success, 4*(2), 147-165.

Wells, S. (1996). *Cultural competence: Preparing for the next millennium* (booklet). Workshop presentation. College of Occupational Therapists 20th Annual conference, University of Leeds.

Finally We Have Arrived

Men in Nursing

VERN L. BULLOUGH

In 1997 some 6.5% of the over 2 million registered nurses in the United States were men. This is still not up to the 6.98% who were men in 1910, but it represents a significant increase from the low point of 1960, when less than 1% of the nurses were men. The increase in men nurses in the last 40 years of the 20th century reflects the changes in nursing and nursing education that have made nursing at the beginning of the 21st century far more attractive to men than it once was. It is also clear that the percentages will continue to increase, since over 10% of both the associate and baccalaureate degrees conferred in 1996 went to men and the percentage of men enrolled in nursing schools continues to rise (American Nurses Association [ANA], 1946, 1994; Hospital and Health Network, 1994; National Center for Education Statistics, 1999; Statistical Abstract of the United States, 1998). To explain the reasons for the change and their implications is the purpose of this chapter.

BACKGROUND

American nursing clearly remains a profession dominated by women and will remain so in the foreseeable future, although men will play an increasing role in the 21st century. Nursing, however, was not always dominated by women and for much of its history men, as they had traditionally done in most jobs outside the home, dominated the field (Bullough & Bullough, 1993a). It was only in the last few decades of the 19th century that nursing in America came to be regarded as a woman's profession, and this was due to the example and influence of Florence Nightingale. Interestingly there was always a higher percentage of men nurses in the United Kingdom than in the United States.

As a general rule, women in the past were always under the legal control of their husbands, fathers, brothers, or sons. Much of modern history can be interpreted as a story of women's efforts to break free of the limitations put on them by a male-dominated society and to be recognized as important persons in their own right. The struggle was not an easy one, since it was necessary to overcome long ingrained beliefs and patterns that weighed as heavily on women as on men. The world was essentially defined by men who simply assumed that they were the high-status sex and that women were supposed to be subordinate to them. Although women had special abilities such as childbearing that made them indispensable, this was seen as simply justifying the male need to protect them. To put it simply, biology was regarded as destiny, and being female slotted a person into a special category; cultural assumptions followed biological beliefs, and simply being a woman put all kinds of restrictions on what a person could do. Economic and social status did have some effect on what was or was not permissible, but regardless of class, women usually had severe restrictions on their ability to act independently. Being a mother and bearing and nursing children, however rewarding this may be, does not in itself mean that women can not do other things as well. Many women aspired to have more diverse opportunities, and some, often with the encouragement of the men in their lives, were successful. Not infrequently the women who broke the "male only" barriers were often described, by themselves as well as by others, as having a manly mind, manly courage, or manly ability; that is, their biology was slightly different from that of other women. Such a comparison allowed a few women to be exceptional but permitted the continual degradation of the inherent abilities of the majority of women.

As Mary Wollstonecraft (1759-1797), the intellectual founder of modern feminism, in her 1792 manifesto, *Vindication of the Rights of Women*, said:

Men complain, with reason, of the follies and caprices of our sex, when they do not keenly satirize our headstrong passions and groveling vices. Behold, I should answer the natural effect of ignorance! The mind will ever be unstable that has only prejudices to rest on, and the current will run with destructive fury when there are no barriers to break its force. Women are told from their infancy and taught by the examples of their mothers, that a little knowledge of human weakness, justly termed cunning, softness of temper, outward obedience, and scrupulous attention to a puerile kind of propriety, will obtain for them the protection of a man, and should they be beautiful, everything else is needless, for at least twenty years of their lives (Wollstonecraft, 1929, p. 23).

One reason a woman like Wollstonecraft could argue for and achieve an audience for change is that the Industrial Revolution was undermining traditional patterns of life and the intellectual movement known as the Enlightenment was encouraging the challenge of long-held ideas. Although the emerging factories, first in England and then elsewhere, employed the village women, this only accentuated the problem of the middle-class women who lacked opportunities to make themselves useful. Even those women who initially worked in the factories were ultimately seen as taking jobs away from men, and so employment increasingly came to be limited to unmarried women or widows, and these jobs were regarded as temporary. Most of the women who worked long term did so as domestics or washerwomen or in similar tasks regarded as belonging to the female world. Such positions were not available to middle-class women, since, as one woman wrote in the middle of the 19th century, a "proper" woman could not:

> work for profit, or engage in any occupation that money can command, lest she invade the rights of the working classes. ... Men in want of employment have pressed their way into nearly all the shopping and retail businesses that in my early years were managed in whole, or in part, by women. The conventional barrier that pronounced it ungenteel to be behind a counter, or serving the public in any mercantile capacity is greatly extended. The same in household economy. Servants must be up to their offices, which is very well but ladies, dismissed from the dairy, the confectionery, the store room, the still room, the poultry yard, the kitchen garden, and the orchard have hardly yet found themselves a sphere equally useful and important to the pursuits of trade and arts to which to apply their too abundant leisure. [Greg, 1969, pp. 315-316]

Many of the more well-to-do women tried to participate in the intellectual ferment by becoming hostesses or par-

ticipating in intellectual discussion. The term "blue stocking" was often used to describe such women because they tended to dress more informally at such literary events.

The problem that women faced was how to break through the barriers yet retain the proper feminine image. An obvious solution was to busy oneself with traditional women's activities in the home and somehow make these activities into a profession. Such activities included caring for the sick, raising and educating small children, visiting and helping neighbors, raising the cultural consciousness of the men in their lives, assisting their husbands in their work or profession, and managing the household. It was from these "wifely" tasks that nurses, elementary school teachers, friendly visitors (who eventually came to be called social workers), librarians, and secretaries emerged, although the last case also coincided with the invention and widespread use of the typewriter (Bullough & Bullough, 1978, 1984).

The first efforts of women in all these fields were essentially charitable ones, and only gradually did these tasks become paying jobs. Whether consciously or unconsciously, women who wanted to challenge tradition seized on the 19th century notion that they constituted a special class; the very biology that made them different and unable to compete with men gave them a weapon they could use. The belief that they were somehow made of finer and more delicate materials than men meant that they had to be protected because life in the real world could more easily destroy or weaken them compared with the hardy, more rugged men, and if this happened, they might end up as prostitutes or other types of "bad" women. It also meant that women were set aside to be the guardians of culture and tradition, even though few fit the stereotype of wan, ethereal, spiritualized creatures that some of the literature of the time tried to make them. In fact, such portrayals bore little resemblance to the real world of lower-class women who operated machines, worked the fields, washed clothes by hand, and took care of large households. Nonetheless, these portrayals were endorsed by the science and religion of the time, at least for middle- and upper-class women. Some male physicians even went so far as to claim that the female biology prevented a woman from cultivating her intellect, since so much of her bodily resources had to be expended on developing her reproductive organs (Bullough & Bullough, 1978, 1984).

Florence Nightingale was in a full-scale, lady-like rebellion against such an image, and this is best illustrated by her essay "Cassandra," which was written before she visited Kaiserworth (Nightingale, 1979). She did not want to marry and turn her fate over to some man; rather she wanted to be her own woman and still be socially useful. Money was of no concern to her, since she was independently wealthy, and so this did not need to be a consideration in what she chose to do. Nursing came to be her answer because it allowed her to fit the image of a proper woman yet still be on her own.

Nightingale was also a member of a class and moved in the social circles that led her to be well acquainted with the important people in British society. When her friend, Sidney Herbert, the Minister of Defense, was attempting to overcome bad publicity about the dreadful care of the sick and wounded during the Crimean war, he (with prompting from his wife, a friend of Nightingale, and from Nightingale herself) conceived of a public relations coup of sending a contingent of women to nurse the troops (Bullough & Bullough, 1978, 1984). Nightingale and her nurses became what in today's term would be called a media sensation and continued to be one because the nurses proved to be extremely effective. The American poet Henry Wadsworth Longfellow made her a mythical heroine in his poem that included the following lines:

A lady with a lamp shall stand
In the great history of the land,
A noble type of good
Heroic womanhood

THE AMERICAN EXPERIENCE

Inevitably, Nightingale became a heroine for all young women, and her life became standard reading material (somewhat highly embroidered) for generations of girls who wanted to make something of themselves (Vicinus, 1990). During the American Civil War, many women seeking to emulate Nightingale's example became nurses, although men served as caretakers for the sick as well. In 1873, in the aftermath of the Civil War, groups of women in New York City, New Haven, Connecticut, and Boston organized training schools for women to become nurses, on the basis of what they believed was the model Nightingale had established at St. Thomas Hospital in London. The organization of these schools coincided with a period of hospital expansion in the United States resulting from the development of aseptic techniques and the growing need for institutional care of the poor and homeless in America's growing urban centers. Medicine itself was also changing. Procedures formerly reserved for the home, including childbirth, began to move into the hospital setting as physicians took over tasks previously performed

by midwives and other nonprofessional healers. Nursing made the growth of hospitals possible, especially when it became clear that nursing students were cheap labor because they could staff the hospitals in return for room and board and a modicum of education. Because the hospital administrators wanted the nurses available, they established homes for them, a concept that also fit in the perceived need to protect women. This also meant that the homes for nurses were restricted to women, and made it more difficult for men to gain entry into nursing training. Moreover the dominance of the hospital diploma schools led to the segregation of nurses from other students, in a sense keeping them isolated from the mainstream of education.

Alternatives to the diploma schools were not easily available, in part because of the fact that nurses were for the most part women and higher education was dominated by men. Colleges and universities, when American nursing developed, were primarily aimed at men, and although there were women's colleges, their purpose was to raise women to be culture bearers, not workers. Even in the existing coeducational schools, all state land grant agricultural and technical schools, and in many state universities, the female equivalent to the male major in engineering was home economics, not nursing. The hospital became the defining educational experience for nurses as it had been for medicine, and it was only after medicine moved into the university, mainly after World War I, that nurses could even contemplate such a move. Medicine, however, moved in on its own terms, that is, with a separate administration and a clearly defined expertise. Nursing, however, did not fit into the traditional college and university subject matter and was unable to dictate its own terms as had medicine, and so when it began to enter into college and universities, it did so through teacher training institutions, where women had already broken barriers but also where education and teaching techniques were emphasized at the expense of a unique nursing knowledge. Even in the best of the institutions—and Teachers College, Columbia University, was the dominant graduate school in the 1930s, 1940s, and even 1950s for nurses—subject matter emphasized not nursing research but educational research, which are not necessarily the same thing. Public health nurses, the one nursing specialty where a baccalaureate degree was often required, were regarded primarily as teachers of public health, and although they carried out the regular nursing duties, their special expertise was in health teaching, so much so that for a time there was debate whether regular teachers should be given more health training instead of giving nurses the educational backgrounds essential for them to enter the public school system. The eventual solution was for nurses to get more education training, but this meant that as nursing initially moved more and more into the university setting elsewhere, almost all the degrees were in nursing education (there were almost no doctorates). Certainly this raised the level of nursing education, and anyone who has read the basic texts for many of the courses in the hospital nursing schools—ranging from history to principles and practices of nursing—during the first part of the century comes away distressed by the simplified and, in nonnursing subjects such as history, erroneous information imparted in many of them. In most of the nursing schools the nonclinical courses such as anatomy, physiology, or pharmacology generally were taught by physicians, while the actual clinical experience was acquired in what can only be called an apprenticeship mode (Bullough & Bullough, 1978, 1984).

This description of the struggle nurses had to mount to overcome the obstacles put in their path, largely because they were women, is not to put down nursing but to emphasize why so few men went into it. Nurse training in many ways was similar to that of apprenticeship in many of the male occupations such as those of machinist, mechanic, or carpenter, but far more confining. Students had to live in nurses' quarters to protect them from the world of men, and the last thing that nursing schools wanted was male students. Until the beginning of World War II, most nurses who continued to nurse after graduation went into home nursing, and this usually entailed living in the home of the patient, taking care of him or her, and often doing household duties as well. The nurse was on the case as long as the patient needed her. When hospitals first began to professionalize their staff in the 1930s, they wanted to have nurses live by or in the hospitals so they could be subject to call, take a split shift, and work nights. Most hospitals set up resident homes for their staff nurses to live in, and many if not the majority of them required their nurses to live there. The wages were not good; the hours were long; and the whole structure was designed to discourage men.

The major exception was in mental hospitals, where it was believed nurses needed greater strength. This led to schools for men only, such as that established by the Department of Mental and Nervous Diseases at Pennsylvania Hospital or the Mills School of Nursing for Men at Bellevue. Although there is no real evidence that women in nursing took a strong stand against men in their ranks, it is clear that nursing was conceived by most of them as a woman's profession where the role of men was limited.

None of the male nursing schools was affiliated with the Associated Alumnae (which became the American Nurses Association), and when the ANA was reorganized between 1916 and 1922, no provisions were made for male nurses. It was not until 1930 that the membership bylaws were revised to include properly qualified male nurses (Nash, 1936). Male nurses quite clearly were on the fringe of mainstream nursing (Bullough & Bullough, 1978, 1984).

Undoubtedly some of the difficulties that men faced were due to their own ambivalence about nursing. One of the issues that many men had to deal with was the public perception of any man who wanted to be a nurse or who thought he might want to be a nurse. Although it was permissible for a woman to strive to be more manlike, for a man to enter a woman's world such as nursing was perceived to mean that he might be labeled as somehow not quite a man. The anxiety and fear over homosexuality meant that the men who did go into nursing had to be willing to take a lot of "guff" about their manliness, and it was not until both the feminist movement and the gay liberation movement of the 1960s that attitudes began to change. This ambivalent attitude toward men who entered nursing had been institutionalized as early as 1901 by the organization of the U.S. Army Nurse Corps, which specifically excluded male nurses (Bullough & Bullough, 1978; Kalisch & Kalisch, 1978). Men were to fight, not nurse; when male nurses were drafted into the military during World War I, they fought in the trenches and were excluded from staffing the hospitals. In fact, the military disregard of male nurses in World War I proved to be a crucial factor in the decline of men in the profession. At a time when nursing school enrollments were increasing radically and a special army school had been established to train nurses, enrollment of men almost disappeared.

This discrimination against male nurses continued in World War II, in spite of the efforts of some segments of organized nursing. Concerned about the repetition of the exclusionary policies for male nurses in mainstream nursing, Leroy Craig, Director of the School of Nursing for Men at Pennsylvania Hospital, and his allies (both men and women) persuaded the ANA at its 1940 convention to set up a section for "men nurses." Although the section focused its attention on many issues including upgrading patient care and raising salaries for nurses, its members were not at all successful in changing the treatment of male nurses in the military. For example, Luther Christman, a 1939 graduate of the Pennsylvania Hospital, was denied enlistment in the Army Nurse Corps at the onset of World War II. He found, much to his dismay, that male nurses were not even given priority enrollment in medical corpsmen schools, perhaps because, as some have argued, their knowledge often intimidated their less well-educated military instructors. Christman tried to bypass the issue by joining the merchant marines as a medical corpsman and then petitioning for appointment to the Army Nurse Corps and for assignment to the front lines (where women nurses were not then assigned). He was unsuccessful. Enrollments of men in nursing schools during this period dropped drastically, from 725 in 1939 to 169 in 1945 (ANA, 1946, 1994).

THE REBIRTH OF THE MALE NURSE

Conditions for men in nursing began to change following the end of World War II, and male enrollments in nursing schools slowly started to build. They did not climb very high, however, until the establishment of the associate degree programs and the decline of segregated diploma hospital schools. Other changes were also necessary within nursing itself. One of the difficulties was that nursing had got into playing the doctor-nurse game, a game that male nurses did not play very well, and until this pathological behavior was challenged, the male nurse would suffer. Recognition and description of the game was the first step, but the rise of the nursing clinical specialties was another. Nurse anesthetists had existed since the end of the 19th century, but they had been more or less excluded from mainstream nursing organizations. The rise in their numbers came after World War II, pushed by, among other groups, the U.S. Army. The development of the nurse practitioner and physician's assistant forced a redirection of nursing, and as one who bears some of the scars of that battle with organized nursing, I know the success of the movement shook nursing to its roots and emphasized something that people like Luther Christman had long been agitating for, namely clinical expertise. As nursing schools began to give their own master's degrees and ultimately their own doctorates, research became a major element in nursing, and it was now research on subjects of importance to clinical nursing, not on how to develop a curriculum. The explosion of nursing journals is indicative of the explosion of research. For a time in the 1950s there were basically only two nursing journals after the *Trained Nurse* had closed its doors, namely the *American Journal of Nursing (AJN)* and *Nursing Outlook*. There was a public health nursing journal, but its subject matter was limited. It was only in the late 1950s that others entered the field and that nurses could claim an increasingly large section of health care as their own, where their expertise

was greater than that of the physician (Bullough & Bullough, 1978, 1984).

As nursing changed, so did the role of men in nursing. A major indicator of change was the granting of military commissions to male nurses through legislation initiated by Frances Bolton. This legislation led to Edward Lyon's becoming the first male RN to be commissioned as a reserve officer in the Army Nurse Corps on October 6, 1955. The change in the military status of male nurses was rapid, and by 1990 approximately 30% of the RNs in the various military Nurse Corps were men, more than four times their ratio in civilian nursing. During the Vietnam War, more than 500 male nurses were drafted and given commissions in the various Military Nurse Corps.

In the long run, the most important factor in attracting men to nursing was the improvement in salaries and working conditions in the profession during the 1950s and 1960s. Although census data indicate that male nurses generally were and still are paid somewhat more than female nurses (Bullough & Bullough, 1975), part of this disparity was due to the fact that a disproportionate number of men were nurse anesthetists, nurse administrators, or held other high-paying nursing jobs. It was also true, however, that men in the past were often paid more than women for doing the same job. This might have been due to the fact that there were more job alternatives open to men than to women, and that men could leave nursing if the salaries were not high enough. Ultimately, however, the disparity tended to reflect the reality in American life where men doing the same jobs were paid more than women simply because it was argued that men had a family to support while the women workers only had to support themselves. This did not correspond with the reality, but it indicates the basic values of a male-oriented society. It was only as the new wave of feminism of the 1960s and the demand for equal pay began that the salary gap between men and women lessened, both in and out of nursing. Undoubtedly, this inequality created some tension between male and female nurses, although many female nurses continued to encourage men to enter the field because they felt that their own salaries might rise as a result.

Tensions came from other directions as well, and these became more noticeable as the number of men entering nursing grew. Nursing educators who had taught only women found the men behaving somewhat differently. They were not as submissive as female students traditionally had been, and they often used different problem-solving methods. Most of the problems with male students required simple adjustments and were soon solved by most teachers (Bush, 1976; Schoenmaker, 1976), but a few influential members of the nursing community did not want to adjust and opposed the growing numbers of men in nursing.

MEN AND NURSING THEORY

Many of those in opposition turned to newly developing nursing theory to justify their opposition (Bullough, 1994). As nursing entered the mainstream of academia, nurses in academic positions became convinced that a nursing theory was necessary to provide a bridge between practice and research, and that theory-based research was the key to broadening nursing knowledge (Dickoff, James, & Wiedenback, 1968). The result was the development of a number of grand theories, particularly at the University of California at Los Angeles and at New York University.

Among the most troublesome of such theories to men were the caring theories, particularly those that emphasized caring as a particularly feminine trait. Although rooted in the work of Johnson, who distinguished between caring and curing (Johnson, 1959), many others also contributed. Kreuter (1957, p. 303) defined caring as the special task of the nurse clinician: "Care is expressed in tending to another, being with him, assisting, protecting . . . providing for his needs and wants with compassion—tenderness." Caring became a major part of Watson's theory and led her to establish an early caring center (Watson, 1979, 1985). The concept of caring was also given special sanction by the ANA in its 1965 position paper, *Educational Preparation for Nurse Practitioners and Assistants to Nurses,* in which the professional role of the nurse was defined as social psychological support, teaching, and sustaining care (ANA, 1965).

There is nothing particularly wrong with emphasizing caring from a man's point of view because caring obviously is one of the basic fundamentals of nursing. The problem, however, was with the implementation. One faction of nursing interpreted caring as a uniquely feminine quality. By implication, caring was something that men (as males) were not especially qualified to do. Although nowhere is this thesis stated quite so baldly, it certainly contributed to male uneasiness. One male graduate student in the mid 1990s, in a letter he wrote to a magazine, reported some of his experience in a graduate course:

[T]here was a cohort of vehement feminists in the program. It became rapidly apparent to me that not only did these

women have strong opinions about traditional science, but they also felt that men had no place in nursing.

These feminists were critical of empirical methodologies and proposed that nursing science should be much more qualitative and based on intuitive knowledge. It was the feminists' contention that traditional science was paternalistic and male-oriented and thus suspect at all levels. They stated that men's and women's minds operated in dramatically different ways. "Men's science" dissected an event and attempted to empiricize it and in the process lost the Gestalt that was essential to understanding the event. It was the feminists' contention that only women could understand a holistic viewpoint.

The next stage of the feminists' argument was that nursing is an eclectic, and holistic science that requires an understanding of each individual patient's gestalt. Because nursing practice required a holistic view of patients and men could not comprehend this view, nursing research and the knowledge base of nursing should be developed by women. Their next conclusion was that caring requires specific mental functions that men are not able to accomplish. Therefore, men are incapable of "caring." [Ross, 1995, pp. 58, 60]

To the extent that such an attitude exists, and Ross was careful to state that the caring views he criticized were not held by the majority of nurses, it is strongly held by many and makes male nurses uncomfortable. In my own experience, I have met a few women nurses who will not recognize me as a nurse because I am a man. The sad part is that most current research would indicate that caring is not particularly confined to women. As one who has specialized in gender research, I can state that it is true that men statistically tend to be more aggressive than women and seemingly have special mathematical skills, but these statistical differences show up at the skewed end of the spectrum. The most interesting finding in gender research is the tremendous overlap in talents between most men and women (Bullough & Bullough, 1993b; Hyde, 1986). Moreover, some of the most obvious differences are as much or more cultural than biological.

NURSING IN THE 21ST CENTURY

Nursing has changed radically in the 20th century and will continue to change in the future. Women will remain the dominant force, however, in the foreseeable future, and if men in nursing are to become a force, they have to recognize some of the anxieties and fears that women have about men. This was emphasized by a study of men in nursing in the United Kingdom, which has a higher percentage of men in the field than there is in the United States. A study done in the United Kingdom in the 1980s found that half of the top posts in nursing within the British National Health Service were held by men (Nuttal, 1983). Men were also found to hold disproportionate strength in the Royal College of Nursing, where 15 of the 31 elected members were men. One female nurse felt that once male power was established, it would tend to be self-perpetuating, making it difficult for women to regain leadership (London, 1987). These fears have carried over into American nursing (Ryan & Porter, 1993). Although there are unique factors in the British system that encouraged what might be called the "disproportionate" power of men and although these are not present in the United States, there is still a real basis for the fears of women in nursing. Even though I feel that with the changing power relationships between men and women in American society such fears are greatly exaggerated, they still need to be confronted openly. As an academician for nearly 50 years, I have observed the rapid change in the role of women, not only in American higher education but also in the business and professional worlds as well. There are still a few isolated campuses where the dean of nursing is the only woman in the higher ranks of administration, but this is rare and becoming rarer as women of all backgrounds hold major administrative jobs.

It might be, as one theory holds, that the problems faced by gender minorities tend to increase as their numbers in a particular occupation grow, until they reach a critical mass, when the barriers more or less disappear. If this is the case, then it is important to determine this critical mass where the barriers collapse. Kanter (1977) estimated that this percentage in any group ranges between 20% to 40%. Testing this theory on nursing was a study comparing women in law enforcement and men in nursing (Ott, 1989). Ott's study supports the theory in law enforcement, where women tended to see increasing resistance to their presence, but not in nursing, where men found greater acceptance in their increasing numbers (Ott, 1989). This tends to illustrate that women, or at least those in nursing, are more willing to share their domain with men than men in typically male occupations and professions such as law enforcement have been with women. It would also indicate that those uncomfortable with men in the nursing profession constitute only a very small minority.

As women seek jobs in other than the traditional women's professions, the major source of potential new recruits to nursing in the future will be men. Those women who do enter nursing will be far more committed to it than those who once entered merely because there seemed to be no alternative. Now women can become engineers, physicians, dentists, auto mechanics, truck drivers, and almost no occupational position is automatically closed to them. This commitment to nursing as a profession, common among the new women students, will undoubtedly be true of the men who enter as well. It is important, however, that every nurse who is a man should be made conscious of the tremendous contribution that women have made to our profession.

Interestingly, although much of the empowerment of women in the marketplace has come through Title IX of the Civil Rights Act, no similar provision exists for men. This only emphasizes that nursing is helping to change itself by recruiting men, an act which is a credit to the profession. Like any minority, men in nursing need occasionally to meet with some of their own, and for this reason the National Male Nurse Association was organized in 1971. The objectives of the organization, as defined in 1981 when it was renamed the American Assembly for Men in Nursing, are:

1. Men and boys in the United States are to be encouraged to become nurses and join together with all nurses in strengthening and humanizing health care for all Americans.
2. Men who are now nurses are encouraged to grow professionally and to demonstrate to each other and to society the increasing contribution made by men within the nursing profession.
3. The American Assembly for Men in Nursing intends that its members be full participants in the nursing profession and its organizations and use their association to achieve these goals.

The association holds that every professional nurse position and every nursing education opportunity shall be equally available to those meeting the entry qualifications, regardless of gender (see various issues of *Interaction*, the newsletter of the group). These are not particularly revolutionary goals, nor should they be. Men today go into nursing because they want to be nurses, and this is the way nursing should be and hopefully will be in the 21st century as it continues to emphasize the caring potential in both genders. It has become a quite different profession from the one Nightingale first visualized, but the caring element remains its foundation.

At the opening of the 21st century the profession has finally rid itself of the handicaps that existed throughout much of the 20th century because it was a woman's profession (a good example being the ghetto of the diploma school), and yet the profession has managed to keep the benefits that our women predecessors have brought to nursing. Men will undoubtedly help change nursing, but they will be joining with the women to do so. Nursing is radically different at the beginning of the 21st century than it was at the beginning of the 20th century, and men have finally arrived at a position where they can help shape its future. Nevertheless the only prediction possible to make is that nursing will continue to change, preserving the best of the past but growing with the future.

REFERENCES

American Nurses Association. (1946, 1994). *Facts about nursing.* Kansas City, MO: Author.

American Nurses Association. (1965). *Educational preparation for nurse practitioners and assistants to nurses.* Kansas City, MO: Author.

Bullough, B. (1994). Nursing theory and critique. In B. Bullough & V.L. Bullough (Eds.), *Nursing issues for the nineties and beyond* (pp. 64-82). New York: Springer.

Bullough, B., & Bullough, V.L. (1975, January). Sex segregation in health care. *Nursing Outlook, 23,* 40-45.

Bullough, V.L., & Bullough, B. (1978). *The care of the sick.* New York: Neale Watson, Prodist Science History.

Bullough, V.L., & Bullough, B. (1984). *History, trends, and politics of nursing.* Norwalk, CT: Appleton-Century-Crofts.

Bullough, V.L., & Bullough, B. (1993a). Medieval nursing. *Nursing History Review, 1,* 217-226.

Bullough, V.L., & Bullough, B. (1993b). *Cross dressing, sex, and gender.* Philadelphia: University of Pennsylvania Press.

Bush, P.J. (1976). The male nurse: A challenge to traditional role identities. *Nursing Forum, 15,* 390-405.

Dickoff, J., James, P., & Wiedenback, P. (1968). Theory in a practice discipline. *Nursing Research, 17,* 415-435, 545-554.

Greg, M. (1969). *Women workers and the Industrial Revolution 1750-1850* (pp. 315-316). London: Frank Case.

Hospital and health network (Computer database). (1994, October 5). *68*(19), 78.

Hyde, J.S. (1986). Gender differences in aggression. In J.S. Hyde & M.C. Linn (Eds.), *The psychology of gender* (pp. 51-60). Baltimore: Johns Hopkins University Press.

Interaction. Newsletter of the American Assembly for Men in Nursing. C/O NYSNA, 11 Cornell Rd., Latham, NY 12110-1499.

Johnson, D. (1959). A philosophy of nursing. *Nursing Outlook, 7,* 198-200.

Kalisch, P., & Kalisch, B.J. (1978). *The advance of American nursing* (2nd ed.). Boston: Little, Brown.

Kanter, R.M. (1977). *Men and women of the corporation.* New York: Basic Books.

Kreuter, E.R. (1957). What is good nursing care? *Nursing Outlook, 5,* 302-305.

London, F. (1987). Should men be actively recruited in nursing? *Nursing Administration Quarterly, 12*(1), 75-81.

Nash, H.J. (1936, August). Men nurses in New York State. *Trained Nurse and Hospital Review,* p. 123.

National Center for Education Statistics. (1999). *Digest of education statistics, 1998.* U.S. Office of Education. Washington, DC: U.S. Government Printing Office.

Nightingale, F. (1979). *Cassandra.* M. Start (Ed.). Old Westbury, NY: Feminist Press.

Nuttal, P. (1983). British nursing: Beginning of a power struggle. *Nursing Outlook, 31*(3), 184.

Ott, E.M. (1989). Effect of the male-female ratio at work: Police-women and male nurses. *Psychology of Women Quarterly, 13*(1), 41-57.

Ross, D. (1995, July-August). Letter. *Skeptical Inquirer, 10,* 58-60.

Ryan, S., & Porter, S. (1993). Men in nursing: A cautionary comparative critique. *Nursing Outlook, 41*(6), 262-267.

Schoenmaker, A. (1976). Nursing's dilemma: Male versus female admissions choice. *Nursing Forum, 15,* 406-412.

Statistical Abstract of the United States. (1998). Washington, DC: U.S. Government Printing Office.

Vicinus, M. (1990). What makes a heroine? Girls' biographies of Florence Nightingale. In V.L. Bullough, B. Bullough, & M.P. Stanton (Eds.), *Florence Nightingale and her era: A collection of new scholarship* (pp. 96-107). New York: Garland.

Watson, J. (1979). *The philosophy and science of caring.* Boston: Little, Brown.

Watson, J. (1985). *Nursing, human science and human care: A theory of nursing.* Norwalk, CT: Appleton-Century-Crofts.

Wollstonecraft, M.A. (1929). *A vindication of the rights of women.* London: J.M. Dent.

Bridging Cultures

African Americans and Nursing

BETTY PIERCE DENNIS

The many immigration patterns in the United States have created a rich and uniquely diverse society. If current demographic trends continue, minority groups will comprise about 51.1% of society by 2050 (United States Bureau of the Census, 1996). Of the many identifiable societal groups, African Americans have the longest tenure, their ancestors having been brought to America over 300 years ago. Their full acceptance and integration, however, lags behind groups that arrived later. African Americans, now 13.5% of the population (United States Bureau of the Census, 1996) are only marginally represented in important arenas of power and influence.

Marginality, or movement away from the mainstream toward the periphery, is a term generalized from the struggles of the vulnerable and the disadvantaged, like the poor, children, the mentally ill, and people of color. Marginalization occurs through the process of social, cultural, and political interaction and produces collective and individual strengths and risks (Hall, 1999). The strengths and risks are clearly evident in health care. Consequently, health is a surrogate and multifaceted measure of the status of a group in society. However, precise assignment of the meaning of health to African Americans as a group requires new ways of interpreting health behavior.

These new ways begin with the reconceptualization of health. Instead of a "state" or point on the wellness-illness continuum, health is viewed as a nonlinear, developmental, and continuously reconfiguring construct. Typically, descriptors of health focus on broadly applicable practices and observable behaviors. This obscures prismatic patterns of experience in which health is actually only one interacting element within the larger cultural and social context. Thus, despite working closely with African American clients, many nurses—regardless of race—fail to recognize how ethnohistory has shaped the perceptions of health and the behaviors that relate to health.

CULTURAL CONTEXT AND NURSING

The cultural and social lives of blacks are interdependent outcomes of history, education, income, and a host of other factors. Taken together, they form a contextual framework that is unique to the group. The philosophy of contextualism embraces the full range of conditions and motivations that are possible in person-environment exchanges. Therefore, nurse and client may, and often do, behave out of dissimilar contexts or theoretical and empirical frameworks (Gergen, 1982). For this reason, interpretive perspective is necessary. Interpretive perspective allows both the nurse and the client to identify points of divergence and, more importantly, points of convergence from their respective cultural perspectives. Without this process, genuine understanding between the African American client and the nurse is altogether elusive or in a permanent nascent state, very much as it is today. The challenge to nursing is not only to include the worldview of the African American client but to merge it with nursing actions. In other words, promote inclusion and competence through a shared vision. An example is the natural tendency to raise one's voice when attempting to communicate with someone who speaks another language. Speaking louder does not compensate for the fact that the languages are different. Majority groups are equivalent to that raised voice. What is really needed is translation that permits mutual understanding.

Three factors will retard or facilitate the progress of nursing toward cultural competence: breadth of perspective, depth of commitment, and evolution of nursing systems. In the care of African American clients, approaches that accept difference and recognize commonalities will question traditional nursing therapeutics. Existing therapeutic approaches are based on ahistorical, acontextual ways of knowing clients. Contrary to the emphasis on objectivity in nurse-client interactions, reaching out to other cultures requires subjectivity born of shared experiences. As used here, *sharing* means acceptance of ethnopluralism without erecting a cultural hierarchy or ranking that places lesser or greater value on each culture. Myers (1991) contends that only through subjective experiences are we able to acquire knowledge that "deepens" what we know of another culture. Therefore, the culturally competent nurse has to have more than a superficial understanding of other cultures. Being a stranger to African American culture will not support an increase in levels of competence in the delivery of culturally sensitive health care to African American clients. Ancient African systems of knowledge, Myers states, were built on subjectivity. When substantive cultural knowledge is the basis of cultural competence, it begins to bridge the chasm between African Americans and the health care system (Myers, 1991).

At its most basic level, culture is an expression of the lifestyles of a collection of individuals belonging to a group or community. Because culture is intelligible only within its own context, comparisons between cultures are neither informative nor valid. Unfortunately comparisons are a common practice leading to stereotypical characterizations. Closely related, yet distinct from culture, is the social system in which that culture exists (Valentine, 1968). The dynamism of the two is implicit in Whitehead's (1992) description of culture as enmeshed in an "ecological system, historically created, intergenerationally reproduced and moderated, to allow humans to meet their basic . . . needs" (p. 95). Through a consideration of history it is possible to uncover the generative layer that is responsible for the attitudes, beliefs, and values unique to African Americans. History does endow cultures and serves as the wellspring of many societal forces that promote, restrain, extend, or limit the options available to black clients.

Explorations of African American culture and nursing from the perspective of a construct or contextualism philosophy raises the following questions: (1) How is the health of Africans determined by their ethnohistorical legacy as well as by their contemporary reality? (2) How can nursing become a proactive force in bringing these facets together within a pattern of culturally competent health care?

HISTORY AND CULTURE

History is critical to understanding African American culture. Africans arrived in America either before Columbus (Van Sertima, 1976) or in 1619 before the Mayflower (Bennett, 1982). Initially their work obligations and conditions of freedom were like those of indentured servants. The rapid expansion of colonial economics, however, escalated the need for manpower and ultimately resulted in the creation of slavery. In 1661 Virginia was the first state to legally convert immigrant Africans from indentured servants to slaves (Johnson, 1982). Trade in humanity exploded.

Before the mid-20th century, historians proposed two main theories about the culture of captured Africans in America. The first theory is that the African culture was destroyed by a repressive system that randomly disbursed them and continually disrupted their lives. It was hypothesized that these practices made order and stability impossible. Communication was hampered by the lack of a common language and the outlawing of the use of drums. The void caused by these circumstances was thought to have been filled by the English language and European culture. The second theory of this "peculiar institution" (Stampp, 1956) was that slaves had acceded to their fate, as evidenced by their tranquil deportment. They were depicted as healthy and robust despite severely deprived living conditions, exhaustive work requirements, and poor nutrition (Byrd & Clayton, 1992). Interpretation of the behavior of African Americans, then as now, was based on outward observations and objective versus subjective assessment.

After the midcentury the institution of slavery was analyzed using actual documents of that era. The findings contradicted earlier theories. Several seminal works attested to the adaptability, resistance, and will to survive displayed by Africans. They were, after all, descendants of ancient societies with well-developed family and clan systems. Gutman's (1976) study of the black family from 1750 to 1925 described the transcendence of this heritage over slavery. Writers today detail how Africans were able to succeed in transmitting their beliefs, values, and social and familial behaviors and rituals from generation to generation. Because mothers and, more often, fathers were sold away from their families, children were socialized by the community in accord with the African adage that "it takes a whole village to raise a child." The few long and stable marriages that did exist provided role models for younger adults (Stampp, 1956). Finally, historians confirmed that the way of life among the slaves had both dimension and purpose. In the slave quarters the designations of the oppressors, such as "field hand" or "house slave" were replaced by status based on the ability to contribute to community life. There were midwives, healers, teachers, nurses, and others. This organized and supportive subterranean community, however, did not stem the many insurrections and almost daily incidences of runaways. Many successful escapees joined the community of free blacks living in "free" states in the north. During the early 1700s, it is estimated that almost one in eight African Americans was a free person (Franklin, 1956).

Slaves as a group represented many cultures. Creating one culture from many and preserving it against formidable odds was a major achievement. What this demonstrates about perceived meaning as a derivative of acontextual versus contextual exploration is a direct correlate of nursing care. For example, the music of slaves, objectively observed, was taken to mean that they were accepting of their lot. From a subjective vantage point, however, the role of music was more of an expressive channel for the hopes, fears, sorrows, and dreams of the slaves, and a way of communicating with one another. Just as history has refuted many myths about the meaning of the behavior of African Americans, nursing must have the courage and audacity to question tradition and devise other ways of knowing and caring for African American clients.

HISTORY AND HEALTH

The ethnohistory of health issues reveals the germ layer of some current practices and attitudes about health among African Americans. For example, high rates of illness, injury, and death among slaves were recorded. According to the 1850 census in Louisiana's Natchitoches Parish, slaves accounted for 63.8% of deaths. The leading cause of death was helminthiasis due to geophagia, or dirt eating. Fever, pneumonia, whooping cough, and cholera were also major causes of death (Rene, Daniels, Jones, & Moore, 1992). For the first time, Africans were exposed to new diseases like tuberculosis, syphilis, and measles. This drove mortality and morbidity figures up by estimates of 15% to 50% (Byrd & Clayton, 1992; Savitt, 1978). The cause of this health problem, according to the medical community, was unalterable pathological differences between African Americans and others. Therefore, their treatment, when it was given, was differential. Additionally, slaves were pressed into serving as subjects for many medical experiments and treatment trials, including repeated and unnecessary surgeries, starvation, and burning (Beardsley, 1987; Jones, 1981; Jordan, 1968; Savitt, 1982). Southern medical journals of the time carried reports of such experiments (Savitt, 1982). Given these conditions, slaves either delayed seeking treatment or avoided it altogether. Instead, there was a growing reliance on their own cultural

healing system where root doctors, spiritualists, and priests addressed health care needs (Charatz-Litt, 1992).

Suspicions about the intent of health care are reinforced by unethical practices such as the 40-year study of untreated syphilis in African American men that was conducted by the U.S. Public Health Service (Jones, 1981) and studies at Johns Hopkins, Chicago Medical College, and the Medical College of Virginia (Beecher, 1966; Newman, Amidei, Carter, Kruvant, & Russell, 1978). The resulting lack of trust continues today, as reflected in a nationwide poll in which 61% of African Americans admitted being wary and distrustful of people of other races versus a 30% unease in whites (Edwards, 1995). Mouton, Harris, Rovi, Solorzano, and Johnson (1997) surveyed women regarding barriers to participation in cancer clinical trials. Only 28% of African American women felt that research was ethical, and about 29% felt that researchers could not be trusted versus 14% of white women for the same issues. A sensitive critique and valuation of the patterns of experience in the African American past must be factored into the development of a credible and reciprocal nurse-client relationship. Slavery has cast a long shadow and closure is not yet realized.

Following the end of the Civil War in 1865 the Reconstruction period opened a window of opportunity that altered the context of African American life. During this time, clinics, schools, soup kitchens, and churches were opened. African Americans entered politics and bought land. Their health status improved. This progress ended abruptly after 10 years, when segregation or Jim Crow laws were passed (Bennett, 1982). These laws placed legal limits on the economic and social progress of blacks for nearly 100 years. Concurrently the health status of African Americans began to decline. The separate-but-equal doctrine actually fostered disparities in health outcomes between African Americans and whites. These inequities are clearly apparent in the infant mortality rates of 1929, with 98.4 deaths per 1,000 live births for African Americans and 60.2 per 1,000 for whites (Cooper & David, 1986; Reed, Darity, & Robertson, 1993).

Attracted by the economic boom of World Wars I and II, many African Americans migrated from the South to the North; but in the North they were largely confined to economically depressed areas or ghettos. Northern housing patterns yielded results similar to southern legal oppression. This is validated by infant mortality and life expectancy rates for African Americans and whites. In 1950, African American infant mortality was 43.9 versus 26.8 for whites per 1,000 live births, and life expectancy was 60.7 versus 69.1 years, for African Americans and whites, respectively (National Center for Health Statistics [NCHS], 1995).

In the 1960s, legislation initiated in the Civil Rights Movement led to improved access to health care for African Americans. This was another window of opportunity that also lasted little more than a decade. Again, African American health status trended upward, reached a plateau, and then steadily declined. From 1960 to 1990, differences in life expectancy between African Americans and whites changed from 8 years in 1960 down to 6.9 years in 1980 and then up to 8.2 years in 1990. In the same years, infant mortality rates followed a similar trend for African Americans from 14.8% to 10.4% to 10.7% (Haynes, 1975; NCHS, 1995).

Today, the excess death rate of African Americans exemplifies marginalization. "Excess deaths" are calculated as actual deaths before 70 years of age minus the number of deaths that would be predicted when death rates of the white population in the United States are applied to the minority populations. In 1990, the excess deaths for African Americans exceeded 59,000 (Thomas, 1992). McCord and Freeman (1990) studied mortality among African Americans in Harlem and found rates double those of whites and 50% greater than those of other African Americans in the United States. Urban ghetto life has an enduring effect. Recognizing differences is only a beginning. Nurses have a transformative responsibility that transcends difference. Its purpose is to change what is to what should be.

CONTEMPORARY AFRICAN AMERICAN CLIENTS

The sense of self of all African Americans begins as an intragroup attitude but is finely and finally shaped by how the world sees them. The term *African American* is a cognitive construct with uncertain scientific merit. In other words, African Americans are African Americans because they are recognized and treated as such. Variation characterizes all racial and ethnic groups, is thought to move on a continuum through all racial groups, and is not contained in neat racial boxes ("Biological Anthropologist," 1995). However, the nature-nurture or genetics-environment concept of disease causation persists as an explanatory model (Anonymous, 1983; Cooper & David, 1986; Langford, 1981; Thomas, 1992). It is this dichotomous perception that we must revisit.

Race is heavily weighted in perceived meanings of "African American." Race is almost always an antecedent of diseases that are defined by genetics or environmental factors (Freeman, 1991). Variations such as income and

education are combined with health measures to form comparative relationships. On the face of it, African Americans do exhibit differences in some morbid conditions. They have a low incidence of multiple sclerosis, cystic fibrosis, and skin cancer ("Biological Anthropologist," 1995) and a high incidence of hypertension, diabetes, and cancer of the prostate and cervix (NCHS, 1995). Validation of genetic variation requires more than a counting of cases, however. Genes, environment, and culture must be synergized to see how they affect health. The pseudoscience of writers like Jensen, Shockley, Herrnsein, and Murray, however, confuses issues by perpetuating flawed propositions about African Americans. Their works encourage theories of genetic deficits in African Americans. They also support the repugnant practice of "blaming the victim" for illness or disease, reminiscent of some 17th and 18th century medical thinking (Charatz-Litt, 1992). Thinking of this kind is a barrier to the development of equitable, open, honest communications between African American clients, nurses, and other health professionals. Racial inequality is not a uniquely nursing phenomenon, but some forms of racism remain in nursing and that is troubling (Vaughn, 1997).

African Americans are a heterogeneous group. Ten percent are in the upper socioeconomic class, 40% middle class, and 50% lower class (Johnson, 1982). In addition to those born in the United States, blacks emigrate from Haiti, Guyana, Brazil, the Caribbean, and Africa. A study by Cabral, Fried, Levenson, Amaro, and Zuckerman (1990) illustrates that these groups vary in language, history, culture, and health practices. These authors investigated perinatal outcomes between foreign-born and native-born black pregnant women and found significant group differences in the mothers' nutrition, the babies' birth weights, and other perinatal outcomes.

Health disparities among poor African Americans are well documented. But African Americans with higher incomes may have similar health problems. Income may not be a protective factor for African Americans. Thomas, Semenya, Neser, Thomas, and Gillum (1990) and Thomas et al. (1985) studied precursors of hypertension in a cohort of African American physicians for over 25 years. The mortality of these physicians matched the mortality of low-income African Americans rather than that of their white peers. Similarly, hypertension in men in low occupational classes increased when they remained in that status or moved to a lower status. Although African Americans and whites experienced elevated blood pressures, increases in hypertension were greatest for African Americans (Waitzman & Smith,

1994). Among African Americans, hypertension develops earlier and with greater severity. Sixty-six percent of all cases of end-stage renal disease due to hypertension occur among African Americans (Reed et al., 1993; Woodhandler et al., 1985).

It is important to note that when health data are partitioned differently, outcomes change. Instead of income, urban density was used as a surrogate for socioeconomic status. Differences in cancer risks between African Americans and whites were shown to be significantly reduced. The study found that areas of high population density have higher incidences of cancer regardless of race. Some of the cancers (e.g., prostate) that have the highest prevalence in African Americans are not correlated with either income or education (Baquet, Horn, Gibbs, & Greenwald, 1991). In this society, violence is assumed to have an African American face. Centerwall (1984) investigated this assumption by considering the prevalence of domestic homicides in Atlanta from 1970 to 1971. Using household crowding as a measure of socioeconomic status, the relative risk of African Americans and whites was nearly identical. Findings like these suggest that the correlation between health outcomes and living conditions is strong and is mediated not only by race. When applied to data, the interpretive perspective is equally important, if not more important, than the actual numbers.

It is estimated that 70% to 90% of recognized illnesses in African Americans are managed outside the formal health care system (Kleinman, Eisenberg, & Good, 1978). Reports like "Mississippi appendectomies" or eugenic hysterectomies performed on African American women (Chase, 1980; Wiesbord, 1975), testing of women for sickle cell anemia without consent (Farfel & Holtzman, 1986), and court-ordered surgical interventions (Kolder, Gallagher, & Parsons, 1987) serve to maintain the breach between African Americans and the health care system. Heart disease is a leading cause of death in African Americans, but whites use significantly more of the available treatments for heart disease, such as coronary angioplasty and coronary artery bypass grafting (Wenneker & Epstein, 1989).

One of the behaviors arising from unpredictable health care system experiences is called "impression management" (Whitehead, 1992). Using impression management the client projects conforming behavior, responds as expected, and avoids appearing self-destructive or unconcerned. The divergence between the client and the provider is never resolved or brokered. The need for impression management or similar coping mechanisms between client and provider should be greatly reduced if not eliminated.

What are the implications for research? One of the roles of research is to inform, thereby improving nursing practice. Therefore, research outcomes must be reliable and valid. Some of the traditional approaches to protocol implementation cannot assure this and change is imperative. As early as 1929, racial differences in drug response were recorded. Recent studies show, however, that the pharmacodynamics of African Americans is ignored in drug clinical trials because of their underrepresentation (Larson, 1994; Svensson, 1989). Being familiar with the culture of study participants is essential, especially when researchers either target that group or deliberately exclude it. In conducting research among the poor, African Americans, and other minorities, the methodology and theoretical constructs used must be applicable and appropriate. Knowledge of the group should be more in-depth than a mere statistical profile because the data collection and data treatment techniques bear directly on the accuracy of study outcomes (Dennis & Neese, 2000; McGraw, McKinlay, Crawford, Costa, & Cohen, 1992). For example, the practice of combining ethnic minorities to generalize cultural variations makes results highly suspect, if not meaningless (Weitzel & Waller, 1990).

NURSES LEADING AND FOLLOWING

Since the 1940s, the nursing profession has recognized the importance of culture and encouraged its inclusion into health care. Success is slow in coming. In 1992 the American Academy of Nursing (AAN) Expert Panel on Culturally Competent Nursing Care concluded that, "there are no excuses for continuing to provide care that is insensitive and [culturally] incompetent" (p. 277).

Nurses are uniquely positioned to exemplify culturally competent care for African American clients. The first consideration is the model of care used. A Eurocentric model of nursing care has been applied to all who enter the health care system. It was never adequate. The limitations of the North American Nursing Diagnosis Association (NANDA) taxonomy is an example. The usefulness of the defining characteristics listed by NANDA for three of its nursing diagnoses were rated by 245 nurses from eight countries. The nurses concluded that for each of the three diagnoses, it was necessary to expand and rewrite a significant number of its characteristics, delete some, and add others (Geissler, 1991). From a cultural viewpoint, many NANDA terms engendered multiple meanings. Social dysfunction and social isolation, state Kelley and Frisch (1992), are two of the labels that must be defined within their cultural context. Nursing diagnoses are a mainstay of the nursing process, but African Americans and other culturally diverse clients may not be well served by their unmodified use.

Several cultural assessment tools have been proposed to capture relevant data. To date, most are comprehensive but too lengthy and time consuming for clinical utility (Giger & Davidhizar 1991; Tripp-Reimer, Brink, & Saunders, 1984). A promising approach is the use of the client's own explanatory system. Included as a fundamental part of the nursing process, the client's cultural parameters can be assessed quickly through the use of open-ended questions, as suggested by Kleinman, Eisenberg, and Good (1978):

> What do you think caused this illness? What concerns you most about this illness? Why do you think it started when it did? How do you feel about it? What did you do about treating it before you came to the clinic? Hospital? What do you think your sickness does to you? How serious is this illness? What kind of treatment do you think you should receive? [p. 256]

These questions are amenable to time and circumstance. They may be asked early or late in a client's contact with the health care system and are easily postponed until after the acute phase of an illness. Importantly, they create the basis for ongoing discussion.

Heurtin-Roberts and Reisin (1992) found that among hypertensive African American women the patients' cultural beliefs about hypertension influenced their acceptance of treatment and, in turn, the control of their blood pressure. Data from Kumanyika et al. (1989) and Kumanyika, Wilson, and Guilford-Davenport (1993) strongly suggest that beliefs may not be modified by the health-promotion campaigns that are so widely used. They can be affected, however, when the message is delivered in a culturally sensitive format (Martin & Henry, 1989; Parks, 1988). Well-intentioned but culturally inappropriate messages appear in the following two situations. First, African American women in abusive relationships, states Campbell (1993), have concepts of independence and female strength that run counter to accepted ways of help seeking and resource utilization. These women are more likely to remain in their relationships and prefer assistance in working through the abuse problem. That is at odds with the Eurocentric model, which places emphasis on leaving the relationship. The deliberate capture of cultural content must precede real changes in nursing approaches. Second, ethnohistorical influences are basic to nurse-client relationships, and whether acknowledged or ignored they frame the interaction. African Americans respond positively to culturally

sensitive therapeutics. A pilot project in which music therapists used African American music to open avenues of expression for psychiatric clients was remarkably successful when compared with programs using Eurocentric music (Campinha-Bacote & Allbright, 1992).

I believe that accepting the role of culture in practice advances the need for nursing expertise. When seeking out cultural patterns is a consistent expectation, the importance of history and social content will emerge. The pervasive concept of culture must be allowed to move up in the curricular hierarchy as nursing students are being transformed into professional nurses. Culture must be as integrated as the nursing process with a permanent, prominent venue.

Nurses too, must identify their own attitudes, beliefs, and values, and examine ways in which their heritage affects their professional behavior. Nurses are pivotal members of the health care team; they personify one culture (their own), convey another (nursing and health care), and broker a third (the client's). Attitudes based on race, however, continue to influence our perceptions of each other. Once nursing brings order to its own house, it can lead the way to cultural plurality. The alternative is to continue limited efforts that fail.

It is a new century, similar to the old and familiar yet remarkably diverse and different. We may argue as to whether health care is a right or a privilege, but there is no disagreement that it is a choice. African Americans make that choice based on how they perceive the system. Health behaviors are retained because they are functional, but they do not stand alone. Health behaviors are embedded in social and economic arrangements (Pappas, 1994; Smith, 1995). When African American clients are entirely validated by the health care system in all their social and cultural dimensions, a reciprocal relationship can develop that is built on mutual trust, acceptance, and respect.

REFERENCES

AAN Expert Panel on Culturally Competent Nursing Care. (1992). AAN Expert Panel Report: Culturally competent health care. *Nursing Outlook, 40*(6), 277-283.

Anonymous. (1983). Genetics, environment, and hypertension. *Lancet, 1,* 681-682.

Baquet, C.R., Horn, J.W., Gibbs, T., & Greenwald, P. (1991). Socioeconomic factors and cancer incidence among blacks and whites. *Journal of the National Cancer Institute, 83*(8), 551-556.

Beardsley, E.H. (1987). *A history of neglect: Health care for blacks and mill workers in the twentieth century south.* Knoxville, TN: University of Tennessee Press.

Beecher, H.K. (1966). Ethics and clinical research. *New England Journal of Medicine, 274,* 1354-1360.

Bennett, L. (1982). *Before the Mayflower: A history of the negro in America 1619-1964* (5th ed.). New York: Penguin Books.

Biological anthropologist pursues her taste for the big picture. (1995, July 28). *The Chronicle of Higher Education,* pp. A11, A16.

Byrd, M.W., & Clayton, L.A. (1992). An American health dilemma: A history of blacks in the health system. *Journal of the National Medical Association, 84*(2), 189-200.

Cabral, H., Fried, L.E., Levenson, S., Amaro, H., & Zuckerman, B. (1990). Foreign-born and US-born black women: Differences in health behaviors and birth outcomes. *American Journal of Public Health, 80*(1), 70-71.

Campbell, D.W. (1993). Nursing care of African American battered women. *AWHONN's Clinical Issues, 4*(3), 407-414.

Campinha-Bacote, J., & Allbright, R. (1992). Ethnomusic therapy and the dual-diagnosed African American client. *Holistic Nursing Practice, 6*(3), 59-63.

Centerwall, B.S. (1984). Race, socioeconomic status, and domestic homicide, Atlanta, 1971-72. *American Journal of Public Health, 74*(8), 813-815.

Charatz-Litt, C. (1992). A chronicle of racism: The effects of the white medical community on black health. *Journal of the National Medical Association, 84*(8), 717-724.

Chase, A. (1980). *The legacy of Malthus: The social costs of the new scientific racism.* New York: Alfred A. Knopf.

Cooper, R., & David, R. (1986). The biological concept of race and its application to public health epidemiology. *Journal of Health Politics and Law II, 19,* 7-11.

Dennis, B., & Neese, J. (2000). Recruitment and retention of African American elders into community-based research: Lessons learned. *Archives of Psychiatric Nursing, 14*(1), 1-10.

Edwards, A. (1995, October). Coming together. *Essence, 26*(6), 99-100, 102-103, 150-152.

Farfel, M.R., & Holtzman, N.A. (1986). Education, consent, and counseling in sickle cell anemia screening programs. *American Journal of Public Health, 74*(4), 373-375.

Franklin, J.H. (1956). *From slavery to freedom.* New York: Alfred A. Knopf.

Freeman, H. (1991). Race, poverty, and cancer. *Journal of the National Center Institute, 83*(8), 526-527.

Geissler, E.M. (1991). Nursing diagnoses of culturally diverse patients. *International Nursing Review, 38*(5), 150-152.

Gergen, K. (1982). *Toward transformation in social knowledge.* New York: Springer-Verlag.

Giger, J., & Davidhizar, R. (1991). *Transcultural nursing: Assessment and intervention.* St. Louis: Mosby.

Gutman, H.G. (1976). *The black family in slavery and freedom 1750-1925.* New York: Vantage Books.

Hall, J. (1999). Marginalization revisited: Critical, postmodern, and liberation perspectives. *Advances in Nursing Science, 22*(2), 88-102.

Haynes, M.A. (1975). The gap in health status between black and white Americans. In R.A. Williams (Ed.), *Textbook of black-related diseases* (pp. 1-30). New York: McGraw-Hill.

Heurtin-Roberts, S., & Reisin, E. (1992). The relationship of culturally influenced lay models of hypertension to compliance with treatment. *American Journal of Hypertension, 5,* 787-792.

Johnson, J.E. (1982). The Afro-American family: A historical overview. In B.A. Bass, G.E. Wyatt, & G.J. Powell (Eds.), *The Afro-American family: Assessment, treatment, and research issues* (pp. 3-11). New York: Grune & Stratton.

Jones, J.H. (1981). *Badblood: The Tuskegee syphilis experiment.* New York: The Free Press.

Jordan, W.D. (1968). *White over black: American attitudes toward the negro 1650-1812.* New York: WW Norton.

Kelley, J.H., & Frisch, N.C. (1992). A transcultural concept analysis of social isolation. In R.M. Carroll-Johnson & M. Paquette (Eds.), *Classification of nursing diagnosis: Proceedings of the tenth conference* (pp. 232-233). Philadelphia: Lippincott.

Kleinman, A., Eisenberg, L., & Good, B. (1978). Culture, illness, and care: Clinical lessons from anthropologic and cross-cultural research. *Annals of Internal Medicine, 88,* 251-258.

Kolder, V., Gallagher, J., & Parsons, M.T. (1987). Court-ordered obstetrical interventions. *New England Journal of Medicine, 316*(19), 1192-1196.

Kumanyika, S., Savage, D.D., Ramirez, A.G., Hutchinson, J., Trenino, F.M., Adams-Campbell, L.L., & Watkins, L.O. (1989). Beliefs about high blood pressure prevention in a survey of blacks and Hispanics. *American Journal of Preventive Medicine, 5*(1), 21-26.

Kumanyika, S., Wilson, J.F., & Guilford-Davenport, M. (1993). Weight-related attitudes and behaviors of black women. *Journal of the American Dietetic Association, 93*(4), 416-422.

Langford, H.G. (1981). Is blood pressure different in black people? *Post-graduate Medical Journal, 57,* 749-754.

Larson, E. (1994). Exclusion of certain groups from clinical research. *Image, 26*(3), 185-190.

Martin, M.E., & Henry, M. (1989). Cultural relativity and poverty. *Public Health Nursing, 6*(1), 28-34.

McCord, C., & Freeman, H. (1990). Excess mortality in Harlem. *New England Journal of Medicine, 322*(3), 173-177.

McGraw, S.A., McKinlay, J.B., Crawford, S.A., Costa, L.A., & Cohen, D.L. (1992). Health survey methods with minority populations: Some lessons from recent experiences. *Ethnicity and Disease, 2,* 273-284.

Mouton, C.P., Harris, S., Rovi, S., Solorzano, P., & Johnson, M. (1997). Barriers to black women's participation in cancer clinical trials. *Journal of the National Medical Association, 89*(11), 721-727.

Myers, M.J. (1991). Expanding the psychology of knowledge optimally: The importance of world view revisited. In R.L. Jones (Ed.), *Black psychology* (pp. 15-32). Berkeley, CA: Cobb and Henry.

National Center for Health Statistics. (1995). *Health, United States, 1994.* Hyattsville, MD: Public Health Services.

Newman, D.K., Amidei, N.J., Carter, B.L., Kruvant, W.J., & Russell, J. (1978). *Protest, politics and prosperity: Black Americans and white institutions; 1940-1975.* New York: Pantheon Books.

Pappas, G. (1994). Elucidating the relationship between race, socioeconomic status, and health [Editorial]. *American Journal of Public Health, 84*(6), 892.

Parks, C.P. (1988). Development of a hypertension educational pamphlet for the black community: A model approach. *Health Education, 10,* 8-10.

Reed, W.L., Darity, W., & Robertson, N. (1993). *Health and medical care of African Americans.* Westport, CT: Greenwood Publishing Group.

Rene, A.A., Daniels, D.E., Jones, W., & Moore, F.I. (1992). Mortality in the slave and white population of Natchitoches Parish, Louisiana, 1850. *Journal of the National Medical Association, 84*(9), 805-811.

Savitt, T.L. (1978). *Medicine and slavery: The diseases and health care of blacks in antebellum Virginia.* Urbana, IL: University of Illinois Press.

Savitt, T.L. (1982). The use of blacks for medical experimentation and demonstration in the old south. *The Journal of Southern History, 48,* 331-335.

Smith, C.A. (1995). The lived experience of staying healthy in rural African American families. *Nursing Science Quarterly, 8*(1), 17-21.

Stampp, K.M. (1956). *The peculiar institution. Slavery in the antebellum south.* New York: Alfred A. Knopf.

Svensson, C.K. (1989). Representation of American blacks in clinical trials of new drugs. *Journal of the American Medical Association, 261*(2), 263-265.

Thomas, J., Semenya, K., Neser, W.B., Thomas, D.J., & Gillum, R.F. (1990). Parental hypertension as a predictor of hypertension in black physicians: The Meharry Cohort Study. *Journal of the National Medical Association, 82*(6), 409-412.

Thomas, J., Semenya, K.A., Neser, W.B., Thomas, D.J., Green, D.R., & Gillum, R.F. (1985). Risk factors and the incidence of hypertension in black physicians: The Meharry Cohort Study. *American Heart Journal, 119*(3), 637-635.

Thomas, V.G. (1992). Explaining health disparities between African-American and white populations. Where do we go from here? *Journal of the National Medical Association, 84*(10), 837-840.

Tripp-Reimer, T., Brink, P.J., & Saunders, J.M. (1984). Cultural assessment. Content and process. *Nursing Outlook, 32,* 78-82.

United States Bureau of the Census. (1996). *Statistical Abstracts of the United States* (116th ed.). Washington, DC: United States Department of Commerce.

Valentine, C.A. (1968). *Culture and poverty.* Chicago: The University of Chicago Press.

Van Sertima, I. (1976). *They came before Columbus.* New York: Random House.

Vaughn, J. (1997). Is there really racism in nursing? *Journal of Nursing Education, 36*(3), 135-139.

Waitzman, N.J., & Smith, K.R. (1994). The effects of occupational class transitions on hypertension: Racial disparities among working-age men. *American Journal of Public Health, 84*(6), 945-950.

Wenneker, M.B., & Epstein, A.M. (1989). Racial inequalities in the use of procedures for patients with ischemic heart disease in Massachusetts. *Journal of the American Medical Association, 261*(2), 253-257.

Weitzel, M.H., & Waller, P.R. (1990). Predictive factors for health-promotive behaviors in white, Hispanic, and black blue-collar workers. *Family and Community Health, 13*(1), 23-34.

Whitehead, T.L. (1992). In search of soul food and meaning: Culture, food and health. In H.A. Baer & Y. Jones (Eds.), *African Americans in the South: Issues of race, class, and gender* (pp. 94-110). Athens, GA: University of Georgia Press.

Wiesbord, R.G. (1975). *Genocide? Birth control and the black American.* Westport, CT: Greenwood Press.

Woodhandler, S., Himmelstein, D.U., Siber, R., Bader, M., Harnly, M., & Jones, A. (1985). Medical care and mortality: Racial differences in preventable deaths. *International Journal of Health Service, 15,* 1-22.

Bridging Cultures

Asians and Pacific Islanders and Nursing

JILLIAN INOUYE

Asians and Pacific Islanders (APIs) comprise one of the fastest growing minority groups in the United States (Lin-Fu, 1988; Pollard & De Vita, 1997; U.S. Department of Commerce, 1991). This group is heterogeneous with diverse cultural and religious backgrounds and immigrant and refugee status, and they speak a variety of languages. Yet these disparate groups continue to be combined for data reporting and analyzing purposes. "*E pluribus unum*," written on the seal of the United States and on every dollar bill, literally translated means "out of many, one" or figuratively, "out of many people, one nation." It does not say or mean "out of many nations, one people" as has been suggested in the "melting pot" analogy used in the past. However welcoming we have been to immigrants, the idea that acculturation and assimilation may or may not occur is prevalent and influences our interactions with people of other races and cultures. Because APIs are easily identifiable as nonwhite, they sometimes are visually clustered into categories of "foreign," "immigrant," or "different." These visual prejudices of identification are as difficult to change as the false assumptions that people from Hawaii still live in grass huts and wear grass skirts or that Asians are the "model minority." This view of the hard-working and achievement-oriented Asian with few of the socioeconomic or other health problems associated with other groups has been shattered with research on mental health concerns (Lin & Cheung, 1999) and findings of undercounting on morbidity and mortality data (Liao, McGee, & Cooper, 1999). Because of their increasing numbers, the general lack of familiarity with and knowledge of these cultures, and the pervasiveness of false assumptions, we need to understand the health, culture, and self-image issues of this group to provide them with competent care. This chapter will focus on who some of the APIs are and who the nurses are who care for them, with suggestions for practice, education, and research.

WHO ARE THE ASIANS AND PACIFIC ISLANDERS?

The Census Bureau forecasts that by midcentury the population of the United States will be 404 million and by 2100, 571 million. Today's minority groups will account for 60% of the population. Asian Americans and Pacific Islanders are the fastest growing ethnic minorities in America (U.S. Department of Commerce, 1991). In 1980 APIs were less than 2% of the U.S. population. In 1996 they accounted for nearly 4% and are projected to be almost 10.7%, or 41 million Americans, by the year 2050 (Kuo, 1997). Immigrants, who comprise 10% of the U.S. population, are predicted to grow to 13% in 2050, with more from countries other than Europe. Because immigrants tend to be younger, the API population will be one of the younger ethnic groups. In 1990, roughly two thirds of all APIs resided in the 25 largest metropolitan areas in the United States (Statistical Bulletin, 1992). Fifty-six percent live in three states: California, New York, and Hawaii (Pollard & De Vita, 1997). For the Pacific Islanders alone, most Native Hawaiians (180,000) live in the state of Hawaii; 50% of Samoans and Chamorrans live in California; 80% of Fijians live in California; and 20% of Tongans live in Utah (U.S. Bureau of the Census, 1993).

Although median income was about 9% higher than for white households, this difference was achieved largely by more workers in the household contributing to the income (Pollard & De Vita, 1997). Despite their higher median income, API families were nearly twice as likely as whites to live in poverty (Pollard & De Vita, 1997), thus creating a bimodal distribution.

Combining Asian Americans and Pacific Islanders disregards the significant cultural differences of the two ethnic groups. The Census Bureau includes 28 Asian countries and 25 Pacific Islander cultures into their definition of API Americans. Within each subgroup is an immense diversity of languages and dialects. To lump together their socioeconomic, historical, and cultural differences is like trying to compare group differences of the Japanese Americans who came to the United States in 1885 as immigrant workers with the Vietnamese Americans who entered as war refugees in 1975 after the fall of Saigon (Uehara, Takeuchi, & Smuckler, 1994). Each group arrived for different reasons with different beliefs, religions, practices, histories, and health problems. Yet they are all classified as Asian American for demographic purposes. Similarly, Pacific Islanders may consist of peoples from Polynesia, Micronesia, and Melanesia. Among the Polynesians, Native Hawaiians are the largest group, followed by Samoans, Tongans, and Tahitians. Chammorans comprise the largest group of the Micronesians, and Fijians represent the largest group in the Melanesians (U.S. Census, 1990). These groups have different histories, values, and cultures, which were influenced by the nations who colonized them. Combining disparate groups increases the likelihood of poor service planning and resource allocation and the provision of insensitive care.

HEALTH ISSUES OF ASIANS AND PACIFIC ISLANDERS

Because a detailed description of this topic has been covered by others (Chen & Hawks, 1995; Inouye, 1999; Louie, 1999; Lum, 1995), only highlights will be discussed here.

Mortality

Table 68-1 compares the 10 leading causes of death among APIs with those of the general populations. The leading cause of death, based on the 1990 U.S. Census, was heart disease followed by malignant neoplasms, stroke, accidents, and diabetes (Braun, Look, Yang, Onaka, & Horiuchi, 1996). Reports outside of Hawaii rarely disaggregate Asian and Pacific Islander groups, yet limited research on Native Hawaiians has found they have higher morbidity and mortality rates compared with those of other races in the state of Hawaii (Braun et al., 1996). APIs have a lower mortality than whites for all age groups among men and for the over 44-year age groups for women. This may be due to undercounting rates for APIs of 2.4% compared with 0.7% for non-Hispanic whites (Hogan, 1993) and to misclassification of Asians at 21.1% versus 0.5% for non-

TABLE 68-1 The 10 Leading Causes of Death Among Asians and Pacific Islanders and Those of the General Population for 1997

Asians and Pacific Islanders	All Persons
1. Malignant neoplasms	Diseases of the heart
2. Diseases of the heart	Malignant neoplasms
3. Cerebrovascular disease	Unintentional injuries
4. Unintentional injuries	Cerebrovascular disease
5. Pneumonia and influenza	Chronic obstructive pulmonary disease
6. Motor vehicle–related injuries	Motor vehicle–related injuries
7. Diabetes mellitus	Diabetes mellitus
8. Chronic obstructive pulmonary disease	Pneumonia and influenza
9. Suicide	Suicide
10. Homicide and legal intervention	Homicide and legal intervention

From National Center for Health Statistics. (1999). *Health, United States, 1999, with socioeconomic status and health chartbook* (pp. 142-145). Hyattsville, MD: Author.

Hispanic whites on death certificates (Poe et al., 1993). Most of those misclassified were falsely reported to be white, thus understating the mortality rate of APIs (Liao et al., 1999). Misclassification or inconsistency in coding of race at birth and at death show the rates of error to be lowest for whites (1.2%) and greatest for races other than white or black (43.2%), with the error rate as much as 33.3% for Chinese, 48.8% for Japanese, and 78.7% for Filipinos. Most of the direction of error was toward classifying infants as white at time of death (Yu & Liu, 1992).

Self-Perceptions of Health

Several studies have reported that as a group, APIs had better self-perceptions of their health than whites but were less satisfied with and perceived less sharing in the doctor-patient relationship (Koseki & Reid, 1995; Meredith & Siu, 1995). Explanations for the difference in doctor-patient relations may be due to the low ratio of Asian clinicians to the patient population, language barriers, a preference for less direct communication by Asians, different expectations for sharing health care responsibility, the desire for formality in the doctor-patient relationship, different ideas about alternative remedies, and less awareness of their problems by patients (Liu, 1989; Meredith & Siu, 1995; Nilchaikovit, Hill, & Holland, 1993; Stavig, Igra, & Leonard, 1988). These differences can also exist for nurse-patient relations and add to the difficulty in understanding and caring for diverse groups.

Risk Factors

Risk factors differed in the API subgroups in a study by Chung, Tash, Raymond, Yasunobu, and Lew (1990). Where Asians had a higher prevalence of physical inactivity compared with other groups, the Hawaiians were at higher risk for being overweight, for nonuse of seat belts, for cigarette smoking, and for alcohol abuse. Those who were more general risk takers tended to be more overweight, used alcohol and cigarettes more, and drove while intoxicated. These behaviors were more prevalent among men and Hawaiians. Physical inactivity was more prevalent among the Filipinos and Japanese. The fact that lack of physical activity was not related to weight for the Asian group was explained by genetic differences in metabolism. Other physical indicators of health related to activity were not obtained in this sample, however.

Dietary changes have posed threats to the Native Hawaiians in terms of obesity and cardiovascular disease (Blaisdell, 1993; Miike, 1987). Similarly, changing diets of Asian Americans has elevated risks of cardiovascular diseases and cancer (Jha, Enas, & Yusuf, 1993; Whittemore, 1989) but very little in terms of obesity.

Compared with all other racial or ethnic groups, APIs are at greatest risk of contracting tuberculosis and parasitic infections (Chen & Hawks, 1995). In addition, respiratory conditions such as asthma are increasing alarmingly in this group (Chen & Hawks, 1995).

Japanese Americans have twice the rate of diabetes as white Americans and four times the rate of Japanese in Japan. Samoans also have a high incidence of diabetes, three times that of white Americans (Kagawa-Singer, Kumanyika, Lex, & Markides, 1995).

Yoon and Chien (1996) summarize why it is difficult to determine specific problems for APIs. They state that although in the United States smoking rates are lowest among APIs (18.2%) as a group, 92% of Laotians and 71% of Cambodians are smokers. Although cancer rates are about the same for whites and APIs, Korean-American men have a fivefold higher incidence of stomach cancer and an eightfold higher incidence of liver cancer. Because of the lack of specific subgroup research, results of health problems in this group are difficult to address in planning risk reduction and health prevention programs.

Mental Health

Further problems of combining ethnic groups into a single category are illustrated in a study by Uehara et al. (1994) of the community functioning status of clients in a public mental health program. When treated as a single group, Asian Americans were identified with lower levels of functioning difficulty than whites. When treated separately, however, only one of five Asian ethnic groups had significantly lower levels of difficulty. The factors that accounted for this difference were refugee versus immigrant status, time of arrival, ethnic minorities in their country of origin, urban verus rural environment of origin, and the stressors of war-related trauma.

Low admission rates to state hospitals and outpatient mental health services seem to reflect late help-seeking behaviors (Lin & Cheung, 1999). Because of high family involvement with care, Asian patients with schizophrenia typically are cared for within the family and community for a long time before they are admitted to the Western health care system and thus are seen when their symptoms are more severe.

Somatization when in distress was thought to be the acceptable symptom presentation for Asian Americans. A new explanation for this phenomenon is that patients are fully aware of their emotional problems but selectively present symptoms according to what they perceive as appropriate to the practitioner (Lin & Cheung, 1999).

CULTURAL BELIEFS, VALUES, AND ORIENTATION

Although there are between-group and within-group differences among Asians and Pacific Islanders, there are similarities too. The notion of a collectivist versus individualist orientation applies to both groups. Both emphasize the importance of the relationship between the self and the social groups, the spiritual unity of the individual with the environment, the spiritual significance of events such as illness, and the relationship between the body and the mind (Hughes, Tsark, & Mokuau, 1996; Lin & Cheung, 1999). The Hawaiian concepts of *mana* (spirituality), *lokahi* (harmony), *'ohana* (extended family), and *kokua* (mutual help, cooperation) are similar to Japanese concepts of *on* (obligation), *giri* (filial piety), *amae* (interdependency), and *gaman* (suppression of emotion to avoid confrontation and as a sign of strength), and Asian religious beliefs of harmony with nature, balance (*yin* and *yang*), and the importance of family, affiliation, and a group and personal orientation versus the individual and impersonal. As is true in most cultures, traditional health beliefs and customs are also used along with standard allopathic medical practices, depending on the disease. The identification with and degree of immersion of the person in his or her culture play an important role in behaviors and should always be assessed and not assumed.

Asian immigrant patients' distrust of Western medical care is based on their long tradition of herbalist or shamanistic healing (Sung, 1999). Their belief of energy flow pervades all aspects of their daily life, and daily well-being is focused on proper nutrients and brewed teas. Sung further speculates that noncompliance with medication is the manifestation of this mistrust in Western medicine. In addition to a basic philosophical difference, language barriers compound the problem. Communication is important in building trusting relationships and understanding the patient's methods of communication, especially since silence is interpreted by Western health care practitioners as resistance, hostility, or lack of intelligence. This in turn leads health professionals to react defensively with frustration and exasperation at not being able to do their jobs. They resort to communication patterns that may be demeaning to the client, such as using slang, colloquialisms, or the vernacular or speaking slowly and loudly as if the patient were hard of hearing.

Other patterns regarding Asian Americans' attitudes toward health care workers reveal that older people prefer older physicians, a physician that appears busy, and for those patients who were not native-born American, that the physician be of Asian ancestry and bilingual (Pertulla, Lowe, & Quon, 1999). They also relied on combined doctor and family input regarding selection of a health care facility.

NURSING ISSUES

Who are the people caring for the APIs and other minority groups? Table 68-2 lists the health professions chosen by Asian Americans in the United States. No information is given separately for Pacific Islanders.

TABLE 68-2   Percent of Asians Enrolled in Selected Health Profession Schools Compared with Non-Hispanic Whites, 1996-1997

Profession	Non-Hispanic White (%)	Asian (%)
Allopathic medicine	65.8	17.6
Osteopathic medicine	79.8	11.4
Podiatry	78.4	14.0
Dentistry	67.7	22.4
Optometry	73.0	20.2
Pharmacy	70.3	18.7
Registered nurse	81.0	4.4

From National Center for Health Statistics. (1999). *Health, United States, 1999, with socioeconomic status and health chartbook* (pp. 274-275). Hyattsville, MD: Author.

Statistics

Asians comprise 4.4% of all registered nurses compared with 81% for whites, 9.9% for blacks, 3.9% for Hispanics, and 0.8% for American Indians (National Center for Health Statistics, 1999). These figures do not reflect the proportion of increase of APIs in the general population nor in nursing education and graduation figures (Wann, 1992). There has been a decline in annual admissions of minority students into basic nursing programs from 15.9% in 1992 to 15.6% in 1993 (National League for Nursing, 1994, p. 4). The enrollment for Asians in nursing programs indicates 4.6% are in generic baccalaureate programs, 3.2% in master's programs, and 3% in doctoral programs. In 1996 56% of Asian health professionals had baccalaureate degrees, but only about 7% of APIs had master's or doctoral degrees (Buerhaus & Auerbach, 1999). In addition, the numbers of all minority faculty have declined during the past decade, with API full-time nursing faculty decreasing by 0.2 % to 1.6% of all faculty (Campbell & Sigsby, 1994). This is much lower than their numbers in the general workforce.

Kuramoto and Louie (1996) report that 84% of API nurses work full-time; 85% work in hospitals; and 6.2% have master's or doctoral degrees. APIs prefer hospital settings (72%) yet had the lowest percentage of management positions such as administrator, supervisor, head nurse, or instructor compared with other ethnic groups (Buerhaus & Auerbach, 1999). Bessent (1989) also found that persons of color in general were underrepresented in leadership and management positions. While Asians and Pacific Islanders stand out because of their high incomes from nursing and their having the highest rate of any group in obtaining a baccalaureate education, Buerhaus and Auerbach relate this to their education in foreign countries, where the baccalaureate degree is the usual requirement for becoming a registered nurse (RN), and the high employment rates in hospitals explain their high incomes. Additionally, more Asians in the workforce come from families in which many members of the family work, and more work full-time than part-time (Lerner, D'Agostino, Musolino, & Malspeis, 1994). APIs rank high socioeconomically (partly because of dual incomes), but in terms of leadership roles in the workforce, the education system, and role modeling, they rank lowest of all the minority groups (Buerhaus & Auerbach, 1999).

Attitudes

Minority cultures often are not understood by health care providers, and traditional ethnic health care practices are not valued or recognized (Williamson, Allen, & Coppens,

1996). A study by Kulwicki and Boloink (1996) found graduating nursing students had generally little or no confidence in caring for five ethnic groups in Michigan, with confidence in caring for APIs the lowest. The other four groups included African Americans, Latinos/Hispanics, Middle Eastern or Arabic persons, and Native Americans. In addition, the means for confidence in caring for APIs on all subscales were lowest except for one. The authors postulate that lack of self-confidence may preclude the provision of culturally appropriate care and that self-efficacy can be related to specific behaviors that can be gained through role modeling as well as through verbal persuasion and practice.

A survey of 3,242 Anglo-American registered nurses practicing in an urban area found that even though nurses knew more about the culture and health care practices of Asian Americans than about those of Hispanics and African Americans (Rhooda, 1993), they had the least positive attitudes toward Hispanics and Asian Americans. Rhooda suggests that this appeared to be a function of cultural attitudes. Interestingly, associate degree (AD) graduates tended to be less biased toward Hispanics than non-AD graduates. These results are in contrast to those of Sharma (1988), who believes that ethnocentrism and a lack of sensitivity in client interactions are due to lack of knowledge of others' cultural beliefs and suggests that educational programs need to examine differences in learning experiences that can contribute to more positive attitudes and acceptance of diversity.

FUTURE DIRECTIONS AND RECOMMENDATIONS

The changes in our population base should be an impetus to recruitment, retention, retraining, and research in the area of ethnic diversity in nursing. Future directions and recommendations are suggested around the three areas of practice, education, and research.

Clinical Practice

Absence of people of color at every level of care is one of the most profound barriers to equity of care (Henry, Tator, Mattis, & Rees, 1995). The remedy would be to increase minority representation in the health care system. Hiring of nursing staff from culturally diverse groups as resource people and possibly as translators can remedy one of the largest barriers to culturally competent care, that of communication. Use of advance practice nurses with transcultural backgrounds—from formal education, personal knowledge, or experience as consultants—could also assist in providing competent care.

For native Hawaiians, incorporation of cultural values and lifestyle practices such as harmony and cooperation is important. Hughes et al. (1996) suggest using traditional diet as a form of intervention in health education and promotion of cancer prevention. "Talk story," or the use of social talk and establishing of relationships, is important in interviewing Native Hawaiians.

Louie (1995) recommends that services need to be located in neighborhoods where clients and families reside. Because API nurses practice mainly in acute care facilities, there is a great need for more APIs in advance practice positions to work in the community, especially in psychiatric and mental health settings, and serve as role models.

Because of the importance of the family for social support as well as in decision making, approaches employed by nurses should include respect for family presence and for their involvement in the care of patients. In addition, nurses need to be accepting of large numbers of visitors in hospital units, of relatives used as translators or go-betweens in communicating with patients, and in the recognition of the importance of special foods and herbs or teas in the patients' daily lives.

A different view, taken by Fuller (1996), is that rather than learning health beliefs and practices of all groups, nurses need to work with ethnic health workers or interpreters as resources and negotiate care with them; in doing this they will learn the culture and beliefs. The use of native healers or elders from the specific groups is consistent with the health care practices of some API cultures.

Chen and Hawks (1995) have proposed a client-practitioner negotiation model of care that includes (1) creating a dialogue with clients on care-related issues, (2) establishing mutual understanding with clients, (3) identifying a common goal in care, and (4) establishing a plan to work toward the common goal. This personalized approach and attention to cultural diversity and individuality can increase the ability of nurses and other health professionals to provide culturally sensitive and competent care. It is hoped there will be less reliance on stereotypical responses and more on understanding broad philosophical commonalities.

Education

Nursing education must become multicultural to provide a core of culturally competent nurse providers, educators, and researchers (American Nurses Association, 1991). Educational goals and strategies to care for the emerging minorities of the United States focus on increasing diversity of the faculty and student body, enhancing cultural relevance of course content, and increasing options for primary care specialties at the master's level (Norbeck, 1995). Increasing API faculty is unlikely because of the limited numbers of students who earn advanced degrees (Campbell & Sigsby, 1994). A remedy would be to focus on facilitating the success of minority nursing students in undergraduate programs and encouraging and facilitating admission to graduate programs. Increasing the number of students in the graduate program will increase the pool of APIs eligible for faculty positions.

Education for the majority can be a catalyst for providing culturally competent care. Andrews (1992) states that most nurses receive little or no formal preparation for dealing with culturally diverse clients. Continuing education is a method that could be used to fill this gap. Other methods to increase student and faculty competency are immersion in a culture, increasing the quantity and relevance of cultural diversity in the content of the curriculum, and pairing students of different cultures. Andrews summarizes a survey showing that only a handful of nursing programs integrated cultural concepts into the curriculum. A few universities have special projects or curricula that integrate cultural concepts or expand learning experiences with specific minority cultures (West, 1993; Williamson et al., 1996). For example, the University of Hawaii's School of Nursing and Dental Hygiene highlights specific ethnic groups for each course as an organizing framework for the undergraduate program. International content and courses featuring travel abroad are also offered and challenge ethnocentric notions. In addition, the development of faculty practice sites in a community with cultural diversity provides an opportunity for student practice with a faculty or mentor role model.

Other ways to increase self-efficacy and influence expectations in transcultural nursing are performance attainment, observation, persuasion, and low-arousal states (Kulwicki & Boloink, 1996). Using these concepts, nursing educators can focus on increased supervised practice and exposure to culturally diverse clients, role modeling of expert nurses interacting and practicing with multicultural clients, positive feedback using computer-assisted learning and low-arousal practice with clients. This can be accomplished with actors, paid clients, faculty role playing, or protégé or mentoring programs. Schools with little cultural diversity on their faculty could also form diversity partnerships with other schools with a highly diverse faculty. With Picturetel or telehealth technology, faculty could serve as resources and consultants for other schools in their areas of expertise and collaborate with others in areas with which they are less familiar. This ex-

perience can expand exposure to students as well as faculty from different parts of the country.

Further strategies to increase general cultural competence include

1. Immersion programs in which students are exposed to a diverse culture by living in that culture for a time.
2. Courses that focus not only on content and knowledge but also on process and attitudes. Students need to be aware of their own values and beliefs about other cultures (Kirkham, 1998).
3. Pairing of students of different ethnic backgrounds to work on case studies of yet another ethnic culture and using interventions from the perspective of each other's cultures.

To facilitate retention of the API students, curricula should integrate knowledge of their culture-specific beliefs, values, practices, and learning styles and their respect for elders and teachers, collectivism, and harmony. Methods include:

1. Teaching-learning methods that reward cohesion and cooperation versus competitiveness and individuation. These may include group projects, problem-based learning methods, and individual portfolios and journals (Ishida, Inouye, & Shimamoto, 1994).
2. Deemphasizing oral classroom participation by giving credit for written or other types of participation such as the use of Internet courses or synchronous and asynchronous chat rooms.
3. Providing a sanctioned participation process, such as soliciting information or answers rather than asking open-ended questions for anyone to answer, as API students prefer to be called on rather than volunteer (Chattergy & Ongteco, 1991).
4. Mentoring and peer-supervision by more advanced students.

Diversity should be not only taught but also experienced. Although knowledge of cultural concepts are important, students need to examine self-paradigms and perceptions while being educated in nursing. Awareness of our own assumptions can lead to taking responsibility for our ideas and values, examining and testing them, and listening and being open to others' perceptions (McLeod, 1996). Those who are not bicultural must learn to appreciate the perspective of others.

Research

Minority research brings a different and unique perspective to the research setting, one that includes insight into a nonmajority culture (Huttlinger & Drevdahl, 1994). Yet Asian Americans are not considered underrepresented in the area of postgraduate research and are often excluded for funding purposes under this category. There is a misperception that the number of Asian Americans and Pacific Islanders pursuing graduate research careers has increased (American Association of State Colleges and Universities [AASCU], 1989). These figures, however, are based on all postsecondary education programs, not simply nursing. A cursory review of 1998 National Institute of Nursing Research (NINR) federally funded grants in the areas particularly needed by APIs, such as cardiovascular risk, diabetes, cancer, infectious disease, and pulmonary and mental illness, revealed that approximately 3 of 94 funded projects were awarded to people with surnames that appeared to be of API origin. Furthermore, although target samples of patients included African Americans, Hispanics, and Native Americans, not one title included the names of APIs in the target population. Although surnames may not indicate ethnic categories, this perfunctory review highlights the need for more research training and mentoring for APIs.

More research needs to be focused on evidence-based practice for the API population using culturally relevant methods and outcomes necessary for this ethnic group. Five critical research categories are culturally influenced:

1. Disease etiology, meanings of major life events, and beliefs about causes of various illnesses.
2. Preferred modality of treatment, symptoms or illness recognition, and choice of traditional versus Western care systems.
3. Accessibility of health care services and availability, affordability, and acceptability of health services.
4. Health behavior, health-related personal lifestyle, knowledge, attitudes, and practices, communication and media utilized, and leaders who can influence health promotion and disease prevention.
5. Social relations and perceptions, stereotypes, prejudices, and preferences affecting positive and negative interethnic relations, social participation, and organized responses to various threats to quality of life (Penn, Kar, & Zambrana, 1995).

SUMMARY

At the eighth East-West Philosopher's Conference held January 2000 in Hawaii, Roger Ames, a professor of philosophy and director of the Center for Chinese Studies at the University of Hawaii, said, "There is no such thing as a Japanese mind or a Chinese mind. What you have is narratives of populations" (Burris, 2000, p. B1). Radhakrishnan, a thinker and writer and past president of India, said, "What we want is neither a conflict between East and West nor a mergence of the two. Each will retain its integrated structure but acquire from the other whatever is of value" (Burris, 2000, p. B4). What these statements and the goals of the conference highlight is that there is no unified philosophy but that one should create greater understanding and appreciation for the various philosophies and how they can help us understand each other and ourselves. This philosophy can be related to our attempt to "bridge cultures" in nursing, especially those as diverse as Asian, Pacific Islander, and Western cultures.

REFERENCES

American Association of State Colleges and Universities/ERIC Model Programs Inventory Project. (1989). *Minorities access to research careers. Fund for improvement of postsecondary education.* (ERIC No. ED306860). New York: Author.

American Nurses Association. (1991). *Position statement on cultural diversity in nursing practice.* Washington, DC: Author.

Andrews, M.M. (1992). Cultural perspectives on nursing in the 21st century. *Journal of Professional Nursing, 8,* 7-15.

Bessent, H. (1989). Post doctoral leadership training for women of color. *Journal of Professional Nursing, 5*(5), 279-282.

Blaisdell, R.K. (1993). Health status of Kanaka Maoli (indigenous Hawaiians). *Asian American and Pacific Islander Journal of Health, 1*(2), 116-160.

Braun, K., Look, M., Yang, H., Onaka, A., & Horiuchi, B. (1996). Native Hawaiian mortality, 1980 and 1990. *American Journal of Public Health, 86*(6), 888-889.

Buerhaus, P., & Auerbach, D. (1999). Slow growth in the United States of the number of minorities in the RN workforce. *Image: Journal of Nursing Scholarship, 31,* 179-183.

Burris, J. (2000, January 9). Hawaii conference will seek philosophical understanding. *Honolulu Advertiser,* pp. B1, B4.

Campbell, D.W., & Sigsby, L.M. (1994). Increasing minorities in higher education in nursing: Faculty consultation as a strategy. *Journal of Professional Nursing, 10,* 7-12.

Chattergy, V., & Ongteco, B.C. (1991). Education needs of Filipino migrant students. *Social Process in Hawaii, 33,* 142-152.

Chen, M.S., & Hawks, B. (1995). A debunking of the myth of the healthy Asians and Pacific Islanders. *American Journal of Health Promotion, 8,* 261-268.

Chung, C.S., Tash, E., Raymond, J., Yasunobu, C., & Lew, R. (1990). Health risk behaviours and ethnicity in Hawaii. *International Journal of Epidemiology, 19,* 1011-1018.

Fuller, J. (1996). Culturally appropriate for all? *Contemporary Nurse, 5,* 40.

Henry, F., Tator, C., Mattis, W., & Rees, T. (1995). *The colour of democracy: Racism in Canadian society.* Toronto: Harcourt-Brace.

Hogan, H. (1993). The 1990 post-enumeration survey: Operations and results. *Journal of the American Statistical Association, 8,* 1047-1060.

Hughes, C.K., Tsark, J.A.U., & Mokuau, N.K. (1996). Diet-related cancer in Native Hawaiians. *Cancer, 78*(Suppl.), 1558-1563.

Huttlinger, K., & Drevdahl, D. (1994). Increasing minority participation in biomedical and nursing research. *Journal of Professional Nursing, 10,* 13-21.

Inouye, J. (1999). Asian American health and disease. In R.M. Huff & M.V. Kline (Eds.), *Promoting health in multicultural populations.* Thousand Oaks, CA: Sage Publications.

Ishida, D., Inouye, J., & Shimamoto, Y. (1994). Learning among ethnically diverse nursing students and faculty. *Nurse Educator, 19*(5), 5.

Jha, P., Enas, E., & Yusuf, S. (1993). Coronary artery disease in Asian Indians: Prevalence and risk factors. *Asian American and Pacific Islander Journal of Health, 1*(2), 163-175.

Kagawa-Singer, M., Kumanyika, S.K., Lex, B.W., & Markides, K.S. (1995). Panel III: Behavioral risk factors related to chronic diseases in ethnic minorities. *Health Psychology, 14*(7), 613-621.

Kirkham, S.R. (1998). Nurses' descriptions of caring for culturally diverse clients. *Clinical Nursing Research, 7*(2), 125-146.

Koseki, L.K., & Reid, S.E. (1995). Health status, life satisfaction and health practices: A study of Pacific Asian and Native Hawaiian elderly cohorts. *Asia Pacific Journal of Public Health, 8*(2), 95-101.

Kulwicki, A., & Boloink, B.J. (1996). Assessment of level of comfort in providing multicultural nursing care by baccalaureate nursing students. *Journal of Cultural Diversity, 3,* 40-45.

Kuo, J. (1997). *Health status of Asian Americans: United States, 1992-1994* (Advance Data from Vital and Health Statistics, No. 298). Hyattsville, MD: National Center for Health Statistics.

Kuramoto, A., & Louie, K. (1996). Asian/Pacific Islander American nurses workforce: Issues and challenges for the 21st century. *Journal of Cultural Diversity, 3,* 112-115.

Lerner, D.J., D'Agostino, R.B., Musolino, J., & Malspeis, S. (1994). Breaking with tradition: The new groups in professional nursing. *Medical Care, 32,* 67-80.

Liao, Y., McGee, D.L., & Cooper, R.S. (1999). Mortality among US adult Asians and Pacific Islanders: Findings from the National Health Interview Surveys and the National Longitudinal Mortality Study. *Ethnicity and Disease, 9,* 423-433.

Lin, K.-M., & Cheung, F. (1999). Mental health issues for Asian Americans. *Psychiatric Services, 50*(6), 774-780.

Lin-Fu, J.S. (1988). Population characteristics and health care needs of Asian Pacific Islanders. *Public Health Report, 103*(1), 18-27.

Liu, M.P. (1989). *Factors associated with premature treatment termination of Asian and white clients at community mental health clinics.* Unpublished doctoral dissertation. California School of Professional Psychology, Los Angeles.

Louie, K. (1999). Health promotion interventions for Asian American and Pacific Islanders. In L. Zhan (Ed.), *Asian voices.* Sudbury, MA: Jones and Bartlett.

Louie, K.B. (1995, November-December). Cultural considerations: Asian-Americans and Pacific Islanders. *Imprint,* pp. 41-46.

Lum, O. (1995). Health status of Asians and Pacific Islanders. *Ethnogeriatrics, 11*(1), 53-67.

McLeod, R.P. (1996). Issues in caring for a culturally diverse population. *Advanced Practice Nursing Quarterly, 2,* viii-ix.

Meredith, L.S., & Siu, A.L. (1995). Variation and quality of self-report health data. Asians and Pacific Islanders compared with other ethnic groups. *Medical Care, 33,* 1120-1131.

Merrill, E.B. (1998). Culturally diverse students enrolled in nursing: Barriers influencing success. *Journal of Cultural Diversity, 5*(2), 58.

Miike, L.H. (1987). *Current health status and population projections of native Hawaiians living in Hawaii.* Washington, DC: Office of Technology Assessment.

National Center for Health Statistics. (1999). *Health, United States, 1999, with socioeconomic status and health chartbook.* Hyattsville, MD: Author.

National Institute of Nursing Research. (1998). *NINR funded grants, fiscal year 1998.* Available: www.nih.gov/ninr/1998grants/1998NINRgrants.htm.

National League for Nursing. (1994). *Nursing data source 1995. Vol. 1. Trends in contemporary nursing education* (p. 62). Division of Research (Publication No. 19-2642). New York: National League for Nursing Press.

Nilchaikovit, T., Hill, J.M., & Holland, J.C. (1993). The effects of culture on illness behavior and medical care: Asian and American differences. *General Hospital Psychiatry, 15,* 41-50.

Norbeck, J.S. (1995). Who is our consumer? Shaping nursing programs to meet emerging needs. *Journal of Professional Nursing, 11*(6), 325-331.

Penn, N.E., Kar, S., & Zambrana, R. (1995). Panel VI: Ethnic minorities, health care systems, and behavior. *Health Psychology, 14*(7), 641-646.

Pertulla, W., Lowe, D., & Quon, N.S. (1999). Asian American health care attitudes. *Health Marketing Quarterly, 16*(2), 39-53.

Poe, G.S., Powell-Griner, E., McLaughlin, J.K., Placek, P.J., Thompson, G.B., & Robinson, K. (1993). Comparability of the death certificate and the 1986 National Mortality Followback Survey. *Vital Health Statistics, 2*(118), 1-53.

Pollard, K.M., & De Vita, C.J. (1997, July-September). A portrait of Asians and Pacific Islanders in the United States. *Statistical Bulletin, 3,* 2-9.

Rhooda, L.A. (1993). Knowledge and attitudes of nurses toward culturally different patients: Implications for nursing education. *Journal of Nursing Education, 32,* 209-213.

Sharma, S.B. (1988). *Bridging the gap: Anthropological brokerage in nursing care.* Unpublished doctoral dissertation, University of South Florida.

Statistical Bulletin. (1992, April-June). *Changing racial composition of metropolitan areas* (vol. 73, pp. 2-9). New York: Metropolitan Life Insurance Co.

Stavig, G.R., Igra, A., & Leonard, A.R. (1988). Hypertension and related health issues among Asians and Pacific Islanders in California. *Public Health Report, 103*(1), 28-37.

Sung, C.-L. (1999). Asian patients' distrust of Western medical care: One perspective. *The Mount Sinai Journal of Medicine, 66,* 259-261.

Uehara, E.S., Takeuchi, D.T., & Smuckler, M. (1994). Effects of combining disparate groups in the analysis of ethnic differences: Variations among Asian American mental health service consumers in level of community functioning. *American Journal of Community Psychology, 22,* 83-99.

U.S. Bureau of the Census. (1993). *We, the American Asians.* Washington, DC: U.S. Government Printing Office.

U.S. Bureau of the Census. U.S. Department of Commerce. (1990). *The 1990 census.* Washington, DC: U.S. Government Printing Office.

U.S. Department of Commerce. Race and Hispanic Origin. (1991). *1990 census profile* (No. 2, June 1991). Washington, DC: U.S. Bureau of the Census.

Wann, M. (1992). Changing the color of nursing. *Nurse Week, 5*(26), 10-13.

Whittemore, A. (1989). Colorectal cancer incidence among Chinese in North America and the People's Republic of China: Variation with sex, age, and anatomical site. *International Journal of Epidemiology, 18*(3), 563-568.

Williamson, E., Allen, B.B., & Coppens, N.M. (1996). Multiethnic experiences enhance nursing students' learning. *Journal of Community Health Nursing, 13*(2), 73-81.

West, E.A. (1993). The cultural bridge model. *Nursing Outlook, 41*(5), 229-234.

Yoon, E., & Chien, F. (1996). Asian American and Pacific Islander health: A paradigm for minority health. *Journal of the American Medical Association, 275*(9), 736-737.

Yu, E.S.H., & Liu, W.T. (1992). U.S. national health data on Asian Americans and Pacific Islanders: A research agenda for the 1990s. *American Journal of Public Health, 82*(12), 1645-1652.

CHAPTER 69

Bridging Cultures

Hispanics/Latinos and Nursing

SARA TORRES, HELEN M. CASTILLO

Hispanics/Latinos and the nursing profession will be faced with a tremendous challenge in the coming decade: to increase the representation of Hispanics/Latinos in the nursing profession at all levels.

The demographic browning of America poses both an issue and a dilemma, that is, meeting the health care needs of an ethnically diverse population in an infrastructure that is philosophically and economically unprepared to do so. Statistics indicate that 90% of all nurses are non-Hispanic whites from middle and working class backgrounds (Health Resources and Services Administration, 1999). It is posited that the only way for the nursing profession to increase the number of Hispanics who are needed to meet existing nursing service demands is to become more culturally diverse. Cultural diversity, however, includes many variables and is not simply a matter of making a choice.

Cultural diversity is not occurring in nursing. Baccalaureate and graduate degree nursing programs are especially challenged to increase the number of new student admissions and to facilitate the admission process for Hispanics. This challenge includes providing flexibility and allowing course credits for registered nurses (RNs) with associate degrees in nursing (ADN) who wish to pursue baccalaureate or master's degrees. The highest education credential of most Hispanic nurses is the ADN, with a significantly lower number of Hispanic nurses attaining baccalaureate, master's, and doctoral degrees than the rest of the RN population in the United States.

Given the financial limitations of Hispanics in this country, most are educated in 2-year ADN programs and in the few remaining 3-year hospital-based diploma schools of nursing. These programs attract students primarily because they provide earning power earlier than the 4-year bachelor of science in nursing (BSN) degree programs and have less stringent entrance criteria requirements. Thus the majority of Hispanics continue to enroll in 2-year programs, limiting their long-term mobility in the nursing profession, unless they continue into baccalaureate education and beyond.

Hispanic nurses who attend 2- and 3-year nursing programs are not appointed to positions of nursing leadership and responsibility because of the lack of specialty preparation in these programs that is provided in higher education. Additionally lacking are Hispanic mentors in higher education and nursing leadership positions who can promote other Hispanics. Hispanics who do hold leadership positions are deluged with requests to participate in activities that demonstrate cultural diversity and visibility of the agency by including an academically prepared Hispanic nurse. Together, selective discrimination and family and financial responsibilities make it more difficult for Hispanics to continue their studies, often precluding them from attaining master's and doctoral degrees.

There have been few Hispanics employed at the level of director or dean in the history of nursing in the United States. The few visible Hispanics in leadership positions further limit opportunities for students to view Hispanics as role models in nursing.

Role modeling is the product of a complex set of social, economic, and educational factors. High dropout rates, poor academic preparation, and inadequate facilities and equipment in underserved communities, together with the low expectations by teachers of Hispanic students, contribute to the small pool of Hispanics who ultimately achieve professional careers and serve as role models. More significantly, these low numbers reflect an education system that remains ill prepared to develop Hispanic students to their fullest potential.

Why are Hispanics/Latinos not entering nursing in correlation to the growing population of Hispanics? According to the National Sample Survey of Registered Nurses in 1996 (Health Resources and Services Administration, 1999), RNs in the United States numbered 2.6 million. Only 40,600 of these nurses were Hispanic, a meager 1.6% of the total. Further, about 7% of the Hispanic nurses had master's or doctoral degrees compared with about 12% of the African American nurses and 10% of the white nurses. These are dismal statistics considering that the number of Hispanic communities and their populations are increasing rapidly, but an increase in the numbers of Hispanic nurses is not occurring. From a nursing leadership perspective, two major questions arise. First, how aware are nursing leaders of this critical issue? Second, what steps are being taken to resolve this issue? Data from both national and state levels are disturbing illustrations that validate the underrepresentation of Hispanics in nursing education and practice. These data support expressed concerns at the baccalaureate and graduate levels, from which most nursing leadership evolves.

Nursing faculty and government agencies must address the recruitment, retention, and attrition problems in nursing schools from a Hispanic/Latino perspective. The U.S. workforce is expected to become more diverse and complex, and nursing must anticipate these effects and their long-term implications in order to prepare accordingly. Recruitment efforts need to be improved dramatically to reflect the cultural diversity of society within the nursing population. Although not consciously intended, health care agency recruiters often select nurses who appear similar to themselves, instead of considering their patient population preferences or needs as the first priority. Thoughtful consideration of patients' needs must be brought to the awareness level of nursing staff members, including recruiters.

OVERVIEW OF THE HISPANIC/LATINO POPULATION IN THE UNITED STATES

The demographic profile of the Hispanic/Latino population is changing in the United States. According to the U.S. Bureau of the Census (1998), Hispanics are the fastest-growing minority group in the country. The Hispanic population grew by 61% between 1970 and 1980 and by 53% between 1980 and 1990. Hispanics now represent 11.1% (29.7 million) of the total U.S. population. By the year 2010, Hispanics are projected to make up 13% of the U.S. population, 17% by 2030, and 23% by 2050. In 1990, about 1 of every 10 Americans was Hispanic, and this number is expected to rise to 1 of every 5 by 2050. This tremendous Hispanic population increase since 1970 has been attributed to several factors. Among these are a higher birth rate than the rest of the population, substantial immigration, and improvements in census-reporting procedures.

The largest group of Hispanics/Latinos in the United States are Mexican Americans (63%), followed by Central or South Americans (14%), Puerto Ricans (11%), and Cubans (4%) (U.S. Bureau of the Census, 1998). Although found in every state, nearly 9 of every 10 Hispanics/Latinos live in just 10 states. California is the home of nearly 1 of every 3 Hispanics; Texas has nearly 1 of every 5; other large concentrations reside in the Northeast states of New York, New Jersey, and Massachusetts. Florida, Illinois, Arizona, New Mexico, and Colorado round out the top 10 states with sizable Hispanic populations. Combined, California and Texas are home to more than half of the nation's Hispanics.

Hispanic Americans are more likely than non-Hispanics to live in metropolitan areas and central cities. Approximately 90% of Hispanics lived in metropolitan areas in 1990, according to the U.S. Bureau of the Census (1995), compared with about 76% of non-Hispanics. In 1997, about 27% of Hispanic families lived below the poverty level compared with about 11% of non-Hispanic white families (U.S. Bureau of the Census, 1998). The poverty rate for Hispanics in 1997 was not statistically different from that in 1980, an indication that essential changes have not taken place. In 1990 (U.S. Bureau of the Census, 1990), nearly 32 million persons (14% of the population) 5 years of age and older spoke a language other than English at home. Of this number, about 6.7 million (less than 3%) did not speak English well or at all. Second to English, Spanish was spoken by over 17 million people (8%) 5 years of age and older. Among Spanish-speaking persons, 8.3 million could not speak English well or at all, and Spanish speakers represented 54% of all non-English speakers in the United States.

THE USE OF HISPANIC/LATINO TERM

The term *Hispanic/Latino* is used interchangeably. Label preferences seem to be geographic, that is, divided by locale. For example, the term *Hispanic* is often used in the Midwest and on the East Coast, while *Latino* is preferred on the West Coast. Yet Hispanics living along the 2,000 mile United States–Mexico border prefer to self-report as Mexican American, Chicano, or Hispanic. It is important to distinguish between these terms because some have a historical base from which negative or positive images and connotations arise. Because of long-standing cultural values and military conflicts such as the historical Battle of the Alamo between Mexico and the United States, Hispanic/Latino terms remain controversial and generate strong feelings and emotions. These labels are distinctive and arise partly from the period of history in which the ethno-cultural label was applied. Perhaps it is also a function of the age of the "labeled" and the stage of their acculturation. Throughout this chapter, Hispanic and Latino will be used interchangeably.

HISPANIC/LATINO WOMEN IN LEADERSHIP ROLES

The question arises why so few Hispanic/Latino women aspire to leadership roles. In the Hispanic culture few women are in leadership roles because leadership has been viewed as a competitive male attribute, especially in business and health care circles. Consider the traditional physician-nurse dyad in which the physician has been male and the nurse has been female. Today, these roles are changing as more women enter male-dominated health care disciplines, law, and business careers. Conversely, more men are also entering nursing and other health care professions. In the past, Hispanic/Latino women were relegated to "ama de casa," which translates as "housewife." The independent, well-educated, entrepreneurial woman has not been readily accepted in the traditional Hispanic family because men have been expected to provide financial and other supports for both wife and family, while the wife remained at home. In the past, Hispanic men were considered poor providers if their wives went to work. The number of Hispanic women who have initiated stronger leadership efforts and sought opportunities for higher education is increasing. Far from representative of the Hispanic population, this group needs to grow significantly. Mentoring by peers and other women leaders is sorely needed, regardless of their ethnicity or culture. The new leadership role of the Hispanic/Latino woman is emerging and needs to be fully addressed.

PROBLEMS FACING HISPANICS/LATINOS IN NURSING

The deteriorating health status of our country's growing Hispanic population is disturbing. Hispanics are disproportionately affected by certain cancers, alcoholism and drug abuse, obesity, hypertension, diabetes, dental diseases, and HIV/AIDS. More Hispanic nurses are needed to care for the specific health and cultural needs of Hispanic patients.

There are few if any data on the career mobility of Hispanics in nursing. The term *career mobility* implies that an individual moves from one career level to another, either laterally or to a higher level. It is important to note that the problems of career development and mobility are applicable to the whole of nursing, and not to Hispanic nurses alone. Historically, however, career advancement in nursing has been difficult and limited for Hispanics, primarily because of their lack of advanced educational preparation in nursing. With the promotion of the BSN, master's, and doctoral degrees in nursing, however, along with the major restructuring taking place in health care facilities today, an ever increasing number of nurses are moving beyond basic ADN and BSN preparation.

The mobility of Hispanics in nursing has been limited for two basic reasons. First, although there has been an increase in the proportion of Hispanics enrolled in nursing schools during the past decade, the increase has been well below the Hispanic population parity. Second, Hispanics continue to enroll in ADN programs, limiting their future mobility and leadership opportunities in the profession. Certainly, while the many options in nursing do allow lateral career moves more easily, mobility into leadership positions is clearly restricted by a "glass ceiling" effect. Research studies (Hickey & Solis, 1990) show this to be true of women in general, specifically women in management and academia (U.S. Department of Health and Human Services [DHHS], 1990; Wilson & Flores, 1992).

As mentioned earlier, the problem of career mobility for Hispanic nurses is intensified by cultural, social, and educational differences. In addition, because Hispanic/Latino nurses lack contact with important professional role models, their opportunities to be socialized in the dynamics of self-advancement are fewer than for their non-Hispanic counterparts. New Hispanic nurses often do not look beyond the prospect of their first position. Instead, they view their "job" as a satisfying career of helping others rather than as a first step in the progression of a lifetime career. If we are to promote career mobility within the existing ranks of Hispanic nurses, we must initiate career development programs that include leadership skills development and provide a variety of resources to guide Hispanics through the educational process. These educational efforts need to begin early and continue through higher education in colleges and universities.

Hispanic nurses must prepare themselves academically and acquire the necessary experience and expertise in clinical areas of specialization. Additionally, Hispanic nurses must develop their leadership skills and other informal skills to increase their competitive edge and success in attaining leadership posts. They need to learn the unwritten rules of success and find out how they "fit" into the organization's culture. These skills are essential to command positions of responsibility and prestige in nursing. Institutions that espouse support need to assist Hispanic/Latino nurses in their career development and mobility by providing opportunities for career planning, addressing professional issues, rewarding nurses for direct patient care and other contributions, and facilitating their education. The nurse should have a personal plan for career development as well. In addition, mutually beneficial plans for career development should be jointly prepared by the nurse and the employing agency to achieve success for both.

Models of career mobility and professional advancement for Hispanic/Latino nurses need to be developed. Nursing organizations such as the American Nurses Association, the National League for Nursing, and the Association of Colleges and Universities must promote and support the advancement of underrepresented Hispanics/Latinos at all levels of nursing practice within the scope of their mission. Needed are strategies that will develop well-prepared leaders among the ranks of nursing practice at state, national, and international levels.

Role socialization is the process by which an individual comes to internalize certain knowledge, skills, behaviors, values, and attitudes that are integral to his or her chosen profession. Role modeling is the method of teaching professional attitudes and behaviors by being the person students emulate; it becomes the process by which a person takes on the values and behaviors of another through identification. For Hispanics/Latinos, the dearth of visible role models is a major contributing factor to a lack of career orientation that exists among the Hispanic nursing population. Dissatisfaction, attrition from nursing, and limited career commitment have been linked to inadequate socialization into nursing as well as insufficient exposure to appropriate role models.

What potential currently exists for career development among Hispanic/Latino nurses in the United States? Hispanics/Latinos must be educated and socialized into professional nursing; their leadership potential must be encouraged through leadership opportunities. The supply of Hispanic/Latino nurses graduating from

nursing programs continues to be disproportionately low compared with the representation of Hispanics in the general population (National League for Nursing, 1997). In 1994, only 3% of all graduates of basic RN programs (including ADN, diploma, and baccalaureate programs) were Hispanic/Latino, too few to respond to the increasing need for Hispanic/Latino professionals as this population grows. Although increasing numbers of Hispanic/Latinos graduate from these programs every year, retention of these students is critical to maintain the number of qualified students eligible to progress into graduate studies. Options are available for Hispanic/Latino nurses. The same factors that influence career development and mobility of Hispanics, such as culture, family support, diplomacy, bilingualism, risk taking, and personal goals, also restrict their leadership opportunities if they are lacking.

With the known available pool of young Hispanics/Latinos in the nation, it is time to capitalize on their abilities by facilitating financial aid and providing new opportunities for higher education. Innovative measures are needed to encourage Hispanic/Latino nurses to pursue graduate education and leadership opportunities that provide career mobility.

FUTURE DIRECTIONS

The factors that will promote successful career development and mobility among Hispanic nurses that have been discussed here include career counseling, career development models, mentoring approaches, networking systems among peers, and role modeling. Career development for Hispanic/Latino nurses should include incentives and recognition for practice, development of clinical and management ladders, and institutional support for their education and professional advancement. Additional incentives should include financial support for nursing faculty such as academic leaves of absence, paid sabbatical opportunities for further study and research, and release time to utilize new knowledge and gain clinical expertise. Institutions need to support the professional development of their members, including their attendance at conferences and participation in professional organizational activities. Career development requires further support for participation in focused programs of personal development, personal financial management, and policy development. Career development also means the inclusion of Hispanic/Latino nurses in agency committees and on policy development boards.

The need to increase the number of Hispanics entering the profession of nursing remains. Educators must provide the basic preparation, information, and incentives to encourage Hispanic/Latino nurses to pursue higher education. Accelerated tracks, including RN options for licensed vocational nurses, BSN options for ADN nurses, and master's options (including specialty completion programs) will increase the opportunity for more Hispanic/Latino nurses to achieve doctoral study. The retention of Hispanic/Latino nurses in generic nursing programs is also critical. Additionally, the voice of Hispanic/Latino nurses in the political arena needs to be heard in order to secure substantial grants for educational programs, stipends for students, faculty development, and curricular change in this time of economic cutbacks. State and federal governments need to develop databases that provide track record information about Hispanic students to appropriate agencies.

Strategies must be developed that inform the public at every level about the comprehensive needs of Hispanic/Latino nursing students in this country. Together, educators can develop strategies that provide pathways of opportunities for the success of Hispanic/Latino nursing students. Participative and cooperative endeavors between the private business sector and nursing schools must be fostered for the recruitment and retention of Hispanic/Latino nursing students in schools, especially in higher education. Additionally, networking systems among peers continue to be a priority for the development of information and centralized key group efforts.

Education has always been an important indicator of success in American society. Studies indicate that Hispanics have not attained an educational level sufficient to compete aggressively in the labor market, especially at the professional levels. Hispanics/Latinos and the nursing profession are faced with a tremendous challenge in the coming decade to increase the representation of Hispanics at all levels in nursing and to provide them with true opportunities for leadership. This leadership will affect the quality of health care delivery of culturally responsive health services, and in the process will enhance the continuing education of professional nursing staffs.

Issues relating to the supply and demand of nursing professionals in the United States continue to change dramatically as major shifts in financial and human resources continue to unfold. Nursing resources have been reallocated from hospitals to community-based facilities and to new structures such as mini-hospitals, elderly care centers, community nursing organizations, and health screening stations in malls and other centers of commerce. Additionally, the critical need is to respond to the growing underserved bilingual and culturally diverse Hispanic population, a need that has not yet been met and continues to be an elusive goal.

The dilemma of poor health care for Hispanics and underrepresentation of Hispanics in nursing is demonstrated by the following issues:

1. A disproportionate number of Hispanics are socioeconomically and educationally disadvantaged. As a result, there is a high attrition rate throughout the educational pipeline.
2. The present and future enrollment of Hispanic secondary education students will continue to represent a large prospective applicant pool for nursing. However, the pool is concentrated in school districts that traditionally have limited educational resources, give little attention to engendering goal-oriented students toward nursing careers, and lack culturally appropriate recruitment models for Hispanics.
3. Hispanic college enrollment is concentrated in community colleges. According to the October 1998 Current Population Survey (U.S. Bureau of the Census, 1999), 53% of all Hispanic college students were enrolled in community colleges versus 31% of white college students and 37% of black college students. Nursing enrollment data also indicate that most Hispanics continue to enroll in ADN programs instead of baccalaureate programs (Health Resources and Services Administration, 1999).
4. Hispanic nurse profession employment data in 1996 illustrate the substantial underrepresentation and general lack of progress in increasing the employment numbers for Hispanics. More than 11% of the total U.S. population are Hispanic, whereas less than 2% of the RN population are Hispanic (Health Resources and Services Administration, 1999). Hispanic nurse enrollment and program completion trends also suggest the lack of significant progress in the representation of Hispanic nurses in the health professions. This continuing disparity is widening between Hispanic enrollments in nursing and degree completion and is not anticipated to increase given the school-age Hispanic student populations.
5. The literature is sparse and documented program interventions few in attempts made to increase opportunities for Hispanics in nursing. Inadequate leadership has been demonstrated by nursing representatives in addressing these important issues, both in the public and private educational institution sectors.

Three central recommendations address these issues:

1. *Recruitment:* Increase the applicant pool of Hispanics/Latinos in higher education programs for prenursing and nursing students.
2. *Retention:* Retain Hispanics/Latinos in nursing education programs for prenursing and nursing students.
3. *Career mobility:* Promote the career mobility and leadership of Hispanic/Latino nurses.

Within the profession, there is a lack of understanding about cultural perspectives and needs, and this leads to conflict. Workforce and workplace conflicts are often silent. Anger that may be present may be difficult to verbalize and is exhibited in other ways, often increasing the intensity of individual and group conflicts. Discussions about cultural differences and similarities are needed to encourage nurses to work together effectively and constructively.

Communication patterns are learned and are culturally based. With Hispanics/Latinos, verbalization may be limited as a result of fear of conflict, reprisal, deference, or feelings of intimidation and violence. Communication and language barriers in health care settings must be recognized and discussed. With the insufficient number of bilingually prepared nurses, the few who are bilingual become overburdened with requests not only to serve as "translators" for an entire institution but also to assist in other similar or greater responsibilities. Language differences that should be viewed as assets often become barriers that serve to further isolate Hispanics/Latinos.

There is a natural affinity and commonality between groups of Hispanic/Latino nurses that draws them together. It is within these groups that they find support and guidance rather than from society as a whole. Likewise, insufficient emphasis is placed on the significant differences among various Hispanic/Latino cultural groups. The tendency is to place all cultural groups together and label them broadly as Hispanic/Latinos without allowing for these differences, especially socioeconomic differences. Institutional ethnocentrism exists. If nurses are to deliver culturally appropriate care, the unique differences among cultures, such as health care beliefs, sick role responses, and the meaning of illness, need to be addressed openly and nonjudgmentally. The institutional racism and discrimination that exist need to be reassessed and eliminated by working together in collaborative environments that foster positive care and nursing outcomes.

Economic, familial, and many other societal factors interfere with the advancement of many Hispanic/Latino nurses. These and other barriers also prevent them from entering the nursing profession or preclude their advancement in the profession. For the majority of Hispanic nurses attaining at least an ADN or BSN, this accomplishment is momentous indeed. Many are the first college or university graduates in their families. This accomplishment is equally important for the many obstacles that they have overcome during the completion of their degrees. Because of these constraints, many Hispanic/Latino nurses complete degree requirements as part-time students.

Hispanics are quickly becoming the largest culturally and linguistically different group in the United States. Hispanic cultural values and family experiences provide the foundation for research and for many positive, culturally based intervention models that can be integrated into efforts for increasing Hispanic student enrollment, retention, career mobility, and leadership in nursing.

The major strides expected of Hispanics were not achieved this decade, partly because systems have informally inhibited such progress with glass ceilings: this obstacle is clearly evident in the lack of educationally prepared Hispanics in nursing and the absence of Hispanics in health care leadership positions regardless of their capabilities. On the other hand, qualified Hispanics may choose not to enter the subtle second-class status afforded them in acquired leadership roles assigned by non-Hispanics, some of whom condescendingly assume that Hispanics/Latinos achieved these positions for reasons of ethnicity alone.

Stronger links between academic and service settings must be established, such as the development of career ladders between hospitals and local colleges or universities. Hospitals and other health care agencies need to build mutually beneficial partnerships with schools and nursing programs via paid preceptorships, adjunct faculty roles, and other alternatives used to provide financial and other assistance to students and the academic programs. The new generation of professional nurses and educators has the tremendous responsibility of opening doors that will secure professional growth, development, and mobility for Hispanic/Latino nurses in education, practice, and research. The process of advocating for access to health care for Hispanics in the United States must continue, and the time for planning strategies has passed. The time for action is now.

REFERENCES

Health Resources and Services Administration. (1999). *Notes from the National Sample Survey of Registered Nurses, March 1996* [On-line]. Available: http://158.72.83.3/bhpr/dn/survnote.htm.

Hickey, L.A., & Solis, D. (1990). *The recruitment and retention of minority trainees in university affiliate programs—Hispanics.* Madison: University of Wisconsin-Madison.

National League for Nursing. (1997). *National League for Nursing final report: Commission on a workforce for a restructured health care system.* New York: Author.

U.S. Bureau of the Census. (1990). *1990 census of population* [Online]. Available: http://www.census.gov:90/population/socdemo/language/table4.txt.

U.S. Bureau of the Census. (1995). *Housing in metropolitan areas—Hispanic origin households* (Bulletin 95-4). Washington, DC: U.S. Government Printing Office.

U.S. Bureau of the Census. (1998). *The Hispanic population in the United States, March 1997.* Atlanta: U.S. Department of Commerce, Bureau of the Census.

U.S. Bureau of the Census. (1999). School enrollment—Social and economic characteristics of students (update). In *Current population reports P20-521.* Washington, DC: U.S. Government Printing Office.

U.S. Department of Health & Human Services. (1990, June). *Minorities & Women in the Health Fields* (Publication URSA-P-DV 90-3).

Wilson, J.M., & Flores, J.H. (1992). *First National Hispanic Nurse Symposium Proceedings: Strategy for change: recruitment, retention, career mobility.* San Antonio: Center for Health Policy Development.

Bridging Cultures

American Indians and Nursing

BETTE KELTNER, DEBRA SMITH, MECHEM SLIM

American Indian culture is both a complex social structure and a deeply embedded, personal life experience. Some American Indian cultural symbols and stories have recently become popular among New Agers and certain groups seeking to incorporate images of diversity into their agendas. Yet culture is much more than art, music, and exotic foods. These facets of culture are vibrant expressions of history, values, beliefs, and resources. It is history, values, beliefs, and resources that shape tradition. Culture guides our behavior and decision making and ascribes meaning to action and circumstance. Culture tells us how to raise our children, treat our mothers-in-law, and spend our time and money. More people will enjoy fry bread than will run to greet the sun each and every morning. At the same time that interest in American Indian culture is increasing, there are concomitant racist advertising in public forums offering bounties for killing American Indian people. Also at the same time are insidious forces inviting the gradual undermining of culture through culturally dissonant programs and services. There exist today contemporary versions of massacre and marginalization. The most remarkable characteristic of American Indian culture is its resilience, thus far, to such assaults.

Bridges can be natural or man made. The purpose of a bridge is access, to directly connect two places separated by substantial barriers. Sometimes the two points of connection can be seen, sometimes they cannot be seen at all or only major landscape features can be seen. Mountains, rivers, and canyons are metaphors for cultural distance. The reason that nurses need the metaphorical bridge is based on their obligation to provide health care for all people. Building bridges involves considerable time and effort. Nurses have been very involved in identifying cultural competence as a critical aspect of practice. Desire or interest in bridge building should be applauded. How-

ever, in concert with the engineering image, good intentions can result in faulty bridges that not only do not work but can cause harm. There are specific skill sets needed to provide good care to culturally diverse people. The issue of culturally competent care is important as a quality indicator for effective nursing practice.

This chapter is written by three American Indian (Indian) nurses who are involved in different professional roles. We represent different tribes, different professional paths, and different contributions to the profession. This diversity reflects the exciting options of our profession and exemplifies a small part of the interesting within-group cultural diversity of American Indians. As Indian nurses we care passionately about cultural competence and our careers as a vehicle to bring the best of dominant science to enhance the spiritual continuity of our culture. Our professional training and the wisdom of our elders point to the possibility of untoward side effects that can arise even from actions filled with good intentions. Side effects can be serious, even fatal. We are eager to embrace technology and its benefits so long as it does not short-circuit the soul. The "missionary mindset" (Keltner, 1994) is not typically brought to Indians by people of faith today, it is brought by people of science and the helping professions streaming onto reservations (in good weather) and urban Indian centers armed with solutions to the many problems they have assessed. The major fault line in achieving cultural competence is the inability to appreciate the different experience and perspective of other people's lives. Looking only at the visible cultural markers—even important things like art, music, food—is insufficient to understand how people live. A discovery that one of your relatives reports "Indian blood" somewhere in your personal lineage may spark interest in the culture but does not convey understanding of a lived experience. The chapter we present provides a framework rather than a blueprint for building bridges between Native Americans and nursing. We seek to give readers information about tools to develop blueprints, the kinds of raw material that will be needed, and where to go to get the material for building bridges. The bridges we support are those that will not desecrate the beauty of the landscape.

BACKGROUND

Approximately 2 million citizens have identified themselves as American Indian in the U.S. Census. American Indians are the only ethnic group for whom self-identification is insufficient for most purposes. To receive benefits as a "real" American Indian, a person must be enrolled in one of the 558 federally recognized tribes. Ethnic identity is authenticated differently for Indian people than it is for other ethnic groups in the U.S. These 558 tribes exist with sovereign nation status in treaty relationship with the United States government. Therefore, while many people claim some Indian heritage, degrees of acculturation are marked not only by life experience but also by specific pedigree. Diversity among tribes can be marked. A pan-Indian perspective will always be limited. Tribes of the Northwest rely on fish as a staple food and fundamental to the economy. In the arid Southwest, some tribes consider fish sacred and would never eat them. A Southeastern tribe developed a popular tourist business but was constantly plagued by tourists wanting to see tipis (tepees). Since few buffalo roamed the heavy forests and mountains, tipis were not part of this tribe's history. However, a tipi was installed for business purposes. If tourists took time to visit the museum, they would learn that the tribal ancestors lived in longhouses made from the abundant wood given to them by their Creator.

As a group category, American Indians are often forgotten or misrepresented. There is a very public image of Indian people, rooted in elementary school history books and Hollywood Western movies. Many Americans who first meet an American Indian person often have precisely this image as an expectation for dress and behavior. When Bill Yellowfeather (who later became a Senator from Montana) first went to Dartmouth College as part of their reclaiming the school's original mission in the 1970s, he was met by a college delegation since he was one of the few entering Indian students perceived to have a "real" Indian name. The highly educated representatives from this Ivy League school were astonished to see that the young man wore jeans and boots, since they were clearly expecting someone exotically attired. In general American culture, specific notions persist about how eth-

nicity among American Indians should be validated. Carrying out the federal government assignation of ethnicity, it is common to question if a person is a "full-blood Indian," a question never asked of people from other ethnic groups.

A current distorted image of casino wealth has become a popular topic for journalists and television personalities. Gaming has operated on some Indian reservations since the early 1980s. Only 198 of the 558 federally recognized tribes have gaming compacts. The top 20 gaming operations (less than 10% of tribes that operate gaming) account for 55% of total gaming revenue (National Indian Gaming Association, 2000). The key indicator for financial success in gaming is proximity to metropolitan areas. Most reservations were selected to be isolated, with few known natural resources when they were established. Urban growth has changed this scenario for some reservations and, consequently, they have some advantages related to developing this type of recreational industry. Just as state governments use taxes to operate programs and services for their constituents, the reservations use casino profits to increase the number of programs and services for tribal members. According to Indian gaming regulations, gaming profits can only be used to improve tribal law enforcement, education, economic development, tribal courts, and infrastructure improvement.

Recent revenue generation from gaming has transformed a few tribal operations, but for the most part has been insufficient to erase centuries of neglect. A public perception that wealth has infused all Indian reservations and enriched Indian people is seriously wrong. The poorest counties in the U.S. encompass primarily Indian reservations, with per capita income as low as $2,637 (U.S. Census, 1990). In 1989, Indians residing in the current Reservation States had a median household income of $19,897 with nearly 32% living below the poverty level, compared with a median income of $30,056 and 13% below the poverty level for all U.S. races. Furthermore, American Indians were the only ethnic group in which median income dropped between 1980 and 1990 (Ambler, 1992). It should be noted that basic income is highly correlated with health and social well-being and, as such, is of concern for Indian people and society at large. Although of course there is within-group variation, Indian cultures are fundamentally non-materialistic. While economic needs profile large for Indian leaders, a position of aggressive acquisitiveness is rare. Pursuit of wealth is different, though, from establishing an economic base for basic needs. Poverty clearly is a major component of disparate health and a prominent issue for Indian people. Economic inequities underlie much of the health disparities.

Social Systems

The formal social structures in the world shape how resources are allocated and services delivered. These structures are symbols of values and history. Many aspects of daily life arise from social systems. One cannot understand how to work with American Indians until one knows about basic structures of social systems, which have powerful effects on Indian health. Indian social structure is rooted in a sense of place as well as people. The actual geography, animal, and plant life can have historic, spiritual, and social meaning. The solution of relocation away from Indian reservations is proposed repeatedly as one way to mediate problems of unemployment and inaccessible services. It is a common, and not necessarily unreasonable question from a dominant culture perspective, to pose the possibility that Indians who are very poor or suffer serious hardship related to isolation move away from their homelands. Moving for advancement is a very entrenched American value. Relocation, however, has a long, unhappy history in Indian country, starting with the reservation system itself.

The 19th century in the United States was one in which the U.S. government fought many battles with Indian people who were determined to preserve their land and way of life. At the conclusion of conquests, tribes were generally sent to live in new places. Typically the places were selected because they were not valuable and generally were known to be insufficient to sustain life. Even in times of peace and posttreaty agreement, Indians could be moved away from their assigned lands if these lands were perceived to be of value to European immigrants. The Indian Removal Act of 1836 forced the fraudulent relocation of Indians in the Southeast by federal troops to an area called "Indian Territory," where, according to the New Echota treaty, the land could never be annexed by another state or territory. Within a generation it became the state of Oklahoma. This relocation is called the Trail of Tears because of the high mortality among Indian people who left their land and belongings at gunpoint to walk from North Carolina, Tennessee, Georgia, and Alabama to Oklahoma. Two quotations remind readers about the values of land to Indians: "They made us many promises, more than I can remember, but they never kept but one; they promised to take our land, and they took it" and "The Great Spirit raised both the white man and the Indians. I think he raised the Indian first. He raised me in this land. It belongs to me. The white man

was raised over the great waters, and his land is over there. Since they crossed the sea, I have given them room. There are now white people all about me. I have but a small spot of land left. The Great Spirit has told me to keep it" (Eagle/Walking Turtle, 1995, p. 10). In the late 1940s and early 1950s, another federal relocation called for Indian people to leave their reservations and allotment lands to move into major U.S. cities. This relocation plan was to entice Indian families into places with more job opportunities. A sense of place is associated with extended family, cultural referents, and spiritual base. Relocation of various types has undermined, sometimes violently, the basic cultural strengths that unite and sustain families and tribes.

To understand the sense of communal grief and pain shared by most Indian communities today, one must first understand relocation that occurred in boarding schools. For many years, Indian children (as young as 4 years old) were routinely removed by the federal government from their parents and homes and sent to boarding schools to be assimilated into the American culture. At the boarding schools, Indian children were not allowed to speak their language or to have contact with their families, were disciplined with beatings, and too often were sexually abused. The removal of Indian children from the home tore the fabric of family life. The children did not learn how to appropriately parent the next generation and did not know their culture or traditions, thus causing a major break between the generations (Morrissette, 1994). In effect, families did not know each other, and within the space of a few generations many functioning family systems became almost extinct. It has been conjectured by Indian people today that the real reason the boarding schools were established was to eliminate Indian people entirely. The effects of the boarding school system are felt today with poor parenting skills, alcohol and drug abuse, and related social ills. Readers can begin to understand, then, why relocation and other external "solutions" may be regarded with suspicion or even hostility.

Self-determination is a nearly sacred value among American Indians for both long-standing cultural reasons as well as for political position. Indian tribes are sovereign governments, meaning that they have an inherent right or power to govern (American Indian Resource Institute, 1993). At the time Europeans "discovered" America, Indian tribes were autonomous and sovereign by nature. Because the Europeans inconsistently treated the Indian tribes as separate governments or foreign nations, the legal status of Indian tribes was uncertain. The United States Supreme Court clarified the situation by establishing the sovereign status of Indian tribes in 1823 (Canby, 1988). American Indians could not vote in U.S. elections until the Indian Citizenship Act of 1924, even though Indian men fought in American wars before that time. While tribal sovereignty has very specific limits, the pledge by the federal government to provide health and education to people in exchange for massive amounts of land make public support for human services among Indian people unique. Government assistance is perceived to be "payment" rather than "welfare." Tribal government structure varies somewhat from tribe to tribe but has its own sets of dynamics and exerts tremendous influence. Tribal leaders may be called chief, president, governor, or chairman. Governing bodies exercise both advisory and decision-making functions for the tribe. If health professionals propose to collaborate with Indian tribes in any way, it is necessary to understand tribal government and its scope of responsibilities. This takes considerable time and effort and absolutely cannot be bypassed. Self-determination does not magically translate to always making the right or "best" decisions. Addressing many complex challenges facing tribes today means that there is, in fact, not a scripted path of best practices. It is essential to note that after centuries of trial and error, federal actions loaded on more error; self-governance may involve some error, but at least it originates directly from the people who are affected. Working within this paradigm communicates respect and mediates many problems of the past.

KEY CHARACTERISTICS OF AMERICAN INDIAN CULTURE

Natural Strengths and Resilience

Indian health and human service summary statements generally focus on needs and deficits related to poverty and disorders. When visiting reservations and Indian communities, many people come away with an image of deficits: substandard roads, public services, and housing. These facts do become prominent for service providers because they are associated with the need for care. However, it is essential to understand important aspects associated with natural strengths and resilience among Indians. The cited abysmal health indicators and markers of poverty and lack of services are, indeed, all too real. These effects stem in large part from both intentional and neglectful social initiatives designed to obliterate Indian culture and Indian people. The fact of survival among Indian people points to cultural strengths worthy of note. Furthermore, Indian culture has been undermined to great extent by "helpers," people who believe that solutions for

perceived problems can be imposed from outside without regard to community values, beliefs, and practices.

Indian family and community supports can be remarkably strong and supportive. The sense of interconnectedness and reliance on family ties mediates many of the visible deficits that visitors to Indian communities remark on. As with any small and close group, there can be tensions and rivalries that play out in many different ways. On the other hand, there are typically strong family obligations and communal identity. Expressions of obligation and identity take a variety of forms. Identity is very much associated with family and tribe. An obligation to assist family and tribe is an important cultural value. This is sometimes perceived as "keeping each other down," but the same values are those that prompt action, such as taking relatives into one's home or writing a chapter together. For many tribes, there is no such thing as an "orphan." There are common examples of multigenerational extended family households and even more common, clusters of houses on reservations that house extensive extended family close together. The American tradition of launching young adult children far away to school or jobs is juxtaposed with Indian traditions such as burying an umbilical cord near a family dwelling so that the child will never go far from home.

A variety of circumstances may cause Indian people to move away from a place where they feel rooted. Economics do impose pressures for some Indians to relocate for jobs. The U.S. Census has found that approximately half of American Indians live in urban areas. This is partly a function of the midcentury federal relocation initiative and is partly due to a pattern that the cross-section census does not detect. Many Indians move "to town" for a job temporarily, for months or a year at a time, after which people return to live again "at home" on the reservation or allotment land. Another major force prompting Indians to move is a need for sophisticated or specialized medical services unavailable on most reservations. This relocation is not based on choice or preference but on fundamental need.

CASE STUDY

A case study in point illustrates this situation. A father, mother, and their four children lived in a small home that was part of a family compound on an isolated section of a large remote Indian reservation. The youngest child in this family was repeatedly misdiagnosed by the nearest Indian Health Service providers, and the child became blind, deaf, and severely mentally retarded as a consequence of untreated meningitis. As the child turned 4 years old, nourished via a gastrostomy and having the developmental level of a newborn, the frequency and nature of specialized medical needs required the family to move to the nearest major city, a distance of 500 miles from their home. Caregiving, which previously was shared among extended family members, now rested exclusively on the parents. Not only were the parents exhausted and overwhelmed (and frightened) by their duties, but also older family members were no longer available for guidance with the older children. The older brothers of the "sick child," who previously played primarily with cousins, fell prey to violence, both as victims and perpetrators. The father could no longer participate in ceremonies and tribal activities. Instead he had a series of low-level jobs that provided constant messages about his low value to society. The young mother suffered from lack of instrumental and emotional support in raising all of her children. She had been a confident and effective mother in her home community but had not grown up with a model or expectation of independent family units. Her attempts to sustain the important traditions and daily family routines were undermined when she was given an overwhelming script from clinics, hospitals, schools, and social service agencies about what she should be doing. The child for whom this upheaval had occurred received surgery and other sophisticated therapies but was missing the daily touch, prayers, and sense of belonging and acceptance the tribe would have given her. This relocation was successful in many terms but came at a price that undermined natural family strengths and family supports.

Characteristics of Resilience

The origins of resilience, a phenomenon of thriving under stress and duress, may be multifaceted but center primarily on family life and spiritual beliefs and practices. Resilience comes partly from individual factors but primarily from collective experience. Families and communities shape experience and response to events and circumstances in ways that are important to the characteristics of resilience. Although risk and resilience are calibrated on an individual basis, Indians who circumvent probable risk regularly identify family and community support and their spiritual traditions and practices as sources of strength. Almost always, American Indians are spiritual people. Faith or "religion" is an integral part of daily life, not separated by time and place. Recently there has been interest among the dominant culture in traditional Native American spiritual practices, meaning particularly those ancient beliefs known to tribes when Europeans first arrived. And while there is clearly a lineage that has sustained these beliefs and practices, there has also been a revival of sorts among Indians who have reclaimed these beliefs after generations of being disconnected from them. Certainly these renewed practices have strengthened many individuals, families, and communities. Spiritual beliefs, however, have a dy-

namic nature, a particularly critical quality as they interact with current circumstances and events. This dynamic nature is characteristic of responses to contemporary issues with enduring core values. It is also important to note that there is a wide diversity of ancient spiritual beliefs among tribes. There are sometimes selected practices from Native American spiritual beliefs incorporated into multigenerational Christian traditions. Diversity of religious practices and beliefs includes the fact that many families have over 300 years of tradition in a Christian faith and deliberately chose to continue with these beliefs. This does not in and of itself make them less "Indian." Therefore, Indians who actively use sweat lodges may also be devout Catholics. Other Indians may adhere to only one or the other system of beliefs and forms of worship. A priori assumptions regarding specific beliefs are inappropriate, even though it is well known that most Indians attribute resilience to being involved in some type of daily spiritual practices.

Another key characteristic of resilience has been the Indian's ability to discern the importance of family and community. This type of collective wisdom is associated with expected behavior and may be symbolized in stories, proverbs, or community rules for etiquette. Respecting and caring for people with disabilities and family role expectations epitomize how important it is for people to have an obligation to others and not only to themselves. Information such as this is passed down through family generations. Nursing homes to care for the elderly have never figured prominently in Indian communities. There is both a sense of obligation to care for the elderly at home and a role for them to play in their families and communities. Cultures that have not been dominated by written information have been more likely to revere elders as keepers of knowledge and wisdom. This has been true of American Indian cultures as well. The tradition of respect and care for elders has been disrupted in those tribes where there is role strain, geographic dispersal, and substance abuse (Maxwell & Maxwell, 1992). Many elders acquired the ability to pass down the most critical aspects of culture that make their people unique and strong. Wisdom is also manifest in knowing what aspects of the dominant culture can be useful, helpful, or congruent with traditional values. Most Indian people use some aspects of Western health care, even if it is combined with traditional healing methods. There are many people, however, who use Western health care only as a last resort, a reverse picture of the white Americans who sometimes turn to native practices when unsatisfied with conventional Western health care.

Traditional knowledge has been documented to be valuable, as in the case of certain common medications, such as aspirin, known to originate with indigenous people of the Americas. In recent research, it was discovered that a Lakota song had been passed down in a family from a grandmother who learned it around 1900. The song was that of a fetus singing to its mother about not drinking alcohol because it causes a "hard time" for children. This song was known decades before fetal alcohol syndrome was a diagnostic category (Keltner, 1994). There have been historic points of discernment about dominant culture attributes that contributed to personal and tribal resilience. Sequoyah (circa 1773) never learned to speak English but created the Cherokee syllabary (or alphabet). He chastised his tribe for taking on the dress of Europeans rather than realizing that it was books, or what he called "talking leaves," that provided the newcomers with important abilities. Some historians have perceived that his interpretation was that books were magic, but Sequoyah stated that anyone could learn to read. He developed written Cherokee materials within a month, and they became widely used.

Resilience has not been without price. There have been high social costs for Indian people associated with the powerful cultural assaults directed toward them. Many of these cultural assaults (such as bounties, boarding schools, relocation programs, explicit termination policies) have aimed at overt extermination. Social costs have come in the form of such pervasive effects as high rates of poverty, domestic violence, and substance abuse (De-Bruyn, Lujan, & May, 1992; Kunitz, Levy, McCloskey, & Gabriel, 1998; Lodico, Gruber, & DiClemente, 1996; Postl et al., 1991). Intergenerational trauma in particular has damaged the cultural rules for appropriate behavior among families and communities (DeBruyn et al., 1992). By recognizing and specifically identifying cultural strengths and sources of resilience, these qualities may be celebrated and leveraged for addressing some of the more difficult challenges now facing Indian tribes. Most importantly, interventions and services should be carefully examined to determine whether giving assistance could undermine aspects of strength and resilience (Keltner & Ramey, 1993).

Health Needs

Standard health indicators of morbidity and mortality point to the extent of health needs among Indian people. Data collection for Indian people is subject to greater error than other ethnic groups due to the fact that raters (health professionals) often take it upon themselves to identify a patient's ethnicity or race based on skin color or surname. Indian people may "look" Hispanic or fail to have what the rater considers to be a "real" Indian surname. A common saying is that people are born Indian but die white because birth certificates are more likely to use self-identified data than do death certificates. Furthermore, Indians are more likely to be born close to home and transferred to mainstream medical centers for dying.

In spite of known underreporting, health indicators for Indian people show a bleak picture. Rates of disease, injury, and death are disproportionately higher among minorities in the United States, and American Indians profile significantly in this differentiation. These epidemiologic ethnic disparities, after decades of documentation, are now being addressed within a systematic plan for a research agenda at the National Institutes of Health (Helmuth, 2000). The research agenda is just beginning to be formulated and funding mechanisms are yet to be determined. It will be years before any systematic plan can be implemented and benefits realized in minority communities. American Indians, as with other underserved minority groups, experience a higher frequency of serious disease, injury, and death. However, also in common with other underserved minority groups, there is extreme suspicion associated with research participation based on a history of exploitation. Specific events vary, but unhappily, examples of using and abusing Indian people in a quest for mainstream knowledge are all too many. Treatment testing for tuberculosis, for example, has a history for Indians similar to that of African Americans in the Tuskegee experiments on syphilis. Therefore an effective research agenda to reduce ethnic disparities is not impossible, but it is complex and not amenable to merely generalizing standard protocols to a new participant population.

The etiology of disorders leading to disease or death can be categorized as having genetic, environmental, infectious, and situational antecedents. As increased understanding for the natural history of disease and injury emerges, it becomes clear that for most disorders there are interactive effects among these etiologic agents. American Indians share a common risk for many disorders with the general population. The leading cause of death for Indians residing in Indian Health Service areas is heart disease, followed by malignant neoplasms. However, Indians have an unusually high risk for diabetes, sudden infant death syndrome (SIDS), alcohol abuse, developmental disabilities, and spinal cord injuries. There are regional and tribal variations in risk for certain conditions (such as SIDS, which is six times higher than average for Indians in the Great Plains). The Indian Health Service (IHS) area age-adjusted death rates in 1992-1994 illustrate that overall Indians experience mortality rates substantially higher than those of the general population in key conditions: alcoholism 579% greater, tuberculosis 475% greater, diabetes mellitus 231% greater, accidents 212% greater, suicide 70% greater, pneumonia and influenza 61% greater, and homicide 41% greater (IHS, 1997). In addition to death, Indian people have a higher frequency of complications and disability associated with common health problems. Besides morbidity and mortality, the burden of disease and disorder is exponentially increased because of poverty and isolation. For example, rehabilitation hospitals assist patients in learning to ride buses and use common assistive devices such as ramps. However, on reservations there is no public transportation. Indian tribes, which have sovereign nation status, do not have to adhere to the federal Americans with Disabilities Act. Ethnic disparities in morbidity, mortality, and burden occur because of many factors, including genetic predisposition, environmental risk and infectious agent exposure, lifestyle, and inaccessible or poor quality—or sometimes even inappropriate—health care.

For all tribes, a traditional belief is that treatment is treatment of the whole person. While this is common rhetoric in health care, it should be an essential premise in the care of Indian people. Many disorders are perceived to have origins that speak to lack of balance or harmony, violating a taboo, or disarray in social relationships. Few Indian people refuse to have any type of conventional medical treatment, but most feel it is necessary or at least important to have traditional healing practices performed as well. Prayers and ceremonies engage major social supports and rely on ancient wisdom. In some tribes, prayers are never for oneself but only for others, a symbolic expression of healthy interpersonal adaptation, avoiding problems of self-absorption common in some people in the dominant culture. Many traditional remedies are characterized by elements of social support, familiarity, and an egalitarian model of treatment, contrasted to the prescriptive model of conventional health care service.

Expectations regarding health and the meaning of health are different in different societies. Good health and optimal functioning are valued in all cultures, and the richness of cultural practices to support health across many different traditions is important knowledge for nurses to have. There are a variety of tribal traditional beliefs that provide a traditional explanation and treatment for certain disorders. For example, in one tribe it is believed that epilepsy is a sign of sibling incest. This creates an overlay of special needs associated with conventional treatment of this disorder. To ignore the stigma assigned to this disorder for particular people is to deny the lived experience and compromise good health care. There are other health disorders, nonspecific in Western terms, that require and respond to traditional treatments. Sometimes these disorders have symptoms that might be described as predominately psychosocial, perhaps a symptom such as sleeplessness commonly associated with depression. Traditional treatments can be highly successful in reducing many such symptoms. It is rare that an Indian person believes that there should be no suffering in life; there are too many visible experiences with suffering and pain. There are many ways to live a healthy life and varied ways among tribes to treat a wide range of disorders. However, meaning and purpose are often ascribed to health problems that cannot be changed. The attribution of meaning and purpose assigned to a serious health disorder, whether terminal or chronic, aids in coping and adaptation (Keltner & Ramey, 1993).

Health Behavior

Behavioral expectation can vary across cultures. Even though human development follows a fairly typical trajectory, the identification of key milestones is known to vary from culture to culture. In some Indian tribes, the age of the first word is a less important developmental marker for social-cognitive development than is the first smile or laugh, and the occasion of a naming ceremony or christening may stand out more in parental memory than does the age of the child's first steps. Child development milestones are recognized by almost all humans and have been cataloged by Western professionals with special emphasis on indicators marking independence from the family unit. These milestones are important, but not all cultures have celebrated them in the same ways. Similarly, role expectations establish some parenting practices. In a study of several different parenting practices among different ethnic groups in the San Francisco Bay area, it was found that American Indian parents expected their children to dress themselves at an earlier age and care for themselves and younger children at an earlier age. It is helpful for nurses to appreciate the meaning associated with developmental milestones.

It is well known that lifestyle, including daily habits, can serve either as a risk or protective function for individual health. Lifestyles develop in many ways but most commonly arise from cultural practices within families.

Routines from teeth brushing to activity patterns are formulated in childhood. Such practices are not immutable but sometimes are value laden. Pima Indians who were experiencing enormous health problems associated with type II diabetes improved their overall health when they reclaimed their tribal tradition of running. Many short-term interventions yield good outcomes but cannot be sustained. The most remarkable feature of the Pima Indian exercise intervention is that it was directly linked to tribal custom, and responsibility for the program became embedded within the tribe rather than as a service provided by external health providers (Wingood & Keltner, 1999). Effectiveness in achieving good health outcomes, particularly in the area of health promotion, is facilitated by honoring rather than ignoring the culture. Issues related to sustainability, an imposing challenge for all health professionals, are also enhanced when culturally competent methods are used.

One of the most well known health risk behaviors is smoking. In many tribes, smoking is directly linked to lung cancer, heart disease, low birth weight, and other known consequences of tobacco use. Smoking is a health behavior that hurts Indian people as much as, and sometimes more than, it harms other people (Helmuth, 2000). Rates of smoking in many tribes are extremely high, making this a serious health concern. In many health arenas, tobacco is abhorred, for good reason, with many health professionals believing that tobacco should be outlawed. It should be noted, however, that tobacco has a different history, and sometime different uses, among Indian people. Tobacco is a New World discovery, a crop that early Europeans learned about when first meeting Indians in America. Tobacco has long been used in different ways and continues to be associated with certain spiritual ceremonies. Tobacco is the appropriate gift for medicine people. Therefore, the dominant culture's war on tobacco, which would ban it, misses the distinction between use and abuse of this substance. It can be hard to make a case to decrease smoking when specific ceremonial uses are not acknowledged.

Alcohol addiction is another health behavior sometimes associated in stereotype with Indian people. Excessive rates of alcoholism and alcohol-related disorders are extraordinarily high in many tribes (Fleming & Manson, 1990). Most reservations are "dry"; that is, they do not sell alcohol, but this does not correlate with a lack of alcohol consumption. Stores and bars are often established on reservation borders with the express purpose of selling to Indians. Although many Indians are teetotalers, it is also true that most Indians have been affected by alcohol in

some way, either personally or with close family members. Motor vehicle injuries and domestic violence are highly correlated with intoxication. The experiences of poverty, isolation, and unemployment interact with a biologic delay in alcohol metabolism among Indians and also with social drinking patterns originally introduced by hard-drinking trappers or traders intending to take advantage of the intoxicated Indians. The effects of these different factors make alcohol abuse an important health behavior concern for many tribes. Binge drinking is especially problematic as both a habitual pattern and when associated with periods when money is available. Increasingly, tribal leaders are implementing successful alcohol treatment and prevention programs, incorporating culture-specific principles and methods. Issues related to health behavior appear to be most amenable to change when solutions come from within the community. Certainly sustaining good health outcomes has been a particular challenge because Indian reservations often have not had the type of formal infrastructure to continue programs that have shown promise. Sustainability is enhanced when programs are "owned" by the local community and continuity is supported from within the group.

Domestic violence is a behavioral phenomenon having serious and pervasive effects on health. There is a public and personal profile associated with domestic violence. The public image exists as data, media reports about an individual situation, and work done by service providers involved in health and social services. The visible parts of domestic violence include epidemiological estimates about nature and frequency, services specific to intervention such as offender treatment, services such as emergency care that require nurses to be alert to signs of unreported abuse, law enforcement involvement, and stories revealed in newspapers and on news programs. Domestic violence is commonly associated with other health and social ills such as alcohol abuse, stress, unemployment, and family dysfunction (Kunitz et al., 1998; Norton & Manson, 1995; Thornton, 1987). These correlates are experienced in higher frequency for Indians. Domestic violence is by no means an Indian problem, but in communities with high numbers of Indian people, the public perception of domestic violence among Indians can be magnified (Deloria, 1982). There is a personal dimension of domestic violence as well. The most enduring effects of this experience are generally psychological and cannot be seen. Potential conflicts in this thorny area became increasingly problematic, since one common solution to child abuse has been the removal of Indian children from their families. In the past, these children have been placed primarily in institutions or in the care of white families, adding to cultural assault. The Indian Child Welfare Act has kept children within their tribal communities unless there is a compelling reason to do otherwise.

Health Services

Indian people are not explicitly excluded from using typical health service options, but the IHS is part of the "agreement" of giving Indian people services in exchange for land. The United States Supreme Court made specific provision for health care for Indians in the 1830s. In 1954 the responsibility for providing health care to Indian people shifted from the Bureau of Indian Affairs (BIA, which is in the Department of the Interior) to the IHS as a branch of the U.S. Public Health Service. IHS is the principal federal health care provider and health advocate for Indian people and its goal is to raise their health status to the highest level possible. Indians often refer in shorthand to either IHS or PHS (Public Health Service, the broader entity in which IHS exists) as their source of health care service. The operation of the IHS delivery system is managed through local administrative units called service units. A service unit is the basic health organization for a geographic area served by the IHS program, just as a county or city health department is the basic health organization in a state health department. The IHS is comprised of 12 administrative units called Area Offices. As of October 1996 the Area Offices consisted of 150 service units, 84 of which were operated by tribes. The IHS operates 37 hospitals, 61 health centers, 4 school health centers, and 48 health stations. In fiscal year 1998 there were 1.46 million American Indians and Alaska Natives eligible for IHS services.

Health system changes abound in today's world and there have been some major changes in IHS as well. Paramount among these changes has been the opportunity to decentralize health care through tribal compacting or contracting. The Indian Self-Determination and Education Assistance Act of 1974 (P.L. 93-638) has been vital in encouraging Indian tribes and people to assume active participation in the program and services conducted by the federal government for Indian people. The Act states that "The prolonged federal domination of Indian service programs has served to retard rather than enhance the progress of Indian people and their communities by depriving Indians of the full opportunity to develop leadership skills crucial to the realization of self-government, and has denied to the Indian people an effective voice in planning and implementation of programs which are responsive to the true needs of Indian communities" (Prucha, 1990, p. 274).

The Indian Health Care Improvement Act of 1976 was developed to lessen or remove the gap between Indian health conditions and those of the total population. Congress provided for increased funding for health services, urban health centers, and the determination of the feasibility of Indian medical schools (Prucha, 1990). The Indian Self-Determination Act (P.L. 93-638) allowed Indian tribes to assume partial control over the provision of their health and social services. Today the IHS is in the process of restructuring. This is the first attempt in 40 years by the IHS to restructure in order to provide better services for Indian people. The need for change was prompted by both external and internal factors. External factors include the change in the general health care industry and its impact on the IHS's ability to provide quality care at a reasonable cost. The "reinvention" of government has included streamlining government from the bottom up, so that downsizing of federal employees within the IHS reduced by approximately 1,000 full-time equivalents (FTEs) a system known to be seriously underfunded already. The possibility of converting federal support to state block grants jeopardizes a focal understanding of Indian health needs. Among the internal forces affecting the need for a system change are sophistication of the Indian health care consumer and increasing abilities of tribal management to assume the delivery of health care for their communities (Design for a new IHS, 1995). The Indian Health Design Team was created in 1995 to examine the issues of Indian health care, IHS, and tribal health care provision and to recommend changes in the IHS structure. In part, the Indian Health Design Team recommendations were to restructure the IHS organization above the local (tribal) level; let tribes determine their own course of action; get support from the IHS for the unique needs of the tribes; authorize, upon request, flexibility to the tribal government in managing its budget; authorize alternative sources for tribal health care agencies' essential business and professional support functions; and authorize the tribes to purchase and develop billing and accounts receivable systems that are equal to those of the private sector. Therefore Indian tribes recently have been able to "compact" or contract directly with the federal government for their portion of the health care monies that would have been retained by the federal government at the IHS level rather than distributed to the tribes. To date, 44 tribes have entered into such a compact with the federal government. Although there is a federal obligation to provide health care for Indian people, the future for Indian health care is often questionable because federal funds for Indian health are appropriated on an annual basis and are frequently challenged and negotiated downward by members of Congress.

BUILDING BRIDGES
Communication

The fundamental resource for building a cultural bridge is communication. Cultural competence is care that respects knowledge and traditions in different cultures and uses both in the pursuit of better health. Verbal and non-verbal communication skills are key to culturally competent care. It is generally true that white professionals talk too much and listen too little. Much may be noted about communication styles among Indians, first and foremost being that there is considerable within-group variation, as one would expect from any large group of people. There are probably many more Indian styles of understated or subtle ways of verbal expression that may be misinterpreted as "slow" than there are in the overall population. Indians are more likely to be comfortable with silence and even use silence as an expression of respect for what has just been said. This communication style can interfere with the current expected pace for health care services. As with any group who has experienced discrimination and marginalization, there is often suspicion or caution when communicating with outsiders. Such barriers cannot be circumvented in a single session. A system is needed that strives for consistency and follow-through of commitments. Two-way communication is the key to constructing such a system.

Some Indian traditions identify self-promotion as bad manners. Indeed, humor—a wonderful human characteristic that Indians also have in abundance—is often self-deprecating among Indians. The particular belief that self-promotion is inappropriate runs counter to many core principles in advocacy groups, including health advocacy groups such as parents of children with disabilities. Relatively few Indians have a college degree, a tool that aids in making system and service change. Nurses and other health professionals are accustomed to advocating for system and service change as a professional responsibility. Nurses also have a tradition of transferring the capacity to advocate to individuals and groups on behalf of their own self care. Advocacy training can empower Indian families who lack formal education with knowledge and skills that combine with their own traditions of resilience to improve health and well-being for themselves and their children. Communicating a skill set that may not have a cultural conceptualization means that nurses will have a different starting point in teaching

advocacy to some Indian groups. It will not come naturally for all Indians to be assertive in this way.

Communication can be impeded simply by the fact that health professionals have a culture almost to themselves. There are words, concepts, and values that are particularly associated with health care. One example of this is the continued search for knowledge and the value of new information. This is a facet almost everyone can appreciate in the abstract but that can become confusing in practice. When a young mother takes her child for a well-baby visit and is advised that feeding strained foods in the first months is "bad" for her child and that her baby should be put to sleep on his back, the information can be interpreted as conflicting. In addition, older women in the family probably were recommending one thing while personnel in the clinic were dispensing opposite advice, which was different from the advice they gave just a few short years ago. The major point of conflict occurs when value judgments are ascribed (feeding a child strained fruit at 4 weeks is "bad"). Rarely are explanations for changes given, and certainly not in the amount of detail necessary for understanding. Grandmothers not only give instrumental assistance and care in childrearing but also rarely change their minds about what is good and appropriate care. Communication therefore becomes a critical part of health care delivery, not just what is said, but how it is said.

When linguistic diversity is spoken about in the U.S., it is rarely recognized that certain tribal languages, such as Navajo, continue to be the primary or only language for some Indian people. For others who do speak English, experience with serious illness may inhibit their understanding of English or require the use of words and phrases of particular intimacy that only native words can provide. When health care providers work with persons who speak a language different from their own, it is always useful to learn as much of that language as possible. There will be times when interpreters are needed. The use of interpreters is a skill in itself (Wingood & Keltner, 1999). Anyone who knows multiple languages knows that precise translations are not always possible. Another aspect of the use of interpreters is to pay attention to who is serving in this role. Young school-age children are often pressed into this duty, but it is, of course, inappropriate for a young child to inquire, for example, about the dates of his mother's last menstrual period. Although this may seem self-evident, such courtesies are routinely violated by many people who use interpreters. In some tribes there are communication customs about when and how men speak to women such as mothers-in-law. Communication is extremely important in building bridges between cultures, but it is essential to recognize the complexity and iterative nature that good communication should have.

Research and Measurement

As the discipline of nursing becomes more empirical, research tools that measure common health phenomena take on a larger profile. As previously mentioned, meaning can be ascribed by context and experience. There is ongoing concern about the validity of measures for ethnic populations that have been underrepresented in research. There is serious concern about abbreviating the careful instrument development process used in dominant research programs through short cuts. Short cuts in this area not only are poor science, but also can lead to faulty conclusions and perpetuation of cycles of misunderstanding and poor practice. There are many examples of popular instrumentation that can be inappropriate for use with Indian tribes. A common question on the Family Resource Scale, for example, inquires about resources to take a "vacation" or "have time alone." In a community with long-standing high unemployment (85% to 95%) and where being with family members is more valued than time alone, the original meaning of these questions is not in concert with the context.

A common problem for American Indian people is that they are "used" by researchers who seek them out for interviews. While this avoids the many pitfalls associated with inadequate instrumentation and outdated research tools to be used among Indians, there are potential problems. It is not uncommon for qualitative methods to be chosen by some researchers less for reasons of interest and more because of their own personal limitations in quantitative skills. This particular motivation does not bode well for meaningful findings through narrative data. Analyses must be just as rigorous using qualitative techniques. Words in English also have particular meanings for people. In a detailed analysis of qualitative data to learn about Indian families' adaptation to children with disabilities in seven different tribes, Keltner (1994) learned that parents of children with disabilities expressed many occasions of "burn-out." Burn-out (stress) is not atypical for family experience with these types of challenges, but this pronouncement simply did not equate with what had been learned in interviews with 150 families. When examining the interview transcriptions more carefully, it was discovered that families were referring to their houses burning down rather than to emotional stress! There are several potential problems of interpretation of data from a researcher's perspective.

American Indians have a long history of exploitation, and marking the perceived problems and deficiencies for a group of people can bring harm, particularly when validity can be reasonably challenged.

Concurrent Challenging Life Circumstances

As a health professional addresses a disorder like diabetes or childhood asthma, the entire context of a patient's experience should be considered. One cannot easily disentangle interactive effects of either of these disorders in the presence of domestic violence, crowded living conditions, a long distance to health care facilities that may be of questionable quality, alcoholism, and diet options that have the variety of commodity or trading post sources. Something as basic as distance and travel can be misunderstood. In the East, many people think of "rural" as a place like Vermont. Distances in Wyoming, Arizona, and New Mexico, where we have lived, are vast and empty by comparison with the rural image that many Americans hold. Comorbid conditions within a family, such as alcoholism or domestic violence, considerably complicate interventions and programs intended to address a disorder such as diabetes. Concurrent challenging life circumstances may impose as serious a threat to well-being as the target disorder itself (Keltner & Ramey, 1992, 1993).

Increasingly, treatment models and systems have become more focused, particularly as payment mechanisms and service systems change to become more efficient. Cost-effectiveness is an attribute that should be beneficial for all people, making resources available to more people with needs. Any health paradigm that neglects the need to acknowledge and address challenging life circumstances in the context of a target disorder, however, is destined to fail. There is no way to circumvent the recalcitrant and pervasive nature of common concurrent challenging life circumstances that many Indians face. Efficiency and cost-effectiveness are worthwhile goals for any health program, but models that work among populations without concurrent challenging life circumstances do not generalize well for people who live in a context that presents multiple interactive variables that impinge on health status.

Partnership Models

The only paradigm for effective health care among American Indians is using some variation of an appropriate partnership model. This is important because involvement is more engaging than commands, exploitation can be minimized, and essential information about history, communication styles, resources, and challenging life circumstances can be more readily discerned. The partnership model also contributes to the overall goal of self-determination.

Partnerships in health care initiatives, both in research and practice, are becoming more popular, at least as they are formulated on paper. There are steady improvements in the development of genuine, functional partnerships in which Indian leaders and health care professionals or outside health systems work together toward common goals. Such partnerships take time and personal effort. An effective partnership model is one that respects and honors the history and traditions of the people being served. Different from this are programs that claim a partnership model but in practice load authority and decisions along conventional dominant lines. A critical indicator to determine whether a program is a real partnership is to follow the money streams: if resources flow primarily to non-Indian personnel, it is likely that the arrangement is not a true partnership. Partnership models are beginning to demonstrate more effective and enduring results (Keltner & Ramey, 1993; Wingood & Keltner, 1999).

AMERICAN INDIANS AND NURSING

Building bridges should be based on seeing both the beginning and the destination associated with a desired connection. There is a common Native American worldview of a circle of life and a circular way of living. Among the many different tribes are terms and images related to a sacred circle, sometimes called a sacred hoop. This image is considered sacred because it epitomizes both family and cultural continuity. Dwellings and ceremonies from most tribes often have employed circular or curved walls or borders that illustrate this perspective. The image of a circle is quite different from the way we typically envision a bridge. Bridges as we know them are linear and direct. Bridges in the physical sense may be seen as essentially unidirectional for different parties. People may pass with different destinations or purposes or perhaps even go back and forth but with a sense that one direction is definitely "to" and the other direction is essentially "from." A linear image is fundamentally different from a circular one. A circular worldview captures a notion of multiple iterations and retains a sense of returning to the beginning time and time again. Within a circular framework there would always be much give and take across the metaphorical bridge, illustrating the partnership paradigm for working with American Indians. The contrasting images of a circle and a straight line serve as a symbolic reminder of how different assumptions and styles of

different cultures can be. From a pragmatic point of view, the pace of interactions is distinctly different in a circular lifestyle. People sometimes comment on "Indian" time, meaning a significantly slower pace. Cultural rhythms for Indians traditionally have been tied to cycles of nature such as seasons, rather than segmented by repeated minutes and hours. There is much benefit to be gained through sharing knowledge and traditions. A metaphorical bridge that encompasses a circular worldview will be a preferred cultural fit with most Indian communities.

Need for Nursing

Health care needs among American Indians are not only extensive but also complex. As major health care providers, nurses are prepared to deliver care to people with a variety of needs and within contexts that may also vary substantively. In earlier times, most nurses may never have met Indians in the course of their practice. As mobility dramatically increases and outreach becomes a health care responsibility in a technological world, nurses are more likely to serve Indians. The epidemiological data document ethnic disparities in risk for both disorders and deleterious outcomes among Indians. Concerns can be grouped according to mortality, morbidity, and burden. Health needs are too often complicated by challenging life circumstances and inadequate community infrastructure to address these needs. Nurses involved in primary care, public health, trauma, and rehabilitation are greatly needed to provide service to diminish the ethnic disparities that are so troublesome in our society. Nursing practice and research must engage in culturally competent actions to provide effective care. Standards for cultural competence have not been well defined.

What Is Culturally Competent Nursing Care for American Indians?

Care and comfort can certainly be provided by Indian to Indian nursing care. There are many merits to such a model, since special sensitivity would increase the likelihood that personal needs would be met. Another good way would include caregivers from a different culture who have acquired a certain level of cultural competence. Nevertheless, it is always reassuring to see visible representation of one's own culture somewhere in the immediate health services. If an Indian person enters a hospital or clinic, seeing other Indians in professional roles communicates some reassurance that the Indian way of life matters to the institution.

The question arises from time to time whether non-Indians can actually provide culturally competent care for Indians. We believe emphatically that they can but that cultural competence is a skill with as much knowledge, sophistication, and the need for continual updating as any other skill within nursing. Cultural competence has three key components: sensitivity, specificity, and synergy. *Sensitivity* is the essential respect afforded to a culture with long-standing strengths and traditions that are positive and sustaining. Being culturally sensitive means possessing a certain humility as an outsider or "nonexpert" in domains that are valuable and beneficial to good health. *Specificity* means assuming a responsibility to learn about specific cultural traditions of a people—words of a native language, knowledge about cultural healers and healing traditions—and an engagement or referral to those experts who can best assist persons in gaining, regaining, or maintaining optimal health. *Synergy* is a characteristic that combines traditions from two life forces and pathways to provide complementary rather than separate or competing health care supports. Cultural competence, therefore, is something that can be taught and learned.

Need for American Indian Nurses

For reasons of philosophy and pragmatism, it is essential that Indians become part of the health care delivery system. There is a fundamental social value in opening education and professional training to people who have long been underrepresented and excluded from participation. Knowledge and professional advancement can be enhanced with a diversity of background perspectives. It is hard to imagine how cultural competence can be articulated or communicated without the participation of Indian health professionals, including Indian nurses. There are a variety of educational preparation models for nurses. Several tribal colleges have nursing programs, mostly at the vocational and associate degree level. Indian nurses are more likely than other Indian health professionals to remain in their own communities, and even within the service systems that provide care for Indians. This permits nurses to have important opportunities in the design and implementation of culturally competent care. There are many nurses who serve on tribal councils and are becoming increasingly prominent in certain arenas as tribes assume more responsibility for their own health care programs. The opportunity to advance nursing practice is especially unique in this context.

Increasingly important is having minority persons in positions of influence in clinical decision making, setting administrative standards, in shaping health services, and, most importantly, in directing health care resources. A persistent barrier to leadership is that the basic, and too often the only, educational preparation Indian nurses have attained has inherent limits. Many, many, more Indian nurses have practical and associate degrees than have baccalaureate or advanced degrees. Among Indian nurses who have standard professional degrees, they are more often from the least selective, least prestigious baccalaureate schools. Education quality and networking opportunities vary according to these parameters of preparation. Nursing has multiple roles and it is important that the best fit for the individual be made. When mere overall numbers are examined, however, minorities are most seriously underrepresented within our professional field in the positions of influence. There are significantly fewer key administrators and policy makers, academic leaders and full professors, senior scientists and nursing leaders who are from any minority group but, most particularly, who are American Indian. There is a need for direct care to be culturally competent, but just as important is that systems of inquiry, program, and service also have the capacity for cultural competence. As the overall presence of nursing dramatically declines in highly selective universities in the United States, there are even fewer opportunities for minority representation in leadership roles in schools with superior education, unparalleled professional networks, and sophistication. At the same time, the best educational institutions in the United States are recruiting many more young Indians into careers other than nursing. Although in important ways this expands opportunities for Indian youth, they are more likely not to return to their home communities than are Indians who choose nursing careers. There is most definitely a need for bright young members of minorities to enter highly selective schools of nursing, as they are being aggressively recruited for other professions. The intellectual vigor and potential scope of influence that minorities can bring to benefit the general public are greatly magnified through this educational stream.

Professional organizations are important networks for support and development. The unity for all nurses through local and national professional organizations fosters such growth. Indian nurses are widely dispersed across the United States but also have a unified organization, the *National Alaska Native American Indian Nurses Association* (NANA-INA). In addition to support and networks, NANA-INA provides a voice to advocate for cultural competence and for addressing special health care needs for Indian people. Although it is a relatively small and young organization, NANA-INA is increasing its public profile and scope of involvement. An annual summit is held for members and supporters who are interested in promoting Indian health and Indian nursing. In the spirit of advancement and collaboration, NANA-INA is a founding member of the new Ethnic Minority Nurse Association Coalition. The coalition is a collective voice for common minority concerns. The coalition is composed of NANA-INA, the Black Nurses Association, Hispanic Nurses Association, Asian American Pacific Islanders Nurses Association, and, more recently, the Philippine Nurses Association. The opportunity to leverage greater political position and support each other's organizations is an important step toward decreasing ethnic disparities in health outcomes.

STORIES

Storytelling is an integral part of learning in American Indian tribes. Recounting events provides exemplars that reflect many complex values. It is a chance to have a "snapshot" from the other side of the bridge. In this section, we will share brief personal stories about an aspect of nursing that has been a meaningful part of our experiences. Using this particular tool in this way provides certain illumination to the content that has been presented in this chapter, but it does not fully engage the diverse utility that storytelling brings to understanding culture. People are generally attracted to stories because they personalize abstract ideas. Our stories are different and yet do not begin to reflect the universe of experiences that Indian nurses have.

Mechem: Leaving the Navajo reservation to come to Georgetown University in Washington, D.C., was a very big decision and change for me. People seemed rushed and rude. Everything seemed so crowded compared to the wide open spaces of home. I had never seen so many people and so many from different ethnic backgrounds before coming here. Even more surprising was meeting so many classmates who had never met an Indian before. My nursing classmates have been very interested in learning about Indian ways and Indian health.

I decided to become a nurse because of my grandmother and the hospice nurse who cared for her when she had cancer. My maternal grandmother was the matriarch and center of our family life. After having her gallbladder removed, we learned that she had non-Hodgkins lymphoma. With her illness came endless trips to the doctors and the treatment center, 4 hours away from home. Each week we had to make several round trips for radiation and chemotherapy. My grandmother spoke little English, so a translator was needed to talk to the doctors and nurses. I noticed the way the nurses were always on top of her care, knowing what she needed and finding ways to communicate. I saw these nurses try their best to learn Navajo so they

could understand my grandmother and take care of her. Five months later her cancer was in remission. Sadly, though, the cancer returned with devastating effects. The nurses in Albuquerque, New Mexico, arranged to have a hospice nurse come out to our home in Sanders, Arizona. Kim was the nurse who drove 3 hours two or three times a week to care for my grandmother. She was more of a family nurse and tended to everyone's concerns. She would listen to us talk, offer advice, play with the small kids, and always tended to my grandmother. Even to this day, on the anniversary of my grandmother's death, she always sends us a simple flower. This happened in my senior year of high school. My grandmother said that Kim was remarkable and made her last days worth while.

Deb: I live and work on the Fond du Lac reservation where I was born. My grandparents were both alcoholics, which prompted my mother to marry a man she hardly knew when she was only 17 years old. When I was barely 2 and my sister a newborn, we returned to live with my maternal grandparents. Even though my grandparents were alcoholics and most of the family and friends who came to our home were also alcoholics, my earliest memories are pleasant and loving ones. I remember sitting in the bars with my grandparents while they drank beer and my sister and I would have orange pop and potato chips. It should be a sad memory, but it isn't. Scenes such as this can be considered child endangerment, neglect, or even abuse today, but to us it seemed normal and secure. Perhaps this is the reason so many Indian people have a hard time understanding why social service agencies are appalled by their behavior, to the point of removing children from their families.

My mother worked in town as a nurse's aid and started to hope that I would become one of the respected "RNs." My role as the eldest of four children and many cousins made caregiving natural for me. As a result of living with drinking and unhealthy relationships, I knew I would never live that way. I was able to attend the small local college because my stepfather taught there in the Indian Studies department. For a while in the 70s it was "cool" to be Indian, and many academic institutions and liberal-minded people were intent on helping Indian people improve their lives. I have worked in different roles, primarily as a public health nurse for Fond du Lac Reservation. I obtained my master's degree in Public Health Nursing from the University of Minnesota while working full time and tending to a family with three adolescent children. I am part of the National Alaska Native American Indian Nurses Association. These women and men are like family to me. Despite the diversity of the group, we all came out of the same background and share common goals.

Bette: My parents grew up on Indian allotment lands within 5 miles of each other, but they actually met as part of the Indian relocation community in the San Francisco Bay area. My father was assigned a job with the bus service in San Francisco. He eventually left the city to work for a lumber mill. Outdoor work associated with forests was more familiar and fulfilling for him than were other opportunities in the city. Therefore, my brothers and I were born in Northern California with many stories about and occasional trips "home." Stories were so vivid and the transplanted community so connected that some of the realities of geographic referents and prominent community members seemed close. A key turning point in our cultural identity, though, occurred with the Indian occupation of Alcatraz in 1969. This event was in response to the government's terminating the prison facility on Alcatraz and activating a statute that said federal lands no longer in use would revert to the original ownership of Indian people in the United States. The political activism that united and showcased several different tribes in a prominent (and valuable) property made an impact on many young Indians.

I have been a public health nurse for nearly 30 years, working in many different places with underserved and marginalized people. It is a wonderful and challenging career. I have been privileged to belong to many excellent organizations. Like Deb, though, I have found that there is no organization as familiar and supportive as my "family" within NANA-INA. As President for two terms, I found the talent, energy, and commitment of this group of nurses to be incredible. Those of us who take on hard jobs, working with complex problems in the context of challenging life circumstances, find special support from our families and the family-like support of NANA-INA.

My father worked for over 30 years (until he died in 1985) for a lumber mill that harvested only redwood trees. Readers may have learned that redwood trees are the oldest living things in the entire world. They tower over skyscrapers. If you have visited a redwood forest, you have seen a car drive through the center of a trunk or perhaps have walked through a reasonably spacious two-bedroom home hollowed from a single log. The wood is unique because of its ability not to warp in the presence of high moisture. One would think that something so enduring and so durable would be deeply anchored in the earth. What you may not know is what my father taught and is so important for families and communities in order to be enduring and durable as well. Redwoods have a very shallow root system. Redwood trees grow in groves wherein the root systems develop intricate interconnections. What cannot be seen below the surface of the earth is that these magnificent trees are holding each other up. The lesson from the Creator, given to us who are willing to learn, is that we are responsible in the same way for each other. It is an important principle to put into practice for improving health care for all people.

REFERENCES

Ambler, M. (1992). The wealth of Indian nations. *Tribal College Journal of American Indian Higher Education, 4*(11), 8-12.

Canby, W.C. (1988). *American Indian law in a nutshell* (2nd ed.). St. Paul, MN: West Publishing.

DeBruyn, L., Lujan, C., & May, P. (1992). A comparative study of abused and neglected American Indian children in the Southwest. *Social Science Medicine, 35*(3), 305-315.

Deloria, V. (1982). Education and imperialism. *Integrated Education*, pp. 58-63.

Design for a new IHS. (1995). *Recommendations of the Indian health design team executive summary.* Unpublished manuscript.

Eagle/Walking Turtle. (1995). *Indian America* (4th ed., pp. 10-11). Santa Fe, NM: John Muir Publications.

Fleming, C., & Manson, S. (1990). Native American women. In R.C. Engs (Ed.), *Women—Alcohol and other drugs* (pp. 143-148). Dubuque, IA: Kendall/Hunt Publishing Co.

Helmuth, L. (2000). NIH, under pressure, boosts minority health research. *Science, 288*(5466), 596-597.

Indian Health Service. (1997). *Trends in Indian health.* Rockville, MD: Available from the Indian Health Service, Office of Planning, Evaluation and Legislation, Division of Program Statistics.

American Indian Resource Institute. (1993). *Indian tribes as sovereign governments.* Oakland, CA: Author.

Keltner, B. (1994). *American Indians and adaptation* (Pub. No. R01HD31863-01). Washington, DC: National Institute of Child Health and Human Development.

Keltner, B., & Ramey, S. (1992). Underserved families affected by developmental disabilities. *Journal of Health Care for the Poor and Underserved, 2*(4), 419-422.

Keltner, B., & Ramey, S. (1993). Family issues. *Current Opinion in Psychiatry, 5*, 638-644.

Kunitz, S., Levy, J., McCloskey, J., & Gabriel, K. (1998). Alcohol dependence and domestic violence as sequelae of abuse and conduct disorder in childhood. *Child Abuse and Neglect, 22*(11), 1079-1091.

Lodico, M., Gruber, E., & DiClemente, R. (1996). Childhood sexual abuse and coercive sex among school-based adolescents in a Midwestern state. *Journal of Adolescent Health, 18*, 211-217.

Maxwell, E., & Maxwell, R. (1992). Insults to the body civil: Mistreatment of the elderly in two Plains Indian tribes. *Journal of Cross Cultural Gerontology, 7*, 3-23.

Morrissette, P. (1994). The holocaust of First Nation people: Residual effects on parenting and treatment implications. *Contemporary Family Therapy, 15*(5), 381-392.

National Indian Gaming Association. (2000, March). Website: Available: http://www.indiangaming.org.

Norton, I., & Manson, S. (1995). A silent minority: Battered American Indian women. *Journal of Family Violence, 10*(3), 307-318.

Postl, B., Gilber, P., Goodwill, J., Moffatt, M., O'Neil, Sarafield, P., & Young, T. (1991). Family violence in the North. *Arctic Medical Research*, pp. 586-589.

Prucha, R.P. (1990). *Documents of United States Indian policy* (2nd ed.). Lincoln, NB: University of Nebraska.

Thornton, R. (1987). *American Indian holocaust and survival* (pp. 175-201). Oklahoma City: University of Oklahoma Press.

U.S. Bureau of the Census. (1990). *1990 census of population* [Online]. Available: http://www.census.gov:90/population/socdemo/language/table4.txt.

Wingood, G., & Keltner, B. (1999). Sociocultural factors and prevention programs affecting the health of ethnic minorities. In J. Raczynski & R. DiClemente (Eds.), *Handbook of health promotion and disease prevention* (pp. 561-579). New York: Kluwer Academic.

Section Eleven

Ethics, Legal, and Social Issues

Ethical, Legal, and Social Concerns in a Changing Health Care World

JOANNE McCLOSKEY DOCHTERMAN, HELEN KENNEDY GRACE

As the world of health care changes and the concerns for cost control escalate, it is increasingly difficult to keep a focus on the needs of people and the underlying legal and ethical issues that surround health care decision making. As the debates over the future of health care continue, much of the discourse is based on an assumption that the problem is one of lack of resources. Therefore, the argument continues, rationing in some form is the only solution. This basic assumption requires examination. Is the problem one of lack of resources, or is it rather a matter of how these resources are spent? Is it fair and just that more than 25% of health care expenditures are spent in processing the paperwork necessary to keep the providers paid and running economically viable businesses? Is it right and just that more than 40 million people in the United States have no health care insurance and are effectively cut out of the health care system? Whose problem is it? The tendency is to blame the victim rather than to accept that this is the responsibility of us all. In the future, ethical, social, and legal questions will be pushed to a new level with the advances that have recently been made in the genetic field and the possibility of detecting genetic problems at a much earlier state. A whole new world of options, each fraught with new legal and ethical issues, is emerging that will further complicate decision making and allocation of resources.

As you read the chapters in this section, we urge you to keep in mind some of the broader issues that have been addressed. Are our problems those of a lack of resources, or are they a reflection of a lack of ability to debate hard issues and reach a reasoned consensus that is fair and just? Much of health care decision making has been pushed out of the clinical domain, which was predominantly a case-by-case approach into the world of "business," which makes decisions on the basis of financial concerns. The general public has been left out of the de-cision-making process. And our problems have been addressed by keeping people out of the health care system. In this section some of the issues are raised that should be a matter of public debate.

In the opening chapter, Corley addresses the ethics of targeting the elderly for health care rationing. This debate chapter presents the arguments for why health care for the elderly should be rationed. In setting up the debate, Corley points out that the elderly constitute 12.7% of the population, and most of the elderly are women. If rationing is the approach used to control costs, the elderly are a prime target. Distributive justice should govern the process of rationing, and the elderly would be a logical target for cost reduction. The arguments are (1) that the elderly are already receiving more than their fair share of health care resources, (2) that persons should be entitled only to their "fair share" of health care resources and that the elderly exceed this, (3) that the elderly have less chance of surviving treatment and therefore could need-lessly consume health care resources, and (4) that too much of the health care dollar is being expended on treating infirmities associated with aging (i.e., Viagra). The arguments against rationing for the elderly are (1) that such an approach drives a wedge between generations, (2) it is impossible to compute a fair lifetime share of health resources to be expended on any one individual, and (3) that health care for the elderly is already being rationed (i.e., long-term care). Corley concludes the debate by arguing that there are alternatives to rationing. These include (1) maintaining the functional abilities of the aging population through health and wellness programs, (2) providing respite care for caregivers who tend to elderly family members, and (3) maintaining bonds between the generations that contribute to a caring society. How we address the issues of health care for the elderly should be governed by a concern for justice for the powerless, vulnerable, and disenfranchised, and any rationing should occur in broad daylight rather than masked, as is currently the case.

In the first viewpoint chapter, Weiler and Clinton address the intertwining of nursing and legal issues. Three specific issues are addressed: nurse licensure, Internet and telecommunication access for nurse-patient interactions, and educational preparation of current and future practitioners in legal aspects of nursing practice. Responsibility for licensure of nurses and its enforcement historically has been a state responsibility. Changes in the practice world brought about by use of communication technology and the mobility of nurses across state lines require accommodating to these new patterns. Different approaches that might be used are described along with their problematic aspects. Use of telecommunications in providing patient care poses others legal difficulties. Elements needed to establish a claim of negligence include the following: duty, breach of duty, harm or injury, and proximate cause. All these aspects of negligence are complicated when care is being provided by means of telecommunication. In light of the legal complexities surrounding nursing practice, the authors advocate greater attention to legal aspects of care at all levels of nursing education.

Next, Zink and Titus address some of the complex issues across the life cycle that are faced by nurses in practice settings. Although institutional ethics committees are in place in most settings, they have limitations, and nurses are in a particularly difficult position. This is complicated by the lack of emphasis on ethical and legal issues in the basic nursing curriculum. Some of the issues faced by nurses in the practice setting with profound ethical implications include cost-containment approaches, end-of-life decisions, pain management, "futile" care, genetic and reproductive issues, informed consent and confidentiality, and incompetent caregivers. The authors advocate nursing ethics committees, clinically based ethics education, and ethical rounds in practice settings.

Although nurses are faced with complexities related to the ethics of clinical decision making, they may also be confronted with problems such as sexual harassment in the workplace. Aiken carefully outlines the specific conditions defining sexual harassment. She then provides information about courses of action that might be taken. The importance of institutional policies for handling sexual harassment is stressed.

The next chapter focuses on one significant social issue that affects especially American children: TV viewing. Children and adolescents in the United States spend more time watching television than doing anything else except sleeping. Chase and Kurtt make a well-researched argument for limiting television for children. They believe that pediatric nurses must use their opportunities to influence the viewing habits of children and youth and their families. The authors present both the positive and negative effects of television, but the negative effects outweigh the positive. A large negative effect is the exposure to TV violence that has been demonstrated to increase the likelihood of aggressive behavior, especially in boys. Other concerns are the viewing of sexual acts, beer and wine commercials, influence in general of commercials, lack of adult supervision and interaction, and inactivity and eating while watching. The authors also discuss the use of television for hospitalized children and use in school and day care settings. TV viewing is a part of our society. The authors believe that the negative effects on children can no longer be ignored by pediatric nurses who care about the health of their patients and the population.

The remaining chapters in this section turn to specific ethical and social issues. Cowen addresses the problem of child neglect. Fourteen of 1,000 children are maltreated. Types of maltreatment that occur include abandonment and supervisory neglect, physical, health care, educational, emotional, and nutritional neglect. Abuse of children is a more blatant type of maltreatment. The author advocates the use of assessment tools to evaluate the status of a child and advocates that the emphasis should be placed on prevention. Teaching of parenting skills and providing support networks are especially important to prevent child maltreatment.

One of the particularly troubling ethical problems confronting nurses who care for the elderly relates to the treatment of Alzheimer patients. Edwards notes that 40% of all elderly older than 80 years of age are diagnosed as having Alzheimer's disease. With a growing population of patients older than 80, this problem will increase in the years ahead. The author advocates that in decision making regarding care of Alzheimer's patients the first step is that of determining the capacity of the individual to participate in decision making and, to the degree possible, to respect the patient's choices. Advance directives are particularly useful. One of the major ethical concerns is that of creating unreasonable burdens for caregivers and weighing the rights of the patient against those of the caregivers. Nurses can be caught in particularly problematic decisions when the proxy for the patient may make decisions, such as that of withholding medication, that the caregiver may feel obligated to refuse to obey. Advance directives and communication with caregivers are advocated in reaching ethically viable decisions.

Kjervik specifically addresses issues related to advance directives. Noting the fundamental value in our society of individualism, advance directives are a way of empowering patients. After describing the main types of advance directives, the author clarifies their ethical aspects. The value of a living will is that it is a clear way of stating what a patient wants at a specific point before a crisis. The major objections to advance directives are (1) the paternalistic view of health care providers that they know best, (2) living wills, which are made at a point when the patient is not in a crisis situation, and (3) the slippery slope between living wills and murder or genocide. Nurses play a key role in the development and implementation of advance directives.

In the final chapter in this section, Zoloth returns to a theme threaded throughout this book, that of ethical decision making in an era of managed care. One of our central cultural myths that influences health care is that "anything created can be repaired." In an era of managed care,

patients are seen as "takers from the pool of money." The business concerns of preserving health plans may be at the expense of patients. Patients are now structured out of the decision-making process. The author notes that health care is currently rationed with the wealthy able to access elaborate and costly care while the poor are able to freely choose inadequate health care. Although this is a de facto form of rationing, full disclosure and rationing in broad daylight is advocated as an alternative.

Nurses stand in the gap between patients and the health-care system. As pressures build from all sides, the profit-making motives of big business at the expense of humane and quality patient care, the escalation of a wide array of social problems inextricably intertwined with health (such as drug abuse and child maltreatment), nurses are obliged to examine the moral, ethical, and legal implications that govern their practice. Never have the challenges been greater. But with challenge comes opportunity, the opportunity to rise to the fore in being a voice for the powerless and the disenfranchised and for speaking out on behalf of patients.

The Ethics of Health Care Reform
Should Rationing Strategies Target the Elderly?

MARY C. CORLEY

Escalating health care costs in the early 1990s and the growing numbers of uninsured citizens in the United States led to efforts by the Federal Government to control these costs and make health care available to the uninsured. Employers sought to limit the cost of health care coverage through contracts with managed care organizations, many of them for-profit. By the end of the 1990s, health care organizations had reduced health care costs through increased efficiency, but the number of uninsured rose to more than 44 million citizens, partly because of reduced coverage by employers and partly because of the underinsured, including the elderly with Medicare coverage who lack supplemental insurance. Difficulties in controlling rising costs include the demand for health care, expensive medical technology, approaches to health insurance and the structure of the health care system, the growing number of elderly, the discriminatory attitude toward the elderly (Hanson, 1994) and defensive medicine to prevent lawsuits (Kapp, 1998). Because no nation can provide for all health care needs of all citizens without neglecting other needs, one approach is to ration care to the elderly.

RATIONING HEALTH CARE AND THE ELDERLY

The elderly are a vulnerable group because of their number, gender, ethnic composition, needs, and costs of care. In 1998 the number of persons 65 years or older was 34.4 million, which is 12.7% of the population in the United States. Those older than 85 number 4 million (a 33 times larger group than in 1990), and most are women (*Health & Aging Chartbook*, 1999). Minorities represent 15% of the elderly population, which is expected to increase dramatically in the next 30 years.

The increasing need for health care is complicated by the limited income of many elderly. The median 1998 income for all older persons reporting an income was $13,768. Older people accounted for 35% of all hospital stays and 49% of all days of care in hospitals in 1997 (AARP, 1999); 88% of those older than age 65 have some type of chronic condition (compared with 17% of adults younger than age 65). In 1965, to reduce the poverty and poor health of the elderly, the federal program of Medicare was developed to cover some medical expenses. Medicare has two components: Part A provides hospital, skilled nursing facility, hospice, and home health care services; Part B provides physician and outpatient medical services. The beneficiary, however, is responsible for Medicare deductibles and coinsurance, charges exceeding Medicare-approved limits, and cost of services not covered such as prescription drugs and long-term care. Many Medicare enrollees have some type of private supplemental health insurance. The Medicare program was never intended to be comprehensive, and current statistics bear this out. The elderly living in the community spend 19% of their income for health care and 17% for prescription drugs, and the poor elderly spend 33% of their income on health care (Gross & Brangan, 1999). Health care costs (currently $200 billion) for the elderly are growing about 4% per year, which is more rapidly than the gross domestic product. Technology is the driving force behind these costs (Fuchs, 1999). Because of both the growth in the elderly population and the cost of their health care, health care rationing is an approach. From an ethical perspective, rationing reflects on the principle of justice.

APPROACHES TO RATIONING

This chapter focuses on approaches to health care rationing, the pros and cons as they affect the elderly, and the ethical implications of various rationing strategies.

These ethical challenges are important to the nursing profession and to the individual nurse (American Nurses Association [ANA], 1995).

Rationing is defined as limiting available interventions or treatments that may have real benefits for patients (Fletcher, Lombardo, Marshall, & Miller, 1997). Allocation is one approach to rationing; it determines the distribution of resources using criteria about the funds to be obtained and expended and the services made available, as well as the methods of distribution and even who will receive them and on what basis (Beauchamp & Childress, 1994). Medicare is an allocation strategy. Three key features of rationing decisions are:

1. The goods we often must provide are not sufficiently divisible to avoid unequal or "lumpy" distribution.
2. When we ration, we deny benefits to some individuals who can plausibly claim they are owed them in principle.
3. The general distributive principles appealed to by claimants and by those doing the rationing do not by themselves provide adequate reasons for choosing among claimants (Daniels, 1994).

Feldstein (1999) identifies two ways to ration: the government limits on access to goods and services and the individual ability to pay. The governmental approach to rationing health care is used by many countries including Great Britain and Canada; in the United States, only Oregon uses this approach. In 1994, Oregon limited access to expensive procedures for those on Medicaid and was thus able to increase Medicaid eligibility to more low-income people. In actual practice a recent review of this program noted that health care professionals made decisions to provide care on the basis of clinical judgment, which was not sanctioned by the Oregon program (Jacobs, Marmor, & Oberlander, 1999). Although health care in the United States has been rationed primarily on the basis of the individual's ability to pay, the general public and policy makers have been reluctant to call this rationing. However, denial of access to treatments of benefit to the patients who cannot pay is by definition rationing. The person's ability to pay is manifested as having access to and being able to pay for health care.

Daniels (1994) poses four key rationing problems that must be addressed: (1) How much should we favor producing the best outcome with our limited resource? (2) How much priority should we give to treating the sickest or most disabled patients? (3) When should we allow an aggregation of modest benefits to larger numbers of people to outweigh more significant benefits to fewer people?

(4) When must we rely on a fair democratic process as the only way to determine what constitutes a fair rationing outcome? Thus, rationing poses major ethical problems. The utilitarian perspective directs the use of resources on the basis of the greatest good to the greatest number. Distributive justice refers to fair, equitable, and appropriate distribution in society determined by justified norms that structure the terms of social cooperation. Distributive justice is challenged under conditions of scarcity and competition. The principle of formal equality asserts that whatever respects are under consideration as relevant, persons equal in those respects should be treated equally. Specifically, unless some difference between them is relevant to the treatment at stake, they would be treated the same. "Material principles identify relevant properties that persons must possess to qualify for a particular distribution" (Beauchamp & Childress, 1994, p. 331). The major tenets of distributive justice direct that the person receive health care on the basis of the criteria of equal share, need, effort, contribution, merit, and free mark exchanges.

Difficulties also arise because of a conflict in the norms used to justify the decision and in what is considered relevant in addressing these major tenets. Who is to determine what norms and what is relevant in the allocation of the scarce good of health care? Where should rationing decisions be made? Although rationing decisions can be made on a case-by-case basis, the approach depends on the values of the individual making the decision and may not be fair.

This debate will be presented with arguments for why health care to the elderly should be rationed, why it should not be rationed, and what approaches are available for nurses to consider as they confront this issue as individual professionals with ethical responsibility and what role the nursing profession should play. The debate will address issues of key stakeholders in these issues. Who will benefit if the elderly are denied health care resources? The stakeholders in this debate include the elderly, their relatives, their caregivers, politicians, other citizens, especially the young, tax payers, and health care providers including nurses.

PRO ARGUMENT

A number of arguments have been proposed to support rationing health care for the elderly. The first point is that the elderly have already benefitted with the advent of Medicare. They receive more than one third of the national annual health care expenditures while representing only 12% of the population (Khandker & McCormack, 1999). The elderly receive health care, but the 44 million uninsured have limited or no access on the basis of their ability to pay. Another argument to support rationing is that from a lifetime perspective; resources should be allocated on a fair lifetime share of health care for each citizen. Daniels, using the fair equality of opportunity approach, argues that the goal should be to achieve a normal life span; thus each would receive resources accordingly. Resources would be allocated for that purpose, not for extending the lives of the elderly. A related argument is that the elderly have less quality-adjusted life-years, and the money should not be spent to achieve less with it than for someone who has more quality-adjusted life-years. Callahan (1989) argues that when the natural life span has been reached in the late 70s or early 80s, the goal should be to relieve suffering rather than to claim life-extending care. Included in a basic minimum of care would be long-term care and support services. Society should guarantee decent and basic care to all individuals, but not unlimited efforts to conquer illness and death.

An additional argument for rationing care to the elderly is that they have less chance of surviving treatment or of surviving after treatment; thus money is wasted on the elderly when others, who could survive, do not have access to treatment. As the number of elderly grows, even more money will be needed than has been spent in the past, making consideration of this issue even more important.

A further argument is that too much technology, including medication, is being developed to treat the infirmities of the elderly. A pertinent example is the development of Viagra, a drug to enhance sexual functioning (Kapp, 1998). Although the initial response of insurance companies was that this drug should not be reimbursed, societal values and the related pressure caused this decision to be overturned. Old age is a natural part of life and the efforts should be directed at interventions that would promote the health of the young. Lamm (1999) says that the elderly should be accepting aging and preparing to die, rather than seeking to live indefinitely. He identifies the importance of focusing on costs of health care, because it is a publicly funded system (50% of health care is funded by the government). Morreim (1995) emphasizes that the common resource pool depends on individual contributions, and justice demands that individuals not make unreasonable demands on collective funds. "While a patient is entitled to rights as an American citizen, these rights do not include publicly subsidized longevity at all costs" (Lamm, 1999, p. 29).

CON ARGUMENT

Many arguments can be made that the elderly should not be targets of health care rationing. The most important impact of focusing on the elderly is that it drives an even greater division between elders and the young than is already prevalent in our country, disrupting societal solidarity and equity (Callahan, 1994).

A second argument is that the inequalities in the larger health care system make the fair lifetime share of health care for each citizen impossible. Age-based rationing violates the approach that would reflect generational equity, in which all generations receive a fair allocation of health care resources. Current inequities in the United States make it difficult to ration care on the basis of age because no system has been developed that provides a decent minimum standard of care.

Another argument is that the elderly should not be blamed for the rising health care costs when many factors have contributed to these costs. These include technology and the practice of defensive medicine, although the costs of the latter are very difficult to quantify (Kapp, 1998).

Elders also make the argument that their taxes have contributed to the development of technologies that would be denied to them under rationing. This argument would continue on through each generation.

In the last 20 years, new initiatives to empower patients have been developed, including the use of advance directives, living wills, and the Patients' Bill of Rights concurrent with concern about brain death, persistent vegetative state, whether health care is a right, the exploding cost of care, and focus on quality. Only limited research has assessed the impact of advance directives, hospice care, futile care restrictions, and do-not-resuscitate (DNR) orders on costs; these studies found little or no impact on costs of care (Emanuel & Emanuel, 1994). And it is important to point out that these approaches were not developed to control costs but rather to respond to problems precipitated by our expanding health care technologies in order to provide for more patient involvement in decision making about treatments. However, their potential impact on costs if required by insurance companies is considered a beneficial byproduct. Another area that has been specifically targeted for saving money is to reduce the costs of end-of-life care; however, it is difficult to use this approach because of the lack of certainty in predicting when someone will die, as well as in distinguishing between care to relieve suffering and care to prolong life. Callahan (1996) warns that the need to control costs because of the great economic burden the elderly impose can lead to a greater willingness to use physician-assisted suicide and to either tacitly or overtly urge the elderly to request it.

Rationing of health care to the elderly is already taking place through the limits on Medicare reimbursement. For example, long-term care and prescriptions are not covered; African Americans and less educated and low-income elders are less likely to receive specialty services under fee-for-service Medicare (Blustein & Weiss, 1998), to be a renal transplant candidate (Varekamp, Krol, & Danse, 1998), or to receive the level of care required in nursing homes where most residents are elderly. Rationing in nursing homes through reduced registered nurse (RN) staffing has been associated with more negative patient outcomes including physical and verbal aggression, greater use of restraints, decubitus, contractures, dehydration, urinary tract infection, and fractures (Anderson, Hsieh, & Su, 1998). In their nationwide study of nursing home resident outcomes, Harrington and Carrillo (1999) found continued quality problems in nursing homes, although the deficiencies identified declined 44% between 1991 and 1997; part of the decline was due to the reduced enforcement process in some states. Rationing health care to elders imposes an additional burden on those in society who already experience discrimination and thus are disenfranchised. These groups include women, who make up a high percentage of those older than 85 years, and the growing percentage of ethnic members who are growing old.

Health care to the elderly is already being rationed by the attitudes of caregivers, who are biased against the elderly or who stigmatize the elderly. For example, Shepardson, Youngner, Speroff, and Rosenthal (1999) found that patients (average age 72) with DNR orders, when matched on the basis of illness and prognosis with a similar group of patients without DNR orders, were more likely to die.

Difficulties in rationing health care are hampered by the lack of public development of resource allocation plans addressing all of health care as has been done in Oregon (Jacobs, Marmor, & Oberlander, 1999) and in a pilot project in Great Britain (Cookson & Dolan, 1999). In the Great Britain study, the citizen groups identified the three main rationing principles of priority to those in immediate need, health maximization, and equalization of lifetime health. Applying these principles would be difficult because of the potential for a wide range of interpretations, a difficulty characteristic of all principles for rationing.

AN ALTERNATIVE TO RATIONING HEALTH CARE IN THE ELDERLY

Rationing may not be the only approach to controlling health care costs. From the perspective of the ethical principle of beneficence, more research is needed focused on what is best for the elderly. Little research has focused on interventions that enhance patient participation in decisions about costly care or improve functional status of the elderly and thus either control or reduce costs. Only a few projects have addressed the approach of involving patients in decision making about end-of-life care. Murphy et al. (1994) found that patients often chose not to have extensive treatments when told their chances of survival. In another study, providing a special elders inpatient unit focused on improving functional outcomes actually resulted in a shorter length of stay, lower use of nursing homes, and only slighter higher cost, more than balanced out by the shorter length of stay (Covinsky et al., 1997). Nurse researchers have developed strategies to maintain or enhance the functional status of the elderly. For example, Jerovec, Wyman, and Wells (1998) and Dougherty et al. (1998) have developed strategies to reduce urinary incontinence in the elderly, a leading predictor of the need for nursing home placement.

A major consideration important to success in care of the elderly is the impact on caregivers. Nursing research had this area as one of its priorities in the 1990s. The research documents the lack of financial or other support available to caregivers of the chronically ill and elderly and the impact on the psychological and physical health of caregivers. They have great need for respite (Strang & Haughey, 1999); experience greater stress when the one being cared for is demented (Levesque, Ducharme, & Lachance, 1999); report fatigue, loss of energy, and sleep difficulty (Teel & Press, 1999); have feelings of grief and loss because of changes in the patient (Lindgren, Connelly, & Gaspar, 1999); want more support (Coe & Neufeld, 1999); have poorer health (Bull, Maruyama, & Luo, 1997; Sparks, Farran, Donner, & Keane-Hagerty, 1998); and believe they are bearing a heavy burden (Houde, 1998). Research on the use of a case manager to reduce the burden to the caregiver had only a limited effect (Newcomer, Yordi, DuNah, Fox, & Wilkinson, 1999), signaling the need for more research on interventions.

The escalating costs of health care are a major impetus for policy makers and health care professionals to seek ways to control these costs. Because the government provides the funds for health care of the elderly through

Medicare, the government has greater control over this program than other sources of funding. Perhaps a compromise is the best approach. Some of the costs could be reduced by more aggressive preventive programs with the elderly. The fact that much of the research in disciplines other than nursing is focused on technological interventions that benefit the elderly should be evaluated with findings used to develop policies that guide the research funded by the federal government.

The current health care system has a number of limitations that make rationing of care for the elderly difficult. For example, health care professionals often do not know the patient's wishes, the health care system lacks an approach to lifelong preventive care and adequate primary care, and underserved and disadvantaged do not trust health care professionals when they say nothing more can be done (Fletcher & Spencer, 1997).

Focusing on the need to ration may produce an approach through the dialogue that it promoted. As Jacobs et al. (1999) point out, "the rhetoric and process of rationing (as opposed to its programmatic application) were crucial in mobilizing support for OHP" (p. 171).

The United States is not the only country facing the growing costs of health care and the increased percentages of the elderly. That social and health care resources for the elderly need to be addressed is at a crisis level in many developed countries, given the growing number of citizens older than 80 years of age. An international panel, including representatives from the United States, made the following six recommendations (Joint International Research Group, 1994):

1. The highest future goal of medicine for the elderly should be a reduction in morbidity and disability and not an explicit effort to reduce mortality or increase average life expectancy.
2. The maintenance of a firm sense of moral solidarity between the generations has become an urgent matter for social dialogue and refinement.
3. An integrated set of priorities for young and old should be pursued as part of an effort to devise a fair and sensible allocation of resources between the generations and within the generations.
4. The burden on women in the care of the elderly that has marked informal caregiving in the past cannot and should not be sustained.
5. Active efforts should be undertaken to help the elderly to organize politically and collectively to define and articulate their major needs.

6. A public dialogue on the significance of old age in the common life of society should be advanced through educational programs, the media, and joint government-private efforts.

The government has a moral duty to distribute resources in a fair and equitable manner, and health care professionals have a responsibility to help define what is fair and equitable.

THE RESPONSE OF THE PROFESSION

In 1991 the American Nurses Association developed a policy to respond to escalating health care costs urging the federal government to define essential health care services and to provide health care to the poor, those at risk because of preexisting conditions, and the medically indigent. The most recent edition of the social policy statement reflects nursing's social contract with society (American Nurses Association, 1995). Nursing has a social contract to "protect the collective values of society as part of being a professional and in the practice of the essence of nursing" (Mohr, 1996, p. 19). But are the collective values of society changing. And is the profession aware of society's values about rationing and their role in guiding decisions about rationing.

Nurses, too, must address the care of the individual. It should be guided by clinical judgment just as has been reported for physicians in the Oregon Health Plan, in which the physicians did not strictly enforce the list of what conditions could be treated because it is difficult to separate the patient's conditions covered from those not covered (Jacobs et al., 1999).

Physicians can be torn between functioning in a medical model with its focus on individual rights in contrast to a public health model with its focus on the health of the population (Reay, 1999). Speaking of the profession of medicine, Kassirer urged action (1997): "Compromising care to control cost is a vexing social issue in which the integrity of the profession is at stake, and medicine must have a clear, strong voice in these public decisions. Before we face far more odious choices, we must come to grips with these difficult trade-offs. So far, except for a few voices in this country, the air is filled with a strained silence" (pp. 1666-1667), creating a void that nursing can be poised to address.

In addition to the nursing profession's need to take some action about rationing, the individual nurse needs to understand how rationing is taking place and should be prepared to help make decisions that do not compromise ethical principles, particularly of justice and beneficence. The nurse has a professional responsibility to be alert to "resource allocation at the bedside." Are the decisions guided by rationale or based only on one's own values about the elderly? Bedside rationing of scarce resources including beds in the intensive care units, organs, blood, other technology (Fletcher et al., 1997), and the nurse's time occurs frequently. Shepardson et al. (1999) suggested additional types of rationing can occur at the bedside: whether to withhold cardiopulmonary resuscitation, less aggressive monitoring of patients, less prompt response to changes in the patients' conditions, or less attention to patients' needs for nutrition and other supportive measures.

Because tension and contradiction will always be present in the professional setting, nurses must be prepared to make "choices . . . about the kinds of contradiction that will shape the patterns of the practice arena and daily life" (Mohr, 1996, p. 21), and these choices must be ethical.

Given that approaches are needed to control costs, Maynard (1999), an economist, outlines six assumptions necessary for the creation, deployment, and use of an efficient system of rationing.

1. The health care system must be efficient (producing health status improvement at least cost).
2. Access to care must be based on need.
3. Need must be determined by the ability to benefit.
4. The decision on how the benefit (need) is achieved efficiently must be weighted by equity goals (fairness).
5. A disinterested group must judge the needs of competing patients.
6. Finally, mechanisms must be in place to manage and monitor the doctor's and nurse's performance.

It is impossible to develop rational and explicit criteria for rationing health care. Mechanic (1995), however, suggests that implicit rationing is more conducive to stable social relations, as does Hunter (1997), who recommends that we muddle through elegantly.

REFERENCES

AARP. (1999). *A profile of older Americans*. Washington, DC: American Association of Retired Persons.

American Nurses Association. (1991). *Nursing's agenda for health care reform*. Washington, DC: American Nurses Publishing.

American Nurses Association. (1995). *Nursing's social policy statement*. Washington, DC: American Nurses Publishing.

Anderson, R., Hsieh, P., & Su, H. (1998). Resource allocation and resident outcomes in nursing homes: Comparisons between the best and worst. *Research in Nursing and Health, 21*, 297-313.

Beauchamp, T., & Childress, J. (1994). *Principles of biomedical ethics* (4th ed.). New York: Oxford University Press.

Blustein, J., & Weiss, L. (1998). Visits to specialists under Medicare: Socioeconomic advantage and access to care. *Journal of Health Care for the Poor and Underserved, 9*(2), 153-169.

Bull, M., Maruyama, G., & Luo, D. (1997). Testing a model of family caregivers perceptions of elder behavior two weeks posthospitalization on caregiver response and health. *Scholarly Inquiry for Nursing Practice: An International Journal, 11*, 231-248.

Callahan, D. (1989, February 10). Old age and new policy. *Journal of the American Medical Association, 26*, 905-906.

Callahan, D. (1994). Aging and the goals of medicine. *Hastings Center Report, 24*(5), 39-41.

Callahan, D. (1996). Controlling the costs of health care for the elderly—fair means and foul. *New England Journal of Medicine, 335*, 744-746.

Coe, M., & Neufeld, A. (1999). Male caregivers' use of formal support. *Western Journal of Nursing Research, 21*, 568-588.

Cookson, R., & Dolan, P. (1999). Public views on health care rationing: A group discussion study. *Health Policy, 49*, 63-74.

Covinsky, K., King, J., Quinn, L., Siddique, R., Palmer, R., Kresevic, K., Fortinsky, R., Kowal, J., & Landefeld, C. (1997). Do acute care for elders units increase hospital costs? A cost analysis using the hospital perspective. *Journal of the American Geriatric Society, 45*, 729-734.

Daniels, N. (1994). Meeting the challenges of justice and rationing. *Hastings Center Report, 24*(4), 27-29.

Dougherty, M., Dwyer, J., Pendergast, J., Tomlinson, B., Boyington, A., Vogel, W., Duncan, R., Coward, R., & Cox, C. (1998). Community-based nursing: Continence care for older rural women. *Nursing Outlook, 46*, 233-234.

Emanuel, E., & Emanuel, L. (1994). The economics of dying. *New England Journal of Medicine, 330*, 540-544.

Feldstein, P. (1999). *Health policy issues* (2nd ed.). Chicago: Health Administration Press.

Fletcher, J., Lombardo, P., Marshall, M., & Miller, F. (Eds.). (1997). *Introduction to clinical ethics* (2nd ed.). Frederick, MD: University Publishing Group.

Fletcher, J., & Spencer, E. (1997). Ethics services in healthcare organizations. In J. Fletcher, P. Lombardo, M. Marshall, & F. Miller (Eds.), *Introduction to clinical ethics* (pp. 239-256). Frederick, MD: University Publishing Group.

Fuchs, V. (1999). Health care for the elderly: How much? Who will pay for it? *Health Affairs, 18*, 11-21.

Gross, D., & Brangan, N. (1999, December). *Out-of-pocket health spending by Medicare beneficiaries age 65 and older: 1999 projections*. Washington, DC: Public Policy Institute, AARP, publication ID: INB14.

Hanson, J. (1994). How we treat the elderly. *Hastings Center Report, 24*(5), 4-6.

Harrington, C., & Carrillo, H. (1999). The regulation and enforcement of federal nursing home standards, 1991-1997. *Medical Care Research and Review, 56*, 471-494.

Health & aging chartbook. (1999). Health, United States, 1999. Available: http://www.cdc.gov/nchs/products/pubs/pubd/hus/99/huschtdes.htm.

Houde, S. (1998). Predictors of elders' and family caregivers' use of formal home services. *Research in Nursing and Health, 21,* 533-543.

Hunter, D. (1997). *Desperately seeking solutions. Rationing health care.* London: Longman.

Jacobs, L., Marmor, T., & Oberlander, J. (1999). The Oregon Health Plan and the political paradox of rationing: What advocates and critics have claimed and what Oregon did. *Journal of Health Politics, Policy and Law, 24*(1), 161-180.

Jerovec, M., Wyman, J., & Wells, T. (1998). Addressing urinary incontinence with educational continence-care competencies. *Image: The Journal of Nursing Scholarship, 30,* 375-378.

Joint International Research Group. (1994). What do we owe the elderly? *Hastings Center Report, 24*(2), S1-S12.

Kapp, M. (1998). *Our hands are tied.* Westport, CT: Auburn House.

Kassirer, J. (1997). Our endangered integrity—it can only get worse. *New England Journal of Medicine, 336,* 1666-1667.

Khandker, R., & McCormack, L. (1999). Medicare spending by beneficiaries with various types of supplemental insurance. *Medical Care Research Review, 56*(2), 137-155.

Lamm, R. (1999). Redrawing the ethics map. *Hastings Center Report, 29*(2), 28-29.

Levesque, L., Ducharme, F., & Lachance, L. (1999). Is there a difference between family caregiving of institutionalized elders with or without dementia? *Western Journal of Nursing Research, 21,* 472-490.

Lindgren, C., Connelly, C., & Gaspar, H. (1999). Grief in spouse and children caregivers of dementia patients. *Western Journal of Nursing Research, 21,* 521-537.

Maynard, A. (1999). Rationing health care: An exploration. *Health Policy, 49,* 5-11.

Mechanic, D. (1995). Dilemmas in rationing health care services: The case for implicit rationing. *British Medical Journal, 310,* 1655-1659.

Mohr, W. (1996). Ethics, nursing, and health care in the age of "reform." *Nursing and Health Care: Perspectives on Community, 17*(1), 16-21.

Morreim, H. (1995). Moral justice and legal justice in managed care: The ascent of contributive justice. *Journal of Law, Medicine and Ethics, 23*(3), 247-265.

Murphy, D., Burrows, D., Santilli, S., Kemp, A., Tenner, S., Kreling, B., & Teno, J. (1994). The influence of the probability of survival on patient preferences regarding cardiopulmonary resuscitation. *New England Journal of Medicine, 330,* 545-549.

Newcomer, R., Yordi, C., DuNah, R., Fox, P., & Wilkinson, A. (1999). Effects of the Medicare Alzheimer's disease demonstration on caregiver burden and depression. *Health Services Research, 34,* 669-689.

Reay, T. (1999). Allocating scarce resources in a publicly funded health system: Ethical considerations of a Canadian managed care proposal. *Nursing Ethics, 6,* 240-249.

Shepardson, L., Youngner, S., Speroff, T., & Rosenthal, G. (1999). Increased risk of death in patients with do-not-resuscitate orders. *Medical Care, 37,* 727-737.

Sparks, M., Farran, C., Donner, E., & Keane-Hagerty, E. (1998). Wives, husbands, and daughters of dementia patients: Predictors of caregivers mental and physical health. *Scholarly Inquiry for Nursing Practice, 12,* 221-234.

Strang, V., & Haughey, M. (1999). Respite—a coping strategy for family caregivers. *Western Journal of Nursing Research, 21,* 450-466.

Teel, C., & Press, A. (1999). Fatigue among elders in caregiving and noncaregiving roles. *Western Journal of Nursing Research, 21,* 498-513.

Varekamp, I., Krol, L., & Danse, J. (1998). Age rationing for renal transplantation? The role of age in decisions regarding scarce life extending medical resources. *Social Science and Medicine, 47*(1), 113-120.

Legal Implications for Professional Practice

KAY WEILER, PATRICIA CLINTON

This edition of *Current Issues in Nursing* again affirms the assertion that the law and nursing are intimately intertwined. The table of contents for this book reflects the issues facing the nursing profession in the new millennium and represents the broad impact that the law has had on nursing practice. Some examples of legal implications of nursing practice are identified in the initial section of this book that debates the question, What is nursing? To answer this question, the nursing profession, currently and historically, reviews, or drafts, state statutory law to assist in examining or defining different aspects of nursing practice (Section One). In addition to the impact of state statutes in defining nursing practice, nursing practice is influenced by governmental and private sector decisions regarding which health care interventions will receive payment, who will pay for the health care, and how much will be paid for the health care services (Section Eight). In response to the decisions regarding health care payments, modifications in the health care system may be made to access the available health care dollars (Section Seven). These changes in access to funding precipitate changing practice settings for nursing care (Section Four). The changes in practice provide an increased demand for quality care in exchange for the expended health care dollar (Section Five).

The reactions to changes in delivery and payment for health care services raise questions regarding the role of nursing in its own professional governance (Section Six). Questions also arise concerning the educational needs of current practitioners and students entering the changing profession (Section Three) and additional legal and ethical implications for nursing practice (Section Eleven). This book, by presenting the current issues facing the nursing profession, also presents the multiple aspects by which the law continues to have a dynamic impact on the nursing profession.

INTRODUCTION TO THE LAW

A careful exploration of the legal implications for professional nursing practice demands that an initial description of the law be presented and then applied to selected aspects of nursing practice. The law is a system of principles and processes by which the people in a society attempt to control each other's conduct in a effort to minimize the use of force in various forms of conflict resolution (Burton, 1995).

The previous edition of this chapter identified how the law governs the relationships between individuals and between individuals and governmental entities. It reviewed various aspects of the law and the sources of American law. The reader is encouraged to review that chapter for general principles regarding nursing and the law or other excellent references that provide more depth and specificity regarding legal aspects of nursing (Aiken & Catalano, 1994; Beckman, 1995; Brent, 2001; Guido, 1997).

EXAMPLES OF THE RELATIONSHIP BETWEEN THE LAW AND NURSING

In the previous edition of this text, three areas of nursing practice were explored: scope of nursing practice, elements of professional malpractice, and the educational preparation of nurses regarding the legal aspects of practice. The intent of this chapter is to provide an overview of two areas of nursing practice that have been dramatically influenced by the legal system and are currently receiving considerable attention: nursing licensure and Internet-telecommunication access for nurse-patient interactions. The third area, educational preparation of current and future practitioners in legal aspects of nursing practice, has received minimal attention from the profession.

NURSING LICENSURE

In 1888 the U.S. Supreme Court held that national licensure laws were not an appropriate use of federal power; however, states could exercise their police powers by enacting medical licensure laws and accompanying criteria for the practice of medicine (*Dent v The State of West Virginia,* 1889). After the Supreme Court's ruling for the regulation of medical practice, states also began regulating the practice of nurses. The early statutes were not ideal and did not prevent a lay person from receiving payment for nursing services; they merely prevented the lay person from providing the care and using the title of nurse. Despite the limitations of the initial nurse practice acts, however, it is clear that these interactions between the law and nursing had a significant role in the emerging definition and recognition of nursing practice (Shannon, 1975).

In 1938, New York enacted the first licensure statute that made it mandatory for persons practicing nursing to have a license (Laws of the State of New York passed at the one hundred and sixty-first session of the legislature begun January fifth and ended March eighteenth, 1938). This allowed each state to define the required educational qualifications, scope of practice, and disciplinary rules for nurses in that state. The independent authority of each state board of nursing was very effective for many years. As computers and telecommunications move more rapidly into the varied health care settings, teleconferencing, interactive video, Internet chat groups, and accredited Internet courses became more readily available, and the scope of nursing practice is dramatically changing.

These changes have forced many state boards of nursing to facilitate the licensure of nurses living in another state but wishing to practice in two or more states concurrently. Some mechanisms include endorsement, mutual recognition, reciprocity, registration, limited licensure, and national licensure. Endorsement is an agreement between or among states in which a state board may grant licenses to professionals who are licensed in other states with essentially equivalent standards. Endorsement provides mobility or dual practice by nursing professionals, while allowing states traditional powers of setting and enforcing standards to protect their citizens (Executive Summary, 1997).

Mutual recognition is an agreement to legally accept the process and policies of the home state. This is an established agreement between state entities in which the licensee by one member state of the agreement is not required to obtain additional licenses to practice in other areas covered by the agreement. For this system to be effective there must be three components, "a home state, a host state, and a harmonization of standards for licensure and professional conduct deemed to be essential to the health care system" (Executive Summary, 1997). Some have compared this with the current driver's license model that allows drivers with a valid driver's license in one state to legally drive in any other state (Hutcherson & Williamson, 1999).

Reciprocity is a different type of relationship between two states in which each state gives the other state certain privileges on the condition that its own subjects will enjoy similar privileges in the other state. This system requires the authorities of each state to negotiate and enter agreements to recognize licenses issued by the other states without an individual ruling regarding each potential licensee's credentials. A license valid in one state would grant privileges to practice in all other states with which the home state has agreements (Executive Summary, 1997).

Registration is a system in which a nurse licensed in one state would inform the authorities of another state that she or he wished to practice part-time in the second state. The registration process would include a statement from the practitioner that she or he would submit to the jurisdiction of the second state. The nurse would not be required to meet the entrance requirements for licensure within the second state. The nurse, however, would be held accountable for breaches of professional conduct in the second state in which she or he is registered (Executive Summary, 1997).

A limited licensure system is a modification of the current system. Under a limited licensure system a nurse would be required to maintain a full and unrestricted license in at least one state. The nurse could then obtain a limited license that would allow the nurse to deliver a limited scope of practice within the second state. The scope of practice would be narrowly defined rather than a broadly defined license being valid for a limited period of time (Executive Summary, 1997).

A national licensure would be based on a standardized national set of criteria. The nationalized set of standards would be monitored and enforced by a national organization or federal agency. In the national licensure system, the license would grant privileges for nursing practice in all states. The individual states would not be able to impose a significant additional set of standards for the professional practice of nursing within that specific state (Executive Summary, 1997).

States historically have assumed primary responsibility for licensing nurses and have based their authority under the police powers reserved to the states by the Constitution. These police powers have allowed states to adopt laws to protect the health, safety, and general welfare of their citizens. Although the federal government has the authority to play a more active role in regulating issues of health and safety, until recently, this authority has rarely been considered appropriate for defining practice standards for health care professionals (The Center for Telemedicine Law, 1997).

PROFESSION'S APPROACH TO MULTI-STATE LICENSURE

In addition to the governmental and societal concerns regarding an arbitrary definition of nursing determined by the physical boundaries of specific states, the nursing profession recognizes that nursing practice is increasingly focused toward a practice that is not defined by face-to-face, nurse-client interactions or arbitrarily limited by physical borders. This professional awareness occurred as a response from health care providers that addressed the changing face of health care delivery in light of recommendations by the Pew Taskforce on Health Care Workforce Regulations. Driven by new technology, such as telemedicine, which facilitates practice in an arena without boundaries and a health care system in which the client base does not confine itself to state borders has led to the reconsideration of how and where nurses practice. The profession has been debating and exploring ways to meet consumer needs for quality care and safety balanced with a model of nursing practice that would eliminate barriers to multi-state practice. While the debate continues, the National Council of State Boards of Nursing (NCSBN) has moved forward and adopted a model that they believe promotes the NCSBN vision for nursing regulation: "A state nursing license recognized nationally and enforced locally" (National Council Publications, 1996).

Nurses would hold a license in their home (nurse's primary state of residence) state but would be able to practice in states that were party states (any state that has adopted the compact) to the compact. The final version of the language of the compact holds that party states possess the authority to hold the nurse accountable while delivering care in the state in which the patient is located (Gaffney, 1999).

By 1998 the Delegate Assembly adopted the strategies for implementation of the Nurse Multistate Licensure Mutual Recognition Model. As the model evolved, professional nursing organizations began raising questions. In particular the American Nurses Association (ANA) and the National Association of Pediatric Nurse Associates and Practitioners (NAPNAP) sought legal opinions

concerning the language of the model. These opinions resulted in serious concerns regarding practice standards among states, disciplinary action, and the implications of the central database. NCSBN continued to dialog with these organizations and responded with a final version of the compact language in November 1998. Although the final language addressed some of the concerns raised by ANA and NAPNAP, doubt continued to linger about the potential impact of the compact on individual nurses, the state boards of nursing, and the consumers once the compact was adopted by individual states (Glazer, 1999a; National Council of State Boards of Nursing, 2000).

As of the summer of 2000, 10 states have formally adopted the Interstate Licensure Compact; one state is awaiting board implementation of rules. Two other states have the compact in state committees (National Council of State Boards of Nursing, 2000).

Questions remain regarding the potential implementation of the Nurse Licensure Compact. King (1999) has identified specific areas of further inquiry that include (1) How compatible are individual state practice standards? (2) What economic impact will the compact have on individual state boards of nursing? (3) Who will determine the informational components of the central database and then compile, update, maintain and protect the confidentiality of the database? and (4) Who will define situations that require investigation and adjudication of disciplinary actions?

Currently, individual states regulate entry level into practice, continuing education requirements, terms of licensure, and other articles of regulation. Under the interstate compact model, states would allow nurses to practice in their state under the practice act of the state holding the license even if those standards were not the same as the party state. Party states, however, reserve the right to limit or revoke the nurses' ability to practice within their state (Gaffney, 1999).

To operate and enforce rules and regulations, state boards of nursing impose fees and fines on nurses who hold a license within that state. Formerly, nurses practicing in a state other than their state of residence were required to hold an additional license from each state. Under the compact, this would no longer be the case. How then would individual state boards recover these lost fees? It has been suggested that the new licensing fees would, by necessity, have to be increased to cover these and other lost costs. In addition, to evaluate allegations of misconduct, states perform investigations of individual nurses. If a state has not collected revenue to fund investigations, the state will have a limited ability to continue this process in an appropriate manner. The compact provides that states may assess the costs of investigation against the individual nurse under review. This would shift the burden of cost from the state administrative review panel to the individual nurse who has been accused of wrongdoing.

Considerable concern lingers over the creation and management of the Coordinated Licensure Information System (CLIS). This is the centralized database that is a repository for all information of licensure and disciplinary action for all registered nurses. Home and party states are required to report adverse actions taken against a nurse and any current "significant investigative information" even if action has not yet been taken. In an increasingly litigious society, unfounded allegations pose serious consequences when implemented against individuals. Under the language of the compact, individual nurses do not have the right to access the database to determine accuracy and further will need legal counsel from each state in which allegations have been made to avail themselves of proper legal representation (Glazer, 1999b).

Other financial burdens may be imposed as the true costs of the compact become apparent. These would include costs associated with compact administration within each state; the creation, management, and maintenance of the CLIS; and costs associated with implementing the compact and necessitating any legislative changes.

It should be made clear that the compact, as it now stands, affects only registered nurses and not advanced practice nursing. However, the stage has been set for this area of practice. Prescriptive authority, hospital privileges, and third-party reimbursement are all issues advanced practice nurses in individual states have fought for and have been successful in achieving to varying degrees. It remains to be seen how these privileges would be interpreted in party states with differing standards. The task before nursing is to critically evaluate the impact of the compact in the states that have adopted it. The full measure of impact may not be realized for several years until the full economic burden is known and any legal proceedings that may occur have been resolved. Barriers to practice in the new health care delivery system deserve attention and resolution. However, it is critical that the nursing profession recognize that any solution must be accomplished in a deliberative manner, or the ultimate cost in independent nursing practice may be much greater than any specific dollar amount (Glazer, 1999a).

INTERNET/TELECOMMUNICATION ACCESS FOR NURSE-PATIENT INTERACTIONS

An early definition of telemedicine is "the use of telecommunication to diagnose and treat a patient" (Kuszler, 1999). A more recent definition offers a broader and more diversified perspective and "clarifies both the characteristics and the functional attributes of modern telemedicine." The basic characteristics of telemedicine include the geographical separation between the provider and patient; the use of telecommunication or computer technology to enable, facilitate, or enhance the interactions between the parties; the development of protocols and normative standards to replace those of the traditional face-to-face contact; and sufficient staffing and infrastructure to support the telemedicine technology (Kuszler, 1999). The functional areas of this growing field are decision-making aids, remote sensing, and collaborative arrangements for the management of patients at a distance (Kuszler, 1999).

Underserved patient populations that could be served are those in remote rural areas, such as American Indians, Alaskans, prison inmates, or the home bound. International applications for telecommunications and nursing care are discussed in Section Twelve of this book. Also, specific at-risk populations that could be served are postsurgical patients, postpartum mothers and newborns, identified or potential victims of child or dependent adult abuse, and patients with chronic mental health problems.

Potential problems associated with nursing by means of telecommunications interaction with patients include concerns about the quality of care or the lack of quality of care. One such concern is the potential for nurses to be negligent in providing nursing care for patients whom they have not met face-to-face or patients that the nurse does not consider his or her responsibility (Kuszler, 1999).

In the fifth edition of this book, this chapter defined nursing negligence and the legal elements that were needed to establish a claim of negligence: duty, breach of duty, harm or injury, and proximate cause (Weiler, 1997). As identified in that chapter, duty has generally been easy to establish for nursing practice. Simply coming to the health care facility and preparing for their responsibilities has been sufficient evidence that nurses have had a duty to care for any and all patients who have required their care. This duty has been established because of the nurse's role as an employee of the health care facility and the facility's responsibility to provide qualified personnel to meet the patient's needs. However, the use of telecommunications may provide an entirely new dimension to the determination of the nurse's duty to the individual or collective group of patients. Qualified nurses may be expected to provide consultation or collaboration for patients located at distant sites within the same state or across other state borders. For example, expert nurses with knowledge and experience regarding ostomy site care, wound healing, and neonatal breastfeeding problems may all offer vital information and consultation to other nurses and patients in remote locations. The nurse's duty is then to be determined by the nurse's obligation or willingness to provide consultation and the components of the consultation. Consultation may be narrowly limited to telephone conferencing. Or the consultation may be broadly described to extend to live audiovisual consultation, an opportunity to examine the patient by means of telecommunication equipment, the transfer of diagnostic information. Whatever the scope of the consultation, the revised definition of duty would not be limited to the traditional face-to-face patient-nurse relationship.

After a determination of duty, the next element has been the determination of whether the nurse has breached his or her duty of care. The determination of a breach of duty is obviously intimately intertwined with the definition of the duty, whatever those parameters may be.

The third element of professional negligence is that the patient must have suffered harm by the nurse's breach of duty. The patient's harm may be physical harm such as pain, suffering, body parts that have been broken, bruised, or burned, or other physical distress. Traditionally, harm has also included loss of income, lost opportunities, or other nonphysical effects that occurred as a direct result of the nurse's breach of duty.

The fourth element of professional negligence involves demonstrating that the patient's injury was the result of the professional's breach of duty. If the first three elements have been proven, this last element may present more difficult challenges than any other step. This element requires that the injury or harm must be linked or related to the nurse's breach of duty. This means that if the nurse breached his or her duty and the patient suffered harm, that direct link must be established between the injury and the nurse's action. This means that if the nurse left a patient's siderail down and the patient fell off the cart while in the x-ray department and broke her leg, a connection between the nurse's actions and the patient's injury must be established. The nurse may have left the patient's side rails down early in the morning, and the patient may have fallen off of the cart in the late afternoon. The breach of duty and injury both occurred; however,

there was no connection between the two events. Without the establishment of the connection, the nurse is not liable for professional negligence.

Additional legal aspects of nursing practice that use telecommunication are significant, yet beyond the scope of this chapter. Concerns not explored in this chapter are the billing agreements among various health care providers, consultants, and third-party payers; potential liability issues of the physically present health care professional and that institution; and the potential liability of the remote consulting professional and health care institution. Additional concerns not addressed in this chapter are the selection of the applicable state's definition of the professional's scope of responsibility. If the nurse is located and licensed in one state and the patient is located in another state, which state nurse practice act applies to the nurse's definition and scope of practice. These are all significant legal aspects associated with telecommunication and nursing practice (Vyborny, 1996).

In examining the extensive impact of legal aspects of nursing practice, we were challenged to narrow the chapter to a manageable scope of content. We, however, were continually reminded that no single chapter could hope to present the depth and breadth of the issue. The sections of scope of practice and malpractice litigation were chosen because these topics have received recent attention with the expanded areas of nursing practice.

In all aspects of developing this, and the previous, chapter, we were consistently facing the question, Which, if any, aspect of nursing practice does *not* have legal implications? The answer to this question has not been more clearly defined in the past several years. The answer has become, instead, increasingly more difficult to describe. The scope, definition of, and physical locations in which nursing services are being delivered have all expanded and become more complex. As each separate element changes, the answer to the question becomes more complicated. Nurses must become more acutely aware of who the patient is, how the nurse is interacting with the patient (that is face-to-face or by telecommunications or Internet), where the nurse and patient are located in relation to each other, and how standards of quality care have been implemented and are maintained.

The topic of nursing educational preparation to resolve some of these two legal aspects has not been addressed in this chapter. Although the legal aspects of nursing are becoming increasingly complex, the profession's approach to including legal aspects of nursing into nursing curricula has become stagnant. This entire book attests to the fact that the nursing profession has met the challenge to identify nursing issues that involve legal aspects. The lack of educational requirements that reflect this recognition, however, indicates that the profession has failed to implement educational requirements that would provide the basic educational background necessary for the nurses to be able to explore these issues. This failure to require educational programs to include basic legal aspects as a portion of any educational curriculum is clearly a nursing issue that must be addressed immediately.

REFERENCES

Aiken, T.D., & Catalano, J.T. (1994). *Legal, ethical, and political issues in nursing.* Philadelphia: F.A. Davis.

Beckmann, J.P. (1995). *Nursing malpractice: Implications for clinical practice and nursing education.* Seattle: University of Washington Press.

Brent, N.J. (2001). *Nurses and the law: A guide to principles and applications* (2nd ed.). Philadelphia: Saunders.

Burton, S.J. (1995). *An introduction to law and legal reasoning* (2nd ed.). Boston: Little, Brown.

The Center for Telemedicine Law. (1997). Telemedicine and interstate licensure: Findings and recommendations of the CTL Licensure Task Force. *North Dakota Law Review,* 109-130.

Dent v The State of West Virginia, 129 U.S. 114 (1889).

Executive Summary. (1997). Telemedicine report to Congress. *North Dakota Law Review,* 131-144.

Gaffney, T. (1999, May 31). The regulatory dilemma surrounding interstate practice. *Online Journal of Issues in Nursing.* Available: http://www.nursingworld.org/ojin/topic9_1.htm.

Glazer, G. (1999a, May 4). NursingWorld OJIN: Legislative column: Legislative and policy issues related to interstate practice: Board position statement. *Online Journal of Issues in Nursing.* Available: http://www.nursingworld.org/ojin/tpclg/leg-7f.htm.

Glazer, G. (1999b, May 4). NursingWorld OJIN: Legislative column: Legislative and policy issues related to interstate practice: Legal opinion. *Online Journal of Issues in Nursing.* Available: http://www.nursingworld.org/ojin/tpclg/leg-7d.htm.

Guido, G.W. (1997). *Legal issues in nursing.* Stamford, CT: Appleton & Lange.

Hutcherson, C., & Williamson, S. (1999, May 31). Nursing regulation for the new millennium: The mutual recognition model. *Online Journal of Issues in Nursing.* Available: http://www.nursingworld.org/ojin/topic9_2.htm.

King, S.E. (1999, May 31). Multistate licensure: Premature policy. *Online Journal of Issues in Nursing.* Available: http://www.nursingworld.org/ojin/topic9_3.htm.

Kuszler, P.C. (1999). Telemedicine and integrated health care delivery: Compounding malpractice liability. *American Journal of Law and Medicine, 25,* 297-326.

Laws of the State of New York passed at the one hundred and sixty-first session of the legislature begun January fifth and ended March eighteenth, 1938. Article 52 §§ 1374-1386.

National Council Publications. (1996). National Council begins revising models for nursing regulation. *Issues, 17*(3), 1-3. Available: http://www.ncsbn.org/files/publications/issues/vol173/msr173.asp.

National Council of State Boards of Nursing. (2000). *State compact bill status.* Available: http://www.ncsbn.org/files/mutual/billstatus.asp.

Shannon, M.L. (1975). Our first four licensure laws. *American Journal of Nursing, 75*(8), 1327-1329.

Vyborny, K.M. (1996). Legal and political issues facing telemedicine. *Annals of Health Law, 5,* 61-119.

Weiler, K. (1997). Legal implications for professional practice. In J.C. McCloskey & H.K. Grace (Eds.), *Current issues in nursing* (5th ed.). St. Louis: Mosby.

Ethical Issues and Resources for Nurses Across the Continuum

MARGO R. ZINK, LINDA M. TITUS

The health care system of today provides an unending supply of bioethical challenges amid its enormous complexity and rapid change. Medical technology has mushroomed, providing an ever-increasing array of diagnostic and intervention modalities that can diagnose and treat illnesses deemed lethal only a few years ago. Life can be sustained, often precariously, for long periods, frequently in an intensive care environment or more often simply through artificial fluid and nutrition or sophisticated pharmacology. The explosion of genetic information has seeded an array of ethical concerns, including threats to confidentiality, misuse of information resulting in discrimination, denial of health care coverage, selective reproduction, and questioning of the value of life with genetic imperfections.

A push for cost containment finds us fearful for those without financial access to service and suspicious of the clinical decisions made by for-profit managed care organizations. Concerns for cost have reduced staffing levels in some health care settings to an extent that may compromise health care workers' duty to patients. Patients entering the health care system have expressed fear that their rights or expectations will be breached with regard to informed consent, use of restraints, medication errors, pain management, or research. Parentalism on the part of providers continues to undermine patient self-determination.

Within this complex health care system, nurses must maintain vigilance and competence to identify and address actions or events, which may ethically compromise them or the patients for whom they are responsible. Sources of assistance in the domain of ethics include professional codes or standards and formal ethics structures.

CODE FOR NURSES

Nurses' involvement in ethical issues has been well documented in the literature and through professional organi-

zational efforts. The *Code for Nurses with Interpretative Statements,* published by the American Nurses' Association, provides a framework from which nurses in any setting can engage in ethical analysis and decision making. The *Code* was originally adapted by the ANA in 1950 and has been periodically revised. A major revision to the 1985 version of the *Code* has been underway for some time. Following are the nine proposed components on the *Code* revisions (ANA, 1999, Draft #8):

1. The nurse, in all professional relationships, practices with compassion and respect for the inherent dignity, worth and uniqueness of every individual, unrestricted by considerations of social or economic status, personal attributes, or the nature of health problems.
2. The nurse's primary commitment is to the patient, whether an individual, family, or community.
3. The nurse promotes, advocates for, and strives to protect the health, safety and rights of the patient.
4. The nurse is responsible and accountable for individual nursing practice and determines the appropriate delegation of tasks consistent with the nurse's obligation to provide optimum patient care.
5. The nurse owes the same duties to self as to others including the responsibility to preserve integrity and safety, to maintain competence and to continue personal and professional growth.
6. The nurse participates in establishing, maintaining, and improving health care environments and conditions of employment conducive of the provision of quality health care and consistent with the values of the profession, through individual and collective action.
7. The nurse participates in the advancement of the profession through contributions to practice, education, policy, and research.
8. The nurse collaborates with health professionals, the public and others in promoting community, national and international efforts to meet health needs.

9. The profession of nursing, as represented by professional associations and their members, is responsible for articulating nursing values, for maintaining the integrity of the profession and its practice and for shaping social policy.

The statements of the *Code* and the interpretation guide nursing practice and maintain high quality in nursing care. Professional codes have a function of self-regulation and are regarded as systems of rules and principles by which a specific profession is expected to regulate membership (Bandman & Bandman, 1995).

INSTITUTIONAL ETHICS COMMITTEES

Recognition of bioethics as an important aspect of health care management spawned the development of institutional ethics committees (IECs) beginning in the early 1980s. With the broadly held purposes of education, policy development, and clinical consultation, these committees provide a forum in which to address difficult patient choices. Staff education and the establishment of clear policies for areas such as informed consent, limitation of treatment, and end of life issues are typical committee topics. Clinical consults are routinely available to health care team members, patients, and families to assist with ethical dilemmas.

Advantages

The IEC provides a more systematic and principled approach to multidisciplinary decision making that can link ethical and social values and medical technology across the health care continuum. "Ethics committees are a necessary resource for all heath care settings: home health, long-term care, psychiatric institutions, clinics, private practices, and hospitals" (Feutz-Harter, 1991, p. 44). Nurses working in long-term care and home care have been in leadership positions in the establishment of ethics committees. Rushton (1994) believes this may be due to the greater practice autonomy in these settings coupled with nurses' increased authority in clinical practice.

Limitations

Institutional ethics committees have a limited membership and do not consistently address the specific concerns of nurses. IECs are able to offer a forum for only a few nurses, leaving the majority of nursing staff in most settings without an opportunity to participate.

Although nurses have been highly visible among the membership, bringing strong clinical voice and patient-focused approaches to committee activity, they have been in the minority of representation. Rushton (1994) advocates expanding nurse membership in IECs in acute care settings to include not only administrators but equal representation of bedside nurses. Bedside nurses focus on the client's response to illness rather than merely on the diagnosis and treatment alone (Rushton, 1994).

Daily nursing practice problems are seldom appropriate topics for discussion at a hospital-wide ethic committee because other discipline representatives may not be prepared or interested in nursing concerns (Scanlon & Fleming, 1990). Edwards and Haddad (1988) found that the unique concerns of nurses, such as nursing dilemmas related to increased high-tech care in acute and home care settings, the allocation of decreasing resources, and changing delivery systems were not believed to be appropriately addressed with IECs. Hospital downsizing, mergers, and the managed care environment across the health care continuum have led to reductions and reallocations of professional staff, creating a highly charged ethical issue of rationing clinical time among many patients. These issues, too, are not generally addressed in an IEC.

Bosek (1993) asserts that medical-surgical nurses face ethical issues and call on either clinical or theoretical resources to solve these issues. Nurses in one study indicated that they often did not know that an IEC existed and that this source would not be their first avenue in dealing with clinical ethical issues (Hoffman, 1991). When they need more information, nurses may consult theoretical resources, including institutional resources, journals, reading groups, and professional publications as available (Bosek, 1993). These avenues, however, do not provide a strong opportunity for discussion of ethical concerns.

NURSES' EDUCATIONAL PREPARATION

Although nurses face ethical issues frequently, they are not prepared educationally to deal effectively with them. A study on ethical issues in the mid 1990s found that most baccalaureate nursing programs did not require a course in ethics (Titus, 1995; Zink & Titus, 1994). "The real tragedy with regard to ethical dilemmas in nursing practice is not that nurses do not recognize that such dilemmas exist; rather it is their lack of preparation to solve these dilemmas using ethical principles" (Fromer, 1982, p. 20).

First, nurses need preparation in ethical concepts, decision making, and pertinent legal standards. This knowledge is necessary to participate articulately in interdisciplinary discussions of an ethical nature. Second, many issues relating to the nurse's role as a patient advocate require a forum in which these issues can be clarified. Appropriate nursing development of the advocacy role has emerged as a crucial element in nursing practice, especially in light of reimbursement declines and managed care.

Specific ethics content in nursing education at the undergraduate or graduate levels is not presently required by state curriculum or nationwide accreditation bodies. Ketefian (1999), however, recommends that ethical content be integrated at all levels of the nursing curriculum in this suggested manner:

Undergraduate Level
- Recognition of relevant ethical theories and principles with application
- Development of decision-making skills
- Development of professional responsibility and accountability
- Skill development in recognition and analysis of ethical issues

Master's Level
- Evaluation of the moral components of the work environment
- Development of strategies to support and reward ethical practice
- Availability as a resource for staff
- Participation in research focused on a better understanding of the determinants of ethical practice

The Division of Nursing at New York University (NYU) has established a separate ethics committee from that of the institutional committee with the purpose of providing education and consultation to students and faculty on ethical and legal issues (Ramsey, 1998). NYU also has Ethics in the Round, a forum allowing students and faculty to meet on a monthly basis to address ethical problems related to clinical practice. The nursing component of NYU provides an elective course in ethics, law, and nursing practice, as well as a palliative care program. Ramsey (1998) indicated that a nurse's competence in clinical ethics education is as critical as an arts and science foundation.

Nurses working in hospital settings are caring for patients with higher acuity, more social stressors (e.g., homelessness, violence, isolation, poverty, and illiteracy), and reduced hospital lengths of stay. These conditions provoke enormous ethical concerns in the area of beneficence. Can effective patient education occur with a short hospital stay? When is a patient ready for discharge? What are the institutional obligations to ensure patient safety after discharge? What if a patient has no financial means for needed posthospital care if the insurance payer limits continued care?

Nurses, however, in direct clinical roles are especially suited to be involved in ethical decision making because of the sustained relationships with patients and families that these roles provide. The nurse in this role is best able to understand the patient's pain, suffering, achievements, and disappointments (Rushton, 1994). The nurse may be the first to become aware of an ethical issue.

ISSUES IN PRACTICE

Although the Code for Nurses provides a framework for critical thinking and adherence to identified core principles, it has limited use in addressing the individual daily practice issues encountered by nurses. Such issues are situational and so often created or influenced by multiple factors, such as clinical status, patient values, family dynamics, institutional policy, organizational culture, and patient outcomes. Erlen (1993) related how emerging economic restrictions, increased technology coupled with more limited resources, and fragmentation of the overall health-care delivery system have created more intense ethical issues, none of which have easy solutions. Nurses do not always have a clear understanding about their role in ethical deliberations or even in the way ethical decisions are made. Nurses frequently feel powerless in these situations.

Surveys have been conducted (Mason, Johansson, Fleming, & Scanlon, 1989; Scanlon & Fleming, 1990; Zink & Titus, 1994) in New York and Connecticut assessing the prevalence of nursing ethics committees, nurses' involvement in ethical decision making, and nurses' educational needs related to ethics. A later survey conducted by the American Nurses Association Center for Ethics and Human Rights (Scanlon, 1994) revealed similar issues identified in the earlier studies cited. The 10 most frequently cited ethical issues were cost, end-of-life decisions, confidentiality, incompetence, pain management, advance directives, informed consent, access, HIV/AIDS, and providing "futile" care.

We believe these 10 ethical issues have changed priority since 1994 and that problems such as HIV/AIDS and advance directives, although still of importance, no longer have the ethical focus they once had. The issues that remain in the forefront are cost containment (managed care and access to health care), end-of-life decisions, confidentiality coupled with informed consent, incompetence, pain management, and "futile" care (related to high-tech options). Genetic and reproductive issues have continued to be fuel for ethical discussions and indecision.

Regulations, incompetence of coworkers, noncompliant clients, termination of home care services (abandonment), racial intolerance of clients, family members, and staff, and truth telling were mentioned across home care providers (nurses, therapists, aides) (Haddad, 1992). Maintenance of professional boundaries can be another challenge in the home setting, the patient's turf. The home care provider who fails to establish and maintain professional boundaries often develops an emotional connection with the patient that may override clinical judgment. There may also be a perception of risk and issues of personal safety in the delivery of home care services (Haddad, 1996).

Cost Containment

Managed care organizations (MCOs) are changing the infrastructure of health care delivery and are placing limitations on access to health care, which has ethical implications for the entire health care continuum. The four fundamental principles underlying the process of decision making in a managed care environment include patient self-determination, well-being, equality, and competence.

The first principle of self-determination is that patients define their values and assume responsibility for their lifestyle and health care practices. A managed care health delivery scheme imposes certain lifestyle practices on patients, whether desired or not. The extreme case scenario would be a patient actually denied care because of certain health care practices, such as a heavy smoker's being denied bypass surgery (Bandman & Bandman, 1995).

The well-being of the patient is a second principle to consider in the decision-making process. The health profession, especially nursing in the community or home setting, has long focused on this through health promotion teaching. Managed care emphasizes health promotion more than the unstructured health care delivery system of the past and promotes prevention rather than merely episodic care.

The issue of equality is an underlying moral principle in ethics. This principle can also be seen as a vital component in the decision-making process; arbitrary decisions about patient care are essentially eliminated in this principle. This, however, also implies that different needs of patients are treated in different ways. This distinction of unique differences of health needs may be more difficult in a capitated managed care environment (Bandman & Bandman, 1995; Zink, 1997).

Other considerations of the decision-making process involve the assessment of the patient's ability and competence to be involved in this process. When managed care guidelines are dictated, how much decision-making ability will either the health professional or the patient have about any desired alternatives?

Although managed care organizations pose many challenges on the ethics of health care delivery, they also minimize some previously existing unethical practices. The focus on maximum quality and cost-effectiveness places more demands on the provider than ever occurred in the past with increased accountability. In the old, unstructured, noncompetitive health care environment, providers were not accountable to the patient for providing the best quality care for the best price. In this managed, integrated market, competition is strong, and so quality becomes a benchmark when alliances and mergers take place.

Futility

With the extreme sophistication of high-tech care, providers and patients struggle with defining the futility of care options. Nurses are central members of the health team participating in identifying the value of particular treatment options and in meeting the desired attainable goals of the patient. Choices with regard to artificial ventilation, chemotherapy, dialysis, artificial nutrition, hemodynamic support, and the like must be made within the context of overall prognosis for recovery. These choices are seldom those of the patient or family alone, rather they are influenced more and more by the insurance payer.

There are now sophisticated catheters and infusion pumps for the delivery of all types of medications to include antibiotics, parental nutrition, and analgesics available for home use. Home ventilator systems and other high-tech equipment can now be adapted to the home setting. Arras and Dubler (1995) refer to this extension of the medical domain into the private sphere of family and friends as the "medicalization" of the home. A feeling of intrusion and loss of privacy can accompany high-tech home care. There are additional burdens placed on caregivers with these technologies. Family and friends must learn about these high-tech needs with sometimes limited instruction before the patient's discharge. "Thus, the transition from hospital to home can be experienced by both patients and family members as a shift from what might be called technological overload to technological isolation at home. In the hospital, patients and families are surrounded by an intensely high-tech environment, including highly skilled support staff always just a call bell away. . . . At home, by contrast, some patients and their families can feel cut off from or even abandoned by this system of intensive medical support" (Arras & Dubler, 1995, p. 7).

Home care nurses with a caseload of all high-tech patients can experience burnout because of the intensity of the care required. No established guidelines outline the qualifications of home care nurses to administer high-tech services such as infusions. Ethical dilemmas arise for the staff and the agency when a nurse is assigned high-tech patients beyond his or her experience level and qualifications. The agency must affirm that nurses are adequately competency tested to ensure safe practice. Nurses, on the other hand, have the ethical obligation to admit to the employing agency any procedure they do not feel qualified to perform. "The 20th century has been described as an era of professional autonomy. Along with autonomy have come regulations and legislation to assist in defining the boundaries of practice. Organizations and staff must be cognizant of the potential liabilities in the home as responsibilities and therapies increase in number and acuteness" (Grace & Tomaseli, 1995, p. 533). Technology in the home setting can create a conflict between the beneficent obligations of the home care provider and the autonomy of the patient and family.

Informed Consent and Confidentiality

Health professionals across settings are now expected to share knowledge with clients and families in the atmosphere of informed consent (Zink, 1997). The right to full disclosure of health care information has become a keen patient right that creates ethical dilemmas in practice. What is full disclosure? When has valid informed consent been given? When is truthtelling secondary to other ethical principles? What is the role of the nurse in the informed consent process? Who is entitled to give information to patients? How has computerization of patient data affected the issue of informed consent?

The patient in any health care setting has the right to be informed of his or her plan of care, any charges the patient may be obligated to pay, and when discharge from services will take place. Patients also have a right to be informed of what staff will be involved in their care and these individuals' qualifications. The patient must be informed of how to voice a complaint through the agency or through a state hotline number.

Information management systems in today's acute care settings are highly computerized. Maintaining security of access to and distribution of information is a re-

sponsibility of nurses not to be taken lightly. The "need to know" standard guides caregivers when friends, family, or high-visibility patients are under care to ensure that medical information is not accessed unnecessarily. Nurses serve as guardians of the medical record for others seeking access.

The mandate of increased data collection in home care has posed additional issues of confidentiality of patient information and the need for the patient's informed consent. The Health Care Financing Administration (HCFA) has mandated that all home care agencies receiving Medicare funding are required to collect the Outcome Assessment and Information Set (OASIS) on patients and transmit these data to HCFA through each state. Ethical issues surrounding the confidentiality of these data, the patient's knowledge of this transmittal, and the initial requirement that all patient information (Medicare and non-Medicare patients) would be transmitted pose potential breaches of confidentiality.

Home telemedicine technology poses additional ethical issues in health care. When care is provided in the home setting, whether in person or interactively on line, ethical guidelines are essential to guide practice with patients and family (Roman, Stickwell, Louvier, & Clements, 1997).

Pain Management

Despite an increasing pharmacological and therapeutic arsenal, patients continue to perceive and fear pain associated with their illness. Nurses are vital in evaluating pain and advocating for effective pain management. Pain control is one of the most common problems with cancer patients. Sixty-seven percent of patients with lower leg ulcers have reported severe pain in previous studies (Gallagher, 1998).

Hospitalizations can be prolonged when appropriate home pain-control measures are not available. A well-designed home care pain management program can effectively deal with concerns such as potential narcotic overdose, poor intravenous access, and complications from a long-term intravenous catheter. Aging, misconceptions, assessment, and an awareness of the nonpharmaceutical alternatives available must be considered in pain program design. Misunderstandings concerning the dimensions of a patient's pain can interfere with adequate assessment and treatment of pain (Gallagher, 1998).

The Joint Commission for Accreditation for Healthcare Organizations (JCAHO) outlines the necessary components to evaluate the pain of the hospice patient (JCAHO, 1998). These measures could be applied to any patient experiencing pain. Although technology and medicine have the ability to control most patient pain, why then does society continue to tolerate people who experience prolonged discomfort with no apparent relief? It is the ethical, moral obligation of the health care staff to continuously assess patients' pain and to intervene appropriately when that pain threshold becomes intolerable.

Pain relief does not equate to euthanasia. Relieving a patient's pain is the humane thing for any health care professional to do within the boundaries of practice. The patient, however, should have the chance to decide for himself or herself whether pain management intervention is needed. Issues of health care rationing and cost containment may be in conflict with degrees of suffering allowed. Ethical dilemmas may arise when nurses are not allowed to implement an effective pain management program because of reimbursement restraints.

Incompetent Colleagues

The nursing profession has the responsibility to demand best practice standards from colleagues. When colleagues are not able to live up to these professional standards and to state practice licensure guidelines, nurses must ethically confront the colleague and report any unethical practice to the appropriate sources. The ethical principle of "do no harm" may be severely hampered if a nurse is impaired or for other reasons not able to perform the duties required. Although this may interfere with the colleague's autonomy, the responsibility to ensure safe practice takes precedence.

Home care nurses practice in a much more independent role than nurses do in other settings. For this reason, it may be more difficult to detect incompetent practice from colleagues. Inconsistency in visit reports, inaccurate recording of patient information, or inability to verbalize and/or report changes in the patient's condition may be suspect.

End-of-life Decisions

Moving from cure to comfort in patient care is often difficult for both patients and providers. Health care workers, by nature and training, want to cure. This strong goal can, at times, inhibit facing a terminal situation squarely and openly for patients. Nurses are key players in moving the health care team toward a recognition of end-of-life situations and the needed comfort care and psychosocial support. Recognizing the individual patient's need for hope while addressing the gravity of a terminal status is an art developed with experience and essential to effective nursing practice in any setting.

Dying at home requires the support of family, the physician, and health care staff. The home care nurse must learn and understand a patient's wishes concerning his or her desires and be aware of whether the patient has developed an advance directive. The agency should know the contents and location of the advance directive. The JCAHO (1998) requires that the patient has the right to formulate advance directives. The standard further states that for Medicare-certified agencies, there must be written policies and procedures addressing any limitations related to the agency abiding by the patient's desires. The nurse has the responsibility to reassess any changes in the patient's wishes during the course of health care services. All staff working with the patient must be informed about the patient's desires. The agency's ethics committee must identify any contradictory types of advance directives that staff would not be able to adhere to; this information must be provided to the patient (JCAHO, 1998).

Genetic and Reproductive Issues

It is clear that our collective social fabric is divided on the moral and ethical issues entwined in reproduction. Nurses are at the forefront of many of these issues, including birth control, abortion, artificial insemination, in vitro fertilization, and fetal tissues use. Selective abortion for multiple pregnancies and embryo implantation in postmenopausal women also raise many new questions. Is it ethical to give birth control information to minors? Should nurses participate in abortions? How should fetal tissues be obtained or used for medical research or treatment? Should any social or sexual condition limit the availability of artificial insemination for an individual? When six fetuses are created by medical manipulation, is it ethical to selectively reduce the number to enhance the chances for survival of those remaining? Should a 60-year-old woman be implanted with an embryo?

The ANA Center for Ethics and Human Rights has issued a comprehensive document entitled "Managing Genetic Information, Implications for Nursing Practice" (Scanlon & Fibison, 1995), which provides a full discussion of ethical issues related to genetics such as consent, privacy, confidentiality, truthtelling, disclosure and nondiscrimination. These issues require nurses to be prepared to respond appropriately in safeguarding patients' rights amid the explosion and use of genetic information (Smith, 1989).

RESOURCES

Studies found that peers were used by more than 85% of nurses in both home care and acute care settings as support when dealing with ethical issues, with additional support involving an immediate supervisor. The referring physician was consulted less often in home care for ethical consultation than in the acute care setting. The use of an ethics committee as a resource was used far more often in the acute care setting and seldom in home care. This is due to the lack of established ethics committees in home care agencies (Zink & Titus, 1996).

Uustal (1993) suggests seven characteristics of ethical principles, which can guide the nurse in formulating "best practice." These characteristics include initially suggesting a direction or proposing specific changes. Through nursing ethics committees and rounds, the nurse can provide guidance in organizing and understanding information associated with an ethical dilemma. The nurse then has the framework for proposing how to resolve competing issues with justification of moral action.

To make critical judgments at this level, it is essential that the nurse has an understanding of the universal nature of ethical principles. This foundation must be part of professional continuing education for nurses and other disciplines involved in patient care and must take into consideration that ethical principles are neither rules (means) or values (ends). Health care workers at all levels must accept the human and unchangeable nature of ethical principles.

Nursing Ethics Committees (NEC)

Although there has been some criticism that NECs compete with institutional ethics committees, it is generally recognized that NECs provide an important forum for nursing-specific issues and also prepare nurses to become involved effectively in IECs (Ross, 1991). NECs allow nurses an opportunity to explore the rich heritage of their profession and to discover tools with which to identify and address ethical issues.

Although the trend in most health care settings is for a multidisciplinary ethics committee, a need remains to provide a specific avenue for nurses to seek advice on ethical issues more unique to the profession. The primary function of a NEC is the identification, exploration, and resolution of ethical issues in nursing practice. The NEC should also provide the availability of the education of nurses in bioethics and nursing ethics. This committee has long been described as a foundation for the preparation of nurses for participation in interdisciplinary decision making about ethical issues.

The committee should also serve as a resource group for other nurses in an institution and be a clearinghouse for the review of nursing ethics materials. Committee members have a responsibility to be involved with review

of departmental policies related to ethics and involvement with nursing ethics research.

Clinically Based Ethics Education

Education in ethics should be provided to the nurse across the continuum during initial orientation and ongoing through continuing education offerings. Specific application of ethical principles to both acute and home care settings should be addressed. Education should also focus on ethical inquiry, reasoning, and decision making unique to these various settings (Scanlon, 1994). The ability to care for patients on line through telemedicine increases the need for up-to-date, ongoing ethics education for nurses.

Nursing Ethics Groups

Forums for ongoing ethics discussions can be established through regular staff meetings, journal clubs, or ethics roundtable discussions (Heitman & Robinson, 1997). The formation of groups composed only of nurses provides the opportunity for the exploration of the viewpoints of nurses and serves to cultivate the knowledge and skills required of nurses to engage in ethical decision making (Scanlon, 1994). Such a group can provide nurses with the opportunity to critique real or situational case studies, test various problem-solving techniques, and assess ethics related to nursing practice (Scanlon, 1994).

Ethics Rounds

This framework provides nurses and other disciplines working with specific patients the opportunity to address current ethical dilemmas involved with care. These discussions can deal with current ethical issues or projected problems in the delivery of care to a specific patient or patient population. Ethical rounds can also prevent ethical dilemmas from surfacing through proactive decision making (Scanlon, 1994).

Other Resources

Methods of increasing ethics resources for nurses in home care needs exploration. Resources are limited to peers, supervisors, and at times, physicians and social workers. Perhaps creative alliances might be forged using representatives of nearby institutions and nursing committees as consultants, involvement with the state nursing ethics committee, or collaboration with nursing faculty with an ethics background. All of these alternative options for support can raise the ethical consciousness of nurses and foster professional confidence in ethical decision making (Scanlon, 1994).

SUMMARY

The *Code for Nurses* provides practicing nurses across settings with a framework for ethical decision making. The *Code*, however, has not been officially updated since 1985 and, therefore, does not speak to the current dilemmas of practice. Telemedicine points to a more obvious need for the current published version of the Code of Ethics for nurses to be updated and comprehensively reviewed (Roman et al., 1997). Although IECs serve a vital role within the broad areas of education, policy, and consultation for the acute care nurse, they do not provide a board resource for the educational and practice issues faced daily by nurses. Significant data show that nurses are inadequately prepared to address the burgeoning complexities of bioethics.

Traditional ethical issues facing nurses today, such as end-of-life decisions, incompetent health care workers, "futile" care, and pain management are taking on added dimensions in the world of cost containment and managed care. Informed consent and confidentiality have taken on more complexity in light of enhanced computerization of patient data and data transmission capabilities. Advancements in technology pose continued ethical dilemmas in the fields of genetics and reproduction.

The academic environment must carefully evaluate the need for more foundation knowledge of ethics at all levels of nursing education. Nurses continue to have a need for an organized avenue to bring forth ethical issues and discuss solutions in a nonthreatening environment. Nursing ethics committees and forums and patient ethic rounds provide the profession with avenues to voice ethical concerns and problem solve on solutions.

REFERENCES

American Nurses Association. (1999). *Code for nurses with interpretative statements.* Draft #8. Washington, DC: Author.

Arras, J., & Dubler, N. (1995). Ethical and social implications of high-tech home care. In J. Arras (Ed.), *Bringing the hospital home.* Baltimore, MD: The Johns Hopkins University Press.

Bandman, E., & Bandman, B. (1995). *Nursing ethics through the life span.* Norwalk, CT: Appleton & Lange.

Bosek, M. (1993). A comparison of ethical resources. *MEDSURG Nursing, 2*(4), 332-334.

Edwards, B., & Haddad, A. (1988). Establishing a nursing bioethics committee. *Journal of Nursing Administration, 18*(3), 30-33.

Erlen, J. (1993). Empowering nurses through nursing ethics committees. *Orthopaedic Nursing, 12*(2), 69-72.

Feutz-Harter, S. (1991). Ethics committees: A resource for patient care decision-making. *Journal of Nursing Administration, 21*(4), 11-12, 44.

Fromer, M. (1982). Solving ethical dilemmas in nursing practice. *Topics in Clinical Nursing, 4*(1), 49-56.

Gallagher, S. (1998). Ethical dilemmas in pain management. *Ostomy/Wound Management, 44*(9), 18-23.

Grace, L., & Tomaseli, B. (1995). Intravenous therapy in the home. In J. Terry (Ed.), *Intravenous therapy—Clinical principles and practice.* Philadelphia: Saunders.

Haddad, A. (1992). Ethical problems in home healthcare. *Journal of Nursing Administration, 22*(3), 46-51.

Haddad, A. (1996). Ethical issues in home care of the oncology patient. *Seminars in Oncology Nursing, 12*(3), 226-228.

Heitman, L., & Robinson, B. (1997). Developing a nursing ethics roundtable. *American Journal of Nursing, 97*(1), 36-38.

Hoffman, D.E. (1991). Does legislating hospital ethics committees make a difference? A study of hospital ethics committees in Maryland, the District of Columbia, and Virginia. *Law, Medicine, & Health Care, 19*(1-2), 105-119.

Joint Commission for Accreditation of Healthcare Organizations (JCAHO). (1998). *CAMHC. 1999-2000 Comprehensive accreditation manual for home care.* Chicago: Author.

Ketefian, S. (1999). Legal and ethical issues—Ethics content in nursing education. *Journal of Professional Nursing, 15*(3), 138.

Mason, D., Johansson, E., Fleming, C., & Scanlon, C. (1989). Ethics committees in health care institutions in the New York City metropolitan region: A report of two nursing surveys. *Journal of the New York State Nurses Association, 20*(4), 13-16.

Ramsey, G. (1998). Nursing and ethical issues. *Imprint, 45*(3), 43-45.

Roman, L., Stockwell, S., Louvier, V., & Clements, F. (1997). Creating an ethical foundation for home telemedicine. *Home Healthcare Management Practice, 9*(8), 58-66.

Ross, J. (1991). Ethics committees for nurses. *Ethical Currents, 25,* 1-2, 7.

Rushton, C. (1994, Fall). The voices of nurses on ethics committees. *Bioethics Forum,* 30-35.

Scanlon, C. (1994). Ethics survey looks at nurses' experiences. *The American Nurse, 26*(10), 22.

Scanlon, C., & Fibison, W. (1995). *Managing genetic information: Implications for nursing practice.* Washington, DC: American Nurses Publishing.

Scanlon, C., & Fleming, C. (1990). Confronting ethical issues: A nursing survey. *Nursing Management, 21,* 63-65.

Smith, J. (1989). Ethical issues raised by new treatment options. *Maternal-Child Nursing, 14,* 183-186.

Titus, L. (1995). CNA ethics survey published. *Connecticut Nursing News, 66*(4), 1.

Uustal, D. (1993). *Clinical ethics and values: Issues and insights.* East Greenwich, RI: Educational Resources in Healthcare.

Zink, M. (1997). Key moral principles applied to managed care. *Home Healthcare Nurse, 15*(6), 423-425.

Zink, M., & Titus, L. (1994). Nursing ethics committees—Where are they? *Nursing Management, 25*(6), 70-76.

Zink, M., & Titus, L. (1996). *The Nursing Ethical Issues Survey: Examination of hospital versus home care settings* (unpublished manuscript).

Zink, M., & Titus, L. (1997). Nursing ethics committees: Do we need them? In J.C. McCloskey & H.K. Grace (Eds.), *Current issues in nursing* (5th ed.). St. Louis: Mosby.

Sexual Harassment

TONIA DANDRY AIKEN

Sexual harassment is a form of sex discrimination; it is a violation of the Civil Rights Act of 1964. Until the 1970s, the term *sexual harassment* was not acknowledged by most people. During the 1970s, sexual harassment started to gain attention but was not seen as a form of sex discrimination under Title VII of the Civil Rights Act. The focus was on male/female work interactions and not on same-sex violations. In the late 1970s, the term was broadened to include any behavior that required sexual favors in exchange for promotions, advancements, or better benefits. Because this broader definition considered sexual favors a condition of employment, sexual harassment fell under the laws and statutes dealing with sex discrimination.

In the 1980s, sexual harassment was defined in more detail. In 1980, the Equal Employment Opportunity Commission (EEOC) defined sexual harassment in its guidelines as (1) unwelcomed sexual advances, (2) requests for sexual favors, (3) verbal conduct of a sexual nature, or (4) physical conduct of a sexual nature. These advances, requests, and types of conduct were considered sexual harassment when they (1) acted as a term or condition of employment, (2) were a criterion for employment decisions, (3) interfered with the victim's job performance, or (4) created a hostile, intimidating, or offensive work environment.

In the mid-1980s, lawsuits began to surface. One notable suit was *Meritor Savings Bank v. Vinson* (1986). In June 1986, the U.S. Supreme Court affirmed sexual harassment as a cause of action under Title VII. The Supreme Court also held that economic losses were not required for a sexual harassment claim. In *Meritor*, the victim alleged that her supervisor made repeated demands for sexual favors, fondled her in front of other employees, forcibly raped her on numerous occasions, and exposed himself to her. The Court in *Meritor* held that the following were true: (1) The allegations were sufficient for a case of sexual harassment based on a quid-pro-quo theory. (2)

Even if a victim engages in sexual relations with a supervisor, the person can still have a claim for harassment if the conduct was *unwelcome*. (3) The "totality of circumstances" rule will be used to determine if there is evidence of sexual harassment. (4) Employers are not necessarily liable for the sexual harassment acts of their supervisors.

WHO SEXUAL HARASSMENT AFFECTS

Sexual harassment affects many people, not just the victims. Employers can lose not only valuable employees as a result of harassment, but they can also lose the trust and productivity of other employees and monetary awards from such lawsuits and litigation costs. Employees can lose dignity, trust, promotions, monetary gains, jobs, and self-esteem. These factors not only affect the employee victims but also their families and coworkers.

Sexual harassment is against the law. Many more claims have been filed since the early 1970s because people are becoming more educated about sexual harassment and are no longer afraid, embarrassed, or intimidated to bring forth such claims.

TYPES OF SEXUAL HARASSMENT
Quid pro quo

As mentioned earlier, since the 1970s the definition of sexual harassment has been broadened to include more than just sexual demands for preferential treatment at work. Sexual harassment also includes unwelcomed sexual advances; requests for sexual favors, and nonverbal, verbal, or deliberate physical behavior of a sexual nature by the offender. With quid-pro-quo sexual harassment, submission to the above conduct is made implicitly or explicitly a condition of the person's employment; employment decisions are based on whether the employee submits to or rejects the offender's conduct. Following are a few examples:

- A supervisor requires sexual favors of an employee as a requirement for the employee to be promoted, hired, or receive raises.
- A male supervisor promises a new male nurse a promotion if he has a sexual relationship with him.
- A hospital administrator tells a nursing supervisor that she looks great in tight dresses and he likes good looks and brains. The nursing supervisor just walks away after the comment and doesn't acknowledge him. The administrator then "finds fault with her work" and fires her.

In the last example, all of the elements of sexual harassment are present: The employee is a member of a protected group. The sexual remarks and advances were unwelcomed. The harassment was sexually motivated. The employee's reaction to the administrator's advances affected an aspect of her employment (e.g., she was fired). The courts have held that "unwelcomed conduct" is conduct that the employee did not solicit or incite and the employee regards as undesirable or offensive.

CASE A

In a recent case, former female employees brought sexual harassment action against the employer's sole stockholder, doctors, and the employer and its insurers. The court ruled that the sexual activities between the stockholder and employees were welcome and, therefore, did not constitute sexual harassment. The employees also failed to establish battery and intentional infliction of emotional distress (*Lawson v. Straus*, 1999).

Causal Connection

To prove sexual harassment, employees must show a causal connection between the harassment and the job benefit in question. They must show that they were qualified for the job benefit in the absence of harassment. The harasser must also play a role in the benefit decision of the alleged victim (*Neidhardt v. D.H. Holmes, Co.*, 1979).

Hostile Environment

The second type of harassment falls under the hostile environment theory. If the offender or the employment conditions create a hostile environment that unreasonably interferes with a person's job performance or creates an intimidating, offensive, or hostile working environment, a claim of sexual harassment can be made. "Hostile environment" can include unwelcomed sexual advances; requests for sexual favors; verbal conduct of a sexual nature; physical conduct of a sexual nature; sexually explicit jokes; offensive language, gestures, or comments; or sexual pictures, calendars, or objects.

More subtle examples of sexual harassment include the following:

- Requesting a person to have dinner after work
- Requesting a person to have drinks after work
- Requesting a person to participate in other social activities after work

The EEOC will determine whether the conduct was unwelcomed by examining the totality of circumstances of each case. Factors that the EEOC will focus on and that should be reviewed by the company or institution include the following:

- Conduct (verbal, physical, or both)
- Frequency of conduct
- Type of conduct (hostile or offensive)
- Category of offender (coworker, supervisor, or other)
- Others who assisted or were a part of the harassment
- Direction of harassment (focused on one or several individuals)
- Consistency of the victim's conduct

Sexual harassment may consist of only one incident if, for example, an employee is denied a promotion because of refusal of a sexual advance by an employer (quid-pro-quo theory). Under the hostile environment theory the single incident or series of incidents usually has to be quite severe to create a hostile environment. Although the incident may not fall under hostile environment, it may be covered by Title VII as a violation.

CASE B

The U.S. Third Circuit Court of Appeals focused on the scope of *respondeat superior* liability for hostile work environment brought under Title VII of the Civil Rights Act of 1964, 42 U.S.C. sub-section 2000 e-2(a)(1). An employee at Sears Roebuck and Co. reported at the end of a 3-week period that an employee was using sexually derogatory language. She only asked the supervisor if "cursing" was permitted in the workplace. The court held that Sears had neither actual nor constructive notice of harassment until the end of the 3-week period. The court reversed the district court's denial of Sears' motion of judgment as a matter of law and entered judgment in Sears' favor (*Kunin v. Sears Roebuck & Co.*, 1999).

Verbal Sexual Harassment

Verbal remarks can constitute sexual harassment. Several factors are examined to determine whether the remarks can be classified as harassment:

1. Were the remarks derogatory?
2. Were the remarks hostile?

3. Did the alleged harasser single out the victim?
4. Did the victim participate in any exchanges with the alleged harasser?
5. What is the relationship between the parties involved?

Sexual Harassment of Men

Title VII protects both men and women. For example, a male general manager pressures two male employees to participate in and observe sex with his secretary. He threatened to blackball them, eliminate medical benefits, and fire them if they refuse to participate in the ménage à trois. The court held the employer liable for quid-pro-quo and hostile environment sexual harassment (*Showalter v. Allison Reed Group, Inc.,* 1991).

Homosexual Harassment

Title VII prohibits sexual harassment by homosexuals against members of the same sex. In an Alabama case (*Joyner v. AAA Cooper Transportation,* 1983), a male employee sued for sexual harassment based on unwelcomed homosexual advances by the terminal manager. The employee was laid off and the employer refused to recall him when a position became available. The employee was entitled to be reinstated with back pay.

Examples of Offensive Conduct

Offensive conduct can be sexual in nature, demeaning, threatening, or hostile. Case examples of conduct that were found by the courts to be "welcomed" include:

1. An employee tells dirty jokes or makes dirty remarks, and the discussions are never complained about by the employee.
2. The employee participates in sexual innuendoes or vulgar story telling.
3. The employee flirts and behaves provocatively and asks the alleged harasser to have dinner at his or her home despite repeated refusals by the harassed.

Conduct does not have to be directed at the victim. It can either be observed, or the victim can have knowledge of incidents involving other employees that affects the plaintiff's psychological and emotional status and well-being. For example, an environment would be considered hostile if a female nurse has to listen to remarks about her anatomy and physical characteristics while she is in the operating room. If a sexually explicit joke about men is shown and passed around the emergency department by female coworkers, and a male nurse is offended and embarrassed by it, the requirements for a hostile environment have been met. If a victim is aware that those employees who have sex with the supervisor receive more benefits, then a hostile environment exists.

WHY PEOPLE SEXUALLY HARASS OTHERS

Power is one reason for sexual harassment. It is an abuse of authority by someone (usually in a supervisory position) who uses power, force, and authority over someone in a lower position. Harassers can be supervisors, subordinates, customers, patients, suppliers, friends, acquaintances, relatives, business associates, or strangers. Harassers are found at all levels and in all occupations. Harassment also takes place among both genders: male to female, female to male, male to male, and female to female.

Dominance

The need to dominate also lends itself to influencing or controlling others. Harassers use dominating behavior to get what they want or need. Some dominate to prevent from being dominated by others. Dominating individuals look for weak traits or spots they can use to control the other individual.

Insecurity is another reason why individuals harass. By harassing or "bullying" others, these people hide their insecurities. Power, dominance, and insecurity needs result in the type of harasser seen in the workplace.

EMPLOYEE/EMPLOYER ACTIONS AFTER HARASSMENT

If you are being harassed, do something about it. Many employers have developed sexual harassment policies and procedures that include guidelines on the administrative process, who should be notified, and penalties for the harasser.

The procedures for a complaint should be confidential and fair to both parties. These policies and procedures should apply to employees, management, and men and women alike. Confidentiality is crucial because of the nature of the complaint. If the complaint is false, it could ruin both the private life and the public life and career of an individual.

If the victim knows that confidentiality will not be maintained, he or she is less likely to come forward because of the implications and effects on his or her public and private life. This is not how a program should be structured. Harassment programs must encourage complaints.

Complaints should be handled promptly, seriously, and sensitively. Programs may provide such things as counseling to victims, publication and publicizing the complaint process, and training employee support groups to aid victims. Employers must maintain an environment that continues to show support and respect for victims after complaints are made.

If you are a victim of sexual harassment, the following actions are crucial:

1. Do not accept your position as a victim.
2. Do something about the harassment.
3. Respond promptly and assertively toward the problem.
4. Make your feelings and position known to the harasser.
5. Communicate directly to the harasser that his or her conduct is unwelcome either through a face-to-face confrontation or through conduct that demonstrates to the harasser that the conduct is unwelcome.
6. Document the times and places of harassment, the people having knowledge of the incidents, and your reactions to and comments about the behavior of the harasser.
7. Document what you have said to the harasser.
8. Report continuing harassment to the appropriate person in your company or institution. If the harasser is your supervisor and the person to whom you report, notify the person with authority over the supervisor.
9. Be assertive and follow through with the process.
10. Do not allow harassment to continue.
11. If these methods are ineffective, contact your local EEOC office as soon as possible.

If you know someone who is being harassed, be supportive and encourage that person to pursue the complaint process. As an employee, know and understand sexual harassment; know how to respond to the harassment and know the process for making a formal complaint. You can also function as a teacher, informing your coworkers about the types of sexual harassment and what to do if harassed.

If you are an administrator, be sure that your institution or company has an effective complaint program and reasonable policies and procedures that can be followed to handle such matters as quickly and confidentially as possible. However, prevention is the best tool. A statement about sexual harassment should be in the institution's policy manual and in the employee handbook.

All personnel in supervisory positions should be notified about the procedures for handling sexual harassment problems. Emphasis should be placed on disapproval of harassers and sanctions for victims. Keep communication lines open with the victim and witnesses. Do not ostracize the victim or make the claim public. Lack of communication and attention given to a claim sends out a message that sexual harassers shouldn't worry because the company or facility does not place such problems high on its priority list. If an employer can prove that the harassment has been eliminated, the victim has been made "whole" again, and future preventive measures have been taken, the EEOC will usually close the case.

EMPLOYER PROBLEMS

Employers face multiple problems when harassers are in the workplace. Following are just a few of the ramifications:

1. Turnover costs of rehiring, recruiting, and retraining employees
2. Dehumanization of employees—humiliation, embarrassment, and physical problems such as headaches or gastrointestinal upsets
3. Increased absenteeism
4. Loss of productivity
5. Inability to concentrate
6. Attorneys' fees
7. Settlement of damage awards

LAWS AFFECTING EMPLOYER LIABILITY

Several state and federal laws pertain specifically to the employer's liability in cases of sexual harassment. These include Title VII of the Civil Rights Act of 1964 and its interpretation by the EEOC; state and local sexual discrimination laws and regulations; and federal or state courts or administrative agency decisions on sexual harassment claims.

PREVENTION OF SEXUAL HARASSMENT IN THE WORKPLACE

To prevent sexual harassment, employers should develop and adopt a strong sexual harassment policy; communicate the policy to all employees; and train supervisory personnel to handle harassment problems in a professional and sensitive manner. The employer can be held liable if the employer knew or should have known of the harassment and failed to take appropriate and immediate action to correct it.

How to Discourage Sexual Harassment

To discourage sexual harassment, every complaint should be investigated. A written policy and procedure specifically prohibiting sexual harassment should be developed. Likewise, a policy and procedure for employee complaints should be developed.

How the Policy Can Be Communicated to Employees

The following venues can be used to let employees know about the sexual harassment policies:

1. Posting information (bulletin boards)
2. Newsletters
3. Institution or company papers
4. Memos (sent out at least once a year)
5. Employee committees/employee meetings
6. Personal communications
7. Employee evaluations
8. Employee disciplinary proceedings
9. Case decisions in court
10. Personnel policy and procedure manuals
11. New employee orientation and training meetings
12. Questionnaires and surveys

Developing a Sexual Harassment Policy

A sexual harassment policy should include the following information:

1. How to lodge a complaint
2. Where to lodge a complaint
3. Whom to speak to about potential complaints or harassing conduct

Developing Policies for the Managerial Level

Procedures for managerial personnel should be developed on the following:

1. How to spot harassment
2. What to do when harassing conduct is detected
3. How to dissolve the problems
4. How to prevent potential lawsuits

Policies for this level should include the following:

1. Types of conduct that constitute sexual harassment
2. Managerial obligations for identifying and handling harassment
3. What is acceptable and unacceptable behavior
4. The complaint process (where to go, whom to see, what to do, and when to do it)
5. The potential for liability and exposure to the employer for such claims

To prevent a breach of contract suit (e.g., do not guarantee absolute confidentiality), nothing should be guaranteed in this policy that cannot be accomplished. Disclaimers may be used (e.g., this policy is not to be construed as a contract between the employer and employee).

Developing the Complaint Procedure

Oral Complaints. Some companies make sexual harassment complaint procedures separate from the usual grievance procedure, whereas others do not. Here are some guidelines:

1. Allow both oral and written complaints.
2. The employer's representative must put the oral complaint in writing.
3. Have the victim read and verify it for accuracy.

Pros and Cons.

1. Grievance procedures may take too long.
2. Confidentiality may be diminished because of the structure of the routine grievance procedure.
3. Harassment claims should be given immediate attention by the upper echelon of a company or facility.
4. Policy language must emphasize that there will be prompt investigation of complaints and appropriate actions taken against persons guilty of harassing.
5. The employer must maintain all information regarding complaint as confidential as possible for both victims and witnesses.

EQUAL EMPLOYMENT OPPORTUNITY COMMISSION (EEOC)

The EEOC provides guidelines that are neither law nor binding in court but do carry considerable weight.

Filing a Charge with the EEOC

A victim can file a charge at any field office located in cities throughout the country. The offices are usually listed under U.S. Government in the phone book.

Time Limits for Filing. A sexual discrimination charge must be filed with the EEOC within 180 days of the alleged discriminatory act *or* within 300 days if there is a state or local employment practices agency that enforces a law prohibiting such discriminatory practices. It is best to contact the EEOC as soon as you believe discrimination has taken place so that you can file a claim in a timely manner.

Laws Enforced

The EEOC enforces Title VII of the Civil Rights Act of 1964, which prohibits discrimination based on race, color, religion, sex, or national origin. It also enforces the Age Discrimination in Employment Act, the Equal Pay Act, and sections of the Civil Rights Act of 1991. Other acts covered include Title I of the Americans with Disabilities Act, which prohibits discrimination in the private sector, state and local government. The ADA prohibits discrimination against disabled persons in the federal government.

Legal Remedies

Actual Damages. With Title VII, the victim can receive actual damages such as promotions, lost benefits, hiring, reinstatement, and back pay that were lost as a result of the harassment.

Injunctive Relief. Injunctive relief is obtained through the courts and orders the employer to stop the alleged harassment and to take steps to prevent such conduct in the future.

Attorney's Fees. Attorney's fees are usually allowed in these cases.

Punitive Damages. Punitive damages are intended to punish the defendant for the egregious nature of the tort. The defendant's actions must be willful and wanton, and the damages are not based on the plaintiff's actual monetary loss. The award is usually doubled or tripled to "punish" the defendant economically to deter this type of behavior in the future. Punitive damages may be awarded if the employer acted with reckless indifference or malice.

Other Damages. Compensation may be given for future pecuniary losses, mental anguish, and inconvenience.

Lawsuit Against Employer. A lawsuit can also be filed directly against the employer and the harasser based on a breach of contract or tort law. Awards can include compensatory damages, economic damages, and actual damages. Tort suits may allow punitive damages.

Intentional Tort Suit. Victims may also sue for such intentional torts as assault, battery, wrongful termination, and intentional infliction of emotional distress.

Criminal Suits. In some cases, the harasser may be charged with a criminal offense such as assault, battery, rape, and attempted rape. The employer usually has no liability under criminal statutes although civil liability still exists.

Many states now have laws that deal with sexual harassment. Victims may use the state court system, claiming a violation of state fair employment laws and are entitled to a jury trial in most states. However, under Title VII there is no jury. In the state courts, awards can include punitive damages, compensatory damages, back pay, and legal fees.

15 Women Will Share $1.2 Million for Ordeal. NEW YORK—Fifteen women who accused their former boss of lewd behavior, including grabbing their breasts and buttocks, going to the bathroom with the door open and conducting business with his fly down, will share a nearly $1.185 [million] settlement.

The $1.185 million sum is more than twice the biggest previous settlement ever obtained by the EEOC in a sexual harassment case.

The women worked as secretaries or executive assistants for a chief executive of Del Laboratories of Farmdale.

As part of the settlement, the company agrees to hold training sessions for its 1,600 employees.

CASE EXAMPLE

In an Ohio Case the court held that to recover on a sexual harassment claim in the workplace, the employee must prove the following:

1. The employee is a protected class
2. Sexual harassment in the form of unwelcomed sexual advances or requests for sexual favors
3. Harassment complained of was based on sex
4. Submission to the advances was an implied or expressed condition of the job or refusal to submit to the employer's sexual demands resulted in problems with the job.

The court found that the alleged actions of the physician who bit a cake shaped like a breast at an office party, told a staff member she looked "really hot today," stated an employee looked sexier after breast surgery, and made unwanted sexual advances to a staff worker did *not support a sexual harassment claim by the nurse who was an employee and a patient (none of the alleged incidents were directed at the nurse)* (Regan Report, 1999).

REFERENCES

Joyner v. AAA Cooper Transportation, (D.C. Ala. 1983).

Lawson v. Straus, 750 S.2d 234; La. App. 4 Cir 1999.

Kunin v. Sears Roebuck & Co., No. 98-1481, 3d Cir. 1999.

Meritor Savings Bank v. Vinson, U.S. Sup Ct, No. 84-1979, June 19, 1986.

Niedhardt v. D.H. Holmes, Co., 21 Fair Empl. Prac. Employment Practice CAS.BNA 452 (E.D. La. 1979), aff'd 624 F. 2d 1097 (5th Cir.).

The Regan Report on Nursing Law. Vol. 40, No. 6, November, 1999.

Tahkach v. Am. Med. Technology, Inc., 715 N.E. 577-OH (1998).

Showalter v. Allison Reed Group, Inc., 767 F. Supp. 1205 (DIR. 1991).

BIBLIOGRAPHY

Aiken, T.D. (Contributor/Editor). (1994). *Legal, ethical, and political issues in nursing.* Philadelphia: FA Davis Company.

How to recognize and prevent sexual harassment in the workplace. (1992). Madison, CT: Business and Legal Reports, Inc.

Howard, J., & Myers, M.S. (1992). *Countering sexual harassment: A handbook for self-defense.* Florida: Choctaw Publishing.

Lloyd, K.L. (1992). *Sexual harassment: How to keep your company out of court.* New York: Panel Publishers, Inc.

RESOURCE

The American Nurses Association—Workplace Information Series—Sexual Harassment. It's Against the Law.

American Nurses Association
600 Maryland Ave., S.W., Suite 100 West
Washington, DC 20024-2571
1-800-274-4ANA

Web site for American Nurses Association: www.nursingworld.org

CHAPTER 75

Pediatric Nursing and TV Viewing

An Opportunity to Affect Children's Health

LINDA K. CHASE, JODY L. KURTT

In the fifth edition of this book the chapter on current issues in pediatric nursing addressed significant changes and advances in health care and pediatric nursing, as well as the status of children's health in the United States as the turn of the century approached. Many of those issues are still relevant today, and the indicators of health for our nation's children have not significantly improved despite a strong U.S. economy and low unemployment. In this sixth edition, our chapter focuses on one significant issue affecting the lives of children today—television—the risks it poses for children's health and development and the opportunities for pediatric nurses to influence and shape the viewing habits of children and families through education and modeling.

TV VIEWING

Children and families are pressured more and more today by the conveniences and technology of modern society. The advent of television and cable networks has been a major influence on the lives of children and families for the past five decades. In recent years the effects of TV viewing on children have attracted significant attention by health care professionals. A growing body of literature documents the negative impact of television on the behavior and health of children and adolescents (Centerwall, 1992; Comstock & Strasburger, 1990; Dietz & Gortmaker, 1985; Hei, Gold, Champman, Qaqundah, & Wong, 1990; Rothenberg, 1975; Somers, 1976; Strasburger, 1992).

In 1984 the American Academy of Pediatrics (AAP) first issued a statement warning parents about the effects of television viewing on children. *"After the family, television is probably the most important social influence on child development in our society. By high school graduation the average teen will have spent more time watching television*

than in the classroom" (AAP, 1984). These statistics and others demonstrate the significant influence that television has on child and adolescent health and behavior (Strasburger & Donnerstein, 1999). Television has a wide range of effects on many aspects of children's lives including their emotional, social, cognitive, and physical development. Although television can have a positive impact on children, the potential negative impact deserves the attention of pediatric nurses, health care professionals, educators, parents, and children.

TV Viewing: Facts and Statistics

In examining the statistics, facts, and related research on television and children, it should be noted that both positive and negative effects exist (see box, p. 584). Age-appropriate television can teach children healthy behaviors and promote positive family values and has unlimited capacity for educational opportunities. Unfortunately, the negative effects of television often outweigh these positive effects. This chapter provides information regarding the specific elements of television that have a negative impact on children's health today. It is critical for pediatric nurses to understand the impact of television on youth, to educate and empower parents and teachers regarding television, and to actively model positive use of TV programming in settings in which children receive health care.

Time Spent Watching Television. Children and adolescents in the United States spend more time watching television than on any other activity except for sleeping (AAP, 1995; A.C. Nielsen Company, 1990). By the time today's children reach age 70, they will have spent a total of 7 to 10 years of their lives watching television (Strasburger, 1993). On average, American children view 23 hours of television per week; children ages 2 to 5 years watch more than 27 hours of television per week (AAP,

EFFECTS OF TV VIEWING

Positive: Age-appropriate television can teach children good behaviors and thinking skills. Appropriate viewing can promote:
- *Imaginary skills:* Television teaches children how to develop and use their imagination.
- *Role playing:* Children will model positive adult-like behaviors.
- *Family values:* Children can learn about family values through TV viewing.
- *Clock skills:* The timing of shows helps to teach the concept of time.
- *Thinking skills:* Children can learn letters, numbers, shapes, and colors through TV viewing.
- *Decision making:* Asking children about what they see and how they will react to situations that they see on television can allow them to make choices and learn to strategize how to cope with difficult situations in appropriate ways.

Negative: Television is not selective in what it teaches children. Along with positive effects, it can give unhealthy, false, or negative messages. Too much or inappropriate viewing can have the following effects:
- *Reality check:* Young children cannot distinguish between fantasy and reality.
- *Violence:* Heavy exposure to television increases the likelihood of aggressive behavior, especially in boys. Weapons appear an average of nine times per hour on prime time programs.
- *Sexuality:* Television may present the young child with mature content and does not promote sexual responsibility.
- *Stereotypes:* Television may present roles based on race, gender, age, and physical beauty. Values of youth and physical attractiveness develop based on these biases.
- *Lifestyle habits:* For the younger child, the television too often becomes a substitute for reading, playing with friends, exercise, and hobbies. Too much viewing leaves the child with little time for other activities that nurture development and creativity.
- *Obesity:* Obesity is linked with television because of inactivity, advertising of low nutrition foods, and snacking during viewing.
- *Alcohol and drugs:* Television promotes unhealthy behaviors such as smoking, drug, and alcohol use.
- *Commercialism:* The young child is not able to distinguish between commercials and reality.
- *Programming:* Special tactics including volume changes, intense plots, suspense, loud music, and rapid-fire commercials are used to grab the child's attention and hold it.

1995; Dowell, 1998) (see box, right). The American Academy of Pediatrics recommends that parents limit their children's time watching television to 1 to 2 hours per day (AAP, 1995).

A heightened awareness regarding the significant amount of time that children spend in front of the television and appropriate limits to viewing is essential for pediatric nurses working in hospitals, clinics, schools, and other agencies. This knowledge should be shared with peers and with the public in an effort to decrease TV viewing time overall and to enhance appropriate selection of programs.

Violence and Television. Numerous studies and reviews attest to the fact that exposure to television violence increases the likelihood of aggressive behavior, particularly in males (Comstock & Strasburger, 1990; Dietz & Strasburger, 1991; Green, 1993). Images and models of violence surround us and are easily available to children: Children watch an average of 8,000 murders and 100,000 other violent acts on television before finishing elementary school. Experts link childhood violence to violence

TIME SPENT WATCHING TELEVISION AND RELATED FACTS

- The average 2- to 11-year-old watches about 25 hours of television per week.
- Today's children spend more time watching television (15,000 hours) than they do in school (11,000 hours).
- During an average year, American children are exposed to more than 15,000 sexual references, yet less than 170 will deal with self-control behaviors.
- During the average year, American children are exposed to between 1,000 and 2,000 beer and wine commercials.
- By high school graduation the average U.S. child will have viewed 18,000 TV murders, many of which are bloodless and painless and depict neither guilt nor remorse in the person who commits the murder.
- A significant negative effect linked to greater than 1 to 2 hours per day of TV viewing has been negative academic performance, especially reading scores.

in the media (Spence, 1995). The existence of a link between what is viewed on the TV screen and subsequent behavior has been demonstrated in children as young as 14 months (Dowell, 1998).

In the past, children admired TV stars who possessed honor, truth, and bravery. Today's television super heroes model aggressive behavior traits and use weapons of powerful destruction. Violent characters are depicted as powerful, exciting, and charismatic. Their violent behaviors are often portrayed as being justified by the use of violence against villains (Dowell, 1998). Children learn from what they see; therefore it should be no surprise that violence on television provokes violent or aggressive behavior in children (Sege & Dietz, 1994).

TV violence is often represented as an effective problem-solving strategy; it ends a confrontation quickly and without the need for patience, negotiation, or compromise (Sege & Dietz, 1994). The rewards that heroes receive for their violent behavior legitimize and endorse violence as a means of problem solving (Sege & Dietz, 1994). The rapidity with which difficulties and conflicts are resolved on television through the use of violence and the absence of negative consequences for those actions increase the likelihood that violence will be among the first problem-solving strategies that a child selects, rather than the last (Sege & Dietz, 1994). Frequent viewing of violence and the lack of recognition of the long-term aftermath for its victims can impair children's ability to distinguish between fantasy and reality and desensitize them to the pain and suffering of others (Sege & Dietz, 1994). This combination of powerful factors influences children to accept violence as an acceptable alternative to life's conflicts and problems.

In recent years the number of children victimized by violence has soared as has the number of teen offenders. Although the escalating violence against and by children is a cumulative manifestation of many serious and neglected societal ills, including child and family poverty, increasing economic inequality, racial intolerance, drug and alcohol abuse, and the disintegration of family values and support, the pervasive violence in our popular culture and television must also be recognized as a major contributing factor (Children's Defense Fund, 1994).

Pediatric nurses can influence the viewing habits of families by sharing with patients and parents, educators, and community groups information about the negative impact of TV violence on children's behavior and health. Pediatric nurses must encourage and support parents in limiting the exposure of their children to violence on television and assist them in selecting age-appropriate, non-

violent programming that provides positive role models for children. Important anticipatory guidance for parents includes limiting children's TV viewing to 1 to 2 hours per day, avoiding or removing televisions in children's bedrooms where viewing is done in isolation, and coviewing of TV programs by parents and children, which provides an opportunity for parents to discuss alternative choices to aggressive and violent behavior.

Sex and Television. The link between viewing sexual acts on television and sexual activity in kids is not as clear as the linkage between viewing TV violence and violent behavior in children. The media provides a major source of sexual content and information for teenagers. Several studies have demonstrated a connection between media with high sexual content and changes in teenagers' sexual behavior (Strasburger & Donnerstein, 1999). Explicit TV messages promoting promiscuous and unprotected sexual activity are cause for concern. American teens see an estimated 15,000 sexual references and innuendoes per year on television, yet only 170 of these references deal with sexual responsibility, abstinence, or contraception (Harris & Associates, 1988). Often TV sex is portrayed as impersonal and exploitative (Dowell, 1998). Music videos, popular with teenagers, are full of sexually suggestive material (75%) and violent acts (56%) (Dowell, 1998).

Teenage pregnancy and sexually transmitted diseases among adolescents and young adults in the United States represent major sources of injury, illness, and death. The United States has the highest teenage pregnancy rate in the Western world despite the fact that American teenagers are not having sexual intercourse at higher rates than teenagers in other countries (Strasburger, 1992). With an absence of appropriate sexual messages from the media and a lack of abstinence and birth control, the high teen pregnancy rate will continue. Young people are learning behavioral cues from the media; the only way to change this is through less exposure (Strasburger & Donnerstein, 1999).

Alcohol, Drugs, and Television. The average American teenager views between 1,000 and 2,000 beer and wine commercials per year (Strasburger, 1993). Numerous studies document that children and adolescents who are exposed to greater amounts of alcohol advertising are more likely to either use or intend to use such products. Although parents, peers, and other environmental influences are important in shaping the beliefs and ultimately the drinking behaviors of children and adolescents, alcohol advertising may also be an important source through which children learn about this drug (Grube & Wallack, 1994).

The effects of alcohol advertising are widespread. In a study by Grube and Wallack (1994), which consisted of fifth and sixth graders from a public school district, it was found that children who were more aware of beer advertisements had more favorable beliefs about drinking, intended to drink more as adults, and had more knowledge about beer brands and slogans. This supports the conclusion that a large amount of alcohol advertising can lead to increased consumption (Strasburger, 1993).

There is a strong link between cigarette advertising and adolescent smoking behavior (Strasburger & Donnerstein, 1999). Despite the fact that tobacco products were banned on television by the Public Health Cigarette Smoking Act of 1969, much passive advertising still exists on television (Strasburger, 1993). There is enormous opportunity for nurses to provide education regarding TV viewing and alcohol and tobacco use through the participation of curriculum development at the primary and secondary grade levels.

Academics, Cognitive Development, and Television. Interaction with children is key to their development; television provides little or none of the interaction that children need. Excessive TV viewing may result in missed opportunities for cognitive and social interaction in imaginary play and all critical components of early childhood development. Television by default becomes the socializer of children if parents are not present. It is a passive way of structuring time that would otherwise be spent in active play with others, in community activities, studying, reading, or thinking (Derksen & Strasburger, 1994).

Academic performance may be affected by too much television. On average, children in the United States spend more time viewing television than they do in school (Strasburger, 1993). Academic studies have demonstrated that greater than 1 to 2 hours of TV viewing per day has a negative effect on academic performance, especially reading scores (Strasburger, 1986). In addition to decreased reading ability, other negative effects of television on academics include decreased Scholastic Achievement Test (SAT) scores, decreased writing skills, decreased attention span, decreased imagination, decreased creativity, and decreased homework completion. Although television can, in the right environment, provide some positive interaction for young children (Dowel, 1998), the potential negative impact on cognitive development and academic achievement is compelling.

Television and Obesity. The United States has experienced alarming increases in obesity among children and adolescents during the past 30 years (Troiano & Flegal, 1998). Obesity is the most common nutritional disorder of the age group 10 to 15 years old. Television has been found to be a major cause of children's overeating in part because of the amount of time spent watching television, resulting in decreased physical activity and the consumption of fatty, calorie-packed foods encouraged by TV commercials (Gortmaker et al., 1996).

The relationship between the hours of television viewed and the prevalence of obesity is convincing. In a major study, Gortmaker et al. (1996) found that the odds of children being overweight were 4.6 times greater for youth watching more than 5 hours of television per day compared with those watching 0 to 2 hours per day. In another study, similar findings showed that children who watched at least 4 hours of television daily were more likely to be overweight than those who watched less television (Anderson, Crespo, Bartlett, Cheskin, & Pratt, 1998).

Inappropriate television viewing (greater than 2 hours per day) has also been associated with hypercholesterolemia (Wong et al., 1992). A second issue is that TV viewing is linked to higher dietary fat intake (Robinson & Killen, 1995). Snacking while watching television often includes foods that are high in fat, calories, sugar, and salt but are also low in nutrients (Vessey, Yim-Chiplis, & MacKenzie, 1998). The average child watches more than 20,000 television commercials per year, approximately two thirds are for food, most frequently high-sugar foods. Advertising influences children's snack selection and families' purchasing habits (Taras, Sallis, Patterson, Nader, & Nelson, 1989).

Television and Commercialism. Young children are especially vulnerable to TV commercial messages because of the low cognitive level of understanding required to understand them (Zuckerman & Zuckerman, 1985). Young people have difficulty distinguishing between program content and commercial messages and are easily influenced by techniques used to enhance the attractiveness of products. Overall, studies on the impact of TV commercials on health-related behaviors suggest that children's attitudes toward food, medicine, and health products are influenced by TV commercials (Zuckerman & Zuckerman, 1985).

Another issue of focus is violent commercials. Violent commercials are frequently shown during nonviolent programming (Anderson, 1997). This is a concern for parents who do not anticipate that their children will be exposed to violence during a family-oriented program.

TV Viewing in Hospitalized Children. The issue of TV viewing by hospitalized children has gained attention in recent decades (Waldner-Guttentag, Albritton, & Kettner, 1981). Hospitalized patients may be exposed to more commercials, excessive daytime programming, and more overall hours of TV programming because of their immobility. This awareness of increased viewing by hospitalized patients creates a challenge for pediatric nurses and health care professionals to provide appropriate viewing selections.

The heavy use of television in the hospital is understandable considering that it is often a means for providing entertainment and diversion to children in a boring or unfamiliar environment (Waldner-Guttentag et al., 1981). Staff and parents should be encouraged to choose appropriate programming, turn off the TV when patients are engaged in other activities, and provide for alternative age-appropriate activities during hospitalization. Another option that is becoming standard in children's hospitals is to have special TV programming available such as a "children's channel" that delivers prescreened, nonviolent, and commercial-free programming. A children's channel is usually provided through a closed-circuit network and is educational and entertaining. Age-specific programs can be made available to various age groups at different times of the day. Another option for hospitalized children is the use of videotapes; this allows for noncommercialized, appropriate selection of content.

Strategies and Interventions

Pediatric nurses need to provide children, adolescents, and parents with the knowledge and skills to "take control" of their TV viewing habits. Equipping parents with the knowledge of the potential positive and negative effects of TV viewing is essential. The impact of too many hours of television and its linkages to aggressive and violent behavior, sexual activity, obesity, and drug, alcohol, and tobacco use must be reinforced. Recommendations to parents, children, and teens for TV viewing can help shape current and future health habits for families (see box, below).

GENERAL GUIDELINES FOR TV VIEWING

- Limit TV viewing to 1 to 2 hours per day.
- Encourage coviewing of television by parents and children.
- Encourage nonviolent, high-quality, age-appropriate programs.
- Educate children regarding commercials.
- Find constructive alternatives to watching television.
- Keep televisions out of children's rooms.
- Turn the television off during mealtimes and when doing homework.

There is also an opportunity to educate hospitalized patients and their families (a captive audience) to the effects of TV viewing. An episode of acute hospitalization may not afford the best timing to ask families to actually change TV viewing habits, but it certainly can be a time for nurses to share information with families about TV viewing and its effects on children's health. A brochure of TV facts can be taken home and families encouraged to evaluate and improve their viewing habits. This opportunity is also available for children and families in ambulatory settings for well-child or specialty service. Waiting rooms, examination rooms, and patient rooms should be stocked with eye-catching posters; literature related to TV viewing should be systematically given to families along with other health information.

School settings provide an excellent avenue for pediatric nurses to deliver education regarding TV viewing issues. Providing classroom curriculum is one method for nurses to present information directly to students and stimulate appropriate TV viewing habits. Another effective strategy for education of school-aged students and families is presentations at school and community heath fairs.

An environment that pediatric nurses and parents must not overlook with regard to TV viewing is children's day care settings. Frequently, licensed day care facilities and in-home day care providers allow children access to televisions. Parents should be concerned about TV viewing in day care settings and evaluate the amount of time that the television is on, when it is used, types of programming allowed, and the amount of adult supervision during viewing times. If the day care setting serves children of various ages, parents should ensure that young toddler and preschool-age children are not viewing TV programs more appropriate for older children. Pediatric nurses must take the opportunity to educate day care providers about the positive and negative impact that television can have on children and emphasize the providers' responsibility to ensure age-appropriate, nonviolent programming for those in their care.

As pediatric nurses, we must recognize the impact of television on children's health and educate other health care professionals, teachers, community leaders, and children and parents. It is important for nurses and other professionals to guide and shape children's viewing habits by modeling positive TV viewing in the home, day care, and health care settings. To do nothing about poor TV viewing habits in the lives of children and adolescents today is no longer acceptable.

REFERENCES

A.C. Nielsen Company. (1990). *Nielsen report on television.* Northbrook, IL: Nielsen Media Research.

American Academy of Pediatrics Committee on Communications. (1995). Children, adolescents, and television. *Pediatrics, 96*(4), 786-787.

American Academy of Pediatrics Task Force on Children and Television. (1984). Children, adolescents, and television. *News and Comment, 35,* 8.

Andersen, R.E., Crespo, C.J., Bartlett, S.J., Cheskin, L.J., & Pratt, M. (1998). Relationship of physical activity and television watching with body weight and level of fatness among children. Results from the Third National Health and Nutrition Examination Survey. *Journal of the American Medical Association, 279,* 938-942.

Anderson, C. (1997). Violence in television commercials during nonviolent programming, the 1996 Major League Baseball playoffs. *Journal of the American Medical Association, 278*(13), 1045-1046.

Centerwall, B.S. (1992). Television and violence. The scale of the problem and where to go from here. *Journal of the American Medical Association, 267*(22), 3059-3063.

Children's Defense Fund. (1994). *The state of America's children yearbook.* Washington, DC: U.S. Government Printing Office.

Comstock, G.C., & Strasburger, V.C. (1990). Deceptive appearances: Television violence and aggressive behavior. *Journal of Adolescent Health Care, 11*(1), 31-44.

Derksen, D.J., & Strasburger, V.C. (1994). Children and the influence of the media. *Primary Care, 21,* 747-758.

Dietz, Jr., W.H., & Gortmaker, S.L. (1985). Do we fatten our children at the television set? Obesity and television viewing in children and adolescents. *Pediatrics, 75*(5), 807-812.

Dietz, W.H., & Strasburger, V.C. (1991). Children, adolescents and television. *Current Problems in Pediatrics, 21,* 8-31.

Dowell, D. (1998). Effects of television on children: A review of the literature and recommendations for nurse practitioners. *American Journal of Nurse Practitioners,* 31-37.

Gortmaker, S.L., Must, A., Sobol, A.M., Peterson, K., Colditz, G.A., & Dietz, W.H. (1996). Television viewing as a cause of increasing obesity among children in the United States, 1986-1990. *Archives of Pediatric Adolescent Medicine, 150,* 356-361.

Green, R.G. (1993). Television and aggression: Recent developments in research and theory. In D. Zillmann, J. Bryant, A.C. Huston (Eds.), *Media, children and the family: Social scientific, psychodynamic, and clinical perspectives.* Hillsdale, NJ: Erlbaum.

Grube, J.W., & Wallack, P. (1994). Television beer advertising and drinking knowledge, beliefs and intentions among schoolchildren. *American Journal of Public Health, 84*(2), 254-258.

Harris, L., & Associates. (1988). *Sexual material on American network television during the 1987-88 season.* New York: Planned Parenthood Federation of America.

Hei, T.K., Gold, K.V., Chapman, B.G., Qaqundah, P.Y., & Wong, N.D. (1990). Television viewing as predictor of elevated blood cholesterol levels in children. *Circulation, 82*(suppl 3), 227. Television in American Society, Lincoln, NE, University of Nebraska Press.

Robinson, T.N., & Killen, J.D. (1995). Ethnic and gender differences in the relationships between television viewing and obesity, physical activity and dietary fat intake. *Journal of Health Education, 26,* 591-598.

Rothenberg, M.B. (1975). Effect of television violence on children and youth. *Journal of the American Medical Association, 234*(10), 1043-1046.

Sege, R., & Dietz, W. (1994). Television viewing and violence in children: The pediatrician as agent for change. *Pediatrics, 94*(4), 600-607.

Somers, A.R. (1976). Violence, television, and the health of American youth. *The New England Journal of Medicine, 294*(15), 811-817.

Spence, A. (1995). Family instability leaves children vulnerable. *AAP News,* 10-11, 144-151.

Strasburger, V.C. (1986). Does television affect learning and school performance? *Pediatrician, 38,* 141-147.

Strasburger, V.C. (1992). Children, adolescents, and television. *Pediatrics in Review, 13*(4), 144-151.

Strasburger, V.C. (1993). Children, adolescents and the media: Five crucial issues. *Adolescent Medicine, 4*(3), 479-493.

Strasburger, V.C., & Donnerstein, E. (1999). Children, adolescents, and the media: Issues and solutions. *Pediatrics, 103*(1), 129-139.

Taras, H.L., Sallis, J.F., Patterson, T.L., Nader, P.R., & Nelson, J.A. (1989). Television's influence on children's diet and physical activity. *Developmental and Behavioral Pediatrics, 10,* 176-180.

Troiano, R.P., & Flegal, K.M. (1998). Overweight children and adolescents: Description, epidemiology, and demographics. *Pediatrics, 101,* 497-504.

Vessey, J.A., Yim-Chiplis, P.K., & MacKenzie, N.R. (1998). Effects of television viewing on children's development. *Pediatric Nursing, 23*(5), 483-486.

Waldner-Guttentag, D.N., Albritton, W.L., & Kettner, R.B. (1981). Daytime television viewing by hospitalized children. *Pediatrics, 68*(5), 672-676.

Wong, N.D., Hei, T.K., Qaqundah, P.Y., Davidson, D.M., Bassin, S.L., & Gold, K.V. (1992). Television viewing and pediatric hypercholesterolemia. *Pediatrics, 90,* 75-79.

Zuckerman, D.M., & Zuckerman, B.S. (1985). Television's impact on children. *Pediatrics, 75*(2), 233-239.

SUGGESTED READINGS

Abelman, R. (1995). *Reclaiming the wasteland: TV and gifted children.* Cresshill, NJ: Hampton Press, Inc.

American Academy of Pediatrics Committee on Communications. (1990). Children, adolescents, and television. *Pediatrics, 85*(6), 1119-1120.

American Academy of Pediatrics Committee on Communications. (1992). The commercialization of children's television. *Pediatrics, 89*(2), 343-344.

American Academy of Pediatrics Committee on Communications. (1995). Children, adolescents, and television. *Pediatrics, 96*(4), 786-787.

American Academy of Pediatrics Committee on Communications. (1995). Media violence. *Pediatrics, 95,* 949-951.

Andrews, N. (1986). Pediatric television [guest editorial]. *CHC, 15*(2), 68-69.

Baden, M. (1977). TV for our children: We can do better [letter to the editor]. *The Journal of Pediatrics, 90*(5), 846-847.

Bordeaux, B.R. (1986). Television viewing patterns of hospitalized school-aged children and adolescents. *CHC, 15*(2), 70-75.

Centers for Disease Control. (1994). *Preventing tobacco use among young people: A report of the Surgeon General.* Atlanta, GA: U.S. Department of Health and Human Services.

Comstock, G., & Strasburger, V.C. (1993). Media violence: Q & A. *Adolescent Medicine, 4*(3), 495-509.

Crocker, E. (1986). In my opinion . . . Television for hospitalized children: The issue of control. *CHC, 15*(2), 76-78.

Dietz, W.H. (1990). You are what you eat—-What you eat is what you are. *Journal of Adolescent Health Care, 11*(1), 76-80.

Dorfman, L., Woodruff, K., Chavez, V., & Wallack, L. (1997). Youth and violence on local television news in California. *American Journal of Public Health, 87*(8), 1311-1315.

DuRant, R.H., Thompson, W.O., Johnson, M., & Baranowski, T. (1996). Official *Journal of the American College of Sports Medicine,* 15-25.

Fosarelli, P. (1986). In my opinion . . . Advocacy for children's appropriate viewing of television: What can we do? *CHC, 15*(2), 79-81.

French, J., & Pena, S. (1991). Children's hero play of the 10th century: Changes resulting from television's influence. *Child Study Journal, 21,* 79-93.

Greenberg, B.S., Graef, D., Fernandez-Collado, C., et al. (1980). Sexual intimacy on commercial TV during prime time. *Journalism Q, 57,* 211-215.

Greenberg, B.S., Stanley, C., Siemicki, M., et al. (1986). *Sex content on soaps and prime time television series viewed by adolescents.* Project CAST, Report No. 2, Michigan State University, Department of Telecommunications.

Harris, C. (1986). Programming for special groups through closed-circuit television. *CHC, 15*(2), 91-94.

Institute of Medicine. (1994). *Growing up tobacco free: Preventing nicotine addiction in children and youths.* Washington, DC: National Academy Press.

Johnson, M.O. (1996). Television violence and its effect on children. *Journal of Pediatric Nursing, 11*(2), 94-98.

Lowry, D.T., & Towles, D.E. (1989). Soap opera portrayals of sex, contraception and sexually transmitted diseases. *Journal of Communications, 39,* 76-83.

Mosedale, L. (1994, March). Putting TV in its place. *Child,* 92-95, 118-120.

Myers, L., Strikmiller, P.K., Webber, L.S., & Berenson, G.S. (1996). Physical and sedentary activity in school children grades 5-8: The Bogalusa Heart Study. *Medicine and Science in Sports and Exercise, 28*(7), 852-859.

Robinson, T.N. (1999). Reducing children's television viewing to prevent obesity: A randomized controlled trial. *Journal of the American Medical Association, 282*(16), 1561-1567.

Sargent, J.D., Dalton, M.A., Beach, M., Bernhardt, A., Pullin, D., & Stevens, M. (1997). Cigarette promotional items in public schools. *Archives of Pediatric Adolescent Medicine, 151,* 1189-1196.

Sege, R.D., Perry, C., Stigol, L., Cohen, L., Griffith, J., Cohn, M., & Spivak, H. (1997). Short-term effectiveness of anticipatory guidance to reduce early childhood risks for subsequent violence. *Archives of Pediatric Adolescent Medicine, 151,* 392-397.

Waldner-Guttentag, D.N., Albritton, W.L., & Kettner, R.B. (1983). Daytime television viewing by hospitalized children: The effect of alternative programming. *Pediatrics, 71*(4), 620-625.

Child Neglect Preventive Interventions

Nursing's Role

PERLE SLAVIK COWEN

If our American way of life fails the child, it fails us all.
— Pearl S. Buck, *The Child Who Never Grew*

Child neglect is the most common form of child maltreatment in the United States. The research, practice, and popular literature have often treated physical abuse and neglect as one entity with the same risk factors, characteristics, recommended interventions, and implications for prevention (Wolock & Horowitz, 1984). Child neglect, however, consists of acts of omission or failures to provide the basic care and protection that human growth requires, whereas physical abuse consists of acts of commission or inflicted injuries. Researchers have indicated that child neglect is strongly correlated with poverty, single-parent caretakers, unemployment, and multifaceted family problems (Cowen, 1999). Treatment for neglectful families requires multidisciplinary efforts to improve family functioning and promote a safe and supportive environment. Nursing, by virtue of the nature of the profession, the variety of its practice settings, and the sheer numbers of its practitioners, can provide leadership in the efforts to combat this form of child maltreatment (Cowen, 1994).

Nurses have a variety of roles in the assessment of and primary, secondary, and tertiary preventive interventions for child neglect, with child safety and optimal family functioning as the desired outcomes (Cowen, 2000). Early identification and intervention have the potential for reducing or preventing the developmental consequences associated with the deprivations of neglect. The nurse's role as child and family advocate is often the critical determinant of whether at-risk families are identified and receive the therapeutic interventions and tangible services they need (Cowen, 1999). In addition, nurses often have direct responsibilities for monitoring and remediat-

ing parenting patterns that have placed the child in hazardous conditions. The different levels of family functioning continually require adaptations in the nursing role, therapeutic approach, and helping activities. The purpose of this chapter is to present an overview of the problem of child neglect. This includes the types and characteristics of child neglect, theoretical perspectives, risk factors, and preventive considerations. In addition, areas of particular relevance to nursing practice are highlighted such as nursing assessment, nursing interventions, and the developmental consequences of neglect for children.

BACKGROUND

Results of the Annual Fifty State Survey (40 states actually provided reporting statistics) indicated that 3,154,000 children were reported as alleged victims of child maltreatment to child protective service (CPS) agencies nationwide in 1998 (Wang & Daro, 1999). The average substantiation rate was 32%, with 14 of every 1,000 U.S. children found to be maltreated after investigation. Most of the substantiated cases were children who had been neglected (54%); the remaining cases were physical abuse (19%), sexual abuse (10%), emotional maltreatment (3%), and other (14%). In reviewing the 1996-1998 child maltreatment fatalities (data from 19 states), the researchers found that 40% of the children who died had prior or current contact with CPS agencies, with 42% of children dying of neglect, 52% of abuse, and 5% of multiple forms of maltreatment. Young children remained at highest risk for loss of life, with 79% under age 5 and 39%

under the age of 1 at the time of their deaths. These figures represent the lowest estimate of the problem and depend on the number of states reporting, the level of involvement of child protective services, and the varying levels of comprehensive investigation into child mortality cases by local authorities and classification variances among the states in reporting deaths due to child maltreatment (Wang & Daro, 1998).

TYPES AND CHARACTERISTICS OF CHILD NEGLECT

Generally, child neglect is defined as the failure of the child's parents or caretakers to provide the child with the basic necessities of life when financially able to do so or when offered reasonable means to do so, including minimally adequate care in the areas of shelter, nutrition, health, supervision, education, affection, and protection. State statutes often classify specific subpopulations of neglect by the type of action that the parent or caretaker fails to take (Crittenden, 1992). Child neglect classifications permit specification of what parents have failed to do or indicate what they need to do. However, such classifications do not provide insight into etiological factors or the severity of the neglect.

Although there is basic agreement as to what constitutes severe child neglect, specific types and individual cases of neglect include variables that create legal and ethical dilemmas that complicate the recognition and reporting of neglect. These dilemmas include but are not limited to (1) legal exemptions related to parental disability, poverty, or religious practices (Johnson, 1993); (2) lack of professional training and guidelines for determining medical neglect of specific diseases (Johnson, 1993); and (3) dilemmas related to the excessive demands of technology-dependent children on their caretakers (Hogue, 1993).

In addition, there are no universal standards for child rearing. What is considered neglect in one culture may not be considered abnormal in another. For example, the norms in Western countries of allowing infants to "cry it out," children to sleep alone at night, and wait for meals may be considered neglect in some cultures (Schakel, 1987). Therefore, some experts suggest that several determinations should be made in culturally informed assessments on the basis of the following questions: (1) Is the practice viewed as neglectful by cultures other than the one in question? (2) Does the practice represent an idiosyncratic departure from one's cultural practice? and (3) Does the practice represent culturally induced harm to children beyond the control of parents or caretakers (Korbin, 1994; National Research Council, 1993b)? In addition to cultural factors, standards for household cleanliness, adequate supervision, child cleanliness, and medical care may be tempered by community and economic factors (Daro, 1988; Rose & Meezan, 1996; Saunders, Nelson, & Landsman, 1993). Nonetheless, practitioners must acknowledge that some cultural beliefs cause harmful outcomes to children, particularly in conditions for which more effective treatment is indicated, and thus should be considered neglectful in concert with state statutes.

Child neglect occurs along a continuum from mild to severe, with many factors blurring the boundaries between these extremes. Because many parents engage in some kind of neglectful behavior, at least occasionally, the issue of severity is critical in assessing the future risk to the child and in designing realistic interventions. Several factors are considered in assessing the severity of neglect including the frequency, duration, and type of neglect; age of the child; potential consequences to the child's development; and the degree of danger to the child. Fatal neglect has been associated with both chronic deprivation of the basic necessities of life (Rosenberg, 1994; Wilkey, Pearn, Petrie, & Nixon, 1982) and with situational failures to supervise the activities of young children (Margolin, 1990; Rosenberg, 1994).

Child neglect also represents multidimensional caregiver problems, and neglecting families demonstrate most or all types of neglect either chronically or situationally. Many children who are reported for neglect experience more than one type of neglect. The general characteristics of different types of child neglect are described in the box on page 592; however, individual cases typically include multiple types of neglect that vary in severity and frequency.

Abandonment and Supervision Neglect

These two types of neglect actually represent different points on the continuum of failure to supervise. Abandonment occurs when parents leave their child without arranging for appropriate substitute supervision (Gaudin, 1993). Infants, particularly those impaired because of the drug addictions of their mothers, may be abandoned immediately after their birth. In these cases the infants become "boarder or resident babies" while attempts, often futile, are made to locate their parents. These infants become wards of the state and are placed in foster care awaiting termination of parental rights so that they can be adopted. Maternal substance abuse during pregnancy has become a pervasive problem with more than 10% of

---

TYPES OF CHILD NEGLECT

Abandonment: Desertion of children on a permanent or temporary basis. This can include failure to take a newborn infant home after delivery, leaving children home to fare for themselves, or failing to retrieve them from "temporary" care with a relative, child caretaker, or health care organization.

Educational neglect: Failure to assure that children attend school on a regular basis or that they receive a planned program of home study under guidelines of their local school district.

Emotional neglect: Failure to provide emotional support to children in ways that are appropriate for the age and development of the child. Psychological unavailability is considered neglectful for children of all ages.

Health care neglect: Failure to provide basic preventive care, adequate care during illnesses, timely visits to health professionals, and maintenance of professionally prescribed health care routines for acute and chronic illnesses.

Nutritional neglect: Failure to provide adequate and age-appropriate food and fluids for infants and children, resulting in inadequate growth, starvation, dehydration, or failure to thrive.

Physical neglect: Failure to provide housing that is safe, dry, and warm; to ensure that children have adequate hygiene; and to provide clean and appropriate clothing.

Supervision neglect: Failure to provide attendance, guidance, and protection to children who, lacking experience and knowledge, cannot comprehend or anticipate dangerous situations. This includes protection from environmental hazards such as poisons, electrical sockets, guns, and standing water. The parent may be in the home but impaired because of substance abuse, physical or mental illness, low intelligence, or immaturity or may delegate their children's care to an inadequate caretaker who is obviously impaired, immature, or abusive.

---

urine toxicology screens in newborns testing positive for illicit drugs in both urban and suburban areas (Gomby & Shiono, 1991).

In supervision neglect, children are left for hours or days at a time. Supervision is often inadequate even when the parents are present because of substance abuse, physical or mental illness, low intelligence, or immaturity. Child care may also be delegated to an inadequate caregiver who is impaired, immature, or abusive. When considering supervision neglect, one needs to consider cultural and community standards as well as the child's age, developmental level, and length of time the child is left alone.

Physical Neglect

Severe physical neglect is characterized by a chaotic family lifestyle with deterioration in most areas of family functioning (Pagelow, 1997; Young, 1981). The children in severely neglecting families do not receive most of the basic necessities of life. There are typically no family routines for accomplishing the activities of daily living including eating, sleeping, bathing, or household cleaning. Substandard housing is common; living areas may be littered with rotting food, garbage, and animal feces with environmental hazards present and accessible. School-age children attend school only sporadically, and their classmates or teachers often complain of foul smells related to their lack of routine hygiene.

In these families, food typically comes into the home on a random basis, and the children must grab it as they can. Infants in these families are often malnourished, have a history of failure to thrive, and may have presented with intestinal disorders possibly due to ingestion of curdled formula, although this cause may be overlooked. Generally these families have many children, not because the parents want children but because they fail to plan. There is a high percentage of mental retardation, mental illness, alcoholism, and substance abuse in these families (Daro, 1988). They often are headed by a single mother. When the parents do live together, however, their behavior tends to be similar, and they often exacerbate each other's problems (Young, 1981). The parents and their older children are conscious that they are considered different from other families, and they often respond with an impotent hostility that only alienates them further (Young, 1981).

Moderate physical neglect is typified by lesser degrees of disorganization in family functioning and with basic functioning demonstrated in at least one area (Young, 1981). These families may have one parent working with some continuity, a happy relationship with an extended family member, or be capable of some responsibility such as sending the children to school regularly or administering a medication. Meals may be erratic and of varying degrees of nutritional value. They are cooked, however, and an effort is made to feed the family, which marks a qualitative difference from severely neglecting families (Young, 1981). Although the children of these families may show the results of poor nutrition, this is often a function of poverty and ignorance and not of indifference (Pagelow, 1997; Young, 1981). Disorder and confusion may be prevalent, but most areas of parental behavior will at least demonstrate some caretaking effort. The children appear dirty, but they will not be encrusted. The parents may leave the children alone; however, it will be for hours and not days (DePanfilis, 1996; National Research Council, 1993a).

Health Care Neglect

The problem of health care neglect has been difficult to characterize. Practitioners vary in their individual opinions as to what constitutes medical neglect by specialty, cultural background, and the population they are serving. In general, a solitary omission in health care is unlikely to cause harm in average children. Nonetheless a pattern of omissions in care, such as failure to immunize, could have detrimental effects for even the healthiest children (Dubowitz, 1994). In addition, there are times when failing to seek or comply with care for a single incidence can have a devastating effect, such as failure to have a severe head injury evaluated.

In cases of severe health care neglect, parents are unable, unwilling, or unmotivated to seek all forms of preventive care, and direct assistance is required to locate a provider and transport families to services (Dubowitz & Black, 1994). Parents are unable, unwilling, or inconsistent in assessing the severity of an illness or accident and may thus seek emergency care on a much delayed basis when the child's problem has advanced to a critical stage (Dubowitz & Black, 1994). They are often unable or unwilling to meet the needs of a child with a chronic condition (Dubowitz & Black, 1994).

In contrast, in families with moderate neglect, children will be taken to an emergency department for acute injuries or illnesses, but the parents will ignore chronic colds, defective vision, or dental care needs. These parents are often inconsistent and inadequate in attempting to care for a child with a chronic condition (Dubowitz & Black, 1994).

Not all instances of health care "noncompliance" should be labeled neglect. Well-intentioned parents may at times fail to comply with health care recommendations as a result of practical problems such as poor communication, a child's refusal to take a prescribed medication, transportation problems, and inability to pay for medication and appointments. There are also times in which the

failure to seek or a delay in seeking health care is simply an error in judgment. Dubowitz (1994) asserts that parents should only be considered responsible for health care neglect if a lay person reasonably could be expected to appreciate the need for health care.

Health care neglect and simple errors in judgment are distinct from the decision to treat children's illnesses by spiritual means. Parents of some religions believe that they are exerting their constitutionally protected religious freedom when choosing spiritual treatment. Most states agree with these parents and have provided exemptions in their child abuse and neglect statutes for spiritual treatment. Courts, however, have not recognized spiritual treatment when a child's life is in danger or the child has died (Lingle, 1996).

Educational Neglect

Educational neglect in its most severe form may include either failure to comply with state requirements for school attendance or failure to provide an approved home-based school curriculum (Pagelow, 1984). This form of neglect also includes the consistently permitted truancy of the child without reason or for nonlegitimate reasons such as to care for siblings or to work (Gaudin, 1993). Educational neglect also involves inattention to a child's special educational needs such as failure to follow through with special interventions or programs recommended by the school without reasonable cause (Erickson & Egeland, 1996).

Emotional Neglect

Parents who emotionally neglect their children may provide adequate physical care but do not provide adequate nurturance. In these families, the parents are detached and uninvolved with their children (Schakel, 1987). Babies and toddlers may be left in their cribs for long periods of time. Children are seldom talked to, cuddled, or hugged (Schakel, 1987). Psychological unavailability has been associated with greater developmental problems than the hostility and anger of abuse or the deprivation of physical neglect (Crittenden, 1996; Crittenden, Partridge, & Claussen, 1991).

Nutritional Neglect

Nutritional neglect is the failure to provide a diet of quality and nutritional balance that is developmentally appropriate (Barnett, Miller-Perrin, & Perrin, 1997). Overdilution of formula may result in insufficient calories, toddlers may be fed "junk foods" with little or no attempt to include the basic food groups, and school-aged and older children may have to fend for themselves with stale or spoiled food the only sustenance available in the home. In healthy children the first effect of malnutrition will be on the child's weight. Moderate malnutrition also affects linear growth and severe malnutrition also affects brain growth as evidenced by microcephaly in young children (Dubowitz, 1991).

THEORETICAL PERSPECTIVES

Theoretical perspectives on the causes and correlates of child maltreatment are many and varied (Cicchetti & Carlson, 1989). The inability of the single dimensional models to adequately address the known characteristics of child maltreatment including neglect has resulted in multidimensional models of child maltreatment. One such attempt in this direction has been proposed by Garbarino (1977; 1980b) in his ecological model of child maltreatment, which in turn derives from Bronfenbrenner's (1977) ecological model of human development (Fig. 76-1).

The Garbarino model is a paradigm for examining the complex interactions among parental and child characteristics, intrafamilial and extrafamilial stressors, and the social and cultural systems that affect families. The model offers a framework for considering available supports and resources in relation to a topology of four levels that have been adapted to include individual, familial, social, and cultural factors (Howze & Kotch, 1984). In addition, the model provides a framework for understanding the relationships among stress, social support systems, and child maltreatment. Stress arising from these domains may be situational, acute, or chronic in nature. However, it should be noted that to date research has not indicated that there are any factors present in all child maltreatment circumstances that are absent in all nonmaltreatment circumstances. Thus there is no litmus test for child maltreatment, only related risk factors whose identification provides the opportunity for preventive interventions to be directed at stressful environments, interpersonal relationships, and parental psychosocial problems

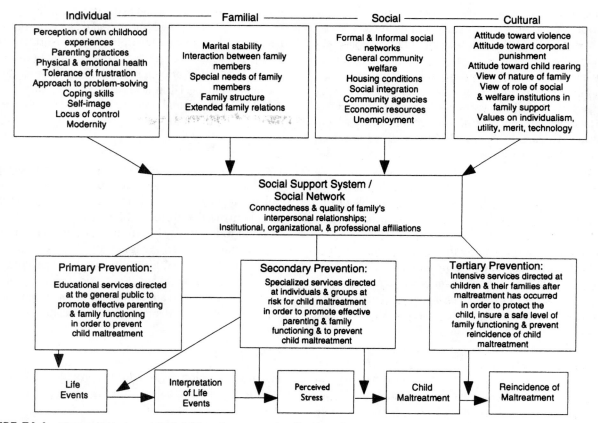

FIGURE 76-1 The ecological model of child maltreatment: implications for prevention. (Adapted from Howze, D.C., & Kotch, J.B. [1984]. Disentangling life events, stress, and social support: Implications for the primary prevention of child abuse and neglect. *Child Abuse & Neglect, 8*[4], 401-409. Copyright 1984 by Elsevier Science, Ltd. Reprinted with permission.)

with securement of the child's safety and optimal growth and development as the desired outcomes.

SOCIOCULTURAL FACTORS

Child neglect has been highly correlated with poverty, with physical neglect found to be concentrated among the poorest of the poor who typically reside in inadequate housing (Pelton, 1985; Wolock & Horowitz, 1979, 1984). Income level has also been associated with the severity of neglect with higher income families generally associated with less severe forms of neglect, presumably because they have more resources at their disposal (Claussen & Crittenden, 1991).

The 1998 official poverty measure indicated that 18.9% of all U.S. children were poor (13.5 million children), with children under age 6 particularly vulnerable, having an overall poverty rate of 20.6% (Dalaker, 1999). Even more startling, related children under the age of 6 living in families with a female householder and no husband present had a poverty rate (54.8%) that was more than five times the rate for their counterparts in married-couple families (10.1%) (Dalaker, 1999).

Child neglect rates have also been found to be higher in poorer neighborhoods with fewer social resources than in equally deprived neighborhoods where social resources (such as respite and crisis childcare) were perceived to be higher (Garbarino & Sherman, 1980a). Although the indirect stress of poverty may lead to child neglect, there is little doubt that poverty is directly hazardous to children. Poor parents are required to be hypervigilant of the environment (deteriorated housing, fires, lead poisoning, crime), manage scarce financial resources, and provide constant supervision of children with little or no margin for error (Pelton, 1994). Poor children are more likely than rich or middle-class children to experience material deprivation and poor health, die during childhood, score lower on standardized tests, be retained in grade or drop out of school, have out-of-wedlock births, experience violent crime, and are more often reported as victims of child maltreatment, including neglect (Brooks-Gunn & Duncan, 1997).

In addition, child neglect has been related to the inaccessibility or unaffordability of health care (Barnett et al., 1997). The number of low-income children who lacked health insurance reached 7 million in 1998, with nearly one of every four low-income children without coverage (Guyer, Broaddus, & Cochran, 1999). The failure to reduce the number of uninsured low-income children results largely from the sharp declines in the number of poor children enrolled in Medicaid, even though virtually all children with family incomes below the federal poverty line ($13,003 for a family of three in 1998) are eligible for Medicaid (Guyer et al., 1999). Several factors have been identified as contributing to this nonparticipation by eligible children and their families. In the past, families with children generally were eligible for Medicaid only if they were receiving welfare, and under those rules state eligibility systems linked the two programs. In 1996 the law changed, and Medicaid eligibility has been "delinked" from eligibility for welfare. Many states, however, have not revamped their systems, and in many cases the two programs remain linked through state computer systems, resulting in Medicaid-eligible families being denied or terminated from Medicaid on the basis of welfare rather than Medicaid rules (Guyer et al., 1999). Additional factors that have been identified include (1) the time-consuming and difficult application process, (2) the stigma attached to a poverty program, and (3) the reality that because most children are healthy, parents may not feel compelled to enroll them proactively (Devaney, Ellwood, & Love, 1997). Health care use research also suggests that nonfinancial barriers such as a lack of transportation also make it difficult for persons, especially poor rural children, adolescents, and women, to obtain both health care and health promotion services (Klerman, 1992).

Family Characteristics

Child neglect has been strongly correlated with both single-parent caretakers and unemployed parents (American Association for Protecting Children, 1988). Although a wide range of family functioning has been reported in neglectful families, observations of family interactions have shown neglectful families to be more chaotic, less able to resolve conflict, less cohesive, less verbally expressive, and less warm and empathetic than a matched comparison group (Gaudin, Polansky, Kilpatrick, & Shilton, 1996). Evidence exists to support the belief that families who are socially isolated and have insufficient social support are more inclined to neglect than matched comparison groups are (DePanfilis, 1996). There is little literature available on the characteristics of emotionally neglectful families. Researchers, however, have characterized such families as having more psychosocial problems, poorer coping skills, and greater levels of perceived stress (Hickox & Furnell, 1989). Researchers have postulated that vulnerable families may also include those in situational crisis related to such life stressors as death, divorce, relocation, and unemployment (Crittenden, 1996).

Parent Characteristics

Although some parents both abuse and neglect their children, research has been conducted to distinguish neglecting parents from those who physically maltreat (Belsky, 1993). Neglectful mothers have been found less likely to have a positive relationship with their own mothers, describing them as less warm and caring and as less able to control their anger than a matched comparison group. The partners of these neglectful mothers were also found to be less likely to live with the mother and to provide less companionship and assistance with child care than a matched comparison group did (Coohey, 1995). Additional characteristics that have been associated with neglecting parents include an immature, childlike personality related to low self-esteem, poor impulse control, substance abuse, increased incidence of maternal depression, limited financial and household management skills, and limited social competencies (Pianta, Egeland, & Erickson, 1989; Polansky, Gaudin, & Kilpatrick, 1992). Poor parental physical health and stress-related symptoms have been related to child physical and emotional neglect (when the parent is physically or psychologically immobilized and unable to provide care) (Brayden, Altemeier, Tucker, Dietrich, & Vietze, 1992; Crittenden, 1966; Hoagwood, 1990; Lahey, Conger, Atkeson, & Treiber, 1984; Whipple & Webster-Stratton, 1991).

DEVELOPMENTAL OUTCOMES FOR CHILDREN

Longitudinal studies have confirmed the relationship between neglectful parenting and severe cognitive and social deficits in the children of neglect (Gaudin, 1995). There are also physical consequences of child neglect identifiable at every stage of child development. The consequences of neglectful parenting are particularly severe in the earliest stages of child development (National Research Council, 1993a). In addition, children may exhibit behavioral indicators of neglect, which often appear as subtle clues that something is amiss. The list of physical, psychosocial, and behavioral outcomes provided are representational and not exhaustive (Table 76-1).

NURSING PROCESS

Nursing roles and therapeutic approaches in supporting families at risk for child neglect have been identified on the basis of Tapia's conceptualization of levels of family functioning (1972) (see box, p. 598). This classic model underscores the need for both the development of trust between the nurse and the family and the use of situational leadership to address the learning and change abilities of families at different functional levels. A specific, stepwise progression toward higher levels of functioning in combination with perceived achievable goals is more effective in enhancing change than a "now and all at once" approach. The initial extensive support required in the early stages of this therapeutic nurse-client relationship tapers off as family members develop competence, confidence, and internalize new values.

ASSESSMENT

Maternal-child nurses, pediatric nurses, visiting health nurses, emergency department nurses, school nurses, and primary care nurse practitioners are the most likely groups of providers to have early, direct contact with parents at risk of neglecting their children. Their role as advocate for the child and family is often the critical determinant of whether at-risk families are identified and receive the services they need. Nurses offer valuable assessments of the physical and developmental manifestations of child neglect and provide information on such topics as parent-child interactions, a parent's ability to care for a child, and parenting stress levels. Nurses are knowledgeable of the range of developmentally appropriate behavior expected of children, and they are quick to notice behaviors that fall outside of this range. In addition, nurses have primary responsibility for monitoring and remediating parenting patterns in families in which neglect has placed the child in at-risk situations.

The importance of early identification and intervention lies in its potential for reducing or preventing the occurrence of child neglect. In the acute setting, several aspects of the presentation should alert the clinician to the possibility of neglect, including child injuries related to environmental hazards, repeated emergency visits, or admissions due to dehydration, noncompliance with medication or care prescriptions, and the rapid departure of parents or caretakers after the admission of a child with an acute or chronic illness in tandem with infrequent visitation during the hospitalization. Initial contact in the community or home setting allows assessment of environmental clues such as inadequate hygiene or physical safety precautions; unused or grossly contaminated assistive equipment for technology-dependent children; inadequate provision for shelter, food, clothing, or care needs; and the absence of nurturing behaviors on the part of the parent or caregiver or frequent lack of adult supervision as observed or reported by neighbors or other relatives.

TABLE 76-1   Developmental Consequences of Neglect

Physical	Psychosocial and Behavioral
Infant	
Inadequate physical development; failure to thrive; "bottle mouth" intestinal disorders; dehydration; diseases related to malnutrition; recurrent and persistent minor infections[5]; severe diaper rash[5]; skin infections related to poor hygiene; delayed psychomotor skills[5]; flexed hips[7]; wasting of subcutaneous tissue[6]; bald patches on scalp related to permanent sensory impairment[6]; unattended physical problems[6]; constant fatigue and listlessness[6]	Developmental delay[5]; lack of social responsiveness[5]; self-stimulatory behaviors (head banging)[5]; negative affect[1]; feeding problems[7]; irritability[7]; difficulty establishing trust and a secure attachment to parent[2]; stiff body, resists being held[6]; apathetic[6]
Toddler	
Inadequate physical development; dental decay; diseases related to malnutrition; wasting of subcutaneous tissue[6]; unattended physical problems[6]; constant fatigue and listlessness[6]	More anxiously attached to mother[3]; negative affect[3]; easily frustrated[3]; delayed or retarded language development[5]
Preschool	
Inadequate physical development; recurrent otitis media (sometimes partial deafness)[5]; dental decay; diseases related to malnutrition; unattended physical problems[6]; constant fatigue and listlessness[6]	Low self-esteem[3]; poor ego control[3]; negative affect[3]; less persistent and enthusiastic, more distractible and impulsive in approach to tasks[3]; limited attention span[5]; decreased ability to play cooperatively[5]
School Age	
Inadequate physical development; dental decay; speech disorders[8]; enuresis[8]; eating disorders[8]; disease-related malnutrition; unattended physical problems[6]; constant fatigue and listlessness[6]	Behavior problems at school[1]; extended stays at school (early arrival and late departure)[6]; frequent absences from school; learning disabilities[5]; poor social, emotional, and academic performance[4]; low self-esteem[5]; poor coping skills[5]; socially aggressive or withdrawn[4]; negative affect[4]; socioemotional immaturity[8]; habit disorders (sucking, biting, rocking)[8]; begging and stealing food[6]; inappropriate attention seeking[6]; assumes adult responsibilities[6]; states there is no care taker[6]
Adolescent	
Inadequate physical development; dental decay; disease-related malnutrition; unattended physical problems[6]; constant fatigue and listlessness[6]	Extrafamilial difficulties such as stress and involvement with deviant peers[9]; social isolation[9]; attention problems[9]; increased risk for juvenile delinquency and runaway[7,10]; increased risk for early initiation of sexual activity and substance abuse[2]

The following references to original studies are representative and not exhaustive: [1]Abramson (1991); [2]Dubowitz & Black (1994); [3]Egeland, Sroufe, & Erickson (1983); [4]Erickson, Egeland, & Pianta (1989); [5]Skuse (1989); [6]Heindl, Krall, Salus, & Broadhurst (1979); [7]National Research Council (1993a); [8]Schakel (1987); [9]Williamson, Borduin, & Howe (1991); [10]Adams (1997).

From Cowen, P.S. (1999). Child neglect: Injuries of omission. *Pediatric Nursing, 25*(4), 401-405, 409-418. Copyright 1999 by Jannetti Publications. Reprinted with permission.

The role of the informed inquisitor is absolutely fundamental to the assessment of child neglect. Accurate documentation in cases of suspected neglect is crucial and should include verbatim information obtained from interviews of the child and parents; health history including any "accidental or environmental injuries"; a detailed description of the physical examination including the child's functional, cognitive, nutritional, and hygiene sta-

tus; parent-child interaction; parental behavior during the interview process; and an environmental assessment either during the initial interview (if occurring in the community setting) or through follow-up. Record keeping or the documentation of evidence is vital because it substantiates the basis for "reasonable belief" and provides the legal basis for state intervention on behalf of the child. Nursing history, assessments, interventions, and re-

NURSING ROLES AND THERAPEUTIC APPROACHES IN SUPPORTING FAMILIES AT RISK FOR CHILD NEGLECT

Family Levels

Infancy: Chaotic family, barely surviving, inadequate provision of physical and emotional supports; alienation from community, deviant behavior, distortion and confusion of roles, immaturity, child neglect, depression, failure

Childhood: Intermediate family, slightly above survival level, variation in economic provisions, alienation but with more ability to trust; child neglect not as great, defensive but slightly more willing to accept help

Adolescence: Normal family but with many conflicts and problems, variation in economic levels, greater trust and ability to seek and use help; parents more mature, but still have emotional conflicts. Family has successes and achievements and are more willing to seek solutions to problems; future oriented

Adulthood: Family has solutions, is stable and healthy with fewer conflicts or problems, very capable providers of physical and emotional supports; parents mature and confident, fewer difficulties in training children, able to seek help; future oriented, enjoy present

Maturity: Ideal family, homeostatic balance between individual and group goals and activities; family meets its tasks and roles well and are able to seek appropriate help when needed

Nurse's Role

Nurturing to provide for health and safety needs of children and family
Collaborating to identify and plan to meet health needs
Facilitating family follow through on health concerns
Enabling family to maintain health
Consulting with families to resolve problems/crises as they arise

Therapeutic Approach and Interventions

Establishment of a trusting relationship using acceptance, patience, warm support, consistency, clarification of role, and limit setting
  • Constant evaluation of relationships and progress; child safety, growth and development, and family violence
  • Mobilization of community resources that address basic needs
  • Multidisciplinary team coordination

Based on trusting relationship; uses counseling and interpersonal skills to help family begin to understand itself and define problems; uses honesty, genuineness, and encourages self-evaluation
  • Frequent monitoring of child safety, growth and development; presence and level of family violence.
  • Referrals to community agencies to address specific needs identified (i.e., substance abuse, marriage counseling).
  • Monitor family compliance with basic needs referrals

Anticipatory guidance and assistance; provide information and teaching, coordinate referrals and teamwork; help family make decisions and find solutions to problems
  • Monitor child safety, growth and development, and family functioning on an enhanced schedule
  • Initiate preventive health services for all family members
  • Make referrals to community agencies that provide specialized services, such as home visitation, parenting education, respite and crisis child care, family counseling, and job training

Preventive teaching that identifies needs and anticipated problem areas and provides information and teaching
  • Monitor child safety, growth and development, and family functioning during routine care
  • Scheduled preventive health maintenance for all family members
  • Provide information on how to access available resources

Assist families to identify relevant factors, potential solutions, and resources for facing situational crises and restoring equilibrium
  • Continue scheduled preventive health maintenance
  • Monitor child safety, growth and development, and family functioning during routine care

These levels reflect family growth and development levels and are not related to the age of the child.

Adapted from Tapia (1972). From Cowen, P.S. (1999). Child neglect: Injuries of omission. *Pediatric Nursing, 25*(4), 401-405, 409-418. Copyright 1999 by Jannetti Publications. Reprinted with permission.

ferrals are considered "germane to the diagnosis and treatment of the child" and therefore qualify as admissible during a court hearing. Entries need to be recorded immediately after contact with the family because they are admissible evidence only if they are recorded at or near the time of the event (Krietzer, 1981). Documentation should reflect accuracy, timeliness, and objectivity and should be devoid of "feelings" or conclusions that are made without documented evidence.

The reporting of suspected child neglect to state authorities enlists the assistance of the Child Protective Services whose professional staff have expertise and resources in this area. Currently, all states mandate that nurses report child maltreatment, including neglect (Fraser, 1986). However, because of the diversity in laws particularly in regard to definitions, nurses should obtain a copy of their particular state's reporting statute and study its provisions carefully.

Assessment Tools

To date, researchers have not indicated that there is any characteristic present in all neglecting parents that is absent in all nonneglecting parents (Wolfe, 1987). No assessment tool incorporates all the elements of child neglect to consider when assessing a child and family. Several tools, however, are available to assist the nurse to assess and identify at-risk families. These tools may be used to examine deficits in the quality of the child-rearing environment, the parent-child relationship, parental caregiving, child growth and development, and the risk for child maltreatment. Results of these assessments taken collectively may be indicative of child neglect. Examples of these tools are described below.

Assessment of the Child Rearing Environment. The *Home Observation for Measurement of the Environment (HOME)*, an observation and interview technique, is available in an infant, early childhood, and middle childhood version for children ages 4 months to 10 years. The purpose of this tool is to assess the quality of stimulation available to the child in the home. Major elements of this tool include parental responsivity and involvement, acceptance of the child, provision of appropriate play and learning materials, organization of the physical environment, and encouragement of maturity (Caldwell & Bradley, 1984). Many of the items contained in this tool relate to the possession of age-appropriate books and toys that appear to bias the tool toward middle and upper income groups (Gaudin, 1993).

The *Checklist for Living Environments to Assess Neglect (CLEAN)* is a tool designed to assess household cleanliness. To evaluate a household, each room is inspected and a score is derived on the basis of whether the room is clean or dirty, the number of clothes or linens in a room, and the number of items not belonging in that particular room (Watson-Perczel, Lutzker, Greene, & McGimpsey, 1988). This tool allows a visiting nurse to identify specific, measurable, and achievable goals for improving the household's cleanliness when this has been identified as neglectful (Gaudin, 1993).

The *Home Accident Prevention Inventory (HAPI)* is a tool designed to assess the safety and hazards in a home environment (Gaudin, 1993; Tertinger, Greene, & Lutzker, 1984). This tool includes five categories of hazards in the home: (1) fire and electrical, (2) mechanical-suffocation, (3) ingested object suffocation, (4) firearms, and (5) solid and liquid poisons. Specific use of this tool measures changes in home safety and hazards after a behavioral intervention.

Assessment of Parent Child Relations. The *Adult-Adolescent Parenting Inventory (AAPI)* is a 32-item questionnaire designed to assess the parenting and child-rearing attitudes of adolescent parent and adult parent populations (Bavolek, 1984). Four parenting and child-rearing constructs associated with dysfunctional parenting formed the foundation from which the items were developed. They include inappropriate parental expectations of the child, lack of empathy toward children's needs, parental value of physical punishment, and parent-child role reversal (Bavolek, 1984).

The *Parenting Stress Inventory (PSI)* consists of 101 items that measure parental competence and stress (Abidin, 1990). This instrument is divided into three domains. The Child domain assesses the degree of stress associated with specific child characteristics separate from the stress associated solely with the parental role. The Parent domain includes measures of personal stress related to depression, attachment, social isolation, spouse (partner relationships), and health. The Life Stress domain provides an index of the amount of stress outside of the parent-child relationship (e.g., death of a relative, loss of a job) (Abidin, 1990).

Assessment of Child Growth and Development. The *Denver II* is a screening test designed to assess a young child's development and is composed of four major categories: personal-social, fine motor-adaptive, language, and gross motor. It is applicable for children from birth through 6 years of age. There are a total of 125 assessment items, and this instrument includes information about standardization sample differences found among ethnic groups, educational levels, and places of residence (Frankenburg, Dodds, Archer, Shapiro, & Bresnick, 1990).

The *Hawaii Early Learning Profile* is a developmentally sequenced "play-based" instrument for children ages birth to 36 months. This tool evaluates cognition, language, gross and fine motor, social, and self-help domains and was developed for lay visitors to use to familiarize parents with normal ranges of growth and development. Results of the test identify current level of skills and suggest developmentally appropriate and challenging activities for the child. The unique advantage of this tool is that it is designed for use with "special needs" or "at-risk" children, as well as the general population (Furuno, O'Reilly, Hosaka, Inatsuka, & Falbey, 1993).

Risk Assessment Measures. Browne (1989) developed a 13-item checklist for home visitors based on known risk and conducted a retrospective study involving a matched sample of 62 known maltreating families and 124 nonmaltreating families. Interestingly, although the tool could correctly classify 86% of the cases, the best predictor of child maltreatment was the health visitor's perception of whether the parent was indifferent, intolerant, or overanxious. The presence of parental mental illness can cause stress and adversely affect the parent-child relationship (Louis, Condon, Shute, & Elzinga, 1997). As such, an assessment of parental mental illness provides an additional avenue to evaluate the risk for child neglect. The *Louis MACRO (Mother and Child Risk Observation)* is a tool that was developed to assess risk by interpreting the relationship between maternal mental illness and its effect on children. There are two versions of this tool designed for use with infant and toddler mother pairs, and it is based on three domains. The first domain relates to three aspects of "proper parenting" and includes safety, care, and emotional responsiveness. The second domain relates to the parent's opinion of child characteristics such as temperament, potential ease of care, and enjoyment. The third domain relates to maternal mental state by evaluating potential for psychosis, depression, and anxiety (Louis et al., 1997).

NURSING CLASSIFICATION SYSTEMS

Nursing classifications, which are specific to the type of maltreatment, victim population (child versus adult), parent or caregiver risks or inabilities, and preventive level (prevention versus protection) would offer the most guidance to both practitioners and researchers. Although nursing diagnoses (NDx) (North American Nursing Diagnosis Association, 1990), Nursing Interventions Classification (NIC) (McCloskey & Bulechek, 1996), and Nursing Outcomes Classification (NOC) (Johnson & Maas, 1997) each demonstrate strengths in some of the preceding areas, they do not allow a seamless connection across classification systems. This requires nurses to customize or develop the nursing diagnoses, interventions, and outcomes they use in documenting the multiple aspects of child neglect.

Within nursing diagnoses, child neglect is primarily addressed through parental or caregiver risks or inabilities (e.g., altered family processes; altered role performance; caregiver role strain; risk for caregiver role strain; family coping: compromised; ineffective management of therapeutic regimen: families; parenting, altered; parenting, risk for altered; and social isolation). Victim symptoms may be addressed through a variety of physical and psychological states that result from maltreatment (e.g., altered nutrition, less than body requirements, pain, anxiety, fear). Nursing diagnoses are available for primary preventive concepts (potential for enhanced community coping) and secondary and tertiary preventive concepts (ineffective management of therapeutic regimen: community); however, they are not specific to the concept of maltreatment or to child and child-rearing populations.

The following nursing outcomes (NOC) associated with neglect are not child specific and include both child and adult victim considerations: neglect cessation; abuse protection: caregiver stressors; caregiver performance: direct care; caregiver performance: indirect care; caregiver emotional health; and caregiver home care readiness (Johnson & Maas, 1997). The addition of population-specific indicators would greatly increase their use in addressing the differing neglect issues of children and adults.

The NIC intervention "abuse protection: child" includes identifiers for child neglect; identifies caregiver risks or inabilities; and provides a variety of primary, secondary, and tertiary preventive activities for all types of maltreatment (McCloskey & Bulechek, 1996). This intervention has been adapted and enhanced to include activities related to child neglect and has been further categorized related to the level of intervention (primary, secondary, or tertiary) (see box, p. 601).

PREVENTIVE INTERVENTIONS

During the last two decades, increasing public concern about child maltreatment has resulted in the development of a diverse base of primary, secondary, and tertiary preventive interventions. Primary preventive interventions are directed at the general population to prevent or reduce child maltreatment, whereas secondary preventive interventions are targeted at high-risk groups, and tertiary interventions are focused on preventing further harm to children who have been maltreated.

Examples of government-sponsored primary prevention programs that address the poverty often associated

NURSING INTERVENTIONS

Primary Preventive Interventions

Conduct public awareness campaigns directed at improving child health, safety, supervision, nutrition, growth, and development

Provide community education workshops that address parent and child needs: parenting survival skills, parenting stress reduction, parent-child nurturing, developmental stimulation exercises for children of various ages in combination with a toy-lending library

Provide training workshops for school nurses, child care workers, recreational center staff and youth workers to assist them in providing education that supports changes in youth behaviors (family life programs, value clarification programs, parenting responsibility, and information programs)

Conduct family health and functioning appraisals at birth of child:

- Determine parent's knowledge of infant/child basic care needs and provide appropriate child care information as indicated
- Determine whether the family has an intact social support network to assist with family problems, respite child care, and crisis child care
- Help families identify coping strategies for stressful situations

Secondary Preventive Interventions

Determine whether the child demonstrates physical signs of neglect, including poor or inconsistent growth patterns, failure to thrive, wasting of subcutaneous tissue, consistent hunger, poor hygiene, constant fatigue and listlessness, bald patches on scalp or other skin afflictions, apathy, unyielding body posture, and inappropriate dress for weather conditions

Identify mothers who have a history of late (4 months or later) or no prenatal care

Refer at-risk pregnant women and parents of newborns to nurse home visitation services

Identify infants/children with high-care needs (e.g., prematurity, low birth weight, colic, feeding intolerances, major health problems in the first year of life, developmental disabilities, hyperactivity, and attention deficit disorders)

Identify parents who have had another child removed from the home or have placed previous children with relatives for extended periods

Identify parents who have a history of substance abuse, depression, or major psychiatric illness

Identify parents who demonstrate an increased need for parent education (e.g., parents with learning problems, parents who verbalize feelings of inadequacy, parents of a first child, teen parents)

Identify crisis situations that may trigger neglect (e.g., poverty, unemployment, divorce, homelessness, and substance abuse)

Provide at-risk families with a Public Health Nurse referral to ensure that the home environment is monitored, that siblings are assessed, and that families receive continued assistance

Instruct parents on problem solving, decision making, and parenting skills or refer parents to programs where these skills can be learned

Engage parents and child in attachment-building exercises

Provide older children with concrete information on how to provide for the basic care needs of their younger siblings

Provide children with positive affirmations of their worth, nurturing care, therapeutic communication, and developmental stimulation

Refer families to human services and counseling professionals as needed

Refer parents with an active substance abuse problem for substance abuse treatment

Provide parents with community resource information that may ameliorate the effects of poverty: addresses and phone numbers of agencies that provide respite care, emergency child care, housing assistance, sliding-fee counseling services, food pantries, clothing distribution centers, health care, human services, hot lines, and domestic abuse shelters

Tertiary Preventive Interventions

Stabilize child's health status, address safety needs

Inform physicians, social worker, or multidisciplinary team designee of observations indicative of neglect

Report neglect or suspected neglect to proper authorities

Collaborate on multidisciplinary teams to establish treatment guidelines and follow-up protocols for neglectful parents and assessment intervals for child well-being determination

Establish a system to flag the treatment records of children who are suspected victims of neglect

Adapted from Cowen, P.S. (2000). Abuse protection: Child. In G.M. Bulechek & J.C. McCloskey (Eds.), *Nursing interventions: Effective nursing treatments* (3rd ed., pp. 549-577). Philadelphia: Saunders.

with child neglect include the Food Stamp Program, the Supplemental Food Program for Women, Infants and Children (WIC), the school nutrition programs (breakfast and lunch), Medicaid, Head Start, and housing assistance programs (Devaney et al., 1997). However, as previously noted, many eligible children are not enrolled in these programs. Nursing, through targeted assessment and referral, could assist in addressing this problem.

Researchers have noted that at-risk families, particularly those headed by young, relatively poor mothers, are most likely to benefit from educational and supportive services (Badger, 1981; Gabinet, 1979; Olds, Henderson, Chamberlin, & Tatelbaum, 1986). In response to this finding, many secondary prevention programs have emerged. Both home-based and center-based programs have demonstrated a wide range of positive client outcomes. A review of randomized trials of prenatal and infancy home-visitation programs for socially disadvantaged women and children indicated that some home-visitation programs were effective in (1) improving women's health-related behaviors during pregnancy, the birth weight and length of gestation of babies born to smokers and young adolescents, parents' interaction with their children, children's developmental status, (2) reducing the incidence of child abuse and neglect, childhood behavioral problems, emergency department visits and hospitalizations for injury, and unintended subsequent pregnancies, and (3) increasing mothers' participation in the work force (Olds & Kitzman, 1990). The authors noted that home-visit programs with the greatest chances of success are based either explicitly or implicitly on ecological models, are designed to address the ecology of the family during pregnancy and the early child-bearing years with nurse home visitors who establish a therapeutic alliance with the families, and are targeted at families with greater risk for maternal and child health problems by virtue of their poverty and lack of personal and social resources (Olds & Henderson, 1990).

Several interventions have been identified as increasing the probability of reducing child maltreatment within diverse populations including those that (Daro, 1996):

1. Initiate parenting support programs before or as close to the birth of their first child as possible
2. Provide parent enhancement services tied to a child's specific development that recognize the unique challenges in caring for and disciplining children of various ages
3. Provide opportunities for parents to model the interactions or discipline methods being promoted through intervention

4. Provide an adequate dosage (i.e., more than 6 months) of interventions focused on changing parental attitudes and strengthening parenting and personal skills
5. Provide parents with community resource information to ensure the safety of children beyond the immediate intervention period
6. Provide a balance of home-based and group-based alternatives for both parents who are not comfortable in group settings and those who desire such interaction
7. Program interventions that recognize the cultural differences in family functioning and parent-child interactions

Research examining tertiary interventions (families who have already been identified as neglectful) has been less promising. One such effort entitled Intensive Family Preservation is a model of crisis care aimed at maltreating families. The goal of programs that operate using this model is to prevent the unnecessary placement of children out of their home while ensuring their safety. The interventions are short-term (4 to 6 weeks) and involve a variety of therapeutic and support services designed for the needs of individual families in crisis (Bath & Haapala, 1993). Bath and Haapala found this model to be significantly less effective in dealing with neglectful families than with their physically maltreating counterparts.

SUMMARY

As described, child neglect represents multidimensional problems that involve the child, parent, family, community, and cultural factors. Community-wide preventive interventions that are directed at each phase of the family life cycle beginning with the prenatal period and continuing through a child's school years have been identified as the most promising child maltreatment preventive interventions (Cohn, 1983; Leventhal, 1996). In addition, interventions need to balance both the parent's problems and needs and the child's developmental needs to be effective (Leventhal, 1996).

Although there has been some progress made in interventions for neglectful families, the problem of child neglect remains difficult to address. This may in part be due to the unidimensional aim of some interventions attempting to address multidimensional family problems. The programs that have succeeded in changing outcomes for high-risk children and their families differ in fundamental ways from prevailing services. Successful intervention programs see the child in the context of the family and the family in the context of its surroundings. They offer (Connell, Kubisch, Schorr, & Weiss, 1995):

1. Support to parents who need help with their lives before they can make use of services for their children
2. A broad spectrum of services including concrete help with basic necessities such as food, transportation, clothing, and respite child care
3. Services that are coherent and integrated with staff crossing traditional professional and bureaucratic boundaries
4. Staff members who are fundamentally flexible and render services ungrudgingly and at a high level of intensity
5. Professionals who are perceived by clients as persons they can trust and who care about and respect them
6. Professionals who are able to redefine their roles and venture into nontraditional settings and provide services at nontraditional hours

Key components of effective nursing interventions include the nurse's ability to:

- Adequately identify indicators of neglect
- Describe the nature of the neglect in a detailed and comprehensive manner
- Identify necessary case management components as a key member or leader of a multidisciplinary team
- Promote maximum independence and self-care of the family through innovative teaching strategies
- Coordinate activities between acute and community settings to ensure continuity of care
- Provide direct care and serve as the child's advocate
- Provide counseling to the family to help them identify coping strategies for stressful situations
- Identify social support resources and assist the family in accessing needed services
- Determine the effectiveness of the parent's ability to meet the child's safety and care needs
- Coordinate efforts with child protective services to ensure the safety needs of the child are met
- Serve as an expert witness in cases involving legal intervention
- Most importantly, Provide guidance in the prevention of child neglect

REFERENCES

Abidin, R.R. (1990). *Parenting stress index.* Charlottesville, VA: Pediatric Psychology Press.

Abramson, L. (1991). Facial expressivity in failure to thrive and normal infants: Implications for their capacity to engage in the world. *Merrill-Palmer Quarterly, 37*(1), 159-182.

Adams, G.R. (1997). Runaway youth. In R.A. Hoekelman (Ed.), *Primary pediatric healthcare.* St. Louis: Mosby.

American Association for Protecting Children. (1988). *Highlights of official child abuse and neglect reporting—1986.* Denver, CO: American Humane Association.

Badger, E. (1981). Effects of parent education program on teenage mothers and their offspring. In K.G. Scott, T. Field, & E. Robertson (Eds.), *Teenage parents and their offspring* (pp. 283-310). New York: Grune & Stratton.

Barnett, O.W., Miller-Perrin, C.L., & Perrin, R.D. (1997). *Family violence across the lifespan: An introduction.* Thousand Oaks, CA: Sage Publications.

Bath, H.I., & Haapala, D.A. (1993). Intensive family preservation services with abused and neglected children: An examination of group differences. *Child Abuse & Neglect, 17*(2), 213-225.

Bavolek, S.J. (1984). Handbook for the AAPI. Eau Claire, WI: Family Development Press.

Belsky, J. (1993). Etiology of child maltreatment: A developmental-ecological analysis. *Psychological Bulletin, 114*(3), 413-434.

Brayden, R.M., Altemeier, W.A., Tucker, D.D., Dietrich, M.S., & Vietze, P. (1992). Antecedents of child neglect in the first two years of life. *Journal of Pediatrics, 120*(3), 426-429.

Bronfenbrenner, U. (1977). Toward an experimental ecology of human development. *American Psychologist, 32,* 513-531.

Brooks-Gunn, J., & Duncan, G. (1997). The effects of poverty on children. *The Future of Children, 7*(2), 55-71.

Browne, K. (1989). The health visitor's role in screening for child abuse. *Health Visitor, 62,* 275-277.

Caldwell, B.M., & Bradley, R.H. (1984). *Home observation for measurement of the environment.* Little Rock, AR: University of Arkansas.

Cicchetti, D., & Carlson, V. (1989). *Child maltreatment: Theory and research on the causes and consequences of child abuse and neglect.* New York: Cambridge University Press.

Claussen, A.H., & Crittenden, P.M. (1991). Physical and psychological maltreatment: Relations among types of maltreatment. *Child Abuse & Neglect, 15*(1-2), 5-18.

Cohn, A.H. (1983). *An approach to preventing child abuse.* Chicago: National Committee for the Prevention of Child Abuse.

Connell, J.P., Kubisch, A.C., Schorr, L.B., & Weiss, C.H. (Eds.). (1995). *New approaches to evaluating community initiatives: Concepts, methods, and contexts.* Washington, DC: Apen Institute.

Coohey, C. (1995). Neglectful mothers, their mothers, and partners: The significance of mutual aid. *Child Abuse & Neglect, 19*(8), 885-895.

Cowen, P.S. (1994). Child abuse. In J.C. McCloskey & H.K. Grace (Eds.), *Current issues in nursing* (4th ed., pp. 731-741). St. Louis: Mosby.

Cowen, P.S. (1999). Child neglect: Injuries of omission. *Pediatric Nursing, 25*(4), 401-405, 409-418.

Cowen, P.S. (2000). Abuse protection: Child. In G.M. Bulechek & J.C. McCloskey (Eds.), *Nursing interventions: Effective nursing treatments* (3rd ed., pp. 549-577). Philadelphia: Saunders.

Crittenden, P.M. (1992). *Preventing child neglect* (pp. 1-23). United States of America: National Committee for Prevention of Child Abuse.

Crittenden, P.M. (1996). Research on maltreating families: Implications for intervention. In J. Briere, L. Berliner, J. Bulkley, C.

Jenny, & T. Reid (Eds.), *The APSAC handbook on child maltreatment* (pp. 158-174). Thousand Oaks, CA: Sage Publications.

Crittenden, P.M., Partridge, M.F., & Claussen, A.H. (1991). Family patterns of relationship in normative and dysfunctional families. *Development and Psychopathology, 3*(4), 491-512.

Dalaker, J. (1999). *Poverty in the United States: 1998* (P60-207). Washington, DC: U.S. Census Bureau, Current Population Reports.

Daro, D. (1988). *Confronting child abuse: Research for effective program design.* New York: The Free Press.

Daro, D. (1996). Preventing child abuse and neglect. In J. Briere, L. Berliner, J. Bulkley, C. Jenny, & T. Reid (Eds.), *The APSAC handbook on child maltreatment* (pp. 343-358). Thousand Oaks, CA: Sage Publications.

DePanfilis, D. (1996). Social isolation of neglectful families: A review of social support assessment and intervention models. *Child Maltreatment, 1*(1), 37-52.

Devaney, B., Ellwood, M., & Love, J. (1997). Programs that mitigate the effects of poverty on children. *The Future of Children, 7*(2), 88-112.

Dubowitz, H. (1991). The impact of child maltreatment on health. In R.H. Starr & D.A. Wolfe (Eds.), *The effects of child abuse and neglect: Issues and research* (pp. 278-294). New York: Guilford Press.

Dubowitz, H. (1994). Medical neglect: What can physicians do? *Maryland Medical Journal, 43*(4), 337-341.

Dubowitz, H., & Black, M. (1994). Child neglect. In R.M. Reece (Ed.), *Child abuse: Medical diagnosis and management* (pp. 279-297). Malvern, PA: Lea & Febiger.

Egeland, B., Sroufe, L.A., & Erickson, M. (1983). The developmental consequences of different patterns of maltreatment. *Child Abuse & Neglect, 7*(4), 459-469.

Erickson, M.F., & Egeland, B. (1996). Child neglect. In J. Briere, L. Berliner, J. Bulkley, C. Jenny, & T. Reid (Eds.), *The APSAC handbook on child maltreatment* (pp. 4-20). Thousand Oaks, CA: Sage Publications.

Erickson, M.F., Egeland, B., & Pianta, R. (1989). The effects of maltreatment on the development of young children. In D. Cicchetti & V. Carlson (Eds.), *Child maltreatment: Theory and research on the causes and consequences of child abuse and neglect.* New York: Cambridge University Press.

Frankenburg, W.K., Dodds, J., Archer, P., Shapiro, H., & Bresnick, B. (1990). *Denver II technical support manual.* Denver, CO: Denver Developmental Materials, Inc.

Fraser, B. (1986). A glance at the past, a gaze at the present, a glimpse of the future: A critical analysis of the development of child abuse reporting statutes. *Journal of Juvenile Law, 10,* 641-686.

Furuno, S., O'Reilly, K., Hosaka, C.M., Inatsuka, T.T., & Falbey, B.Z. (1993). *Helping babies learn.* San Antonio, TX: Therapy Skill Builders.

Gabinet, L. (1979). Prevention of child abuse and neglect in an inner-city population: II. The program and the results. *Child Abuse & Neglect, 3,* 809-817.

Garbarino, J. (1977). The human ecology of child maltreatment. *Journal of Marriage and the Family, 39,* 721-735.

Garbarino, J., & Sherman, D. (1980a). High-risk neighborhoods and high-risk families. *Child Development, 51,* 188-198.

Garbarino, J., & Sherman, D. (1980b). High-risk neighborhoods and high-risk families: The human ecology of child maltreatment. *Child Development, 51,* 188-198.

Gaudin, J.J. (1995). *Defining and differentiating child neglect* [newsletter]. Chicago: American Professional Society on the Abuse of Children (APSAC).

Gaudin, J.M. (1993). Child neglect: A guide for intervention. In U.S. Department of Health and Human Services, Administration for Children and Families, Administration on Children, Youth, and Families, & National Center on Child Abuse and Neglect (Eds.), *The user manual series* (pp. 1-84). Washington, DC: Westover Consultants.

Gaudin, J.M., Jr., Polansky, N.A., Kilpatrick, A.C., & Shilton, P. (1996). Family functioning in neglectful families. *Child Abuse & Neglect, 20*(4), 363-377.

Gomby, D.S., & Shiono, P.H. (1991). Estimating the number of substance-exposed infants. *The Future of Children, 1*(1), 17-25.

Guyer, J., Broaddus, M., & Cochran, M. (1999). *Missed opportunities: Declining Medicaid enrollment undermines the nation's progress in insuring low-income children.* Washington, DC: Center on Budget and Policy Priorities.

Heindl, C., Krall, C., Salus, M., & Broadhurst, D. (1979). *The nurse's role in the prevention and treatment of child abuse and neglect.* Washington, DC: U.S. Department of Health, Education, and Welfare.

Hickox, A., & Furnell, J. (1989). Psychosocial and background factors in emotional abuse of children. *Child: Care, Health, and Development, 15*(4), 227-240.

Hoagwood, K. (1990). Parental functioning and child sexual abuse. *Child and Adolescent Social Work, 7*(5), 377-387.

Hogue, E.E. (1993). Child neglect in home care: Weighing legal and ethical issues. *Pediatric Nursing, 19*(5), 496-498.

Howze, D.C., & Kotch, J.B. (1984). Disentangling life events, stress, and social support: Implications for primary prevention of child abuse and neglect. *Child Abuse & Neglect, 8,* 401-409.

Johnson, C.F. (1993). Physicians and medical neglect: Variables that affect reporting. *Child Abuse & Neglect, 17*(5), 605-612.

Johnson, M., & Maas, M. (1997). *Nursing outcomes classification.* St. Louis: Mosby.

Klerman, L.V. (1992). Nonfinancial barriers to the receipt of medical care. *The Future of Children, 2*(2), 171-185.

Korbin, J.E. (1994). Sociocultural factors in child maltreatment. In G. Melton & F. Barry (Eds.), *Protecting children from abuse and neglect* (pp. 182-223). New York: Guilford Press.

Krietzer, M. (1981). Legal aspects of child abuse. *Nursing Clinics of North America, 16,* 149-160.

Lahey, B.B., Conger, R.D., Atkeson, B.M., & Treiber, F.A. (1984). Parenting behavior and emotional status of physically abusive mothers. *Journal of Consulting and Clinical Psychology, 52*(6), 1062-1071.

Leventhal, J.M. (1996). Twenty years later: We do know how to prevent child abuse and neglect. *Child Abuse & Neglect, 20*(8), 647-653.

Lingle, E.A. (1996). Treating children by faith: Colliding constitutional issues. *Journal of Legal Medicine, 17*(2), 301-330.

Louis, A., Condon, J., Shute, R., & Elzinga, R. (1997). The development of the Louis MACRO (Mother and Child Risk Observation) forms: Assessing parent-infant-child risk in the presence of maternal mental illness. *Child Abuse & Neglect, 21*(7), 589-606.

Margolin, L. (1990). Fatal child neglect. *Child Welfare, 69*(4), 309-319.

McCloskey, J.C., & Bulechek, G.M. (1996). *Nursing interventions classification.* St. Louis: Mosby.

National Research Council. (1993a). Consequences of child abuse and neglect. In *Understanding child abuse and neglect.* Washington, DC: National Academy Press.

National Research Council. (1993b). *Understanding child abuse and neglect.* Washington, DC: National Academy Press.

North American Nursing Diagnosis Association. (1990). *Taxonomy I revised.* St. Louis: Author.

Olds, D.L., & Henderson, C.R. (1990). The prevention of maltreatment. In D. Cicchetti & V. Carlson (Eds.), *Child maltreatment: Theory and research on the causes and consequences of child abuse and neglect* (pp. 722-763). New York: Cambridge University Press.

Olds, D.L., Henderson, C.R., Jr., Chamberlin, R., & Tatelbaum, R. (1986). Preventing child abuse and neglect: A randomized trial of nurse home visitation. *Pediatrics, 78*(1), 65-78.

Olds, D.L., & Kitzman, H. (1990). Can home visitation improve the health of women and children at environmental risk? *Pediatrics, 86*(1), 108-116.

Pagelow, M.D. (1984). *Family violence.* New York: Praeger.

Pagelow, M.D. (1997). Child neglect and psychological maltreatment. In K. Barnett, C. Miller-Perrin, & R. Perrin (Eds.), *Family violence across the lifespan* (pp. 107-132). Thousand Oaks, CA: Sage Publications.

Pelton, L. (1985). *The social context of child abuse and neglect.* New York: Human Science Press.

Pelton, L.H. (1994). The role of material factors in child abuse and neglect. In G. Melton & F. Barry (Eds.), *Protecting children from abuse and neglect* (pp. 131-181). New York: Guilford Press.

Pianta, R., Egeland, B., & Erickson, M.F. (1989). The antecedents of maltreatment: Results of the mother-child interaction research project. In D. Cicchetti & V. Carlson (Eds.), *Child maltreatment: Theory and research on the causes and consequences of child abuse and neglect* (pp. 203-253). New York: Cambridge University Press.

Polansky, N.A., Gaudin, J.M., & Kilpatrick, A.C. (1992). Family radicals. *Children and Youth Services Review, 14*(1-2), 19-26.

Rose, S.J., & Meezan, W. (1996). Variations in perceptions of child neglect. *Child Welfare, 75*(2), 139-160.

Rosenberg, D. (1994). Fatal neglect. *APSAC Advisor, 7*(4), 38-40.

Saunders, E.J., Nelson, K., & Landsman, M.J. (1993). Racial inequality and child neglect: Findings in a metropolitan area. *Child Welfare, 72*(4), 341-354.

Schakel, J.A. (1987). Emotional neglect and stimulus deprivation. In M.R. Brassard, R. Germain, & S.N. Hart (Eds.), *Psychological maltreatment of children and youth* (pp. 100-109). Elmsford, NY: Pergamon Books.

Skuse, D.H. (1989). ABC of child abuse. Emotional abuse and delay in growth. *British Medical Journal, 299*(6691), 113-115.

Tapia, J.A. (1972). The nursing process in family health. *Nursing Outlook, 20,* 267.

Tertinger, D.A., Greene, B.F., & Lutzker, J.R. (1984). Home safety: Development and validation of one component of an ecobehavioral treatment program for abused and neglected children. *Journal of Applied Behavior Analysis, 17*(2), 159-174.

Wang, C.T., & Daro, D. (1998). *Current trends in child abuse reporting and fatalities: Results of the 1997 annual fifty state survey* (Working paper number 808). Chicago: National Committee to Prevent Child Abuse.

Wang, C.T., & Daro, D. (1999). *Current trends in child abuse reporting and fatalities: Results of the 1998 annual fifty state survey* (Working paper number 808). Chicago: Prevent Child Abuse America.

Watson-Perczel, M., Lutzker, J.R., Greene, B.F., & McGimpsey, B.J. (1988). Assessment and modification of home cleanliness among families adjudicated for child neglect. *Behavior Modification, 12*(1), 57-81.

Whipple, E.E., & Webster-Stratton, C. (1991). The role of parental stress in physically abusive families. *Child Abuse & Neglect, 15*(3), 279-291.

Wilkey, I., Pearn, J., Petrie, G., & Nixon, J. (1982). Neonaticide, infanticide, and child homicide. *Medicine, Science, & the Law, 22*(1), 31-34.

Williamson, J.M., Borduin, C.M., & Howe, B.A. (1991). The ecology of adolescent maltreatment: A multilevel examination of adolescent physical abuse, sexual abuse, and neglect. *Journal of Consulting & Clinical Psychology, 59*(3), 449-457.

Wolfe, D.A. (1987). *Child abuse: Implications for child development and psychopathology.* Newbury Park, CA: Sage Publications.

Wolock, I., & Horowitz, B. (1979, June). Child maltreatment and maternal deprivation among AFDC-recipient families. *Social Service Review, 53,* 175-194.

Wolock, I., & Horowitz, B. (1984). Child maltreatment as a social problem: The neglect of neglect. *American Journal of Orthopsychiatry, 54*(4), 530-543.

Young. (1981). *Physical child neglect.* Chicago: The National Committee for Prevention of Child Abuse.

Alzheimer's Disease

Legal, Ethical, and Moral Considerations

NANCY EDWARDS

As we enter the 21st century, the growth of the elderly population, the cost of health care, and the advances in medical technology and science will continue to have a profound impact on the health care system. This transformation in the health care system will raise ethical, legal, and moral issues. The special nature of persons with Alzheimer's disease (AD) and the natural trajectory of their disease require special care on the part of the health care team to meet the ethical challenges and to establish health care goals that result in consistent, reasoned, and compassionate care.

It is estimated that 4 million people in the United States have AD. In a 1993 national survey, approximately 19 million Americans responded that a family member had AD, and 37 million people reported that they knew someone with AD (Alzheimer's Association Facts, 1999). Furthermore, it is estimated that, barring prevention or a cure, 14 million Americans will have AD by the middle of this century. The incidence of AD increases with age. The prevalence of AD is less than 1% at age 60 to 65 but appears to exceed 40% in individuals older than 85 (Katzman & Saitoh, 1991). In light of the increase in absolute numbers of elderly, it is obvious that dementia will be a national health problem of increasing proportion.

The cost of AD care is astronomical. The Alzheimer's Association reported that at least $100 billion a year is spent in the United States on AD (Alzheimer's Association Facts [AAF], 1999). In most cases, neither Medicare nor most private health insurance covers the necessary long-term care that is frequently required. The indirect cost of AD is difficult to measure, but it is estimated that the disease annually costs U.S. businesses more than $26 billion in lost productivity of the caregivers and $7 billion related to health costs, totaling $33 billion (AAF, 1999). The average lifetime cost per patient is estimated to be $174,000. With limited health care resources, issues related to care must be examined.

The progressive decline in cognitive functioning and physical abilities that characterize AD raises numerous issues, which vary and evolve throughout the course of the illness. Those who are afflicted with the disease, their families, and health care providers will have to face these issues. These issues must be examined in light of patient autonomy, justice, veracity, beneficence, and nonmaleficence.

DETERMINATION OF CAPACITY

One of the first issues to be considered is respecting patient choice in regard to the right to know the diagnosis, participation in treatment, and informed consent. The principle of autonomy is fundamental to the U.S. legal system; that is, individuals are entitled to make their own decisions. To the extent possible, the legal and health care communities support the concept of self-determination. Loss of competency, or decision-making capacity, is an inevitable consequence of AD, but nurses must remember that the diagnosis of AD is not an automatic declaration that the patient has lost all decision-making capacity. In a 1914 decision, it was noted that "Every human being of adult years and sound mind has a right to determine what shall be done with his own body" (*Schloendorff v Society of New York Hospital*). Each adult is presumed competent to make personal decisions unless the evidence demonstrates that the person is incompetent. The words "competent" and "incompetent" are legal terms and should be relegated to the legal setting; however, the reality of the health care setting compels professionals to make competency judgments on a daily basis. Some have suggested that the term "capacity" would be more appropriate when referring to the health assessment necessary to determine the ability to make health decisions (Caralis, 1994; Weiler, 1994).

"Capacity" is not an all-or-none thing. Individuals with AD may be unable to make complicated, detailed decisions such as estate or financial matters, but they may well maintain the ability to make decisions regarding their health care. Marson and Harrell (1999) identified five standards necessary for competency. First is the expression of treatment choice, or being aware of what treatment is being offered. Second is the ability to make a reasonable choice. Third is having the capacity to appreciate the emotional and physical consequences of the choice. The fourth standard is that the person can appre-

ciate rational reasons for the treatment choice. The fifth standard is that the individual can understand the treatment situation and the associated risks and benefits. Therefore, assessment of capacity must be considered in light of the preceding standards.

Numerous tests are used to assess capacity, from simple interviews to objective measures such as the Folstein Mini-Mental State Examination. The difficulties with the objective tests presently used are that the tests do not contain capacity-specific assessment measures. It is important to remember that the concepts of "cognition" and "judgment" are not synonymous. It is essential that the individual be assessed for the ability to understand treatment options and consider treatment alternatives in light of all the risks and benefits. If the person is able to do that, either alone or with support, the person must be given the opportunity to determine the course of medical treatment.

ADVANCE DIRECTIVES

The 1994 Advisory Panel on Alzheimer's Disease noted that patients with AD who are diagnosed at an early stage more often than not retain their ability to make health care decisions. In light of this information, they recommend that health care workers who are dealing with these persons should provide information so that the person can pursue voluntary transfers of decision making, such as to a health care representative (Stratton, 1995). This allows the person to maintain autonomy when loss of capacity can be anticipated. This can be accomplished through the completion of estate wills, living wills, and durable powers of attorney for health care. These documents allow individuals with AD who maintain competency to determine what health care measures they would like carried out as their disease progresses.

One area of difficulty that often occurs is that the person who makes the prospective directives (decisional autonomy) will most likely not have the ability to carry out these decisions (executional autonomy). In many situations the consequences of these decisions fall on the family and caregiver. It may be the child of the person with AD who now has to expend a large amount of time, energy, and money to follow through with the directives. Rhymes (1995) states that the presumption in favor of autonomy assumes that persons possess the capacity to decide, to carry out decisions, and to manage and be accountable for the consequences of their decisions. If there comes a time when they are not able to carry out and manage their decisions, the presumption of auton-

---

DEFINITIONS

Autonomy: The capacity to think, decide, and act on the basis of thought and decision freely and independently (Purtilo, 1999). The right of independence and self-determination.

Beneficence: The requirement to do good. Includes a holistic approach to the individual, including the patient's beliefs, thoughts, values, and judgments.

Health Care Representative: An individual appointed to make health care decisions on your behalf if you become unable to make such decisions.

Incapacity: Being incapable of either managing property or providing self-care or both. Incapacity may stem from infirmity, insanity, mental illness, alcoholism, excessive use of drugs, or neurological deterioration. Although these conditions may contribute to incapacity, an individual who has one or more of these problems is not necessarily incapable.

Justice: Equitable distribution of burden and benefits. It is the obligation to be fair to all individuals regardless of race, creed, religion, gender, or socioeconomic status.

Living Will: A document in which you state your wishes and desires to have or not to have life-prolonging procedures such as respirators, surgery, or feeding tubes, which may delay but would not prevent imminent death.

Nonmaleficence: The principle to do no harm either intentionally or unintentionally.

Power of Attorney: A document that gives another person the authority to handle your personal matters.

Veracity: The principle to tell the truth. It requires that the health care worker be honest and not intentionally deceive or mislead patients.

omy must be reconsidered. This is especially true when the execution of those decisions create unreasonable burdens on the caregivers or other persons who have a legitimate interest in avoiding undue stress and demands on their time and resources. Rhymes (1995) contends that "Guidelines which advocate that decisions that can be articulated should be accepted, may abrogate the rights of an entire class of others who are affected by those decisions" (p. 1437). What may occur is that when caregivers decide to meet the predetermined guidelines, it may be at the expense of others in terms of financial, emotional, and social resources. Often caregivers are required to use financial resources needed by other family members, invite outside caregivers into the home to assist in the caregiving tasks, and split limited time between family and the care recipient. If caregivers decide that they cannot meet the predetermined guidelines, they often live with the guilt that accompanies such decisions. One must consider that long-term care decisions involve not only the autonomy of the person with AD but also those who are expected to provide the caregiving support.

DO NO HARM

In addition, ethical and moral conflicts can appear when a person who is delegated to make health care decisions (proxy) follows a course of action that seems not to be in the patient's best interest. One must be careful to avoid the paternalistic route; that is, if the patient or proxy decides on a course of treatment that is not recommended or that threatens the patient's well-being, it must not automatically be dismissed for the AD patient's "own good." For example, if the proxy decides that antibiotics will not be given in case of pneumonia, one must look at all sides of the situation and not just insist that antibiotics be given.

On the other hand, the health care provider has the duty to act as the patient's advocate if necessary. If the course of treatment decided by the proxy is not considered in the patient's "best interest," the health care provider has a moral obligation to take into account possible motives. Such motives may be caregiver burden, either emotional, physical, or financial; financial gain such as inheritance, pension or disability payments; or possibly abuse or neglect. The principle of nonmaleficence requires health care workers to do no harm. This does not imply that every time proxies disagree with health care providers that they are acting for their own gain but that

each case must be investigated on its own merits with an open mind. One must consider all aspects of the case to reach an ethical decision. In most institutions, ethics committees are available as sounding boards to consider both the positive and negative aspects of such decisions and to provide support and feedback to the health care provider.

DISCLOSING DIAGNOSIS

Protecting patients from harm while respecting their autonomy sometimes creates difficult ethical dilemmas that health care providers must confront. Post and Whitehouse (1995) support the concept of disclosing the diagnosis to the individual even if the family does not support the decision. It is the right of the patient to know the diagnosis in enough time to be able to make the appropriate advance decisions for his or her health care. The principle of veracity requires the health care worker to be honest. It states that the truth must always be told. The family, on the other hand, may contend that withholding information is not the same as being dishonest. At this point, the family must be informed that the person with the diagnosis of AD has a moral and legal right to be present and to receive a specific diagnosis unless he or she waives it. If the dementia is advanced at the time the diagnosis is made, disclosure may no longer be an issue.

The disclosure should occur in a setting that encourages the person and his or her support system to be present so that the information can be presented to all simultaneously and so that emotional support can be given. In this type of setting the expectations of the patient and family and their perceptions of the disease can be discussed in an open forum. The health care provider can advise the person with AD and the family to discuss and agree on a plan of care that incorporates the personal values and resources of all involved.

DRIVING

In protecting the person with AD and the community from harm, one must consider when driving privileges should cease. The diagnosis of AD in itself is not sufficient reason to revoke driving privileges. One difficulty in the decision is that there is no precise test to indicate that the person with AD is no longer capable of driving. During the first 3 years after diagnosis, the risk of persons with AD wrecking their cars is well within the range of that of persons the same age without AD (Trobe, Waller, Cook-Flannigan, Teshima, & Bieliauskas, 1996). Yet, it is clear that 3 years cannot be a concrete marker for revocation of license because the rate of declining abilities varies with each person. Therefore, subjective factors must be taken into consideration when this decision is made.

Consideration has been given to reporting people with the diagnosis of AD to the motor vehicle department. This mandated reporting would compromise patient confidentiality and might even deter an individual from seeking diagnosis and treatment. What is vital is that communication lines remain open between the person with AD, caregivers, and health care professionals.

If restriction of driving becomes necessary, negotiation with the person with AD and the family may result in the person's agreeing to limit driving, such as driving only in the daytime hours. Later the decision can be made as to when the driving privileges should be fully terminated. The family must consider that when driving ceases, other arrangements should be made to ensure that transportation will be available when necessary. It is important that the person with AD does not feel that he or she is a burden to others and thus unnecessarily restrict his or her freedom.

RESTRAINTS

Ethical dilemmas related to behavior control may occur as the disease progresses. Wandering occurs in 26% of homebound persons with AD and in 59% of institutionalized patients with AD. In addition, many persons with AD have episodes of aggression and agitation. Many methods have been tried to manage these behaviors, including chemical and physical restraints. Any restraint should be a last resort. Instead, efforts should be made to try to determine whether there is an underlying cause for the behaviors and to correct those causes. For example, sometimes individuals act out because they are in pain or they are constipated or hungry, and they cannot make their needs known. As health care providers, we have the responsibility to do no harm and to look for the least invasive intervention. Medications are necessary in some instances, but ethical problems arise when behavior-controlling medications are given at doses that interfere with what cognitive function remains. The person with AD should be given the lowest effective dose of medication for the shortest duration possible. These medications should only be given for specific purposes, such as control of anxiety, and should be used cautiously. Medications

should be used in the lowest possible doses and increased only when all other interventions have been exhausted.

Physical restraints are usually not necessary and, in fact, may be hazardous to the person. A physical restraint is considered anything that restricts or controls an individual's freedom of movement. In many instances, the person with AD does not understand the purpose of the restraints, and in most instances the restrained person becomes more agitated. Often as the person is attempting to get free from the restraint, a fall occurs, resulting in an injury. For example, a person may fall trying to crawl over a side rail and, as a result, fall from a higher distance than if the rail had not been raised. The ethical dilemma that occurs is the person's right to freedom and autonomy and the health care provider's duty to prevent harm. In many instances, the health care provider is fearful of liability if the person with AD falls. Physical restraints are rarely a necessity and then should only be used for a brief period, and the person must be carefully monitored while being restrained.

END OF LIFE ISSUES

Although AD is a progressive disease, death usually occurs from pneumonia, sepsis, or other infectious diseases that may result from the immobility that frequently occurs. Therefore the person with AD may want to consider what life-prolonging procedures he or she would want. A living will can be made to help health care professionals determine what the patient wishes when the patient becomes incapable of making his or her wishes known. In addition, a living will helps the health care representative make decisions on the basis of the family's wishes. The document allows the health care professional to support the family or health care representative as they make the difficult end-of-life decisions. Goals for end-of-life care should be discussed between the person with AD, the family, and the health care professionals. It should be clarified whether the long-term goal is that of comfort and emotional well-being or that of prolonging life. A cohesive decision about the goal will make future health care decisions clearer.

It is important to remember that health care professionals and caregivers should not equate the right to refuse treatment with assisted suicide or euthanasia. If a person with AD requests no life-prolonging procedures and this wish is not followed, the community may begin to lose trust in the health care system. If this occurs, persons may erroneously believe that they do not have concrol of their future health considerations and view suicide or assisted suicide as a viable alternative.

An important end-of-life issue that must be addressed by our legislators and policymakers is the availability of hospice care to families of persons with AD. The present difficulty is that to qualify for hospice care, the physician must certify that death is imminent and will likely occur within 6 months. Persons with AD need hospice care for extended periods, and hospice workers need to be prepared for the long-term demand of the care of the person with AD. In a recent study, 71% of family caregivers of persons with AD preferred hospice care in cases of end-stage dementia (Post & Whitehall, 1996).

GENETIC TESTING

The progress being made in the area of genetic testing to predict AD makes the exploration of ethical and moral implications a necessity. Early-onset AD in persons younger than 50 has been linked to either chromosomes 14 or 21 (Mayeux & Schupf, 1995). Early-onset AD represents less than 1% of all cases of AD. An association of apolipoprotein E (APOE) with the onset of the most common familial late-onset AD is only a beginning of what is to be learned (Roses, 1996).

APOE, a protein located on chromosome 19, is found in three variations in the population. These variations are called alleles. The alleles are named APOE ε2, ε3, or ε4. Each person inherits one allele from his or her mother and one from the father, resulting in one of six combinations (ε2/ε2, ε2/ε3, ε2/ε4, ε3/ε3, ε3/ε4, ε4/ε4). The APOE ε3/ε3 allele combination is the most common, occurring in 59% of the population. Roses (1996) found that the inheritance of two specific combinations of the ε4 allele (ε3/ε4 or ε4/ε4) is associated with an increased risk and earlier age of onset of AD compared with the other genotypes. The combination ε3/ε4 is found in 21% of the Caucasian population, whereas the combination ε4/ε4 is found in only 2% (Roses, 1996). The presence of the allele indicates an increased risk for AD, although factors that indicate which persons with the ε4 allele may actually have AD develop are under investigation but are presently unknown. Mayeux and Schupf (1995) state that "while the apolipoprotein E genotype may be undeniable as a genetic risk factor for AD, it does not provide sufficient information to be an adequate predictive genetic test" (p. 1281).

Several issues arise from this. First, the question must be asked whether this is a health care need or a health care desire. With the high costs of health care, the principle of justice must consider health care for all. For example, cosmetic surgery in most cases is considered a health care desire. In these cases an individual who had such desires but did not have the economic resources to access those desires would have no basis for claiming unjust treatment. Therefore one must assess the new technological advances as to what benefit they will have and who will benefit.

The second issue arises from the prospect that genetic information may be entered into a computer, where it may become accessible to others. This presents problems with the issue of privacy. If genetic testing becomes more prominent, issues of job or insurance discrimination may arise. In addition, if this is used as a type of genetic testing, a protocol must be in place to ensure that the appropriate counseling and support systems are available.

One suggested use is that of an older individual who has dementia. The additional information gained by the testing would be a benefit if as a result it would reduce the cost of evaluation or if the diagnosis could be confirmed. Also, this predictive testing could be used for the purposes of family planning issues once the testing has been refined and the meaning associated with the presence of the gene has been determined and solidified.

With the increasing incidence of AD, the ethical, legal, and moral issues affect nurses as we deal daily with the patient with AD, his or her family, and other caregivers. Care must be provided in a way that is compassionate not only for the patient but for the entire support system. Nurses must be forward-thinking enough to help facilitate the discussion and planning of future health care needs. The principles of autonomy, justice, veracity, beneficence, and nonmaleficence must be considered as we counsel, educate, and provide care for persons with AD and their caregivers.

REFERENCES

Alzheimer's Association Facts. (1999). Available: http://www.alzheimers.org/facts//rtstats.htm.

Caralis, P. (1994). Ethical and legal issues in the care of Alzheimer's patients. *Medical Clinics of North America, 78*(4), 877-893.

Katzman, R., & Saitoh, T. (1991). Advances in Alzheimer's disease. *FASEB Journal, 5,* 278-286.

Marson, D., & Harrell, L. (1999). Executive dysfunction and loss of capacity to consent to medical treatment in patients with Alzheimer's disease. *Seminars in Clinical Neuropsychiatry, 4*(1), 41-49.

Mayeux, R., & Schupf, N. (1995). Apolipoprotein E and Alzheimer's disease: The implications of progress in molecular medicine. *American Journal of Public Health, 85*(9), 1280-1284.

Post, S.G., & Whitehouse, P. (1995). Fairhill guidelines on ethics of the care of people with Alzheimer's disease: A clinical summary. *Journal of the American Geriatric Society, 43*(12), 1423-1429.

Purtilo, R. (1999). *Ethical dimensions in the health professions.* Philadelphia: Saunders.

Roses, A. (1996). Apolipoprotein E and Alzheimer's disease: A rapidly expanding field with medical and epidemiological consequences. *Annals of the New York Academy of Science, 802,* 50-57.

Rhymes, J. (1995). When the bill comes due for the autonomy of demented older adults, who pays? *Journal of the American Geriatric Society, 43*(12), 1437-1438.

Schloendorff v Society of New York Hospital, 211 N.Y. 125 (1914).

Stratton, W. (1995). Legal implications of Alzheimer's disease. *Kansas Medicine, 96*(2), 44-45.

Trobe, J., Waller, P., Cook-Flannigan, C., Teshima, S., & Bieliauskas, L. (1996). Crashes and violations among drivers with Alzheimer's disease. *Archives of Neurology, 53,* 411-416.

Weiler, K. (1994). Legal aspects of nursing documentation for the Alzheimer's patient. *Journal of Gerontological Nursing, 20*(4), 31-40.

Advance Directives

Challenges for Nurses and Patients

DIANE K. KJERVIK

A commitment to individualism (autonomy) is one of the fundamental values in the United States. Individual freedom is seen as the hallmark of a democratic political system. Soldiers have fought and died for freedom from governmental oppression and for freedom of the individual to say and do what is desired. The Bill of Rights in the United States Constitution promises freedom to speak one's own mind, to associate with persons and groups with whom one wishes to associate, the right to practice one's own religion, and the right of privacy.

Concomitant with the orientation to individual freedom is a corresponding right to make decisions about where one lives, what one does with one's property, and in terms of health care, what one will allow to be done with one's body. As Justice Cardozo stated, "Every human being of adult years and sound mind has a right to determine what shall be done with his own body; and a surgeon who performs an operation without his patient's consent commits an assault, for which he is liable in damages" (*Schloendorff v Society of New York Hospital*, 1914). Assumed in this statement of the law is the necessity of a "sound mind" and the belief that without an affirmation to the opposite, consent is not present. Interestingly, the health care system presumes more often than the legal system that consent is present unless refusal is noted in do-not-resuscitate orders (DNRs), advance directives, and communications with providers.

The concept of informed consent has become widely accepted in health care and legal circles as the standard for entering into a patient-health care provider contract for services. Part of the reason for implementing informed consent in health care is to empower the patient by providing information about services to be given so that the patient is able to make a more meaningful choice among the options available (Kjervik & Grove, 1988). With knowledge of the options presented in a clear and consistent fashion, the patient becomes aware of his or her ability to participate actively and with authority in the decision-making process. In this way the patient becomes an active participant in the health care decision-making process, and the power imbalance created by the lack of information is redressed (Katz, 1984). A corollary of the right to consent to treatment is the right to refuse treatment (*Cruzan v Director, Missouri Department of Health*, 1990). Advance directives in the health care context usually state what the patient does not want done and, in effect, refuses to have done. Nurses are considered by some to be among the best qualified to discuss advance directives with patients and their families (Henderson, 1997; Silverman, Fry, & Armistead, 1994). Patients trust nurses, and as studies have shown, patients consider quality at the end of life to include feeling a sense of control and avoidance of inappropriate prolongation of dying (Cameron, 1999; Singer, Martin, & Kelner, 1999). Nurses and their patients are challenged to achieve the goals of peaceful death for the patient even in circumstances in which others prefer to prolong the patient's life.

TYPES OF ADVANCE DIRECTIVES

Advance directives are legal mechanisms that enable a person to make decisions about financial arrangements or health care services before the occurrence of a situation in which the person is unable to make such decisions. Advance directives enhance individualism by providing a written document signed by the person that indicates what that person wants done under certain specified circumstances. When properly legally executed, these documents serve as a valid statement of the person's wishes and cannot be invalidated without compelling reasons.

Advance directives include those relating to financial affairs such as wills, trusts, representative payeeships, powers of attorney, and joint tenancy (Weiler, 1989). These financial advance directives provide that a substitute decision maker, such as a personal representative in the case of a will or a trustee in the situation of a trust, is empowered to act on behalf of the person who executed the document. The purpose of articulating these wishes in advance is so that the individual's wishes will be predominant, rather than the wishes of persons who are likely to receive direct benefit from the estate of the individual. These legal arrangements have been available for a considerable period of time to handle financial matters. Directives can also be given to a third party about care for oneself rather than one's property such as those relating to health care: the living will and the durable power of attorney for health care.

The living will is a document that states that under certain circumstances, such as terminal illness, an individual prefers to have certain choices exercised on his or her behalf. In 1976, California became the first state to enact legislation that allowed advanced decision making for end-of-life situations (Fade, 1995). The typical direction of the living will is that life-sustaining activities such as the provision of food, fluid, and cardiopulmonary respiration are to be withheld so that the person may die a peaceful death. Without this kind of direction, a hospital or independent health care provider would feel obligated to maintain life for fear of a lawsuit alleging wrongful death. Mental health directives are also becoming more common. For instance, North Carolina enacted a statute that allows a patient to develop an advance instruction for mental health treatment (NC, 1998), and the New York Office of Mental Health issued a policy encouraging the use of written statements by psychiatric patients who would identify the types of treatments they prefer to receive during crises (18 Deaths, 1994). A psychiatric crisis can precipitate life-death consequences as with other illnesses, and many patients who have been through emergency episodes can identify what works well for them.

The durable power of attorney for health care enables the person to name another person to be a substitute decision maker under the circumstances of impaired functioning on the part of the person executing the document. If the person is impaired to the point of being unable to decide what to do, the substitute decision maker can do so. Most states have enacted laws that provide for the living will and durable power of attorney for health care (Cate & Gill, 1991; Choice in Dying, 1992). All states but Massachusetts, Michigan, and New York have laws governing living wills, and all states but Alaska and Alabama have statutes that allow appointment of a durable power of attorney for health care (Fade, 1995). The usefulness of these advance directives in assisting clinical decision making is not yet clear. One team of researchers concluded that advance directives were irrelevant to decision making regarding resuscitation of seriously ill patients (Teno et al., 1994). Another study showed that family members of dying patients perceived that 10% of patients did not receive the care they preferred at the end of life (Lynn et al., 1997).

A recent development is the portable DNR document that patients carry with them or the provider sends with the patient to the hospital, for example, from a nursing home. Forty-one states now use out-of-hospital DNRs that are especially helpful in situations in which emergency medical service (EMS) personnel are called to help and must follow the physician-ordered DNR (State initiatives, 1999).

ETHICAL ASPECTS OF ADVANCE DIRECTIVES

Although advance directives are legal mechanisms to support substitute decision making, ethical principles underlie the development of the statutes and the practice related to advance directives. The concept of autonomy, which is a fundamental ethical principle, is closely related to the freedom of the individual to choose what is to be done with his or her body. Likewise, as Faden and Beauchamp (1986) have pointed out, the principles of justice and beneficence are also served by the implementation of informed consent. Katz (1984) discusses the history of silence between physicians and patients that has led to the doctrine of informed consent. Nurses and patients have not experienced the same degree of silence in relation to nursing care. This could be because nursing care involves patient participation and discussion about the implementation of nursing tasks. In addition, nurses have long espoused the importance of mutuality between nurse and patient.

Caring for patients (beneficence) is manifest in the concern for the individual's decision-making capability and the importance of empowering the individual to be part of the decision-making process. To give patients a voice in what happens with their health care is a beneficent act that is respectful of varying human values and recognizes differences among human beings regarding life and death matters. To feel compassion for the person who is facing difficult choices exemplifies the ethic of care, a new orientation to ethics that attends to feelings that hold relationships together (Beauchamp & Childress, 1994).

The principle of justice is served by giving all individuals a fair share of attention to their wishes about the prolongation of their lives. Whether a person is rich or poor, African-American or Caucasian should make no difference in the decision about whether to end one's life. Deontologically, the rules to be served by advance directives are those relating to the freedom of the individual to choose what will be done with his or her own body and the value of the individual's life and death. Teleologically, the goal to be served is that of peaceful and dignified death for all patients within the health care system.

Empowerment is also an ethical concern from the vantage point of coerciveness by a more powerful party in the decision-making process. Coercion or manipulation makes the choice of less powerful individuals meaningless. Cooperation and conflict resolution among human beings is enhanced by empowering all persons in the relationship. In the case of advance directives for health care, empowerment of both nurse and patient is an ethical matter. If the nurse has far more power than the patient in the interactions, the decisions made by the patient are suspect as lacking autonomy. Therefore the patient must be empowered to speak his or her mind with the nurse as they discuss the decisions to be made. Responsible assertiveness is a communication technique that can assist and empower a client to speak. As Lange and Jakubowski (1976) point out, "responsible assertion means not deliberately using personal power to manipulatively overpower weaker people in conflict situations" (p. 58). Therefore, the more powerful individual has the responsibility to encourage and teach assertive behavior to a less powerful person. An advance directive can strengthen the patient's ability to speak her or his own mind by providing a visible, concrete form of the statement of preference. The nurse too is empowered by advance directives, because information is made available to the nurse about the patient's orientation to life and death. This information assists the nurse to implement the nursing process. In one study, nurses indicated that working with patients to help them with advance directives promoted communication among patients, families, and health care providers and increased staff knowledge about advance directives (Silverman et al., 1994).

The living will is a clear way of stating what the patient values at a point in time that is outside the framework of the time of crisis (i.e., when a patient is admitted to a hospital or a nursing home). It is under circumstances of these critical admissions to a health care facility that decisions often must be made by the staff and family of the patient without benefit of prior consideration and decision by the patient. Effective December 1991, federal law mandated that hospitals and other health care facilities inform patients of their rights under state law to have living wills and durable powers of attorney for health care (*Patient Self-Determination Act,* 1990). Although it is useful for incoming patients to be informed of these rights, the time of admission is not the most fruitful time for development of this thought and emotion-provoking document. However, the federal mandate to agencies and health care workers raises their awareness of the importance of these documents to patients, families, and society, and the effect of this attitudinal change is presumably passed on to patients.

Another fundamental ethical issue underlying advance directives is the value placed by society on life. In *Cruzan v Director, Missouri Department of Health* (1990) it became apparent that United States Supreme Court justices were divided on the importance that could be attached to life per se in relation to quality of life. Most of the justices in the Cruzan case believed that life per se was worth preserving and that a state had the right to set the parameters for using advance directives. The minority opinion emphasized the quality of life and the right of an individual to determine when that quality of life had deteriorated to the point that intrusive measures were no longer justified.

Considerations of the quality of life must always address the question of who is to determine the quality of life. Living wills and durable powers of attorney for health care are premised on the belief that the patient determines what quality of life means for herself or himself. Other individuals who are willing to be more paternalistic in their orientation say the quality of life is to be determined by health care providers or the government. In reality, the quality of one's life can only clearly be ascertained by oneself on the basis of an evaluation of whatever criteria the individual decides constitutes quality. One's values are a critical element in ascertaining the quality of one's life and can be evaluated by use of a values history such as that developed by the Center for Health Law and Ethics at the University of New Mexico (Cate & Gill, 1991). One study showed that older persons often continue to rely on others to make decisions and so lack enthusiasm about creating advance directives even when they receive written information about them (High, 1993). The trend toward surrogate decision-making laws (Fade, 1995) responds to the need some persons have to rely on others to make difficult choices.

OBJECTIONS TO ADVANCE DIRECTIVES

Several arguments are raised in opposition to advance directives. The first is the paternalistic belief that the health care provider, usually physician, knows what is best for the patient. This notion has been eroded by consumer activism and by other health care providers who are interested in sharing power with other members of the health care team and their patients. The designation of "patient" is even undergoing challenge and revision because of its emphasis on a one-up/one-down position between doctor and patient. As consumers become more active and interested in their own health care, they expect to be part of the decision-making process and ultimately to make their own decisions. Certainly there are rare cases in which individuals do not want to be bothered with decisions about their health care. These cases, however, are less frequent as consumers become more sophisticated about health care alternatives and therefore interested in asserting their own voice or relying on a relative who knows their preferences. One reason they are interested in asserting their own voice is their experience with inadequate diagnostic and treatment decisions by health care providers that have resulted in injury to patients and corresponding large medical malpractice awards.

Another argument against living wills asserts that these directives do not reflect an incompetent patient's interests accurately. Because these documents are formulated when the person is competent and presumably has different interests, it is argued that later when the person becomes incompetent, the best interests are served in entirely different ways than what the patient long ago envisioned (Robertson, 1991). Following this line of reasoning, one's will and choice would have to be recorded continuously for a living will or any other form of advance directive to be considered valid. Contracts, wills, and trusts would all have to be invalidated because they were developed before the time that they are acted on. Clearly this is an absurd result that would create tremendous dysfunction in several areas of the law.

A third argument points to research that shows patients are willing to grant their surrogates leeway in the way the living will is interpreted and do not expect strict adherence to wishes they have stated in their living wills (Sehgal et al., 1992). The response to this argument is that specification as to areas of leeway and principles to be followed can be enumerated and, indeed, should be enumerated in the living will itself. Alternatively the proxy decision maker acting under the durable power of attorney for health care can be instructed orally by the patient

as to the leeway to be given. Decisions of the surrogate thus can reflect an accurate and full discussion with the patient.

Probably the most vociferous argument against living wills has been raised in legislative sessions in which opponents warn of a slippery slope between living wills and murder or genocide. This argument can be rebutted by the realization that the law examines carefully any coercion or manipulation involved in entering into this as with any other legal contract. Therefore, only documents that are the will of the patient are to be followed. No independent judgment by health care professionals that a given patient or a given group of patients should die would control the situation in which a living will is in effect. The law would not want to reach the absurd result that no contract or other legal document could be entered into if there were any possibility of coercion or manipulation. Ethical and legal rules must be adopted on the basis of their ability to organize human behavior. These rules cannot be controlled by the fear of numerous possibilities of human evil. As far as coercion and manipulation go, to not allow a person to determine what will be done with his or her body during a terminal illness is a form of coercion as well, one in which the outside person decides that the life of another should be preserved at all costs. This argument against living wills also overlooks the fact that some persons indicate in their living wills that they wish every possible means to be used to keep them alive (request directives). A slippery slope in the other direction could be imagined in which a patient's wish overrules resource allocation decisions, an equally absurd result.

ADVANCE DIRECTIVES IN RELATION TO NURSING PRACTICE

The nursing process can be enhanced by use of advance directives. As part of the assessment of the patient's goals in relation to severity of health care status, the nurse can discuss provisions that exist in the patient's living will or durable power of attorney for health care. Members of the health care team must respond to provisions of the living will, so they need to understand the meaning of the document to the patient, and they need to understand what the law within their state requires for the document to be considered valid. In a much publicized 1992 case in Texas the patient and his family were distraught when the patient's living will was not followed by the facility because state law requires that two physicians certify the patient as terminally ill and only one physician had done so (Gamino, 1992). Other legal cases have been brought in Ohio and North Carolina when patients' express wishes were not followed (Martin, 1997). Close work with the attorney for the facility is necessary to make the legal mandates clear to staff and administrators.

A values history can give a picture of the patient's beliefs about organ donation, respirators, and independent functioning, for instance. If the patient has no advance directive, discussion of personal values may assist the patient to make a choice to execute a living will. Knowing the patient's belief about artificial extension of life, the nurse can plan and implement care that is respectful of the patient. Care can be evaluated according to standards developed by the patient in addition to those imposed from the outside that have to do with technical choices such as which antihypertensive drug to prescribe. If the patient chooses to have no heroic measures exercised, the nurse will be present to assist with comfort measures. Interventions in the direction of this goal rather than the goal of preserving life might create moral conflict for some nurses. In the future, nurses may be called on to take a more active role in assisting with death (Johnson & Weiler, 1990). Nursing must take an active part in the debate about aid-in-dying because without doubt, nurses will be called on to play a close, active role in the process (Kjervik, 1997). The American Nurses Association issued a statement about nurse-assisted suicide that makes clear that direct assistance with suicide is not an accepted standard in nursing (American Nurses Association, 1994). Interestingly, however, carrying out the patient's wishes for withdrawal of treatment as specified in a written advance directive is legally and ethically acceptable as previously argued.

Nurses are moral agents who are responsible for their own conduct. As Theis (1990) has noted, "To conceive of the nurse as one who simply follows directives without moral reflection concerning the treatment being rendered fails to recognize the moral status of the nurse as an individual with standards of personal conscience and professional ethics." The nurse cannot assist the patient to examine values without having a sense of her or his own values. Therefore part of the process of caring for the patient involves self-reflection and decision making about how one views one's own life and death. Nurses can act as role models for behaviors considered valuable for the patient to demonstrate, for example, by having their own living wills (Weber & Kjervik, 1992). Because the range of persons with advance directives ranges from less than 10% of the public to 28% of AIDS patients (Crisham,

1990; Teno et al., 1994), nurses' role modeling is especially important.

Patients who have advance directives demonstrate health-promoting behaviors. By stating values and preferences manifestly in writing, the patient shows the strength to be an active participant in the maintenance of health rather than a passive observer and recipient of the preferences of others. In the process of preparing an advance directive, the patient imagines his or her own possible incapacitation. Through the use of this imagery the patient is able to consider all alternatives, including the opportunity to have choice over life and death options. The act of imagining and then creating a written statement of choice is strengthening to patients who often feel like victims in the health care setting.

Advance directives also act as preventive measures. Because primary prevention in health care means the practice of health-promoting and disease-preventing behaviors, risk management in the law means preventing legal difficulties. Advance directives prevent legal problems in the future when the viewpoint of the patient may be at issue. Economically, respecting the patient's choice may reduce escalating heath care costs by ruling out a number of expensive procedures. As Katz (1984) suggests, "first patient opinions" may be less costly than "second medical opinions."

The encouragement of advance directives may also provide an opportunity for nurses to apply a relational ethic of care. Parker (1990) describes this ethic as a process of sharing relational stories of caregiving. This process is based on reciprocity and interconnectedness among human beings. To talk with patients about their stories of the meaning of life and death to them assists them in making decisions about advance directives. Self-disclosure by the nurse enriches the process and contributes to mutual understanding and concern. Deliberate conversations about death and dying issues are recommended by Badzek, Leslie, and Corbo-Richert (1998). Requests for assisted suicide or euthanasia have been withdrawn after support is received from nurses and family members and pain management and treatment of depression are introduced (Severson, 1997).

An important foundation on which the realization of an ethic of care, the principles of justice, beneficence, and autonomy, and the legal goal of self-determination is based is the relationship between the nurse and patient. Trust is imperative to this relationship and can be enhanced by the execution of advance directives. Katz (1984) poses several assumptions that are part of a trusting, mutual relationship in the context of informed consent:

1. There is no single right or wrong answer for how life, health and illness should be lived. Numerous treatment options exist and suffering can be alleviated in a variety of ways.
2. Health care providers and patients both have vulnerabilities and conflicting motivations, interests and expectations. Sameness of interests cannot be presumed; it must be confirmed in conversation.
3. Both parties relate to each other as equals and unequals. Professionals share professional expertise and patients their personal expertise. At the outset, neither knows what each can do for the other.
4. Human behavior contains both rational and irrational elements. These elements must be accepted in health care providers and patients. Incompetence should not be presumed for either when signs of irrationality appear.

The assumptions enumerated by Katz indicate that the physician must engage in dialogue with patients about health care choices, options, and decisions. Although nurses do not demonstrate the silence referred to by Katz, the assumptions still are important for nurses to consider. Nurses should recognize the variety of "right" answers available to patients, should be aware of their own vulnerabilities and be able to discuss these with patients, should recognize their equalities and inequalities with patients, and should become comfortable with their own irrational sides. As Katz (1984) states, "trust must be earned through conversation." It is in the face-to-face encounter with the patient that mutual understanding develops. With the understanding comes more effective decision making about health care choices.

SUMMARY

Nurses play a key role in the development and implementation of advance directives. Nursing values of mutuality, open and direct communication, caring, and health promotion and prevention support the use of advance directives for health care. A shared decision-making model is a natural for nurses and patients and is helpful during the dying process (Hiltunen, Medich, Chase, Peterson, & Forrow, 1999). The challenge to patients is honest and forthright expression of their wishes. The skill nurses have in developing trusting relationships with patients can be used as a model for other health care professionals who are burdened with silence or unsupportiveness in their relationships with patients. The Patient Self-Determination Act of 1990 provides the impetus for nursing involvement with patients on the topics of living wills and durable powers of attorney for health care. Now, nurses must engage patients, their families, and other health care providers in deliberate discussions about the end of life.

We help our patients speak.
We help them look deep within
For truth, conflict and decision.
Then we accept their paths
As we accept our own.

REFERENCES

American Nurses Association. (1994). *Position statement on assisted suicide.* Washington, DC: Author.

Badzek, L.A., Leslie, N.S., & Corbo-Richert, B. (1998). End-of-life decisions: Are they honored? *Journal of Nursing Law, 5*(2), 51-63.

Beauchamp, T.L., & Childress, J.F. (1994). *Principles of biomedical ethics* (4th ed.). New York: Oxford University Press.

Cameron, M.E. (1999). Completing life and dying triumphantly. *Journal of Nursing Law, 6*(1), 27-32.

Cate, F.H., & Gill, B.A. (1991). *The Patient Self-Determination Act: Implementation issues and opportunities* (pp. 65-73). Washington, DC: Annenberg Washington Program of Northwestern University.

Choice in dying: Right-to-die case & statutory citations. (1992, March 17). New York: Author.

Crisham, P. (1990). Living wills—Controversy and certainty. *Journal of Professional Nursing, 6*(6), 321.

Cruzan v Director, Missouri Department of Health, 110 S. Ct. 2841, 111 L. Ed. 2d 224, 58. USLW 4916 (US Mo., June 25, 1990).

18 Deaths in NY psychiatric facilities instigate changes: Ethical concerns about restraints apply equally to mental patients. (1994). *Medical Ethics Advisor, 10*(12), 162-163.

Fade, A.E. (1995). Advance directives: An overview of changing right-to-die laws. *Journal of Nursing Law, 2*(3), 27-38.

Faden, R.R., & Beauchamp, T.L. (1986). *A history and theory of informed consent.* New York: Oxford University Press.

Gamino, D. (1992, May 15). A living will fails to ensure dignified death. *Austin American-Statesman,* pp. A-1, A-12.

Henderson, M.L. (1997). Advance directives for patients with cancer. *Cancer Practice, 5*(3), 186-188.

High, D.M. (1993). Advance directives and the elderly: A study of intervention strategies to increase use. *The Gerontologist, 33*(3), 342-349.

Hiltunen, E.F., Medich, C., Chase, S., Peterson, L., & Forrow, L. (1999). Family decision making for end-of-life treatment: The SUPPORT nurse narratives. *The Journal of Clinical Ethics, 10*(2), 126-134.

Johnson, R.A., & Weiler, K. (1990). Aid-in-dying: Issues and implications for nursing. *Journal of Professional Nursing, 6*(5), 258-264.

Katz, J. (1984). *The silent world of doctor and patient* (pp. xiv, 28-29, 47, 102-103, 228). New York: Macmillan.

Kjervik, D.K. (1997). Assisted suicide: The challenge to the nursing profession. *Journal of Law, Medicine & Ethics, 24*(3), 237-242.

Kjervik, D.K., & Grove, S. (1988). A legal model of consent in unequal power relationships. *Journal of Professional Nursing, 4*(3), 192-204.

Lange, A.J., & Jakubowski, P. (1976). *Responsible assertive behavior: Cognitive behavioral procedures for trainers* (p. 58). Champaign, IL: Research Press.

Lynn, J., Teno, J.M., Phillips, R.S., Wu, A.W., Desbiens, N., Harrold, J., Claessens, M.T., Wenger, N., Kreling, B., & Connors, A.F. (1997). Perceptions by family members of the dying experience of older and seriously ill patients. *Annals of Internal Medicine, 126*(2), 97-106.

Martin, R.H. (1997). Advance directives: Legal implications for nurses. *Journal of Nursing Law, 4*(2), 7-15.

NC ST sec. 122C-72, GS sec. 122C-72 (1998).

Parker, R.S. (1990). Nurses' stories: The search for a relational ethic of care. *Advances in Nursing Science, 13*(1), 31-40.

Patient Self-Determination Act of 2990, 42 U.S.C.A. § 1395 cc (f) (1) (A) (I)(1991 Supp. pam.), PL 101-508 § 4206, 104 Stat. 1388-115 (1990).

Robertson, J.A. (1991). Second thoughts on living wills. *Hastings Center Report, 21*(6), 6-9.

Schloendorff v Society of New York Hospital, 211 N.Y. 125, 129-30, 105 N.E. 92, 93 (1914).

Sehgal, A., Galbraith, A., Chesney, M., Schoenfeld, P., Charles, G., & Lo, B. (1992). How strictly do dialysis patients want their advanced directives followed? *Journal of the American Medical Association, 267*(1), 59-63.

Severson, K.T. (1997). Dying cancer patients: Choices at the end of life. *Journal of Pain and Symptom Management, 14*(2), 94-98.

Silverman, H.J., Fry, S.T., & Armistead, N. (1994). Nurses' perspectives on implementation of the Patient Self-Determination Act. *The Journal of Clinical Ethics, 5*(1), 30-37.

Singer, P.A., Martin, D.K., & Kelner, M. (1999). Quality end-of-life care: Patients' perspectives. *Journal of the American Medical Association, 281*(2), 163-168.

State initiatives in end-of-life care. (1999, April). Implementing end-of-life treatment preferences across clinical settings. *National Program Office for Community-State Partnerships to Improve End-of-Life Care,* Issue 3.

Teno, J.M., Lynn, J., Phillips, R.S., Murphy, D., Youngner, S.J., Bellamy, P., Connors, A.F., Jr., Desbiens, N.A., Fulkerson, W., & Knaus, W.A. (1994). Do advance directives affect resuscitation decisions and the use of resources for seriously ill patients? *The Journal of Clinical Ethics, 5*(1), 23-30.

Theis, E.C. (1990). Life-sustaining technologies: Ordinary or extraordinary? *Focus on Critical Care, 17*(6), 445-450.

Weber, G., & Kjervik, D.K. (1992). The Patient Self-Determination Act—The nurse's proactive role. *Journal of Professional Nursing, 8*(1), 6.

Weiler, K. (1989). Financial abuse of the elderly: Recognizing and acting on it. *Journal of Gerontological Nursing, 15*(8), 10-15.

Just Managing

Ethical Obligations and the Managed Health Care Marketplace

LAURIE ZOLOTH

As the American health care system moved toward the dramatic reorganization known as "managed care," nurses have been increasingly faced with ethical conflicts that range far beyond the familiar ethical dramas of withholding and withdrawing life support (Krieger, 1995). Indeed, in the last 5 years, the conflicts that have emerged at the bedside and in the clinic and that have spilled over into courts and legislative sessions have been dominated by a new set of concerns. In case after case, even for patients with health care insurance, nurses are being asked to do more care with fewer resources. At stake are the deepest ethical decisions about the meaning and intent of medicine itself and the responsibility of the nurse toward her or his patient. When we speak of a health care system that is just, what is the place for advocacy for a decent climate for care? When we call for a health care system that is effective, what is the cost of compassion? How do ethical principles and precepts help when the nurse feels that instead of managing with justice, she or he is just managing? At the heart of this question is a search for the values that ought to guide the provision of medical care in the new world of health care delivery. What are the mechanisms that will be necessary both to protect patients and to articulate provider standards in a health care system increasingly regulated by the marketplace? How can the development of such ethical standards help to define parameters in the evolving health care system?

This chapter will make reference to such core issues as how the necessity for justice, the creation of desire, the construction of need, and the historical formulation of a basic demand for health care services have driven the present structure of health care. The main focus, however, will be on how the specific ethical issues are created in a system of "negative reward." This system, used to contain costs in a managed care health care delivery system creates special problems for the nurse who often is the one "standing at the gate" in the organization. This chapter will argue that only a robust and publicly accessible discourse before the onset of crisis can create a just encounter over the issue of health care intervention and that as part of such a system all participants must have access to the truthful data, the lucid process, and the clarity of the financial relationships that are suggested by each medical choice. Burdens and benefits of such a system must be mutually borne. It is only by opening the process up to such disclosure that the power differential can begin to be equalized and that both infinity of desire for medical care and the capacity for fiduciary abuse be examined. This chapter will argue that if we are to take the dominance of medicine by the managed care system as a first premise, we are then obligated to create a system in which a strong moral agency is encouraged and supported and patient advocacy is a normative structure of the nursing role.

THE CASE

"The case has brought the unit nearly to a standstill," said Sheila Fuentes, the clinical nurse specialist in the cardiac care unit, shaking her head slowly at the ethics committee meeting. The other nurses from the unit watched her quietly, their arms folded, waiting for their turn to present their side of the story. "Mr. McGill is a 27-year-old laborer from a poor rural family in the dusty California coastal range. He drifted down to Los Angeles for a construction job about 4 years ago, got on our HMO plan, and then got sick. He tried to keep working, but finally he came home, so his family could take care of him, which is how he landed up here, because our hospital was just bought by his HMO. He was really sick—advanced endocarditis—and because he had insurance, the University hospital was only too happy to give him a transplant. But our HMO will only pay for 4.5 days inpatient care, and they sent him home. His wound was not even closed—the drains were still in. Now "home" is his parent's trailer on 15 acres of scrub land. So he got a massive wound infection. He needs twice daily sterile dressing changes, antibiotics, and still his wound is not healing. But here is the dilemma. His wound infection care is not covered by his HMO. The heart transplant is, but not the 4 × 4's he needs every day." She turns to her colleagues, some of whom are looking at their laps; others look defiantly at the committee. "Mr. McGill has begun to show up on our floor asking for 4 × 4's because he knows us. Sometimes his mother or his little sisters come. Some of the nurses have even done a few changes themselves, in the treatment room." One of the other nurses interrupts. "But some of us feel that it is just not fair to do this for *him* and not for the rest of our patients!" she says. "I am always sending home frail elderly women with no one to care for them! How can we use resources this way—steal them, really—for one patient and not for all?" Another nurse raises her voice. "I snuck McGill into the treatment room," she admits. "One day on pms. You could see that snazzy new heart beating underneath a mass of necrotic tissue. How can you ignore the needs of your patient, just because he can't pay? Have we really come to that?"

Sheila Fuentes is silent. She is facing an irony of her own. This is the last case she will bring to the ethics committee as a CNS: the hospital, in another cost-containment measure has elected to phase out all CNS positions next month, and she will be looking for work. She used to be an unequivocal advocate for her patients, at whatever cost; now she wonders if the sum of this attitude has finally come home to roost.

DESIRE AND THE PRODUCTION OF HEALTH CARE SERVICES

Fundamental ethical questions about the dynamics that drive the desire for good health care services and the corresponding health system are in part historical and in part cultural (Daniels, 1985). We need to ask, What are the ethical justifications for resolving the conflict between explicable desire and just health care delivery, and to what moral appeals are we obligated to be accountable as institutions and as citizens of a good society?

THE GOOD SOCIETY AND GOOD HEALTH

One can think of a variety of ways in which to describe such a society. Many of the measures are descriptions of what we mean by fairness in the allocation of basic social goods such as health care (Menzel, 1990). In reflecting on how nurses committed to caring ought to describe a just allocation several contending perspectives emerge. At the heart of each lies a theory of justice. Traditional ways to

describe a theory have been based in libertarianism, utilitarianism, and egalitarianism. Each of these depends on giving different weight to the importance of such issues as desert, equality, or desire.

American health care is based on an amalgam of these different theories. Institutions develop and provide for their participants a particular narrative that is rooted in a belief structure based in these theories (Moreno, 1995). Yet because these narratives attempt to reconcile significantly different vantages, there is a discrepancy in their underlying themes.

Hence, although we have a commitment to the relationship between hard work and rewarding outcomes, we are troubled by stark differences in the quality of health care for the poor and health care for the wealthy (Aaron, 1990; Daniels, 1985; Rhodes, 1992). Although we speak of autonomy and consent as centrally important, we are concerned about our ability to set limits when the needs of the one threaten to obscure the needs of the many. Although we retain a concern for the vulnerable, we are uneasy in an open-ended commitment, and we are troubled by the links between lifestyle and disease.

Furthermore, into this theoretical confusion has been thrust a central cultural myth of the late twentieth century: anything that is created can be repaired, all problems have a solution, and that medical power and progress are infinite. The rewards for this promise have been lucrative for physicians, for pharmaceutical companies, and for the vast network of subsidiaries (Aaron, 1991). Even the insurance companies, despite the rising costs of medical care, have made substantial profits; in fact, one of the cautionary impulses that mitigated against reform is the fear of upsetting this powerful and robust industry.

HEALTH CARE REFORM

But the rising costs of medical services and the difficulty in access forced a rethinking of how Americans received their care. The subject of health care became first a campaign issue and then a matter of national policy in the period 1988 to 1992. Fierce struggles erupted over the best way to address the moral dilemmas presented by the kind of case that the nurses faced in the California hospital described previously. The Clinton administration and Congress disagreed and ultimately did not find consistent legislative solutions to the problem. Since this discourse effectively ended in 1992, the number of uninsured Americans has risen to 44 million.

After the failure of Congress to resolve the much-discussed health care system crisis, in many states the market forces have already stepped in to reconstruct the health care marketplace. In these states, most of the population (both private payers and Medicaid beneficiaries) is organized into managed care organizations, physicians are organizing into networks, and hospital and health care systems consolidate into ever larger health care conglomerates every week.

What does this all mean for the clinical nurse, and how ought a nurse seek to resolve ethical dilemmas raised by a larger social crisis in health care? One thing is certain. It means that nurses and their patients are participating in a vast social experiment (albeit without prior consent) on how a population is served by such a medical care delivery system. How is this experiment faring and is such a system fair? As the preceding case shows, the answer to this question depends on where in the power relationship one stands.

CONFLICTS OF INTEREST

Ethical conflicts between stakeholders are inherent in any system of health care delivery that relies on relationships between strangers as the basis of a contract for care (Arras & Steinbock, 1995). This is not a new feature of American health care. Although the provision of health care is a compassionate and necessary gesture, it is also a business, a way that millions earn their living, a product that is sold in a marketplace. In the current climate of economic downturn, the nurse is being told about the marketplace with greater vigor. Ethics raises the question, What of the older organizing principles of nursing and medicine? In a marketplace-driven system, what protection is there for the vulnerable, the frail, the patients without the ability to compete as "customers?"

In a fee-for-service plan, ethical conflicts arose in the structure that asked a third party to pay for medical care in an unregulated relationship. The more medical intervention, the more money the third party payer had to throw toward the problem: overtreatment and overtesting were rewarded in such a system. In fact, the earliest cases in the clinical ethics literature reflect the need to protect patients, the Quinlans, the Cruzans, for example, from burdensome overtreatment in situations that their families considered hopeless.

In a sense, the fee-for-service system "taught" a generation of patients and staff that more was better, that the best medicine was the most expensive medicine. Health insurance, once the complexities of access could be assured, allowed for most patients, most of the time, a generous stay, tertiary care, and a recovery that included ro-

bust teaching, progressive ambulation, and at least a few days of bedbaths (Daniels, 1985). Hence most patients did what they were told, accepting whatever the doctor said was needed for recovery. And the doctor, and the nurse, had a fiduciary interest in the most abundant treatment plan. The third-party payer had an interest in paying out less, of course, but in a system in which most health care dollars were generated by union contracts, huge premiums were assured.

THE PATIENT AS CUSTOMER

But managed care has changed this model. Conflicts of interest between the patient and the physician are structured into the essential relationships of managed care. It is how the system creates incentives for providers in a capitated plan. The providers, doctors, and hospitals are paid a capitated fixed amount per patient, or they are paid a salary that is influenced by their behavior. In such a system, the more treatment that is given out and paid for, the less the providers will take home to their families. Imagine a fixed pile of money, paid by patients, now called "customers" when they buy their health care every year. Now imagine that every time a visit is made, a computed tomography scan taken, a drug provided, a few coins are taken away from the pile. If that money is now your own, if there will be no more added until next year, and if the third-party payers are being told by the people who buy health care for their workers that next year they want premiums to go down 5%, then you have a picture of how managed care works. Each provider's interest in retaining the pile is in a conflict with the patient's interest in using more services to support their health. Patients are seen in this system as revenue centers: this is not new but is more stark in the system of managed care, in which the fewer care gestures that a capitated physician offers and that a nurse provides, the more profit is generated.

At this juncture in the nursing literature a new language emerged: the language of the patient as "customer." The image of the healthy, immunized, bran-eating (or soy-eating) purchaser of health care replaced that of the needy ill person as the object of interest. (Efficient telephone advice replaced afternoon skin care as the expectation.) The goal, and it is not a bad goal, was reformulated as keeping people healthy. It is a goal that keeps people as payers into the system rather than as takers from the system. No ethical conflicts emerge until the payee is struck by illness or accident. Then, as a vulnerable person, a patient and not a customer, his needs must be fully and truthfully met by the system that he has in essence supported, or a violation of an essential promise will have been made. It is a promise made not only by the doctor but by every nurse who works in the system, whose wages are paid in advance, as it were, by our patient, in trust for the time when he will need our care.

The case described earlier develops the themes of the moral meaning and the moral worth of our medical interventions. Any concrete cases of allocation will raise issues of the role and the duty of the health care provider and the nursing leadership of the health care institution (Menzel, 1990). Should the role of the nurse be gatekeeper, visionary, businessperson, or citizen? Because the provision of this particular social good is so critical, does the provider stand outside normative concerns of the marketplace or of justice considerations, or is this just a business relationship like any other? Do nurses have to be accountable to considerations of justice for a whole society or just to their patient? Is the ethical choice that is required by a nurse to remain a part of a managed care organization an ethical compromise of her promise to serve the patient selflessly?

BEYOND COMPLAINT

When such autonomous wishes, the real need of the patient, and the beneficent acts toward the patient all argue for treatment that is costly and that will directly affect the income of the provider, some of the staff argue that asserting "good business practices" is merely a way of preserving the income of the health plan at the expense of the patient. But all of the nurses involved in the McGill case had a keen sense of the crisis in private fee-for-service medicine. (That was in large part why they were committed to managed care models in the first place.) All agreed that "too much is spent on medicine" in general, and all were strong proponents of alternative solutions to high technology. In the case they brought to the ethics committee, all reported feeling as though they were being coerced to act wrongly, even unethically. What is distinctive about such admissions is not that they are unique instances of patients not getting what they needed, but that there were no checks and balances for what the patient needed in the new system. There was no one who told Mr. McGill that the recovery phase of his surgery would be unsupported. There was no one who told the nurses the limited parameters of available care until after the fact, and there was no plan for involving either the patient or the nurse in how such limits are set.

Patients are not presented with the consequences of their health care choices as customers: most in fact have no idea of the compromises that their practitioners are agonizing over. Although a story of grotesque abuse is occasionally revealed in public testimony (on *60 Minutes* or *Frontline* or in *The New York Times*) it is impossible to monitor every detail of one's own plan. Patients expect that if a serious compromise is being made about their bodies, they would, of course, be made aware of such a problem. This is the essential trust relationship of the gesture of stranger medicine, made morally coherent and physically safe only by a reliance on the oaths and the obligations of the physician and the role-specific duties of the nursing professional.

Who should decide about the limits of care if the traditional Hippocratic oath is no longer the keystone of medical practice and to whom do such decision makers answer, to what code of honor? Many nurses spoke in the McGill case of the need to advocate for the patient in this system but were frustrated about who to turn to. In the past the care could theoretically be given long past efficacy, but not long past desire, because it is only a fringe number of patients who would eagerly seek appendectomies capriciously. Hence patients themselves often called the medical question in a treatment plan. The traditional conflict had the patient and provider allied against a third party: the government, the employer, or the insurance company. This new era creates stranger bedfellows, more uneasy allies, leaving the patient not only in practice but also by theoretical design as the one who is structured out of the decision process by virtue of his prepayment status.

The organization of managed care in California has advanced to a fairly complex stage, with the presence of well-developed health maintenance organizations that have been in practice since the 1940s. Now operating in anticipated advance of health care reform, the system according to those who brought this case is capricious: serving many well and many poorly, marketplace driven and subject, especially in the smaller managed care organizations, to the possibility of abuse. At issue is how to act fairly in the actual present, how to operate more justly in an unjust world.

RATIONING IN BROAD DAYLIGHT: THE ETHICAL OBLIGATIONS OF THE NURSE AS CITIZEN

One solution to such problems begins in the promise of absolute full disclosure to patients as they face medical crisis. If cost-cutting mechanisms are to be used, the true cost—meaning the social cost to all—must be publicly explained, and the burdens and the benefits jointly shared. The one who bears the brunt of the burden is entitled to the heft of the financial benefit goes this argument. For such choices, all of which involve some elements of risk, the patient could elect to save the money, pay for her own care with it, or choose another social good. If sending the patient home days earlier than has been the case saves money for the plan ($3,200 to $1,000 per day), then that money may rightly belong back in the hands of the patient, who could then use it to buy his own 4 × 4s. One could argue that there would be some secondary social gain as a result of such a process. It would be perhaps true that earlier forms of care would reappear at the American sickbed: family, neighbors, and the like would again have to function as primary caregivers, with a corresponding increase in general lay knowledge about illness, childbirth, and death, and a corresponding sense of the limits of the medical enterprise. The notion that one's health care insurance company, whose revenues are wielded by the hand of the physician, can and ought to solve the social and the medical facts of illness is a relatively late concept in American society after all. It is most assuredly not a useful one. This solution is occurring, in any case, it must be noted, but with the considerable cost savings being passed on elsewhere. It is occurring with only provider incentive and patient burden, hardly an ethical solution. In several large managed care organizations outpatient mastectomy is becoming standard, and childbirth stays are normatively 6 to 12 hours postpartum. Yet the process is sold and delivered as a "new standard of care," not as the cost-saving (and hence revenue-generating) move that it truly is.

The plan suggested earlier, however, is fraught with the familiar potential horrors of all stark marketplace schemes: when any individual is given the brunt of choice, in the context of all that surrounds such a choice, the individual has a "liberty" that is bogus, based now fully on his social economic status, like housing, food, and clothing. The wealthy will be able to contend for elaborate care, whereas the poor will merely have the ability to "freely" chose inadequate care.

There is of course an alternative model of a full social and a priori discourse that affects all equally (Danis & Churchill, 1991). Rather than the model of car salesmanship (full disclosure, individual incentive) this model more closely parallels the model of the public police or library system (full disclosure, citizen response). In this case, all members of a managed care organization can debate the reasonableness of limits and the allure of benefits gained by strict adherence to such limits. Because taxes are intended to reflect a democratic assessment of what it is just to pay for as citizens, insurance premiums and the rationing of health care benefits could reflect such shared democratic decision making. Such decision making would have to occur in a widely publicized public discourse with the first premise being that care is being rationed covertly now and that such rationing would be made visible and debatable. The conversations that seek to answer such ethical dilemmas must take place before the clinical bedside decisions raised by actual cases can be made. Such conversations must be face-to-face and specifically focused. Such discourse needs to begin at all levels and will have to include testimony about the widest range of outcome measures, in addition to the full range of costs and the cause of such costs. It will be critical to ensure that all outcome measures of such subjective factors as "utility" or "satisfaction" be applied equally to both physicians and patients. Any determination of the outcome of such a plan needs to resist efforts that ground success in merely instrumental terms of cost containment or utilization, although such measures will surely have their place. One of the early epistemic problems that any evaluative tool will have to address is who sets the criteria for the evaluation itself.

Not only patients but also nurses and physicians will need to expand the fullness of the informed consent process to include honest disclosure of the fiduciary re-

---

ETHICAL CONFLICTS

In California, one state in which managed care is virtually hegemonic, a pilot grant project has begun that will design a curriculum to address the ethical conflicts that practitioners face in such bedside delivery. I am a consultant ethicist for this grant. The project, funded by the Pew Charitable Trust (principal investigators Dr. K. Marten and Dr. L. Sommers of the Center for the Development of the Health Care Professions), could function as a much needed support system if the curriculum is fully implemented, but the primary goal would be to address the main issue for the clinician: the problem of limits, the new reality of external limits, and the increasingly understood structural limits in the practice itself. In the interviews that I conducted for this grant I was moved by the depth of despair that the clinicians expressed in their work. The subjective feeling that I heard expressed was of new responsibility for that which had not been their problem: the issues of justice and allocation on a public scale. There is no flight from this, of course. A curriculum must teach the tools of the honest discourse.

sponsibility that is at stake. It is only through a thorough and comprehensive reflection on the significant desire that undergirds the meaning of health care that reform can be constructed that is both comprehensible and congruent with our deepest social values. In such a system the nurse will have to address the ethics of managed care not only as "citizen" but also as a citizen with special knowledge: such a role ought not buy access to more privilege, but to more responsibility.

Such discourse is based on the language of the common good rather than the language of need-based or liberty-based autonomy (Danis & Churchill, 1991). And the language of the common good is based on the premise that there is a basic decent minimum of social goods that is owed to all and that such a just share should be democratically arrived upon. And such language presumes that societies exist, in large measure, to bear the burden of the vulnerable who cannot obtain such social goods on their own. It is true that, in any system like this, in any one individual case the person before you may not get what he or she needs to be well. The point of such conjunct responsibility, however, is that, given the tenuous equilibrium of the current era, such choices would even out over the long term. Unlike a strictly marketplace, liberty-based solution, such a priori discourse would create open reflection on the meaning of such choices long before they were made.

WHAT IS NEEDED FOR ETHICAL PRACTICE: TRUTHTELLING AND INDEPENDENT MORAL AGENCY

For such a citizen-based program to work, it will need the nurse to pursue a clear course of moral agency and the straightforward adherence to the principle of veracity. Patients not only must be told the truth about their diagnosis and prognosis, as in all informed consent relationships, but also must be told whether the treatment options they are offered are influenced by financial considerations. All conflicts of interests must be fully disclosed (Veatch, 1991). Nursing staff that witnesses such conflicts must be supported to uncover and open the process of true informed consent to the patient without any fear of reprisals.

Nurses must be counted on to identify conditions of unsafe practice: areas in which the drive to cut costs endangers the health and safety of patients, areas in which the teaching role of the nurse is compromised, and areas in which the standard of care is unacceptably altered. Such objections must be documented and reported, and it must be a part of ethical professional practice to refuse to work without objection in such venues. Patients may well be unaware of previous standards and may simply accept situations that are untenable. The role of the nurse as moral agent must be to reflect on all aspects of current

ETHICAL IMPLICATIONS

Such discourse must also make a commitment to the full and frank exploration of the ethical implications of the managed care environment without undue hesitancy about problems of external judgments. The development of such curriculum is key.

Over the last several years my colleague Susan Rubin and I have taught the theory and practice that surround the ethical issue of distributive justice in the clinical setting. We have used several models. The most successful was based on the encounter between physician–direct care providers and administrators and utilization personnel over the issue of scarce resources. We have developed a curriculum that teaches intensive review of (1) classic justice theory, (2) challenges to these theories, and (3) extensive case review that involves explicit rationing. Included in this curriculum is a prioritization project based on the Oregon health care model that uses the work of Larry Churchill as a theoretical frame. Our experience, based on provider reports, is that such sessions have been extraordinarily useful in the clinical arena.

We have also developed a teaching module that examines in depth the issue of medical futility from a broad theoretical overview of the topic to detailed case review, which has been offered to ethics committees throughout our practice. In actual clinical case reviews we have observed, we have seen a rapid learning curve about this information affect the way the case reviews are conducted. Our experience is that success with this model is based on the strongest possible theoretical ground and the consistent use of case review in the work. Another feature that is uniquely successful is the opportunity to directly address the concerns of a multidisciplinary group in an academic rather than an adversarial setting.

A third important part of the ethics curriculum that we have recently developed is a research project and teaching tool that examines the problem of truthtelling in the physician-patient relationship. Based on a model that stresses a strong theoretical base and a focus on actual case encounters, the more than 150 initial respondents have reported the immediate usefulness of the curriculum in their practice.

practice and insist on the maintenance of standards that are defensible.

The uncovering of financial considerations and the explicit dynamics of the marketplace as metaphor and social construct will have profound implications for the most privatized of relationships, that of physician and patient. Such a shift, or rather such an overt naming of the centrality of the need for considerations of social justice, is at the heart of the need for reflections on the competing moral appeals and theories of justice that underlie health care reform.

At stake in such a discourse will be the reframing of the method and the power in the medical decision-making process. Bioethics has stressed the necessity of the informed consent relationship, but it does not as yet have a robust theory of informed consent in a time of scarcity. The model of autonomy is itself strained by the necessity to make public policy on the basis of more generalized notions of the good. This underlying philosophy will have to be carefully examined to be clear about a number of troubling ethical issues.

First among these are the justice considerations concerning the place of the powerless, the vulnerable, and the disenfranchised (Zoloth-Dorfman, 1995). Here the issue of power and relationality will have to be addressed clearly. Second, the use of outcome data as a tool carries with it all the complexities of unilateral decision making by the health care provider, a particularly problematic history, and serious epistemological problems as well. At issue in many uses of outcome data will be not only the choice of instrument but also the community that sets the goals for the evaluative standards. Finally, the discourse must reflect on the reality of significant ethical and value conflicts over such questions as the ultimate worth of a human life, the meaning of quantitative assessment of life quality, and the plurality of religious and cultural perspectives on the goal and meaning of the person in health and in illness.

Such a conversation held before the passion and loss of the bedside will not forestall all despair in the actual world any more than after-the-fact remorse over poor social choices is avoided entirely by public discourse. But the patient in such a system can at least be assured of one thing: whether for harm or for good, the rationing that all such choices represents will be done in broad daylight, with all the goods bartered for and beckoned for on the table between us all.

The nurse in the new era of managed care will confront ethical dilemmas that will test the limits of courage (McClinton, 1995). Moral agency is hard to maintain in a climate in which nurses themselves feel threatened. Layoffs and diminishing contractual benefits have been some of the subsidiary effects of cost cutting in the clinical setting, and nurses will have to remember that in many situations they must act despite their fear. Ultimately, moral responsibility in the system of managed care rests where it has always resided: in the heart and hands of the clinical provider.

REFERENCES

Aaron, H. (1991). *Serious and unstable condition: Financing America's health care.* Washington DC: The Brooklings Institution.

Arras, J., & Steinbock, B. (1995). *Ethical issues in modern medicine.* Mountain View, CA: Mayfield.

Daniels, N. (1985). *Just health care.* Cambridge, MA: Cambridge.

Danis, M., & Churchill, L. (1991, January-February). Autonomy and the common weal. *Hastings Center Report,* 12-19.

Krieger, L. (1995, January 17). Family doctors are disappearing. *San Francisco Examiner,* p. A1.

McClinton, D. (1995, June). Balancing the issue of ethics in case management. *Continuing Care,* 13-16.

Menzel, P. (1990). *Strong medicine: The ethical rationing of health care.* New York: Oxford.

Moreno, J. (1995). *Deciding together: Bioethics and moral consensus.* New York: Oxford.

Rhodes, R. (1992). *Health care politics, policy and distributive justice: The ironic triumph.* Albany: State University of New York.

Veatch, R. (1991). Allocating health resources ethically: New roles for administrators and clinicians. *Frontiers of Health Services Management, 8*(1), 3-44.

Zoloth-Dorfman, L. (1994, December). Standing at the gate: Managed care and daily ethical choices. *Managed Care Medicine,* 1-7.

Section Twelve

International Nursing

Nursing Around the World

JOANNE McCLOSKEY DOCHTERMAN, HELEN KENNEDY GRACE

Beginning with the third edition published in 1990 we have included international chapters about nursing and health care in other countries. In past editions, we attempted to include one international chapter at the end of each section. In this edition we continue this tradition, but we have grouped the chapters together in this final section of the book. As the globalization of health care grows, a review of nursing and health care issues around the world seems a fitting way to end the book. Space limitations allow us to include only a small number of countries, selected for diversity and because we knew of someone who had knowledge of the country who would write a good chapter. There is no debate chapter in this section, but reading about health care in different countries raises several topics for debate, for example, the debate about whether health care should be nationalized or privatized or the debate about whether health care should be paid for by the government or the consumer.

The chapters are ordered alphabetically by country, beginning with Africa. In her chapter, Tlou discusses the health care issues of fourteen African countries that make up the Southern African Development Community. These are Angola, Botswana, Democratic Republic of Congo, Lesotho, Malawi, Mauritius, Mozambique, Namibia, Seychelles, South Africa, Swaziland, Tanzania, Zambia, and Zimbabwe. Major constraints to health care in these countries include conflict and war, poverty, lack of autonomy for women, especially related to use of contraceptives, and the HIV/AIDS epidemic. Many pregnant women are HIV positive and have great chances of passing on the infection to their children. This disease is wiping out the gains made in life expectancy during the past decades in some of the countries. Other adverse effects of the disease are an increase in infections, unavailability of hospital beds, and increases in suicide rates. Nurses in Africa are extending their traditional roles to respond to the needs of the communities, and nursing education has integrated the concepts of primary care, public health, and community

health. Tlou concludes her chapter by outlining present and future challenges for nursing in the Southern African Development Community. These include shortages of nursing personnel, limited nursing research opportunities, risk of HIV/AIDS, and the need to mainstream a woman's perspective in health care. For development of nursing in each country, Tlou recommends a strong national nurses association as well as proper legislation relating to nursing and nurse midwifery. This is a fact-filled chapter that demonstrates well the enormous challenges facing nurses in this part of the world.

Next is a chapter about the neighbor to the north of the United States, Canada. Ross-Kerr provides an overview of the Canadian health care system, which is neither free enterprise medicine nor socialized medicine. Provisions of the Canadian plan include universality of coverage to all people, comprehensiveness of medically necessary services, accessibility of health services to all segments of the population, portability of coverage from one province to another, and public administration of the program at the provincial level. Ross-Kerr traces the development of health care in Canada from the 1800s and gives an overview of the tax-supported system that has evolved over the last 40 years. Today there is recognition that there are limits to the system and that some reform is needed. Approximately 75% of health expenditures are paid for by Medicare. The Canadian system has been built primarily around medical service in hospitals. There is a growing emphasis, however, on maintaining patients in community-based settings, stressing prevention and health promotion. An escalating nursing shortage is predicted. One in ten graduates migrate to the United States, where salaries, benefits, and the working environment are better. The Canadian education system for nurses is much like, but lags behind that in the United States, with a total of five doctoral programs now available. While health care systems of the United States and Canada have some similarities, there are several important differences.

In Great Britain, nursing continues to face turbulent times. Clark overviews the past and present changes in health care and in nursing. Her chapter demonstrates two great influences on health care and nursing in Great Britain: the past and the political party. According to Clark, many of the organizational anomalies and traditions that shape the present day system are relics of the past. The National Health System (NHS), formed in 1948, nationalized many existing services. The core values of the NHS are universality, comprehensiveness, and no cost at the point of use. Changes in the reigning political party bring sweeping reforms in health care. Changes opposed by strong groups often result in compromise, and several of the compromises are due to the opposition of the medical profession. Since 1983 there has been an enormous change in health care. Clark says that the British health care system of 2000 is in transition. Most health care is provided through the NHS, but there is a private hospital sector and a private nursing home sector. Most nurses work for the NHS, but a growing number work in the private sectors. Nursing education is undergoing many changes with slow movement toward baccalaureate education. Nursing specialization has increased with, for example, eight different types of community nurse. Interestingly there are no practice acts that define the work of nurses in Great Britain, but regulation of health care providers is currently under review. Some nurses can prescribe drugs, but the formulary that they must use is limited. A new nurse-run telephone help line available to all citizens and paid for by the NHS is opposed by medicine but is creating new career opportunities for nurses. Clark's chapter, filled with many interesting facts, is a good overview of the changes and challenges faced by the nursing profession in a country where history is a major influence.

In Japan the aging of its population, a movement toward community-based nursing, and the increasing numbers of nurses with baccalaureate and graduate degrees are improving the status of nursing. Takahashi and Brandi begin their chapter with an overview of the health care environment and the Japanese health care system. Japanese citizens lead the world in life expectancy. Public and community health centers are integral parts of the health care system. The extended family system has shifted to a smaller nuclear family, and more elderly are living independently. The hospital average length of stay is one of the highest in the world, over 30 days, primarily because of elderly hospitalizations and free care. There are three types of nurses, each with separate licensure. The nursing educational system is complex; there is, however, a major push for baccalaureate and higher degree

education. In 2000, there were 12 doctoral programs in nursing; all graduate programs had a shortage of qualified faculty. The authors state that the changes in the population, health care, and nursing are improving the status of nursing in Japan. Their chapter is an excellent overview of these exciting times for nursing in this rapidly changing country.

In the next chapter, de Villalobos provides an overview of another rapidly changing health care system in Latin America. Since the 1980s, Latin America, a collection of several countries, has been immersed in crises involving politics, disasters, and violence. Every country in Latin America has made or is planning to make sweeping change. Some progress has been made including a decline in maternal and neonatal morbidity, reduction in childhood disease, and an increase in family planning. Nursing in Latin America varies by country, but in all countries the challenges for the nursing profession are great. Nurses who are in short supply are being replaced by assistants. de Villalobos overviews the differences in the various nursing education programs. Education is the most advanced in Brazil and Columbia, with Brazil having the largest number of undergraduate and graduate programs. There is a great need for more continuing education programs throughout all the countries. The author ends her chapter citing three challenges for the immediate future; each involves change. She urges nurses to take charge before the opportunities are lost.

In the closing chapter in this section and in the book, Smith describes in fascinating detail the current political and economic situation in Russia and, within this context, health care and the role of nursing. Russia, the largest country in the world, has a negative growth rate and a declining population. Life in Russia is difficult and may be dangerous. Inflation, poverty, crime, and rising rates of communicable diseases are destroying the hope of the people. Salaries for health care workers, especially nurses, are dreadful. Tax evasion is a major problem, so there is no money for government reform. As many as 15 families living in public housing may share kitchen and toilet facilities. Smith details these and many other problems, including the oppression of Russian women. Despite the general oppression of women in Russian society and of nursing as a women's profession, nursing is making some advances. Nursing organizations are beginning to develop, and nursing educational programs are being strengthened. Master's programs have been developed in the past decade, and continuing education, hospital-wide programs have been initiated. East-West collaboration is being promoted. Introduction of the nursing process is being considered. The chapter written by Smith about the hardships and courage of our Russian colleagues is a sad but inspiring conclusion to this book. Despite enormous odds against it, the nursing profession in Russia is improving itself. What a great example for the rest of us.

The chapters is this section and others indicate that nursing the world around is challenged on many fronts.

In spite of the differences in the health care systems and the conditions under which nurses work, nurses worldwide share common concerns about patient welfare and struggle to advance the profession and the views of nursing to make a positive impact on patient care. We salute those nurses in so many countries who are helping to make a difference.

An Overview of Health Care and Nursing Education and Practice in Southern Africa

SHEILA DINOTSHE TLOU

This chapter provides an overview of the current challenges and issues facing nursing education and practice within the primary health care system of Southern Africa. An analysis is made of the opportunities and current and future challenges for nurses in Southern Africa.

Because Africa is a vast continent with diverse cultures and nursing programs, this chapter cannot possibly cover them all. This chapter therefore confines itself to analyzing health care, nursing education, and nursing practice within the Southern Africa Development Community (SADC).

The SADC is a group of 14 countries in Southern Africa that agreed to collaborate on matters concerning the development of their region: Angola, Botswana, Democratic Republic of Congo, Lesotho, Malawi, Mauritius, Mozambique, Namibia, Seychelles, South Africa, Swaziland, Tanzania, Zambia, and Zimbabwe. Each country is responsible for the improvement of a particular sector to benefit the whole region; for example, South Africa has the responsibility for the health of the region and therefore has to initiate research and interventions that will improve the health status of all the citizens of the SADC.

HEALTH CARE IN SADC

To appreciate the important role of nursing in the SADC, one needs to understand the health care system of each country, each of which is at a different stage of development.

All SADC countries, or their colonial rulers, were signatories to the Alma-Ata Declaration of 1978, which committed members to attaining socially acceptable and productive primary health care strategies (WHO-UNICEF, 1978). Primary health care includes the provision of curative, preventive, and rehabilitative care to in-dividuals and families at an affordable price. This care should be accessible to all age groups, from birth to death.

MAJOR CONSTRAINTS TO HEALTH CARE DELIVERY

Conflict and War

Conflict and war situations in some countries in the SADC such as Angola and the Democratic Republic of Congo have diverted funds from national health and social service programs to national defense. As a result these countries have been "plunged into debt, and foreign reserve levels have not enhanced investment. Developed countries whose economic and business investments would help create jobs and boost national economies have lost confidence in countries in the region and consider them more of a liability than an asset. This has not only affected the cash flow and food security at the household level. It has also shifted family health seeking behaviours and practices to food gathering and income generation activities" (Ngcongco, 1995, p. 3).

The impact of conflict on the national health care system has been so great that formal health care is almost nonexistent in these countries.

Poverty

Poverty is another major health challenge for Southern African countries, and for some it is exacerbated by inter-country and intracountry strife. All the SADC countries are still at the level of development where the disease patterns are predominantly determined by poverty, poor nutrition, low levels of education, and conditions inconsistent with health such as poor sanitation and pollution. Even where health services are relatively free, poor families experience real problems when they or a dependent is

TABLE 80-1   Health and Development Indicators: Southern Africa Development Community (SADC)

SADC Country	% Population with Access to Health Services, 1990-1995	Contraceptive Prevalence (%)	Deliveries by Skilled Personnel (%)	Maternal Mortality Rate (per 100,000), 1993	Total Fertility Rate
Angola	30	—	17	1,500	7.2
Botswana	89	33	77	250	4.9
Lesotho	80	23	45	610	5.2
Malawi	80	22	55	560	7.2
Mauritius	100	75	97	120	2.4
Mozambique	39	—	30	1,500	6.5
Namibia	62	29	68	370	5.3
South Africa	—	50	82	230	4.1
Swaziland	—	20	56	560	4.9
Tanzania	80	18	44	770	5.9
Zambia	75	26	51	940	6.0
Zimbabwe	85	48	69	570	5.2
Sub-Saharan Africa	57	22	58	929	6.1

Data from the World Health Report, 1996, and the Human Development Report, 1998 (United Nations Development Programme, 1998).

referred to a major hospital in another village or town. A survey among elderly village women in Botswana, for example, revealed that lack of money was the major deterrent to their seeking health care. The elderly are not expected to pay consultation and drug fees; however, there are many expenditures connected with:

1. Drugs unavailable at the health facility that have to be bought at a private pharmacy.
2. Referrals for treatment to other health care facilities. The dilemma then is lack of transportation, which is compounded by the need for food and lodging at the referral center.

These expenditures for some people, especially older women, have meant delaying treatment or not undergoing needed treatment at all (Tlou, 1994).

Gender and Health Aspect

The gender and health aspect involves especially reproductive health. In most SADC societies women do not have the right to decide on when to have children, on the number of children they want, or on whether to have children at all. Motherhood is seen as destiny, a social responsibility, and a passport into the world of womanhood. The following all contribute to women's relatively poor health status: lack of autonomy, discrimination in law enforcement such as the criminalization of abortion, inadequate allocation of health resources, and failure by

governments to implement remedial measures sanctioned by international agreements.

Table 80-1 shows the health and development indicators of the SADC region, among them contraceptive prevalence rate, or the percentage of women ages 15 to 49 who currently are using a modern method of contraception. The term *modern* refers to the methods often offered by family planning programs and includes male and female sterilization, intrauterine devices (IUDs), the pill, injectable hormonal contraceptives, male and female condoms, and female barrier methods such as diaphragms, cervical caps, jellies, creams, and spermicidal foams.

In ideal conditions, all women would have access to quality, reliable and affordable methods of contraception, but in no SADC country are the conditions ideal. Family planning services usually are not woman friendly and are "demographic targets" to be used by politicians and administrators for seeking rewards for services and targets accomplished. For example, in most countries the number of children that women desire to have is less than the total fertility rate (i.e., the total number of children that a girl will bear if her childbearing follows the current fertility patterns and she lives through her entire childbearing years). Observation indicates that for some countries the total fertility rate approximates the number of children that men desire, showing it is they who control and decide on women's fertility. Indeed in most SADC countries a woman cannot be sterilized (have a tubal ligation) without the written consent of her husband, but the husband does not need his wife's consent to have a vasectomy. This marital power and control is so firmly established that even when the woman is not married, her future husband's rights to her fertility are protected and she is simply advised to use another form of contraception because she might marry and the future husband may desire children (Tlou, 1997).

On the whole, trends indicate improved provision of services for women in all the SADC countries compared to 10 years ago. For example, Mauritius has one of the highest levels of contraceptive use in Sub-Saharan Africa, estimated at 75% of all women. Accessibility, availability, and affordability of contraceptives are good, and all health care facilities provide family planning services. Also in most SADC countries the fertility rates (births per woman) have declined considerably (United Nations, 1995). The decline in fertility rate has also been due to higher educational achievement by women, their increased opportunities for employment outside the home, and improved child survival rates. All these have contributed to declining family size and better child spacing.

Adolescent Fertility. Adolescent fertility is on the increase in some SADC countries, where about 23% of the births are to girls under 18 years of age whose bodies are not yet well developed for childbearing, let alone child-rearing. Adequate care for teenage mothers before and after birth is still lacking, especially in the areas of information dissemination, education, and counseling concerning reproductive health.

What is needed in the SADC are nurses and health care workers who are trained to reach teenagers, both boys and girls, to educate them on responsible sexual behavior and the postponement of childbearing until they are physically, psychologically, and financially ready to raise a child. At the moment the attitudes of some health care personnel toward teenagers who need contraceptive services are so discouraging that most teenagers shy away from health facilities and end up having unwanted pregnancies or, worse still, sexually transmitted diseases.

HIV/AIDS Epidemic

The HIV/AIDS epidemic is already having a major impact on the quality of life of citizens in the SADC. As Table 80-2 indicates, Southern Africa has some of the countries in the world most affected by HIV/AIDS, and its negative impact on development is already being felt as more and more people infected by HIV several years ago are now developing AIDS, becoming critically ill, and dying. Probably 250,000 people in the SADC are at the moment living with AIDS, and a further 6 million are living with HIV infection, assuming a general prevalence of 6% to 10% in any adult population. Many pregnant women are HIV positive and are at high risk of passing on the infection to their children in utero, during birth, or through breastfeeding. In Botswana and other SADC countries, for example, between 25% and 50% of pregnant women in various localities are HIV positive.

HIV/AIDS is systematically wiping out the gains made in life expectancy during the past several decades in some of the SADC countries, as indicated in Table 80-3 showing the trends in life expectancies of men and women in some countries. The general trend in all the countries is higher in the years 1990 to 1995, mainly because of improvements in the socioeconomic environment and the standards of living. The present declines in life expectancy are mainly a result of the impact of the HIV/AIDS epidemic.

Following are other adverse effects of the HIV/AIDS epidemic in the SADC:

1. Increases in infections, especially pneumonia, meningitis, and tuberculosis. Drugs for these illnesses are expen-

TABLE 80-2   HIV/AIDS in Selected Southern Africa Development Community Countries

	South Africa	Botswana	Namibia	Lesotho	Swaziland
Population (000s)	43,336	1,518	1,612	2,131	906
Population ages 15-49 (000s)	21,717	743	752	985	439
% of total population with HIV	7%	13%	9%	4%	9%
HIV-infected people (000s)	2,900	190	150	85	81
Adult prevalence rate of HIV	13%	25%	20%	8%	19%
Female HIV population: % of total	50%	49%	50%	48%	51%
Pregnant HIV-infected women, prevalence	16%	36%	24%	21%	27%
AIDS orphans	180,000	25,000	7,300	8,500	7,200

Data from UNAIDS (1996).

TABLE 80-3 Indicators of Health: Life Expectancy at Birth (Years) of Selected Southern Africa Development Community Countries: 1970-1995

Country	1970-1975		1990-1995		1995 Average
	Males	Females	Males	Females	
Botswana	51	56	60	66	52
Lesotho	48	53	58	63	58
Namibia	48	50	58	60	56
South Africa	51	57	60	66	64
Swaziland	45	50	56	60	58
Zambia	46	49	43	45	43
Zimbabwe	50	53	54	57	49

Data from United Nations Data, 1995, 1998.

sive, and money is being diverted from other health services that are equally important but not deemed urgent.

2. Availability of hospital beds. About 50% of hospital beds in the medical and pediatric wards of urban and rural areas are occupied by persons with HIV-related illnesses. This situation is likely to continue even with the setting up of home-based care programs because of relapses and repeated admissions of patients.

3. Increases in suicide rates as more infected and affected people struggle to cope with the disabling effects of the scourge. The mental health care system and social support system are finding it difficult to face up to the challenges of the HIV/AIDS epidemic.

4. Loss of trained personnel, including health personnel. The impact of the HIV/AIDS epidemic on the development of human resources for the SADC is being felt as more people are dying. Future effects of the virus on the economy will be enormous and definitely will retard or threaten most of the socioeconomic gains that have been achieved so far.

Studies in Botswana have shown no impact of HIV/AIDS on the recruitment and retention of nurses (Tlou, 1998). In fact more and more young men and women are entering the nursing profession every year, and some have to be turned away because there are too few training facilities.

NURSING EDUCATION AND NURSING PRACTICE

SADC health care systems are organized in several levels of increasing sophistication, starting from the most basic (the health post or the mobile health stop) to the major referral hospital. In all these facilities, nurses are the backbone of health care delivery. Health consultations, nutrition care, health education, maternal health, patient education, and immunization of infants and children against communicable diseases have all been functions and responsibilities of nurses and subsumed under the discipline and practice of nursing. Nursing has therefore earned for itself a unique place in the national health care system in the Southern African region.

Nursing Practice

Nursing practice is seen as a broad-based service that should meet the health care needs of individuals, families, and communities in all sorts of settings such as hospitals, schools, community centers, homes, and workplaces. The latter include mines, factories, farms, and construction sites. Even in these settings, however, nursing roles vary greatly from country to county. As Moores (1998) puts it,

> In one country a nurse may be effectively a medical assistant, in another, the only health care professional who provides a comprehensive health care service to a community. Nurses and midwives may work in hospital, in smaller first line health care centres, in towns and villages, or more remote locations, bringing care directly to individuals who need it. Some may be able to use the latest medicines, equipment and specialist skills, while others may have only the most primitive of facilities and supplies. In countries where there is a shortage of doctors, people would often have no access to preventative, curative, palliative or continuing care if it were not for the skills and expertise of nurses. [p. 2]

Indeed nurses are extending their traditional roles to respond to the needs of their communities; for example, in Botswana, community health nurses run sewing classes for youth, horticultural programs for women, and workshops for traditional healers and primary school teachers.

Nursing Education

Nursing education in the SADC has responded to the changing needs of patients and communities by integrating concepts of primary health care, public health practice, and community health care in basic, postbasic, and graduate programs, and nursing practice has continued to redefine and expand the scope and parameters of nursing to meet the requirements and dictates of primary health care–oriented national health care systems. Conceptual frameworks for both nursing and midwifery programs were broadened to include concepts and content of primary health care (PHC). Postbasic and graduate programs have been developed for nurse clinicians, family nurse practitioners, advanced midwifery and maternal and child health and family planning practitioners, and community health and community mental health practitioners to prepare nurses for providing quality nursing care and health care to individuals, families, and community groups with a variety of nursing and health care problems and needs. Because of the need for nursing leadership and management in the provision of patient care, clinical nursing research programs have also been developed and implemented at the basic, postbasic, and graduate levels (Ngcongco, 1995).

Formal education for nurses in SADC countries is similar to the model presented for Botswana in Figure 80-1. Most nurses are trained at the diploma level for 3 years and then undergo 1 year of concentrated study to enable them to practice in that area. After at least 2 years of nursing practice as registered nurses (RNs) they have the opportunity to study for a baccalaureate degree in nursing as RN completers for a further 2 to 3 years.

Generic baccalaureate programs in nursing science admit high school graduates for a 4-year training program, after which they have the opportunity to specialize in any field of nursing at the master's degree level. Currently the number of baccalaureate- and master's degree–prepared nurses in all the SADC countries is few, but their impact is being felt, as they provide leadership in all areas of nursing care and nursing research.

PRESENT AND FUTURE CHALLENGES FOR NURSING IN SADC

Changing educational patterns, economic development, technological advances, and sociopolitical trends have resulted in the trend for better educated nurses in SADC countries, but nurses still face some challenges in the delivery of health care. Among these are shortages of nursing personnel, limited nursing research opportunities, HIV/AIDS, and implementing recommendations related to women in health care.

Shortages of Nursing Personnel

In most SADC countries, nursing is a popular profession for both men and women, but the number of facilities requiring nurses is growing at a faster pace than the number of trained nurses to staff them. Every graduating class is absorbed into the health care system months before commencement exercises, but nursing shortages still persist. Some of the shortages are also due to poor working conditions and inadequate information and support systems for nurses, resulting in their looking for "greener pastures" in neighboring countries or overseas. This brain drain has had a negative impact on the health care systems of both the sending country and the receiving country, where the recruited nurses may not be familiar with the language and culture of the people they are supposed

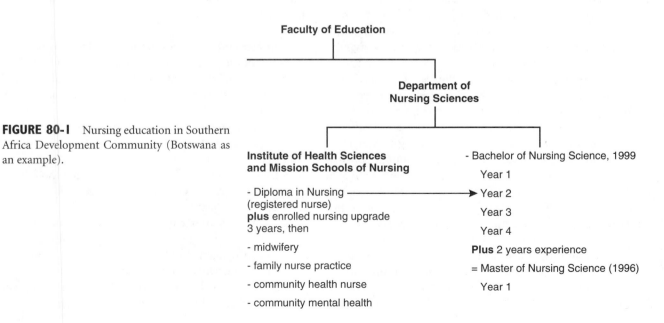

FIGURE 80-1 Nursing education in Southern Africa Development Community (Botswana as an example).

to serve. A possible intervention is for SADC countries to collaborate with each other in expanding the training of professional nurses and to improve working conditions of nurses to alleviate the problems of nursing staff shortages and turnover.

Nursing Research in SADC

Nursing research in the SADC is still in its infancy, but there are initiatives to encourage research, especially at university schools of nursing. Nurses prepared at higher levels, however, need to come down from the ivory tower of academic research and simplify the process so that the real implementers of care (diploma nurses) can do research to gain reliable information on which to base their decisions. Funding for nursing research is a major problem, and it is not even seen as a priority in any of the SADC countries.

HIV/AIDS

Nurses in all the SADC member states have provided leadership in HIV/AIDS prevention and control and in caring for people living with AIDS and their families. Although there is no real research on the phenomenon, HIV/AIDS seems to be having little impact on the recruitment and retention of nursing personnel. Indeed, young people are joining the profession in increasing numbers. Nurses as human beings, however, are at risk of HIV infection from their own sexual behavior and their behavior at the workplace. Most of the nurses are women, and they have the same biological and sociocultural vulnerability to HIV/AIDS as all women in this society. They may therefore feel powerless to protect themselves and experience anxiety and fear of contagion, which interfere with their ability to care for people living with AIDS.

The International Council of Nurses (ICN) has appealed to governments to take appropriate measures to reduce the negative impact of HIV/AIDS on nursing and midwifery personnel. The ICN has released position statements on AIDS (1996) and on reducing HIV/AIDS risks to nursing personnel (1998). National nurses associations in the SADC have provided information to their members on HIV/AIDS prevention and care of people living with AIDS and have disseminated the universal precautions to take to minimize the risk of HIV transmission in the health care setting. The nurses association in some countries, Botswana, for example, also stress the importance of responsible sexual behavior and run workshops to teach nurses skills on condom use and negotiating safer sex with partners.

Implementing Recommendations Related to Women in Health Care

In the followup to the Fourth World Conference on Women (1995) and the International Conference on Population and Development (1994), countries in the SADC have started to implement the recommendations related to women and health and have endorsed them in their health policies. Major constraints imposed by civil unrest and reforms in the economic sector in most countries, however, make it difficult to design comprehensive national health plans that are gender sensitive. Nurses are still not proactive in this matter and need to be in the forefront in introducing equity for women in all aspects of health.

For health care delivery, applying a fully comprehensive gender perspective would require that all health statistics be segregated and that a comprehensive women's health profile be constructed. The ICN (1995) has issued guidelines to the national nurses associations for countries to use in developing such a profile covering demographics, socioeconomics, health status, lifestyle, environment, health care services, health service use, sexuality, and policy development. The ICN's guidelines include eliminating negative cultural practices such as female genital mutilation, supporting programs to reduce violence against women, and promoting women's access to comprehensive health services and health education of girls and elderly women.

OPPORTUNITIES FOR NURSES IN SADC

The most important opportunities for SADC nurses are that each country has

1. A **nurses and midwives act** that provides for the regulation of the practice of nursing and midwifery for the training and registering of nurses and midwives and for the establishment of a nursing and midwifery council.
2. A **nursing council,** a statutory institution, that:
   - Issues registration
   - Represents the state
   - Lays down minimum requirements for the education of nurses to ensure safe practice
   - Issues certification
   - Protects the public from professional malpractice by laying down minimum requirements for practice and ensuring that only those practitioners who meet such requirements are licensed to practice

Nursing councils are concerned with issues of accountability and the quality of nursing care.

3. A **national nurses association** that ensures that nursing education, nursing research, and nursing practice respond to the dictates of primary health care and that nurses assume leadership roles in health care delivery. Its activities allow for
   - Definition and nature of nursing practice
   - Development of education necessary for practice
   - Development, promotion, and maintenance of high standards of practice
   - Professional growth and development of individual practitioners
   - The maintenance of the honor and status of the nursing profession
   - Improving the social and economic welfare of the profession

Through bodies such as the East, Central, and Southern African College of Nursing (ECSACON), uniform standards of nursing education, legislation, and nursing practice are being formulated as part of having a common or similar nursing curriculum in all the countries. Reviews of current curricula or programs for nurse training are being undertaken in a number of countries, providing the opportunity for ensuring that developments in health care are reflected in the curricula and that nurses and midwives are prepared for their developing roles. Leadership training is also important. In Botswana, for example, basic nurses training includes management and leadership courses; the university offers master's degree courses in nursing administration; and in-service education for nurse leaders in administration is offered on an ongoing basis. Some of the students are from SADC countries, and some are from as far away as Kenya, Uganda, and Sierra Leone.

SUMMARY

This chapter has outlined the important roles that nurses and nurse-midwives play in the provision of health care in the Southern Africa Development Community (SADC). It also has outlined present and future challenges for health care and for the nursing profession, as well as opportunities that will in the long run enable nurses of SADC to achieve their common objective: enhancing the health and well-being of their communities. A strong national nurses association as well as proper legislation relating to nursing and midwifery are essential to the growth and development of the nursing profession in any one country.

REFERENCES

ICN. (1995). *Women and health: Nurses lead the way.* Information package. Geneva: Author.

ICN. (1996). *Acquired immunodeficiency syndrome.* Position statement. Geneva: Author.

ICN. (1998). *Call for action to reduce HIV/AIDS risks to nursing personnel.* Position statement. Geneva: Author.

Moores, Y. (1998). *Health sector reforms: The nursing and midwifery contribution.* Paper presented at the Commonwealth Health Ministers Meeting, Barbados, November 15-19.

Ngcongco, V. (1995). *Nursing practice in the African region.* WHO Expert Committee on Nursing Practice. Geneva: World Health Organization.

Tlou, S.D. (1998). *Caring for the carers: The impact of HIV/AIDS on nursing personnel in Botswana.* Unpublished research report. University of Botswana.

Tlou, S.D. (1997). Indicators of health. In Botswana Society (Eds.), *Poverty and plenty: The Botswana experience* (pp. 303-315). Gaborone: Macmillan.

Tlou, S.D. (1994). The elderly and their use of the health care system. In F. Bruun, Y. Coombes, & M. Mugabe (Eds.), *The situation of the elderly in Botswana* (pp. 93-99). Gaborone: National Institute of Research.

UNAIDS. (1996). *The status and trends of the global HIV/AIDS pandemic.* Report presented at the XI International Conference on AIDS, Vancouver, July 7-12.

United Nations Development Programme. (1998). *Human development report, 1998.* New York: Oxford University Press.

United Nations. (1998). *Women and health.* Report of the Expert Group Meeting, Tunisia, 1998. New York: Division for Advancement of Women.

United Nations. (1995). *Beijing declaration and platform of action.* New York: Author.

United Nations. (1995). *The world's women 1995.* New York: Author.

WHO-UNICEF. (1978). *Alma-Ata Declaration: Primary health care.* Geneva: Author.

An Overview of Health Care and Nursing Education and Practice in Canada

JANET C. ROSS-KERR

Canadians believe passionately in health insurance coverage as a right of citizenship, and the tax-supported Medicare program remains as one of the most highly valued and popular initiatives of the Canadian government. Public opinion polls have reflected this support, which has been reported to be consistently high (Inglehart, 1990; Wilson & Ross-Kerr, 1998). Even though costs have spiraled in recent years, Canadians are unsympathetic to the possibility of a return to the private arrangements for health care that were common before federal legislation for hospital care over 40 years ago. Despite the high level of public support for Medicare, several provinces have challenged the provisions of the Canada Health Act by allowing private clinics to operate under contract from health authorities. These private clinics have come under fire from citizens concerned about the assault on Medicare for charging patients extra fees for expensive upgrades on items such as cataract implants, for generally higher operating costs than are found in the public system, and for the potential for creation of a two-tiered health system. There has also been loud public criticism of the fact that physicians working in private clinics are allowed reimbursement for their services through publicly funded Medicare, a federal program that is administered jointly by the federal and provincial governments.

While the high cost of federal health care expenditures has led to a rethinking and reconsideration of funding arrangements by successive federal governments, the Liberal government, reelected in 1997, has continued to affirm its fundamental commitment to the principles of Medicare. Alberta has been somewhat of a renegade province in that it has challenged the federal government in terms of its move to privatize various components of the Alberta health system. Specifically, the Klein government has attempted to pass legislation allowing the private clinics to keep patients overnight following procedures such as hip replacement. A vociferous and negative public reaction to the first two versions of the bill resulted in their withdrawal from the respective sessions of the legislature in which they had been introduced. A third version of the bill was introduced in March 2000 and engendered possibly the most critical reaction of all. Opponents of the legislation emerged from across the country indicating that passage of the bill under Alberta law could jeopardize Medicare as it is known in Canada under the terms of the Free Trade Agreement with the United States and Mexico. The reason given for this potential violation was that, if one province was allowed to offer private health care, the others would have to make it available as well under the terms of the agreement.

Although the National Forum on Health chaired by the prime minister championed the publicly financed system of Medicare over a private health system (National Forum on Health, 1995), the federal government has yet to wade into the current debate over health care financing with concrete proposals to ensure that renegade provinces are not allowed to jeopardize Medicare in their own provinces or in others. At the present time, the call for federal assistance in the fight against private health care has become the rallying cry for those who hold the future of Medicare near and dear to their hearts. However, this battle over the fundamental structure of the health system is a historic one that has been played out over the last century. As Northcott (1994) has reflected: "And so the debates continue. Canada's health-care program is currently neither free-enterprise medicine nor socialized medicine. Rather it is something in between." It is defining that "something in between" that has presented challenges to practitioners, policy makers, and the Canadian public alike.

PHILOSOPHICAL BASIS OF THE CANADIAN SYSTEM OF UNIVERSAL HEALTH CARE

The rationale for the evolution of the federal health legislation program in the way that it has, can be found in five basic principles of health care from which the standards for the legislation are derived. The first principle, *universality,* refers to the fact that under any provincial plan, 100% of insured residents must be entitled to insured services provided by the plan on uniform terms and conditions; therefore coverage must be offered to the population as a whole rather than to selected population groups. The principle of *comprehensiveness* ensured that the provincial health insurance plan must insure all insured services provided by hospitals, physicians, or dental surgeons, and similar or additional services given by other health care practitioners in provinces where legislation permits. Although extra billing and user fees were allowed prior to 1984 and facility fees by private clinics up to 1994, since that time differential charges may no longer be applied on a private basis for services covered by the plan. *Accessibility* is perhaps the most difficult principle to satisfy, particularly with a sparse population scattered over a vast amount of territory. However, reasonable access to services is seen as essential even in view of the need to constrain costs. *Portability* or coverage for residents of one province when they require services just after a move or during a visit to another province must be assured in plans. *Public administration,* nonprofit operation by an organization fiscally responsible to the provincial government, is also required. In the various acts passed by the federal government relative to health insurance since 1957, progressive refinement of the standards applicable to provincial health plans based on the basic principles has been evident.

The incorporation of a system of health care in legislation ensures that certain defining characteristics will emerge from the philosophy and principles on which it is based. Because the system itself is entrenched in law, if change is desired, full legislative review is required. This might be either an advantage or a disadvantage depending on the issue of concern and the nature of any change deemed necessary. Approximately 75% of health care expenditures in Canada come under Medicare, while about 25% fall outside it in services not reimbursed by the plan. At the outset the Canadian health care system evolved in a manner not unlike systems in other Western countries. The fact that the provincial plans insure hospital care and physicians' services means that the hospital and physician are paramount in the system. It is not surprising to find

that the number of hospital beds increased at a rate much higher than the rate of population increase until legislation appeared to end the 50/50 federal/provincial cost sharing. Outpatient care, home care, and community health services were areas not eligible for federal cost sharing at the outset. The exclusion of these forms of care from federal financing encouraged the physician-centered, in-hospital care that have been dominant features of the system that evolved over 40 years (Ross Kerr, 1996, pp. 224-225). The high cost of these methods of providing care has led to a search for more effective and efficient lower-cost alternatives. The consumer movement has also heightened awareness of the need for consumers to be active participants in matters pertaining to their health. The Alma Ata agreement by countries who are members of the World Health Organization of health for all by the year 2000 has carried with it an implicit challenge to encourage genuine community involvement in planning for health in ways that have not been either recognized or explored previously in health care delivery systems. The challenge for health care in Canada is to tailor the legislative arrangements for health care to encourage community-based measures facilitating health maintenance, health promotion, and prevention of disease and to balance these with measures to restore health. Thus,

> Many believe that it will not be possible to sustain the current system without major modifications. Task forces and commissions in most provinces are looking at ways to shift the heavy focus on physician and institutional care to "community based" alternatives and non-physician providers. [Deber, Hastings, & Thompson, 1991, pp. 73-74]

THE ESTABLISHMENT OF THE CANADIAN HEALTH INSURANCE SYSTEM

In a society in which life is deeply valued, the health of people becomes an issue of fundamental importance. Responsibility for health was granted to the provinces in the British North America Act, which established the Canadian Confederation in 1867. Health was reserved as a federal prerogative for marine and quarantine hospitals and for aboriginal peoples. The Constitution Act of 1982 superseded the original legislation and confirmed and continued this division of powers. Social democratic traditions along with Canada's growth and development as a colonial empire were undoubtedly important in public acceptance of the need to ensure the availability of health care for the population. In the aftermath of social upheavals created by the Great Depression and two world wars, many factors converged to create a receptive climate for consideration of public financing of individual health care expenditures. Federal and provincial agreements emerged from public debate and culminated in a system of national health insurance to cover health care costs for all Canadians.

Although the Canadian program of insurance for hospital services at the federal level was not enacted until 1957, the stage was set for the federal legislation through developments in the provinces. The province of Saskatchewan was clearly in the forefront and, after World War I, passed legislation enabling municipalities to raise taxes to support the employment of physicians (the municipal doctor plans), the establishment of hospitals, and the development of hospitalization plans. The window of opportunity created by the Canadian Medical Association's (CMA) firm support for publicly financed health insurance in 1934 was lost through government inaction, and the CMA later withdrew its support in favor of private plans initiated by physicians in several provinces. Saskatchewan decided to "go it alone" when it became the first jurisdiction in North America to enact legislation establishing a prepaid plan of hospital insurance in 1947. Although it fell short of the objective of establishing a prepaid hospital insurance plan, the first legislation dealing with health was passed by the federal government in 1948. The National Health Grants Act included funds for hospital construction, professional training, public health and other provincial services, areas seen as providing the basis for the later establishment of national health insurance.

When the Hospital Insurance and Diagnostic Services Act was passed in 1957, it provided for comprehensive in-hospital patient care services with universal coverage for residents of participating provinces. Because health fell within provincial jurisdiction, the government of each province had the right to decide whether or not to develop a plan to insure hospital services conforming to the federal guidelines outlined in the legislation. However, because the plan involved 50/50 cost-sharing with the provinces, any province deciding to opt out of the arrangement would forego tax dollars the federal government would otherwise contribute to health care in that province and would, in opting out, effectively subsidize the plans of other provinces. Initially five provinces agreed to participate when the act came into force in 1958, and by 1961 all provinces were full participants in the program. Excepted from the national hospital insurance program were tuberculosis, mental hospitals, and certain other institutions.

In adding prepayment for medical services to the hospitalization plan in 1962, the province of Saskatchewan again became the first jurisdiction to implement such legislation. It did so over the loud protestations of Saskatchewan physicians who went on strike for 23 days beginning July 1, 1962, the date the legislation was implemented. In the face of vehement opposition from physicians, the Saskatchewan government was forced to make concessions to the medical profession in the form of allowing opting out of the plan and extra billing. Implementation of the federal agenda to add medical services to its program of prepaid health insurance was undoubtedly hastened and facilitated by the lessons learned from the Saskatchewan experience. The federal Medical Care Act was thus passed in 1966, and the controversial nature of the legislation may explain the participation of only two provinces at the time the legislation came into force on July 1, 1968, as well as the 5-year length of time required for all provinces to enter into an arrangement with the federal government for the prepayment of medical services. The plan allowed for coverage of physicians' services in and out of hospital, but did not prevent the provinces from allowing physicians to opt out of the plan, bill patients directly, or impose surcharges on the established fee for a particular service.

In the early part of the 1970s the escalation of expenditures and the growing size of the federal deficit caused concern over the open-ended nature of some health expenditures, in particular those for physicians' services. In 1977 the system of federal-provincial cost sharing was amended with the passage of the Fiscal Arrangements and Established Programs Financing Act. This ended the open-ended 50/50 cost sharing and introduced block funding, which involved transfer of tax points to the provinces and reduced the federal contribution to health care to 25% with additional federal contributions based on increases in the gross domestic product (GDP). In the years following the passage of this legislation concern mounted over the increased use of copayments termed user fees for institutional services and extra billing practices among physicians in provinces where this was allowed. The Liberal federal government responded to these perceived erosions of Medicare by disallowing extra billing and user fees in the Canada Health Act of 1984. Physicians mounted a strong and vocal campaign to prevent the prohibition of extra billing to no avail. A similarly perceived erosion of Medicare in the charging of facility fees by private clinics established in some province a decade later was disallowed by the federal government in 1994 and provinces contravening the federal legislation were penalized by lowering their federal transfer payments.

NURSING PRACTICE IN CANADA

As the largest group of health professionals, nurses form the backbone of the health system in Canada. In 1998 the nursing workforce comprised 254,964 registered nurses practicing in acute care facilities (62.4%), while 11.8% of this total worked in nursing homes, 7.1% in public health, 4.4% in home care, and 2.6% in physicians' offices. A further 2.2% were employed in educational institutions (Statistics Canada, 1999). The fact that the number of nurses working in tertiary care has dropped by about some 20% over the past decade is perhaps somewhat surprising since this is a rather large change in a short period of time. However, seen in the context of the health reform movement of the mid-1990s where hospital-based care was deemphasized and newer community-based approaches to care were implemented, a shift of this nature was predictable. Perhaps more surprising is the fact that the increase in the number of nurses working in home care is as low as it is because day surgery programs and shorter hospitals stays have created an increasing need for expansion of the home care sector.

The Canadian Nurses Association predicts an escalating shortage of nurses over the next decade if new nursing graduates continue to seek employment out of the country at the rate of the past decade. According to the Canadian Council of Social Development's recent study, nearly one in ten nursing graduates migrated to the United States between 1995 and 1997 (Canadian Council on Social Development, 2000). Perhaps at the root of the problem are low salaries, inadequate benefits, and a need to enhance the quality of the working environment. Of the 227,651 registered nurses employed in nursing in 1998, 50.8% indicated that they worked full time, while 47.6% stated they worked on a part-time basis (Statistics Canada, 1999). Although some nurses may choose part-time work to allow them to cope with their family responsibilities, many others would like to have full-time work but are unable to secure full-time positions because a great many full-time positions have been converted to part-time and casual positions.

Specialization in nursing has grown exponentially with the increase in knowledge and technology in health care and the demand for nurses with advanced preparation in particular specialty areas. Specialties have tended to parallel medical specialization, and such areas as occupational health nursing and neurosciences are among those that have gained recognition under the Canadian Nurses Association Certification of Nursing Specialties program. This is a program where there are specified requirements for sustained as well as current practice in the specialty as well as basic preparation in nursing and a specialty examination set by the Canadian Nurses Association Testing Service in consultation with the specialty group. Baccalaureate or master's level education is not required for achieving certification in a designated nursing specialty under the Canadian Nurses Association program. Nursing specialization has also occurred at the graduate level, however, with the emergence of the advanced practice nursing role incorporated into master's programs throughout the 1990s. The health reform movement across the country has led to a rationalization of the roles of all health professionals, and it is clear that nurses educated in advanced practice can deliver high-quality care at a fraction of the cost of physicians. While specialty roles for advance practice nurses are well developed in the United States, these are just developing in Canada, where until relatively recently, health care financing arrangements may not have been as open to this development. Provincial health legislation has been amended in some jurisdictions to provide a legal framework within which advanced practice nurses may function.

Nurses have been on record as supporting health care reform for decades. It has been clear that the health system as it has developed in Canada under a system of national health insurance has been relatively costly. It should be noted, however, that health system costs in Canada are far less than in the United States, where since the full implementation of Medicare in Canada, health spending as a percentage of the GDP has consistently been several percentage points higher. While many other countries have established national health systems that are publicly funded, the Canadian system employs a private overlay on a public system. Excess capacity in certain sectors including acute care, remuneration for certain categories of health professionals on an expensive fee-for-service basis, and overdevelopment of some services with little attention to whether or not these were needed have characterized the system. In addition, financial incentives to the provinces to develop systems based on hospital and physician-centered care have added considerably to the overall cost of the system. Because of these incentives, the total cost of the system has been higher than would have been the case if certain other policy directions had been taken.

The political will to reform the system has not been there until recently, and whether true reform will occur or just window-dressing remains to be seen. Since political will is driven by the ability to garner votes from the electorate, the shape of reform may be such that a publicly funded health system may be less attractive to the politicians than one with more privately funded services than previously. Politicians have historically found it much easier to support the high cost elements of the system such as physicians' services since these individuals constitute a powerful pressure group in society. Politicians ultimately responsible for health policy have always found it difficult to address the aspects of the system that most need reform in order to ensure that the publicly funded system of health care remains viable. Among these are included the need for shifting the acute care focus of the system to a focus that is based in community health centers; streamlining the method of payment for health to exclude fee-for-service and include remunerating health professionals on a salary or contract basis; identifying how many professionals are needed in the system and limiting the number practicing in the system to the number required; and limiting the facilities where the work of the health system is carried on to those that are required and closing those not needed. Rationalization of the system could lead to the establishment of community health centers where a range of services provided by health professionals could be offered and in which nurses would figure prominently. This could potentially facilitate coordination of care and achieve efficiencies through common use of facilities and interdisciplinary teamwork. The need to address these matters in order to preserve a publicly funded and effective health system is critical.

Health care reform as envisioned by nurses would see the primary focus of health care moving to the community in primary health centers from its traditional base in tertiary care hospitals. The movement of health care policy development and decision making relative to health care delivery to health authorities in regionally based systems has occurred in several provinces and has required major transitions in a relatively short period of time. The closing of acute hospital beds was accompanied by a promise to shift care to the community with the development of community health centers. This is reflected to a certain extent in the nursing statistics quoted earlier, but most would agree that there will be a greater shift in the future. Nevertheless, true reform of the system requires hard decisions about care and the best ways of providing it to people by qualified professionals. If the hands of the health authorities are tied by a lack of jurisdiction over all services required for care, those services will continue to be fragmented and expensive.

To date, nurses have not been engaged in substantial numbers for the delivery of primary health care, but it is entirely possible that this will occur in the future with the development of community health centers. It is likely that changes in the way in which nursing is practiced will continue as society becomes more aware of the benefits of health promotion and the need to develop healthier lifestyles to prevent disease. Alternatives to hospitalization for tertiary and long-term or continuing care, in the form of home care and ambulatory care, appear attractive at both the personal and societal levels. It must be recognized, however, that all levels of hospitalization will continue to be required to meet the needs of people. In the rhetoric about downsizing the tertiary care hospital and moving services to the community, it must be recognized that high-quality tertiary care services are critical to a well-functioning system. Nurses have been preparing for their new roles in community and long-term care settings and have the knowledge and the communication and interactional skills to assist consumers in meeting health goals. They are thus well poised and positioned to serve society in a health system that is centered in the community and based on the primary health care model.

NURSING EDUCATION

The history and traditions of nursing education in Canada are long and impressive. A system of diploma nursing education developed following the establishment of the Mack Training School in association with the St. Catharines General and Marine Hospital in 1874. The first university courses in nursing in Canada were offered in public health nursing at the University of Alberta in 1915. Subsequently the University of British Columbia offered the first degree program in nursing in the country in 1919 under the direction of Ethel Johns. The system of diploma nursing education in hospitals and later community colleges has undergone further changes with the drive to establish the baccalaureate degree in nursing as the entry level for the profession since it is widely believed that increased availability of baccalaureate programs in nursing will provide a stronger basis for the practice of nursing. Collaborative baccalaureate degree programs offered jointly between the community colleges and the universities have been developed in a number of provinces, and students now entering initial programs in nursing are able in many areas of the country to study for a baccalaureate degree in nursing whether they enroll initially in a nursing program at a community college or at a university. Baccalaureate nursing programs have been available to diploma-prepared nurses dating from the time of the early degree programs in nursing. More recently distance programs have allowed registered nurses in more remote centers to study for their degrees even though they do not live in a major university center. The development of a context-based learning program or problem-based learning as it is termed in some centers is an innovative response to providing high-quality baccalaureate nursing education that encourages critical thinking and problem solving in nursing graduates.

Graduate programs at the master's level have been available in Canada since the establishment of the first master's degree program in nursing at the University of Western Ontario in 1959. Since then, master's degree programs have developed in every region on the country so that today they are widely available to students. The first fully funded doctoral program in nursing was established at the University of Alberta on January 1, 1991, and there are now five doctoral nursing programs across the country. The initiation of doctoral education has been an important milestone for the profession, since preparing nurses to contribute to the discovery of nursing knowledge through theory and research will lead to improved care.

Nursing has made great progress in improving its standards. It would appear that the long and difficult campaigns by the provincial professional associations as well as the Canadian Nurses Association have not been in vain, for nursing education programs in Canada have moved from the jurisdiction of hospitals to the general educational system. Programs are generally of high quality, and the collaboration between community colleges and universities to develop joint baccalaureate programs has been positive both for students and health care. It is apparent that there has been a progression in thinking over time about schools of nursing and about the system of nursing education. Nevertheless, certain principles have continued to characterize the approaches that the profession and those engaged in the educational system have taken to the improvement of standards and monitoring the quality of education in programs. The importance of engaging well-qualified instructors, selecting appropriate content, retaining a strong clinical focus, and maintaining appropriate admission standards have been elements that have been concerns over time. The concern for standards of education and practice has been a fundamental one in view of the responsibility for providing safe and competent care to clients. However, dynamic leadership will be required to provide direction to new generations of skilled practitioners and to ensure that their talents are used to the fullest extent for the benefit of the public.

With the development of the discipline and the expansion of the knowledge base, the appropriateness of the environment in which learning takes place is at issue. The fact that nursing is one of the last sex-segregated professions has led to attention to the potential for differential treatment, with improvement in the status of women as they gradually gained fundamental rights and privileges previously accorded only to men. Systematic undervaluing of the contributions of the profession continue to be common and are evident in the published histories of many health care institutions where nurses have played significant roles in the implementation and management of care. However, the gender balance of the profession is changing, albeit slowly, and this transition forms an important part of new perspectives on the roles of men and women in society generally.

FUTURE DIRECTIONS

The tax-supported system of health care that has evolved in Canada over a period of some 40 years, while not flawless, is nevertheless highly regarded by consumers who react negatively to any suggestion that the system is imperiled. Such suggestions are the order of the day and simply part of business as usual in a not-for-profit system operated in the public sphere where interest groups and institutions alike have the opportunity to put forward their views freely. It is recognized today that there are limits to the nature and amount of care that can be provided and limits to growth of the system. In order to ensure the continuation of the system, measures must be taken to ensure that universal availability and access to needed services are balanced by the provision of reasonably comprehensive services in a publicly funded, nonprofit, and affordable system.

The system must respond to perceptions of a need for change in the nature and context of health care. It has been pointed out that Canada "provides a test case in the limits of medical care *per se,* and the health problems which still confront Canadians cannot, in general, be improved merely by improving access to medical care" (Deber et al., 1991, p. 74). Canada has had a hospital and physician centered system of health care entrenched in its universal health care legislation for some 40 years. The social determinants of health such as income, education, and the environment are important elements in the health of a nation. Universal health insurance has provided some assistance to vulnerable population groups, but other measures to address some of these problems are needed. Health is increasingly seen more broadly than simply the absence of illness, and in the presence of new approaches to the meaning of health, the nature and context of health care must change as well.

REFERENCES

Canadian Council on Social Development. (2000). *The labour market integration of new nursing graduates in Canada (1986-1998)*. Ottawa: Author.

Deber, R.B., Hastings, J.E.F., & Thompson, G.G. (1991). Health care in Canada: Current trends and issues. *Journal of Public Health Policy, 12*(1), 72-82.

Inglehart, J.K. (1990). Health policy report: Canada's health care system. *New England Journal of Medicine, 315*(12), 778-784.

National Forum on Health. (1995). *The public and private financing of Canada's health system: A discussion paper*. Ottawa: Government of Canada.

Northcott, Herbert A. (1994). Threats to Medicare: The financing, allocation, and utilization of health care in Canada. In B.S. Bolaria & H.D. Dickinson (Eds.), *Health, illness, and health care in Canada* (2nd ed., pp. 198-219). Toronto: Harcourt Brace.

Northcott, Herbert A. (1994). Alternative health care in Canada. In B.S. Bolaria & H.D. Dickinson (Eds.), *Health, illness, and health care in Canada* (2nd ed., pp. 487-503). Toronto: Harcourt Brace.

Ross-Kerr, J. (1996). The organization and financing of health care. In J. Ross-Kerr & J. MacPhail (Eds.), *Canadian nursing: Issues and perspectives* (2nd ed., pp. 216-227). Toronto: Mosby–Year Book.

Statistics Canada. (1999). *Registered nurses management data*. Ottawa: Policy, Regulation and Research Division.

Wilson, D.M., & Ross-Kerr, J.C. (1998). An exploration of Canadian social values relative to health care. *The American Journal of Health Behavior, 22*(2), 120-129.

An Overview of Health Care and Nursing Education and Practice in Britain

JUNE CLARK

Almost everything in the present day social structures of Britain, including its health care system, can be explained by history. In the first edition of *Nursing and Social Change,* one of the classics of the history of nursing in Britain, Monica Baly wrote:

> The development of nursing is like the weaving of a cloth, with social change as the warp, and running to and fro with the weft is the shuttle of care. Sometimes the shuttle moves slowly . . . then as new knowledge and ideas develop, the shuttle moves faster and a number of threads are woven together to form a new pattern. The new pattern forms the basis for the health services of the next generation, but the warp changes again and the shuttle moves on faster, and the nearer we come to the present day the more complicated becomes the design. Only by tracing the threads to their historical origin can we begin to understand the confusion and profusion of the health services of the twentieth century. [Baly, 1973]

In the last decade of the twentieth century the shuttle has moved faster than ever, and nursing and health care in Britain have been subjected to more change than is comfortable. The warp of social change has included major political shifts to the right (Thatcherism) and then back to the left (New Labour), the rise of consumerism, changes in the position of women in society and in the economy, and the information revolution. The shuttle of care has included the introduction of new technologies and treatments, a shift from care in hospitals to care in the community, and the effects of cost constraint. The new pattern retains some of the old core values, and issues such as cost constraint and nurse shortages are perennial, but there are new challenges and new (not always successful) solutions.

There is also an old saying that "When America sneezes, Britain catches the cold." Many of the new patterns in nursing and health care in Britain reflect what has previously happened in the United States. The incubation period seems to be about 20 years, but is getting shorter!

HEALTH CARE IN BRITAIN

Most people date the beginning of the British health care system to the introduction of the National Health Service (NHS) in 1948, but formal forms of health care have existed in Britain for several hundred years. The oldest hospital in Britain (which is still in use and still uses some of the original buildings) is St. Bartholomew's Hospital in London (known as "Barts"), which was established in 1123. "Madhouses" had similarly existed for centuries, although they were not formalized as mental hospitals until late in the 19th century, and the training of mental health nurses did not begin until 1891. Community health services for the poor had been provided by the public authorities since the time of the first Queen Elizabeth. The major development of our formal health care system, however, took place in the 19th century when Britain was at the peak of its imperial power, when the Industrial Revolution changed Britain from an agricultural society to an industrial society in which the growth of cities created health problems that politicians could no longer ignore, when scientific medicine was beginning and medicine and later nursing were becoming organized as professions. Every nurse has heard about Florence Nightingale and her work on hospitals and nursing education, but Florence Nightingale was a product of her time, and there were many other pioneers developing services that were to become a century later the "new" National Health Service. Edward Chadwick's *Report on the Sanitary Conditions of the Labouring Population of Great Britain* (1842) provided the seedcorn for the organization of a proper system for public health, which led in turn to the establishment of health visiting (public health nursing) in Manchester in 1862 and district nursing (home care nursing) in Liverpool in 1863. These services reflect a feature common to many of the British health and social welfare services (which can still be seen in much later developments such as the development of the hospice movement in the 1960s and 1970s), namely that the local effort of a group of volunteers was gradually recognized, encouraged, and eventually taken over by the public authorities. By the turn of the century the shift of emphasis toward the development of personal health services (and recognition of the appallingly high infant mortality rate) brought the formalization of midwifery and the regulation of midwives in 1902, the establishment of the school health service (triggered by the Boer War) in 1905, and an insurance-based system of primary medical care in 1911.

Many of the organizational "anomalies" and the cultural traditions that shape our present-day health services are the living relics of this history. For example, one of the most important features of the present British health care system that is derived from history is the arrangement by which direct access to specialist (hospital) services is not permitted (except for accident and emergency services) but is dependent on a referral by the primary care physician (general practitioner). This arrangement was originally negotiated during the 19th century by the physicians themselves as a means of protecting the respective financial interests of those who worked in hospitals and those who worked in what became primary care. While people in other countries may interpret this as a limitation on the consumer's individual choice, it has not been perceived as such (at least until recently) by the British public, and it is undoubtedly a major factor in the relatively low cost of the NHS.

By the time of the inception of the NHS in 1948, therefore, there already existed in Britain an extensive and complex pattern of health services, although it was fragmented, patchy in its coverage, and financially unsustainable. What the National Health Service Act of 1946 did was to take the existing services and rationalize and nationalize them. That is, all services were to be made available to all citizens free of charge at the point of use, provided through public authorities (of various kinds), and financed through direct government funding derived from taxation. Over the past 50 years some of these principles have been eroded in various ways (e.g., some services now require copayment, and access [as distinct from eligibility] for all citizens remains an important issue), but what has persisted are the core values of:

- Universality (services available to everyone as a citizens right)
- Comprehensiveness (all types of services: hospital and community-based, preventive as well as curative, from "cradle to grave")
- Free at the point of use (access to services on the basis of need regardless of ability to pay)

These values remain dear to the hearts of the British people (as many governments who have tried to make changes in the NHS since 1948 have discovered to their cost) and are still clearly visible in the structures and processes of the NHS today.

The achievement of the 1946 act was the culmination of a great political battle in which many compromises had to be made. In particular, the service could not run without the cooperation of the medical profession, yet at the time the medical profession was opposed to several aspects of the plan. For example, they were adamantly opposed to control by the local authorities (which they interpreted as political interference with their clinical freedom), and they were worried by the threat to their personal income derived from private practice. The compromises that were agreed with the medical profession in 1946 and that have been fought for by sections of the medical profession ever since explain many of the organizational and financial "anomalies" of the NHS today. For example, the resistance to working for local authorities explains the existence of Health Authorities, variously named in the years since 1946; the right of senior hospital doctors (called "consultants") to undertake private practice alongside their salaried work in NHS hospitals explains the coexistence and pattern of private sector health care in Britain; and the fierce battle by primary care physicians (general practitioners) to work as "independent contractors" rather than as salaried employees explains the present organization of primary care services.

THE FINANCING OF HEALTH CARE

The NHS is funded primarily (approximately 95%) from taxation, including a small proportion from the national insurance scheme that is compulsory for all employers and employees; approximately 5% is derived from copayments, mainly for drugs (but not drugs prescribed in hospital) and dental and ophthalmic services. In the NHS the only third-party payer is the government. The amount to be spent each year is determined in the annual Public Expenditure Survey, which is the process by which public expenditure is divided among the various government departments responsible for functions such as defense, education, and law and order. Currently health services consume about 15% of public expenditure and about 6% of the gross domestic product (GDP). The health budget is managed by the Department of Health in England and the parallel government departments in Scotland, Wales, and Northern Ireland. After "top-slicing" for various centrally provided services, the money is devolved on a weighted per capita basis to geographically defined Health Authorities who spend it on providing health care services for their populations. Before 1990 the Health Authorities used the money to run and finance the hospitals and community-based agencies; since 1990 (see below) they have used the money to purchase services through contracts with provider agencies called NHS Trusts. Primary care is provided, also free of charge, by general practitioners whose contracts include a fixed annual payment for each person on their "list" plus a variety of item-of-service and incentive payments and reimbursement of the costs of support services (including the employment of practice nurses).

The assumption made in 1946 that once the backlog of disease had been dealt with, the costs of the NHS would become less, turned out to be a major mistake. As in all Western countries, the costs of health care have risen inexorably, and in Britain as in most countries cost constraint is a major preoccupation.

STRUCTURE AND ORGANIZATION OF THE NATIONAL HEALTH SERVICE

Between 1946 and 1974 the NHS was organized in three branches that reflected the structures that existed previously: hospital services were run by Regional Hospital Boards; public health, the school health service, and community nursing services continued to be run by the local authorities; and the general practitioners operated independently with contracts administered by executive councils. The three distinct organizational cultures can still be seen in present day services. Through the 1950s and 1960s there were many initiatives to bring the three branches together, and in 1974 the hospital and community services were brought together under newly created Health Authorities, although the general practitioners fought successfully to remain outside as independent contractors administered locally through Family Practitioner Committees.

In 1979, however, the election of a new right-wing conservative government under the leadership of Margaret Thatcher began a series of changes in the health care system (and many other aspects of British society) that were ideological as well as organizational and more radical than anything that had happened since the end of the second world war. The 1980s saw a sequence of changes that were introduced as "efficiency improvements" but that in their effects constituted radical cultural as well as organizational changes. The most significant for nursing was the introduction in 1983, on the recommendation of Sir Roy Griffiths, of the concept of general management to replace the system of functional management by the traditional "triumvirate" of doctor, nurse, and administrator; many senior nurses lost their jobs, provoking a loss of leadership from which the nursing profession has only recently begun to recover. At the same time the view that care in the community was cheaper as well as better than hospital care led to major reductions in the number of hospital beds, especially in psychiatric hospitals and hospitals providing long-term care. Health care began to be redefined as acute medical care. The long-term care of frail, elderly people was gradually transferred to private-sector nursing homes, which expanded dramatically in number, causing a reconfiguration of the nursing workforce, which previously had been employed almost exclusively in the NHS.

The culmination of these changes was the publication in 1989 of proposals for reform of the NHS in two government documents, *Working for Patients* and *Caring for People,* which were implemented by the NHS and Community Care Act of 1990.

THE 1990 REFORMS

The core component of the 1990 NHS reforms was the introduction of an internal market through changes in the roles of the Health Authorities and the hospitals and community agencies that provide health care to create a "purchaser/provider split." Instead of using their money to run facilities themselves, the Health Authorities were to use it to purchase services for their resident population from the provider agencies that were now reconstituted as self-governing, not-for-profit organizations called NHS Trusts. Some of the money was made available to general practitioners who chose to become "fundholders" to purchase certain services directly for their patients from Trusts and other agencies; from 1993 the range of services included community nursing services. Trusts would compete with one another (and with the private-sector agencies) for contracts with Health Authorities and Fundholders, and it was expected that this competition would drive down costs and improve quality.

These changes produced a great change in the organizational culture of the NHS. On the one hand it undoubtedly became more cost-conscious at all levels and therefore probably more efficient. Quality assurance and outcome measurement became much more important. On the other hand, the market could not be allowed to behave as a "normal" market because Trusts that failed financially could not be allowed to close down. Clinicians of all disciplines complained that commercial pressures interfered with clinical freedom. Community nurses found that their clinical priorities were now determined by "fundholder" physicians. Services that were regarded as "uneconomic" were cut or responsibility transferred to other sectors. Commercial competitiveness prevented the sharing of good practice. Most seriously, the negotiation of contracts by some fundholders with preferential terms for their patients produced for the first time in the history of the NHS a two-tier service that violated the basic principle of access on the basis of need alone.

In the 1997 general election, in which the NHS was a major election issue, the Conservative government was heavily defeated, and power moved to the New Labour government led by Tony Blair, among whose election commitments was "restoration" of the NHS.

THE NEW NHS—MODERN DEPENDABLE

Within a few months of the election the new government's proposals were published in a White Paper entitled *The New NHS—Modern Dependable* (Department of Health, 1997). In line with the government's commitment to political devolution, parallel papers that differed in detail but not in their central policy were published for Wales, Scotland, and Northern Ireland. The proposals were followed by further documents that detailed specific policies and implementation strategies and were implemented by the 1999 Health Act.

The main changes are:

• The competitive internal market is abolished, but the split between Health Authorities as purchasers (renamed "commissioners") and Trusts as providers is retained. Short-term contracts are replaced by longer term "service agreements."
• A new performance framework has been introduced, based on "clinical governance" in which chief executives of Trusts (and other staff) are personally accountable for the quality of services as well as for financial management. New organizations have been established to set standards and monitor quality.

• Fundholding is abolished, but new local organizations (called Primary Care Groups in England, Local Health Groups in Wales) composed of general practitioners, community nurses, representatives of the local authority, and lay representatives, are created who will initially act as advisory committees to the Health Authorities for commissioning services but will eventually provide community and primary care services for their local population (approximately 100,000).
• A duty is placed on Health Authorities, Trusts, and Primary Care Groups to collaborate and work in partnership with local authorities within jointly agreed health improvement programs.
• New ways of delivering services are being established, including a national telephone help line staffed by nurses, called NHS Direct.
• A program of "modernization" is being introduced based on the use of information technology.

THE BRITISH HEALTH CARE SYSTEM IN THE YEAR 2000

The British health care system in the year 2000 is therefore a service in transition but one that continues to reflect some of the organizational structures of the past and is based on strong cultural values that were established in the immediate postwar period when the NHS was established. Most health care is provided through the NHS, but there is a relatively small private hospital sector (supported mainly by private insurance) that provides mainly nonemergency surgical services and a large private nursing home sector that provides long-term care for frail, elderly people. The NHS is a *national* service, conforming to national standards, centrally funded and monitored, but managed operationally at the local level by local public authorities. Within the overall financial allocation, responsibility for managing services is devolved to the newly established governments of Scotland, Wales, and Northern Ireland, and there are some differences in local terminology and management arrangements. Services are free at the point of use, although copayment is required for a few services; children, elders, and people in receipt of social security benefits are exempt from these charges.

Geographically defined Health Authorities receive money from central government to commission health services for their resident population (approximately 300,000 to 500,000); from 1999 onward part of this responsibility is being transferred to the new local health authorities (called Primary Care Groups in England, Local Health Groups in Wales), who will eventually also become responsible for the provision of primary care and community services to their populations (approximately 100,000).

Hospital and community health services are provided through self-governing not-for-profit organizations called NHS Trusts. In Wales, Trusts provide the full range of hospital, community, and mental health services to their geographically defined population; in Scotland each health authority (called Health Boards in Scotland) has an acute (i.e., hospitals) Trust and a primary care Trust; in England there are various combinations.

Primary care services are provided by family physicians called general practitioners, based in primary care centers that usually are called surgeries. They work in close association with community nurses who are employed by Trusts and may also employ their own nurses who usually work only in the surgery. Every citizen has the right to register with a general practitioner of his or her choice. About 96% of the population is registered with a general practitioner, but there are difficulties for some mobile or homeless people. The general practitioner contracts with the government to provide medical services to all the people on his or her list whenever needed. Usually members of a family register with the same general practitioner and may remain registered with the same general practitioner from birth until death or until they move to another locality; this enables considerable continuity of care, which is one of the strengths of the system. The general practitioner is usually the point of first contact for people needing health care and acts as gatekeeper to other services to which he or she refers patients as necessary. This position is, however, currently being challenged by new services such as NHS Direct.

Hospital services are similar to those in any developed country, but one of the particular strengths of the British system is its long tradition of community-based nursing services, which, like hospital services, are provided free at the point of contact to all who need them. In the British system the term "community-based services" is preferred to "ambulatory care." District nurses provide nursing care to people suffering from chronic illness and following discharge from hospital; health visitors provide preventive health care and support to all families with young children; preventive health services are provided through the school health service to children at school. Mental health services and services for those with learning disabilities (mental handicap) are nowadays mainly community based and are run in close collaboration with the local authority's social services, as are community-based services for elderly people. Long-term care for elderly people is nowadays provided mainly in private-sector nursing homes (often paid for by public funds), but district nurses provide nursing care when needed for people living in residential care. Occupational health is not included in the National Health Service but is independently provided by some large employers.

NURSING PRACTICE

Nursing practice in any country is shaped by the health care system, by nurses' educational preparation, by the system for professional regulation, by the organizational framework in which nurses work, and by the shape of the health care workforce (e.g., the number of qualified nurses relative to the number of physicians and other health care personnel). Most nurses in Britain work within the NHS, although the recent expansion in private-sector nursing homes for elderly people means that about a third now work in the private sector. They work in hospitals (mainly), community-based clinics, people's homes, schools, workplaces, and many other settings, so that what constitutes nursing practice varies greatly.

Specialization

As in many highly developed health care systems, nursing has become highly specialized, in Britain to the extent that nursing is described in legislation as consisting of three distinct professions: nursing, midwifery, and health visiting. Health visitors are always and midwives are usually also registered nurses (although direct entry to midwifery through separate educational preparation is growing). Even within nursing there are four different branches at the basic level (adult nursing, children's nursing, psychiatric nursing, and learning disabilities nursing). At postbasic level there is a wide range of specialties in both hospital and community practice. In community nursing, for example, there are eight different kinds of community nurses, each requiring specific educational preparation: health visitors (public health nurses), district nurses (home care nurses), school nurses, practice nurses, community psychiatric nurses, community pediatric nurses, community learning disability nurses, and occupational health nurses. In addition there are many specialties that operate in both hospital and community, sometimes specifically working across the interface to provide continuity of care to patients, for example, stoma nurses, continence nurses, and palliative care (hospice) nurses.

In Britain there are no nursing practice acts that define the work of nurses. The competencies required for registration as a nurse are specified by the United Kingdom

Central Council (UKCC) (see below). Beyond this, what nurses were allowed to do was largely a matter of custom and practice until 1992 when the UKCC published a seminal document entitled *The Scope of Professional Practice* (UKCC, 1992). This document stressed that every nurse is personally accountable for his or her practice and that it is the nurse's professional judgment that determines what to do. It set out six guiding principles: In deciding what to do, the nurse must:

1. Be satisfied that the patient's needs are uppermost
2. Keep up to date and develop knowledge, skill, and competence
3. Recognize the limits of his or her personal knowledge and skill and remedy deficiencies
4. Ensure that existing nursing care is not compromised by new developments and responsibilities
5. Acknowledge personal accountability
6. Avoid inappropriate delegation

In essence this means that the only limit on the nurse's practice is his or her own competence. Since 1992 this principle has facilitated the development of advanced practice and many new nursing roles.

Regulation of Nursing

The organization responsible for the regulation of nursing, midwifery, and health visiting in Britain is the United Kingdom Central Council for Nursing, Midwifery and Health Visiting. The UKCC, established in 1979, brought together the several regulatory bodies that had developed since the first Nurses Act established nursing registration in 1919. The UKCC maintains the register of nurses, specifies the standard and content of the basic nursing education that is required for entry to the register, and maintains the disciplinary process under which professional misconduct may lead to the removal of a nurse's name from the register. Being "on the register" constitutes the nurse's license to practice. To continue to practice, nurses are required to renew their registration every three years, and this requires evidence of continuing education to ensure continuing competence. As part of its disciplinary function the UKCC also issues guidance documents such as the Code of Professional Conduct (1992) and the Scope of Professional Practice (1992).

In the wake of several high-profile failures of the system (mainly in medicine), however, the regulation of both medicine and nursing is currently under review. In 1997 consultants appointed by the government recommended that the present regulatory organizations (the UKCC and its subsidiary National Boards) should be replaced by a new statutory body to be called the Nursing and Midwifery Council. The principle of self-regulation will be retained but the system and structures are to be streamlined, and the Council will be given new powers to protect the public. The new bodies are scheduled to be in place by the end of the year 2001. Separate legislation is being introduced to achieve the registration of support workers (assistive personnel).

Levels of Practice

In spite of the high degree of postbasic specialization, little consideration has been given until recently to differentiated *levels* of practice. For many years discussion centered on the extended role of the nurse (which was taken to mean the transfer of certain tasks from doctors to nurses) as opposed to the expanded role of the nurse (which was taken to mean a greater depth of nursing decision making) (Hunt & Wainwright, 1994). The main driver for change has been the need to reduce the working hours of junior hospital doctors. The professional lead, however, has been taken by those nurses who have developed the role of nurse practitioner in primary health care, whose work is seen as complementary to, not a substitute for, the primary care physician. There is currently no system in Britain for the certification or regulation of advanced practice, and the indiscriminate use of titles such as nurse practitioner and clinical nurse specialist has increased the confusion.

A recent government initiative is the development of new posts for consultant nurses, which are presented as equivalent to the role of hospital consultants (i.e., the most senior hospital doctors), although at much lower salaries. Specific criteria have been agreed upon that include a commitment to clinical practice alongside education, research, and leadership roles.

One indicator of advanced practice that has been achieved—after some 15 years of strenuous political lobbying by organizations such as the Royal College of Nursing—is prescriptive rights (known in Britain as nurse prescribing). The formulary from which (specially trained) nurses may prescribe is limited, however; it does not, for example, include antibiotics or oral contraceptives.

NHS DIRECT

NHS Direct is a new telephone help line staffed by nurses that is available to all citizens for the price of a local telephone call (which in Britain is cheap but not free). The idea is similar to the many telephone help lines that are available, usually for specific services, in other countries; the difference is that it is an integral part of the NHS, linked with other parts of the health care system and subject to the same standards and controls. If the caller wants advice the call is transferred to a nurse who uses an algorithmic decision support system to make a decision about whether and where to refer the caller for further help or to give advice about treatment and self-care; it is therefore much more than a triage system. The service is popular with patients and nurses (for whom it opens exciting new career opportunities) but unpopular with doctors who see it as an "unnecessary" service for the "worried well" or as a threat to their own role (Clark, 2000).

BASIC NURSING EDUCATION

Britain is famous for the first school of nursing established at St. Thomas's Hospital, London, by Florence Nightingale in 1858. However, as Monica Baly has shown (Baly, 1986, 1995), the reality is somewhat different from the myth, and the strength of the Nightingale tradition, based on the concepts of obedience, discipline, and vocational training by apprenticeship, has not helped more recent attempts in Britain to achieve a proper professional education for nurses. Over a period of more than 50 years from the 1930s onward, many attempts were made to reform nursing education, but as Miss Nightingale herself once wrote, "Reports are not self-executive." Moreover nurses themselves still strongly disagree about the kind of education that is appropriate, some favoring the Nightingale model of vocational training, others the university model developed in the early days by Mrs. Bedford Fenwick.

Until the early 1990s nurse training in Britain consisted of a 3-year hospital-based program in one of four separate specialties (general hospital nursing, children's nursing, mental nursing, and mental handicap nursing). A 2-year program was available for licensed practical nurses, known in Britain as Enrolled Nurses. In 1988, however, the government accepted in principle the recommendations of the UKCC report entitled *Project 2000: A New Preparation for Practice* (UKCC, 1986), and programs based on these recommendations began in 1989, although they were not universally introduced until 1993. In addition, from the 1960s onward, programs at the baccalaureate level were run by a few universities, which also began to develop programs to enable registered nurses to obtain degrees and work at master's and doctoral level. The current nursing workforce therefore includes nurses who have qualified by all four routes.

Since 1979 European Union requirements for mutual recognition of qualifications across Europe specify the length of the program as 3 years or 4,600 hours and a balance between theory and practice. These requirements are incorporated into the UKCC requirements that specify that programs must last 4,600 hours and have a 50:50 ratio of theory to practice.

"Project 2000" recommended:

• That there should be only one level of registered nurse and that training for the second level (the enrolled nurse, equivalent to the licensed practical nurse (LPN) in the United States should be discontinued

• That students should no longer be considered as hospital employees but during their period of training should be supernumary to the labor force

• That schools of nursing should develop links with institutions of further and higher education

• That the basic program should consist of a 2-year common foundation program followed by a "branch" program in adult nursing, children's nursing, mental health nursing, mental handicap nursing, or midwifery and should lead to a diploma in higher education.

These recommendations represented a series of compromises designed to resolve continuing conflicts within the profession (for example, between those who wanted a university-level, generalist preparation and those who wanted to continue the traditional model). Further compromises were made during the period of negotiation with the government that preceded and accompanied implementation.

At the time of writing (June 2000), all programs conform to the Project 2000 model:

• A 3-year program consisting of an 18-month common foundation program, followed by a "branch program" in one of four specialties (adult nursing, children's nursing, mental health nursing, or learning disabilities nursing; midwifery would not agree to be defined as a branch of nursing and succeeded in establishing separate programs leading to registration as a midwife (RM).

• Students are supernumary during most of their program but must complete 1,000 rostered hours during their third year; unlike other students, they do not have to pay fees, and they are supported financially by a bursary.

• Schools of nursing are now organizationally established within higher education institutions (universities), although many remain physically located in their original hospital premises.

• Clinical practice education is undertaken in the hospital and community settings of the NHS Trusts.

• The program leads to professional qualification as a registered nurse, plus a Diploma in Higher Education.

The number of degree-level programs has expanded, and currently about 10% of nurses qualify by this route. Enrolled nurse training has been discontinued, and most Enrolled Nurses have "converted" to first-level registration.

The period of implementation has been fraught with difficulties. Funding for basic nursing education remains with the NHS and not with the Department for Education, which funds all other higher education, so integration with the university sector is incomplete; this difference is exacerbated by the diploma level of the program and by the inability of nursing programs to conform to the "normal" academic year. Implementation coincided with çost constraint and the rapid changes in the NHS that followed the 1990 reforms, so the provision of support during clinical placements has often been less than adequate. The internal market that was applied to NHS service provision was also applied to nursing education; the purchasers or commissioners are consortia of employers who contract with the universities to train a defined number of students in each of the four branches. Most significantly, traditional attitudes to students persist; many service managers and many nurses who qualified under the "old" system continue to expect high levels of practical skill early in the program and complain that the Project 2000 nurses are "too academic."

However, in many areas great progress has been made. Project 2000 nurses are demonstrating a more thoughtful approach to practice and improved decision-making skills. Nurse teachers who were themselves prepared and practiced as teachers in the "old" environment have worked hard to respond to the challenges of teaching in the university environment. More teachers (faculty) are achieving master's and doctoral qualifications. Basic nurse training is becoming nursing education.

FITNESS FOR PRACTICE

Under pressure to remedy some of the perceived deficits of Project 2000, in 1998 the UKCC established a Commission for Nursing and Midwifery Education, whose report *Fitness for Practice* (UKCC, 1999) was published in September 1999. Many of its recommendations support the original aims of Project 2000, stressing in particular

the need for greater support for students in the clinical areas and better collaboration between clinical areas and the academic departments. It suggests that some of the contentious and unresolved issues such as the funding of students and the four specialist branches should be further examined. One recommendation, however, constitutes a major change in the Project 2000 program: the common foundation program that Project 2000 recommended should last 2 years and that was reduced during the implementation negotiations to 18 months is to be further reduced to 1 year; programs based on this recommendation will begin in autumn of 2000.

MAKING A DIFFERENCE

The commission's proposals were to some extent preempted, however, by proposals contained in the government's strategy for nursing, *Making a Difference* (Department of Health, 1999), which was published in July 1999. Driven by the acute shortage of nurses, especially in London (which was attributed to the "overacademic" nature of Project 2000 programs but which was actually caused by the major reduction in the number of training places commissioned following the 1990 NHS reforms), the government committed itself to making nursing education "more responsive to the needs of the NHS" by widening the entry gate to include more candidates without formal educational qualifications, enabling students to "step off and on" at the end of the first year of training, and increasing the practical component during the first year. Planning for the new programs was begun even before *Fitness for Practice* was published. This strategy, however, applied only to England; the Welsh strategy, *Realising the Potential,* retains the commitment to expanding nursing education at the baccalaureate level with the aim of achieving all graduate entry as soon as feasible.

POSTBASIC AND ADVANCED NURSING EDUCATION

Postbasic education has been much less contentious. Evidence of continuing professional development (CPD) is required for renewal of registration. Programs leading to a specialist practice qualification are required to last a year and to be at the level of a first degree. Master's-level programs are developing rapidly, although there are relatively few clinical master's programs. The number of nurses achieving doctorates is also increasing rapidly.

CHALLENGES FOR THE 21st CENTURY

These are turbulent times for nursing in Britain. There are many challenges, risks, and opportunities. Whether and how nursing continues to develop as a profession only time will tell.

REFERENCES

Baly, M.E. (1973). *Nursing and social change.* London: Heinemann Medical Books Ltd.

Baly, M.E. (1986). *Florence Nightingale and the nursing legacy.* London: Routledge.

Clark, J. (2000). Old wine in new bottles: Delivering nursing in the 21st century. *Journal of Nursing Scholarship, 32*(1), 11-15.

Department of Health. (1989). *Working for patients.* London: The Stationery Office.

Department of Health. (1989). *Caring for people.* London: The Stationery Office.

Department of Health. (1997). *The new NHS—Modern dependable.* London: The Stationery Office.

Department of Health. (1999). *Making a difference.* London: The Stationery Office.

Hunt, G., & Wainwright, P. (1994). *Expanding the role of the nurse: The scope of professional practice.* Oxford: Blackwell Scientific Publications.

National Assembly for Wales. (1999). *Realising the potential.* Cardiff: The Stationery Office.

United Kingdom Central Council for Nursing Midwifery and Health Visiting. (1986). *Project-2000: A new preparation for practice.* London: Author.

United Kingdom Central Council for Nursing Midwifery and Health Visiting. (1992). *Code of professional conduct for nurses, midwives and health visitors.* London: Author.

United Kingdom Central Council for Nursing Midwifery and Health Visiting. (1992). *The scope of professional practice.* London: Author.

United Kingdom Central Council for Nursing Midwifery and Health Visiting. (1999). *Fitness for practice: The UKCC Commission for Nursing and Midwifery Education.* London: Author.

An Overview of Health Care and Nursing Education and Practice in Japan

TERUKO TAKAHASHI, CHERYL L. BRANDI

During the 20th century, Japanese society was confronted with dramatic challenges. Japan is recognized as a nation that experienced the most rapid demographic and economic changes following World War II. An aging population, a low birthrate, and an emphasis on health and quality of life are all causing health system changes. In addition, Japan is a highly industrialized country with strong cultural traditions. These factors are all significantly influencing nursing practice and education.

HEALTH CARE ENVIRONMENT

Demographic Trends

In October 1998 the population of Japan was approximately 126,486,000. This is 2.2 times the population taken in the first national census in 1920. Birthrates have been decreasing since 1973, however, resulting in a higher proportion of people over 65 years of age. In 1998 the elderly comprised 16.2% of the total population (Health and Welfare Statistic Association, 1999a). This proportion is expected to increase to 30.4% by 2050 (Health and Welfare Statistic Association, 1999b).

Japan presently leads the world in life expectancy. In 1998 the average life expectancy for women was 84.01 years of age compared to 79.1 years in the United States in 1996. The average life expectancy for men was 77.16 years compared to 73.1 years in the United States in 1996 (Health and Welfare Statistic Association, 1999b).

Recently, diseases associated with lifestyle have replaced infectious diseases such as tuberculosis as leading causes of death. In 1997 the top three causes of death were carcinoma, heart disease, and cerebral vascular disease, which account for 60.7% of all deaths in Japan (Health and Welfare Statistic Association, 1999a).

The Japanese Health Care System

In 1961 a system of social security and health insurance was established (Health and Welfare Statistic Association, 1999b) that covers all Japan's citizens under a compulsory universal health insurance program. Depending on their age and employment status, citizens enroll either through their employers or local societies. The program is universal in that any insured citizen can seek medical help in any hospital or clinic. Reimbursement for all medical services is made according to a set fee schedule, with a separate schedule for pharmaceuticals. Patients pay a small copayment at the point of service, the amount determined by the type of insurance (Yoshikawa, Bhattacharya, & Vogt, 1996). In 1973, medical insurance systems changed to cover all medical costs for patients over 70 (Health and Welfare Statistic Association, 1999b; Yoshikawa et al., 1996). Recently, because of the increasing aging population and the concern for the financial burden on society, the elderly have been required to pay a part of their medical expenses according to income.

Public health and community health centers are integral parts of the health care delivery system. Public health centers are managed by the Japanese Ministry of Health and Welfare. In 1999 there were 641 public health centers throughout Japan. They serve as administrative headquarters for disease prevention, health promotion, environmental sanitation, and so forth (Health and Welfare Statistic Association, 1999a). In comparison, the number of community health centers in 1999 was 1,909. Community health centers are managed by cities and towns. Their main purpose is to provide direct and personalized services for health promotion (Health and Welfare Statistic Association, 1999a). In both types of centers, public health nurses (hokenfu) play essential roles.

Current Trends in Health Care

A rising elderly population combined with changes in the traditional family structure is posing severe challenges for Japan's health care system. More elderly also means an increased number of people with dementia, chronic illnesses, and functional limitations. These people were traditionally cared for in their homes.

Since 1960 the conventional extended patrilocal family has shifted to a smaller, nuclear family consisting only of husband, wife, and children. In the traditional system the family assets were inherited by a single successor, with the stipulation that the successor would become responsible for his or her parents (Sonoda, 1988). Usually this meant the eldest son and his wife would care for his parents at home. Family roles are changing, however, with an influx of women into the workforce and a decrease in family-owned enterprises (Sonoda, 1988). Many nuclear families have migrated to urban areas in search of work, and high urban housing costs have precluded the inclusion of elderly parents in one household.

Additionally, in recent years, parents have been demanding less of their children and not expecting so much support from them (Sonoda, 1988). They plan to live apart from their children on their savings and pensions (Sonoda, 1988) and take care of each other. Therefore the need for community-based care, including preventive and rehabilitative services, has become socially mandated as the elderly try to maintain an independent and high quality of life. In 1994 the Japan Visiting Nursing Foundation (JVNF) was established by the Japanese Nursing Association (JNA) to develop and advance home care services (Japan Visiting Nursing Foundation, 1999a).

Appropriate service utilization and cost control have become important issues in Japanese health care. In 1996 the average length of stay in hospitals was 32.8 days (Health and Welfare Statistic Association, 1999a; Nakahara, 1997), and it is still one of the highest in the world, primarily because of elderly long-term care hospitalizations (Ikegami & Campbell, 1999). Because of free medical care after 1973, many elderly hospitalizations have been for social rather than medical needs (Yamauchi, 1999).

In 1997, legislation was passed to establish a new type of insurance (kaigo hoken) for the purposes of providing care to elderly and handicapped persons and reducing insurance costs. Under this plan, any person aged 40 to 64 is covered for any age-related disease, and all people over 65 are covered, regardless of disease. Beginning in April of 2000, all citizens over age 40 were required to enroll in the plan and pay premiums. The insurance covers all medical costs and home care services as directed by a case manager (Japan Visiting Nursing Foundation, 1999b).

Case managers are either nurses (kangofu), public health nurses (hokenfu), or persons with extensive experience in elderly patient care. All are certified after completing a special training program and passing an examination. A case manager assesses, plans, coordinates, and monitors cost-effective care for eligible patients after consultation with patients and families. Of the 90,000 people who passed the first case manager examination, 44.1% were nurses (Yamazaki, 1999a).

The government of Japan is trying to control medical costs in other ways. Until recently, hospitals had a financial incentive to add beds to attract more patients. In 1985 a law was passed to reduce the number of hospital beds (Chiyo & Kuroda, 1999). Hospitals have also had a financial incentive to maximize patient length of stay, but the government is seeking ways to implement standards somewhat similar to diagnosis-related groups (DRGs) in the United States. A replication of the United States DRG model, however, will not work in Japan because of different systems for hospital reimbursement and hospital record-keeping policies (Ikegami & Campbell, 1999). Finally, the government is supporting the use of medical technology to reduce length of inpatient hospitalization, such as using less invasive surgical techniques for cholecystectomy patients (Chiyo & Kuroda, 1999).

In 1977 the concept of hospice was introduced in Japan, but as of 1999 there were only 63 palliative care institutions with a total of 1,140 beds throughout the country. Slow hospice development stems from a cultural tradition in Japan of not telling a patient he or she has cancer. The physician does tell the family, and both parties try to protect the patient from learning the diagnosis (Kashiwagi, 1996). Kashiwagi (1996) claims this nondisclosure is the result of a moya moya culture. The Japanese word moya moya is defined as "ambiguity," but in a fuller sense it is a lack of clarity about a situation intended to give an impression to all involved parties that things are going well.

Despite cultural traditions the hospice movement is growing. With rising consumerism, citizens are supporting hospice development. Also, medical insurance covers palliative care. About 50 palliative care institutions are scheduled to open in the next 2 to 3 years (Takamiya & Kojima, 1999).

NURSING PRACTICE

Kangofu, Hokenfu, and Zyosanpu

The understanding of "nurse" in Japan is different than it is in the United States and Canada. Many Japanese people use the word "nurse" to facilitate international understanding, but there are really three separate occupational titles to describe health care workers with basic nursing preparation: *kangofu, hokenfu,* and *zyosanpu.* Among Japanese people, the differences are clear, and members of each category maintain a distinct identity. *Kangofu* is translated as "nurse" in English, *hokenfu* as "public health nurse," and *zyosanpu* as "nurse midwife." Many *hokenfu* and *zyosanpu,* however, prefer not to be called *kangofu.* There is a separate licensing examination for each type of practitioner, but each must first hold a license as a *kangofu.* The law governing the scope of practice for *kangofu, hokenfu,* and *zyosanpu* was established in 1948 and has essentially remained unchanged (Nakayama, 1999).

All groups are initially prepared as *kangofu. Kan* means "to observe." It is written using symbols for a hand and an eye. *Go* means "to protect." After graduating from a nursing program, *kangofu* may choose to remain *kangofu* or become *hokenfu* (public health nurses) or *zyosanpu* (nurse midwives). The law defines *kangofu* as one who cares for sick people and postpartum patients and who assists with medical practice and cure (Inoue, Shimizu, & Yamaguchi, 1984). Only *kangofu* with baccalaureate degrees are eligible to take the licensing examinations for both *kangofu* and *hokenfu* without further specialized education. The words *kangofu* and *hokenfu* represent both males and females, but the titles change to *kangoshi* and *hokenshi* for men. Only women may become *zyosanpu.*

Practice settings and role functions vary among the three types of health workers. In 1999 there were 565,918 *kangofu,* 81% of whom worked in hospitals and 12% in clinics. There has been a shift in work setting from hospital to outpatient clinics and visiting nursing stations for this group. The focus of *hokenfu* is health education. In 1999 there were 35,566 *hokenfu,* with 44% working in community-based settings, 25% in public health centers or companies, and 22% in hospitals, clinics, or visiting nurse stations. *Zyosanpu* care for prenatal, perinatal, and postpartum patients. They independently manage uncomplicated deliveries and newborn care. In 1999 there were 24,129 *zyosanpu,* with 83% working in hospitals and clinics and 10% in private birthing centers (Inoue et al., 1984; Minami, 1999).

Nurse-Physician Relations

For many *kangofu, hokenfu,* and *zyosanpu,* relationships with physicians present the biggest practice dilemmas. One reason is that Japan is a strongly male-dominated society. Second, physicians are perceived as authority figures with a much higher socioeconomic status than

nurses and similar workers have. Health care is therefore doctor centered. The third factor is an outdated legal definition of *kangofu* that stresses dependent practice. Recently some change has occurred in physician thinking. As more *kangofu* attain baccalaureate degrees, physicians are thinking of them more as coworkers and less as paramedical workers.

Continuing Education

The JNA and the Ministry of Health and Welfare have created many new continuing education opportunities, mainly for *kangofu.* There are many special courses for *kangofu* desiring to specialize in fields such as pediatric nursing, nursing administration, and nursing education. Since 1990 the JNA has focused on advanced practice nursing. A *kangofu* can be certified as a certified nurse specialist (CNS) or a certified expert nurse (CENC). CNS certification requires a master's degree, 5 years of clinical experience, and passing an examination. CNS certification is available for cancer, mental health and psychiatric nursing, and community nursing. CENC certification requires 5 years of experience, completion of a 6-month training program, and passing an examination. CENC programs exist for emergency, intensive care unit (ICU), cancer and pain care, and wound, ostomy, and continence nursing (Takamiya & Kojima, 1999). CNS certification was first granted in 1994, and CENC certification in 1997 (Sato, 1999).

NURSING EDUCATION
History of Nursing Education

As previously mentioned, *kangofu, hokenfu,* and *zyosanpu* are first educated as *kangofu* (nurses). The history of modern nursing education in Japan began in 1885, with the establishment of the first school of nursing by Kanehiro Takagi, a Navy physician. In the late 1880s, Linda Richards, the first graduate of an American nursing school, taught at the Kyoto Kanbyofu School (Hisama, 1996). The first nurse licensing examination was given around 1900. In 1950 the first junior college nursing program was instituted, followed by the first baccalaureate program in 1952. The first assistant nurse program (*junkangofu*) began in 1951 in response to a critical nursing shortage (Sugimori, 1999).

Although diploma programs outnumber baccalaureate and associate degree programs, there has been a major push for baccalaureate and higher education for *kangofu, hokenfu,* and *zyosanpu* in the last 10 years. Table 83-1, based on information from the Japanese Nursing

TABLE 83-1 Number of Nursing Programs in Japan

	1997	1998	1999
Bachelor of science in nursing	52	64	75
Junior college	72	73	73
Diploma program	496	503	506
Total	620	640	654

Data from the Japanese Nursing Association.

Association (1999a), shows the number and types of nursing programs in Japan. In 1991 there were only 11 baccalaureate programs compared to 86 programs as of April 2000. There were 34 master's degree programs and 12 doctoral programs in 2000 (Sugimori, 1999; JNA, 2000). A major limitation for more rapid growth of graduate programs is a severe shortage of qualified faculty. Recently, qualified foreign nurse educators have been recruited as faculty for graduate programs.

Educational Systems

Japanese systems of nursing education are complicated. As illustrated in Figure 83-1 (Takahashi, 1995), there are seven ways to become a *kangofu* registered nurse (RN). Most commonly, high school graduates enter a baccalaureate, junior college, or diploma nursing program. The Ministry of Health and Welfare regulates these three programs in order to ensure students are uniformly prepared to take the national RN *(kangofu)* examination. The Ministry of Education also governs all baccalaureate and junior college programs and some of the university-affiliated diploma programs. Before a baccalaureate, junior college, or university-affiliated diploma program is opened, the curriculum, the academic credentials of all faculty members, facilities, and so forth must be reviewed by the Ministry of Education. The Minister of Education must accredit the school. With the recent increase of baccalaureate programs, some nurse leaders are insisting that a professional nursing organization should examine and accredit any kind of new nursing program, similar to the National League for Nursing (NLN) in the United States.

THE FUTURE OF NURSING IN JAPAN

In this discussion, whenever the word "nurse" is used, it represents *kangofu, hokenfu,* and *zyosanpu.*

Community-Based Nursing

The trend toward community-based nursing presents one of the best opportunities for nurses in Japan (Ya-

mazaki, 1999b). The government's goal is to create 5,000 visiting nurse stations throughout Japan. The goal of the JNA (Project 500 Task Force) is to create and manage 500 of these stations so that by having 10% control, nurses working in the field will gain increased power in community health care delivery (Yamazaki, 1999a). Nurses can also be independent owners of visiting nurse stations. Furthermore the role of the *hokenfu* (public health nurse) will expand in order to ensure the availability of visiting nursing services for everyone, establish and maintain illness prevention programs, and support family caregivers (JVNF, 1999b). The increased emphasis on community and public health nursing will give nurses much greater responsibility and autonomy.

Politics in Nursing

The changing social needs of Japanese citizens, the movement toward community-based nursing, and the increasing numbers of baccalaureate and graduate schools are improving the status and influence of nurses in Japan. Nurses must now think about increasing their political power to make system-wide changes.

The political voice for nurses in Japan is the JNA. Before 1946, *kangofu, hokenfu,* and *zyosanpu* interests were represented by three separate organizations. In 1946 these organizations were integrated into one organization, the JNA (Aso, 1998). Approximately 460,000 nurses belong to JNA, which is about half the total number of working nurses. The JNA represents the largest number of medical and welfare professional workers in Japan (Tanino, 1999). Out of necessity the JNA has focused on occupational issues of nurses such as status, hospital working conditions, and salary instead of addressing health policies (Ikegami, 1999). Recently the organization has recognized the importance of political power.

The JNA is also working to stop the assistant nurse *(jun-kangofu)* training programs in order to upgrade overall nursing practice. A *jun-kangofu* is similar to a licensed practical nurse (LPN) in the United States. The greatest opposition comes from the Japan Medical Association (JMA), the strongest political group in Japan regarding any decisions related to medicine or welfare. Most JMA members are physicians who own their own hospitals or clinics. Their opposition stems from personal interests rather than a concern for health care quality. They can pay a *jun-kangofu* less than a *kangofu.* To complicate matters, the Ministry of Health and Welfare has decided to start a new type of *jun-kangofu* to *kangofu* bridge training program in 2002 without eliminating the

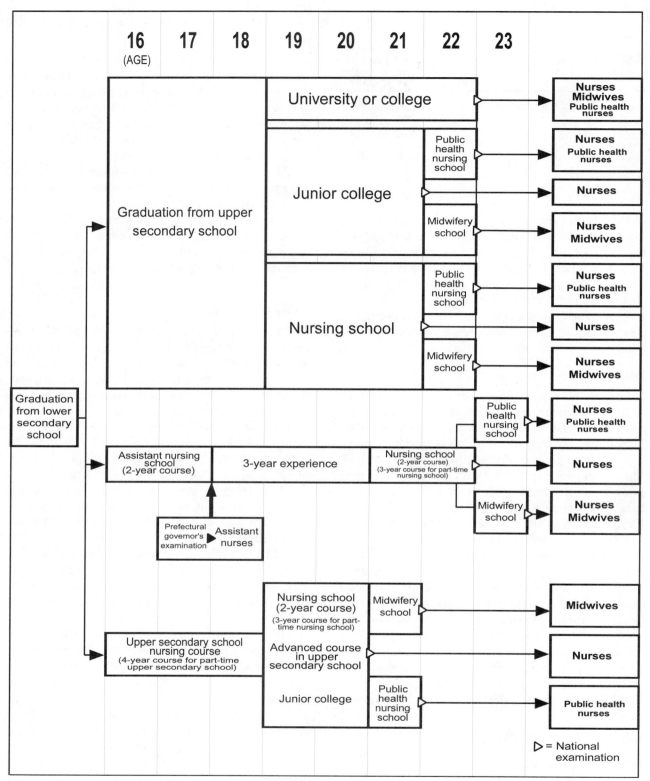

Lower secondary school is equal to junior high school.
Upper secondary school is equal to senior high school.

FIGURE 83-1 Nursing education in Japan. (From *Nursing in Japan* [p. 15], Japanese Nursing Association, 1993, Japanese Nursing Association Publishing Company. Copyright 1993 by Japanese Nursing Association. Reprinted with permission.)

jun-kangofu program as requested by the JNA (Japanese Nursing Association, 1999b).

The other major political issue facing the JNA is the need to change the outdated 1948 law for *kankofu, hokenfu,* and *zyosanpu.* Japanese nurses must organize to change the definition of a *kangofu* from one who assists with medical care and cure to one who works for patients receiving medical care and cure, and who cares for all people who have actual or potential health problems.

Ethics in Nursing

Medical practice in Japan is becoming more complex. Organ transplants are becoming more common. Nurses face new dilemmas regarding brain death and gene therapy. Nurses must support patients and families and also clarify their own ethical positions. The JNA Investigation Committee for Ethics (1999) has outlined six topics for further investigation:

1. Support for patients' rights to make their own decisions
2. Responsibility for maintaining confidentiality about medical care
3. Roles and responsibilities of the nursing profession in terminal care, visiting nursing, and pediatric nursing
4. Role of the nurse as patient advocate in nurse and physician relations
5. Roles of nurses in organ transplant
6. Consideration of patients' rights in clinical examinations and research

Education and Research

With steadily increasing numbers of baccalaureate and graduate programs, master's and doctoral programs in particular, the need for qualified nurse educators, administrators, and researchers is growing fast. Curricula must change from hospital-oriented to community-based, with an emphasis on social changes and citizens' needs. Research activities are increasing to support advanced nursing practices. There are approximately 60 research groups in Japan, 11 of which have been authorized as academic societies by the Science Council of Japan. They include the Japan Academy of Nursing Science and the Japan Academy of Nursing Education (Personal communication, Nozaki, H., editor at *Igakusyoin,* February 1, 2000).

SUMMARY

These are exciting times for nursing in Japan. Japanese nurses have opportunities to advance nursing practice and influence health care as never before. With careful preparation, increased political power, and a strong sensitivity to individual and social needs, they can greatly influence health care in Japan in the 21st century.

REFERENCES

Aso, Y. (1998). Kango no rekishi [History of nursing]. In M. Matuki (Ed.), *Kangogaku gairon* (pp. 27-58). Tokyo: Hirokawa-syoten.

Chiyo, H., & Kuroda, K. (1999). *Igaku gairon [Introduction to medicine].* Tokyo: Igakusyoin.

Health and Welfare Statistic Association. (1999a). *Kousei no Shihyou [Journal of Health and Welfare Statistics], 46*(9), 35.

Health and Welfare Statistic Association. (1999b). *Kousei no Shihyou [Journal of Health and Welfare Statistics], 46*(12), 11.

Hisama, K.K. (1996). Florence Nightingale's influence on the development and professionalization of modern nursing in Japan. *Nursing Outlook, 44*(6), 284-288.

Inoue, Y., Shimizu, K., & Yamaguchi, J. (1984). *Kango hourei youran [Handbook of laws related to nursing].* Tokyo: Japanese Nursing Association Publishing Co.

Ikegami, N., & Campbell, J.C. (1999). Health care reform in Japan: The virtues of muddling through. *Health Affairs, 18*(3), 56-75.

Ikegami, N. (1999). *Nihon no iryou seisaku ha dou kimaruka [How to decide medical policy in Japan]. Kango, 51*(6), 24-28.

Japan Visiting Nursing Foundation. (1999a). *5-nenkan no Ayumi to jisseki [Processes and Results for 5 Years].* Tokyo: Author.

Japan Visiting Nursing Foundation. (1999b). *Seturitu 5-syuunen Kinen Kouenkai [Memorial Lecture Meeting for 5-year Anniversary].* Tokyo: Author.

Japanese Nursing Association. (1999a). *Kango kankei toukei shiryousyuu, Heissei 11-nen [Statistical data on nursing service in Japan, 1999].* Tokyo: Japanese Nursing Association Publishing Co.

Japanese Nursing Association. (1999b). *Kouseisyou "jun-kangofu no ikou kyouiku ni kansuru kentou-kai" houkoku-syo heno Nihon kango kyoukai no kenkai* [JNA's opinion of the report of the "Investigation Committee for Bridge Education of Assistant Nurses" by the Ministry of Health and Welfare]. *Kango, 51*(8), 67-72.

Japanese Nursing Association. (2000, January 15). *Kyoukai nyuusu [Association Newspaper],* 391.

JNA Investigation Committee for Ethics. (1999). *Nihon kango kyoukai rinri kentou iinkai tyuukan toushin [The middle report of the JNA Investigation Committee]. Kango, 51*(8), 83-89.

Kashiwagi, T. (1996). *Aisuru hito no shi wo mitoru toki [Caring for the loving person].* Tokyo: PHP Institution.

Minami, H. (1999). *21-seiki ni muketeno kangosyoku no kyouiku ni kansuru seimei Nihon kango-kei daigaku kyougikai* [Statement of education for nursing professions in the 21st century]. In Japan Association of Nursing Programs in the University (JANPU) (Ed.), *Kango hakusyo* (pp. 127-133). Tokyo: Japanese Nursing Association Publishing Co.

Nakahara, T. (1997). The health system of Japan. In R.W. Raffel (Ed.), *Health care and reform in industrialized countries* (pp. 105-133). University Park, PA: Pennsylvania State University Press.

Nakayama, Y. (1999). *Nihon no genzyou to syourai no tenbou* [Present and future of nursing in Japan]. In the Japanese Nursing

Association (Ed.), *Kango hakusyo* (pp. 3-11). Tokyo: Japanese Nursing Association Publishing Co.

Sato, N. (1999). *Senmon kango seido [Systems for professional nursing].* Tokyo: Igakusyoin.

Sonoda, K. (1988). *Health and illness in changing Japanese society,* 2nd printing. Tokyo: University of Tokyo Press.

Sugimori, M. (1999). *Kango kyoikugagu [Science of nursing education].* Tokyo: Igakusyoin.

Takahashi, T. (1995). *Professional socialization of baccalaureate nursing students in Japan.* Unpublished doctoral dissertation, University of Illinois, Chicago.

Takamiya, A., & Kojima, M. (1999). *Ippan byouin ni okeru kanwa kea to senmon kangoshi no hataraki* [Palliative care in a general ward and roles of the certified nurse specialist]. *Taaminaru Kea, 19*(6), 404-411.

Tanino, H. (1999). *Kangosyoku to seiji* [Nursing professions and politics]. *Kango, 51*(6), 33-36.

Yamauchi, T. (1999). Healthcare system in Japan. *Nursing and Health Sciences, 1,* 45-48.

Yamazaki, M. (1999a). *Kaigo hoken seido no hossoku ni mukete* [Toward starting a new insurance system]. In the Japanese Nursing Association (Ed.), *Kango hakusyo* (pp. 38-46). Tokyo: Japanese Nursing Association Publishing Co.

Yamazaki, M. (1999b). *Seisaku kettei purosesu heno kanyo to senryaku* [Participation and strategy in the policy-making process]. *Kango, 51*(6), 37-41.

Yoshikawa, A., Bhattacharya, J., & Vogt, W.B. (1996). *Health economics of Japan. Patients, doctors and hospitals under a universal health insurance system.* Tokyo: University of Tokyo Press.

CHAPTER 84

An Overview of Health Care and Nursing Education and Practice in Latin America

MARÍA MERCEDES D. DE VILLALOBOS

No aspect of Latin America lends itself to generalization. The vast expanse of the American continent known as Latin America extends from México to Tierra del Fuego (Argentina) and is home to a host of ethnic, ecological, and economic contrasts, health being no exception. This extreme diversity dates from before the discovery of the New World and continues to this day, with regional emphasis, and even exists among countries, despite an attempt to homogenize their culture on the basis of little more than certain common roots and problems, which according to the experts are also common. Yet, nothing could be further from reality. For example, what bigger contrast is there in Latin America than the wealth and development of southern Brazil compared with that of Haiti, which has one of the lowest standards of living in the world.

Having said as much, I should point out that the following observations on health care and nursing education and practice in Latin America are general assessments within the scope of this diversity. They should be analyzed critically and are applicable to a greater or lesser degree, depending on the circumstance. I have tried to portray the situation as it exists and what is anticipated for the future, since current conditions and decisions are basic to what could happen in the years ahead, even though this is impossible to predict.

GENERAL ASPECTS OF THE ECONOMY AND HEALTH

Since the 1980s, Latin America has been immersed in the worst political and economic crisis of its history: one that has affected every country to some extent (Boletín del Banco Mundial, 1999). The reasons for the crisis are many, but it has been aggravated during the last 10 years by several specific factors, such as the indiscriminate ap-

plication of neoliberal policies, globalization of the economy and trade, and other policy decisions that have deepened the already serious social inequalities found within the region and intensified the extent of human poverty (Bustelo, 1992). In addition to these problems, some parts of the continent have been devastated by natural disasters and violence. It is said, for example, that the four countries hit by Hurricane Mitch in 1998 (Nicaragua, Honduras, El Salvador, and Guatemala) were set back 50 years in terms of their economic development and suffered more than 2.3 billion dollars in losses (Boletín del Banco Mundial, 1999; Bustelo, 1992).

As would be expected, the crisis has had a profound impact on health. In a generic sense, every country has made sweeping changes in its health system or will do so in the future. The idea is to cut expenses and place responsibility for health in the hands of the market and people themselves. There is nothing wrong with this, and these changes are sure to bring tremendous long-term benefits. But, for the moment, they have caused a great deal of concern among health workers and consumers alike.

The last 30 years have witnessed important developments in health throughout Latin America. Progress toward controlling infant morbidity and mortality is obvious, without the need to mention figures, and although statistics on maternal and neonatal morbidity remain high, they have declined by almost 40%. Figures on the control of transmittable childhood diseases and on family planning are also promising. However, these changes in the right direction have yet to eliminate the problems associated with the appearance of degenerative illnesses, chronic diseases and aging, those caused by violence of every type, drug addiction and the physical and emotional consequences of natural disasters, which have produced health problems that were thought to be controlled and created a series of complex phenomena such as those derived from human migration and displacement, with the all too familiar social consequences (Pan American Health Organization [PAHO], 1994). The Latin American countries also face the urgency of coping with funding problems and developing infrastructure and human resources in keeping with the demands of the time. Although now the subject of major debate, these issues have not been addressed decisively enough, especially by health professionals (Manfredi, 1999a).

WHAT HAS HAPPENED TO NURSING?

Nursing in Latin America has developed in a context shaped by differences and similarities. Each country must be regarded differently and, by the same token, nursing cannot be viewed as a homogeneous whole. Situations vary from country to country and basically merit individual analysis. Yet, we can generalize about the progress and development achieved in the nursing profession as a result of policies and strategies that have given it strength and proved sound and flexible, according to the particular characteristics of the countries. The lessons they provide are replicable and effective. Latin American nursing has received valuable contributions within the framework of regional policies, PAHO/WHO, UNICEF, and the Dutch government, international support from the W.K. Kellogg and Ford foundations, and institutional support from nursing institutions, such as the Canadian nursing association and the International Council of Nurses, to name a few (Kisil & Chaves, 1994; Manfredi, 1999b). This does not mean, however, that the plight of the profession has been resolved. In fact, nursing faces a difficult and contradictory situation like none in its history, but one that is tremendously stimulating (PAHO & WHO, 1999).

The challenge to nursing is difficult because this is a time of sweeping change. Economic and health legislation has been modified, altering economic conditions in the health sector as well. This change in health legislation has undermined the traditional stability of the job market for health professionals, especially nurses. Despite the growing demand for health care and a shortage of nursing professionals, the profession is plagued by unemployment (unfortunately, there are no precise figures per country). This was something that was virtually unknown in the past. The new economic reality in the health sector took the nursing profession by surprise. It was unprepared to modify certain aspects of nursing practice quickly and in an aggressive way. Nevertheless,

the situation is encouraging because it gives nursing a unique opportunity to play an active role in these changes and to evolve toward a new type of practice that responds to the growing needs of a population that is involved in health decisions and more conscious of the need for quality health care. This new type of practice is far more independent and active than what was traditional in health systems of the past (de Villalobos, 1999a, 1999b).

Accordingly, nursing is being shaped by several predominant trends. The first is the strong tendency of the market to influence decisions on the modus operandi of health systems. This eliminates the stability of programs and personnel, and fosters competition to satisfy market needs. The second trend concerns the growing challenge posed by the balance between the individual health care needs of consumers, in uncontrolled contexts (as opposed to traditional centralism and individual decisions in the private sector), and the need for cost-effective but quality intervention that improves people's health through the use of resources organized in a sophisticated way. The third tendency is the promise of better health and the use of resources for health care at less cost. This is essentially an illusion, since the possibility of having systems like this in operation does not exist at present, and there is discontent on both sides: among health personnel and administrators who provide service and among consumers. A fourth tendency, derived from the other three, is an uncertainty about direction and a breakdown in a number of basic parameters that guided the system in the past (de Villalobos, 1999b).

In short, the future of nursing practice in Latin America is patterned by market forces, by changes in practice, and by the redefinition of health institutions. These are significant transformations and pose important challenges to a profession that has not been sufficiently strong in the past and has taken a rather immature approach to what this uncertain future holds in store. We must ask ourselves what will happen to nursing and how it will deal with the challenges that lie ahead. The next question is, Will Latin American nursing stay tied to tradition and struggle to maintain the status quo, or will it be capable of adapting to the need for creative and effective mobilization in response to the new needs? It is impossible to know the answer, but we can analyze the behavior of nursing today. In doing so, we see that, in spite of the limitations, nursing has been a vital survivor in the field of health. Were it not for this definitive force in solving health care problems, Latin America would be in an even more precarious situation. In other words, nursing has an important heritage, a wealth of experience, and can produce strategies to bolster its strength in the years ahead and to continue its role in health care maintenance.

LABOR FORCE AND PRACTICE

Series 16: "Enfermería en la Región de las Américas: Organización y Gestión de Sistemas de Salud" (Nursing in the Americas Region: Organization and Management of Health Systems), published by the Pan American Health Organization and the World Health Organization (1999), offers a general overview of profiles, distribution, and legislation concerning the nursing labor force. According to the introduction to that document: "Nurses comprise 80% of the health labor force in most countries of the Americas. This means nursing is important to the development of health services and systems in every country. However, in most countries, there is a serious and persistent shortage of nursing professionals and these limited resources are distributed inadequately. The challenge for countries in the region is to make better use of their limited resources to provide safe care, until a medium and long-term improvement in quality can be achieved with a nursing labor force that is better prepared" (PAHO & WHO, 1999).

Demographic changes, the availability of resources, and models for health service delivery are basic to identifying the demand for nursing personnel and the supply nursing could generate to care for the population. The demand will probably grow in most Latin American countries. However, estimates indicate it will not be covered. Part of the difficulty in maintaining coverage is due to the shortage in nursing personnel, especially professionals (PAHO & WHO, 1999).

According to Bucham, in this context the general tendency among countries is to regard auxiliary nursing personnel as a solution to the "shortage." Guaranteeing quality care, however, implies maintaining a balance between the various categories of nursing. This balance can be achieved only with optimum ratios of nurses at the primary level, support personnel, and nursing assistants and auxiliary personnel (Bucham, 1993).

The skill mix (nurse/auxiliary ratio or combination of personnel categories) has declined steadily during the last 10 years. It does, however, vary within a relatively broad range (from 209.7 in Cuba to 0.11 in Brazil). And, due to the differences that separate countries in the Americas, it is extremely difficult to arrive at a definite picture of the whole.

Although the total labor force has grown as a result of an absolute and relative increase in professional and non-professional personnel, it is not enough to resolve the critical situation most countries face in terms of coverage per 10,000 inhabitants (12 countries have less than 20 nurses per 10,000 inhabitants, 7 have between 20 and 40, and no country except Cuba has more than 40 nurses for every 10,000 inhabitants) (PAHO & WHO, 1999).

The ratio of physicians to nurses and the condition of health facilities also provide an indication of the problem. The health labor force is totally distorted, with most health workers situated at either end of the skill and education line. The ratio of health personnel with more years of education (physicians) is the same as those with the least amount of schooling (nurse's aids and similar personnel). Between these two extremes, the number of nursing professionals with specialized skill and knowledge appears "strangled." This relatively low number makes it extremely difficult to ensure generalized coverage and to provide the quality demanded of health services (some countries have 8 to 10 physicians for every nurse, and most have between three and five physicians per nurse) (PAHO & WHO, 1999). This is an indication that health care models are maintaining orthodox forms of health care, which may be the case for quite some time. These emphasize curing disease through medical treatment of choice, with little attention to health care management strategies. This also obliges the more trained members of the labor force to concentrate in the major cities, leaving large pockets of the population in rural areas and urban poverty belts without coverage. These people are served by auxiliary personnel.

EDUCATION

The increase in the number of nurses and auxiliary personal is a clear indication of the increase in training. And, at places where this is not the case, their numbers have at least been maintained. But, again, the differences in education are broad, and there is little or no standardization in the names of programs. Bachelor's degrees or the equivalent are awarded at the university level (a 4- to 5-year program, depending on the school) and the regional tendency is to teach nursing at the university. There are a number of technical or technological programs (2 to 3 years), many of which are attached to health ministries and schools for nurse's aids. They train personnel of this type in 12 or 18 months, besides offering complementary studies for aids, promoters, and attendants (the name given in Brazil to personnel who do not have a formal certificate). Most of these schools are sponsored by health ministries or the private sector (de Sena, 2000). Generally

TABLE 84-1 Types of Programs to Train Nursing Personnel in Latin America

Type of Program and Location	Duration	Degree
Additional or complementary training for aids, attendants, and promoters; health ministries and the private sector; full secondary education required for admission	8 to 12 months	Certified
Nursing assistant; health ministries and the private sector; full secondary education required for admission	12 to 18 months	Certified
Secondary education with an emphasis on health (diversified secondary schooling, Venezuela, Nicaragua, Cuba, Brazil)	Last 2 to 3 years of secondary education	Technical secondary diploma
Technicians or nurses with a degree; private or public universities or technological institutes	2 to 3 years	A technical degree or diploma in nursing
General nurses or technologists; public or private universities	3 years	A nursing or general degree
Bachelor's degree in nursing and advanced studies; public or private universities	4 to 5 years	A bachelor's degree in nursing or a professional nursing degree

Data from PAHO & WHO. (1999). La enfermería en la región de las Américas (series 16, pp. 14 & 15). Geneva: Authors; and de Sena. (2000). La educación de enfermería en América Latina. Santa Fe de Bogota: Gráficas Ducal.

speaking, the education subsystem trains nursing personnel to respond to the traditional needs of health systems and, although the names of the programs are different, most have traditional curriculums, even those established in recent years (de Villalobos, 1999c). A summary of the various programs available in the region is provided in Table 84-1.

The development of postgraduate education has been mixed, as illustrated in Table 84-2. Like basic education, postgraduate programs are structured in a traditional way, taught at universities, and vary widely (Wright & Garzón, 1995). They are oriented more toward specialization than a master's or doctoral degree. This may imply some risk for the future, considering the need for a disciplinary buildup and innovative proposals to encourage professional development. Brazil and Colombia are the countries where postgraduate studies at the master's and doctoral level are most developed. This could lead to serious differences, not only in postbasic professional training but also in the amount and quality of research being done.

An interesting phenomenon revealed by the Wright and Garzón study (1995) concerns the large number of postgraduate degrees held by nurses in Latin America (up to three specializations and one master's degree for the same person), most of which are only incidental to nursing. This suggests adequate postgraduate preparation but weak education in the disciplinary component of nursing. The result is a limited emphasis on aspects particular to the profession and to research, both of which are essential if nursing is to develop with the priorities required to guarantee the short-term changes that are needed.

Continuing education is the Achilles heel of nursing education in the region. It is impossible to give a fair estimate, since there are no programs at the service level or in schools or universities that respond to the continuing education needs of health personnel. Programs for continuing education are casuist, short-term, and sporadic. This is a serious problem, given the speed at which changes in service occur, the adoption of new technology, and the current demand for personnel (de Villalobos, 1999c).

Fortunately, Latin American nursing has not been discouraged by this complex and confusing panorama. On the contrary, for more than three decades it has tried to find

TABLE 84-2 Postgraduate Nursing Programs in Latin America and the Caribbean

Countries	Specialization	Master's Programs	Doctoral Programs
Colombia	14	6	
Ecuador	3	2	
Peru	...	1	
Venezuela	1	3	
Chile	3	1	
Brazil	102	19	7
Panama	6	2	
Mexico	5	1	
Jamaica	1	1	
Total Region	135	36	7

Data from Wright, M. da G., & Garzón, N. (1995). Study of specialization and master's degree programs in nursing in Latin America. Presentado en Bogotá, Colombia, en Conferencia de Postgrado en Enfermeria.

ways to solve persistent problems through regional and country proposals, with the help of organizations like PAHO and WHO and the W.K. Kellogg Foundation, which were mentioned earlier and have played a fundamental role in the development of continuing programs for improvement and innovation, and with the advice of numerous international organizations, such as the International Council of Nurses and nursing associations (the Canadian Nurses Association, the Danish Nurses Association), working through alliances among countries, strengthening the associations, both professional and academic, and the Latin American federations (Chompre & de Villalobos, 1995).

PROPOSALS FOR A PROMISING FUTURE

A number of plans, innovative projects, and programs that demonstrate nursing's capacity to promote changes in service and education have been advanced in the wake of the 1986 Caracas Conference, the conclusions of which played an important role in producing strategies for regional development (Federation Panamericana de Facultades de Medicina, 1985). These actions have strengthened nursing by encouraging its power to negotiate with political and executive levels and by creating successful experiences, many of which have proven effective enough to be adopted as models for care. The case of Colombia's Santander province, educational development in Minas Gerais in Brazil, and the case of Patagonia in Argentina are examples (Chompre & de Villalobos, 1995; W.K. Kellogg Foundation, 1998, 1999).

Yet, these strategies must go even further. Nursing in Latin America faces three challenges in the immediate future. The first is to generate continuing practice for the services nurses offer. This implies differentiating functions to make sure the skill mix guarantees quality coverage. Otherwise, who can guarantee that care achieves the desired result? Examples of this possibility are many. They can be found in the evaluations of UNI-Kellogg projects (a new initiative for educating human resources in health) (W.K. Kellogg Foundation, 1996, 1997, 1998), in the community-based projects sponsored by PAHO and WHO, and in experimental initiatives that have become sustainable over time in a number of countries. These innovative projects have done much to overcome many of the problems associated with resources and are proof that creativity and political will can produce changes in the right direction (Chompre & de Villalobos, 1995; W.K. Kellogg Foundation, 1998, 1999).

The second challenge is to have this continuity reflected in education for nurses overall, as an independent analysis for each type of personnel is virtually impossible This integration must insist on a link between teaching and service, since the changing nature of nursing practice and the opportunities that lie ahead will originate with a different structure. Integration will facilitate the transition from school to the workplace. Associated work must do more than ensure the skill and mobility of resources (de Villalobos, 1999a). It must steer nursing research toward new avenues of investigation into care, the results of which can be used more effectively in the new continuing practice, with an eye toward lowering the cost of care and improving its outcome. Promoting creative changes in nursing education is no easy task. But Latin America has innovative experiences in the educational field. These can be coordinated appropriately and strategies created to cope with the continuing crisis in the countries (de Sena, 2000). Today's organizational resources, such as the associations of schools and faculties in each country, the federations, the Latin American Nursing Network (REAL), and many others, are available and are extremely important to this effort.

The final challenge is just as intrepid as the first two. New rules are required for those who deliver service. This is not a call to eliminate the associations and interest groups that have emerged over time but a call to analyze the traditional modus operandi. From now on there will be periods of flexibility, creativity, and experimentation. Much of what made sense in the past will no longer seem important or necessary. What will predominate are measures to ensure continuity: job security, participation in decision making, opportunities for training and advancement, development of new skills required to stay in the right place, and recognition of the need to change certain roles on the job, according to age.

The fact of change, which is so complex, hints at two situations: (1) quality care must be guaranteed and (2) the process of change must be appropriated by nurses themselves. It is not health institutions that should decide how nursing care can be improved in terms of cost-benefit. As an important part of human resources in the health sector (80%), nurses must maintain a strong position and have sufficient capacity for self-criticism and flexibility to produce the desired results.

These proposals for coping with the situation as it exists today do not imply blind acceptance of what is happening in the health sector. They do, however, suggest that changes are taking place and must be dealt with. Obviously, if the new rationalization of nursing practice in Latin America is to be relevant, it must be linked to the organizational forms and systems that emerge from health services.

This broad overview of Latin American nursing raises questions that will have to be answered carefully. The conditions for progress are in place. Educational and service components have been strengthened steadily and systematically in virtually every country, and the change in health systems facilitates opportunity. So, why not respond to today's challenges in a more consistent and decisive way? Latin America is a vast region where every effort is needed to complement its development. Nursing can and will do the job, but there can be no waiting on decision and strategies for action. Change is quick in coming, and the opportunity could be lost.

REFERENCES

Boletín del Banco Mundial. (1999). Oxford University Press for the World Bank.

Bucham, J. (1993). *World nursing "shortages" and human resource planning.* A study group on nursing beyond the year 2000. Geneva: World Health Organization.

Bustelo, S.E. (1992). *La producción del estado de malestar: Ajuste y política social en América Latina.* Salud Internacional, Un debate norte-sur. Washington, DC: Pan American Health Organization, Human Resource Development Series No. 95.

Chompre, R.R., & Villalobos, M.M. de (1995). A cooperative effort: Nursing leadership development and the W.K. Kellogg Foundation. *Nursing and Health Care Perspectives, 16,* 192-203.

Federation Panamericana de Facultades de Medicina. (1985). *La enfermería en Latinamerica: Estrategias para su desarrollo.* Caracas: Fondo Editorial FEPAFEM. W.K. Kellogg Foundation (A new initiative).

W.K. Kellogg Foundation. (1998 & 1999). Cluster evaluation reports on the Leadership Development Program to train nursing resources in Latin America. Confidential documents.

W.K. Kellogg Foundation. (1996, 1997, & 1998). Cluster evaluation reports on the UNI Program (a new initiative to educate human resources for health).

Kisil, M., & Chaves, M. UNI Program. (1994). *Una nueva iniciativa para la educación de los profesionales de la salud* (W.K. Kellogg Foundation). Sao Paulo: Ediciones Loyola.

Manfredi, M. (1999a). *El recurso humano de enfermeria: Retos en la práctica y educación para el siglo XXI.* Santo Domingo: I Institute for Human Resource Development, Central American Nursing Group.

Manfredi, M. (1999b). *Los grandes retos de enfermería al aproximarse el siglo XXI.* Managua: II Institute for Human Resource Development, Central American Nursing Group.

Pan American Health Organization. (1989). Análisis prospectivo de la educación en enfermería. *Educación Médica y Salud, 23,* 2.

Pan American Health Organization. (1994). Las condiciones de salud en las Américas. Scientific Publication No. 549.

Pan American Health Organization and World Health Organization. (1999). La enfermería en la región de las Américas. HSO, HSR, and HSP Programs, Series 16.

Pan American Health Organization. (1998). *Health care reform and capacity building in health professions: The nursing contribution.* Washington, DC: Background Paper.

Sena, R.R. de (Ed.). (2000). *La educación de enfermería en América Latina.* Santa Fe de Bogota: Gráficas Ducal.

Villalobos, M.M. de (1999a). *Educación de los recursos humanos de enfermería.* IV Institute for Human Resources and Leadership Development in Latin America. Comodoro Rivadavia, Argentina: Universidad de Patagonia, San Juan Bosco.

Villalobos, M.M. de (1999b). *Contexto socioeconómoco y el cuidado de enfermería.* Managua: II Institute for Human Resource Development, Central American Nursing Group.

Villalobos, M.M. de (1999c). *Estrategias para la educación de enfermería en América Latina. Simposium report: Impacto de la política social en la educación y la práctica de enfermería.* Santa Fe de Bogota: Universidad de la Sabana.

Wright, M. da G., & Garzón, N. (1995). Study of specialization and master's degree programs in nursing in Latin America. Presentado en Bogotá, Colombia, en Conferencia de Postgrado en Enfermeria.

An Overview of Health Care and Nursing Education and Practice in Russia

LINDA S. SMITH

UPHEAVAL IN RUSSIA

As the largest country in the world, Russia's 6.5 million square miles is about 1.8 times the size of the United States and laments a declining population of only 147.4 million people. Thus Russia is one of the most sparsely populated nations on earth. Although literacy rates are close to 100%, life expectancy is just 58 years for men and 72 years for women. Presently, Russia is in a negative (–6%) growth rate with a productivity level (gross domestic product [GDP]) that fell 38.5% between 1992 and 1997 (U.S. Dept. of State, 1997). By December 1998 the GDP was about 55% of the 1989 level, with an annual national inflation rate of 30% (CSIS, 1999).

The Independent Republic of the Russian Federation (a federation government system) became a reality on August 24, 1991, with an official, newly approved constitution on December 12, 1993 (U.S. Dept. of State, 1997). As Russia struggles now to enact social reforms and a market-driven economy, however, inflation, poverty, crime, and a disintegrating infrastructure are destroying hope for the Russian people (CSIS, 1999; Plant, 1993). Consequently Russians, who were 15% poorer in 1999 than in 1998, with the number living below the poverty line growing to 50 million (Russians poorer, 2000), lament the loss of the stability of the old Soviet system.

Many problems exist. When Mikhail Gorbachev, former President of the Soviet Union, returned from forced exile after the aborted coup in August of 1991, he returned to a changed nation. Soviet Union Republics de-

---

It is with the greatest admiration that I dedicate this chapter to my nursing friends and colleagues in Russia. On a daily basis, they show all of us the ideals for which our beloved profession stands. Let us share of ourselves toward one goal and purpose: international health, love, and peace.

clared their independence, and the communist party disintegrated (Ryan, 1992). Unfortunately, deeply ingrained social attitudes such as the lack of respect for and acknowledgment of the contributions of health care professionals continued. Salaries for health care workers, especially nurses, were then and continue to be dreadful (Curtis, Petukhova, & Taket, 1995; Gulland, 1998). Health care was a centrally ordered, government-controlled, hierarchical system (Curtis et al., 1995) in which patients did not pay directly for care and health care professionals were state employees. This status permitted little autonomy or authority.

Although between 1970 and 1989 the number of hospital beds increased from 30 to about 48 per 10,000 population (Curtis et al., 1995) and the number of physicians per capita was high by U.S. standards, only 2.4% of the GDP was spent on health care, indicating it had a much lower priority than industrial and military endeavors. This low rate of expenditure led to chronic underfunding, rationing, and, even in Russia's major cities, a health care quality far below Western standards (U.S. Dept. of State, 1997). Because the purpose of all health care was to increase worker productivity, the elderly and disabled became vulnerable. Long waits and medical supply shortages impaired access. To circumvent these problems, informal bribing and tipping and separate elitist facilities were introduced. Primary health care principles weakened, and individual patient needs were mostly ignored.

Politics

Prices for almost all goods and services have skyrocketed. Police are considered corrupt, and safety at night, especially for women, is a major concern. Even so, few Russians wish to turn back Glasnost reforms and return to a totalitarian regime. Unfortunately, since 1993 quiet legislation has rolled back some of Russia's most important and hard-won gains in human and civil rights. Although official government positions on human rights demonstrate some progress since 1993, the institutionalization of safeguards for these rights has lagged (U.S. Dept. of State, 1997). For example, in January of 2000, Russian police threatened to take journalists who report on corrupt officials to remote psychiatric institutions (Cockburn, 2000). Furthermore, although the Russian government proclaims a respect for religious freedom and that the separation of church and state has been in place since 1054, Yeltsin signed into law a 1997 bill to recognize officially the Russian Orthodox Church and restrict activities of other religious groups (Holmes, 1997). Minority faiths are out of favor with local authorities, and therefore overt demonstrations of prejudice and societal discrimination (e.g., anti-Semitic hate crimes) have not been prosecuted (U.S. Dept. of State, 1997).

In a 1998 opinion survey of 1,500 Russians, fully half reported an existence so bad that they could not think of how they would live. Today, Russian savings, hope, and trust are gone (Dahlburg, 1998). One reporter for *USA Today* (Babakian, 1998) quoted Russians as predicting a national coup. In this article, one Russian plumber, stating that he could barely feed his family on a monthly salary of $85, declared, "And what if there is another coup, that doesn't bother me. Things can't get much worse for us" (p. 7A). Yeltsin and now Putin, Russia's president since Yeltsin's surprise resignation December 31, 1999, have vowed to "curb all plans for seizing power" (Babakian, 1998). When taking office, however, Putin promised to reinstitute a strong central government. There is speculation that Putin, an ex-KGB officer (the Soviet equivalent to the CIA and FBI) and as of January 2000 the most popular Russian politician, will crack down even further on hard-won yet tenuous civil liberties. Although Putin has vowed in writing not to return to a Soviet state (Wines, 2000), he continues to be a powerful and visible proponent of the military campaign in Chechnya. Thus, Russia's military continues to demolish Grozny (Chechen capital) apartment houses and, by so doing, experiences multiple casualties inflicted by highly motivated, armed Chechen rebel forces (Gordon, 2000). But Russia's military, as with other government factions, has been severely impaired. One out of three potential soldiers are turned away for health reasons, and of those recruited, 25% need special diets to regain normal weight (Ronalds, 1998).

Russians have seen a 75% drop in their living standard since 1991; that is double the plunge felt by Ameri-

cans during the Great Depression. Since October 1997 the Russian stock market lost nearly 75% of its value (Aron, 1998). Not surprisingly, Russia has a 200 billion dollar debt (Dahlburg, 1998). Moreover, debts among businesses in Russia have increased to $45 billion, causing factories to lay off workers, skip payrolls, or pay employees with goods such as glassware and tampons. Nearly 50% of all consumer goods and services are imported (Longman & Caryl, 1998). Older Russians, raised on Soviet ideals now destroyed, find their savings and pensions worthless. Three thousand of Moscow's homeless died on the streets in 1998 (Johnstone, 1999). Thus, not surprisingly, as many as 30% of Russians pledge their support to the Communist Party, and Lenin's tomb is still a major attraction among those who look back at the Soviet state as a lifetime security blanket (Zuckerman, 1999a). Democratic dreams fade as crime runs rampant; thus the concern now is that Russian nationalism will force a change.

Crumbling Infrastructure

Tax evasion is a major problem in Russia, and without a reliable income, Russia's government may truly be helpless. In 1997 the Russian government collected only 10.8% of its GDP in taxes yet spent 18.3% (Aron, 1998). Yet, since 1993, Russians were required by law to pay income taxes on April 1 of each year. Under communism, taxes were automatically deducted from each pay check. Now, with state services desperately limited or missing, Russians believe they should not pay anything, and they don't (Coleman, 1997). Only 8% of taxes due are paid in cash, and they are never paid on time (Zuckerman, 1999a). And because business must often barter goods (over 50% of all transactions) rather than use rubles, "income" is not easily taxed. Combine this problem with an incomprehensible system of over 200 overlapping national and local tax rules and regulations, an off-the-books underground economy, overt and covert bribing of officials, and 25% to 40% of all workers in second, undocumented jobs, fair tax collection in Russia becomes impossible without major tax reform, which has been opposed by Russia's Duma (lower parliament) (Aron, 1998).

Life in Russia is difficult and often dangerous. On January 7, 2000, the U.S. State Department warned Americans not to live or travel in the Caucasus region of Russia. Throughout this region, local criminal gangs routinely kidnap and even murder foreigners for ransom. Furthermore, unexplained acts of terrorism to government buildings, hotels, tourist sites, and public transportation sites cause the U.S. State Department to recommend travel only in groups and only with organized, reputable tour agencies. Thus throughout Russia, crimes against foreigners are a major problem. Picked pockets, assaults, and robberies are frequent regardless of time or place. Furthermore, "skinhead" groups and local militia harass and attack persons of African and Asian descent. Russian roads are poor and there is no roadside assistance (U.S. State Dept., 2000). Russian communications, with about 12 phone lines per 100 people (the United States has 56 lines per 100 people) makes using a telephone in Russia painful. Connections are uncertain or full of static; there are no telephone books or directory assistance. Furthermore, Watkins and Rees (1999) noted the dreadful condition of public housing. Urban dwelling Russians live in high-rise apartment blocks, a legacy of the Soviet era, with as many as 15 families sharing kitchen and toilet facilities.

In July of 1995 the ruble hit an all-time low of 4,900 rubles per dollar (Easterly & Wolff, 1996). (In July of 1989, 1 ruble was worth 6 U.S. dollars.) In contrast, in January 2000 the official currency exchange was 1 U.S. dollar for each 28.48 Russian rubles (Xenon Labs, 2000). For the elderly, this inflation often means they must sell their most prized possessions or beg in order to live. Russian elders are also vulnerable to crime and fraud. Crime doubled between 1990 and 1994, yet laws remain outdated and courts overcrowded, ill prepared, and ill funded. Police answering distress calls must carry automatic weapons and wear bulletproof vests (Moscow cops feeling, 1995; Nelan, 1995). In 1999 to further complicate Moscow's crime problem, the Moscow police chief admitted that 95% of his force was "on the take" (Zuckerman, 1999a). This rising violence has led to growing pessimism over democratic reforms. It seems likely that Russians, overwhelmed with hopelessness, will follow any politician who can guarantee law, order, and stability, regardless of the loss of civil rights.

Pollution

Russian industries, unable and unwilling to install quality water and air treatment devices, continue to pollute the environment. In line with the old Soviet ideology, industry intends to survive at any cost. Untreated waste is commonplace. Pesticides contaminate over 30% of the food eaten. The prevalence of respiratory diseases is 1.5 times higher for children living close to industrial plants and 1.5 to 2.5 times higher for children living near chemical, petrochemical, or metallurgy plants (Revich, 1999). Obviously Russia's ecological situation is growing worse. Currently over 70 million Russians drink water and

breathe air exceeding permissible pollution standards by 5 to 10 times, and more than 75% of the nation's water supply is contaminated. The reason: a federal budget for pollution control that is too little and too late (Kunin, 1997; Zuckerman, 1999a). Russian women downwind from industrial plants are encouraged not to breastfeed because of high levels of dioxin in breast milk. Thus Russian people have endured ever higher rates of respiratory disease, mental retardation, and congenital deformities. Of course, new laws impose fines on polluters, but Russia's environmental inspectors remain impotent (Environment still bleeds, 1993). Nuclear accident coverups, nuclear smuggling, and nuclear safety violations also have led to increases in environmental disasters (Yeltsin's secret nuclear, 1995).

Increasing Morbidity and Mortality

Russia's youth have suffered. Nearly 40% of Russia's children are chronically ill; without safety matches or flame-retardant clothing, burns are common in children. Domestic violence and suicide are also rising dramatically (Zuckerman, 1999a). The most common causes of death for Russian children ages 5 to 9 years were accidents and drownings. Drowning alone accounted for almost 20% of deaths; accidental poisonings in Russia for children ages 1 to 9 far exceed those of the United States. Mortality rates for Russian children between 1 and 4 years was 2.7 times higher than the U.S. rate (CDC, 1999), and an infant mortality rate of 23.5 deaths per 1,000 live births was reluctantly reported. Psychological disorders—aggressiveness, anxiety, depression—have also increased as a result of the destabilized Russian society (Smirnov & Beznosuk, 1995). Birth rates continue to drop as mortality climbs; Russia's death rate outstrips the birth rate by 1.6 times (PHRI, 1997), with an average life expectancy for men of 57 years. Half of this increased mortality is related to cardiovascular disorders, which reflect social habits of smoking, alcohol abuse, obesity, and poor diet, and to the inadequate diagnosis and treatment of this disease (Burger, 2000). Interestingly, a good portion of cardiovascular deaths, especially for young men, is due to acute alcoholism and binge drinking (Watkins & Rees, 1999). For example, rotgut vodka killed 32,000 Russians in 1998 (Zuckerman, 1999a).

Ever increasing pollution, crime, inflation, and unemployment and the virtual collapse of the Russian health care system have led to increasing morbidity and mortality. Fewer women are bearing children; it is estimated that Russia's population will shrink by 1 million people per year over the next decade (Ronalds, 1998).

RUSSIA'S DISORDERED HEALTH CARE SYSTEM

As mountain factories encase downwind cities in soot and the Chernobyl nuclear accident continues to take its toll, the incidence of diseases such as diphtheria, hepatitis, tuberculosis (TB), syphilis, gonorrhea (CDC, 1999), and AIDS is rising in children ages 0 to 17. Childhood diseases are increasing because of malnutrition (especially in the first year of life as evidenced by rickets, stunted growth, and obesity) and the fear parents have regarding immunizations. Apprehensive parents have seen evidence that diseases such as AIDS and hepatitis are transmitted through contaminated needles and vaccines. Unfortunately there was a tremendous growth in syphilis in 1997, with 376,000 new cases; within that number the rate of syphilis infection for girls between 10 and 14 years has increased 30 times in the past 5 years (Ronalds, 1998).

Concurrently, in the past 10 years, viral hepatitis morbidity in Russia doubled, largely because of contaminated blood transfusions (Komarov, 1994), drug use, and sexual promiscuity. TB mirrors social life, economic conditions, and health policy. TB spreads rapidly among prisoners (25% of all prisoners are considered infected), alcohol and drug abusers, the homeless, and Russian mountain dwellers. Nearly 2 million Russians are believed to have been exposed to TB, with 150,500 new cases reported yearly. To complicate this problem, TB drugs and diagnostic supplies are difficult to access for local districts, and thus Russians with TB are poorly diagnosed and ineffectively treated as a result of budget cuts for public health (WHO, 1997; Zuckerman, 1999a). This is especially true of the homeless (most are former prisoners), who must prove residence to receive the standard free health care offered to citizens. Besides TB, present and former prisoners are also infected with AIDS. In 1 year the number of AIDS (pronounced "speed" in Russian) cases in Russia increased 650% (Kunin, 1997) because of IV drug use, an escalation in prostitution, contaminated blood supplies, and contaminated needles. Between 1998 and 1999, cases of HIV infection more than trebled as 14,980 new cases were recorded (Russian official criticizes, 2000).

Substance abuse is a concern for Russian youth, who abuse chemicals such as alcohol, homemade drugs, opiates, and cannabis. The number of drug addicts rose by 50% among the total Russian population and by 100% among teens. This contributes to the spread of AIDS, which is believed to have reached 800,000 in 2000 (Kunin, 1997; Stanley, 1993). Because of inadequate financing of health care services and facilities, equipment and phar-maceutical shortages are severe. Russia's inability to produce pharmaceuticals and medical devices is of major concern. And when medicines are available, they are believed to be ineffective, weak, or contaminated.

Another concern is the illness-treatment focus rather than a primary prevention focus (Maksimova, 1998). Most of Russia's health care budget is spent on secondary care, with only 2.2% allocated for prevention of health problems. Therefore follow-up care is rare for children and adults discharged from acute care institutions. As evidence of this, most hospital stays are at least 21 days long (Watkins & Rees, 1999). Interestingly, according to Douglas and Mannino (1997), hospitalized patients were compliant and tolerant of a near total lack of privacy; 4-, 8-, 12-, and even 24-bed wards are common. Clinics and hospitals have no money for food, medicines, equipment, or utilities (PHRI, 1997), and many medical institutions have been closed because of lack of funding.

All industry is divided into four categories, and salaries are paid accordingly. The first and highest paid are the workers in heavy industry, metallurgical endeavors, and machine manufacturing. The second level includes light industry and textiles. Health care workers, educators, and entertainers are in this third class (L. Filatova, personal communication, September 28, 1995). Additionally, physicians are divided into three categories, with the highest—physician—receiving only about $80 per month (D. Chikh, personal communication, September 18, 1995).

Below physicians are middle-level workers including feldshers (four years of training beyond the tenth grade), pharmacists, and medical nurses. Nurses with the most training and status earn $35 to $40 per month (average Russian salary is about $100 per month). Dreadfully, in 1995 only about 1% of Russia's GDP was devoted to health care (D. Chikh, personal communication, September 18, 1995). The Duma has promised to make health and education top priorities. But will salaries for nurses improve? Will nurses be paid their back wages? Certainly the Duma will need to move quickly. Specialists, scientists, artists, educators, and highly skilled personnel including physicians and nurses are leaving Russia or their professions, taking with them the contributions they could make to Russian life. Within the Ministry of Health the 1996 federal budget debt included wage arrears to medical workers of 3.5 trillion rubles (PHRI, 1997). Although wages are a huge problem, numbers of professional health care workers are not. According to 1994 statistics, for every 100,000 people the Russian Federation boasts 380 physicians, 44 dentists, and 659 nurses or midwives. This compares with 245 physicians, 63 dentists, and 878 nurses or midwives for every 100,000 people in the United States (WHO, 1999).

Each Russian hospital has two parts. The first part or corridor is for people without money or insurance. Their care is free, but they receive no medications and limited attention. The second corridor is reserved for patients who can pay. Medications are available for a price, and health care quality improves (L. Filatova, personal communication, September 28, 1995). Paying new mothers are in semiprivate rooms, hold and feed their babies at will, receive care by the physician of their choice, have televisions, telephones, and family visits. On the other side of the doors rest eight women to a room as they wait for a physician they have never met to deliver their babies. Babies are fed on a rigid schedule. Here, women have no contact with husbands or family until discharge. This side of the facility is dirty but free, as guaranteed in the new Russian Constitution (Kunstel & Albright, 1994).

OPPRESSED RUSSIAN WOMEN

Gender discrimination is a powerful Russian force. Under Soviet rule, most employees in nonindustry categories were women, and thus women received lower wages. The disparity in wages became even greater after the collapse of communism, as inflation rose (Ryan, 1992). Although most physicians and teachers are women and Russian women are well educated, these women lack authority and responsibility. Women are denied opportunities and continue to be relegated to menial labor (Boe, 1993), especially in the home. Thus unemployment is highest among women and young people (U.S. Dept. of State, 1997).

Life is hard for Russian women. This is especially true for women working for state enterprises (such as nurses, teachers, doctors), where salaries have not increased proportionately to prices. Russian men, generally loathe to participate in child care and housework, become indolent. This nearly total responsibility for home and family is even worse if one considers there are no Western conveniences such as garbage disposals, dishwashers, microwave ovens, or large capacity washers and dryers; even electric irons are scarce (Zagalsky, 1994). To add to the insult, many Russian men leave their families for younger, more attractive wives. A sign that adultery is common is the proliferation of young, unattached Russian mothers (L. Filatova, personal communication, September 28, 1995).

In seeking men who will stay employed, avoid alcoholism, and assist with children, Russian women turn to foreign marriage brokers, prostitution, and pornography

in the hopes of finding love and stability. *Penthouse, Playboy,* and Internet sources all purport the virtues of "beautiful" Russian women. Using a mega search engine, one need only type "Russian and women" to locate hundreds of Internet pornography and marriage brokering sites. Most sites include biographies and photographs. Unfortunately, foreign men want beautiful, subservient wives and may be surprised by the independence of Russian women (Russian women want, 1994), the result of years of defending themselves and surviving in the midst of hostile conditions. Russian women have been called "drill sergeants" by men seeking fragile femininity.

It is no wonder that violence against Russian women has increased dramatically. Appropriately, this secret violence has been called the "undeclared war" and represents the deep contempt of Russian men for women. As evidence, women who leave their husbands lose their legal status and their property rights. Women are often expected to give sexual favors to employers and landlords. Partly because women do not press charges against abusing partners (they fear severe retaliation), Russian police have been loathe to exhibit empathy or even file reports when witnessing violence against women in the form of rape or domestic battles. During the Soviet rule, authorities could be consulted when battering occurred. Women could report abuses to their employer, their local party, or their trade union representatives. Now they say there is no one to listen. Clearly, Russian women face a more stressful living environment with desperate financial constraints, violence, unemployment, and alcohol abuses (Bennett, 1997).

Russian women also have pregnancy, labor, and delivery concerns Russian men never face. Abortion as a right became popular when the Soviet state needed women in the workforce. Now, few women have the time, money, social support, or living space to have more than one child. Poor Russian women cannot get contraceptives (only 18% use them), condoms are unpopular, difficult to obtain, and of poor quality. Thus the average Russian woman has three to eight abortions, increasing to 4 million the number of Russian abortions performed in 1994. This number would seem accurate given that official numbers reported by the Russian Ministry of Health do not include abortions performed in nongovernment facilities and clinics. Under new health care changes, abortions for fetuses older than 5 weeks are no longer free, and often Russian women are told to go to private or regional clinics too costly for many.

In contrast to the estimated total, official Ministry of Health statistics indicate that within 1 year, Russian women had 2,753,000 abortions (compared with less than half that number in the United States), and nearly 75% took place on fetuses older than 6 weeks. Although the official number of abortions in Russia has declined 35% from 1990 to 1995, the rate of abortions per 100 live births declined by only 3% (CDC, 1999). Not surprising, Russian maternal morbidity and mortality is seven times greater than in other developed countries. Over 20% of all pregnant Russian women are diagnosed with anemia. Maternal deaths are due to sepsis, toxemia, hemorrhage, abortion (25%), and ectopic pregnancy. Not surprisingly, maternal mortality increased by 12% during the 1990s (CDC, 1999), and with 90% of Russian women in the workforce, workplace conditions become health risks.

OPPRESSED RUSSIAN NURSES

Russians view nursing as a low-prestige job. The noun "nurse" (as a separate profession) does not even exist. Instead, Russian nurses are called medical sisters, similar to the title given a domestic servant (Douglas & Mannino, 1997). As health care providers, Russian nurses are dependent on physicians, unable to make independent decisions regarding clinical care. Physicians give orders and nurses carry them out (Watkins & Rees, 1999). Hard physical labor and shift work are familiar burdens to Russian nurses. In many hospitals, nurses work double shifts, second and third jobs, and take increased patient loads just to bring wages high enough to survive. When they do get paid, the salaries are among the poorest in Russia. Nursing is a woman-based (about 5% men), physician-dominated (Perfiljeva, 1997), task-oriented profession. Physicians believe strongly that they, not nurses, are best able to assess patients and plan care. Thus nurses often carry out roles of technical (e.g., setting up and maintaining all respiratory equipment), dietary, laboratory, janitorial, and clerical personnel.

CHANGES FOR RUSSIAN NURSING
Nursing Education

Before the Russian Revolution of 1917, nursing practice blended the physical, social, psychological, and spiritual aspects of human life and death. After the rise of communism, however, nursing education moved to procedure-oriented technical schools (referred to as medical schools), with little attention paid to the social sciences and humanities (Edwards, 1994; Picard & Perfiljeva, 1995). The job of nursing "still remains dependent on and subordinate to medicine. Most doctors believe this is right and proper" (Perfiljeva, 1997, p. 8).

Russian nursing education generally is a 2-year program with candidates entering after the completion of the tenth grade (high school graduate). Feldsher education also takes place in technical schools. Feldshers have been compared to the U.S. physician's assistant. They learn advanced techniques such as suturing and birthing and may apply these techniques without physician presence. Feldshers ride in ambulances and work in polyclinics (Edwards, 1994). Feldshers and midwives are more heavily relied on in rural areas (CDC, 1999).

Despite the problem that Russian physicians do not believe nurses need any additional schooling (V. Sarkisova, personal communication, December 17, 1997), progress has been made in the area of Russian nursing education. A new curriculum was formulated and circulated to all basic nursing education institutions. "Following the recommendations of the first World Health Organization Conference on Nursing, this curricula is focused not only on hospital nursing, but also on community nursing" (Perfiljeva, 1997, p. 9). This community focus translated into reality when a United States–based $20 million health reform project was implemented. One of its health care reform goals (subscribed to by Russia's Ministry of Health) was to enhance medical and nursing school curricula in such a way that quality, family focused, preventative, population-based, and community-based health care would be promoted and enhanced (Maksimova, 1998; Milburn, 1997; Perfiljeva, 1997). In 1996, intensive work was underway in Russia to create standards for all branches of nursing education. Thus one important advantage for Russian nursing schools has been the exchanges of faculty, students, and nursing administrators on a regular basis between Russia, the United States, and other countries (Y. Filan, personal communication, December 23, 1996; Mikheeva, 1997).

As with nursing, educating Russian physicians is the responsibility of the Russian government, as all medical schools follow the established Ministry of Health curriculum. Medical school takes 6 years, with an additional year of internship and 3 years of mandatory service. Russian physicians are highly specialized, and only 25% of Russian physicians specialize in general practice or internal medicine (CDC, 1999).

Before 1991, Russian nurses had little hope of advancement other than becoming a physician because nursing education was considered a lesser version of medicine (Wallen & Cammuso, 1997). Therefore for decades nursing journals were authored, edited, developed, and directed by physicians. During a 1991 meeting with representatives from Russia's only nursing journal,

Meditsinskaya Sestra, other delegates and I faced an editorial board and administration composed entirely of physicians. We discussed the complete lack of manuscripts authored by nurses and were told that "nurses cannot write." We discussed the lack of nursing representation on their board and were told, "Nurses cannot be leaders. Physicians are the ones who must lead and inform nurses." Without government funding, this journal disappeared shortly after our meetings.

As with journal authors, nurse educators were almost always physicians; supervisors of patients and nurses were physicians, and government standards for nurses were and continue to be established by physicians. Now this physician dominance may be changing. In 1991 the Ministry of Health in Russia developed the first college of nursing designed to promote baccalaureate nursing education with a 3-year curriculum following Western models. By 1997 there were 48 such nursing colleges and an additional 10 programs planning to offer graduate nursing education (Douglas & Mannino, 1997). Additionally, also beginning in 1991, the Moscow Medical Academy, through the vision of Dr. Galina Perfiljeva, initiated a master's program in nursing. This prestigious educational facility also collaborated with Nursing College No. 1 to offer a baccalaureate-in-nursing program. The master's program emphasized nursing theory, leadership, research, and education (Picard & Perfiljeva, 1995). Hence, achieving formal, postgraduate nursing education has been an 8-year effort designed to "advance nursing through development of master's programs in nursing, which now include 14 universities throughout the country. The first, at the I.M. Sechenov Moscow Medical Academy, has so far graduated three classes [as of 1998] of students who are now faculty and leaders in major health care facilities" (Perfiljeva & Picard, 1998, p. 108). Certainly the hope of a national nursing system developed and implemented by nurses rather than physicians rests with these graduates who have been taught to write, speak, and teach about the values of the nursing profession (Picard & Perfiljeva, 1995).

As nursing education and patient advocacy improved, the need to develop continuing education programs for new and currently practicing nurses became more evident (Mikheeva, 1997). Postgraduate, ongoing specialty training for nurses includes periodic continuing education for 1 to 4 months, after which a certificate is awarded and, depending on the specialty, additional salary. Work analyses have demonstrated the efficacy of such ongoing continuing education for nurses (Mikheeva, 1997), which enhances professional skills via a continuous educational

patient care focus. Importantly, hospital-wide continuing education programs have been developed through American partnerships since 1993 (Kirgetova, 1997).

Even with additional continuing education the nursing process was not emphasized clinically until now. Valentina Sarkisova, president of the newly formed Russian Nurses Association (RNA), explained in her December 26, 1999, correspondence that "we hope to gradually introduce the nursing process into all hospitals as we hope this technique will improve the quality of nursing care in all hospitals and give nurses increased status and prestige."

Nursing Practice

It has been said that Russian nurses must carry the health care burdens with their bare hands. Despite almost overwhelming oppression by physicians and an unyielding system, Russian nurses continue to struggle for authority and dignity within their practice. They are trying now to improve the quality of the care they provide, but there is little time (about 30 patients per nurse) and little equipment. Through their professional organization, Russian nurses continue to appeal to the Russian Ministry of Health asking for enough equipment (such as gloves, disposables, and goggles) to remain safe from blood-borne pathogens and to care adequately for their patients. Russian nurses believe that the quality of nurse-patient communication has improved as a result of the nurse exchanges. They have seen the benefits of American nurses spending time listening to patients, and they hunger to use these skills but need the time and resources to do so.

In addition to dreaming of independent practice, Russian nurses dream of improved working conditions in hospitals, especially of lowering the high nurse/patient ratios. They look for ways to finance medical equipment and pharmaceuticals to avoid shortages and maldistribution. Last, they wish to impose employment standards for hospitals so that only dedicated, qualified, hardworking nurses receive positions. As in the United States, Russian nurses love their profession and care deeply for their patients (Barron, 1994). Russian health care facilities have shortages of everything from soap, sutures, gloves, pharmaceuticals, anesthesia, diagnostic equipment, and nearly all other imaginable amenities U.S. nurses take for granted, such as a sink and running water in which to wash hands and clean instruments. V. Sarkisova proclaims in nearly all communications her honest appraisal of the hard work and many burdens of Russia's nurses.

Nursing Research

The master's in nursing program at the Moscow Medical Academy includes nursing research as a studied and supported endeavor. But funding is precarious. As proof, faculty at this federally funded academy received no salary for 4 months because of budget problems (Picard & Perfiljeva, 1995). Therefore publishers of U.S. nursing research journals have been encouraged to donate subscriptions to the academy. Practice-based nursing research endeavors have surfaced in the area of home health care, where Russian nurses have been taught by Western colleagues to measure health outcomes and thus validate their profession (Bjornsson, Dalgard, Fonn, & Kjeldsen, 1998). Perfiljeva (1997) explained the implementation of joint research endeavors among Russian and U.S. nurse colleagues. Additionally, specially trained Russian nurses are now actively participating in scientific research efforts through the assistance of the American International Health Alliance (Mikheeva, 1997).

Nursing Organizations

Before 1992, professional nursing organizations were already in place in Russia. For example, the Moscow City Nurses Association, whose members I met during two visits to Russia, was officially registered in 1992. Nationally, in 1990, nurses from each Soviet republic met and discussed education and practice standards (Perfiljeva & Picard, 1998). Early that year each Soviet republic sent nurses to a Ministry of Health–sponsored meeting. They met because of the perceived need to standardize nursing education and practice throughout the Soviet Union (Picard & Perfiljeva, 1995). (These goals were expressed to me during my meeting at the Soviet Ministry of Health on July 4, 1989.) The breakup of the Soviet Union slowed but never stopped these standardizing efforts. In 1993, as evidence of a continued effort to improve nursing care, I met RNA President Sarkisova, along with regional representatives from over 36 Russian districts. (Representative regions are loosely connected subgroups of this national organization.) Members of these nursing groups are the leaders of nursing in Russia: education, practice, research, and administration. During these meetings they were willing to come together to explain their problems and their concerns for the purpose of improved nursing care. Our Russian colleagues asked wonderfully challenging questions regarding nursing practice models, theories, and decision-making tools. Clearly, knowledge and information from the United States that has been shared with Russian nurses have been used significantly. They told me, "We are all very interested in the medical and nursing practices in the USA." In 1998, the RNA boasted 7,000 members who must pay individual membership fees either through a 10% allocation of their regional nurses' association's fees or as individual members with a fee of 1% of their salary (Bjornsson et al., 1998).

Several endeavors can be credited with assisting Russian nurses to organize. These include World Vision International, which provided its first of three grants in 1992 and assisted in the RNA's growth (Milburn, 1997). World Vision monies were channeled through the Agency of International Contacts in Moscow and in 1996 prolonged their grant for an additional 6 months. Valentina Sarkisova, the RNA's president, proclaimed, "thanks to the financial support, we have made many improvements for nurses" (personal communication, 1996). Importantly, besides computers, telefaxes, and copiers, Sarkisova was able to initiate a new nursing journal produced and written by Russian nurses for Russian nurses. In Volume 1, issue 1 of *Nurses Work*, I wrote of my initial 1987 contacts with Chairman Gorbachev and the Ministry of Health, as well as of my great honor and privilege in meeting and working with beloved Russian colleagues. Thanks to an outpouring of interest from Russian nurses, a moral Code of Russian Nurses was formulated and published during two Russian nursing conferences.

In addition to World Vision International assistance, RNA President Sarkisova has sought advice and thereby prepared necessary documents for RNA inclusion into the International Council of Nurses (ICN). Certainly, President Sarkisova has taken her leadership position seriously. She is an inducted Sigma Theta Tau (STT) member and hopes to bring STT chapters to Russia. In November and December of 1999, President Sarkisova presented two seminars with Swedish nursing colleagues, gave a presentation to the Russian Ministry of Health (27 December) regarding the problems of nursing, and participated in a week-long health program in Louisville, Kentucky. On December 26, 1999, Sarkisova asserted that "the most important thing is that nurses need to understand that they need to unite. Sure, we have professional associations on the state and regional levels, but we still have a long way to go to reach a totally national Russian nursing organization." Sarkisova spent time in 1997 attending the Swedish Congress in Stockholm. The topic was nursing and computer science, another indication that Russian nurses continue to be interested in learning needed technology to advance their profession. Consequently in late 1999 President Sarkisova recognized the Swedish Association of Health Workers for their generous offering of materials and assistance.

I have had several opportunities to speak before the Moscow Nurses Association in Moscow, Russia, during the beginnings of the RNA. On these occasions I was struck with the strength and fortitude of this visionary group. Love for our beloved profession of nursing remains as the binding force for us all. Watching these nurses struggle with almost overwhelming obstacles—yet making progress politically and professionally—was inspirational. In closing impromptu remarks I explained that, "We are nurses. We are the ones who heal the hurts of the world. We have seen and experienced great suffering, yet we survive. As sisters we'll join you as you've joined us—in one united profession. I honor and respect your courage. I love you all."

EAST-WEST COLLABORATION
What We Will Learn

Many Western nurses lack the knowledge our Russian colleagues have regarding holistic, homeopathic health care, including herbal medicines and leech therapy. In a nation suffering severe pharmaceutical shortages, Russian nurses understand the art and science of massage therapy, contactless massage, acupuncture, magnetic therapy, and acupressure. With advanced training, they perform these techniques to promote patient relaxation and noninvasive pain relief. Furthermore, in the absence of mechanical tools and diagnostic workups, Russian nurses have become expert clinicians. They have truly learned to treat with their hands. For decades, Russian nurses have practiced contactless massage, hands-on massage, and the application of hot wax treatments to promote analgesia and circulation. Bjornsson et al. (1998) wrote of the practice of "blood therapy," in which venous blood is drawn and then reinjected into muscle in order to bolster immune systems. I also witnessed the teaching of leech therapy to student nurses. During episodes of angina, nurses were taught to place 6 to 8 leaches in a semilunar fashion around the left chest wall. The saliva of the leech emits a nearly perfect combination of anticoagulation, analgesia, and vasodilation, the effects of which can last up to 6 hours.

What We Will Teach

The Russian health care system gives patients a passive, subordinate position in the health care culture. This dependency presents problems regarding patient rights and responsibilities (Curtis et al., 1995). Additionally, palliative care concepts for the treatment of terminally ill patients are new and doubted philosophies (Novikov et al, 1995).

One reason for this reluctance is the concern medical professionals have for honesty with dying patients. Nurses are taught that under no circumstance should the patient be told of an incurable disease (Salmon, 1999). For this reason, Russian nurses were alarmed during discussion sessions that stressed openness with dying patients. Additionally, dying patients are often feared so much that families and health care workers abandon them.

Western nurses share with Russian colleagues research-based nursing care that is sensitive to patients' physical and psychological distress. Head nurses learn to use informatics systems for data entry and retrieval (Kirgetova, 1997), and knowledge and skills regarding occupational therapy and nursing management are implemented. A nursing management program and manual were developed jointly between the faculty of nursing of the University of Western Ontario and Volfograd Medical College (CIDA, 1999).

The Aid to Russia Controversy

Multitudes of Russian financial and health care problems can cause Westerners to believe that giving aid to Russia is like pouring money into a huge black hole. Doubts remain over the efficacy of such endeavors. A report by the U.S. Senate Foreign Relations Committee concluded that the average Russian is "unaware of or affected by international assistance or the reforms that it is supposed to foster" (U.S. aid trickles, 1994, p. 1a). Many believe that no amount of foreign aid will help until Russia can put inflation, increasing financial deficits, and skyrocketing crime in check. The frightening side of Russia's economic turmoil is the tendency for high-level, underpaid Russian scientists to leave the country for more lucrative employment or to supplement meager salaries by selling sensitive knowledge and materials. This Russian brain-drain is a major threat to world peace efforts and has become a complex problem given the 30,000 nuclear weapons in the possession of desperate Russians residing in over 39 separate Russian districts (Rescuing Russia, 1999; Zuckerman, 1999b). Nuclear, chemical, and biological weapons could easily enter black markets. Thus a stable Russia is in the interest of U.S. foreign policy.

Yet even with $22 billion in aid in 1998, Russia was in default on its nearly $347 million debt. Billions of dollars have vanished within a corrupt and powerless system (Troubled Russia, 1998). Russia's external debt amounted to $149.9 billion on January 1, 1999 (CSIS, 1999).

Health care is inextricably linked to all other social concerns in Russia, and foreign intervention is essential (Vaile, 1993). For example, mass media teaching projects need to be funded that would convince Russians to immunize their children. These aid benefits would be tangible and far-reaching. For example, one of the more productive joint projects has been through the United States–Russia Joint Commission on Economic and Technological Cooperation. The commission's charter runs from 1994 to 2004 and includes helping Russian health officials control the spread of infectious diseases (TB, AIDS, and sexually transmitted diseases), improve access to quality health care (primary and preventive medicine), and promote maternal and child health including programs for nutrition, alcohol abuse, diabetes, and pollution of the environment (U.S.-Russia Joint, 1999). Unfortunately, not all Russians (especially ultranationalists) welcome Western help, even for health programs (Ronalds, 1998).

NURSE-TO-NURSE EFFORTS

Assistance to Russian nurses from American colleagues is and will continue to be accomplished through the efforts of many nursing groups such as the American International Health Alliance, Project Hope, World Health Organization, and U.S.-Russian Nurse Exchange Consortium of Racine, Wisconsin. The consortium, with members in multiple U.S. states and Russia has hosted U.S.-Russian exchanges of health care professionals since 1989.

Russian health professionals propose that education scholarships, people-to-people exchanges, and quality health care research be financially supported (Komarov, 1994). Russian nursing education can be supported through the LEMON Project (Learning Education Materials on Nursing), a curricular package of nursing materials developed by European nurses and a World Health Organization (WHO)–sponsored activity (Perfiljeva & Picard, 1998). With the help of foreign money, nursing materials are translated, packaged, printed, and distributed (Picard & Perfiljeva, 1995).

Nurse-to-nurse efforts need to focus on teaching the teachers and leaders so they may teach each other. This is easy. Russian nurses are hungry to learn from Western peers. They are well educated, quick to grasp concepts, and creative in their attempts to implement new knowledge (Barron, 1994, p. 59; V. Sarkisova, personal communication, December 26, 1999). Milburn (1997) wrote that

[O]ur role in Russia was that of catalysts to facilitate the reform movement and its partnerships, ambassadors of our country in a country that until recently viewed the US as a dreaded enemy, role models of market economic principles

in an environment that is just learning the meaning of competition, teachers of nurses . . . on management principles needed to sustain reform, liaisons with the government health care leaders to promote changes at the local and national levels and advocates for Russia's health care consumers who today face challenges of a broken-down health care system and society. [p. 6a]

Dr. Yevgeny Filan, nursing school director in Moscow, wrote in June 1998, "Our colleagues from the USA have given us and our faculty a powerful impulse for creativity and we are really anticipating the continuation of this cooperation."

RUSSIA'S FUTURE

New freedoms will help Russian nurses and other health care professionals identify and track health care issues and indexes without forced data embellishment. Computer systems are in place that will restore the true health care picture in Russia. Reform programs started under Yeltsin will it is hoped continue to move forward under President Putin's regime. Especially important will be the Russian government's budget prioritization in the area of health care and education of health care professionals.

Fortunately, as Perfiljeva (1997) wrote, the need to improve nursing care quality has been well supported throughout Russia. Nurses, once docile and subservient, are finding new political and professional savvy as they confront old, worn traditions of medical authority. They are showing officials that nursing decision making and independent practice can and will move Russian health care forward. "Join us now as we struggle for our identity," Russian nurses have said; "We are strong and we will survive these difficult times; we are one with you as nurses. Our profession is our hope and our voice."

REFERENCES

Aron, L. (1998, Summer). *AEI Russian outlook.* American Enterprise Institute for Public Policy Research. Retrieved March 16, 1999, from AEI data base on the World Wide Web: http://www.aei.org.ro/ro9464.htm.

Babakian, G. (1998, July 14). Fraying economy feeds rumors of a coup in Russia. *USA Today,* p. 7A.

Barron, S. (1994). A nursing experience in Russia. *Neonatal Network, 13*(2), 59.

Bennett, V. (1997, December 6). Violence against women in Russia grows worse. *LA Times.* Dimensional. Retrieved January 23, 2000, from dimensional.com database on the World Wide Web: http://www.dimensional.com/~randl/russ.htm.

Bjornsson, K., Dalgard, P., Fonn, M., & Kjeldsen, S.B. (1998). Nursing and health in Russia. *International Nursing Review, 45*(3), 89-93.

Boe, B. (1993). Boe knows Russia. *The Carthaginian, 72*(4), 6.

Burger, E.J. (2000, January 2). An unhealthy Russia (letter). *Washington Post*. Retrieved January 3, 2000, from Johnson's Russia List #4005, davidjohnson@pop.erols.com.

Canadian International Development Agency (CIDA). (1999). *Canada-Russia Health and Social Development Project*. Author. Retrieved August 18, 1999, from the queensu (Queen's University) home page links on the World Wide Web: http://www.queensu.ca/crhsd/can-rus.htm.

Center for Strategic and International Studies (CSIS). (1999, February 18). *Net assessment of the Russian economy*. Author. Retrieved March 16, 1999, from the csis database on the World Wide Web: http/www.csis.org/ruseura/rus_econ.html.

Centers for Disease Control and Prevention (CDC). (1999). *Vital and health statistics: Maternal and child health statistics: Russian Federation and United States, selected years 1985-1995* (DHHS publication no. [PHS] 99-1486). Hyattsville, MD: Author.

Cockburn, P. (2000, 21 January). Russians threaten to incarcerate 'dissident.' *The Independent* (UK). Retrieved January 21, 2000, from Johnson's Russia List, davidjohnson@erols.com.

Coleman, F. (1997, April 14). Meanwhile, in Russia. *US News & World Report, 122*(14), 10.

Curtis, S., Petukhova, N., & Taket, A. (1995). Health care reforms in Russia: The example of St. Petersburg. *Social Science and Medicine, 40*(6), 755-765.

Dahlburg, J.-T. (1998, November 8). As Russian economy crumbles, many despair of better life. *Arkansas Democrat Gazette*, p. 18A.

Douglas, J., & Mannino, J.F. (1997). Postconference tour highlights challenges facing Russian nurses. *Journal of Transcultural Nursing, 9*(1), 40-41.

Easterly, W., & Wolf, C.H. (1996). The wild ride of the ruble. New York University, Leonard N. Stern School of Business. Retrieved October 8, 2000, from the Ideas at UQAM RePEc database on the World Wide Web: http://www.esq.uqam.ca/ideas/data/papers.

Edwards, D.J. (1994). Transcultural nursing: A view of the Russian health care system. *Orthopaedic Nursing, 13*(2), 47-51.

Environment still bleeds in Russia. (1993, August 29). *The Journal Times* (Racine, Wis., KR), p. 2A.

Gordon, M.R. (2000, January 23). Putin sacks commander in Grozny. *The Sunday Oregonian*, p. A9.

Gulland, A. (1998). Economic fallout. *Nursing Times, 94*(40), 12-13.

Holmes, C.W. (1997, September 27). Yeltsin OKs restricting some faiths. *The Atlanta Journal/Constitution*, p. B3.

Johnstone, A. (1999). Homelessness: Cold feat in Moscow. *Nursing Times, 95*(7), 30-31.

Kirgetova, G. (1997). *Improving nursing training through partnerships*. American International Health Alliance (AIHA). Author. Retrieved August 20, 1999, from the AIHA database on the World Wide Web: http://www.aiha.com/english/pubs/nursbook/p26.htm.

Komarov, Y.M. (1994). Quality assurance in health care: Lessons for others. *International Journal for Quality in Health Care, 6*(1), 27-30.

Kunin, V. (1997, March 5). *Russian medicine on verge of crisis*. Public Health Research Institute. Retrieved August 20, 1999, from PHRI database on the World Wide Web: http://www.russia.phri.org/b3597.htm.

Kunstel, M., & Albright, J. (1994, May 9). Gap widening in Russian health care. *Atlanta Constitution*, p. A8.

Longman, P.J., & Caryl, C. (1998, August 31). Russian roulette. *US News & World Report, 125*(8), 55-57.

Maksimova, L. (1998, January). *Major medical projects in Russia*. Business Information Service for the Newly Independent States (BISNIS). Retrieved May 29, 1999, from BISNIS database on the World Wide Web: http://iepnt1.itaiep.doc.gov/bisnis/isa/9801medi.htm.

Mikheeva, T. (1997). *Continuous training of nursing staff as an integral part of improving the quality of medical care*. American International Health Alliance (AIHA). Author. Retrieved August 20, 1999, from the AIHA database on the World Wide Web: http://www.aiha.com/english/pubs/nursbook/p27.htm.

Milburn, L.T. (1997, June-August). Health reform in Russia: Challenges and success. *Prairie Rose, 66*(2), 5a-7a.

Moscow cops feeling blue. (1995, March 25). *The Journal Times* (Racine, Wis., AP), p. 2A.

Nelan, B.W. (1995, March 20). Crime and punishment. *Time, 145*(11), 54.

Novikov, G.A., Osipova, N.A., Starinsky, V.V., Prokhorov, V.M., Benenson, L.I., & Gazizov, A.A. (1995, October). Prospects in the development and improvement of palliative care of cancer patients. *Russian Medical Journal, 1*(1), 13-17.

Perfiljeva, G. (1997). Progress in Russia: Working together for change. *Reflections, 23*(2), 8-9.

Perfiljeva, G., & Picard, C. (1998). Clarification about nursing in Russia. *Image: Journal of Nursing Scholarship, 30*(2), 107-108.

Picard, C., & Perfiljeva, G. (1995). Nursing education in Russia: Visions and realities. *Nursing & Health Care: Perspectives on Community, 16*(3), 126-130.

Plant, F. (1993). Next stop Moscow. *Nursing Times, 89*(34), 44-45.

Public Health Research Institute (PHRI). (1997, June 7). Russia is dying doctors warn. *Reuter*. Retrieved August 20, 1999, from PHRI database on the World Wide Web: http://www.russia.phri.org/b6797.htm.

Rescuing Russia. (1999, November 21). *Parade Magazine*, p. 20.

Revich, B.A. (1999). *Environmental epidemiology in Russia: Some results and prospects*. Centre of Demography and Human Ecology Institute of Forecasting. Retrieved August 20, 1999, from friends-partners database on the World Wide Web: http://www.friends-partners.org/oldfriends/welling/revich.htm.

Ronalds, F. (1998, February 10). *The health crisis in Russia*. Voice of America. Retrieved August 20, 1999, from PHRI database on the World Wide Web: http//www.russia.phri.org/b21098.htm.

Russian official criticizes government over HIV. (2000, January 29). *Reuters*. Retrieved January 30, 2000, from David Johnson's Russia List #4079 on davidjohnson@erols.com.

Russian women want foreign men. (1994, January 6). *The Journal Times* (Racine, Wis., KR), pp. 1A, 9A.

Russians poorer in 1999, official figures show. (2000, January 11). *Reuters*. Retrieved January 12, 2000, from Johnson's Russia List #4028, davidjohnson@erols.com.

Ryan, M. (1992). Russian report: Perspectives on strikes by health care staff. *BMJ (British Medical Journal), 305*(6848), 298-299.

Salmon, I. (1999). To Russia with cling film. *Nursing Times, 95*(18), 35.

Smirnov, I.V., & Beznosuk, Y.V. (1995). Prospects in the solution of problems in psychoecology and psychohygiene. *Russian Medical Journal, 1*(1), 30-35.

Spiral. (1999). *AIDS in Russia.* Spiral, AIDS infoshare. Retrieved November 13, 1999, from the spiral database on the World Wide Web: http://www.spiral.com/infoshare/article1.html.

Stanley, S. (1993). Bringing mental health care to Russia. *American Nurse, 25*(2), 12, 14.

Troubled Russia needs a New Deal. (1998, September 17). *USA Today,* p. 14A.

US Aid trickles down to ordinary Russians. (1994, March 28). *The Journal Times* (Racine, Wis., AP), p. 1A, 7A.

U.S. Department of State. (1997, June). *Background notes: Russia, June 1997.* Office of Russian Affairs. Author. Retrieved March 16, 1999, from state.gov database on the World Wide Web: http://www.state.gov/www/background_notes/russia_0697_bgn.html.

U.S. State Department. (2000, January 7). *Russia—Consular information sheet.* Retrieved January 30, 2000, from state.gov database on the World Wide Web: http://travel.state.gov/russia.html.

U.S.-Russia Joint Commission on Economic and Technological Cooperation. (1999, March 23). *Joint report of the 8th Health Committee Meeting.* Washington, DC. Author. Retrieved August 20, 1999, from the dhhs database on the World Wide Web: http/odphp.osophs.dhhs.gov/russia/jr8eng.htm.

Vaile, M.S.B. (1993). Health and health care in the former Soviet Union. *The Lancet, 341*(8840), 310-311.

Wallen, A.J., & Cammuso, B.S. (1997). Healthcare in the new Russia: A Western perspective. *Nursing Forum, 32*(3), 27-32.

Watkins, D., & Rees, C. (1999). Healthcare crisis in Russia: A public health issue. *Nursing Standard, 13*(22), 33-35.

Wines, M. (2000, January 2). Putin's acts hint at agenda addressing graft, economy. *The Sunday Oregonian,* p. A19.

World Health Organization (WHO). (1997). *Annual report 1997—Country profiles: Russia.* WHO Tuberculosis Site. Retrieved January 10, 2000, from WHO database on the World Wide Web: http://www.who.int/gtb/publications/tbrep_97/countries/russia.htm.

World Health Organization (WHO). (1999). *Statistical information: Evidence and information for health policy.* WHO. Retrieved January 10, 2000, from WHO database on the World Wide Web: http://wwwnt.who.int/whosis/statistics/health_personnel.cfm.

Xenon Labs. (2000). *The universal currency converter.* Retrieved January 23, 2000, from Xenon Labs Incorporated database on the World Wide Web: http://www.xe.net/ucc/convert.cgi.

Yeltsin's secret nuclear survey finds problems, reveals cover-ups. (1995, August 7). *The Journal Times* (Racine, Wis., AP), p. 3A.

Zagalsky, L. (1994, August). Lifestyles of the not-so-rich. *Popular Science, 245*(2), 42-44, 70, 72.

Zuckerman, M.B. (1999a, February 8). Proud Russia on its knees. *US News & World Report, 126*(5), 30-36.

Zuckerman, M.B. (1999b, February 8). Coming to Russia's rescue. *US News & World Report, 126*(5), 68.

Concluding Notes and Future Directions

JOANNE McCLOSKEY DOCHTERMAN, HELEN KENNEDY GRACE

As we have said in previous editions, there is no "ending" for a book on issues in nursing. Given the purpose of the book, "to provide a forum for knowledgeable debate on today's nursing issues so that intelligent decision making can occur," an ending is, in fact, inappropriate.

An issue is an issue for one of two reasons: either (1) what is known is not well understood or (2) there is not enough known. What is needed is debate on what is known to foster understanding and ongoing search for knowledge about what is not known. Thoughtful debate and research are the keys to understanding a professional issue.

Yet, searching and debate are not enough for continued growth. Decisions have to be made, and sometimes they have to be made in the absence of full knowledge. In this case, it is even more important to understand what is known and to be able to put this knowledge into a broader perspective.

The broader perspective requires that one keep current on the changes in the profession and health care field. Many things have changed since the first edition of this book was published in 1981. Recent changes in nursing include the downsizing of hospitals, expansion of ambulatory and home care, more use of nurse practitioners, the emergence of new roles for nurses, replacement of nurses with unlicensed assistants, a decline in applicants to nursing programs, a beginning of a severe nursing shortage, more use of the computer and recognition of a standardized nursing language for documentation, more concern with costs and delivering a quality product, movement to a managed care environment, more nurses desiring participation in policy making, more concern by all nurses with the care of the elderly and those with chronic illnesses, more inclusion of consumers in health care policy making, more community-based care, and more interest in nursing and health care in other parts of the world.

Yet, despite the many changes, the dilemmas faced by nursing remain much the same as in the past. Stating them in the debate format, the dilemmas, in alphabetical order, are:

- Client focus versus economic focus
- Collaboration versus competition
- Independence versus dependence
- Inside control versus outside control
- Quality versus cost
- Safety versus risk
- Standards versus access
- Unity versus diversity

Our recommendations to aid resolutions are:

- Become more involved professionally and politically
- Become more proactive
- Celebrate our successes
- Concern ourselves with costs
- Conduct and use nursing research
- Create new roles that fit the emerging system
- Document our care with nursing's standardized languages
- Learn how to work in teams but don't give up the nursing identity
- Make ethical decisions
- Perform our jobs well
- Participate in the creation of a global nursing community
- Produce more and better prepared leaders
- Promote flexibility and diversity
- Realign education and service
- Support each other
- Take some risks and initiate needed changes
- Widen our horizons to include relevant issues outside the profession

Our authors report that we are making progress on many of these suggestions. The general tone of this edition is a bit more positive than the previous one. Despite the continued challenges related to managed care, financial cutbacks, and a nursing shortage, there is a growing positive regard for the contributions of nurses and the nursing profession. We must continue to identify and work to resolve the important issues facing our profession. We must also recognize when an old issue is no longer an issue and turn our energies to the new issues.

We believe that continuous thought and debate on important issues can lead to effective decision making and professional growth, both for the individual and the profession. With our learning and growth will come important benefits for our patients and, we believe, for society in general. This book, now in its sixth edition, has been our contribution to that process.

Index

Note: Page numbers in *italics* refer to illustrations; page numbers followed by t refer to tables.